Volume 2

25 Years Silver Jubilee Edition

# Manipal Manual of SURGERY

As per the latest **NMC** Guidelines | **Competency Based Medical Education (CBME)** Curriculum under Graduate Medical Education Regulation

**Seventh Edition**

Book Shaped by the Students

Read in Over 20 Countries

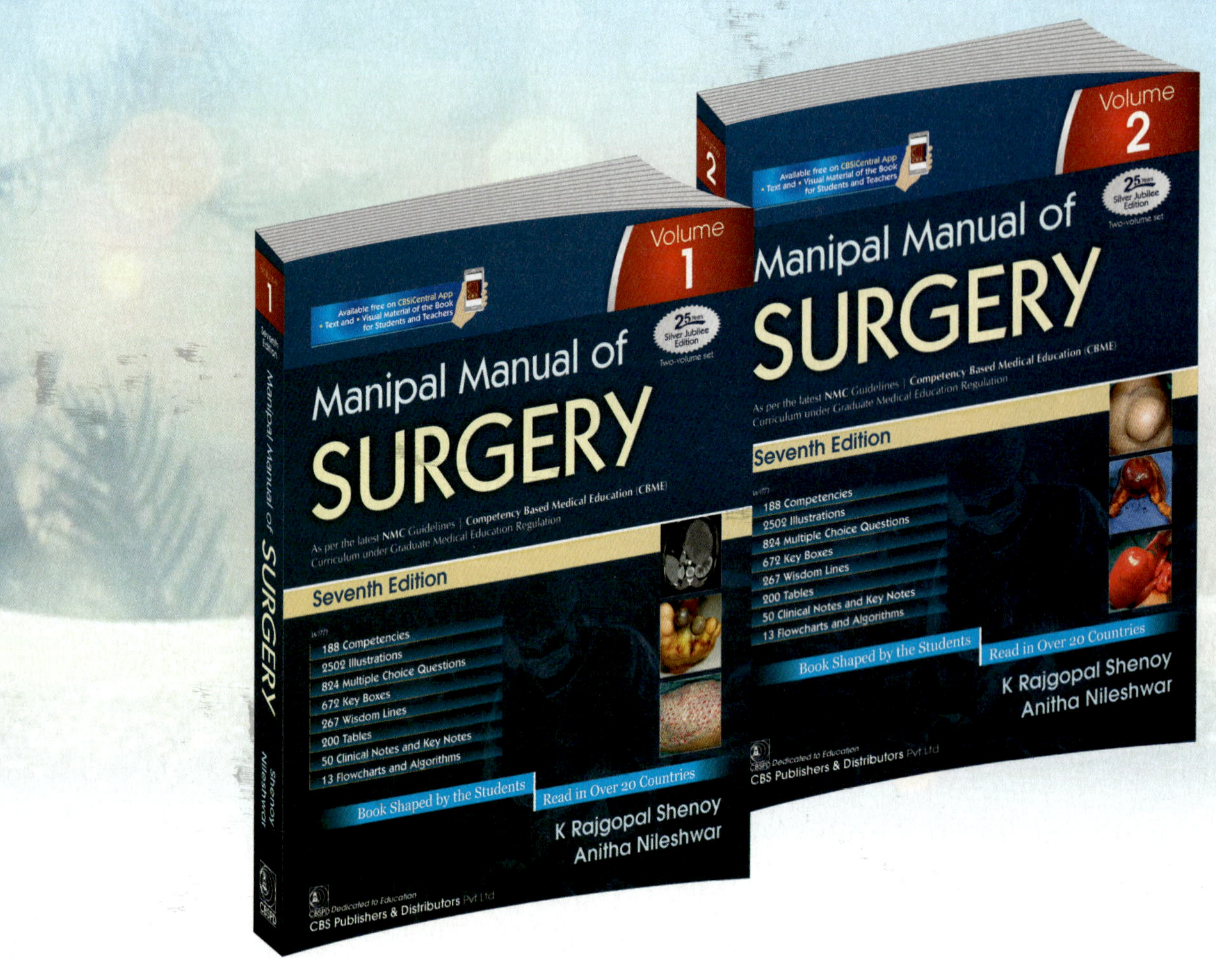


## Other CBS Titles by the Same Authors

- *Manipal Manual of Clinical Methods in Surgery*
- *Manipal Manual of Instruments,* Second edition
- *Manipal Manual of Surgery with Clinical Methods for Dental Students,* Fourth edition
- *AETCOM Attitude, EThics and COMmunication*

Volume

2

25 Years Silver Jubilee Edition

# Manipal Manual of SURGERY

As per the latest **NMC** Guidelines | **Competency Based Medical Education (CBME)** Curriculum under Graduate Medical Education Regulation

## Seventh Edition


*Chief Editor*

**K Rajgopal Shenoy** MBBS, MS, FRCS (Glasgow)
Professor
Former Associate Dean–Academics and Head, Department of Surgery
Kasturba Medical College, and
Consultant Surgeon, Kasturba Hospital, Manipal 576104
Karnataka, India
Manipal Academy of Higher Education (MAHE)
email: kallyarajgopalshenoy@gmail.com

*Coeditor*

**Anitha Shenoy (Nileshwar)** MBBS, MD, FRCA
Professor and Former Head
Department of Anaesthesiology
Kasturba Medical College, and
Consultant Anaesthesiologist, Kasturba Hospital, Manipal 576104
Karnataka, India
Manipal Academy of Higher Education (MAHE)
email: anitharshenoy@gmail.com


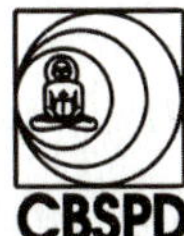



**CBS Publishers & Distributors** Pvt Ltd

New Delhi • Bengaluru • Chennai • Kochi • Kolkata • Lucknow • Mumbai
Gujarat • Hyderabad • Jharkhand • Nagpur • Patna • Pune • Uttarakhand

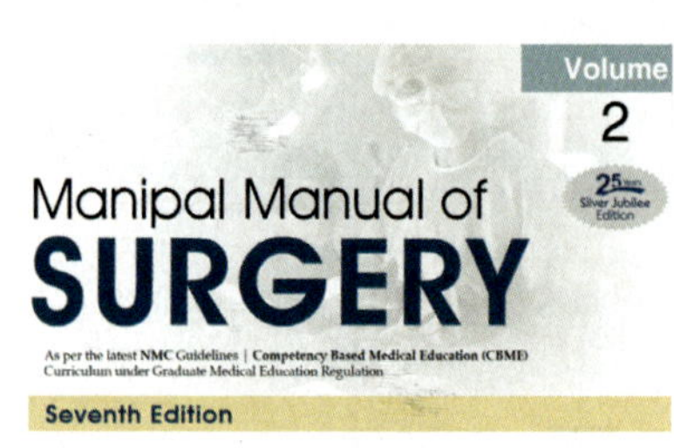


**ISBN:** 978-93-48385-70-3


**Seventh Edition: 2025**
First Edition: 2000
*Reprint: 2001, 2002, 2003, 2004*
Second Edition: 2005
*Reprint: 2006, 2007, 2008, 2009*
Third Edition: 2010
*Reprint: 2011, 2012*
Fourth Edition: 2014
*Reprint: 2016, 2017, 2019*
Fifth Edition: 2020
Sixth Edition: 2023
*Reprint: 2024*

*Disclaimer*
Science and technology are constantly changing fields. New information, research and experience broaden the scope of knowledge. The editors and contributors have tried their best in giving information available to them while preparing the material for this book. Although, all efforts have been made to ensure optimum accuracy of the material, yet it is quite possible some errors might have been left uncorrected. The editors, the contributors, the publisher and the printer will not be held responsible for any inadvertent errors or inaccuracies.

Book Shaped by the Students | Read in Over 20 Countries

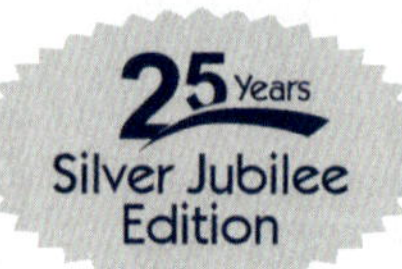




Published by **Satish Kumar Jain** and produced by **Varun Jain** for

**CBS Publishers & Distributors** Pvt Ltd

4819/XI Prahlad Street, 24 Ansari Road, Daryaganj, New Delhi 110 002, India
Ph: 011-23289259, 23266838 Website: www.cbspd.com
e-mail: delhi@cbspd.com

***Corporate Office:*** 204 FIE, Industrial Area, Patparganj, Delhi 110 092, India
Ph: 011-49344934 Fax: 011-49344935 e-mail: publishing@cbspd.com; publicity@cbspd.com

***Branches***

- **Bengaluru:** Seema House 2975, 17th Cross, K.R. Road, Banasankari 2nd Stage, Bengaluru 560 070, Karnataka, India
  Ph: +91-80-26771678/79 Fax: +91-80-26771680 e-mail: bangalore@cbspd.com
- **Chennai:** 18/8B, Subbarayan Street, Shenoy Nagar, Chennai 600 030, Tamil Nadu, India
  Ph: +91-44-42032115, 26681266 e-mail: chennai@cbspd.com
- **Kochi:** 42/1325, 1326, Power House Road, Opposite KSEB, Power House, Ernakulum 682018, Kochi, Kerala, India
  Ph: +91-484-4059061–65 Fax: +91-484-4059065 e-mail: kochi@cbspd.com
- **Kolkata:** 147, Hind Ceramics Compound, 1st Floor, Nilgunj Road, Belghoria, Kolkata 700056, West Bengal, India
  Ph: +91-33-25330055/56 e-mail: kolkata@cbspd.com
- **Lucknow:** Basement, Khushuma Complex, 7 Meerabai Marg (behind Jawahar Bhawan), Lucknow 226001, UP, India
  Ph: +91-522-4000032 e-mail: tiwari.lucknow@cbspd.com
- **Mumbai:** PWD Shed, Gala No. 25/26, Ramchandra Bhatt Marg, Next JJ Hospital, Gate No. 2, Opp. Union Bank of India, Noorbaug, Mumbai 400009, Maharashtra, India
  Ph: +91-22-66661880/89 e-mail: mumbai@cbspd.com

***Representatives***

- **Gujarat** 0-9879558667
- **Hyderabad** 0-9885175004
- **Jharkhand** 0-9811541605
- **Nagpur** 0-8692091830
- **Patna** 0-9334159340
- **Pune** 0-9664372571
- **Uttarakhand** 0-9716462459

*Printed at:* Manipal Technologies Limited, Manipal

# Contents

## VOLUME 2

### SECTION V: GASTROINTESTINAL SURGERY

## SECTION VI: *VIVA VOCE* EXAMINATION

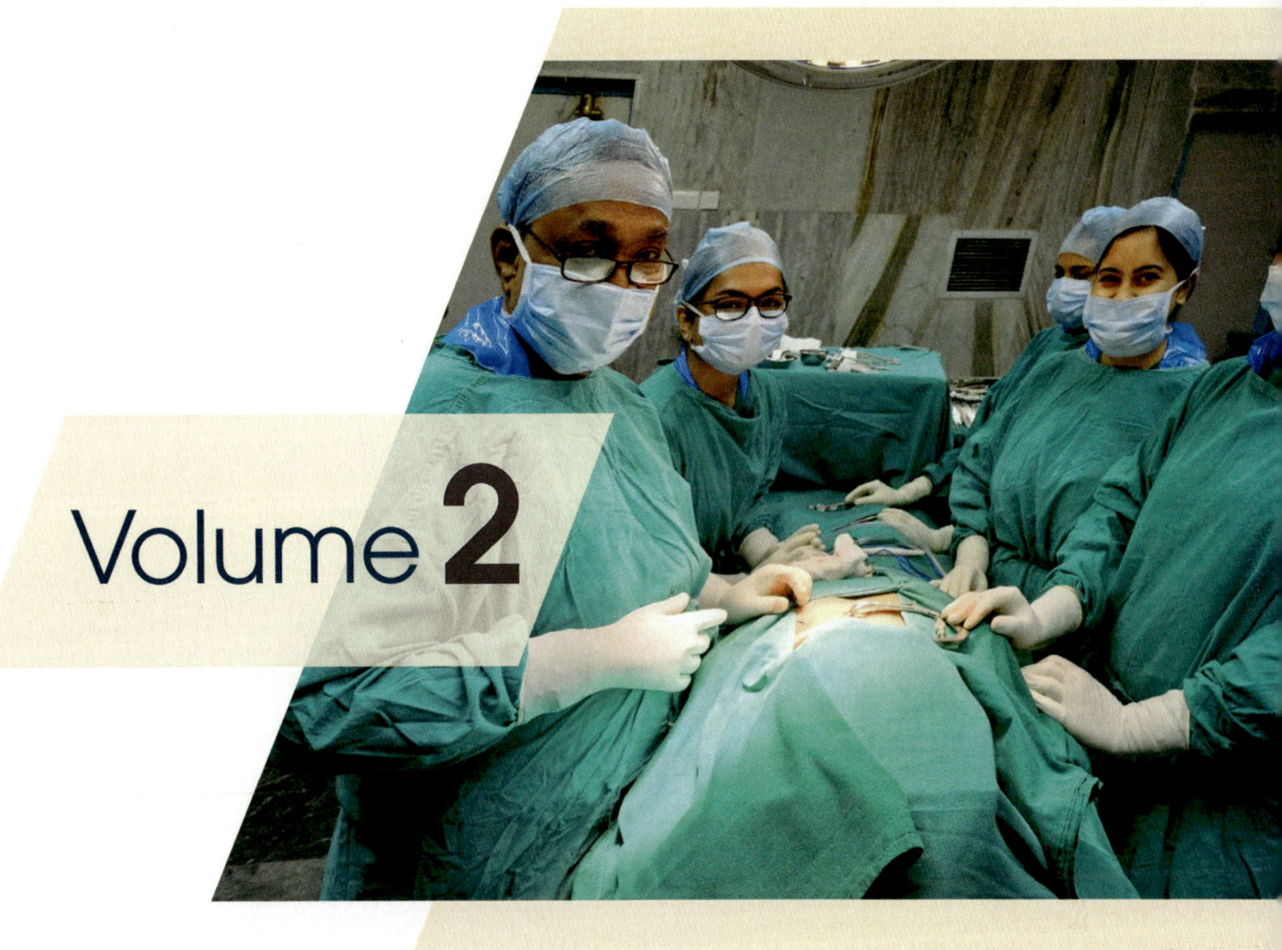

# Volume 2

## Gastrointestinal Surgery
## *Viva Voce* Examination

Section

V

# Gastrointestinal Surgery

52. Oesophagus and Diaphragm
53. Stomach and Duodenum
54. Gallbladder and Pancreas
55. Liver
56. Spleen
57. Peritoneum, Peritoneal Cavity, Mesentery and Retroperitoneum
58. Small Intestine
59. Large Intestine (Colon)
60. Intestinal Obstruction
61. Rectum and Anal Canal
62. Lower Gastrointestinal Bleeding
63. Appendix
64. Hernia
65. Umbilicus, Wound Dehiscence, Wound Closure and Abdominal Wall Swellings
66. Trauma—Initial Management, Blunt Abdominal Trauma, War and Blast Injuries and Triage

Chapter 52

# Oesophagus and Diaphragm

- Surgical anatomy
- Physiology
- Gastro-oesophageal reflux disease (GORD)
- Barrett's oesophagus
- Motility disorders of the pharynx and oesophagus
- Achalasia cardia
- Nutcracker oesophagus/Jackhammer oesophagus
- Carcinoma of the oesophagus
- Corrosive oesophageal stricture
- Oesophageal perforations
- Diverticulum of oesophagus
- Differential diagnosis dysphagia
- Surgical anatomy of the diaphragm
- Diaphragmatic hernia
- Tracheo-oesophageal fistula

**SU28.5:** Describe surgical anatomy of oesophagus.

## SURGICAL ANATOMY

- Oesophagus is 25 cm in length, extending from the cricopharyngeal sphincter to the cardio-oesophageal junction (Fig. 52.1).
- It runs in the posterior mediastinum as a continuation of pharynx. 2 cm of this tube lies below the diaphragm.
- Cardio-oesophageal junction lies to the left of T11 vertebra. It is identified at endoscopy by a Z-line.
- It is a jagged line where the oesophageal mucosa changes to gastric mucosa.
- **Collar of Helvetius:** It is the site at which the circular muscles of oesophagus turns to oblique muscles of the stomach at the incisura.
- **Physiological constrictions** (Table 52.1).

### Muscle Layers (Figs 52.2 and 52.3)

- It has an inner circular layer and an outer longitudinal layer.
- Upper 1/3rd has striated muscle fibres.
- Lower 2/3rd has smooth muscle fibres.

### Mucosa

- The entire oesophagus is lined by squamous epithelium except last 3 cm which is lined by columnar cells. The columnar cells are similar to gastric mucosa but oxyntic and peptic cells are absent.

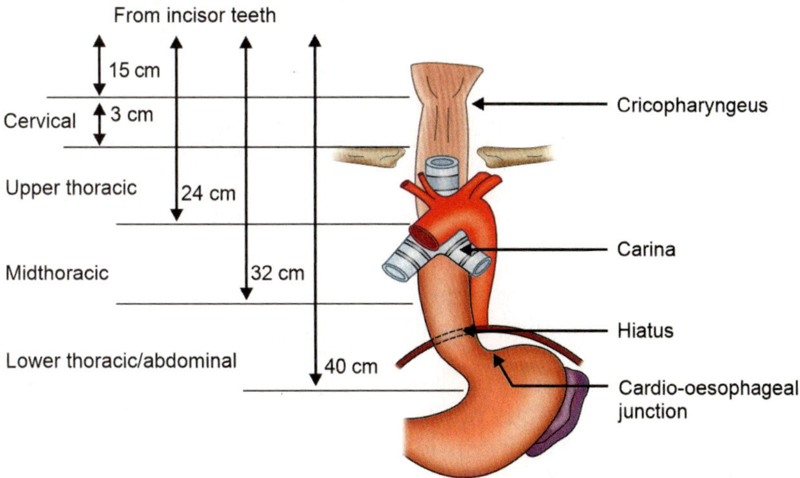


**Fig. 52.1:** Division of oesophagus into 4 parts based on distance from incisor teeth

| TABLE 52.1: Physiological constrictions | | | |
|---|---|---|---|
| **Constrictions** | **Distance from incisor teeth** | **Diameter of oesophagus** | **Problems** |
| Cricopharyngeal | 15 cm | 14 mm | Foreign body lodgement |
| Aortic and bronchial | 25 cm | 15–17 mm | Perforations during endoscopy |
| Diaphragmatic sphincter | 40 cm | 16–19 mm | Malignancy |

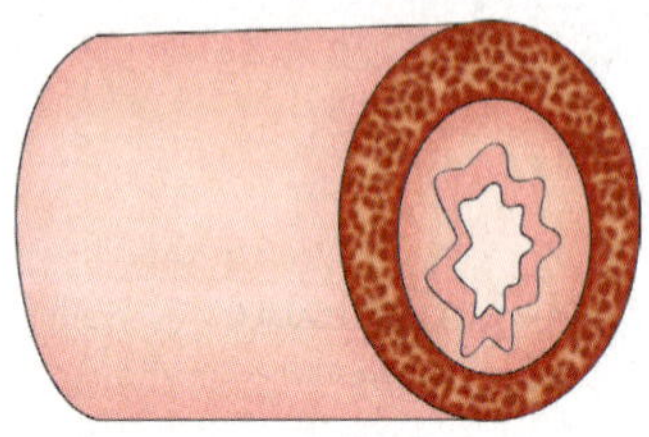

**Fig. 52.2:** You can see the multilayered structure. Endosonography detects all these layers

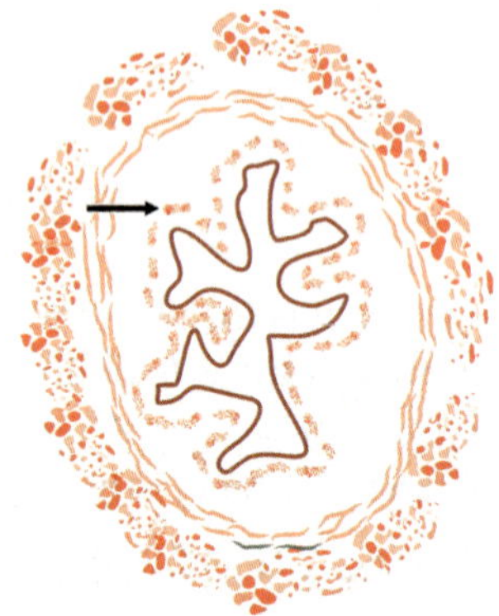

**Fig. 52.3:** Helicoidal muscle (arrow)

- **Mucosa is the toughest coat of oesophagus.**
- The smooth oesophageal mucosa gets transformed into rugal folds.

*Pearls of Wisdom*

Clinically significant motility disorders affect lower two-thirds (smooth muscle) of oesophagus. Squamous cell carcinoma in the upper two thirds- upper and mid-oesophagus and adenocarcinoma in the last 3 to 4 cm of the oesophagus, because of nature of the epithelial lining.

## Lymphatic Drainage (Key Box 52.1)

- Upper oesophagus drains into the left and right supraclavicular nodes.
- Middle oesophagus drains into the tracheobronchial nodes and paraoesophageal nodes.
- Lower oesophagus drains into lymph nodes along the lesser curvature of stomach and then into coeliac nodes. Involvement of coeliac nodes indicate inoperability.

## Nerve Supply

The parasympathetic nerve supply is by vagus nerve through extrinsic and intrinsic plexuses. The intrinsic plexus has **no Meissner's network** and **Auerbach's plexus is present only in the lower two-thirds**.

Key Box 52.1

### Lymphatic Drainage of Oesophagus

- Extensive lymphatic plexus in the submucosa which explains the easy spread
- Like in the colon they are classified as perioesophageal, paraoesophageal and lateral oesophageal lymph nodes
- Thus, throughout the entire length of oesophagus various groups of lymph nodes are enlarged such as deep cervical, mediastinal, subcarinal, hilar, diaphragmatic, para- and peri-oesophageal, gastric, coeliac, etc.
- Presence of coeliac nodes indicates inoperability
- **Longitudinal lymphatics are 6 times more than transverse.** Hence, distant spread occurs fast—satellite nodules occur proximal and distal to the growth. This is the reason why 10 cm margin must be given in resection of the oesophagus
- These are advantages of transhiatal resection over Ivor-Lewis operation

## Blood Supply (Figs 52.4 and 52.5)

### *Arterial*

- **Cervical oesophagus:** Mainly from branches of the inferior thyroid artery.
- **Upper thoracic oesophagus:** Mainly from branches of the inferior thyroid artery and less consistently from anterior oesophagotracheal branch from aorta.

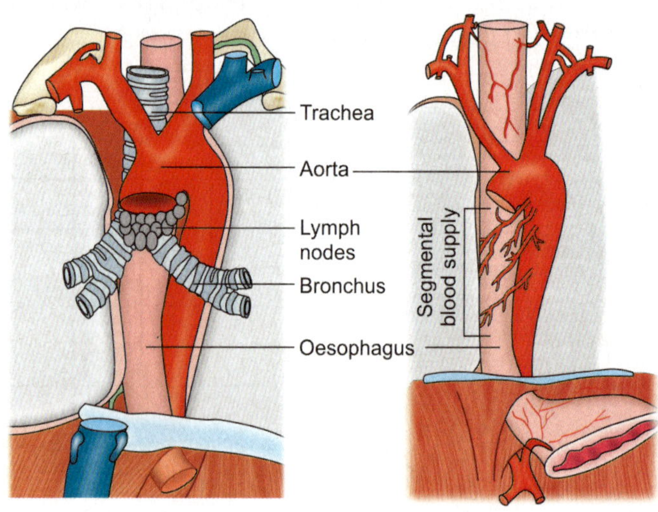


**Fig. 52.4:** Oesophageal anatomy—relationships

**Fig. 52.5:** Oesophageal anatomy—segmental blood supply

- **Mid and lower thoracic oesophagus:** Supplied by bronchial arteries.
- **Lower oesophagus:** Small branches of the left gastric artery.

Rich internal arterial anastomosis is present in the oesophagus and in the stomach. Hence, extensive mobilisation of oesophagus can be done without compromising viability.

### *Venous Drainage*

Veins accompany corresponding arteries. Importantly, thoracic oesophagus drains into azygos and hemiazygos veins. Key points of surgical anatomy are given in Table 52.2.

## PHYSIOLOGY (Deglutition–Swallowing)

The main function of the oesophagus is to transfer food from the mouth to the stomach. Voluntary contraction of the oropharynx pushes food into the upper oesophagus through a relaxed cricopharyngeal sphincter (Key Box 52.2). Then, due to primary and secondary peristalsis, the food bolus is transferred to the stomach (Fig. 52.6).

- **Cricopharyngeal sphincter** is closed at rest. It helps in preventing regurgitation of oesophageal contents into the respiratory passage. Killian's dehiscence (also known as Killian's triangle) is **a triangular area in the wall of the pharynx between the cricopharyngeus and thyropharyngeus** which are the two parts of the inferior constrictors—site wherein Zenker's diverticulum can occur (Table 52.2).
- **Lower oesophageal sphincter (LOS):** It is a physiological sphincter at the gastro-oesophageal junction. It is 3–4 cm long with a resting pressure of 20–25 mmHg. Hence, it is known as **high pressure zone (HPZ)**.

Key Box 52.2

**The Pharyngeal Stage—Reflex**

- Food stimulates mechanoreceptors
- Soft palate is pulled upwards so that food will not enter nasal cavities
- Vocal cords adduct and larynx is pulled upwards against epiglottis so that food will not enter trachea
- Cricopharyngeal sphincter opens
- Muscular wall of the pharynx then contracts from above downwards

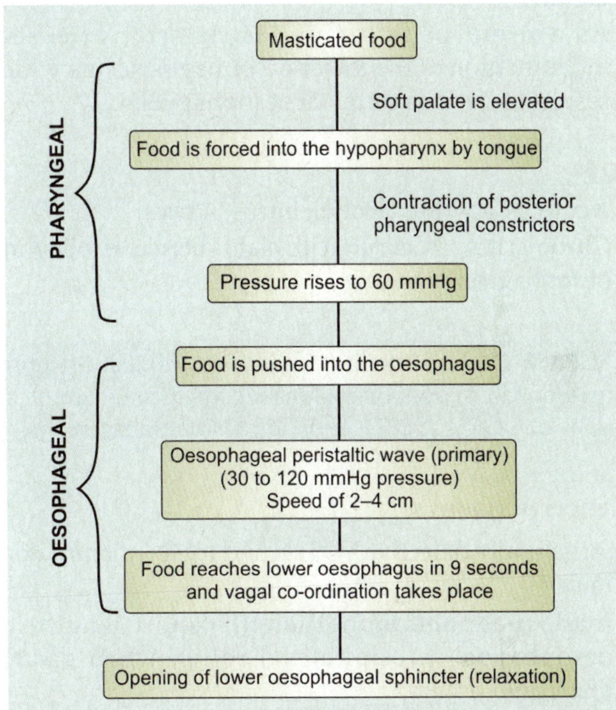


**Fig. 52.6:** Mechanism of swallowing—two phases

**TABLE 52.2:** Surgical anatomy of the oesophagus—key points

| Surgical anatomy | Significance | Surgical points of interest |
|---|---|---|
| Upper oesophageal sphincter | Dense cricopharyngeus muscle | Zenker's diverticulum through Killian triangle |
| Lower oesophageal sphincter | High pressure zone at gastro-oesophageal junction | Weakness causes reflux oesophagitis |
| Oesophageal mucosa | Toughest coat of oesophagus | Important in oesophageal anastomosis |
| No serosa, no mesentery | Requires mobilisation | Leak rate is high, easy spread of carcinoma |
| Helicoidal muscle | Helps in peristalsis but it recoils due to elasticity | Hence, once resection takes place—specimen 'shortens' or retracts—anastomosis may become difficult especially in abdominal anastomosis |
| Segmental arterial supply | Extensive mobilisation can be done without compromising blood supply | Hence, transhiatal oesophagectomy (THE) is done with ease |
| Lower end of oesophagus—veins | Rich intercommunicating veins between portal and systemic veins | Oesophageal varices occur here |
| Azygos vein crossing oesophagus in thorax | Can get injured and bleed | Resection of midoesophageal tumours |
| Mucosal and submucosal lymphatics out number capillaries | Oesophageal tumours extend over a long distance within oesophageal wall | Need for total oesophagectomy and cervical anastomosis + lymph node clearance |

- This HPZ prevents reflux of gastric contents into the oesophagus. Cigarette smoking affects this zone and so, smokers have a high incidence of reflux oesophagitis.

## GASTRO-OESOPHAGEAL REFLUX DISEASE

- Loss of competence of LOS leads to gastro-oesophageal reflux disease (GORD, also called GERD). The competence of LOS can be affected by obesity, smoking, excessive eating, etc. Sliding hernia is associated with GORD.
- As a result of reflux of gastric acid, extensive inflammation of the lower oesophagus occurs which results in various forms of oesophagitis.

### Types

1. **Acute:** Following alcohol, burns, stress.
2. **Chronic:** It is associated with hiatus hernia or following oesophagojejunostomy.

**SU28.5:** Describe aetiopathogenesis, clinical features, investigations, principles of management and complications of GORD (GERD) and Barrett's oesophagus.

### Aetiopathogenesis

1. Structurally defective LOS secondary to inflammatory injury.
2. Inadequate abdominal length (short length) of oesophagus—precipitates a reflux when gastric distension occurs.
3. Ineffective oesophageal pump affecting clearance of food into stomach. This is influenced by following factors:
   - Gravity
   - Oesophageal motility
   - *Salivation*—saliva neutralises the minute amount of acid that is left following a peristaltic wave.

   When salivary flow is decreased (following radiotherapy), the reflux can get exaggerated.
4. **Increased gastric pressure:** Can occur due to pyloric stenosis and diabetic gastroparesis. Following vagotomy, loss of receptive relaxation occurs resulting in increased intragastric pressure.
   - Acid refluxes into the lower oesophagus and produces diffuse inflammation with multiple ulcers.
   - The symptoms are worse when the patient lies down.
   - Due to vagal hyperactivity, inflammation and ulcers develop which produce severe longitudinal muscle spasm. Consequently, the cardia is drawn up into the thorax, leading to an increase in the oesophagocardiac angle. This increases the reflux. Later, fibrosis causes shortening of the oesophagus.
   - Thus, it becomes a vicious circle of *oesophagitis—longitudinal muscle spasm—displacement of oesophagus—increased regurgitation.*

### Clinical Features

Most common presentation of GORD is history of heart-burn and regurgitation. Heartburn is confined to epigastrium and retrosternal areas, does not radiate to the back. Clinical presentation of the GORD can be classified as follows: Atypical symptoms can be so many and can thus confuse the picture.

| | | |
|---|---|---|
| Oesophageal | : | Dysphagia, regurgitation, heartburn |
| Gastric | : | Early satiety, belching, bloating, nausea |
| Pulmonary | : | Asthma, wheezing, aspiration, cough, dyspnoea, bronchitis, hoarseness of voice due to damage to vocal cords, etc. |
| Ear, nose, throat | : | Waterbrash, globus, hoarseness |
| Cardiac | : | Chest pain |

**What is globus? Sensation of a substernal lump (globus).** When this occurs during fasting, it is termed 'globus hystericus'. It is a neurotic symptom in patients with emotional instability.

- **Retrosternal pain:** It is burning in nature and becomes worse on lying down. The pain reduces in the sitting position. The pain is described as *heartburn and can be confused for angina pectoris.* It is relieved on taking antacids.
- **Heartburn** is otherwise called **pyrosis**.
- **Occult blood in stools** and streaks of blood in the vomitus are common.
- **Anaemia** and weakness are uncommon features.
- **Dysphagia:** Transient difficulty in swallowing results from spasm due to inflammation of the lower end of oesophagus. Late dysphagia is due to stenosis or stricture of the oesophagus. Belching is not uncommon.

### Complications

- **Benign:** Oesophageal ulcers, bleeding and peptic strictures. Peptic strictures are not common nowadays due to the treatment of acid peptic disease with proton pump inhibitors.
- **Barrett's oesophagus and adenocarcinoma:** Chronic reflux will bring metaplasia in the lower and mid-oesophagus resulting in Barrett's oesophagus which progresses to adenocarcinoma oesophagus (Fig. 52.7).

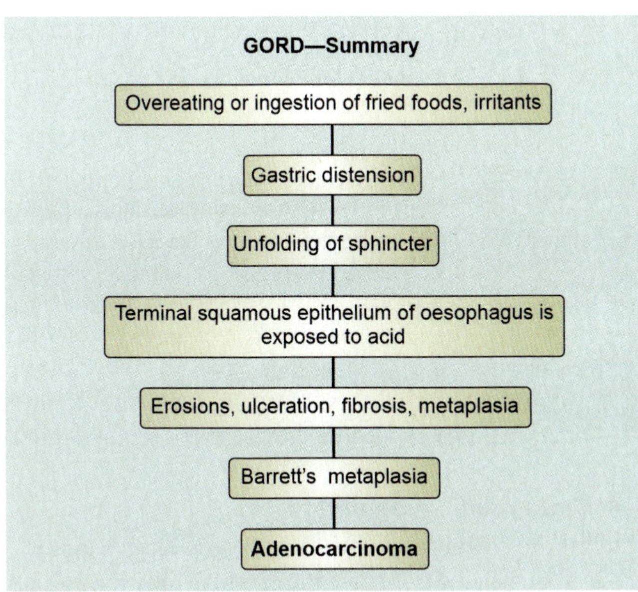


**Fig. 52.7:** Carcinogenesis due to GORD

## Scoring Systems/Classification of GORD

### *Johnson-DeMeester Scoring System*

Three important symptoms are taken into consideration.

| Grade | Features |
|---|---|
| | **Heartburn** |
| 0 | None |
| 1 | Minimal—occasional episodes |
| 2 | Moderate—medical therapy visits |
| 3 | Severe—interferes with daily activities |
| | **Regurgitation** |
| 0 | None |
| 1 | Minimal—occasional episodes |
| 2 | Moderate—on position or straining |
| 3 | Severe—features of aspiration |
| | **Dysphagia** |
| 0 | None |
| 1 | Minimal |
| 2 | Needs fluid to clear |
| 3 | Causes food impaction |

### *Modified Savary-Miller Classification of Reflux Oesophagitis*

Grade I: Single or isolated erosion at or above GE junction.

Grade II: Multiple non-circumferential erosions above GE junction.

Grade III: Circumferential erosions above GE junction.

Grade IV: Chronic lesion—stricture, ulceration/short oesophagus.

Grade V: Columnar epithelium in continuity with Z line (Barrett's oesophagus).

## Investigations (Table 52.3, Key Boxes 52.3 and 52.4)

- **Barium swallow**[1] in the Trendelenburg's position (head down position) can demonstrate the reverse flow of barium into the lower end of the oesophagus (from the stomach).
- **Oesophagoscopy** may reveal red, angry looking mucosa in the lower end of the oesophagus.
- **Oesophageal manometry** to detect motility disorders. A thin catheter is passed through the nose which contains pressure sensors.
- **24-hour pH monitoring is the gold standard.**

Key Box 52.3

**Oesophageal Manometry**

- Information about LOS
  - Resting pressure
  - Length
  - Relaxation
- Quality of oesophageal peristalsis
- **Manometry is essential. To place the pH probe 5 cm above upper border of LOS for ambulatory pH monitoring.**

Key Box 52.4

**24-hour pH Monitoring is the Gold Standard**

- Indications: When symptoms are certain but endoscopy is normal, atypical symptoms
- It involves the transnasal placement of a pH measuring electrode in the lower oesophagus. The pH electrode monitors the changes in intra-oesophageal pH over 24-hour
- A 24-hour pH profile is thus obtained that provides information on frequency, duration and pattern of reflux
- A reflux episode is defined as a pH drop to below pH 4
- Thus, identification, type and duration of reflux is noted.

**Summary of the investigations and the utility of these have been summarized in Table 52.3.**

## Treatment

It can be classified as medical, endotherapy and surgical line of management. Conservative treatment or medical line of treatment should be attempted in all these patients. Majority of the patients respond to conservative line of treatment.

[1]Barium swallow: Thick paste to see the oesophagus. Barium meal: A thin paste to see the stomach. Both are radio-opaque.

**TABLE 52.3:** Investigations of GORD

| To detect structural abnormalities | To detect increased exposure to gastric juice | To detect functional abnormalities |
|---|---|---|
| ***A. Barium swallow***<br>• Detects hiatus hernia (prone position)<br>• Detects stricture or any rings<br>• Extrinsic compression can be detected<br>• Can also detect small carcinoma<br>***B. Flexible endoscopy***<br>• Can detect hiatus hernia or diverticulum, etc.<br>• Can detect oesophageal abnormalities | ***A. Flexible endoscopy and to biopsy—the Barrett's oesophagus***<br>***B. Grading of oesophagitis by endoscopy***<br>Grade I: Small, circular, nonconfluent erosions<br>Grade II: Linear erosions lined with granulation tissue that bleeds on touch<br>Grade III: Erosions with circumferential loss of the epithelium—cobblestone oesophagus<br>Grade IV: Stricture | ***Oesophagus manometry***<br>• It is indicated when motor abnormality is suspected such as achalasia, diffuse spasm<br>• Can also detect scleroderma polymyositis<br>• Average LOS pressure <6 mmHg, suspect GORD<br>• High resolution manometry is more accurate |

## A. Medical Management

**Treatment of uncomplicated GORD** can be discussed under the following headings:

**I. Lifestyle modification** (Key Box 52.5)

- Stop smoking
- Stop alcohol
- Control obesity
- Small meals
- Avoid coffee, chocolate and coke
- Head up—propped-up position
- Avoid stooping
- Avoid tight garments.

Key Box 52.5

**Medical Management of GORD**

- **A**lcohol to be minimised. Also stop smoking
- **L**ose weight
- **C**offee/tea to be minimised
- **O**esophageal mucosa protectors—antacids, $H_2$ receptor blockers
- **H**ead—up tilt
- **O**ily and spicy food must be avoided
- **L**arge meal to be avoided at night times

*Remember as* **ALCOHOL**

**II. Drugs**

- Antacids with alginate—antireflux floating alginate.
- **Proton pump inhibitors:** Pantoprazole 40 mg, esomeprazole till 20 mg may have to be given for one or two months or full symptoms are controlled. These are antisecretory drugs.
- **Prokinetics:** Itopride 50 mg can be given 2–3 times a day for 8 weeks on empty stomach. Prokinetics enhance motility. Cisapride and mosapride are not favoured because they can cause cardiac arrhythmias.

**III. Mucosa protective agents**

- Sucralfate colloidal bismuth—cytoprotective agent.
- It is a sucrose sulphate–aluminium complex which binds to the mucosa. Thus, it protects mucosa of GI tract against hydrochloric acid.
- Colloidal bismuth compounds.

## B. Endoscopic Management

**I. Endoscopic plication/suturing or enteryx injection**

- **Plexiglass microspheres (PMMA):** Through an endoscopic needle, microspheres suspended in gelatin are injected. Gelatin is absorbed and spheres cause tissue bulking.

**II. Endoscopic treatment of GORD:** Three types:

1. **Radiofrequency energy to LES:** It changes sphincter compliance.
2. **Barrier at GE junction:** An ethylene vinyl alcohol copolymer is injected into submucosa 1–2 mm caudal to Z line.
3. **Direct endoscopic suturing and tightening of LES**

## C. Surgery: Indications

- Intractable pain—heartburn and dysphagia
- Recurrent aspiration, cough respiratory infections.
- Complications such as haemorrhage or stricture
- The results of antireflux surgery are good with a small mortality rate (0.1 to 0.5%). However, careful selection of patients depending upon their symptoms and lifestyle are important factors.

### Types of Surgery

1. **Nissen's total fundoplication** (Figs 52.8A and B): The aim is to restore 2–4 cm of intra-abdominal oesophagus by reducing the hernia, followed by repair of the hiatus.
   - In this operation, fundus of the stomach is mobilised by dividing short gastric arteries.
   - Fundus is brought behind the oesophagus and wrapped in front of oesophagus. It is a ***loose wrap (Floppy Nissen)***.

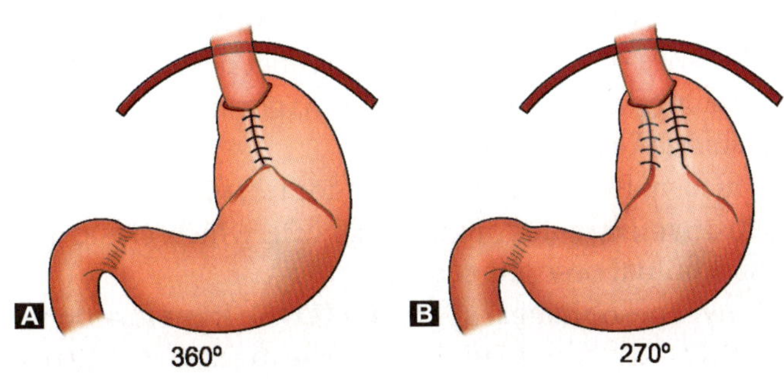


Figs 52.8A and B: Nissen's fundoplication

- Diaphragmatic defect is repaired by using non-absorbable sutures such as nylon or silk. This is the operation which serves all aims.

### Laparoscopic fundoplication

- It is the gold standard
- Most popular today
- Minimal morbidity and mortality
- Early discharge, within 1–2 days
- Early recovery
- All operative steps that are performed in open surgery are carried out here with a 'better vision' in laparoscopic method.

**Principles of fundoplication**

- 360° gastric fundoplication should be no longer than 2 cm.
- It should be constructed over a 60 F bougie.
- Fundoplication should be placed in the abdomen without tension.
- Only 'fundus' should be used to wrap (fundus relaxes—body does not relax on swallowing).
- Vagus should not be damaged because it may result in failure of sphincter to relax.
- Lengthen the oesophagus with a Collis gastroplasty (in cases of short oesophagus).
- Patients with normal peristaltic contractions do well with 360° Nissen's fundoplication—for others, two- thirds partial fundoplication may be the procedure of choice.

### Complications

- Too tight a plication may result in dysphagia or gas bloat syndrome wherein belching is prevented.

2. **Partial fundoplication (Toupet)** solves the above problem wherein fundus is sutured around the back of oesophagus (Fig. 52.9) or Dorr's, where fundus is sutured anterior to the oesophagus.
3. **LINX device treatment**

- It is a ring of interlinked titanium beads with magnetic cores.
- It is indicated in patients who have **GORD but without hiatus hernia**. Patients with weak oesophageal peristalsis or large hiatal hernias about 2 cm or more are not candidates for the LINX procedure.
- These are magnetic beads placed around oesophago-gastric junction.
- These beads will stretch with increased pressure in the oesophagus.
- This is called magnetic sphincter augmentation. Magnets keep the LES tight enough to allow food to enter into stomach but will not allow reflux to happen. Success rates of 95% has been mentioned in the Western patients.

## HIATUS HERNIA

### Definition

Abnormal protrusion of abdominal viscus through the oesophageal hiatus into the chest.

### Types (Key Box 52.6)

I. **Sliding hernia or oesophagogastric hernia:** It is the commonest type of hiatus hernia, accounting for about 80% of cases (Figs 52.10 and 52.11). It may be associated with GORD.
II. **Rolling or paraoesophageal hernia**
III. Mixed hernia
IV. Massive herniation.

1. **Type I** hernias are sliding hiatal hernias, where the gastroesophageal junction migrates above

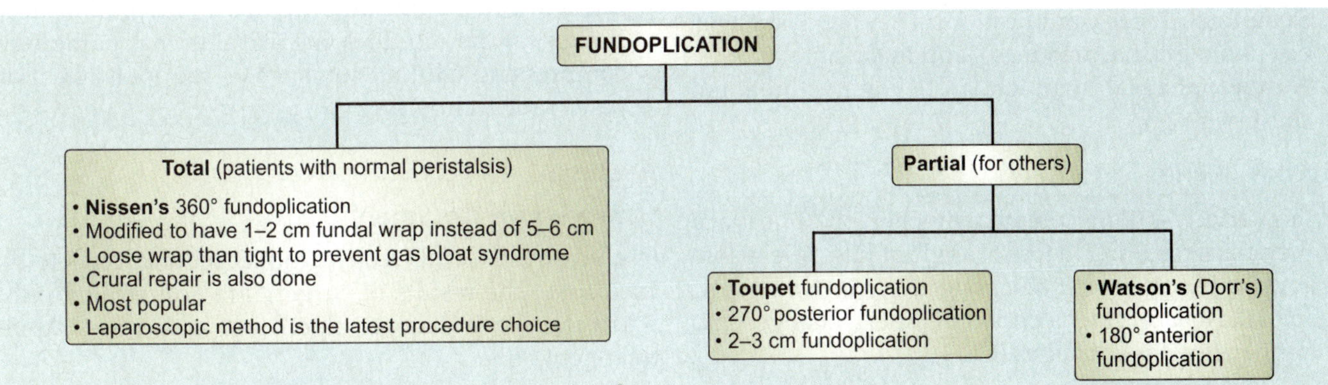


Fig. 52.9: Types of fundoplication

Key Box 52.6

**Types**

| | | | | |
|---|---|---|---|---|
| I | : | $H^0$ | : | Normal |
| II | : | $H^1$ | : | Sliding |
| III | : | $H^2$ | : | Paraoesophageal |
| IV | : | $H^3$ | : | Mixed |
| V | : | $H^4$ | : | Massive herniation |

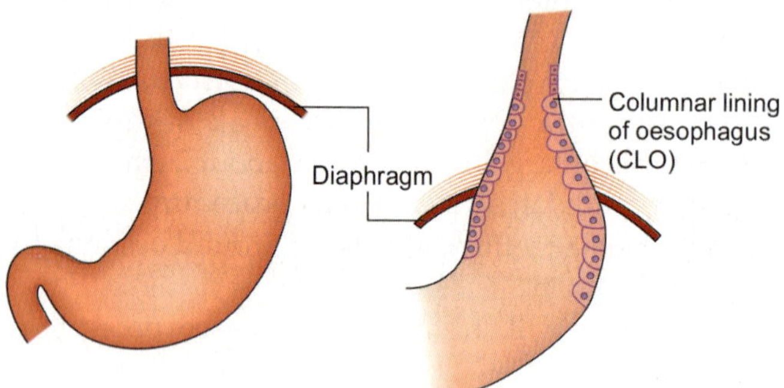


**Fig. 52.10:** Normal position **Fig. 52.11:** Sliding hernia

the diaphragm. The stomach remains in its usual longitudinal alignment and the fundus remains below the gastroesophageal junction.

2. **Type II** hernias are pure paraoesophageal hernias (PEH); the gastroesophageal junction remains in its normal anatomic position but a portion of the fundus herniates through the diaphragmatic hiatus adjacent to the oesophagus, through a defect in the phreno-oesophageal membrane.
3. **Type III** hernias are a combination of Types I and II, with both the gastroesophageal junction and the fundus herniating through the hiatus. The fundus lies above the gastroesophageal junction.
4. **Type IV** hiatal hernias are characterized by the presence of a structure other than stomach, such as the omentum, colon or small bowel within the hernia sac.

## Common Symptoms

1. **Symptoms due to reflux:** Regurgitation and heart burn are the two most common symptoms.
2. **Symptoms due to complications:** They are dysphagia, odynophagia, haematemesis and melaena.
3. **Nonoesophageal symptoms:** They are asthma and chest pain.

## SLIDING HERNIA

In this variety, squamocolumnar junction or Z line is at a higher place resulting in loss of angle of His. Due to loss of angle of His and lower oesophageal sphincter activity, reflux takes place. Over a period of time, it changes into columnar-lined oesophagus (CLO).

**Anatomical factors which prevent sliding hernia**

- Presence of 2 cm of intra-abdominal oesophagus.
- **The angle of His:** The oesophagocardiac angle of about 45° has valvular effect.
- Mucosal folds at the oesophagocardiac junction.
- Positive intra-abdominal pressure which closes the abdominal oesophagus.
- **Lower oesophageal sphincter (LOS):** It is a functional sphincter which increases the pressure during coughing, straining, etc.

## Causes of Sliding Hernia[1]

- Deposition of **fatty tissue** in the hiatus leads to weakening of the hiatus in obese individuals.
- Advancing **age** resulting in muscular degeneration can predispose to hernia.
- Raised intra-abdominal pressure due to lower **abdominal tumours**, pregnancy, etc.
- **Saint's triad:** Gallstones, diverticulosis and hiatus hernia can occur together in a patient.

## Clinical Features

- In many patients, there may not be any symptoms. Symptoms are like that of reflux oesophagitis—heart-burn, chest pain, bloating sensation.
- More common in women, especially if obese.
- Symptoms are exaggerated after a heavy meal or binges of alcohol.

## Investigations

- **Oesophagoscopy** reveals varying degree of inflammation. During oesophagoscopy, when the patient is asked to strain (Valsalva's manoeuvre), the sphincter is seen to be more patulous and herniation of gastric mucosal folds can be seen. **Reflux of the gastric acid is the most valuable sign. Biopsy should be taken from suspicious areas of metaplasia.**
- **Barium meal** demonstrates gastroesophageal reflux in the Trendelenburg position.
- **Ultrasound** of abdomen to rule out gallstones. Reflux can be due to some extraluminal pathology compressing GE junction such as retroperitoneal or pancreatic tumours.

## Treatment

### *Conservative Treatment*

In all cases of GORD, conservative treatment has to be tried first. The results of surgery are appreciated only when the symptoms are significant and conservative treatment fails.

[1]Causes can be remembered as FATTY (F: fat, A: age, T: tumour, T: triad (Saint's triad), Y: yielding hiatus.)

*Principles—You can remember mnemonic LORD*

1. **Lifestyle changes**
   - Decrease in weight
   - Diet control with increased intake of proteins and decreased consumption of fat and sugar.
   - Decreased alcohol and tobacco consumption.
2. **Oesophageal mucosa protection**
   - *Antacids:* Preparations containing alginates, cytoprotective agents.
   - $H_2$ blockers: Ranitidine.
   - Proton pump inhibitors: Omeprazole or esomeprazole.
3. **Reflux prevention**
   - Oesophageal reflux: Cisapride, metoclopramide
   - Gastric reflux: Domperidone, metoclopramide
4. **Decision of surgery:** When all measures fail, surgery should be done—reduction of hernial sac, repair of hiatus and reduce reflux by fundoplication—laparoscopic fundoplication.

*Pearls of Wisdom*

Oh LORD, save me from GORD!

## ROLLING HERNIA

- This is also called as paraoesophageal hernia. A paraoesophageal hernia is characterized by an ascent of the gastric fundus through a defect in the phrenoesophageal membrane. In this condition, cardio-oesophageal junction is normal. Thus, there are no features of reflux oesophagitis but the sac containing stomach in the thorax causes compression of the heart and lung.
- Volvulus of the stomach is a dangerous complication in this variety.
- It is an uncommon type of hiatal hernia that mainly affects older adults, with a median age of presentation between 65 and 75 years. Loss of elastic fibres as in advancing age or increased intra-abdominal pressure or multipara are the few causes mentioned.
- As the hernia enlarges, the greater curvature of the stomach rolls up into the thorax. Because the stomach is fixed at the GE junction, the herniated stomach tends to rotate around its longitudinal axis, resulting in an organoaxial volvulus. Infrequently, rotation occurs around the transverse axis resulting in a mesenteroaxial volvulus.

### Clinical Features

- No retrosternal burning pain because no reflux
- Discomfort after a small meal
- Feeling of fullness after a meal or dysphagia due to large sac
- Palpitations due to compression on the heart
- Respiratory tract infection and hiccough due to irritation of phrenic nerve.

### Investigation

- Barium meal shows the sac in the thorax containing stomach. Sometimes, it can be upside down.
- Contrast CT scan is the investigation of choice. Patients who come with features of volvulus with obstruction are evaluated with plain X-ray and CT scan as shown in Figs 52.12A and B—grossly dilated stomach and duodenum showing a large gas fluid level on the right side with partial volvulus.

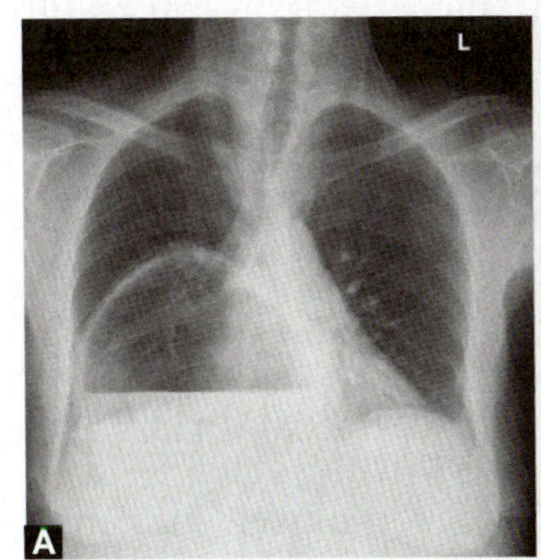

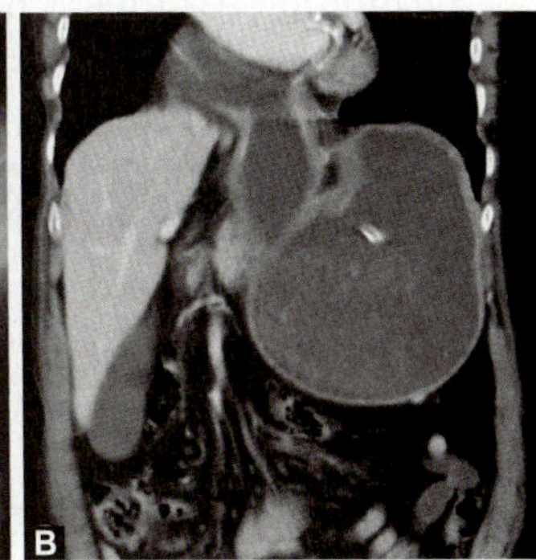


**Figs 52.12A and B:** (A) A large gas fluid level on the right side caused by obstruction of the duodenum by the defect in the diaphragm through which stomach is herniated and with partial volvulus; (B) CT scan showing grossly dilated stomach and duodenum showing partial volvulus.

### Treatment

- Reduction of the sac and repair of the hiatus by using nonabsorbable suture material to approximate the right crus of the diaphragm.
- When the defect is large, nonabsorbable mesh such as prolene, is used to cover the defect.

## MIXED HERNIA

In this, both sliding and rolling hernias are present. Symptoms are mixed—features of reflux esophagitis and compression on the mediastinal structures. Treatment is also mixed and is done for both sliding and rolling hernias.

### Complications of GORD

1. **Stricture oesophagus:** It is seen in middle-aged and elderly patients. Due to repeated reflux, ulcers, fibrosis and stricture develop in the lower end of the oesophagus. Early diagnosis by endoscopy followed by **frequent dilatation** and **proton pump inhibitors** will help the situation.

   Peptic strictures are difficult to manage surgically. Surgery is indicated in refractory cases of dilatation, in the form of **gastroplasty**.

2. **Oesophageal shortening** is also treated by Collis gastroplasty by using stomach (short oesophagus).
3. **Barrett's oesophagus:** Also known as columnar-lined oesophagus (**CLO**) (details are given below).
4. **Gastric/oesophageal ulcers**—can give rise to bleeding. **Cameron ulcers** are the ulcers in the stomach of a patient with haitus hernia. They are seen in about 3 to 5% of the patients. These ulcers occur at the site of extrinsic compression of the diaphragm on the stomach in patients with large hiatal hernias. It can be easily missed. Cameron ulcer is one of the causes of occult upper GI tract bleeding.
5. **Aspiration pneumonitis, asthma and pneumonia** are common features. Chronic aspiration can result in fibrosis of lung and bronchiectasis.

## BARRETT'S OESOPHAGUS

### DEFINITION

- When columnar mucosa extends at least 3 cm into oesophagus or when it shows intestinal metaplasia, it is described as Barrett's oesophagus.
- Ulcer in the Barrett's CLO is called **Barrett's ulcer**.

### Pathogenesis

Repeated reflux results in shifting of the oesophagogastric junction upwards, which further increases the reflux resulting in intestinal metaplasia of **middle and lower oesophagus**.

### Pathological Types

- **Gastric type** with chief and parietal cells.
- **Intestinal type** with ***goblet cells*** is a marker of intestinal metaplasia. This mucosa is smooth (unlike gastric folds).
- **Junctional type:** It has mucus glands and resembles gastric cardia.

### Prague classification for Barrett's oesophagus

- The lower measurement boundary is formed by the proximal cardiac notch (optimally with moderate insufflation), and the two upper measurement boundaries are marked by the proximal limit of the circumferential Barrett's segment (C) and the longest tongue of Barrett (M).

In Fig. 52.13, the circumferential segment (C) is 3 cm and the tongue an additional 2 cm, so that M is 5 cm (3 cm circumferential + 2 cm tongue = 5 cm maximum Barrett's extent, M). The length of the Barrett is thus C3M5. A short Barrett segment only forming a 1 cm tongue is reported as C0M1. A circular Barrett's that is 2 cm long without tongues, i.e. with a relatively straight proximal boundary is reported as C2M2.

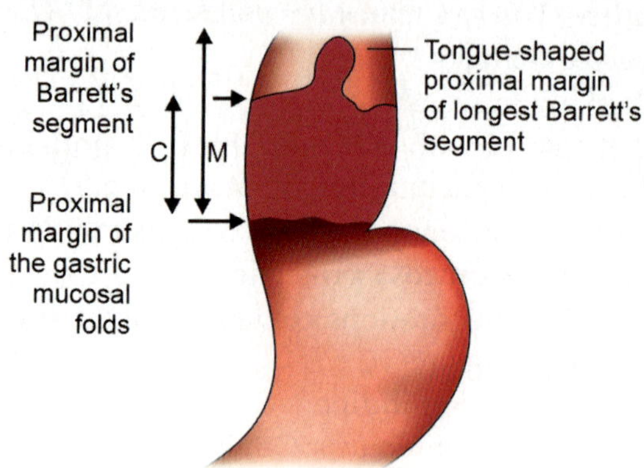


**Fig. 52.13:** Prague classification

### Clinical Types

- **Long segment:** Metaplastic changes involving more than 3 cm.
- **Short segment:** Metaplastic changes involving less than 3 cm.

### Incidence of Malignancy

40 times more prone to carcinoma of the **lower and middle oesophagus** as compared to the general population (Key Boxes 52.7 and 52.8).

**Key Box 52.7**

**Risk Factors for Carcinoma**

- CLO >8 cm
- Smoking
- Reflux due to previous gastric surgery
- High grade dysplasia—indication for oesophagectomy

**Key Box 52.8**

**Carcinoma in Barrett's Oesophagus**

- It will be invasive
- It is more proximal
- Carries poor prognosis
- 40 times increased risk compared to general population

### Types of Dysplasia

- Low grade: Negligible risk of carcinoma
- High grade: Very high-risk of carcinoma.

### Endoscopy and Screening Programme

It is important to screen these patients regularly with **repeat endoscopies and multiple biopsies to find dysplasia. Few endoscopy pictures are given here** (Figs 52.14 to 52.17).

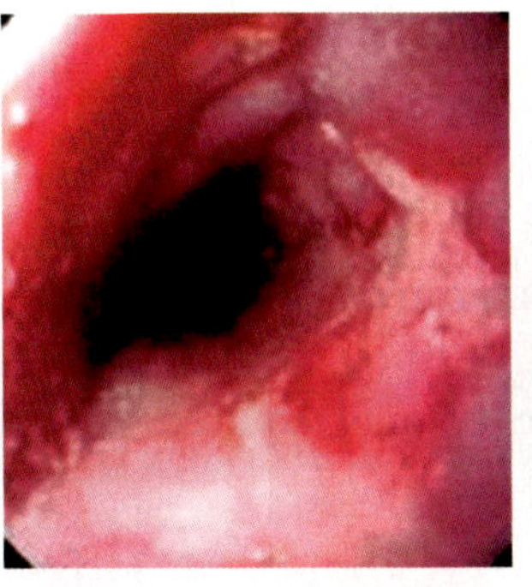
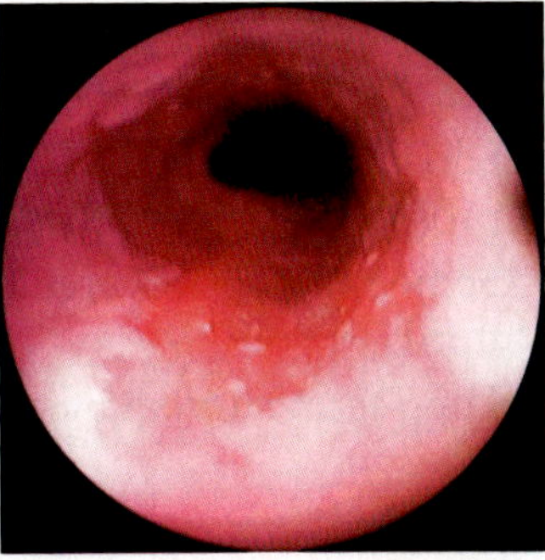

**Figs 52.14 and 52.15:** Endoscopic view of reflux oesophagitis and Barrett's oesophagus

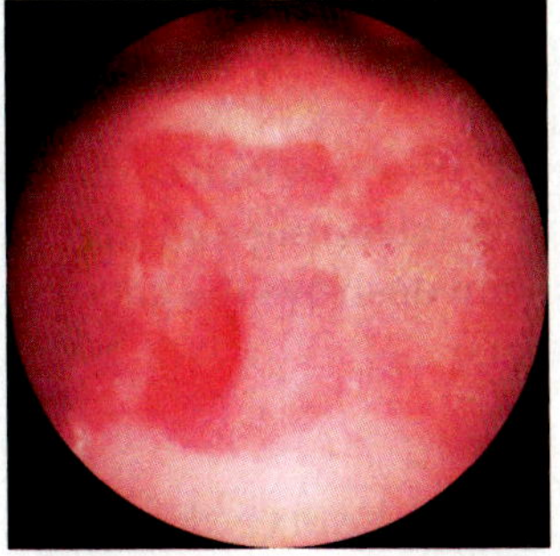

**Fig. 52.16:** Barrett's oesophagus with stricture

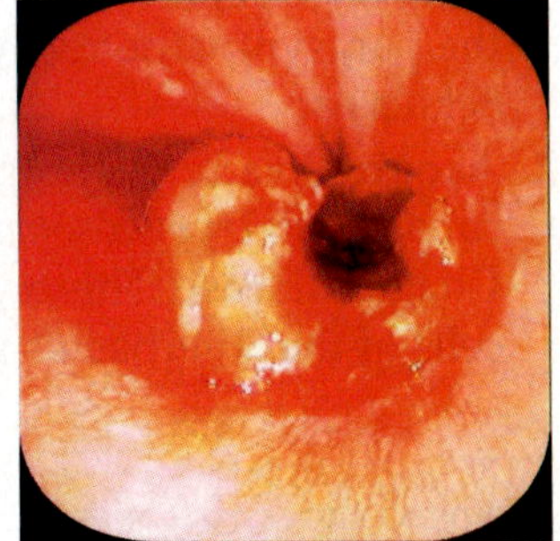

**Fig. 52.17:** Carcinoma GE junction in Barrett's oesophagus

## Treatment

- High dose proton pump inhibitors for 8 weeks.
- Radiofrequency ablation (RFA) is better than photodynamic therapy and very effective. RFA produces heat and destroys superficial tissue. Ablation pulses of two double pulses of 125/cm$^2$.
- Laser photodynamic therapy.
- Argon beam plasma coagulation.
- Asymptomatic, symptomatic Barrett's oesophagus respond well to laparoscopic antireflux surgery. Antireflux surgery also prevents progression to high grade dysplasia or adenocarcinoma.
- Endoscopic mucosal resection for Barrett's oesophagus with low grade dysplasia.
- Oesophagectomy in cases of high grade dysplasia.

*Pearls of Wisdom*

Antireflux surgery may protect mucosa against development of dysplasia in patients with Barrett's oesophagus.

## Complications of Barrett's Oesophagus

1. **Oesophageal ulcers:** Barrett's ulcer—pain, bleeding and perforation.
2. **Oesophageal stricture:** Usually located in the middle or upper oesophagus.
   - **Peptic stricture occurs in the distal oesophagus.**
3. **Dysplasia and adenocarcinoma.**

## *Nonreflux Oesophagitis*

This is also a condition which occurs due to several factors such as corrosives, drugs, chemoradiation, AIDS, etc. They are summarised in Table 52.4. Basic treatment is similar to that of reflux oesophagitis. Avoid the causative agents.

**TABLE 52.4:** Types of nonreflux oesophagitis

| | Agents causing | Clinical features |
|---|---|---|
| 1. Corrosive | Lye, acid, alkali | Burns, stricture |
| 2. Infective | Candida, herpesvirus | Chronic illness, AIDS |
| 3. Radiation | 20–40 Gy units to mediastinum | Ulceration and stricture |
| 4. Chemotherapy | Adriamycin | — |
| 5. Drug induced | NSAIDs, doxycycline | ↑reflux |

**SU28.5.4:** Describe the various symptoms associated with oesophageal disorders.

**SU28.5.5:** Describe the various investigations used in evaluation of oesophageal disorders.

## MOTILITY DISORDERS OF THE PHARYNX AND OESOPHAGUS

**Introduction:** Motility disorders of the oesophagus is an important chapter for postgraduate students. There are many classifications. However, Chicago classification has been widely accepted. Few important lesions have been discussed here.

**Classification:**

**A. Disorders affecting lower oesophagus (oesophagogastric junction)**
- Achalasia
- Diffuse oesophageal spasm
- Nutcracker oesophagus or Jackhammer oesophagus

**B. Disorders affecting upper oesophagus and pharynx**
- Plummer-Vinson syndrome

**C. Disorders affecting body**
- Diffuse oesophageal spasm.

## PLUMMER-VINSON SYNDROME

**Introduction:** It is also called Paterson-Kelly syndrome. It is a precancerous condition in which there is a severe spasm of circular muscle fibres at the cricopharyngeal sphincter level or pharyngo-oesophageal junction, and it is associated with **development of postcricoid web**.

### Aetiopathogenesis

- Aetiology is not known.
- It is seen in women who have worries and anxiety.

- As a result of the spasm and web, dysplasia occurs and leads to features of anaemia later. The proximal mucosa is constantly irritated due to stasis. It undergoes hypertrophy, hyperkeratosis and desquamation. This, over a period of years, predisposes to carcinoma oesophagus (carcinoma oropharynx).

### Clinical Features

- Women in the middle age group are affected.
- Increasing **dysphagia** for solids and liquids due to spasm.
- Features of **anaemia**—pallor, stomatitis, ulcerations, bald tongue (without papillae), koilonychia, splenomegaly and microcytic hypochromic anaemia.
- As a result of obstruction, the fluid tends to spillover into the larynx giving rise to recurrent aspiration, respiratory tract infection, cyanosis or choking.

### Treatment

- Reassurance
- Improving anaemia: Iron tablets or blood transfusion and correction of nutritional deficiencies.
- Regular dilatation by using gum elastic bougies.

**Summary:** Refer Key Box 52.9.

Key Box 52.9

**Summary**

**P**ost cricoid web
**L**ow haemoglobin–anaemia–correction by iron supplements
**U**pper cricopharyngeal sphincter spasm
**M**iddle aged woman
**M**alignancy is a complication
**E**lastic bougie—dilatation
**R**espiratory complications

**You can remember as PLUMMER**

## ACHALASIA CARDIA

- Achalasia means failure to relax.
- It is a primary oesophageal motility disorder.
- It is also called cardiospasm because of severe spasm of the circular muscle fibres of the lower end of the oesophagus. The contracted segment does not relax during the act of swallowing (achalasia = failure of relaxation). As a result of this, there is dilatation, tortuosity and hypertrophy of the oesophagus above.
- Incidence: 6 in 1,00,000 population/year.
- Importantly it is a pre-cancerous condition for carcinoma oesophagus.

### Achalasia and Carcinoma Oesophagus

- 8% chances of carcinoma over 20 years period.
- Squamous cell carcinoma is the most common due to prolonged stasis and irritation.
- Sometimes adenocarcinoma can occur in the middle third.
- Long-term surveillance program is required.

### Aetiopathogenesis

1. **Idiopathic:** This occurs due to absence or degeneration of Auerbach's plexus throughout the body of the oesophagus leading to improper integration of the parasympathetic impulse. This is called primary achalasia.
2. **Acquired variety** is seen in South American countries caused by *Trypanosoma cruzi* (sleeping sickness)—**Chagas disease**. This organism destroys the ganglion cells of the Auerbach's plexus.

*Pearls of Wisdom*

*Trypanosoma cruzi* causes megaoesophagus, megaduodenum, megacolon and megaureter. Can we call it a 'mega'organism?

3. Stress and emotional factors and vitamin deficiencies are also associated with this disease.

### Pathophysiology

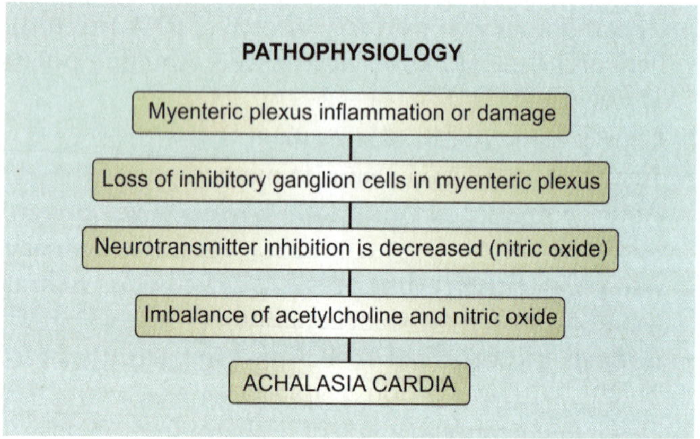


### Types of Achalasia Cardia

- Classical achalasia: Loss of ganglion cells and neural fibrosis occurs (**Type I—classic**)
- Achalasia with oesophageal compression (**Type II**)
- Vigorous achalasia: No loss of ganglion cells but ganglionitis occurs **(Type III/spastic achalasia)**.

### Clinical Features

- Women around 30–40 years of age are commonly affected. The ratio of affected females to males is 3:2.

- Most patients find eating slow and they drink large volume of fluid. As a result when peristalsis starts retrosternal pain develops.
- **Dysphagia** develops slowly, and it is progressive. Solids, by forming a bolus and aided by gravity, as they touch the contracted segment, may partially open up the sphincter. Thus, there is no dysphagia for solids. Dysphagia for liquids is an important feature and it results in **regurgitation** (oesophageal pseudovomiting). The regurgitant material contains foul-smelling oesophageal contents. Malnourishment, ill health and weight loss follow soon. **Dysphagia, regurgitation and weight loss form the triad of achalasia cardia**.
- **Recurrent respiratory tract infection** due to spillage of liquids can also occur.
- **Features of anaemia**—glossitis, stomatitis, pallor, bald tongue.
- **Retrosternal discomfort** and radiation of pain to the interscapular region may be present.
- **Pseudoachalasia:** Tumours of cardia mimicking achalasia. Often patients present with features of recent achalasia (dysphagia). During endoscopy, some difficulties are encountered and once the scope enters the GE junction, growth will be seen.

*Pearls of Wisdom*

Inhalation of amyl nitrite leads to sphincter relaxation in achalasia but not in pseudoachalasia.

## Investigations

1. **Barium swallow:**
   - Uniformly dilated oesophagus above, with a smooth tapering segment below—**cucumber oesophagus**.
   - In chronic cases, it may be sigmoid-shaped (Figs 52.18 and 52.19).

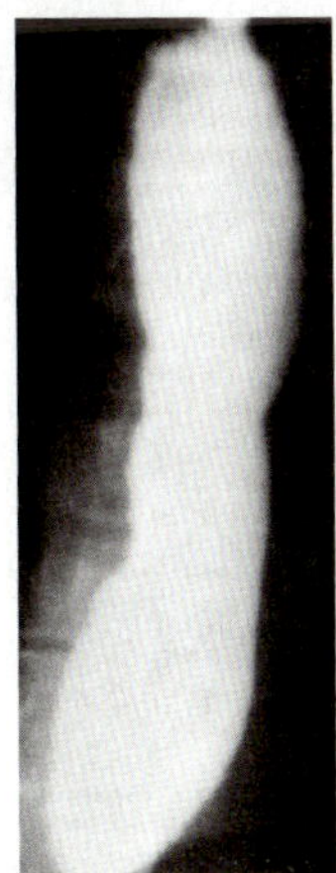

**Fig. 52.18:** Barium swallow showing dilated oesophagus

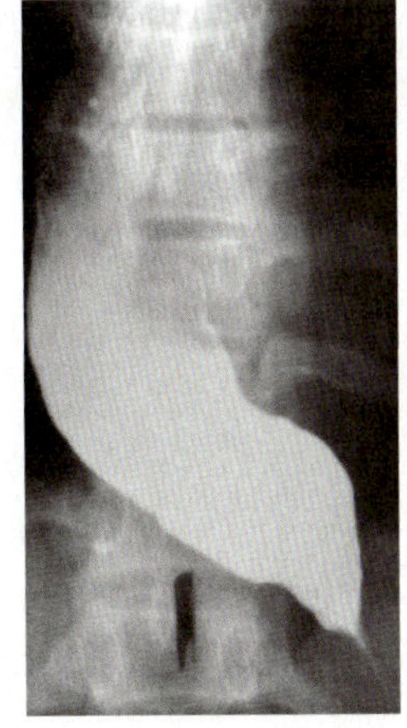

**Fig. 52.19:** Barium swallow showing sigmoid oesophagus

2. **X-ray chest:**
   - Mediastinal mass (pseudotumour)[1] produced by dilated oesophagus can be seen (Fig. 52.20).
   - **Retrocardiac air-fluid level is seen in the lateral view.**
   - Aspiration pneumonitis can be diagnosed.
3. **Plain X-ray abdomen erect:** Fundic air bubble is absent because of the stasis of fluid in the oesophagus.
4. **Oesophagoscopy:** It reveals a dilated sac containing stagnant food and fluid due to stasis which splashes out with each heartbeat and with each respiratory movement.

   **LES:** Lower oesophageal sphincter is closed, with air insufflation. It has a 'rosette' appearance (Fig. 52.21).
   - Oesophagoscopy is also done to rule out proximal malignancy.
   - Also done to evaluate oesophagitis, stricture or a tumour at cardia.
5. **Oesophageal manometry:** Following features are characteristic of achalasia cardia:
   - Hypertensive lower oesophageal sphincter (LOS): It does not relax on swallowing.
   - **Aperistalsis in the body** of oesophagus
   - Increased resting pressure in the oesophagus
6. **Ultrasound:** It may detect subepithelial tumour infiltration in secondary achalasia due to a distal carcinoma.

*Pearls of Wisdom*

You suspect achalasia by clinical features
You support achalasia by barium swallow
You confirm achalasia by manometry
You exclude carcinoma by UGI scopy
You treat by dilatation or POEM or surgery

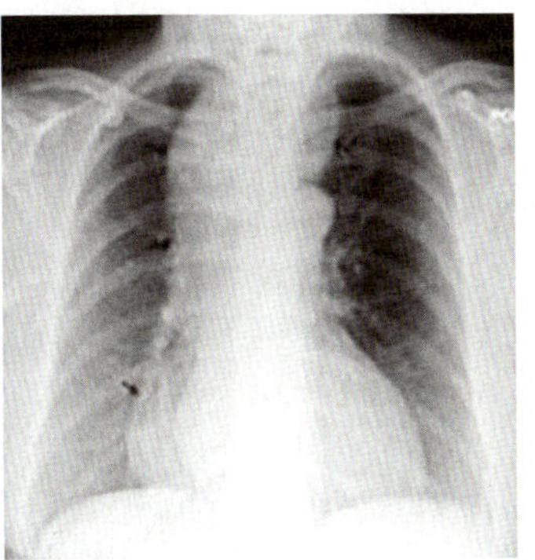

**Fig. 52.20:** Achalasia—chest X-ray

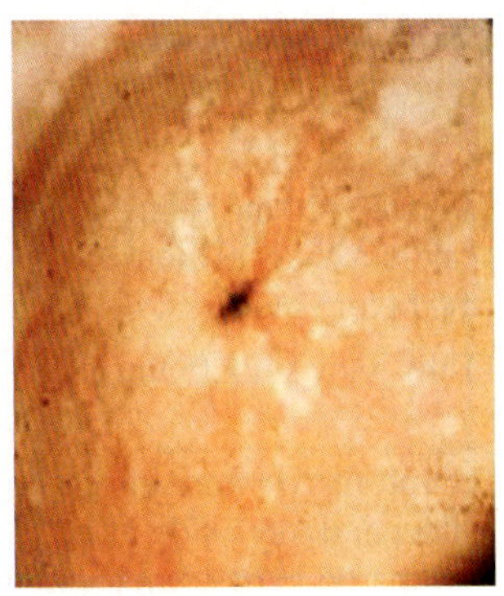

**Fig. 52.21:** Endoscopy showing rosette appearance

[1]Aortic aneurysm, cold abscess (paravertebral), scoliosis are the other pseudotumours in the chest X-ray.

**Treatment** (Table 52.5—four choices)

- Aim of the treatment is to cure the disease.
- **More importantly, the obstruction at the lower end of oesophagus must be relieved.**
- **Modified laparoscopic Heller's cardiomyotomy is the choice of surgery now.**

1. **Heller's cardiomyotomy:** The aim is to reduce outflow resistance at the lower oesophageal sphincter.
    - With a left thoracoabdominal incision, the oesophagus and the stomach are completely mobilised.
    - The contracted segment is felt between the fingers.
    - A 7–10 cm long incision is made through the lower end of the oesophagus and carried over to the stomach. The muscles are cut till the mucosa bulges out. **The myotomy should extend proximally up to the aortic arch and distally up to the stomach to 1–2 cm below the junction.** Success rate is around 90%. About 3 to 5% of the patients develop reflux oesophagitis which needs to be treated conservatively.
2. **Forceful dilatation:** By using **pneumatic balloon**—the balloon is positioned under fluoroscopic control within LOS. It should be rapidly inflated to a pressure of 300 mmHg for 15 seconds. Success rate is around 70%. 20% chances of reflux are present. Oesophageal perforation can also occur. Recurrences are common (Figs 52.22 and 52.23).
3. **Injection treatment: Inj. botulinum toxin A** is injected into the lower oesophageal sphincter (LOS) endoscopically. It is temporary and repeat injections are necessary (Key Box 52.10).

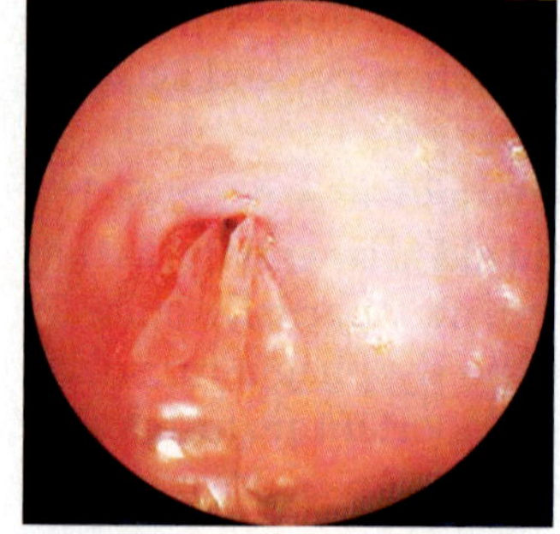

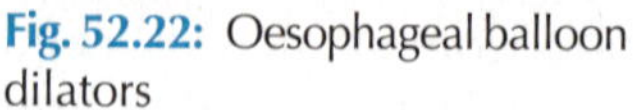

**Fig. 52.22:** Oesophageal balloon dilators

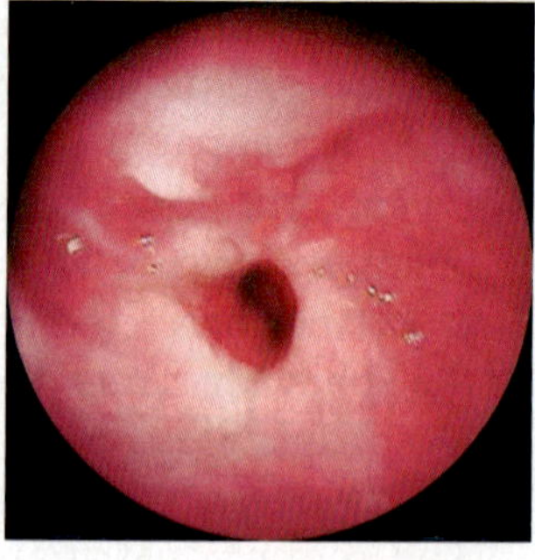

**Fig. 52.23:** Oesophageal narrowing of lower end

Key Box 52.10

**Injection Botulinum Toxin A**

- Endoscopic botulinum toxin is the most common initial treatment of achalasia cardia in USA.
- It is a neurotoxin.
- 8 different types of toxin are available. Most common being type A.
- Injection acts by interfering with cholinergic excitatory neural activity at LOS and blocking acetylcholine release from nerve terminals.
- It is an excellent endotherapy for short-term treatment of achalasia cardia.
- In about more than 50% cases, relapse occurs within few months and repeat injections are necessary.

4. **Drugs:** Sublingual nifedipine can produce short-term relief.
5. **Per oral endoscopic myotomy—popularly called POEM:** In this, through endoscope, a submucosal injection of a mixture of indigo rouge, epinephrine,

**TABLE 52.5:** Treatment of achalasia cardia

| Pharmacological therapy | Botulinum toxin injection | Pneumatic dilatation | Surgery |
|---|---|---|---|
| Sublingually used | BoTx A 80–100 units are injected in one sitting | Most effective nonsurgical option | Modified lap. Heller's cardiomyotomy is the gold standard |
| Nitrates and calcium channel blockers | 20–25 IU are injected into each quadrant | It disrupts the circular muscle fibres of LES | 6 cm of lower oesophagus and 1–2 cm of proximal stomach myotomy is done |
| Nitrate 5–20 mg before meal and calcium channel blockers 10–30 mg before meal | Use 5 mm sclerotherapy needle | Polyethylene balloon is used | 90% success |
| They relax smooth muscle | It acts by blocking acetylcholine release | Dilators are 3, 3.5 and 4 cm | 3% reflux oesophagitis |
| Nitrates have more intense effect and more side-effect as compared to calcium channel blocker | Repeat injections are necessary as effect is temporary | 70% permanent relief | **POEM:** Per Oral Endoscopic Myotomy is popular now |
| Headache is the side-effect | Pregnancy, hypersensitivity to albumin are contraindications | Side-effect is perforation, gastro-oesophageal reflux, haemorrhage | |

and saline is done. A 2 cm long incision is made and submucosal tunnel is created. Then circular muscle bundle is cut slowly, beginning from 7 to 8 cm above GE junction to 2–3 cm below GE junction. Mucosa is sutured with absorbable sutures or clips.

### Complication of Achalasia Cardia

- Reflux is the most common complication. As a result of which recurrent aspirations and lung complications including pneumonia are the features.
- Due to prolonged stasis and chronic irritation, it can predispose to **carcinoma** of the mid and lower oesophagus (due to metaplasia). Hence, it is a precancerous condition. Squamous cell carcinoma is the most common type identified in a patient with achalasia.
- Nutritional deficiencies—anaemia and weight loss.

## DIFFUSE OESOPHAGEAL SPASM

- An entity of unknown aetiology, presents with dysphagia and chest pain. It is a hypermotility disorder of the oesophagus.
- Motor abnormality affects body of the oesophagus.
- Degeneration of branches of vagus nerve has been documented.

### Aetiology

Exact cause is not known. *Stress* may be one of the factors.

### Symptoms and Signs

- Discomfort in the chest (chest pain) or spasmodic pain, dysphagia, weight loss.
- Regurgitation is common. But no acid reflux is found.

### Investigations

1. **Barium swallow:** It is typically described as corkscrew oesophagus—segmental spasms, area of narrowing and irregular uncoordinated peristalsis.
2. **Manometry:** It is the diagnostic test. Findings are normal lower oesophageal sphincter, alteration of oesophageal peristalsis and contractions. Contractions of high amplitude >120 mmHg of long durations (>2.5 seconds) are findings.
3. **Ambulatory 24-hour pH monitoring:** This is an important test to rule out GORD.

### Treatment

- It is directed in the similar lines of achalasia cardia—medical therapy, pneumatic dilatation intrasphincteric botulinum toxin injection, Heller's myotomy and partial fundoplication.
- Long oesophageal myotomy may be required.
- These patients need counselling. Depression, anxiety status to be ruled out.
- Sedation, nitrates, calcium channel blockers are used.

## NUTCRACKER OESOPHAGUS OR JACKHAMMER OESOPHAGUS

- Aetiology is not known.
- Chest pain is the most common symptom followed by painful dysphagia (odynophagia).
- Barium swallow is usually normal. An epinephric diverticulum is usually present.
- Majority of the patients have normal propagation of peristaltic waves. However, in the distal oesophagus, peristaltic waves have very high amplitude (>180 mmHg) and duration (>6 seconds).
- Dilatation, myotomy, proton pump inhibitors, calcium channel blockers are used with limited success.
- Regurgitation and reflux are uncommon.

> **SU28.6:** Describe the clinical features, investigations and principles of management of benign and malignant disorders of oesophagus.

## CARCINOMA OF THE OESOPHAGUS

### Introduction

- Majority of oesophageal cancers are squamous cell carcinomas, worldwide. However, in most Western countries, more than 70% are adenocarcinomas. This shift is mainly due to smoking, alcohol and Barrett's oesophagus. More than 50% of patients present with locally advanced carcinomas. Some improvement has taken place now because of early diagnosis, detection and multimodality treatment.
- **Oesophageal cancers have poor prognosis because of the following reasons:**
  1. More lymph vessels are present in the submucosa than blood capillaries and hence, spread is fast.
  2. Lymph flow in submucosal plexus runs in a longitudinal direction. Hence, primary tumour can extend for a considerable length both superiorly and inferiorly.
- Cervical oesophagus has direct spread to regional nodes and there are less lymphatics in the submucosa. Hence, prognosis is better.

### Carcinoma Oesophagus—What is Changing?

- Squamous cell carcinoma is more common in Africans and Asians. Adenocarcinoma is more common in whites and Americans. Adenocarcinoma is increasing.
- Survival is improving.
- There is improvement in detection and staging.
- Detected more frequently in younger patients.
- Detected at an early stage also.

## AETIOPATHOGENESIS

### I. Precancerous/Predisposing Conditions

A. GORD with Barrett's oesophagus (*see* page 676). Malignancy in Barrett's oesophagus is curable if detected at an early stage. Hence, endoscopic surveillance is recommended.

B. Plummer-Vinson syndrome with squamous metaplasia (*see* page 683)—upper oesophagus.

C. Achalasia cardia (*see* page 684)—lower oesophagus.

D. Corrosive strictures (*see* page 697). **Lye strictures up to 30%:** Squamous cell carcinomas may arise in lye strictures, often developing 40–50 years after caustic injury. The majority of these cancers are located in the middle third of the oesophagus.

### II. Carcinogens

A. Tobacco, heavy smoking and abuse of alcohol increase incidence of both squamous cell carcinoma and adenocarcinoma by almost 20–25%.

B. **Dietary carcinogens and squamous cell carcinoma**
- Elevated nitrates in drinking water.
- Food (pickles, corn) containing fungi—*Geotrichum candidum* as in endemic areas of China.
- Baked bread
- Protective: Fruits and vegetables have a varieties of vitamins and minerals that may protect against developing cancer.

### III. Viral

**Human papillomavirus (HPV) infection increases squamous cell carcinoma.** This oncogenic virus has been associated with cervical and oropharyngeal cancers also.

### IV. Hereditary

A. Hovels-Evans syndrome or tylosis—40–60% of the patients develop cancers. Also called familial keratosis plantaris.

> Tylosis (focal nonepidermolytic palmoplantar keratoderma) is a rare disease inherited in an autosomal dominant manner that is characterised by hyperkeratosis of the palms and soles and oesophageal papillomas. Patients with this condition exhibit abnormal maturation of squamous cells. They also cause inflammation within the oesophagus and are at extremely high risk of developing oesophageal cancer.

B. Patients with head and neck cancers—field cancerisation.

### V. Bacterial

***Helicobacter pylori* infection:** Infection with *Helicobacter pylori*, and particularly with cag A+ strains, is inversely associated with the risk of adenocarcinoma of the oesophagus. Mechanism is not clear. In fact, it should not have been a factor responsible because *H. pylori* infection can cause chronic atrophic gastritis leading to decreased acid production, which negates the effects of chronic reflux, including the potential for development of Barrett's oesophagus.

### VI. Miscellaneous

**Factors for adenocarcinoma**
- **Obesity:** Increased body mass index is a risk factor for adenocarcinoma of the oesophagus, and individuals with the highest body mass index have up to a sevenfold greater risk of oesophageal cancer than those with a low body mass index. Probably, the linkage between obesity and gastro-oesophageal reflux disease is presumed to be a chief factor.
- **Economic status:** Low socioeconomic status as defined by income, education, or occupation is associated with increased risk for oesophageal squamous cell carcinoma, and adenocarcinoma to a smaller extent.

## SITES

- 50%—middle 1/3rd of oesophagus
- 33%—lower 1/3rd of oesophagus
- 17%—upper 1/3rd of oesophagus.

## TYPES

### I. Squamous Cell Carcinoma

- Epitheliomatous ulcer (carcinomatous) with raised edges and flat base.
- Proliferative growth (cauliflower) with surface ulcer which commonly bleeds.
- Infiltrative variety or annular stenosing variety with a 5-year survival of 10%, gives rise to early dysphagia due to circumferential and longitudinal spread.
- Polypoidal lesions (5 years survival 70%).

### II. Adenocarcinoma

Mostly lower end and middle oesophagus (in Barrett's oesophagus).

**Comparison of squamous cell carcinoma and adenocarcinoma** is given in Table 52.6.

## CLINICAL FEATURES

- Men more than 60 years.
- **Dysphagia** which is **progressive** and mainly for solids (it takes 18 months for dysphagia to develop).
- It means 60% of the circumference of the lumen is involved by the growth. By the time, the patient presents with dysphagia, the disease is fairly advanced. Hence, it has a poor prognosis. **Dysphagia is a late symptom because smooth muscle of oesophageal wall can dilate with ease due to lack of serosal layer on the oesophagus**.
- **Regurgitation** of the food contents. Haematemesis is not very common. Vomitus may contain streaks of blood and melaena is rare.
- Loss of appetite, loss of weight and cachexia
- Backache indicates enlarged lymph nodes (coeliac).

**TABLE 52.6:** Comparison of two types of oesophageal cancer

| | Squamous cell carcinoma | Adenocarcinoma |
|---|---|---|
| Site | Upper two-thirds | Lower one-third |
| Predisposing factors | Smoking alcohol | Barrett's oesophagus—GORD |
| Corrosive stricture (Lye stricture) | Definite premalignant condition | Not a premalignant condition |
| Behaviour | Less aggressive | More aggressive |
| Incidence | Less common | More common |
| Achalasia cardia | Is the predisposing factor | Does not give rise to adenocarcinoma |
| Chemoradiation | It can be an alternate treatment | Not alternate to surgery |
| Surgery | Can be the first choice or chemoradiation | Surgery is the first choice—unfit patient, chemotherapy |
| Dietary carcinogens | A. Elevated nitrates in drinking water<br>B. Food containing fungi—*Geotrichum candidum*—pickles<br>C. Baked bread | Consumption of meat<br>Alcohol |

- Abdominal findings are normal in upper and middle third of carcinoma oesophagus patients. Left supraclavicular node enlargement (Troisier's sign) should be looked for. Lower third carcinoma patients (in advanced stages), may have palpable liver due to metastasis, epigasric mass can be due to enlarged para aortic lymph nodes. Rectal examination may reveal pelvic deposits.

## SPREAD

### 1. Local Spread or Direct Spread

- To start with, it is a mucosal ulceration which spreads to the submucosa. Later, it causes fibrosis and the lumen gets narrowed. The spread occurs transversely and longitudinally. Once, it spreads to all the layers, the structures in the vicinity are involved. Factors responsible for early spread and aggressive behaviour of carcinoma oesophagus are lack of serosal layer, proximity of vital structures, extensive mediastinal lymphatic drainage and late presentation.
- When the trachea is involved, tracheo-oesophageal fistula develops from carcinoma upper 1/3rd of oesophagus.
- Broncho-oesophageal fistula from carcinoma middle 1/3rd.
- Oesophago-aortic fistula results in massive bleeding (one of the causes of death).
- All these complications are contraindications for surgery and radiotherapy.

### 2. Lymphatic Spread

Studies have showed that **patients having metastasis to 5 or fewer lymph nodes** have a better outcome. Palpable left supraclavicular nodes indicate advanced disease. This sign is described as **Troisier's sign.**

### 3. Blood Spread

It results in secondaries in the liver, which clinically appear as nodular enlarged liver. Later, ascites and rectovesical deposits occur.

## INVESTIGATIONS

1. **Hb%** is low, which is the cause of generalized weakness.
2. **Liver function test (LFT)** is affected, if secondaries in liver occur (increased ALP).
3. **Ultrasound** is done to rule out liver secondaries, lymph nodes in the porta hepatis, coeliac nodes, etc.
4. **Barium swallow** demonstrates irregular, persistent, intrinsic filling defect (Figs 52.24 to 52.27)—**shouldering is characteristic**. Barium can also detect

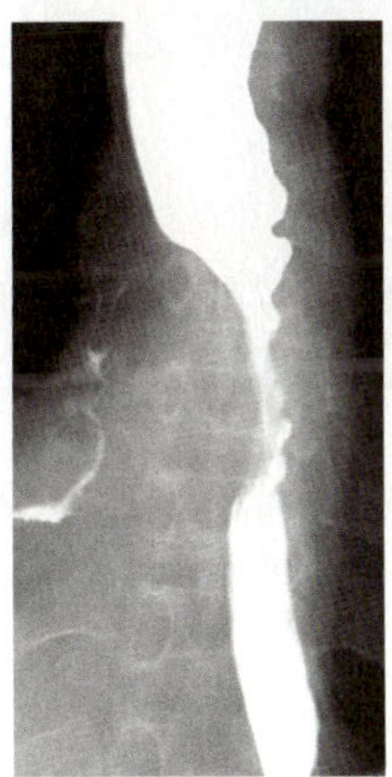

**Fig. 52.24:** Barium swallow—carcinoma middle oesophagus

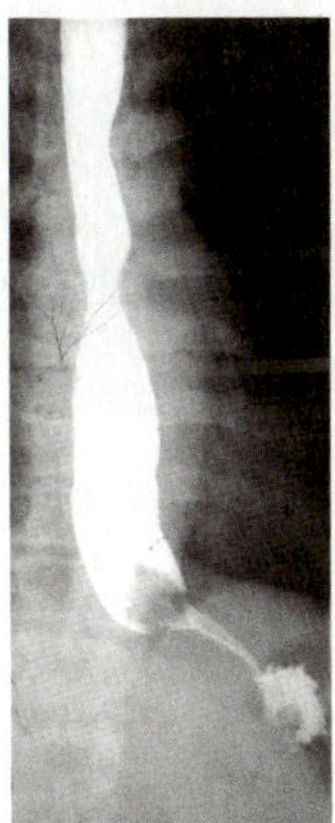

**Figs 52.25 and 52.26:** Carcinoma lower end of the oesophagus. Observe proximal shouldering

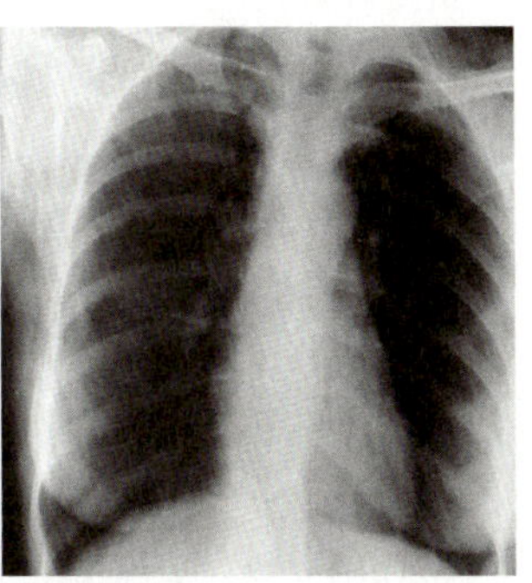

**Fig. 52.27:** Barium swallow showing straight axis—inoperable sign

abnormal 'axis'. It can also demonstrate fistula. Both these features suggest that 'CURE' is not possible.

5. **Oesophagoscopy** to visualise the growth and to take biopsy (Figs 52.28, 52.29 and Key Box 52.11).
   - **Multiple biopsies** may be necessary. In high-risk areas like China, **endoscopic staining with supravital dyes** (indigo carmine) is done to identify dysplastic epithelium. If found, some advocate endoscopic mucosal resection.
6. **Chest X-ray** to rule out aspiration pneumonia, mediastinal widening and posterior tracheal indentation.
7. **Bronchoscopy** to rule out involvement of bronchus, as in carcinoma middle 1/3rd. If involved, it can confirm that tumour is locally unresectable.
8. **CT scan** (Figs 52.30 and 52.31) of the chest and abdomen to detect local infiltration and to stage the disease. It is a very useful investigation before contemplating for total oesophagectomy. It is useful to assess involvement of vital structures such as bronchus, airway, pericardium, aorta, etc. Obliteration of fat planes gives the clue.
9. **Endoscopic ultrasound** to know the depth of wall involvement, to detect mediastinal lymph nodes, etc. (Fig. 52.32 and Key Box 52.12).

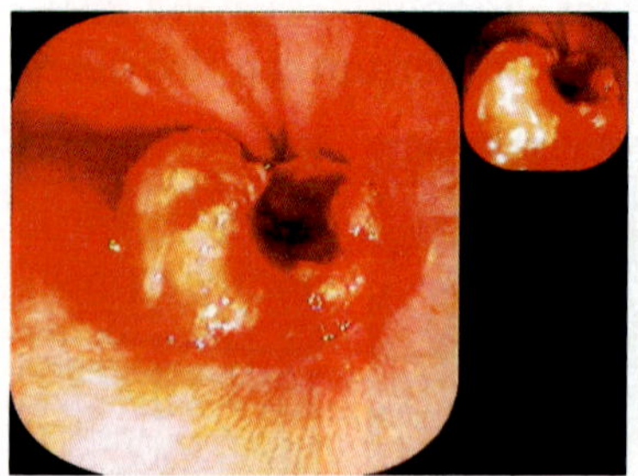

**Fig. 52.28:** Biopsy taken—observe the bleeding—friable growth

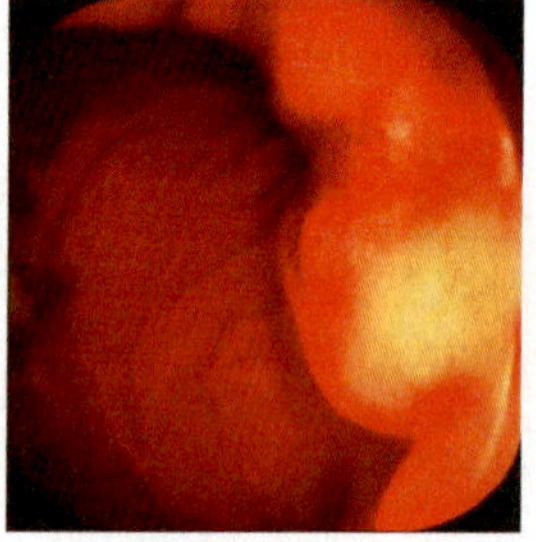

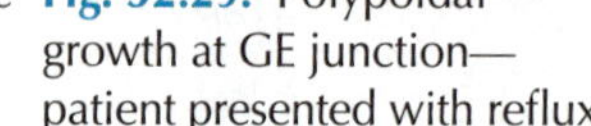

**Fig. 52.29:** Polypoidal growth at GE junction—patient presented with reflux

Key Box 52.11

### Chromoendoscopy

- Chromoendoscopy involves the topical application of stains or pigments to improve tissue localisation, characterisation, or diagnosis during endoscopy.
- Several agents have been described that can broadly be categorised as absorptive (vital) stains, contrast stains, and reactive stains.
- Absorptive stains (e.g. Lugol's solution and methylene blue) diffuse or are preferentially absorbed across specific epithelial cell membranes.
- Contrast stains (e.g. indigo carmine) highlight surface topography and mucosal irregularities by permeating mucosal crevices.
- Reactive stains (e.g. Congo red and phenol red) undergo chemical reactions with specific cellular constituents, resulting in a colour change.

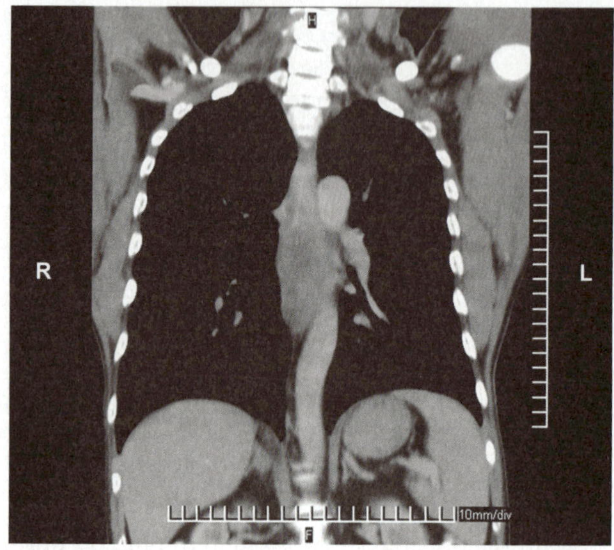


**Fig. 52.30:** Contrast CT showing a large mid-oesophageal growth

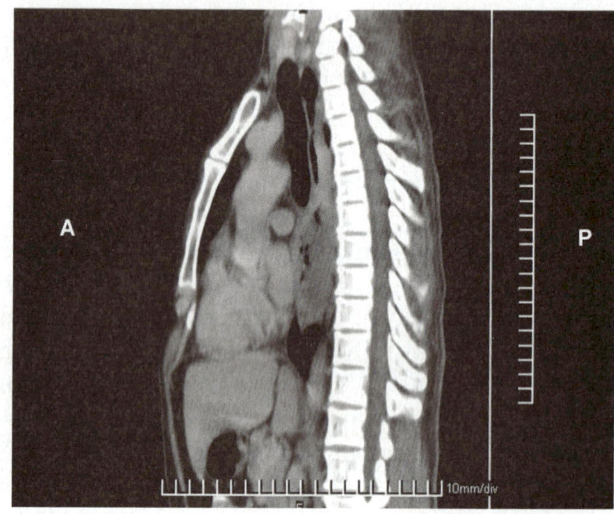


**Fig. 52.31:** Contrast CT lateral picture showing total occlusion of mid-oesophagus

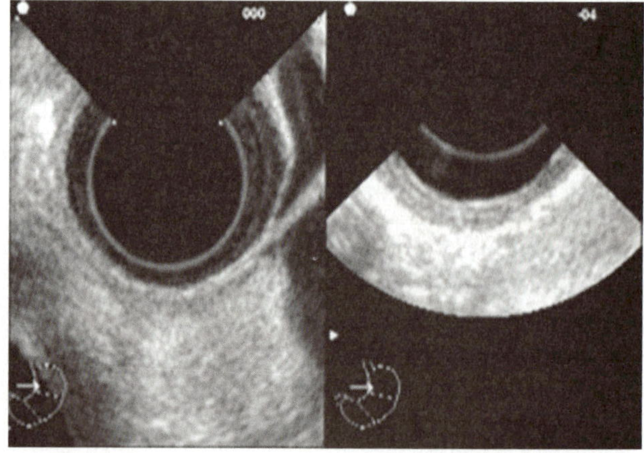

**Fig. 52.32:** Endosonography showing oesophagus and stomach layers. (*Courtesy*: Prof Ganesh Pai, Head, Department of Medical Gastroenterology, KMC, Manipal)

Key Box 52.12

**Endoscopic Ultrasound (Endosonography)**

- It relies on a high frequency (5–30 MHz) transducer
- To determine the depth of spread of a malignant tumour through the oesophageal wall
- Involvement of adjacent organs
- Metastasis to lymph nodes
- Also detects contiguous spread **downward into cardia**
- Can detect metastasis in the liver
- Can also detect small lymph nodes which are less than 5 mm (which cannot be detected by CT scan also)
- If 'endosonography' detects more than **5 lymph nodes**, it is not a case for curative resection.

10. **Positron emission tomography (PET)/computerized tomography scanning:** PET scan is based on the principle that metabolically active tumour cells can be visible once radiopharmaceutical agent 18F-fluorodeoxyglucose (FDG) is given intravenously. These lymph nodes, if malignant, are clearly visible thus differentiating them from nonmalignant enlargement (Fig. 52.33). Applying the same principles, PET can be used to know the 'response' after radiotherapy or chemotherapy.
11. **Thoracoscopy and laparoscopy:** At the end of all investigations, it is important to decide, whether one can resect this tumour or not? Is it worthwhile resecting? Can patient tolerate the procedure? Is palliative major resection worth doing? Even in the absence of systemic spread, some features will suggest surgical cure is unlikely. Check these key boxes (Key Boxes 52.13 to 52.15).
12. **Laparoscopic ultrasound:** It is an extended investigation (Key Box 52.16).

Key Box 52.13

**Investigations and their Importance in Carcinoma Oesophagus**

- **Haemoglobin:** If it is low, wound healing is delayed
- **Albumin:** If it is low, anastomotic leak rates are high
- **Barium studies:** Straight axis of oesophagus indicates inoperability
  Fistula can be detected
- **Chest X-ray:** If it shows coin lesions, it is an advanced disease
- **Bronchoscopy:** Infiltration of bronchus indicates inoperability
- **CT scan:** Investigation of choice, helps in deciding the type of treatment
- **Endosonography:** To know the involvement of different layers of oesophagus for TNM staging
- **PET scan:** Is not done in the initial stage for evaluation, done for recurrent disease.
- **Diagnostic laparoscopy** before radical surgery, if peritoneal metastases are present—avoid radical surgery.

**CECT—PET SCAN OF CARCINOMA OESOPHAGUS**

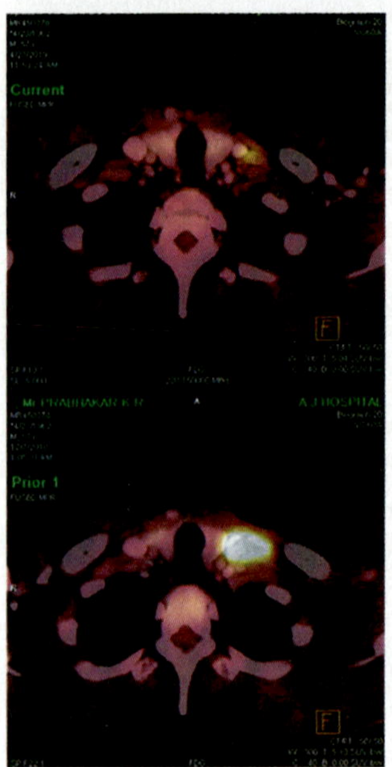

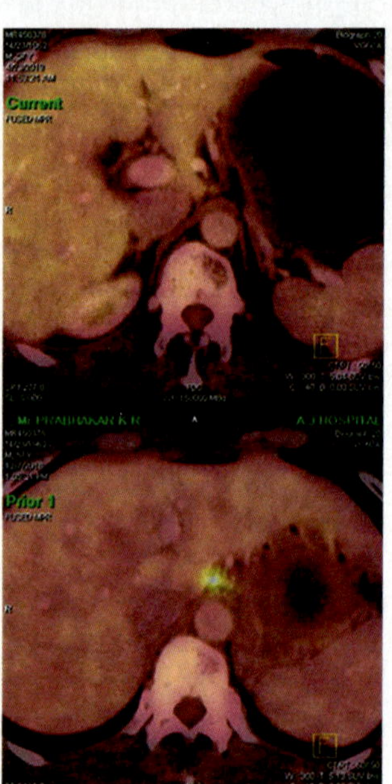

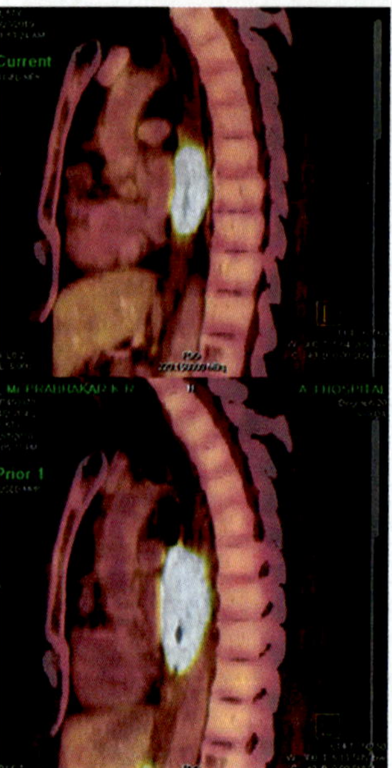

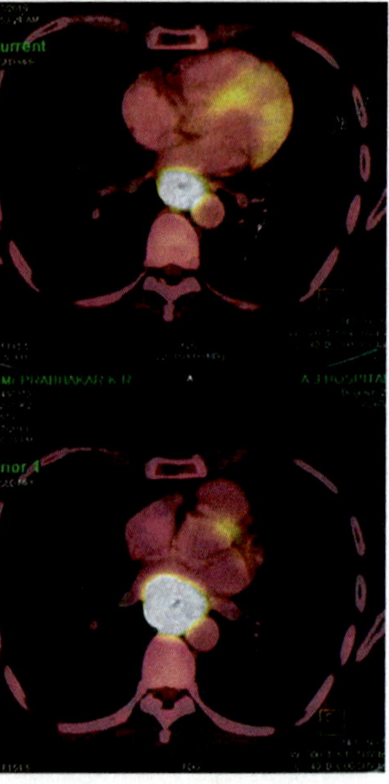


**Fig. 52.33:** CECT—PET scan of carcinoma oesophagus. Increased FDG uptake is noted in the circumferential wall thickening involving the mid and lower oesophagus (max wall thickness 1.9 cm, length 6.6 cm, SUVmax 24.43) causing near total occlusion of lumen and dilatation of proximal oesophagus. Increased FDG uptake is noted in the left supraclavicular nodal mass measuring 3.1 × 2.2 cm, SUVmax 13.12. (*Courtesy*: Dr Anant Pai, Associate Professor, Medical Oncologist, KMC, Manipal).

Key Box 52.14

**Thoracoscopy and Laparoscopy**

- Staging tools in oesophageal cancer.
- More accurate in determining nodal status than non-invasive techniques and helpful in evaluating the extent of local invasion and metastatic disease.
- Thoracoscopy is accurate in 93% and laparoscopy in 94% of patients in identifying metastatic disease.
- Studies have proved that 6 cases of unsuspected coeliac nodal disease were identified in 19 patients despite preoperative CT and EUS.

Key Box 52.15

**Unlikely Surgical Cure in the Absence of Systemic Spread**

- **L**oss of weight more than 20%
- (O)**E**sophageal 'axis' is abnormal on barium test
- **N**odes—multiple on CT scan
- **G**rade—invasive, poorly differentiated
- **T**umour length more than 8 cm
- **H**orner's syndrome

*Remember as* **LENGTH**

Key Box 52.16

**Laparoscopic Ultrasound (LUS)**

- LUS is also a staging modality and may provide improved accuracy in T and N staging.
- LUS may also be more accurate for staging coeliac nodes because EUS probe is more distant and does not provide direct inspection.

**Depth of invasion**

- For T1 lesions, conservative oesophageal resection such as vagal-sparing, transhiatal or minimally invasive oesophagectomy can be opted.
- For localised intramucosal tumours of limited extent, EMR or ESD are an acceptable alternative.
- There is almost no role for chemoradiotherapy for treatment of T1 lesions.
- Surgical or endoscopic resection alone carries a good long-term survival, as high as 88% in some series.

**Depth of tumour *vs* lymph node involvement (LNI)**

| | |
|---|---|
| 1. T1 lesion (intramucosal) | 18% LNI |
| 2. T1 lesion (submucosal) | 55% LNI |
| 3. T2 lesion | 60% LNI |
| 4. T3 lesion | 80% LNI |

## General Assessment for Staging

- Once the diagnosis is confirmed and staging (TNM) is done by metastatic work-up, performance status is done by using ECOG (Eastern Cooperative Oncology Group) criteria.
- General health of the patient, co-morbid conditions, fitness for anaesthesia—all these factors decide the choice of therapy.

**TNM STAGING: AJCC, 8th edition**

**Tumour**

| | |
|---|---|
| **T0** | No primary tumour |
| **Tis** | Carcinoma in situ—high-grade dysplasia |
| **T1a** | Tumour invades lamina propria, muscularis mucosa |
| **T1b** | Tumour involving submucosa |
| **T2** | Tumour involving muscularis propria |
| **T3** | Tumour with paraoesophageal spread |
| **T4** | Involvement of recurrent laryngeal nerve, phrenic nerve, sympathetic chain, azygos vein; malignant effusion (adjacent structures) |
| **T4a** | Resectable structure |
| **T4b** | Tumour invades unresectable structure |

**Nodal Status**

| | |
|---|---|
| **Nx** | Lymph nodes cannot be assessed |
| **N0** | No regional lymph node metastasis |
| **N1** | Regional lymph node metastasis—1 to 2 nodes |
| **N2** | Metastasis in 3–6 regional nodes |
| **N3** | Metastasis in 7 or more regional nodes |

**Metastasis**

| | |
|---|---|
| **M0** | No distal spread |
| **M1** | Upper thoracic oesophageal carcinoma with spread to other nonregional nodes or distant spread. Middle thoracic oesophageal carcinoma with spread to neck nodes/coeliac nodes or other nonregional nodes. Lower thoracic oesophageal carcinoma with spread to other nonregional nodes or distant spread. |
| **Mx** | Distant metastasis cannot be assessed |

**TNM Stage Grouping**

| | |
|---|---|
| **Stage 0** | : Tis N0 M0 |
| **Stage I** | : T1 N0 M0 |
| **Stage IIA** | : T2 N0 M0, T3 N0H0 |
| **Stage IIB** | : T1N1N0, T2N1, M0 |
| **Stage III** | : T3N1M0, T4 and N1N0 |
| **Stage IV** | : A—Any T and N, M1a<br>B—Any T1 and N, M1b |

| | |
|---|---|
| GX | Grade cannot be assessed—stage grouping as G1 |
| G1 | Well differentiated |
| G2 | Moderately differentiated |
| G3 | Poorly differentiated |
| G4 | Undifferentiated—stage grouping as G3 |

## TREATMENT WITH CURATIVE INTENT

- Once diagnosis and accurate staging is done, the histological diagnosis is also considered for treating carcinoma oesophagus.
- Incidence of lymph node positivity is around 5% even when the disease is confined to submucosal region—early cases. Depending upon the location of

the tumour, lymph node stations have to be removed. Example: Classical 3 field lymphadenectomy is done for patients with carcinoma mid-oesophagus. 3 field include cervical, mediastinal, and abdominal lymph nodes.

- Tumour location is also important because of close proximity of oesophagus to pleura, pericardium azygos vein, aorta, etc.

**While treating, cancers in the oesophagus can be broadly classified as follows (Fig. 52.34):**

- **Cervical oesophagus:** It is from hypopharynx to thoracic inlet (at sternal notch). Upper thoracic oesophagus is from thoracic inlet to azygos vein.
- **Midthoracic oesophagus** tumours arise from lower border of azygos vein to inferior pulmonary vein (IMV).
- Lower oesophageal tumours distal (IMV) to gastro-oesophageal junction.

## A. Carcinoma Cervical and Upper Thoracic Oesophagus

- In vast majority of cases, treatment of carcinoma oesophagus is aimed at to relieve dysphagia by palliative resection/palliative radiotherapy/metallic stenting.
- **Tumours that have not penetrated** through oesophageal wall and have not metastasised to regional lymph nodes are **potentially curable**.
- **Decision of surgery/radiotherapy** also depends upon location of the tumour, histology, site of the tumour, staging and cardiopulmonary reserve. Nutritional status has to be improved to raise albumin levels from 3 to 3.4 g/dl to decrease complications such as anastomotic leak.
- **Cervical oesophageal cancers** (Fig. 52.35) are almost always squamous cell carcinomas. Upper thoracic is also squamous cell carcinoma. Involvement of thoracic nodes, early spread to trachea, bronchus and great vessels is common.
- Concurrent chemoradiotherapy (CCRT) is the first line of treatment for cervical and upper oesophageal cancers.
- Cisplatin, 5-fluorouracil (5-FU), calcium folinate or cisplatin, 5-FU and paclitaxel are the drugs used.
- Radiotherapy: 50 to 60 Gy units.
- Patients who have recurrence after CTRT can be considered for total oesophagectomy with gastric pull up as palliative intent provided they are fit candidates for surgery.

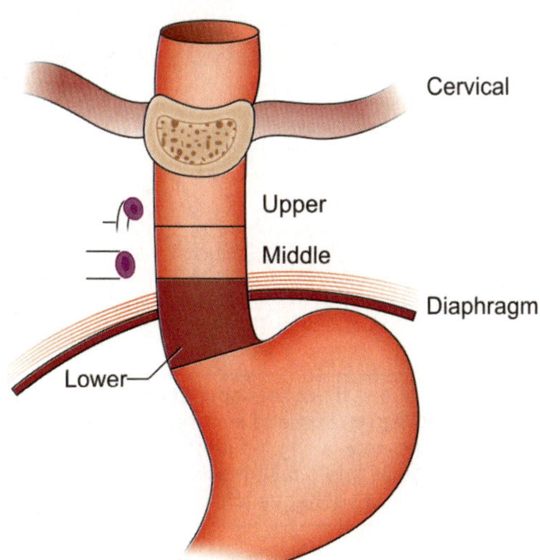

Fig. 52.34: Division of oesophagus for resection purposes

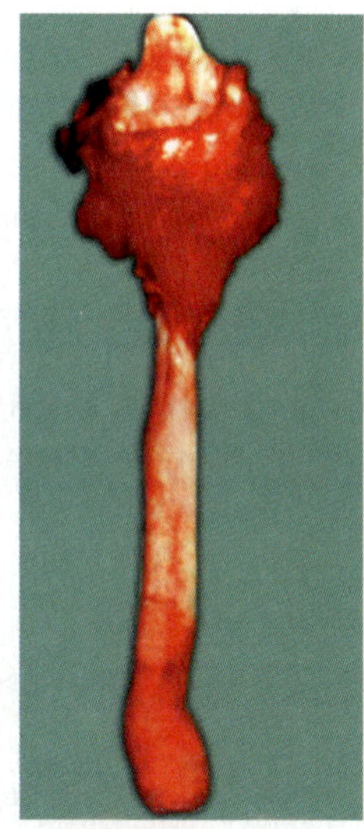
Fig. 52.35: Total pharyngolaryngo-esophagectomy—followed by gastric pull-up

## B. Tumours of the Thoracic Oesophagus

They are usually **adenocarcinomas**. These tumours have a tendency to spread for long distances submucosally and the lymphatic flow is in the longitudinal direction (Table 52.7).

### I. Ivor Lewis operation

- In this operation, abdomen is opened first, stomach is mobilised and the wound is closed. The patient is put in left lateral position, and right thoracotomy is done through 6th intercostal space. **The growth is removed and oesophagogastric anastomosis is done inside the thorax, above the level of aortic arch**. Hence, it is described as a two-stage Ivor Lewis approach (Figs 52.36 to 52.38).
- However, a few surgeons do not advocate this surgery because of the following reasons:
  1. Higher incidence of **pulmonary complications**.
  2. Higher morbidity associated with **anastomotic leak**.
  3. Higher incidence of **oesophagitis**.
  4. Higher chances of **local recurrence** due to inability to resect long length of oesophagus. Hence, the alternate procedure (McKeown) is a better choice.

### II. McKeown's three-stage *en bloc* oesophagectomy

This surgery can be done in all levels of carcinoma oesophagus. However majority of the cases are from middle and lower third of oesophagus. These 3 incisions help in not only doing total oesophagectomy, but also in extensive 3 field lymphadenectomy. *En bloc* resection is the best treatment with removal of all lymph nodes (abdominal and thoracic). Hence, three incisions are

**TABLE 52.7:** Total oesophagectomy—comparison of two types (*see* Fig. 52.39)

| *En bloc* oesophagectomy—McKeown | Transhiatal resection—Orringer |
|---|---|
| **First choice**<br>• Three incisions: Consequently, mobility is restricted and post-operative pain is more. Hence, morbidity and mortality are higher<br>• Under vision, all lymph nodes in the thorax, neck and the abdomen can be removed<br>• Surgery takes longer period of time<br>• However, long-term survival is better than THE<br>• When lymph nodes involved are less than 8 in number, survival is better than THE | **Alternate choice**<br>• Two incisions: Abdominal and cervical. Hence, mobility is better and postoperative pain is less<br>• Pulmonary complications are less as chest is not opened. Hence, mortality and morbidity are less than *en bloc* resection<br>• Some mediastinal lymph nodes get cleared if proper dissection is done through hiatus<br>• Surgery takes much shorter period of time |

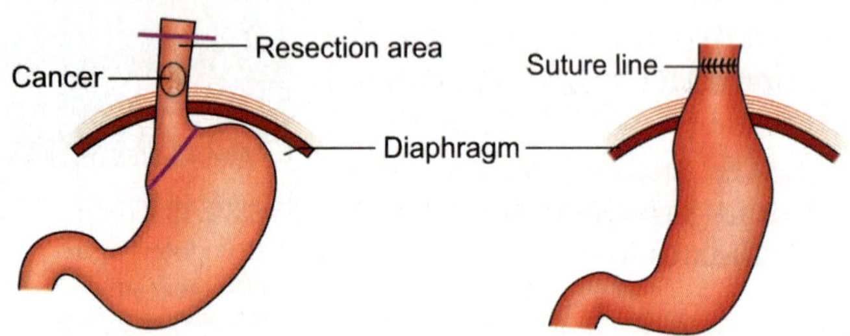


**Fig. 52.36:** Ivor Lewis operation **Fig. 52.37:** Anastomosis in the thorax

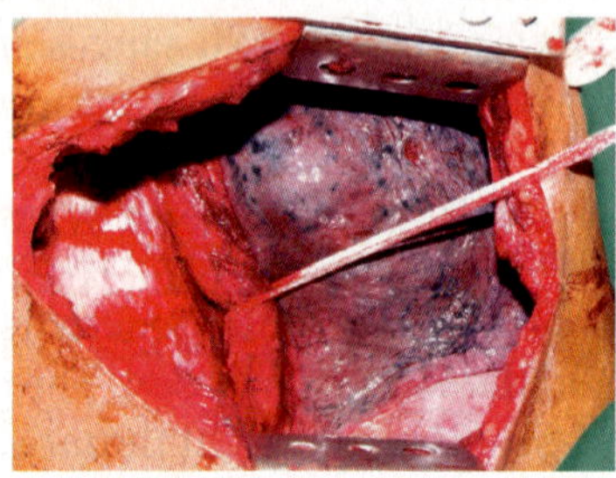

**Fig. 52.38:** Oesophagus is mobilised in the thorax

required: (1) Abdominal, (2) right posterolateral thoracotomy through the fifth space, and (3) left cervical incision. Local recurrence at the anastomosis is not a problem because of wide clearance (by obtaining a 10 cm margin of normal oesophagus above the tumour). Gastrointestinal continuity is obtained by **gastric tube anastomosis to cervical oesophagus**.

## C. Carcinoma Lower Oesophagus and Cardia

- They are adenocarcinomas.
- Surgery is the best method of treatment and palliation.
- *En bloc* resection is the best treatment with removal of all lymph nodes (abdominal and thoracic).
- An alternative method is **transhiatal oesophagectomy** (THE) without thoracotomy. Figure 52.39 shows various types of oesophageal surgery done for carcinoma oesophagus.

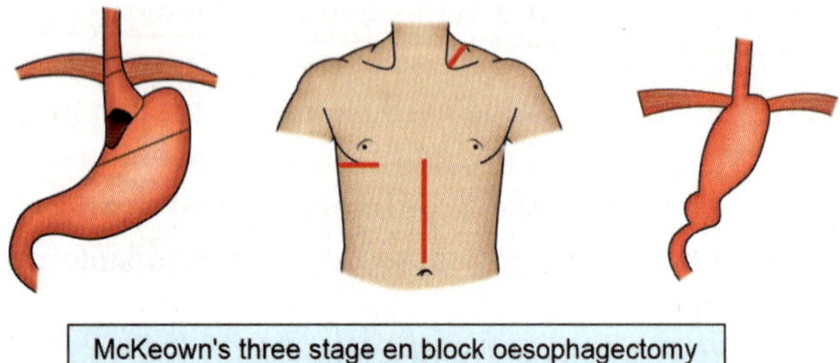


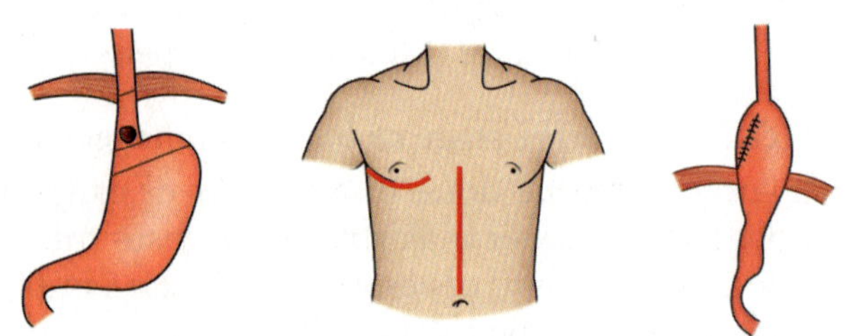


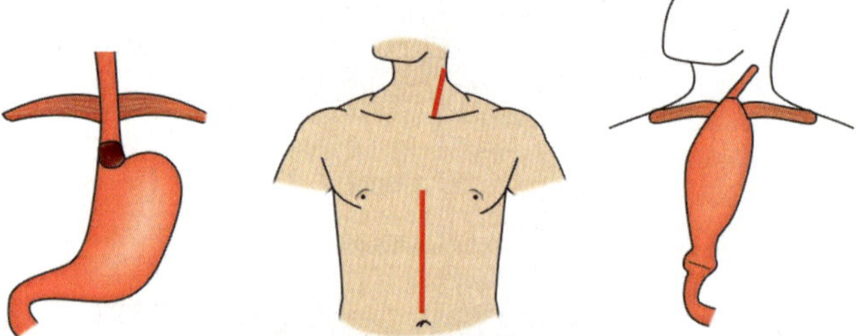


**Fig. 52.39:** Various incisions for oesophageal surgery

## TRANSHIATAL OESOPHAGECTOMY (THE)—WITHOUT THORACOTOMY—ORRINGER (Figs 52.40 to 52.42)

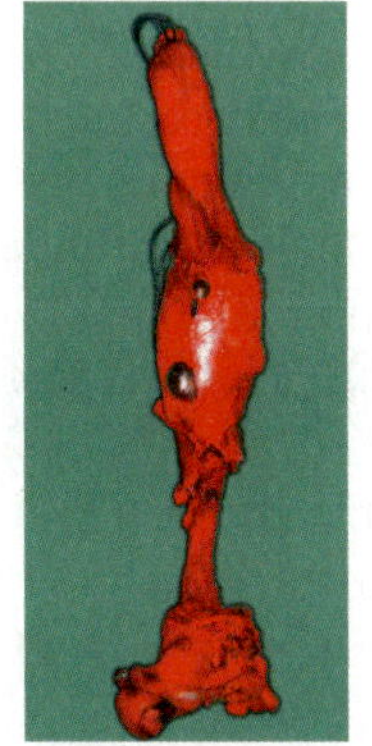
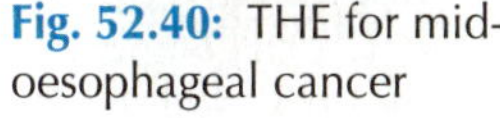

**Fig. 52.40:** THE for mid-oesophageal cancer

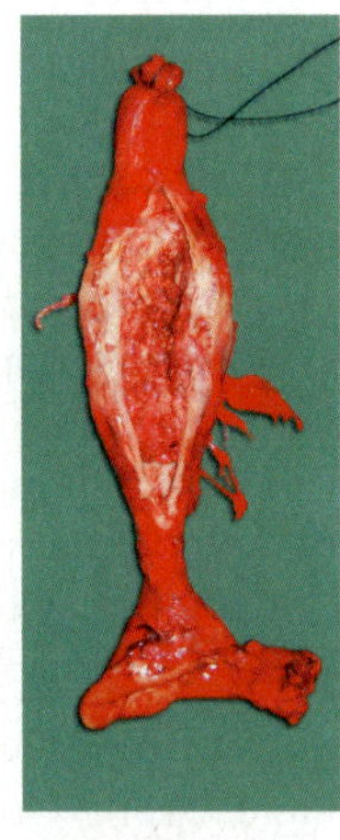

**Fig. 52.41:** Opened specimen showing extensive ulceration and nodularity—minimum 10 cm clearance for oesophageal cancer is important. Hence, THE is better than Ivor Lewis operation to get this length. (*Courtesy*: Dr Basavananda Hartimath, Associate Professor, Department of Surgery, KMC, Manipal)

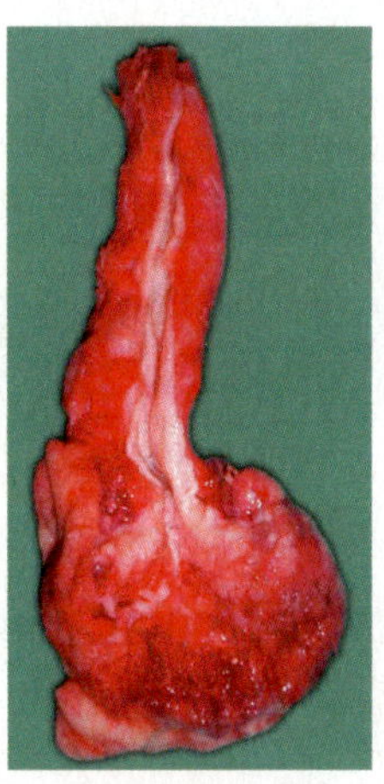

Carcinoma lower end of oesophagus—without opening the thorax by mobilisation from above and below, the oesophagus with the growth can be removed.

**Fig. 52.42:** Transhiatal (Orringer) total oesophagectomy. (*Courtesy*: Dr Sachidanand, Associate Professor, Karnataka Institute of Medical Sciences, Hubli, Karnataka)

**Comments:** Transhiatal oesophagectomy is a very good alternative (almost as good as en bloc) to lower oesophageal and GE junction tumours. No specific attempt is made to remove lymph nodes. Patients tolerate the procedure very well. No mediastinal complications related to leak are seen because of anastomosis in the neck. It gives a reasonably good relief from dysphagia and survival. It is not blind oesophagectomy. With good retraction of the hiatus, mobilisation can be done under vision. It is not the type of operation that influences survival but rather the stage of the disease at the time of the operation.

- Prophylactic vagal sparing is indicated in severe dysplasia and intramucosal lesions.

## GASTRO-OESOPHAGEAL JUNCTION (GEJ) CANCERS

**Definition:** The TNM Classification of Malignant Tumors, 8th Edition, defines GEJ adenocarcinoma as adenocarcinoma with an epicenter within 5 cm of the GEJ and extending into the oesophagus. Smoking, obesity and consumption of red meat rich diet are important risk factors. GEJ tumours are classified as follows.

### Siewert classification of GEJ tumours (Fig. 52.43)

**Type I:** It represents tumours arising from lower oesophagus which has changed to metaplastic columnar epithelium. They are oesophageal adenocarcinomas. Today, preoperative chemoradiotherapy has been considered as standard care for GE junction Type I tumours. Chemotherapeutic drugs used are:

- Cisplatin and paclitaxel—5 cycles
- Radiation—41.4–23 Gy fractions of 1.8 Gy each

  This results in lower rate of lymph node positivity, good R–O resection rates and high chances of complete pathological response. They are treated like oesophageal cancer—total oesophagectomy.

**Type II:** They are actually from GE junction and they are from stomach adenocarcinoma.

**Type III:** Gastric adenocarcinoma: They are treated like gastric cancer—gastrectomy.

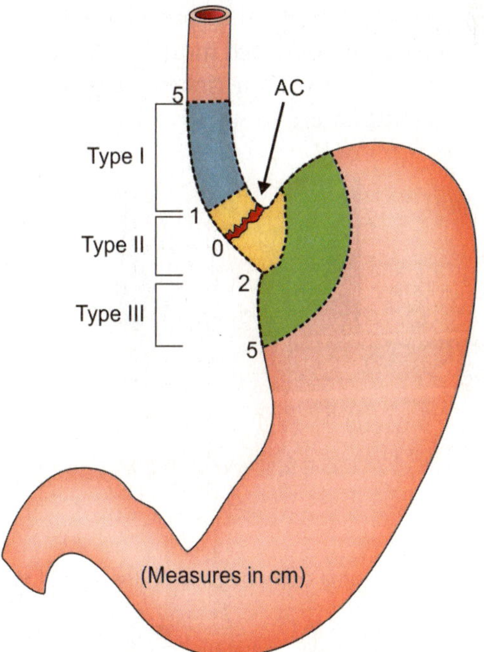


**Fig. 52.43:** Types of GE junction tumours

## PALLIATIVE INTENT TREATMENT/PROCEDURES

- In spite of endoscopy and other investigations, the treatment of carcinoma oesophagus is palliative in more than 75% of cases, especially in our country. By the time the first symptom of dysphagia appears, it is too advanced. Also, the location of the tumour, adjacent structures in the mediastinum, widespread lymphatic drainage alters the overall prognosis to a very low percent of survival.
- A few considerations before treatment of carcinoma—since they often present at an advanced stage, 5-year survival is very low in the majority of cases.

The following factors are considered for *palliative treatment.*

1. Comorbid conditions: Cardiac diseases, bad chest
2. Blood spread metastasis: Para-aortic lymph nodes
3. Contiguous organ: Trachea, aorta, pericardium invasion (CT scan)
4. Diagnostic laparoscopy: Peritoneal spread, omental nodules, ascites
5. CT scan or laparoscopic ultrasound: Lymph nodes metastasis: Para-aortic lymph nodes, supraclavicular lymph nodes.

- Palliation is done to relieve dysphagia or to control bleeding lesions or for feeding purposes.
- Palliation to control pain.

1. **Intubation:** The choice of the intubation material is self-expanding metallic stent (SEMS, Key Box 52.17). Two types are available—covered and noncovered. The stent is deployed by endoscopy under fluoroscopic guidance. It is collapsed during insertion and once confirmed radiologically by position, it is expanded. Minimal dilatation of the oesophagus (8 mm) is required to place the stent (Figs 52.44 to 52.46). On the other hand, the plastic tubes which were used earlier, required more than 8 mm dilatation and there was always a risk of perforation. If the patient is expected to survive beyond 3 months, SEM stent can be considered. Complications include aspiration, feeling of tightness in the chest, bleeding, food blockage, etc.
   - This is the choice in cases of tracheo-oesophageal fistula due to carcinoma oesophagus.

Key Box 52.17

**SEMS**

Self-expanding metallic stents (SEMS) are the best choice of stents in the palliation of malignant strictures and tracheo-oesophageal fistulae. Coated SEMS are now the device of choice for the management of tracheoesophageal fistulae.

They have 2 layers of superalloy monofilament wire with a layer of silicon between them. This prevents tumour growing within the lumen.

Although, SEMS placement is simple, inadequate insertion and positioning occurs. Complications can be dangerous too. However, in vast majority cases, it gives a best palliation.

**Complications**

- Severe chest pain is due to expansion of the stent
- Acute perforation rate reported in less than 1–2% of the cases.
- Bleeding is rare but can give rise to death by exsanguination.
- Recurrent dysphagia (10%).
- Occlusion of the stent by tumour (8%).

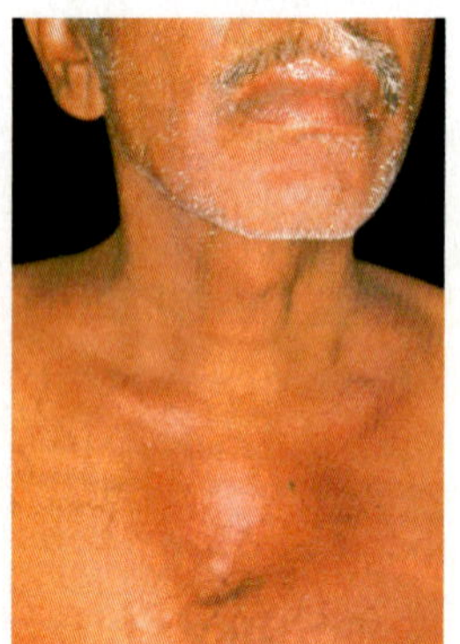

**Fig. 52.44:** Carcinoma oesophagus with the sternal secondary

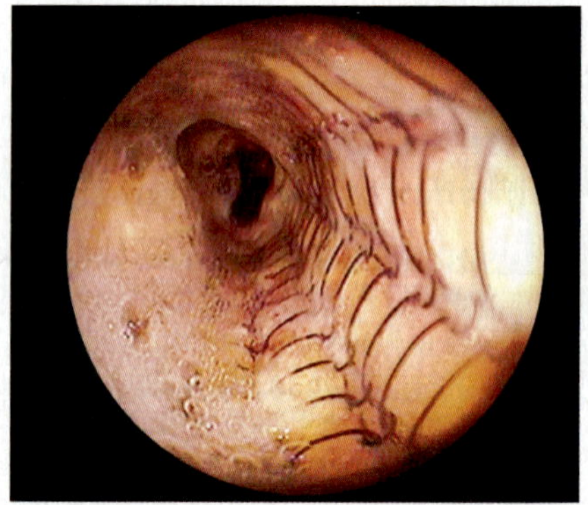

**Fig. 52.45:** Oesophageal stenting with metallic stent

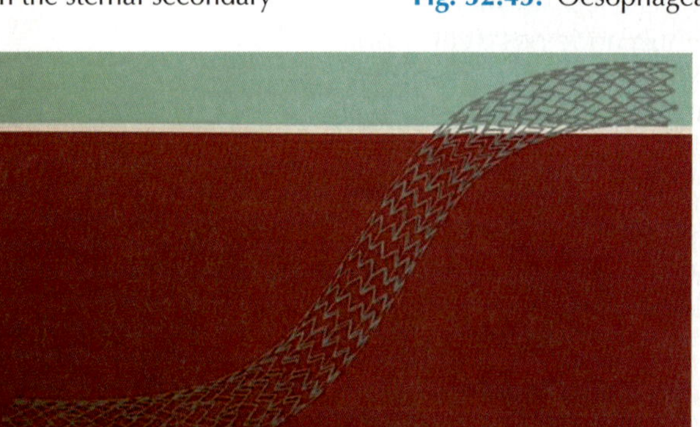

**Figs 52.46A to C:** Stent—SEMS (*Courtesy*: Dr Shirren Shetty, Head, Department of Gastroenterology, KMC, Manipal)

2. **Laser therapy:** Endoscopic laser treatment is used to core the tumour and widen the lumen to relieve dysphagia. Principle is thermal destruction of the tumour. The procedure has to be repeated. Laser used is Nd:YAG laser or diode laser. Infiltrative lesions are not suitable for laser treatment but exophytic lesions are ideal—less than 6 cm. Success rates are 80–90% in relieving dysphagia.
   - Perforation, fever, chest pain, fistula are complications.
3. **Photodynamic therapy:** It is used in early carcinomas—mucosal lesions wherein patients are not willing for surgical procedures including endoscopic mucosal resection. In this procedure, a photosensitiser (porfimer sodium) is given. It will be taken by dysplastic cells and malignant cells.
   - Perforation, fever, sunburn, pleural effusion are the complications.
4. **Radiotherapy, brachytherapy:** It is intraluminal radiation (RT) with short penetration distance 1500 cGy radiation is given. No systemic side effects. Palliative external beam radiation to doses of 50 to 60 Gy is successful in 50 to 70% of patients.
5. **Feeding gastrostomy or jejunostomy:** In very late advanced cases, where all other treatment feels.

### Causes of Death in Carcinoma Oesophagus

- Cancer cachexia
- Complications such as bronchopleural fistula, aspiration pneumonia, haematemesis due to erosion of aorta, perforation of the growth and mediastinitis.

### Summary of Treatment of Carcinoma Oesophagus

- Majority of oesophageal cancers are advanced at the time of diagnosis.
- 5-year survival rates after curative resections are around 10%.
- **The best results are obtained after surgery—radial oesophagectomy.** Curative resections are major surgeries and should be undertaken by an experienced surgeon. Curative resections can be attempted at all levels of carcinoma oesophagus (upper, middle and lower) provided vital structures are **not involved** (assessment by CT scan and endosonogram).
- **Chemoradiotherapy may cure the disease** in selected patients—these are squamous cell cancers.
- **Palliation:** Radiotherapy, chemotherapy, dilatation and stenting also can give palliation. As majority of the patients with carcinoma oesophagus have dysphagia, all the methods of palliation are aimed at relieving dysphagia. Endoscopy followed by dilatation using guidewire is a simple procedure with rate of complications such as perforation around 2–3%. However, the results are only for a few weeks. Self-expandable metal stents are regularly used nowadays as a palliation.
- **Endoscopic laser therapy** relieves obstruction and bleeding. It can be carried out as an outpatient treatment but needs multiple sittings.
- **Radiotherapy** alone has been tried for squamous cell carcinoma of the oesophagus—dose is 6,000 cG units. No survival advantage is seen with this method.
- **Combination chemotherapy** using cisplatin and 5-fluorouracil with radiotherapy has been tried in patients who are not fit for surgery. Paclitaxel achieves high response rate in metastatic oesophageal cancer and it also acts as a radiation sensitiser.
- **Endoscopic intraluminal brachytherapy** is used in, cases of recurrent tumour growing inside the lumen and causing obstruction.

**SU28.6:** Describe the clinical features, investigations and principles of management of corrosive strictures, oesphageal perforations, diverticulum (benign disorders).

## CORROSIVE OESOPHAGEAL STRICTURE

These caustics are taken accidentally or in attempted suicide. The agents are sodium hydroxide, sulphuric acid, household bleach (Key Box 52.18).

- The acids affect acidic stomach mucosa.
- The squamous epithelium of oesophagus is relatively resistant to acids (also due to rapidity of flow of fluids).
- The alkali—sodium hydroxide affects oesophageal mucosa more than gastric mucosa. Alkali ingestion is more common than acid ingestion.
- Alkali ingestion is more devastating than acid.
- Alkali ingestion almost always leads to significant destruction of oesophagus.
- The corrosive injuries may involve oropharynx, larynx, oesophagus, stomach and sometimes intestines also.

Key Box 52.18

**Causes of Stricture**

1. **C**orrosive (caustic) injuries
2. **C**arcinoma
3. **C**olumnar lined oesophagus—Barrett's oesophagus
4. **C**apsules of tetracycline group of antibiotics
5. **C** vitamins—potassium compounds
6. **C**hronic reflux due to GORD, results in **Schatzki ring**—a stricture at lower oesophagus at squamocolumnar junction. It is a circular ring consisting of fibrous tissue and cellular infiltrates.

### Classification of Injuries

- **Superficial:** Erythema, oedema, blisters, etc. Re-epithelialisation of mucosa is complete by 6th week.
- **Deep:** Circumferential ulcers, produces scarring and contractures. Major injury of the stomach produces gastric outlet obstruction.

### Clinical Features

- Severe pain, drooling of saliva, inability to swallow.
- Retrosternal burning, abdominal guarding and rigidity.
- Hoarseness, stridor, laryngeal oedema, if there is laryngeal injury.
- Dysphagia occurs later due to stricture.

### Important Examinations in Corrosive Injury

- Examination of the oral cavity, chest and abdomen.
- Auscultation of the lungs
- Examination of upper airway
- Abdominal examination—guarding and rigidity of the abdomen indicate perforation.

*Pearls of Wisdom*

- What should not be done: Stomach wash or induced vomiting, as it will aggravate oesophageal injury or it may result in aspiration. No role for corticosteroids in cases of deep injuries or acid injuries.
- What should be done: Verification of the aetiologic agent and accurate assessment of depth and extent of injury.

### Investigations

- Early endoscopy—within 12–24 hours—to grade the injury (*see* below ten commandments for detail).
- CT scan can reveal any perforation in the thorax or in the abdomen.

### Treatment

Can be divided into acute and chronic cases. In acute cases, treatment depends upon the severity of the injury or burn.

**Acute cases:** Any surgical intervention should be done only in selected referral centres. Kindly follow the instructions given below.

**Chronic cases** present with **stricture** that need regular dilatation. This is ideally done after 6 weeks (the time for re-epithelialisation of oesophagus) (Figs 52.47 and 52.48 and Key Box 52.19).

- **Colonic pull-up** is the choice for impassable strictures, only after adequate nutrition is achieved through feeding jejunostomy.

### Complications of Stricture

- **Development of malignancy** (3 to 5%)
- Progressive nutritional deficiency
- Recurrent respiratory tract infection.

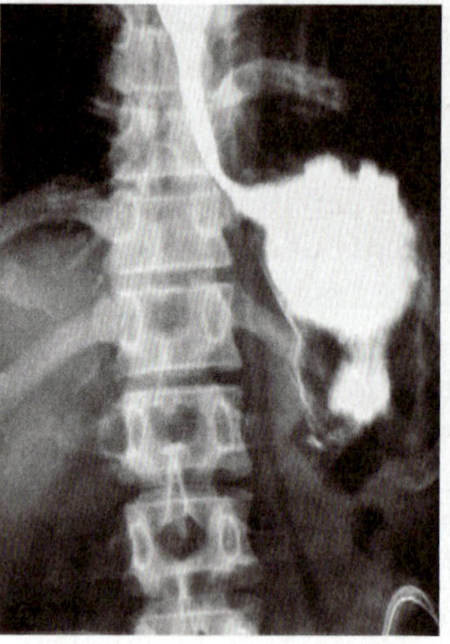
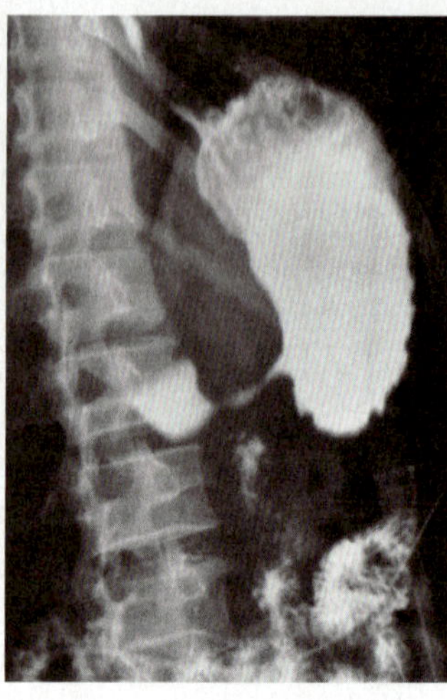

**Figs 52.47 and 52.48:** Corrosive strictures of lower end of oesophagus and pyloric antrum of stomach. Oesophageal stricture was dilated. However, antral stricture could not be dilated. Hence, he underwent vagotomy and gastrojejunostomy

Key Box 52.19

**Dilatation of the Stricture**

- Indicated in all cases of symptomatic oesophageal stricture.
- Peptic strictures, corrosive strictures, anastomotic strictures following oesophagogastric anastomosis in the neck after 'THE' or following oesophagogastrectomy for lower oesophageal cancer.
- Flexible oesophagoscopy is done and a guidewire is passed. The scope is withdrawn. Solid dilators of increasing diameter are passed over the guidewire.
- A stricture should be dilated to at least 16 mm in diameter to restore normal swallowing.
- Peptic strictures are easy to dilate as they are short.
- Beware of a GE junction stricture. It may be malignant. Once it is dilated, a growth may be seen. Take a biopsy.
- Pneumatic dilatation can also be used.

**TEN COMMANDMENTS OF ACUTE CORROSIVE INJURY**

1. Neutralisation of the ingested material
2. Alkalis are neutralised by half strength vinegar, citrus juices
3. Acids are neutralised by milk, egg white, antacids
4. Avoid emetics and sodium bicarbonates
5. Stabilise the patient and arrange upper GI scopy—classify the degree of injury.
6. **No burns:** Observe, small amount of clear fluids may be allowed orally
7. **First degree burns:** Observation for 48 hours. If he can swallow saliva, clear fluids can be started. Repeat endoscopies after a month, 3 or 6 months later to rule out stricture.
8. **Second degree burns:** Intravenous fluids, nil per oral, acid suppression, relieve airway obstruction, parenteral nutrition
9. Cervical oesophagostomy, staple the GE junction, feeding jejunostomy. 6 weeks later, gastric pull up and oesophagogastric anastomosis, in cases of perforation.
10. Call for senior surgeon's help.

## OESOPHAGEAL PERFORATIONS

- Oesophageal perforation is a serious, acute emergency carrying a very high mortality rate. Fortunately it is not common. There are many causes and are totally different from gastric or duodenal perforations.
- Instrumentation perforations are the most common cause of perforation.
- **Cervical oesophagus** is the most likely site of perforation.
- **Cricopharyngeal** region is the most common site.

### Causes

- **Instrumentation:** Endoscopy, dilatation of strictures, injection sclerotherapy and laser treatment are the common causes.
- **Operative:** Thyroidectomy, vagotomy, spine surgery, mediastinoscopy.
- **Traumatic:** Caustic injury, sharp and blunt trauma.
- **Oesophageal diseases:** Carcinoma, Barrett's oesophagus.
- **Spontaneous rupture:** Boerhaave's syndrome.

### Clinical Features

- **Severe pain in the neck,** chest or abdomen, stiffness of the neck depending upon the site of perforation.
- Haematemesis, dysphagia, dyspnoea, hypotension, **tachycardia, shock** and pleural effusion are the other features.
- **Mackler's triad:** Chest pain, vomiting and subcutaneous emphysema. It is present only in 10–15% of patients.
- **'Hamman's sign'** escape of air into the mediastinum resulting in "mediastinal crunch" which is produced by the heartbeating against air-filled tissues.

### Investigations

- The investigation of choice is plain chest X-ray which can demonstrate **pneumomediastinum,** subcutaneous emphysema and mediastinal air fluid levels. When in doubt, **CT chest** is diagnostic.
- **Contrast swallow** can also be done.

### Treatment Principles

- Infection is polymicrobial: *Staphylococcus, Streptococcus, Pseudomonas* and *Bacteroides.*
- **Early surgery** should be done within 24 hours. Closure of perforation and external drainage is the treatment.
- Perforation older than 24 hours—treated by temporary cervical oesophagostomy, ligation of oesophagus proximal to GE junction and feeding jejunostomy. After 6–8 weeks, oesophagectomy and gastric or colonic pull up is done.
- **Conservative treatment has risk of continuing leak,** sepsis and mediastinitis.

## BAROTRAUMA—BOERHAAVE SYNDROME

### Spontaneous Perforation

It occurs when a person vomits against a closed glottis.

**Historical:** First reported by Professor Hermann Boerhaave—a case of grand admiral who was a glutton and practising autoemesis.

### Aetiopathogenesis

- Rupture is due to sudden rise in oesophageal pressure during vomiting, combined with negative intrathoracic pressure.
- Excessive eating as in bulimia/excessive alcohol has been thought to be responsible.
- It is a serious condition because of large volume of material realised under pressure.

**Spontaneous Perforation of Oesophagus—Causes**
- Vomiting—the most common cause
- Weight-lifting
- Defecation
- Epilepsy
- Childbirth

### Site of Perforation

- Posterolateral wall of the lower third of the oesophagus.
- Typically a middle-aged man after a bout of alcohol first vomits food contents followed by blood.
- He complains of lower thoracic pain—typically about 10 hours from thoracic perforations.
- Pain in neck is due to cervical perforation.
- Tachycardia, tachypnoea, fever are present.
- **Hamman's sign is positive.**

### Differential Diagnosis

- Myocardial infarction
- Acute pancreatitis.

### Investigations

- **Chest X-ray:** Air in the mediastinum, air in the pleura, air in the peritoneum, pleural effusion
- **CECT scan:** It is the investigation of choice to detect the exact site of perforation
- Barium meal (Fig. 52.49).

### Treatment Principles

- **Conservative:** It is indicated in small ruptures without any contaminations and they are contained rupture.
- **Endoscopic stent:** It is indicated in case of early cases without much contamination. In delayed cases, it will help in preventing fistula formation.

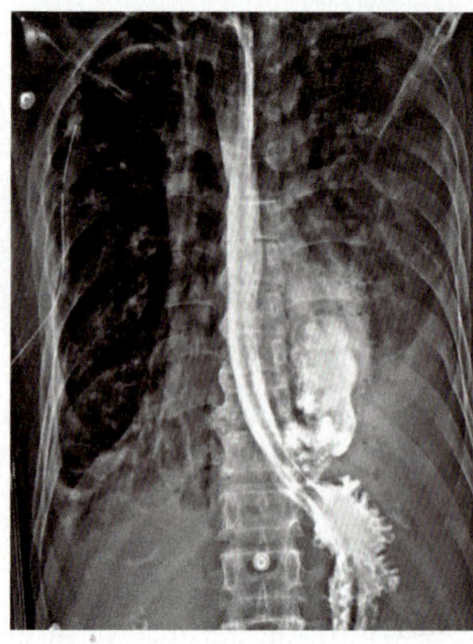

**Fig. 52.49:** Barium meal showing extravasation of barium—Boerhaave syndrome

- **Surgery:** Indicated in case of early perforations either open thoracotomy, repair or video-assisted thoracoscopic surgery (VATS) with reinforcement by using gastric fundus.

## DIVERTICULUM OF OESOPHAGUS

### Types of Diverticulum

Table 52.8 describes types of diverticulum.

**Cervical diverticulum** (Fig. 52.50) is the commonest type of diverticulum which can present with regurgitation of meals, aspiration of food contents into the lungs or recurrent respiratory tract infections. It is treated by excision of the sac and repair of the defect along with cricopharyngeal myotomy—**posterior midline.**

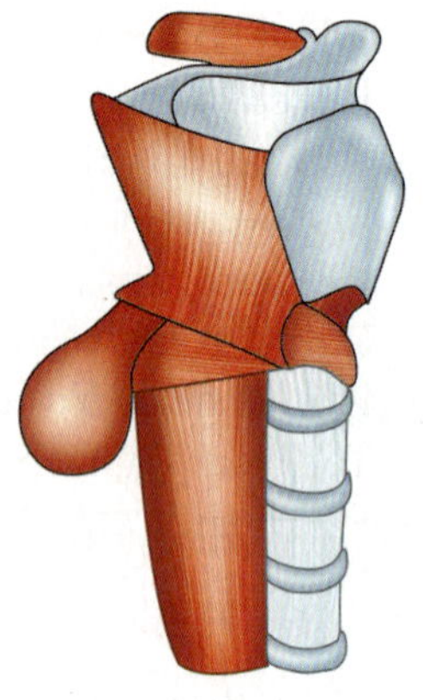

**Fig. 52.50:** Diverticulum

## DIFFERENTIAL DIAGNOSIS OF DYSPHAGIA (Fig. 52.51)

I. Causes from outside (extraluminal) oesophagus
   1. Thyroid swellings
   2. Cardiomegaly
   3. Aortic aneurysm
   4. Mediastinal nodes: Tuberculosis, lymphoma or secondaries
   5. Rolling hiatus hernia

II. Causes in the wall of oesophagus (luminal)
   1. Oesophageal stricture
      - Corrosive acid poisoning
      - Tuberculous stricture
   2. Carcinoma oesophagus
   3. Oesophageal diverticulum
   4. Muscular spasm: Plummer-Vinson syndrome and achalasia cardia.
   5. Tetanus

III. Causes in the lumen of oesophagus
   1. Foreign body: Dentures, coins, etc.

### History

1. **Acute dysphagia:** Common in children. Foreign bodies are common causes. Acute dysphagia with pain suggests tonsillitis or pharyngitis.

> *Pearls of Wisdom*
>
> In the absence of usual causes mentioned above, acute dysphagia in an old man may be a manifestation of vertebrobasilar insufficiency.

2. **Chronic dysphagia:** Stricture, achalasia, Plummer-Vinson syndrome and carcinomas produce chronic dysphagia. The increasing difficulty to swallow, first to solids and later to liquids is typical of carcinoma oesophagus (in achalasia cardia, it is the reverse).
3. **Age and sex:** Achalasia and Plummer-Vinson syndrome is common in females, carcinoma in men and foreign body in children.
4. **Change in voice** or even hoarseness with dysphagia suggests advanced laryngeal carcinoma.

> *Pearls of Wisdom*
>
> Dysphagia means difficulty in swallowing. Odynophagia means painful swallowing as in quinsy, retropharyngeal abscess, tonsillitis, etc.

**TABLE 52.8:** Types of diverticulum

| Name | Situation | Aetiology |
|---|---|---|
| **Zenker's** diverticulum (**cervical** or pulsion) | Proximal to the upper oesophageal sphincter | Protrusion of oesophageal mucosa between cricopharyngeus muscle inferiorly and thyropharyngeus muscle superiorly |
| Epiphrenic diverticulum | Proximal to the lower oesophageal sphincter | It is due to some kind of motility disturbance, wherein protrusion occurs in the lower end |
| Parabronchial diverticulum | Mid-oesophagus | Tuberculosis, by causing enlargement of mediastinal nodes, fibrosis and adhesions produce traction on the oesophagus, which results in the diverticulum |

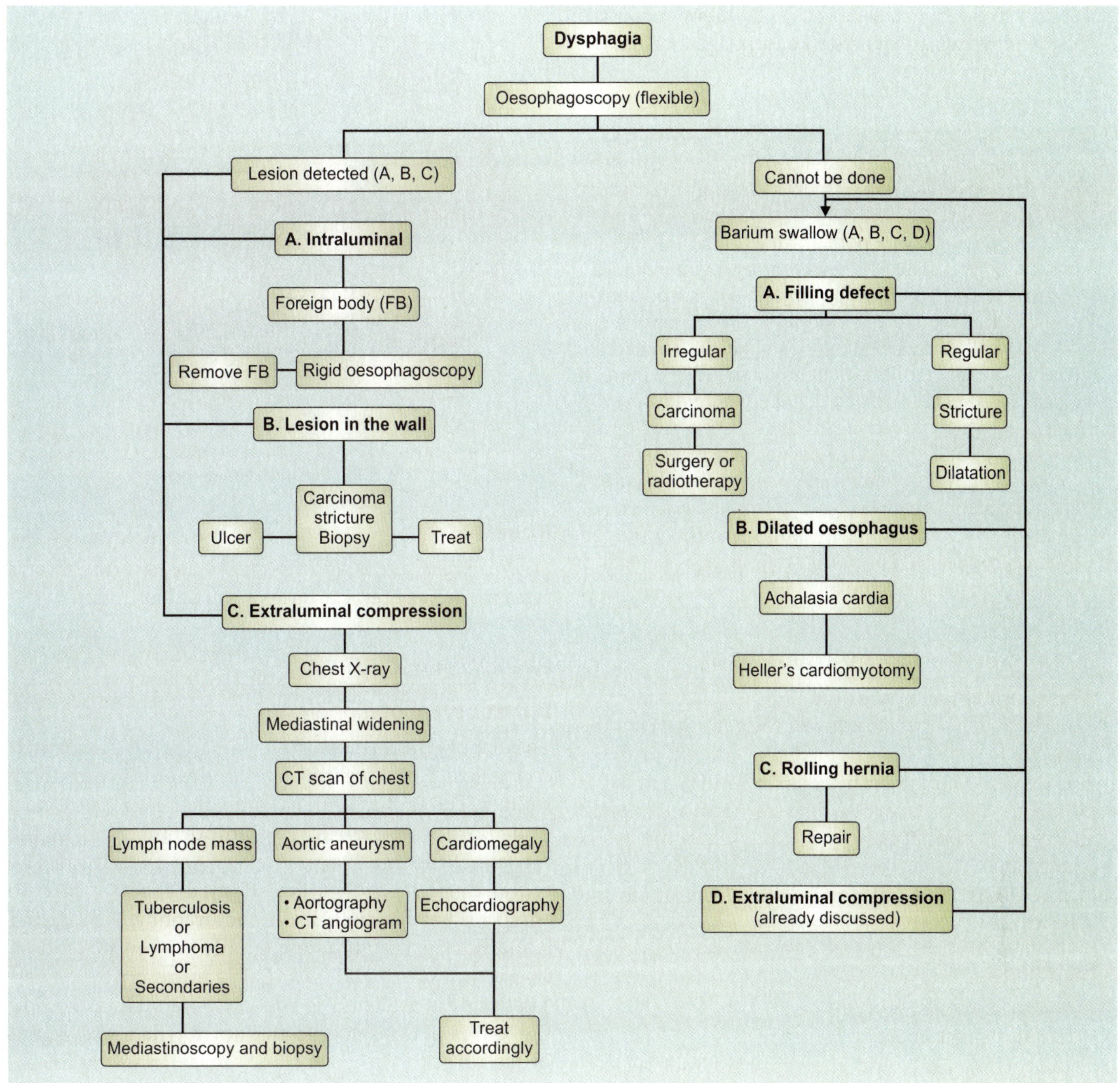


**Fig. 52.51:** Investigations of a case of dysphagia

## RARE CAUSES OF DYSPHAGIA (RINGS, SLINGS AND WEBS)

1. **Vascular slings and pulmonary artery slings:** These occur due to developmental anomalies of great vessels causing dysphagia. More common is aortic arch anomaly wherein the right subclavian artery arising from the descending aorta travels behind oesophagus creating incomplete vascular ring to complete the course. Pulmonary artery sling is due to left pulmonary artery arising from right pulmonary artery causing anterior compression of oesophagus.
2. **Oesophageal ring (Schatzki's ring):** It is located at the squamocolumnar junction with oesophageal squamous epithelium above and columnar epithelium below. There is a concentric symmetrical narrowing with restricted distensibility of lower oesophagus. It presents as dysphagia and episodic aphagia. Diagnosis is by barium oesophagography.

   It is treated by repeated bougie dilatation. The cause is obscure but there is strong association with reflux disease. Many rings are incidental findings in radiology. They do not have any symptoms.

3. **Webs:** Oesophageal webs are uncommon causes of dysphagia. They are treated by oesophageal dilatation. *Refer to* clinical notes.

**Clinical Notes**

- A 60-year-old agriculturist was referred to the department of ENT for dysphagia of 3–4 days duration. A registrar who saw the case did rigid oesophagoscopy under GA. The findings were normal. Later in the evening he was called to see this patient who had rigid abdomen. A general surgeon was consulted. He suspected a perforation. An X-ray abdomen (erect), however, was normal. A senior faculty surgeon was consulted who examined the case properly and gave a correct diagnosis. It was a case of tetanus with mild trismus. The patient had injured his left thumb a few days back. The anaesthesiologist acknowledged later that there was some difficulty in opening the patients mouth during endotracheal intubation.
- Occasionally, patients undergo gastroscopy for dysphagia which will be normal only to realise later that what he is having is a stroke!!!

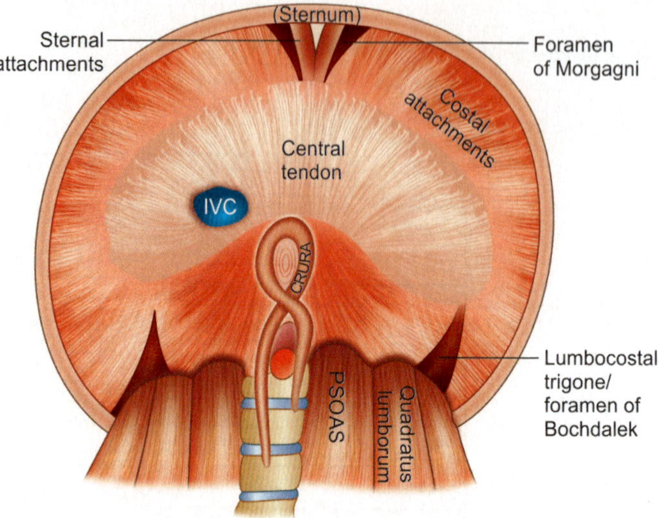


**Fig. 52.52:** Diaphragmatic hiatus

## SURGICAL ANATOMY OF THE DIAPHRAGM

- The diaphragm is a dome-shaped thin sheet of muscle which separates the thoracic cavity from the abdominal cavity.
- It is derived from the innermost layer of the muscles of the body. Hence, it arises in continuity with transversus abdominis fibres from within the costal margins.
- It has a right and left dome with a central tendon (Table 52.9).

### Attachments

- Anteriorly: Lower sternum
- Laterally: Costal margin
- Posteriorly (crura): First three lumbar vertebrae.

### Nerve Supply

The muscles of the dome on its abdominal surface is supplied by phrenic nerve (C4). The crura are supplied by the lower intercostal nerves.

### Blood Supply

Lower five intercostal arteries, subcostal arteries, and right and left phrenic arteries supply diaphragm.

## DIAPHRAGMATIC HERNIA

### Development of Diaphragm

The diaphragm develops from—muscle and its associated connective tissue, central tendon develops from three sources: The septum transversum, the pleuroperitoneal folds, and the somites. Two important parts of the muscle of the diaphragm are—costal and crural. The costal diaphragm is a thin domed sheet of muscle composed of a radially arranged myofibers extending laterally from the ribs and medially to a central tendon. The crural part of diaphragm is more posterior and thicker. It is attached to the vertebrae. Here we find the hiatus of oesophagus and aorta. The muscles and fibres of both the costal and crural muscles insert into the central tendon medially. The central tendon is located at the apex of the domed diaphragm. Caudally, it attaches to the liver via the falciform and coronary ligaments. Maldevelopment of the septum transversum results in diaphragmatic hernia.

**TABLE 52.9:** Diaphragmatic hiatus (Fig. 52.52)

| Hiatus | Location | Structures passing through |
|---|---|---|
| Aortic hiatus (median arcuate ligament) | Posteriorly opposite 12th thoracic vertebra | Aorta, thoracic duct, azygos vein |
| Oesophageal hiatus (formed by right crus) | Anterior at the level of 10th thoracic vertebra 1 inch to the left side | Oesophagus, vagus nerves, oesophageal branches of left gastric artery, veins and lymphatics |
| Caval opening | Just to the right of the midline, opposite 8th thoracic vertebra | Inferior vena cava, right phrenic nerve |

### Types of Diaphragmatic Hernia

It is of two types: Congenital and acquired.

1. **Congenital:** Majority of congenital hernias present shortly after birth. However, a few cases present late to the hospital, and most of such children are treated for recurrent respiratory tract infection elsewhere, without a proper diagnosis. 80% of congenital diaphragmatic hernias occur on the **left side**.
2. **Acquired:** The acquired diaphragmatic hernias are very often (almost always) due to road traffic accidents or due to stab injuries of the abdomen. They are discussed in blunt abdominal trauma.

### Sites of Congenital Diaphragmatic Hernia

1. **Hernia through the foramen of Bochdalek:** This is the most common diaphragmatic hernia in children. These hernias occur through the persistence of the pleuroperitoneal canals. The defect is posterior. It occurs due to failure of closure of diaphragm posteriorly during development. Respiratory distress, shift of mediastinum and scaphoid abdomen clinch the diagnosis (Fig. 52.53). It can also occur in adults. Incidence is one in 5000 persons.
2. **Hernia through the foramen of Morgagni (parasternal hernia):** Failure of fusion of few fibres from going to xyphoid process with fibres from several costochondral arches result in a defect which is muscle free—it is called foramen of Morgagni—both right and left. The defects are anterior (Fig. 52.54). These hernias present in late childhood or in adult life with features of partial (subacute) intestinal obstruction, pain in the right hypochondrium or tightness in the chest (Fig. 52.54). This is because majority of them contain transverse colon.

*Pearls of Wisdom*

Anterior diaphragmatic defect—foramen of Morgagni: Posterior (posterolateral) diaphragmatic defect-foramen of Bochdalek.

3. **Herniation through the central tendon:**
   - This can affect the right or the left apex of the cupola or the central portion. The contents may be fundus of the stomach on the left side and a portion of the liver on the right side.
   - These cases are very often diagnosed accidentally by routine chest radiograph.
4. **Eventration:** Due to paralysis or atrophy of the muscle fibres, one or both hemidiaphragms are weak and they are elevated in position. Truly speaking, this is not a hernia, but signs and symptoms are almost like other types of hernia.

### Diagnosis

- Chest radiograph: Gas and fluid level is within the chest. Left dome of the diaphragm can be elevated as you see in Fig. 52.55.
- The thin rim of the diaphragm, as seen in a plain radiograph, is broken or shows a defect.
- CT chest and abdomen is the gold standard investigation (Figs 52.56A and B).

### Treatment

- The repair of the defect is done by using non-absorbable sutures. If the defect is more than 20 mm, mesh is used to close the defect.
- Eventration of the diaphragm is repaired by plicating the redundant diaphragm. A mesh can be used to reinforce the defect.

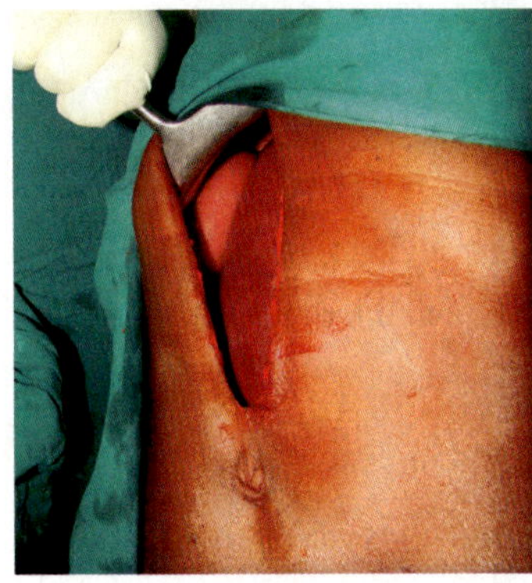

**Fig. 52.53:** Bochdalek hernia showing intestine above the liver as soon as laparotomy is done. The defect was two fingers (5 cm)

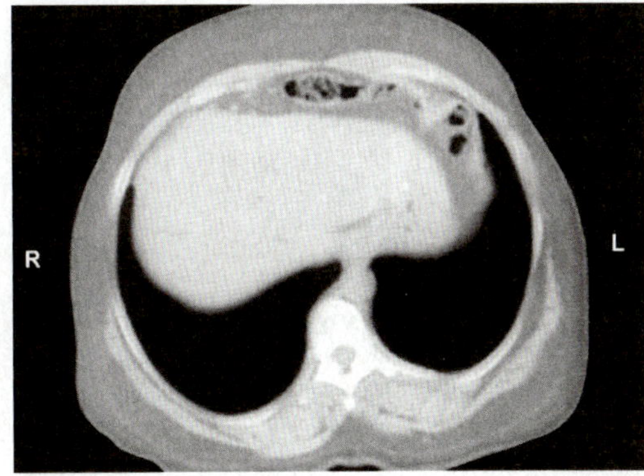


**Fig. 52.54:** Morgagni hernia—CT scan showing intestine (colon within the thorax). (*Courtesy*: Dr Srinivas Pai, Dr Nitin Nagpal, Dr Rohith Jain, Department of Surgery, KMC, Manipal) in diameter. Nonabsorbable sutures were used to close the defect (*Courtesy*: Dr Balakrishna Shetty, Surgeon, Chinmaya Hospital, Kundapur)

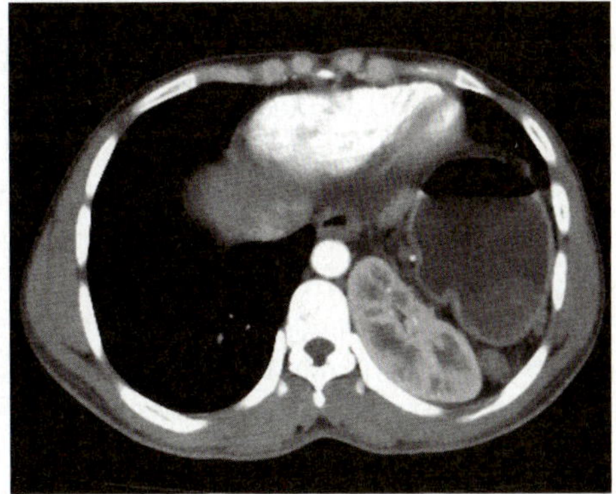

**Fig. 52.55:** CT chest revealed left Kidney is in the thorax with colon and stomach. Contents were reduced, eventration repaired with prolene mesh. (*Courtesy*: Dr Vijayendra, Dr Kalyan Reddy, Dr V. Vivek, KMC, Manipal)

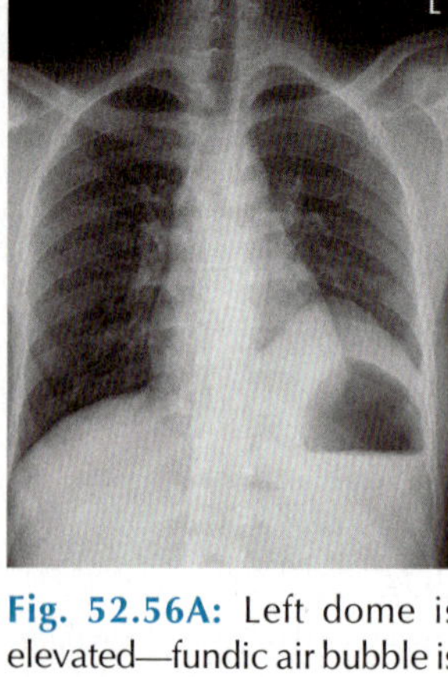

**Fig. 52.56A:** Left dome is elevated—fundic air bubble is separated. In fact this patient had spleen in that area

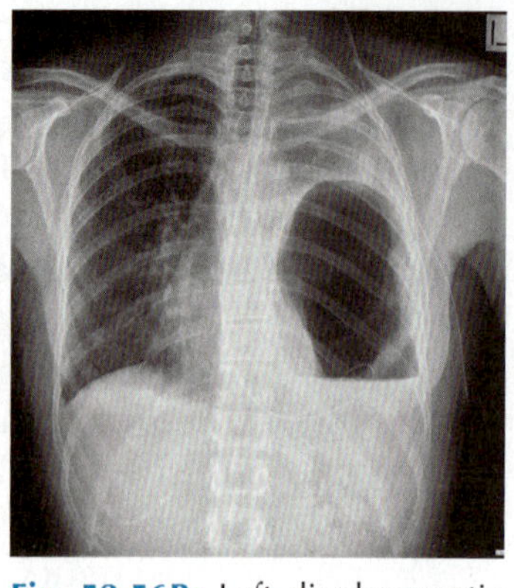

**Fig. 52.56B:** Left diaphragmatic hernia. (*Courtesy*: Dr Santhosh John Abraham, Chief Surgeon, Director, Lourde Hospital, Cochin)

## TRACHEO-OESOPHAGEAL FISTULA

### Types

In majority of the cases (85%), lower end of the oesophagus communicates with the trachea and upper end is blind.

### Associated Anomalies (Key Box 52.20, VACTER)

### Clinical Features

- Continuous pouring of saliva from the mouth in the newborn baby is a diagnostic feature.
- Newborn baby regurgitates all feeds.

Key Box 52.20

**Associated Anomalies**

| | | |
|---|---|---|
| **V** | : | Vertebral defects |
| **A** | : | Anorectal malformation |
| **C** | : | Cardiac defect (PDA/VSD) |
| **TE** | : | Tracheo-oesophageal fistula |
| **R** | : | Radial hypoplasia and renal agenesis |

- Aspiration, cough and cyanosis are other features.
- It is commonly associated with maternal hydramnios (50%).
- TOF should be recognised and diagnosed within 24 hours of birth—by introducing a red rubber catheter.

### Management

- Right thoracotomy, ligation of TOF and primary anastomosis of oesophageal ends.
- Feeding gastrostomy and oesophagostomy in type III fistula.
- In difficult cases, where there is a long atretic segment, colonic or gastric transposition is required.

### Complications

Pneumonia, reflux, dysphagia, anastomotic leak.

## CLINICAL CASE CAPSULE 6: Management Oriented Discussion in Surgery (MODS)

**Interesting Case of Acute Abdomen**

A 32 year old male, was admitted with severe upper abdominal pain and breathing difficulty of 1 day duration following a large meal. There was no history of alcohol intake preceding the event. He had 3 episodes of vomiting food particles. Similar episode was present 6 months back which was relieved with medication. On examination, he was tachypnoeic and tachycardic. Tracheal and mediastinal shift to the right were present. Decreased air entry was noted in the left lower zones of lungs on auscultation. Chest X-ray (Fig. 52.57) revealed intestines inside the thoracic cavity. CECT (Fig. 52.58) confirmed the diagnosis of diaphragmatic hernia. He underwent emergency laparotomy. The caecum, ileocaecal junction, ascending colon, part of jejunum, ileum and stomach were present in the left hemithorax. An 8 × 6 cm oval shaped defect in the left hemidiaphragm was noted extending on to central tendon. There was no hernial sac. The contents were reduced. A 15 × 10 cm prolene mesh was placed and sutured to the structures available in the surrounding area. **The final diagnosis was adult Bochdalek's hernia.** It usually presents in neonates as emergency – it is a congenital posterolateral hernia of the diaphragm and is rare in adults.

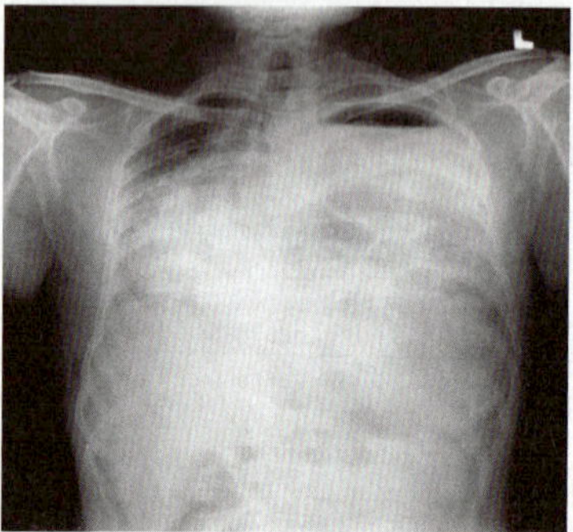

**Fig. 52.57:** Chest X-ray showing gas filled loops of intes-tines within thoracic cavity and gross deviation of trachea and mediastinum to the right side

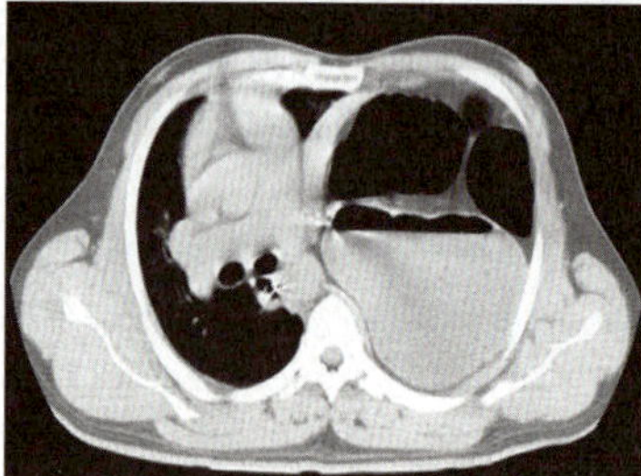

**Fig. 52.58:** Contrast enhanced CT scan showing gas filled loops of intestines in the thoracic cavity

(*Courtesy:* Professor B Srinivas Pai, SDM Medical College, Dharwar, Karnataka)

## MULTIPLE CHOICE QUESTIONS

**1. Following are disorders of the pharyngo-oesophageal junction, *except*:**
A. Stroke
B. Myasthenia
C. Cricopharyngeal achalasia
D. Nutcracker oesophagus

**2. Following are true for oesophageal lymphatics, *except*:**
A. Extensive lymphatic plexus in the submucosa
B. They are classified as perioesophageal, paraoesophageal and lateral oesophageal lymph nodes
C. Presence of coeliac nodes indicate inoperability
D. Longitudinal lymphatics are 6 times less than transverse

**3. Which one of the following is highest percentage of premalignant condition, for carcinoma oesophagus?**
A. Tylosis
B. Lye strictures
C. Achalasia
D. Oesophagus

**4. Factors for adenocarcinoma oesophagus are following, *except*:**
A. Barrett's oesophagus
B. Obesity
C. Reflux oesophagitis
D. Oesophageal web

**5. Factors for development of reflux disease of oesophagus include the following, *except*:**
A. Obesity
B. Absence of intra-abdominal length of oesophagus
C. *Helicobacter pylori* infection
D. Defective angle of His

**6. Clinical features of reflux disease of oesophagus include the following, *except*:**
A. Heartburn
B. Vomiting
C. Epigastric pain
D. Regurgitation

**7. Gold standard for the treatment of reflux disease is:**
A. Barium meal
B. Oesophagoscopy
C. 24-hour pH monitoring
D. Endosonogram

**8. The most effective drugs for reflux disease are:**
A. Alginates
B. Antacids
C. $H_2$ receptor antagonists
D. Proton pump inhibitors

**9. The most effective curative treatment for carcinoma oesophagus is:**
A. Radiotherapy
B. Oesophagectomy
C. Photodynamic therapy
D. Chemotherapy

**10. Following are features of Barrett's oesophagus, *except*:**
A. 3 cm or more of columnar epithelium
B. Cardiac metaplasia
C. Development of squamous cell carcinoma
D. Presence of mucus secreting goblet cells (intestinal metaplasia)

**11. Which of the following conditions predisposes to volvulus of the stomach?**
A. Sliding hernia
B. Para-oesophageal hernia
C. Following gastrojejunostomy
D. Wide hiatus

**12. Following are true for PET scan, *except*:**
A. Drug used is oral fluorosodeoxycholic acid
B. Combining PET with CT is better for diagnosis
C. Can be used after chemotherapy to see the response of the tumour
D. High metabolic activity—glycolytic pathway

**13. Following are true for transhiatal oesophagectomy, *except*:**
A. Thoracotomy is a must for completion of the procedure
B. Anastomosis is in the neck
C. Ideal for lower oesophageal cancers
D. Upper oesophagus mobilisation is blind

**14. About achalasia cardia following are true, *except*:**
A. It affects lower oesophageal end
B. It is due to loss of inhibitory neurons
C. Dilated oesophagus above contains normal ganglion cells
D. In vigorous achalasia, normal ganglion cells are present

**15. About treatment of achalasia cardia following are true, *except*:**
A. Balloon dilatation is ideal for patients above the age of 45 years
B. Botulinum toxin injection gives permanent relief from dysphagia
C. Sublingual nifedipine can relieve symptoms
D. Myotomy with anterior fundoplication is a good surgical procedure

**16. Schatzki's ring is associated with:**
A. Proximal oesophagus
B. Carcinoma oesophagus
C. Reflux oesophagitis
D. Congenital ring

**17. For normal swallowing stricture should be dilated to at least:**
A. 12 mm diameter
B. 14 mm diameter
C. 16 mm diameter
D. 18 mm diameter

**18. Following are true for Mallory-Weiss syndrome, *except*:**
A. The vertical split occurs in the lower end of oesophagus in majority of cases
B. Surgery is rarely required
C. Endoscopic sclerotherapy is very useful treatment
D. More often, it is a mucosal tear than rupture

**19. For the diagnosis of intraperitoneal metastasis, which is the ideal investigation?**
A. Ultrasound B. CT scan
C. MRI D. Diagnostic laparoscopy

**20. Following are true about Heller's cardiomyotomy, *except*:**
A. It is best done by laparoscopic method
B. Many surgeons add fundoplication
C. Myotomy should be more in length in the stomach side than oesophagus
D. Reflux is a major complication

**21. Most accurate method for the diagnosis of T stage for oesophageal cancer is by:**
A. Upper gastroduodenal scopy
B. Barium swallow
C. CT scan
D. Endosonogram

**22. The typical defect in Bochdalek hernia is:**
A. Posterior B. Posterolateral
C. Anterior D. Anterolateral

## Answers

| | | | | | | | | | |
|---|---|---|---|---|---|---|---|---|---|
| **1.** D | **2.** D | **3.** A | **4.** D | **5.** C | **6.** B | **7.** B | **8.** D | **9.** B | **10.** C |
| **11.** B | **12.** A | **13.** A | **14.** C | **15.** B | **16.** C | **17.** C | **18.** A | **19.** D | **20.** C |
| **21.** D | **22.** B | | | | | | | | |

Chapter 53

# Stomach and Duodenum



## Introduction

The oesophagus continues from the oesophagogastric (OG) junction as a muscular tube—the stomach.

> **SU28.7:** Describe applied anatomy and physiology of stomach.

## SURGICAL ANATOMY

### Fundus

Part of the stomach which projects upwards and lies in contact with the left dome of diaphragm. It is usually full of gas.

#### *Significance*

- To identify the side (right or left) of the body in a plain X-ray abdomen.
- In achalasia cardia, fundic air bubble is absent.
- Fundic **'Wrap'** is used in hiatus hernia.
- During mobilisation of the fundus as in splenectomy or other upper gastric surgery, short gastric arteries need to be divided. If ligatures are too close to the stomach near the fundus, gastric fistula may occur due to **necrosis of the stomach**.
- Gastrointestinal stromal tumours (GISTs) are common in fundus.

### Body

Extends from fundus to *incisura angularis*. It has a lesser curvature and a greater curvature.

#### *Significance*

- Ability to have a large meal is due to receptive relaxation of the body of the stomach.
- Greater curvature is located at the level of umbilicus.
- Classical gastrojejunostomy (GJ), anterior or posterior, involves using body of the stomach.
- Posteriorly, it is related to the lesser sac and pancreas. Carcinoma of the body may infiltrate pancreas—necessitates careful dissection to separate from pancreas (sometimes not resectable).

### Pyloric Antrum

It extends from incisura till pylorus. Pylorus is thicker than the rest of the stomach. It is a sphincter of circular muscle fibres. Its canal is usually closed.

#### *Significance* (Table 53.1)

- Pyloric antrum is a common site for gastritis, ulcer and carcinoma.
- Incompetence of pyloric sphincter results in severe duodenogastric reflux.
- It is in close contact with the head of pancreas. During gastrectomy, extreme care has to be taken to mobilise the antrum to avoid bleeding in the pancreatic head region.

### Greater Omentum

It lies in contact with transverse colon and gastrocolic omentum (Fig. 53.1 and Key Box 53.1). This has to be divided from transverse colon during gastrectomy for carcinoma or ulcer.

**TABLE 53.1:** Anatomy and surgical significance

| **2 Orifices** | **Recognition** | **Pathology** | **Result** |
|---|---|---|---|
| Pyloric orifice | Recognised by prepyloric vein of Mayo | Incompetence causes duodeno gastric reflux | Biliary gastritis |
| Cardiac orifice | Lower end of oesophagus | Incompetence causes acid reflux into lower end of oesophagus | Barrett's oesophagus |
| **2 Curvatures** | | | |
| Lesser curvature | Concave lesser omentum is attached to it | Site of benign gastric ulcer | Hour-glass contracture |
| Greater curvature | Convex greater omentum is attached to it | Site of carcinomatous ulcer | Carcinoma stomach |
| **Part** | **Common pathology** | **Commonly used for** | **Nature of the condition** |
| Fundus | GIST | Fundic wrap | Hiatus hernia |
| Body | Carcinoma | Gastrojejunostomy | Erosive gastritis |
| Pylorus | Pyloric stenosis, carcinoma | Pyloric myotomy in idiopathic pyloric stenosis | Pyloric stenosis |

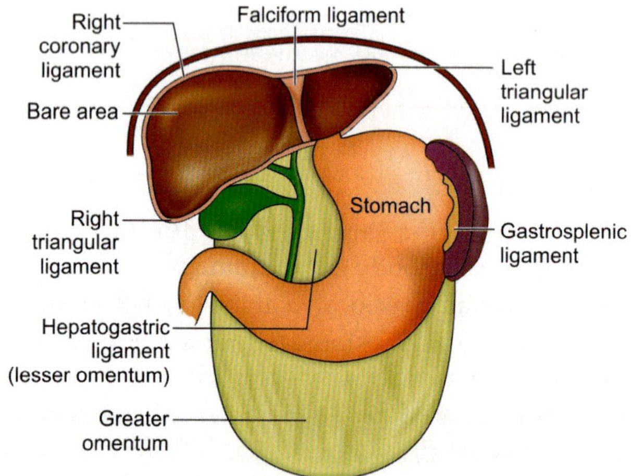


**Fig. 53.1:** Stomach, omentum and ligaments

Key Box 53.1

**Greater Omentum is a Friend and Sometimes Enemy of the Patient and the Surgeon**

- The greater omentum is the **policeman** of the peritoneal cavity. It exhibits protective action in inflammatory processes and perforations.
- **Omentoplasty** (omental wrapping of anastomosis) may decrease the occurrence of anastomotic leakage when oesophagogastric anastomosis is performed for cancer of oesophagus or as in closure of duodenal perforation.
- It has many **important applications** and can be used in colorectal surgery, reconstruction of the irradiated pharyngeal wound and packing of bleeding liver wounds.
- It was used to **treat peripheral vascular disease** such as TAO wherein direct arterial surgery was not possible.
- It becomes an enemy when involved with metastasis or directly by malignant neoplastic process from ovary or colorectal cancer. Omentum is one of the common sites of involvement in tuberculosis also. Omentum itself can act like a **band** and can cause intestinal obstruction.

## Lesser Omentum

- The lesser omentum is a double-layered structure.
- It is suspended between the lesser curvature of the stomach and the proximal 0.5 inch (2 cm) of the first part of the duodenum inferiorly, and the porta hepatis and the fissure of the ligamentum venosum superiorly.

The lesser omentum is divided into two ligaments:

1. **Hepatogastric**
2. **Hepatoduodenal:** Located within the lesser omentum are the **hepatic triad**, branches of the anterior vagus nerve, some lymph nodes, and the right and left gastric arteries.

## Vagus Nerves

- The left and right vagus nerves descend parallel to the oesophagus and form oesophageal vagal plexus between the level of the tracheal bifurcation and level of the diaphragm.
- From this plexus, two vagal trunks, anterior and posterior, form and pass through the oesophageal hiatus of the diaphragm **(mnemonic LARP: Left trunk—anterior gastric wall; right trunk—posterior gastric wall).**

## Blood Supply of the Stomach (Fig. 53.2)

It is mainly supplied by coeliac trunk and its branches:

1. **Left gastric artery** is a direct branch of coeliac trunk. It ascends up to oesophageal hiatus and turns to the right along the lesser curvature of stomach. It branches and anastomoses with branches of right gastric artery and supplies anterior and posterior wall of the stomach. There is true anastomosis between branches of left gastric artery and branches from other arteries.

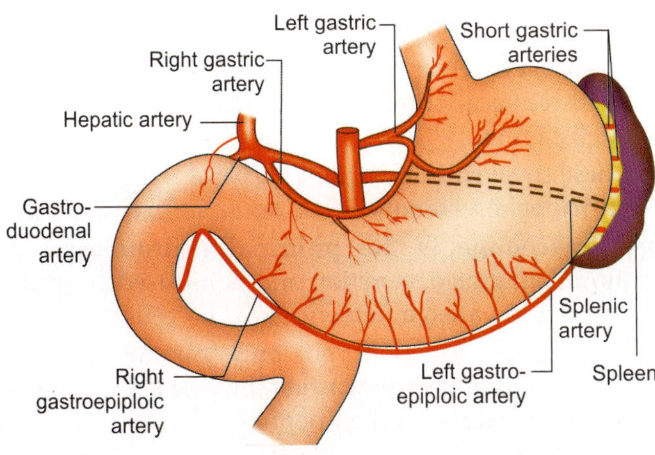


Fig. 53.2: Blood supply of the stomach arteries

2. **Right gastric artery** is a branch of hepatic artery which comes from coeliac trunk. It also supplies lesser curvature and body of stomach, along with left gastric artery.
3. **Left gastroepiploic artery** arises from splenic artery and supplies greater curvature of stomach and anastomoses with right gastroepiploic artery.
4. **Right gastroepiploic artery** is a branch of gastro-duodenal artery, which is a branch of hepatic artery.
5. **Short gastric arteries** are the branches of splenic artery. They supply the fundus of the stomach. They are also called *vasa brevia*.

## Venous Drainage

- Veins run with the corresponding arteries.
- Right and left gastric veins drain into the portal vein directly.
- Right gastroepiploic vein joins superior mesenteric vein.
- Left gastroepiploic vein and *vasa brevia* join splenic vein.
- **Prepyloric vein of Mayo** is a useful guide to the junction between stomach and duodenum.

## Surgical Importance

- Because of extensive anastomoses of blood vessels (extramural and intramural collateral vessels), stomach can survive with right gastric and right gastroepiploic arteries only. Thus stomach can be used to replace the entire oesophagus after oesophagectomy—gastric pull up.
- The order of ligation of blood vessels in gastrectomy is as follows: Left gastroepiploic, right gastroepiploic, right gastric (then stomach is divided) and lastly, left gastric arteries.
- Gastroduodenal artery, a branch of hepatic artery runs behind first part of duodenum and divides into right gastroepiploic artery and superior pancreatico-duodenal artery.
- It is this artery which bleeds when a posterior duodenal ulcer erodes into it.

## Lymphatic Drainage (Fig. 53.3)

It is an important pathway for spread of carcinoma of the stomach. The spread occurs both by emboli and permeation.

1. Right gastric nodes/suprapyloric nodes mainly drain the pyloric antrum.
2. Subpyloric nodes/gastroepiploic nodes (right) drain the greater curvature of stomach and pyloric antrum.
3. Left gastroepiploic nodes (splenic nodes) drain the upper portion of stomach, mainly the fundus (carcinoma of fundus).
4. Left gastric (superior gastric) nodes drain the lesser curvature and body of the stomach (anterior and posterior wall).
5. Coeliac nodes receive lymph from the entire foregut (including stomach) and drain directly into the *cisterna chyli* and the thoracic duct. Later, mediastinal nodes and left supraclavicular nodes (**Virchow nodes**) are involved. **Lymphatic zones are discussed under carcinoma stomach**.

## Lymphatics of the Stomach

The lymphatics of the stomach are formed from two networks: Intrinsic and extrinsic.

**Intrinsic network:** The submucosal lymphatic plexus is perhaps the richest in anastomoses.

- Upward invasive spread of gastric cancer to the oesophagus is common but downward mucosal or submucosal invasion of the duodenum is not common.
- Hence, gastrectomy with distal oesophagectomy is done for carcinoma of the proximal stomach.

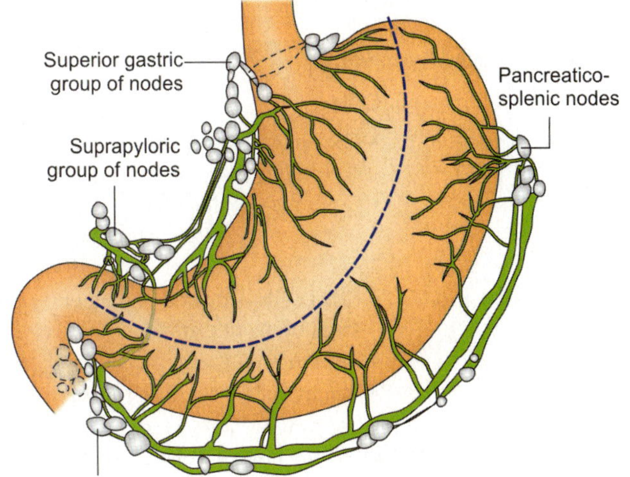


Fig. 53.3: Lymphatic drainage of the stomach

**Extrinsic network:** The extrinsic lymphatic vessels of the stomach follow the gastric veins.

- They drain to perigastric lymph nodes, which in turn drain to the lymph nodes located at the coeliac axis.
  1. **The superior gastric group** drains lymph from the upper lesser curvature into the left gastric and paracardiac nodes.
  2. **The suprapyloric group** of nodes drains the antral segment on the lesser curvature of the stomach into the right suprapancreatic nodes.
  3. **The pancreaticosplenic group** of nodes drains lymph high on the greater curvature into the left gastroepiploic and splenic nodes.
  4. **The inferior gastric and subpyloric group** of nodes drains lymph along the right gastroepiploic vascular pedicle.
- All four zones of lymph nodes drain into the coeliac group and then into the thoracic duct.

## GASTRIC PHYSIOLOGY

### HYPERGASTRINAEMIA

Various causes of surgical interest are given in Key Box 53.2.

Key Box 53.2

**Causes of Hypergastrinaemia**

| Ulcerogenic causes | Non-ulcerogenic causes |
|---|---|
| ○ Antral G cell hyperplasia or hyperfunction | ○ Antisecretory agents (PPIs) |
| ○ Retained excluded antrum | ○ Atrophic gastritis |
| ○ Zollinger-Ellison syndrome | ○ Pernicious anaemia |
| ○ Gastric outlet obstruction | ○ Acid-reducing procedure (vagotomy) |
| ○ Short-gut syndrome | ○ *Helicobacter pylori* infection |
| ○ Chronic renal failure | |

### Gastric Acid Secretion (Table 53.2)

- Gastric acid secretion by the parietal cells is regulated by three local stimuli: 1. Acetylcholine, 2. Gastrin, 3. Histamine.
- These three stimuli account for basal and stimulated gastric acid secretion.
- **Acetylcholine is the principal neurotransmitter** modulating acid secretion and is released from the vagus and parasympathetic ganglion cells.
- Vagal fibres innervate not only parietal cells but also G cells and enterochromaffin-like (ECL) cells to modulate release of their peptides.
- **Gastrin has hormonal effects on the parietal cell** and stimulates histamine release.
- **Histamine has paracrine-like effects** on the **parietal cell**. Its release from ECL cells plays a central role in the regulation of acid secretion by the parietal cell.

  Ingestion of a meal stimulates vagal fibres to release acetylcholine ***(cephalic phase)***. Binding of acetylcholine to parietal cell and G cell results in the release of histamine, hydrochloric acid and gastrin, respectively (Fig. 53.4).

  Acetylcholine also inhibits somatostatin release by inhibiting ECL.
- Following a meal, G cells are also stimulated to release gastrin, which interacts with receptors located on ECL cells and parietal cells to cause the release of histamine. Somatostatin from D cells decreases histamine release and gastrin release from ECL cells and G cells, respectively. In addition, somatostatin inhibits parietal cell acid secretion (not shown). The principal stimulus for activation of D cells is **antral luminal acidification** (not shown).
- As depicted, somatostatin exerts inhibitory actions on gastric acid secretion.

**TABLE 53.2:** Gastric secretion

| | Cells | Location | Function/mediators |
|---|---|---|---|
| 1. Acid secretion 150–160 mEq/L | • Oxyntic glands, principal cell type is parietal | • Fundus and body | • Cephalic—vagus<br>• Gastric—gastrin<br>• Intestinal—not clear |
| 2. Mucus | • Columnar epithelium | • Entire stomach | • Luminal cytoprotection from acid, pepsin and ingested substances |
| 3. Pepsinogen I and II | • Chief cells—located in deeper areas of oxyntic gland | • Body and fundus | • Vagal stimulation |
| 4. Mucus, gastrin | • Antrum | • Antrum | • Cytoprotection |
| 5. Bicarbonate | • Mucus cells | • Stomach | • Vagal stimulation increases $HCO_3^-$ secretion<br>• Prostaglandin $E_2$ |
| 6. Intrinsic factor | • Parietal cells | • Fundus | • Necessary for absorption of vitamin $B_{12}$ |
| 7. Peptides, histamine | • Enterochromaffin like (ECL) cells<br>• D cells (delta) | • Fundus<br>• Antrum | • Release of peptides<br>• Somatostatin inhibits acid secretion |

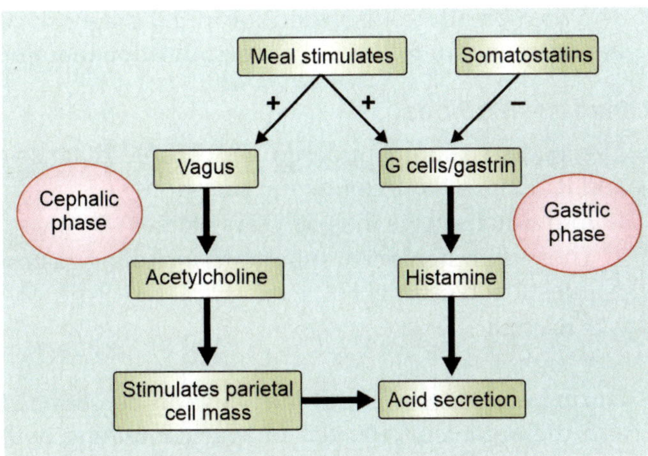


**Fig. 53.4:** Physiology of acid secretion

- Release of **somatostatin from antral D cells** is stimulated in the presence of intraluminal acid to a pH of 3 or less.
- After its release, somatostatin inhibits gastrin release through paracrine effects and also modifies histamine release from ECL cells.
- In some patients with peptic ulcer disease (PUD), this negative feedback response is defective.
- Consequently, the precise state of acid secretion by the parietal cell is dependent on the overall influence of the positive and negative stimuli.

### Functions of Gastric Acid

Key Box 53.3 describes the functions of gastric acid.

Key Box 53.3

**Functions of Gastric Acid**

- Gastric acid plays a critical role in the digestion of a meal.
- It is required to convert pepsinogen into pepsin, which is necessary for hydrolysis of proteins into polypeptides.
- Gastric acid also elicits the release of secretin from the duodenum, which results in pancreatic bicarbonate secretion.
- In addition, gastric acid functions to limit colonisation of the upper GI tract with bacteria.

### Gastric Emptying

Vagus not only increases secretion but also increases motility of the stomach. Vagotomy produces decreased gastric motility. Decreased gastric motility or atony is called gastroparesis. It can be seen in patients who are taking narcotic drugs, severe anorexia, diabetes, etc. Following Whipple's pancreaticoduodenectomy, gastric motility is also affected. Erythromycin helps in gastric emptying. Refer Key Box 53.4 for other details.

Key Box 53.4

**Promotility Agents that Accelerate Gastric Emptying**

| Drug | Mechanism |
|---|---|
| Metoclopramide | Dopamine antagonist |
| Domperidone | Dopamine antagonist |
| Erythromycin | Motilin agonist |
| Bethanechol | Cholinergic agonist |
| Neostigmine | Cholinergic agonist |

## *HELICOBACTER PYLORI* INFECTION

- It is now established that 90% of duodenal ulcers and 75% of gastric ulcers are associated with *H. pylori* infection.
- **Warren and Marshall** were the first to identify and isolate the organism, originally referred to as ***Campylobacter pyloridis***.
- The organism is a **spiral or helical gram-negative rod** with **4 to 6 flagella** and resides in gastric-type epithelium within or beneath the mucus layer, which protects it from both acid and antibiotics.
- Its shape and flagella aid its movement through the mucus layer, and it produces a variety of enzymes that help it adapt to a hostile environment.
- Most notably, it is one of **the most potent producers of urease among any bacteria yet described.**
- This enzyme is capable of **splitting urea into ammonia and bicarbonate,** creating an alkaline microenvironment in the setting of an acidic gastric milieu, which facilitates establishing a diagnosis of this organism by various laboratory tests.
- The organism is microaerophilic, and the optimal temperature for isolation is 35°C to 37°C, with growth occurring after 2 to 5 days.
- Interestingly, *H. pylori* **can only live in gastric epithelium** because only gastric epithelium expresses specific adherence receptors *in vivo* that can be recognized by the organism. Thus, it can also be found in **heterotopic gastric mucosa in proximal oesophagus** and **Barrett's oesophagus,** in gastric metaplasia in the duodenum and Meckel's diverticulum, and in heterotopic gastric mucosa in the rectum.
- **The mechanisms responsible for *H. pylori*-induced GI injury** are not very clear but three potential mechanisms have been proposed:
  1. Production of toxic products to cause local tissue injury
  2. Induction of a local mucosal immune response
  3. Increased gastrin levels with a resultant increase in acid secretion.

### Locally Produced Toxic Mediators

1. Urease activity, i.e. ammonia
2. Cytotoxins
3. Mucinase that degrades mucus and glycoproteins.
4. Phospholipases that damage epithelial cells and mucus cells.
5. Platelet-activating factor, which is known to cause mucosal injury.

### Mediators of *Helicobacter Pylori*-induced Injury

(Key Box 53.5)

- Most *H. pylori* strains express—**vacuolating cytotoxin**.
- **The VacA exotoxin** causes the release of cytochrome *c* from mitochondria and induces apoptosis.
- *H. pylori* infection is accompanied by an **abnormal T cell response** which may be partially responsible for the long-term persistence of *H. pylori* infection.

Key Box 53.5

**Mechanism of *Helicobacter Pylori*-induced Injury—Summary**

**H**elical gram-negative rod
**E**nzyme produced is urease, which splits urea. Resulting bicarbonate creates alkaline environment. Another enzyme mucinase degrades mucus
**L**ives only in gastric epithelium
**I**njury is due to:
- Toxins such as vacuolating cytotoxin
- Increased gastrin levels
- Phospholipases
- Platelet-activating factor
- Increased immunoglobulin response (host response)

**C**ytotoxins
**O**ther factors
- Local tissue injury
- Local ischaemia

*Remember as* **HELICO**

### Diagnosis (Table 53.3)

*H. pylori* infection can be diagnosed by both noninvasive and invasive means.

#### I. Non-Invasive Methods

- They are **urea breath test, serology, and detection of antigen in stool samples**.
- The urea breath test is based on production of urease by *H. pylori* in the gastric mucosa.
- $^{14}$C-labelled urea is ingested and $^{14}$C-labelled $CO_2$ is produced and excreted in the breath.
- This test has a sensitivity and specificity of greater than 90% and indicates ongoing infection.
- The urea breath test is useful for initial diagnosis of infection and for follow-up after eradication therapy.

#### II. Invasive Methods

- The patient should undergo endoscopic diagnosis and it is indicated in following situations:
  - Individuals more than 50 years of age
  - Those with significant symptoms including gastrointestinal bleeding
  - Anaemia
  - Weight loss.
- During endoscopy, antral biopsies can be obtained and the organism cultured in agar containing both urea and a pH-sensitive colorimetric agent.
- *H. pylori* hydrolysis of urea causes a diagnostic change in colour.
- The sensitivity of this test varies from 80 to 100% and specificity exceeds 90%.
- Biopsy also permits histologic examination with visualisation of the organism.

Culture of *H. pylori* is not routine and is usually reserved for recurrent infection and for antibiotic sensitivity testing when second-line therapy has failed.

### Treatment

- To be effective, antimicrobial drugs must be combined with gastric acid secretion inhibitors or bismuth salts.
- Cure rates of 80–85% are achieved using combination therapy, usually proton pump inhibitors, ranitidine, or bismuth citrate with two antibiotics.
- The most common antibiotics used are **clarithromycin, amoxicillin, and metronidazole or tinidazole**.
- Metronidazole has been a mainstay of *H. pylori* treatment.
- Eradication therapy with a proton pump inhibitor, metronidazole, and amoxicillin decreases the prevalence of metronidazole-resistant *H. pylori* strains.

#### Different Regimens

*Bismuth triple therapy*

Bismuth, 2 tablets four times daily + Metronidazole, 250 mg three times daily + Tetracycline, 500 mg four times daily.

*PPI triple therapy*

PPI twice daily + Amoxicillin, 1000 mg two times daily + Clarithromycin, 500 mg two times daily or metronidazole, 500 mg two times daily.

*Quadruple therapy*

PPI twice daily + Bismuth, 2 tablets four times daily + Metronidazole, 250 mg three times daily + Tetracycline, 500 mg four times daily.

**TABLE 53.3:** Test for *Helicobacter pylori*

| Test | Indication | Advantages | Disadvantages |
|---|---|---|---|
| **1. Serologic test** | When the patient has not received treatment for *H. pylori* infection, test of choice is serological test | Non-invasive; sensitivity of >80%, specificity of about 90% | Does not confirm eradication, because serologic positivity remains for indefinite period after microbiologic cure |
| **2. Urea breath test:** Based on ability to hydrolyse urea | This test is to confirm cure of *H. pylori* infection, but no sooner than 4 weeks after completion of therapy | Simple; sensitivity and specificity of 90 to 99% | False-negatives possible, if testing is done too soon after treatment for *H. pylori* infection. Small radiation exposure with $^{14}C$ method, cost and availability are disadvantages |
| **3. Histologic test** is done by staining with silver, Giemsa, etc. | Presence of *H. pylori* in biopsy material taken during endoscopy establishes the diagnosis | Sensitivity of 80 to 100%, specificity of >95%; Giemsa stain has sensitivity of >95% and specificity of 99% | Requires laboratory facilities and experience; when haematoxylin-eosin stain is nondiagnostic, other stains have to be used |
| **4. Rapid urease test** | Simplest method. However, endoscopy is required | Simple; rapid (once biopsy specimen has been obtained); sensitivity of 80 to 95%, specificity of 95 to 100% | Invasive; false-negatives possible, if testing is done too soon after treatment with proton pump inhibitors, antimicrobials or bismuth compounds |
| **5. Culture** (not routinely done) | When antimicrobial resistance is suspected after many drug failures | Allows determination of antibiotic susceptibility. Sensitivity is 80% and specificity is 100% | Time-consuming; expensive; usually not necessary unless resistance is suspected |

### *New drug therapy*

Vanoprazan, is a drug, which is potassium competitive acid blocker. This can be combined with other drugs.

### Complications of *Helicobacter Pylori* Infection

- Chronic duodenal ulcer
- Gastric carcinoma
- Gastro-oesophageal reflux disease
- Barrett's oesophagus
- Chronic gastritis
- Gastric maltoma
- Oesophageal cancer
- Idiopathic thrombocytopenic purpura.

## GASTRITIS

- Various forms of gastritis have been depicted in Table 53.4.
- Type B gastritis and erosive gastritis are common.
- Endoscopy and biopsy are the key investigations in all forms of gastritis.
- The treatment depends upon the type of gastritis.
- Rarer forms of gastritis include granulomatous gastritis, lymphocytic gastritis, etc.

## NONULCERATIVE DYSPEPSIA

- Dyspepsia is characterised by symptoms related to upper abdominal viscera. Symptoms may include abdominal pain, bloating, indigestion, nausea and

**TABLE 53.4:** Gastritis

| Type A | Type B | Reflux | Erosive |
|---|---|---|---|
| Autoimmune—antibodies to parietal cell | *H. pylori* associated | After cholecystectomy, gastric surgery | It occurs due to NSAIDs |
| Fundus and body are affected | Antrum is affected | Antrum is affected | It affects entire stomach |
| Atrophy of parietal cell mass. Hence, hypochlorhydria and decreased intrinsic factor | Predisposes to peptic ulcer disease | Usually does not give rise to peptic ulcer disease | It occurs due to defective gastric mucosal barrier |
| Hypochlorhydria stimulates antral gastrin. Predisposes to development of gastric cancer | Can give rise to intestinal metaplasia, dysplasia and predisposes to development of gastric cancer | Treated by prokinetic agents or bile chelating agents | Treated by $H_2$ blockers or proton pump inhibitors |

heart burn. Heart burn as a single symptom suggests gastro-oesophageal reflux disease and excludes the diagnosis of dyspepsia.

- Nonulcerative dyspepsia is considered when no anatomic or biochemical abnormality is discovered to explain the patient's symptoms.
- After *H. pylori* infection, ingestion of nonsteroidal anti-inflammatory drugs (NSAIDs) is the most common cause of nonulcerative dyspepsia and PUD.
- *H. pylori* infection is always associated with histologic gastritis which is absent in cases of nonulcerative dyspepsia.
- Hence *H. pylori* eradication therapy is not recommended in the treatment of nonulcerative dyspepsia.
- For surgeons, the importance of nonulcerative dyspepsia relates to its place in the differential diagnosis of epigastric pain. There is no role for surgery in the treatment of this disorder.
- Some of these patients, who have been diagnosed as nonulcerative dyspepsia, may have gallstones or oesophageal reflux disease. Hence, abdominal ultrasound and oesophageal manometry are required to rule out these diseases.
- Before we start discussion on peptic ulcer disease, we will discuss nonulcerative dyspepsia (commonly mistaken as peptic ulcer disease) and Zollinger-Ellison syndrome which is one of the rare causes of peptic ulceration. Oesophagogastroduodenoscopy should be done in all the patients with nonulcerative dyspepsia followed by biopsy from stomach to rule out *H. pylori* infection. One important cause of peptic ulcer disease—Zollinger-Ellison syndrome is being discussed first.

## ZOLLINGER-ELLISON SYNDROME

### Introduction

- Zollinger-Ellison syndrome (ZES) is a **clinical triad consisting of gastric acid hypersecretion, severe PUD, and non-islet cell tumours of the pancreas.**
- The tumours are known to produce gastrin and are referred to as gastrinomas (Fig. 53.5).
- These tumours are usually localised to the head of the pancreas, duodenal wall or regional lymph nodes. The majority (90%) of gastrinomas are thought to arise in gastrinoma triangle, also known as Passaro's triangle.
- About one-half of these gastric tumours are multiple and two-thirds are malignant.

### Association with MEN

About one-fourth are associated with **multiple endocrine neoplasia syndrome (MEN 1)**. Other tumours in MEN 1 are pituitary adenoma and parathyroid adenoma.

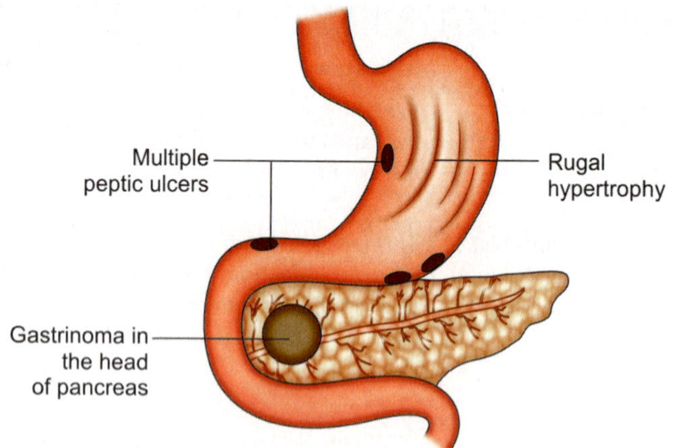


**Fig. 53.5:** Pictorial representation of gastrinoma (refer to page 806 also)

### Pathophysiology

Pathophysiologic features of ZES that distinguish it from duodenal ulcer are present and are all explained either by the actions of **gastrin to stimulate gastric acid secretion** and **mucosal growth** or by the action of other associated hormones in the MEN 1 syndrome.

### Clinical Features

- Abdominal pain and PUD are the hallmarks of the syndrome and typically occur in more than 80% of patients.
- About one-half of patients have diarrhoea secondary to increased gastric acid secretion.
- Weight loss and steatorrhoea also occur secondary to decreased duodenal and jejunal pH, and inactivation of lipase.
- Oesophagitis from gastro-oesophageal reflux is also common.

### Investigations

#### *I. Endoscopy*

- **Demonstrates prominent gastric rugal folds, reflecting the trophic effect of hypergastrinaemia on the gastric fundus in addition to evidence of PUD.**
- Gastrinoma and ZES are always considered and ruled out in patients who have:
  1. Recurrent or intractable PUD despite eradication of *H. pylori* and appropriate antisecretory therapy.
  2. Multiple or atypically located ulcers.
  3. PUD associated with significant diarrhoea.
  4. PUD associated with symptoms of MEN 1 such as hyperparathyroidism or kindred of MEN 1.
  5. Large gastric rugae on endoscopy.
  6. **In those patients with other pancreatic endocrine tumours.**

7. Patients undergoing elective surgical intervention for PUD have the possibility of gastrinoma included in their preoperative evaluation.

### *II. Serum Gastrin Levels*

Most patients with gastrinoma have **elevated fasting levels (>200 pg/ml), and values greater than 1000 pg/ml may be diagnostic**.

### *III. The Secretin Test*

- It is the most sensitive and specific provocative test for gastrinoma and aids in the differentiation between gastrinomas and other causes of ulcerogenic hypergastrinaemia.
- Secretin (2 mg/kg) is administered intravenously and serum gastrin samples are measured before and after secretin administration at 5-minute interval for 30 minutes.
- An increase in serum gastrin of greater than 200 pg/ml above basal levels is specific for gastrinoma.

### Treatment

- Acid suppression therapy with a proton pump inhibitor.
- Localisation of the gastrinoma is performed before operative intervention is made.
- **Noninvasive methods** include computed tomography (CT) scanning, MRI, endoscopic ultrasound, and $^{111}$In-octreotide scintigraphy (somatostatin receptor imaging).
- In patients with **resectable gastrinomas**, surgical resection is performed that includes tumour resection from the duodenum, pancreas and regional lymph nodes.
- **Total gastrectomy is rarely indicated** and is reserved for patients who are noncompliant with acid suppression therapy or when the tumour cannot be localised.

> **SU28.9:** Describe and discuss the aetiology, the clinical features, investigations and principles of management of peptic ulcer disease.

## PEPTIC ULCER DISEASE

### Definition

Acid peptic digestion of the alimentary mucosa resulting in an ulcer is called peptic ulcer disease (PUD). The corrosive effects of acid with proteolytic effect of pepsin are responsible for PUD. Duodenum and stomach are the common sites of peptic ulcer disease. Rarely, they can occur in the jejunum and in Meckel's diverticulum when it contains ectopic gastric mucosa.

### Types of Peptic Ulcer

#### *I. Depending on the Site*

A. **Chronic duodenal ulcer:** Typically occurs in the first inch of the first part of the duodenum.
B. **Chronic gastric ulcer:** Occurs in the lesser curvature adjacent to acid secreting parietal cell mass.
C. **Combined:** Gastric ulcer type II—Zollinger-Ellison syndrome
D. **Anastomotic ulcer**

#### *II. Depending on the Duration*

A. Chronic peptic ulcer, and B. Acute peptic ulcer.

## CHRONIC DUODENAL ULCER (CDU)

Hyperacidity is the chief cause of duodenal ulcer. **No acid, no ulcer** still holds good for CDU.

1. **Neurological causes:** Stimulation of vagus increases secretion of acids. This is brought about by **anxiety, worry, hurry and curry**.
2. **Nonsteroidal anti-inflammatory drugs:** They are responsible for gastric ulcer rather than duodenal ulcer by altering mucosal defence.
3. **Genetic causes:** Family history of duodenal ulcer may be present in a few cases which suggests a genetic cause. Patients with blood group **'O'** are more prone, for the development of CDU because of **increased parietal cell population**.
4. **Food habits:** Spicy food, diet poor in vitamins, smoking and alcohol, alone or in combination precipitate the development of chronic duodenal ulcer.
5. **Bacteriological causes** (Fig. 53.6): ***Helicobacter pylori***, a spirochaetal bacterium, has been demonstrated in the submucosa of the antrum and duodenum, from the biopsies of the ulcer. **It increases pH levels by splitting urea and releasing ammonia.** Rise in pH results in proliferation of bacteria. This is the most important cause of chronic duodenal ulcer today.
6. **Endocrinal causes**
   - Zollinger-Ellison syndrome is a non-β cell tumour of the pancreas with hypergastrinaemia.
   - Hyperparathyroidism causes increased levels of calcium which stimulates the parietal cell mass resulting in hyperacidity.

### Pathophysiology of Duodenal Ulcer

- Duodenal ulcer is a disease of multiple aetiologies.
- The only absolute requirements are acid and pepsin secretion in combination with either infection with *H. pylori* or ingestion of NSAIDs.
- **Duodenal ulcer patients have an increase in mean parietal cell number. Thus, they secrete more acid,** whereas gastric ulcer patients do not.

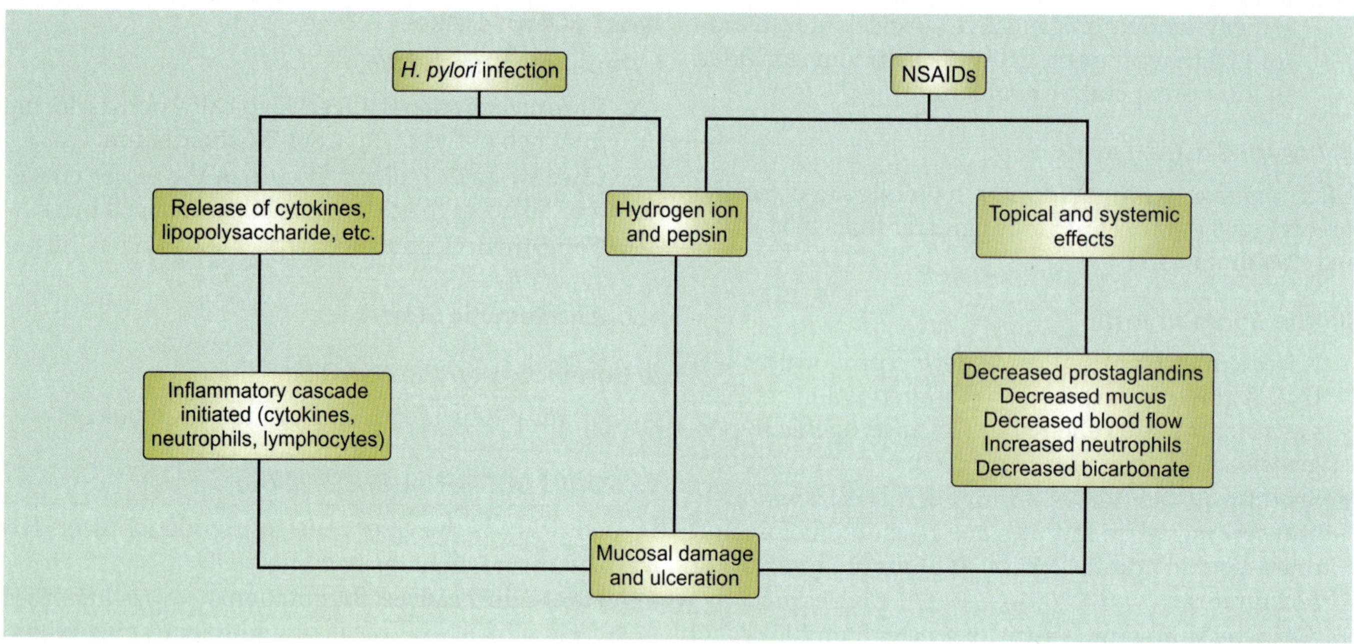


**Fig. 53.6:** Peptic ulceration

## CHRONIC GASTRIC ULCER

- In majority of the patients, there is no **hyperacidity**. Many patients have hypoacidity, or normoacidity.
- Ulcer occurs due to a defective gastric mucosal barrier. This barrier is a coat of thick mucus which is impermeable to pepsin (Key Box 53.6).
- Prostaglandins, normally present in the gastric mucosa, do not allow back diffusion of hydrogen ions from the lumen.
- Nonsteroidal anti-inflammatory drugs inhibit the production of prostaglandins causing a loss of protective activity.
- This can also be damaged by smoking, spicy food, alcohol and reflux of bile into the stomach.

Key Box 53.6

**Some Conditions that may Predispose to Gastric Ulceration**

- Age older than 40, sex (female to male ratio of 2:1)
- Ingestion of barrier-breaking drugs such as aspirin or nonsteroidal anti-inflammatory drugs (NSAIDs)
- Abnormalities in acid and pepsin secretion
- Gastric stasis through delayed gastric emptying
- Coexisting duodenal ulcer
- Duodenal gastric reflux of bile
- Gastritis, and infection with *H. pylori*
- Chronic alcohol intake, smoking
- Long-term corticosteroid therapy
- Intra-arterial chemotherapy

### Classification (Johnson) Types of Chronic Gastric Ulcer (Figs 53.7 to 53.11)

#### *I. Acute Superficial*

These may be single or multiple (erosions).

#### *II. Chronic*

**Type 1:** Primary gastric ulcer on the lesser curvature in the antrum near the junction of oxyntic cells and central mucosa.

**Type 2:** Gastric ulcer with duodenal ulcer.

**Type 3:** Prepyloric or channel ulcer.

**Type 4:** High gastric ulcer (cardia, proximal stomach) <2 cm from gastro-oesophageal junction.

**Type 5:** NSAIDs-induced gastric ulcers.

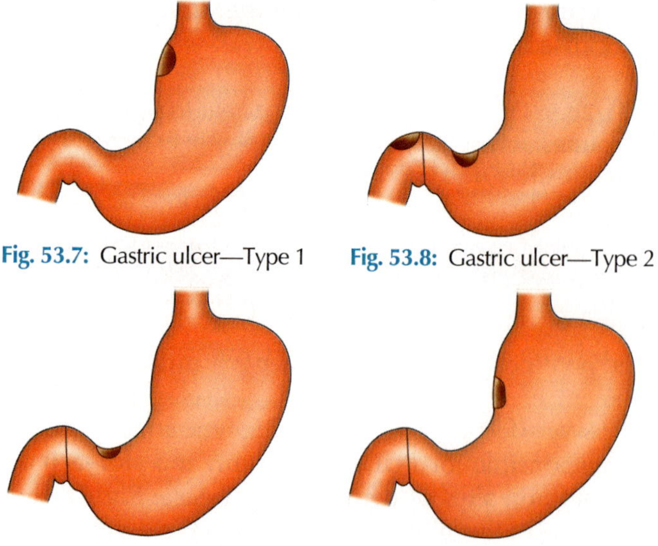

**Fig. 53.7:** Gastric ulcer—Type 1

**Fig. 53.8:** Gastric ulcer—Type 2

**Fig. 53.9:** Gastric ulcer—Type 3

**Fig. 53.10:** Gastric ulcer—Type 4

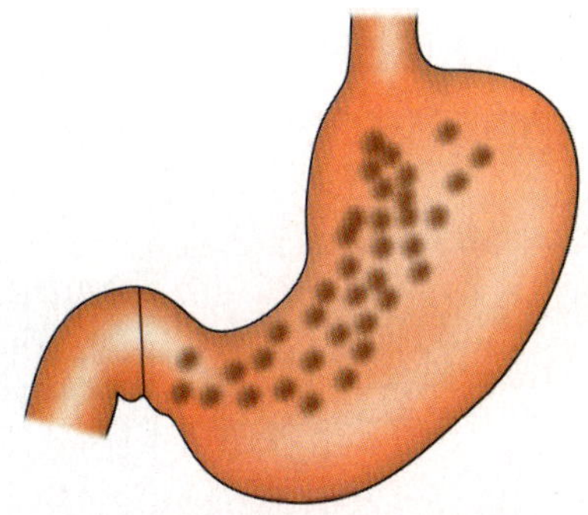

Fig. 53.11: NSAIDs-induced gastric ulcer—Type 5

*Pearls of Wisdom*

Types 2, and 3 gastric ulcers are to be treated like duodenal ulcer because they are associated with hyperacidity.

**Giant gastric ulcers:** These are important because they are more prone for perforation and malignancy. Incidence may vary from 10 to 20 cm (Key Box 53.7).

Key Box 53.7

**Giant Gastric Ulcer**

- Diameter >2 cm
- Typically, lesser curvature at incisura angularis
- Incidence of malignancy—10%
- High chances of perforation and bleeding
- Medical treatment heals majority of cases (80%)
- Re-endoscopy biopsy is a must to look for healing and also to rule out malignancy
- Gastrectomy including ulcer bed. Add vagotomy for type 2 and type 3 gastric ulcers

## Investigations (Figs 53.12 to 53.18)

1. **Oesophagogastroduodenoscopy (OGD):** Ulcer appears as a crater with/without slough or bleeding in their typical locations. In gastric ulcers, routine biopsy is advised to rule out malignancy. In duodenal ulcers, biopsy is done in recurrent cases to rule out *Helicobacter pylori.*
   - In long-standing duodenal ulcers, there may be narrowing of the pylorus, with stasis of food in the stomach suggestive of pyloric stenosis.
   - Other uses of OGD is given in Key Box 53.8.

Key Box 53.8

**Oesophagogastroduodenoscopy (OGD)**

**Diagnostic** (Figs 53.12 to 53.18)
- Peptic ulcers—acute and chronic
- Gastritis
- Carcinoma stomach
- Oesophageal varices, ulcers, oesophagitis
- Biopsy to rule out *H. pylori* infection
- Brush cytology and biology, yield is better

**Therapeutic**
- Injection of adrenaline into the bleeding vessel
- Variceal injection
- Snaring of polyps
- Electrocoagulation of bleeders
- Endoscopic cystogastrostomy
- Foreign body removal
- Percutaneous endoscopic gastrostomy (PEG)
- Endoscopic mucosal resection for early carcinoma stomach

## Clinical Features (Table 53.5)

**TABLE 53.5:** Classification of clinical features

| | Chronic duodenal ulcer | Chronic gastric ulcer |
|---|---|---|
| Incidence | Common | Less common |
| Site | 1st inch of 1st part of duodenum | The lesser curvature or prepyloric region |
| Pain | It is due to the acid irritating the ulcer (hunger pain). It is relieved on taking food. After 1–2 hours of food, the pain becomes severe. It is burning in nature with retrosternal radiation (heartburn) and increased salivation (water brash) | Pain occurs on taking food and it is relieved by induced vomiting. Pain is of burning nature as in duodenal ulcer |
| Vomiting | Never occurs in duodenal ulcer till the patient develops pyloric stenosis | Frequent and it occurs immediately after patient takes food |
| Weight | Weight gain | Weight loss |
| Periodicity | Common | Less |
| Haematemesis and melaena ratio | 40:60 | 60:40 |
| Incidence of malignancy | Never becomes malignant | 0.5–5% (2%) |
| On examination | Tenderness in the right hypochondrium | Tenderness in the epigastrium |

## ENDOSCOPIC PICTURES

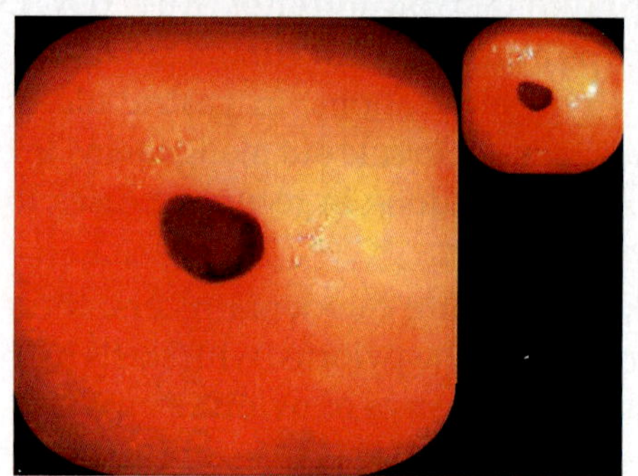

**Fig. 53.12:** Normal pyloric opening

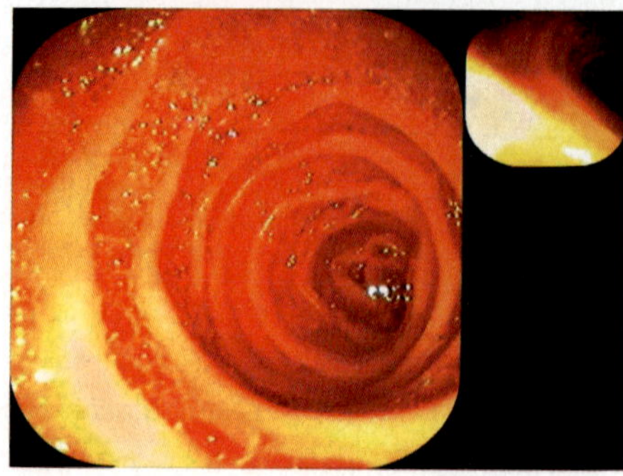

**Fig. 53.13:** Normal 2nd part duodenum

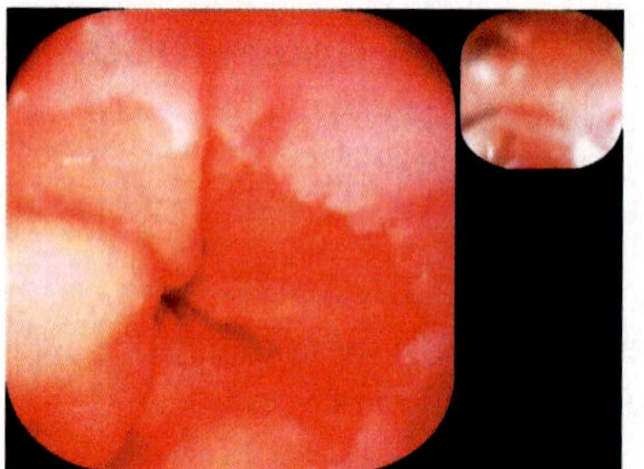

**Fig. 53.14:** Normal squamocolumnar junction—Z line

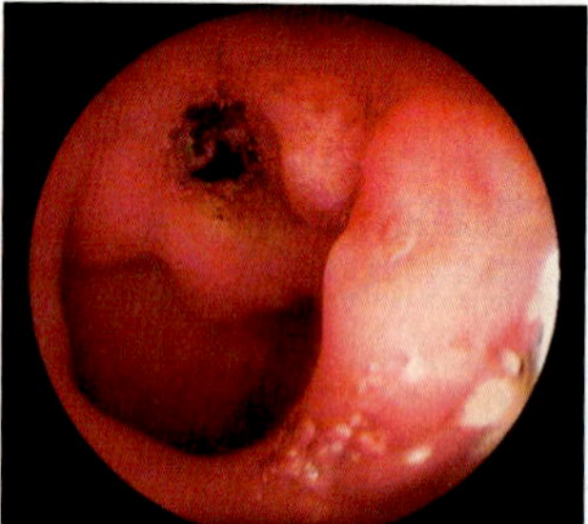

**Fig. 53.15:** OGD showing bleeding duodenal ulcer

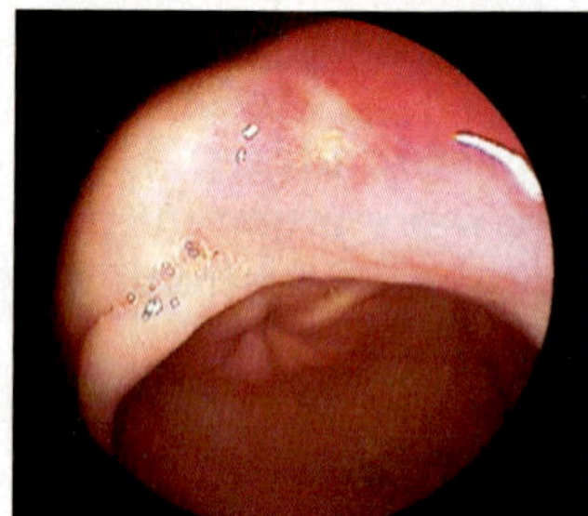

**Fig. 53.16:** OGD showing chronic gastric ulcer

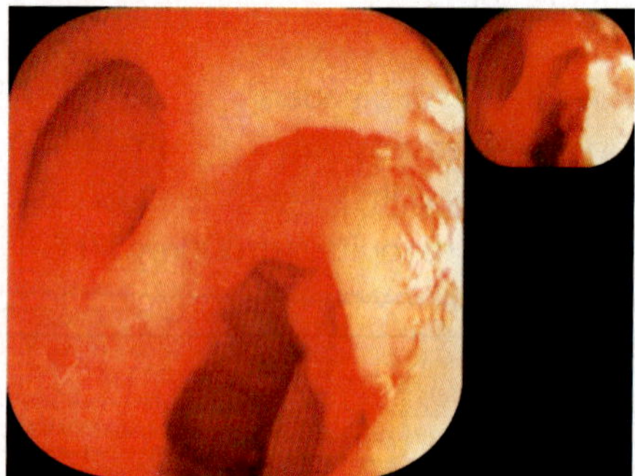

**Fig. 53.17:** OGD showing bleeding duodenal ulcer and diverticulum due to ulcer

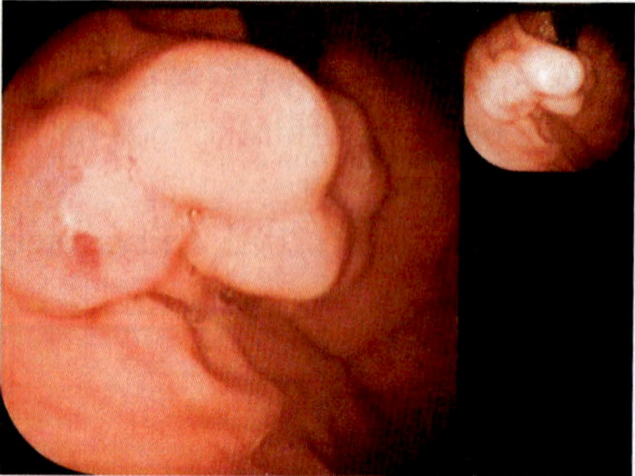

**Fig. 53.18:** Large gastric varices—this patient also had duodenal ulcer

(*Courtesy*: Prof Ganesh Pai, Head, Department of Gastroenterology, KMC, Manipal)



2. **Barium meal study** (historical—obsolete now)
   - **Duodenal ulcer:** Deformed duodenal cap.
   - **Trifoliate deformity** is seen when secondary duodenal diverticulum occurs.
   - **Gastric ulcer** appears as a niche in the lesser curvature due to ulcer crater and as a notch on the greater curvature due to the spasm of stomach (Fig 53.19).
   - In general, benign ulcers are smoother, more regular, with rounded edges and a flat, smooth ulcer base. In malignancy, the mass protrudes into the lumen or has folds surrounding ulcer crater.
   - To detect **hour glass stomach** and **gastric outlet obstruction** (Figs 53.20 and 53.21).
3. **Test for *Helicobacter pylori*** (already discussed).

## Treatment

### A. Treatment of Chronic Duodenal Ulcer (CDU)

**Aim** is to decrease the pain because of its severity (by reducing acidity) and to prevent relapses (Key Box 53.9).

Key Box 53.9

**Aims of the Treatment**

- To relieve symptoms
- To heal the ulcer
- To prevent recurrence
- To prevent complications

### I. Medical Line of Management

- **Pantoprazole in a dose of 40 mg/day for 4 weeks has become the first line of treatment for chronic duodenal ulcer.** Other drugs are esomeprazole: 40 mg/day, lansoprazole: 30 mg/day,
- Lifestyle modification: Stop smoking, decrease alcohol, avoid spicy food, minimize coffee.
- Discontinue aspirin or NSAIDs and other gastric irritants.
- **Eradication therapy if biopsy is proved for *Helicobacter pylori*.**

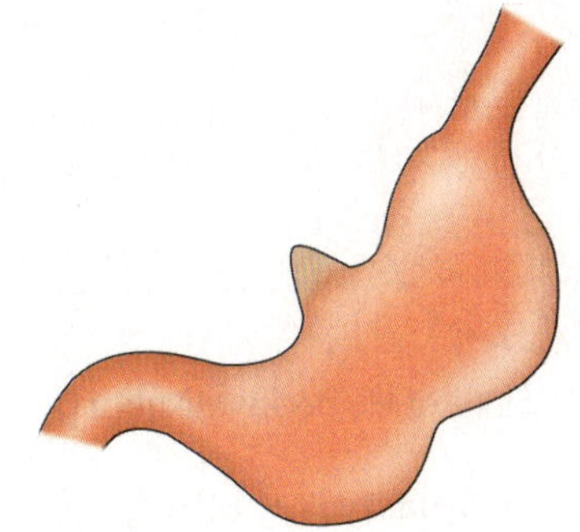

Fig. 53.19: Diagram showing niche and notch

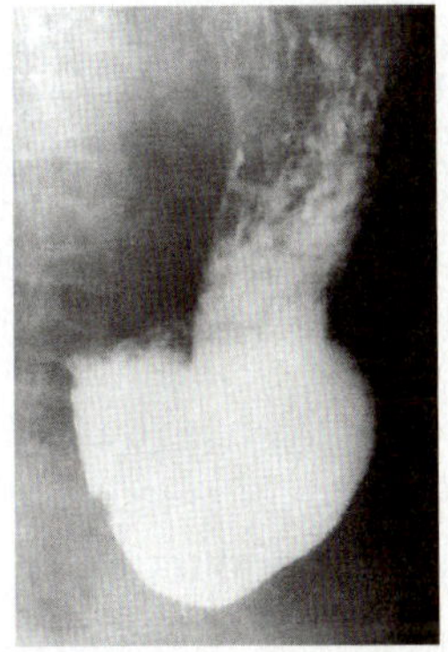

Fig. 53.20: Gastric outlet obstruction. Barium meal can detect dilated stomach

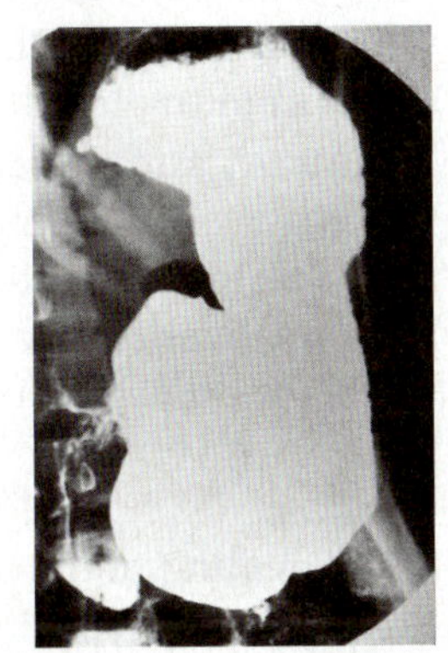

Fig. 53.21: Hugely dilated J-shaped stomach

### II. Surgical Line of Management

***Surgery:*** Indications for surgery is given in Key Box 53.10.

Key Box 53.10

**Indications for Surgery**

1. Frequent relapses, *H. pylori* negative
2. Complications of duodenal ulcer:
   - Gastric outlet obstruction
   - Haemorrhage

1. **Highly selective vagotomy (HSV):** It is also called PCV (parietal cell vagotomy) or PGV (proximal gastric vagotomy) (Fig. 53.22).
   - In this operation, **vagi are not divided at the trunks.** Both anterior and posterior vagi are identified,

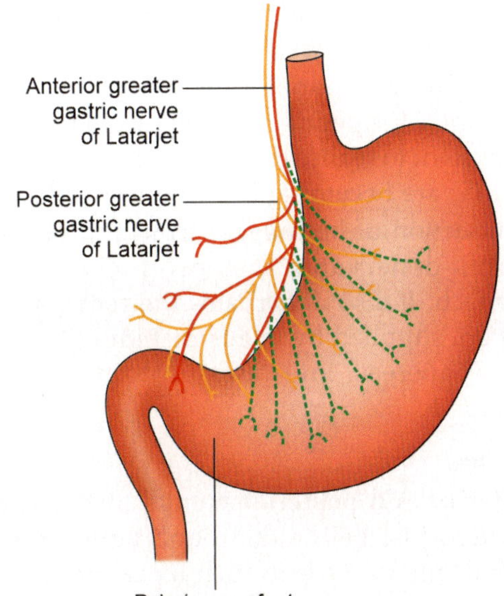


Fig. 53.22: Highly selective vagotomy—pyloric crow foot is preserved. Hence, drainage procedure is not required. Red colour indicates blood supply. Watch carefully–blood supply to the parietal cell mass is also cut which helps in isolating and dividing nerve fibres supplying parietal cell mass

isolated and preserved. Their branches which run along the lesser curvature are isolated. They are anterior and posterior greater gastric nerves of Latarjet. The branches of the nerves of Latarjet supplying parietal cell mass are divided. Hence, it is called parietal cell vagotomy. The terminal fibres of the nerve of Latarjet which supply pylorus are preserved (5–7 cm of 'Crow foot').

#### *Advantages of HSV*

1. More physiological, with **minimal disturbances.**
2. No drainage procedure is required because pyloric functions are preserved.
3. Nerve supply to gallbladder and liver is not disturbed.
4. No diarrhoea as that can occur in 5–8% of cases of truncal vagotomy which can be morbid.

**Pearls of Wisdom**

It is important to note that experience of many surgeons today with HSV is 'minimum'. Hence, it is safe to do 'vagotomy and gastrojejunostomy (GJ)'.

#### *Disadvantages of HSV*

- This is not the procedure for prepyloric ulcer as there is a high recurrence rate.
- Complicated procedure—needs an experienced surgeon.
- Recurrence rate: 10–15%
- Rare chance of lesser curvature necrosis.

2. **Total truncal abdominal vagotomy with gastro-jejunostomy of Mayo** (Fig. 53.23) **or pyloroplasty**
   - This is the most popular and most commonly done operation for peptic ulcer disease. However, it is important to realise that **indications for vagotomy and GJ are becoming less and less today**.
   - Transection of both vagal trunks at oesophageal hiatus denervates acid producing fundus of stomach. It also denervates the remainder of the viscera supplied by vagus including liver, biliary tree, pancreas, intestines up to mid-transverse colon.

*Procedure*

- **Anterior and posterior trunks of the vagus are divided** just below the diaphragm followed by a drainage procedure such as gastrojejunostomy (GJ). **Vagus is secretomotor to stomach and after vagotomy the motility of the stomach is lost and gastric stasis occurs. Hence, drainage procedure is done.**
- Posterior GJ is preferred because it gives a dependent drainage of the food contents by gravity. Classically, it is described as "posterior, vertical, retrocolic, isoperistaltic, no loop (short loop), no tension, GJ of Mayo **(PVRING)**".
- Alternatively, pyloroplasty is preferred by a few surgeons instead of GJ.
- In **Heineke-Mikulicz pyloroplasty,** pylorus is incised longitudinally and sutured vertically. Thus, the pyloric ring becomes incompetent and wide open. Bile reflux gastritis and diarrhoea are major problems after pyloroplasty (Fig. 53.24).

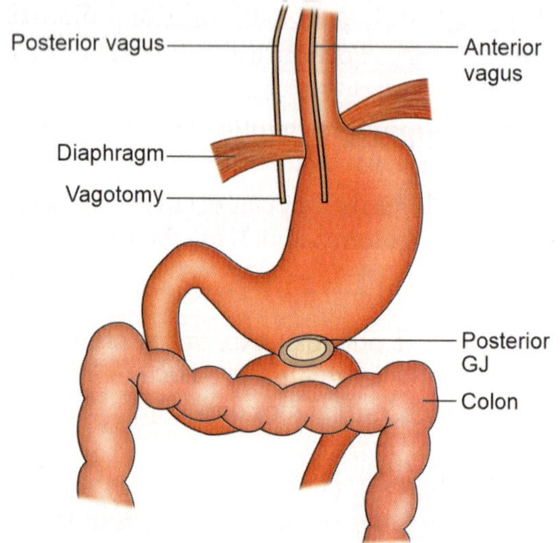


**Fig. 53.23:** Posterior GJ **(Mayo)**[1] with vagotomy—motility of the stomach is lost after vagotomy. Hence, drainage procedure (GJ in this picture) is required (vagus is secretomotor of the stomach)

[1]About Mayo—Mayo's scissors, Mayo's forceps, Mayo's GJ, Mayo's vein, Mayo's umbilical hernia repair to be remembered.

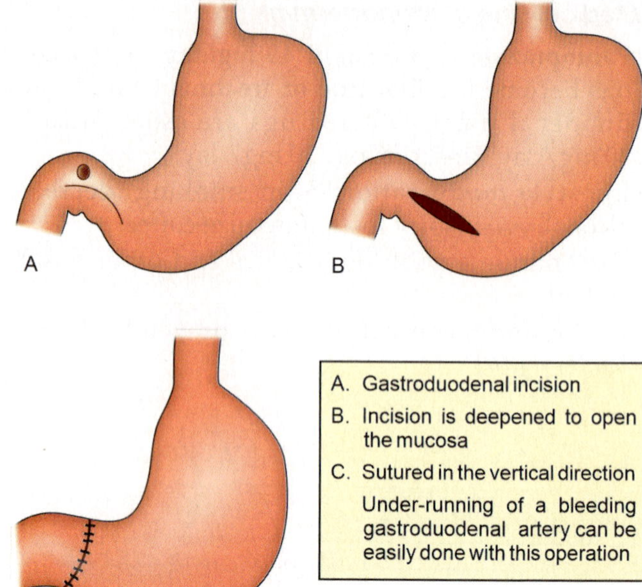


**Fig. 53.24:** Steps of Heinecke-Mikulicz pyloroplasty

- **Finney pyloroplasty** is another procedure wherein inverted U-type of incision is given involving distal stomach and duodenum and a gastro-duodenal stoma is created. This type of pyloroplasty is indicated when duodenum is dilated (Fig. 53.25).

3. **Vagotomy and antrectomy** (Fig. 53.26): By removing the vagal stimuli and the antral gastrin, the entire stimulus to acid secretion is lost. Hence, it carries the **least recurrence rate (1%)** but carries 3–4% mortality rate. Not done routinely.

## B. Treatment of Chronic Gastric Ulcer

- Aim: Healing of the ulcer and relief of symptoms.
- Frequent biopsy is done to rule out malignancy.

I. **Medical line of treatment** can be given for duodenal ulcer, in the form of ranitidine or omeprazole. Cigarette smoking should be stopped. Drugs such as NSAIDs and aspirin are to be avoided. If an ulcer

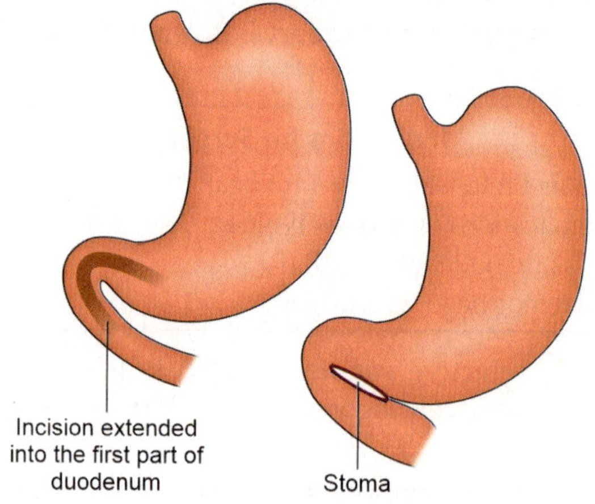


**Fig. 53.25:** Finney pyloroplasty

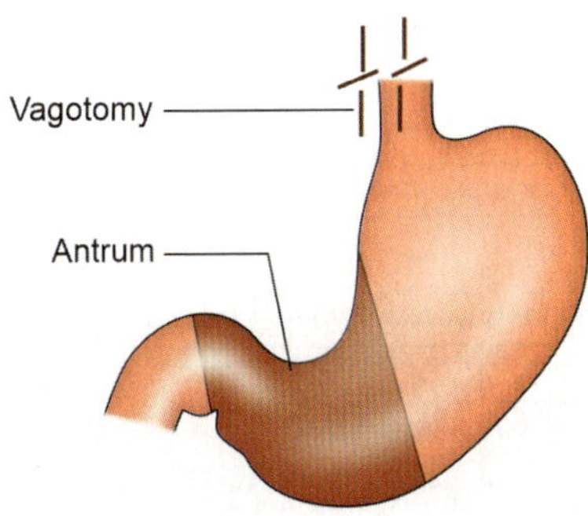


Fig. 53.26: Vagotomy with antrectomy

persists after 6 weeks, the aim is to eradicate *H. pylori* **provided malignancy is ruled out**.

II. **Surgery** is indicated in case of gastric ulcer persisting in spite of medical treatment.
   1. **Billroth I partial gastrectomy** (Fig. 53.27): Partial gastrectomy is done including removal of the ulcer followed by gastroduodenal anastomosis. It has the least recurrence rate of less than 1% but mortality rate is around 1–2%.
   2. **Billroth II gastrectomy** (Fig. 53.28): It is indicated when the gastric ulcer is located on the lesser curvature. Here the gastrectomy is done below the ulcer and remnant of the stomach is anastomosed to a jejunal loop (gastrojejunal anastomosis). This is also described as Polya gastrectomy.
   3. **HSV with excision of the ulcer** can be done, if the experience of surgeon is good.

## TYPE 4 GASTRIC ULCERS

- The type 4 gastric ulcer presents a difficult management problem.
- The surgical treatment depends on the ulcer size, distance from the GE junction and the degree of surrounding inflammation.
- Whenever possible, the ulcer should be excised.
- The most aggressive approach is to perform a gastrectomy that includes a small portion of the oesophageal wall and the ulcer followed by a Roux-en-Y oesophagogastrojejunostomy to restore intestinal continuity.

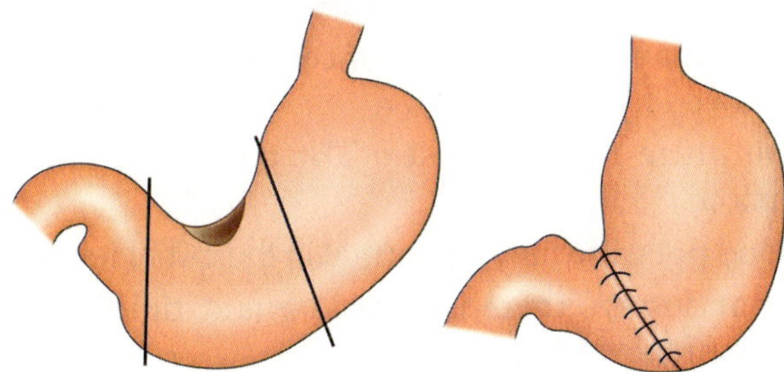

Fig. 53.27: Billroth I gastrectomy followed by gastroduodenal anastomosis

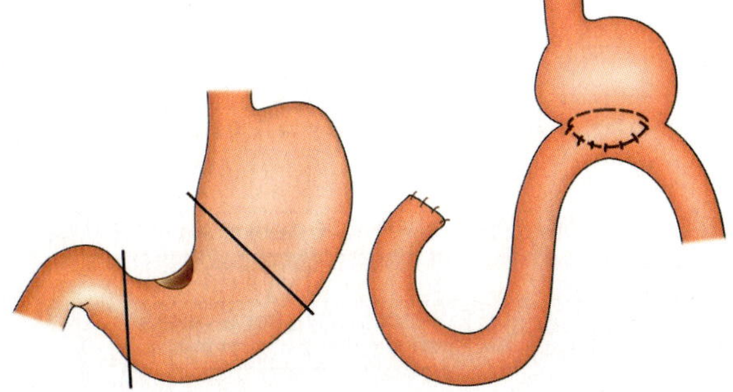

Fig. 53.28: Billroth II gastrectomy followed by gastrojejunal anastomosis

- For type 4 gastric ulcers that are located 2 to 5 cm from the gastroesophageal junction, a distal gastrectomy with a vertical extension of the resection to include **the lesser curvature with the ulcer can be performed (i.e. Pauchet procedure).** After resection, bowel continuity is restored with an end-to-end gastroduodenostomy.
- **The Csendes procedure may be useful in stable patients or the Kelling-Madlener operation in unstable ones** (Fig. 53.29).

### Summary of the Management of Peptic Ulcer

Figure 53.30 depicts the summary of management of peptic ulcer.

### Complications of Peptic Ulcer

**A. Acute**
- Perforation
- Haematemesis and/or melaena

**B. Subacute—residual abscess**

**C. Chronic**
- Gastric outlet obstruction (pyloric stenosis)
- Teapot deformity
- Hour glass contracture of the stomach

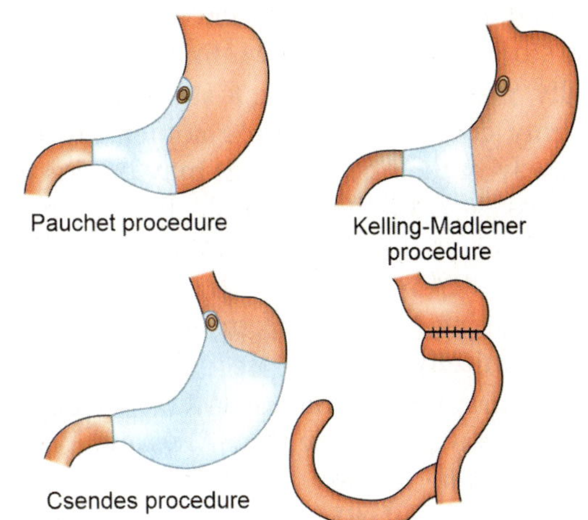


Fig. 53.29: Other types of resections for gastric ulcer

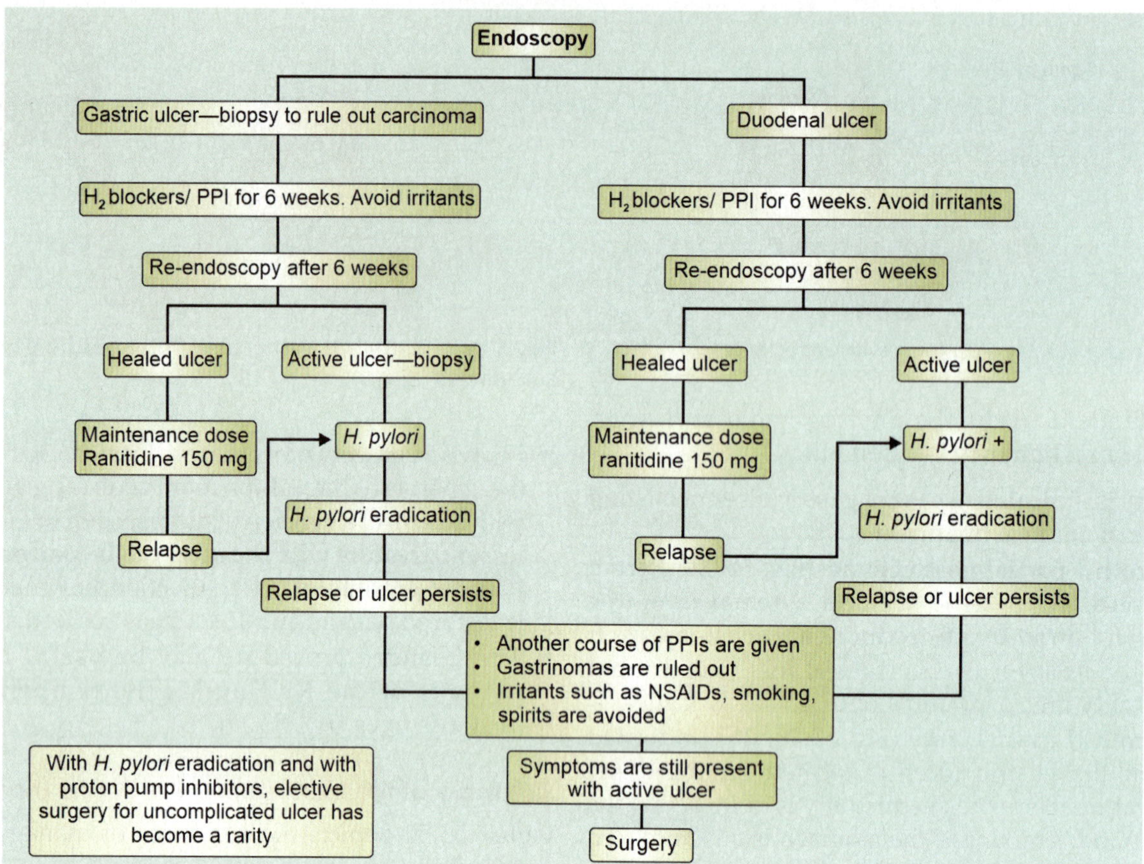


**Fig. 53.30:** Management of peptic ulcer

- Penetration into the pancreas
- Carcinoma of stomach.

## ACUTE COMPLICATIONS OF PEPTIC ULCER

### PERFORATED PEPTIC ULCER

#### Introduction

- More common in males. The ratio is 8–10 men to 1 woman in India.
- **Anterior duodenal ulcer perforates and posterior duodenal ulcer bleeds.** An ulcer on the posterior wall of the stomach can perforate into the lesser sac.
- Usually, patients with a **long history of peptic ulcer**, suddenly complain of feeling something that has given way in their abdomen. It may be precipitated by excessive smoking, alcohol, drugs, etc. Rarely a **'silent' ulcer** can also perforate (especially those patients treated with cortisone).
- Patients taking NSAIDs (often elderly) can present less dramatically.
- **Two factors** are associated with most perforated peptic ulcers: Chronic use of NSAIDs and *Helicobacter pylori* infection.
- Patients with ***H. pylori* infection** and perforated peptic ulcers tend to be **younger, with a male preponderance** and more prolonged period of dyspepsia. However, NSAIDs category of patients are elderly with equal proportion of both sexes being affected.
- Perforated peptic ulcers have a mortality rate of 5–10%.
- Perforated gastric ulcers in the elderly have 10–20% mortality rate.
- Golden time to operate is within 6 hours.

#### Stages of Duodenal Ulcer Perforation

##### *1. Stage of Chemical Peritonitis*

- Immediately after the perforation, gastric and duodenal contents leak into the peritoneal cavity and produce severe agonising pain in the right hypochondrium. It is mainly HCl which produces pain.
- There may be an episode of coffee-ground vomitus, followed by melaena later.
- The pulse rate increases. The patient is pale and anxious.
- Blood pressure may be normal in the initial few hours.
- *Per* abdomen, there is guarding and rigidity of the abdominal wall.
- Rebound tenderness is present all over the abdomen. This sign is called **Blumberg's sign**.

- On percussion, liver dullness is obliterated because of collection of free air (gas) under the right dome of diaphragm. This stage is seen for about 2–4 hours from the time of perforation.
- Bowel sounds are usually absent.

### 2. Stages of Reaction

- The peritoneum reacts to the chemical irritants by secreting peritoneal fluid. As a result of this, HCl and bile are diluted by the peritoneal secretions (reaction of peritoneum to the insult) resulting in an **improvement of symptoms**. Hence, it is also called **stage of dilution or stage of illusion.** This stage lasts for 3–6 hours. However, the signs are worse. Pulse is feeble, more than 120/min, hypotension persists, dehydration due to loss of fluid into peritoneal cavity, shifting dullness is present, abdominal distension is due to fluid and paralytic ileus.[1]
- Bowel sounds are absent and guarding and rigidity are worsened.

### 3. Stage of Bacterial Peritonitis

- The peritoneal contents get contaminated with gram-negative organisms resulting in bacterial peritonitis (the organisms are from the intestine itself and not from the peritoneum).
- The patient becomes severely ill, dehydrated, toxic with drawn in cheeks. The tongue is dry and coated but with bright eyes (**Hippocratic facies,** Fig. 53.31).
- Features of hypovolaemic and septicaemic shock such as feeble thready pulse, cold peripheries, shallow respiration, high grade fever and persistent hypotension are present. Gross abdominal distension, guarding, rigidity, abdominal tenderness all over suggest generalised peritonitis.

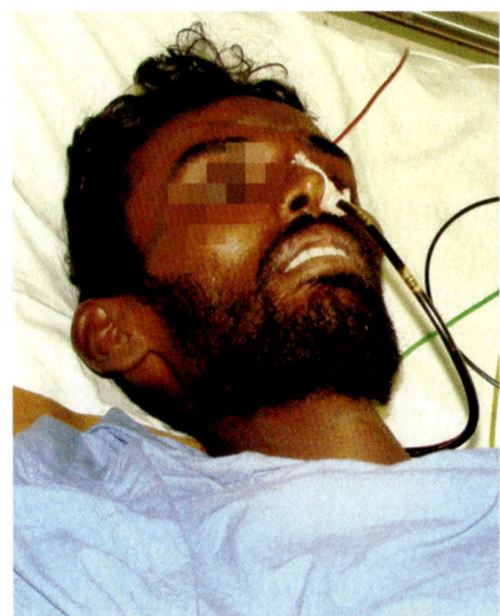

**Fig. 53.31:** Peritonitis—Hippocratic facies—sunken eyes, jaundice due to sepsis, nasogastric tube showing altered blood

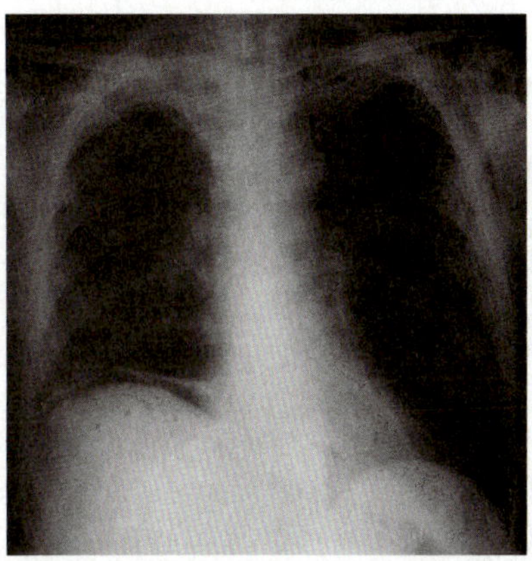

**Fig. 53.32:** Chest X-ray PA view showing collection of free gas under the right dome of the diaphragm

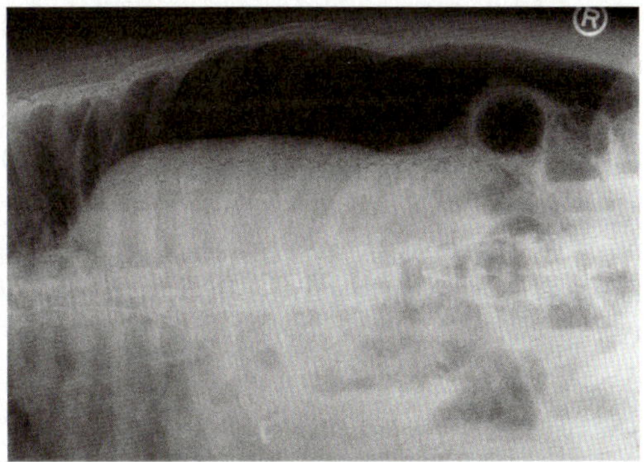

**Fig. 53.33:** Lateral decubitus X-ray showing free gas under abdominal wall suggestive of perforation.

## Investigation of Perforated Duodenal Ulcer

- Complete blood picture and electrolyte study. Immediate correction with Ringer's lactate to be started because of significant abnormalities in the electrolytes.
- Plain X-ray chest or abdomen (Fig. 53.32) in **erect position** shows collection of free gas under the right dome of diaphragm, in majority of cases. If patient is unable to stand, left lateral decubitus films are taken (Fig. 53.33). It can show signs such as appearance of gas on both sides of the bowel wall (**Rigler's sign**). Large volume of free gas resulting in a large round black area (**Football sign**).
- When in doubt, request a CT scan with contrast which can demonstrate pneumoperitoneum, fluid in the abdomen, site of perforation and some surprises also.

[1]It resembles a strike by employees paralysing the work of a factory in response to an insult.

### Treatment (ABCDEF)[1]

A: Aspiration of stomach contents with Ryle's tube to reduce further contamination and to decrease biliary and pancreatic juice.

B: Blood grouping and cross-matching may be necessary for surgery.

C: Charts: Temperature, pulse, BP, respiration, urinary output (urinary bladder is catheterised using a Foley's catheter).

D: Drugs:
- Injection cephalosporins 1 g IV stat and 12th hourly against gram-positive organisms.
- Injection gentamicin 60–80 mg IV, 8th hourly or amikacin 700 mg stat against gram-negative organisms (Check creatinine—if high, the dose needs to be monitored or another drug has to be chosen).
- Injection metronidazole 500 mg IV, 8th hourly to treat anaerobic organisms.

E: Exploratory laparotomy is done through a midline incision. The perforation is identified and closed with interrupted nonabsorbable silk sutures, which is strengthened by **placement of pedicled omentum** (Figs 53.34A and B). In Graham's repair, three interrupted sutures are placed but not tied. The defect is not sutured but a tongue of vascularised omentum is kept over the defect to seal the defect. This is followed by tying the knots. Peritoneal toilet/wash is given to avoid residual abscess. Abdomen is closed with a drain which is removed after 3–5 days. If it is a large gastric ulcer, it is better to do a gastrectomy, if condition of the patient permits.
- Vagotomy and GJ is not done at this stage as the general condition of the patient is very poor and there is peritoneal sepsis.
- Postoperatively, the patient is put on anti-ulcer drugs. An endoscopy is done after 2 months. If the ulcer persists, it may be worthwhile giving a course of *H. pylori eradication treatment*. However, it should be remembered that *H. pylori* eradication and simple suturing cures vast majority of acute ulcers.

F: Fluids are given preoperatively to treat dehydration and postoperatively for 3–4 days till the paralytic ileus settles down (soft abdomen and bowel sounds present).

#### Early Cases of Perforation

It can also be managed by laparoscopic closure of perforation with peritoneal drainage. In fact, a thorough wash is really possible with a laparoscope.

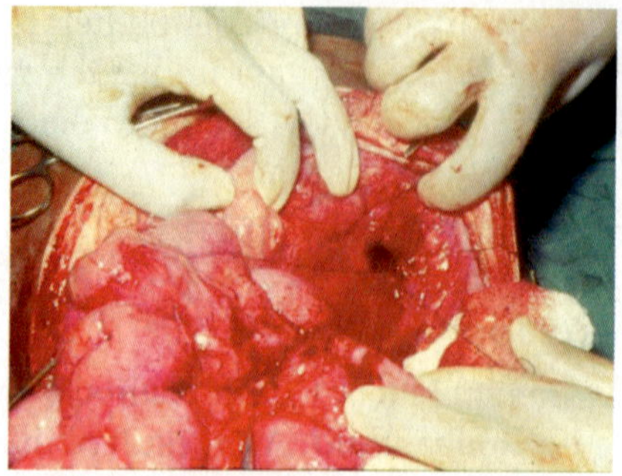

**Fig. 53.34A:** Duodenal ulcer perforation—closure

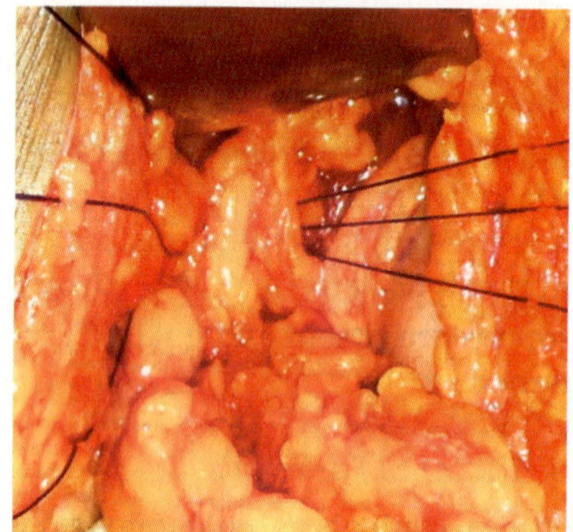

**Fig. 53.34B:** Pedicled omentum is used here

#### Subacute

Perforation with abscess. Some patients present late to the hospital with features of sealed perforation.

#### Non-operative Treatment of Perforated Duodenal Ulcer

It was first proposed by Herman Taylor called as **Herman Taylor regimen.**

- Initial steps of ABCD remain the same. There are few indications for non-operative line of treatment for perforated duodenal ulcer:
  A. Patients who are not fit for surgery due to severe comorbidities
  B. CECT shows no leak or no extravasation of the dye.
  C. Small perforation with no signs of peritonitis
- However, following precautions should be taken during non-operative treatment.
  1. **R**adiologically undetected leak
  2. **R**epeated clinical examination
  3. **R**epeated blood investigations
  4. **R**espiratory and renal support
  5. **R**esources for monitoring
  6. **R**eadiness to operate

  *Observe* **6 Rs**.

[1] Students should remember that ABCDEF are the basic principles of treatment of any acute abdomen. In majority of cases of acute abdomen, these principles can be applied with minor modifications.

## HAEMORRHAGE FROM PEPTIC ULCER

- Haemorrhage from peptic ulcer can be chronic which causes anaemia, or acute, resulting in massive haematemesis and melaena.
- It is the **posterior duodenal ulcer which commonly bleeds,** because it erodes into the gastroduodenal artery which runs posterior to the duodenum. A gastric ulcer on the lesser curvature erodes into one of the branches of left or right gastric artery.

### Precipitating Factors for Haemorrhage

- **Chronicity,** results in destruction of the layers of the stomach, exposing the vessel.
- Sudden, severe acid peptic digestion brought about by **irritants** such as alcohol, drugs, etc.
- **Atherosclerosis:** Sclerotic artery does not contract, resulting in massive haemorrhage.

### Characteristics of Individuals at an Increased Risk of Developing Acute GI Bleeding

- Increased age
- Male sex
- Cardiovascular disease
- Diabetes mellitus and renal disease
- Increased number of medications
- Oral anticoagulant use.

### Clinical Features of Bleeding Peptic Ulcer

- Previous history of abdominal pain of peptic ulcer disease.
- History of haematemesis or melaena (black tarry stools), one or more attacks.

There may be features of haemorrhagic shock such as feeble, thready pulse, hypotension, syncope. Oliguria, due to inadequate renal perfusion. Brainstem hypoxia results in change in rate and depth of respiration. There may not be any abdominal signs. However, due to accumulation of blood in the intestines and stomach, mild distension may be present.

**Perforation produces abdominal signs and haemorrhage produces systemic signs.**

### BLEAD Risk Classification

The following are some of the factors associated with increased morbidity and mortality (Key Box 53.11).

Key Box 53.11

**BLEAD Risk Classification**

- **BL**ood pressure low
- **E**levated prothrombin time
- **A**ltered mental status
- **D**ysfunction—myocardial, renal, comorbid disease

**Forrest classification of endoscopic appearance of bleeding ulcers**

| Type | Description |
|---|---|
| Ia | Spurting, bleeding |
| Ib | Nonspurting, active bleeding |
| IIa | Visible vessel |
| IIb | Nonbleeding ulcer with overlying clot |
| IIc | Ulcer with haematin—covered (black) base |
| III | Clean ulcer base |

As previously mentioned, endoscopy provides the opportunity not only for diagnosis but also for therapy.

### Management

- Emergency upper OGD is done to confirm the diagnosis. If the source cannot be detected due to large clots or massive bleeding, it can be repeated a few hours after a stomach wash and blood transfusion.
- Emergency upper OGD should be done within 12–24 hours of bleeding depending upon condition of the patient.
- Resuscitation is more important than an urgent endoscopy.
- Since elderly patients cannot tolerate shock well, decision to control bleeding surgically must be taken early.

### *I. Conservative Line of Management*

- Emergency replacement of blood, after initial resuscitation with a plasma expander.
- Ryle's tube is passed and cold saline stomach wash is given to produce vasoconstriction.
- Cold antacids are given every 2nd hourly, about 10–20 ml.
- IV Pantoprazole 40 mg is given to reduce acidity.
  - Majority of cases respond to conservative line of management within 48 hours.

### *II. Nonsurgical Treatment*

1. **Laser coagulation**
   - It can arrest the bleeding without direct tissue contact. Nd:YAG laser has been used more commonly because it can penetrate tissue more deeply compared to argon laser which penetrates very superficial tissues. The success rate of laser coagulation is around 80%.
2. **Sclerotherapy** (Key Boxes 53.12 and 53.13)
   - Epinephrine (1:10,000) arrests bleeding by vasoconstriction
   - 2% ethanolamine, a sclerosant, causes dehydration and shrinkage of surrounding tissues.
   - It also produces inflammation and thrombosis of the bleeding vessel (Fig. 53.35).
   - This is the most popular method. The success rate is around 80–90%. It is a cheap and easy treatment.

Key Box 53.12

**Endotherapy**

- Bipolar electrocoagulation—failure rate—50%
- Inj. sclerotherapy—failure rate—20%
- Haemoclip application

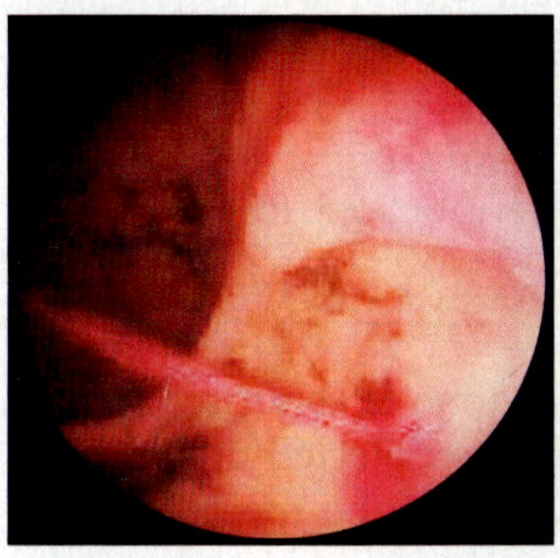

**Fig. 53.35:** Bleeding vessel **Fig. 53.36:** Haemoclip applied

3. **Haemoclip application** (Fig. 53.36)
4. **Bipolar electrocoagulation**—failure rate is 50%.
   - Surgical eradication of *H. pylori* prevents rebleeding.

### *III. Surgical Control of Bleeding Peptic Ulcer*

(Key Boxes 53.13 and 53.14)

Key Box 53.13

**Endoscopic Prognostic Factors**

- Visible level: 40–60% rebleeding ulcer >2 cm
- Adherent clot: 20% rebleeding
- Flat pigmented spot: 10% rebleeding
- Clean ulcer base: Rarely bleeding

Key Box 53.14

**Role of Surgery**

- Explore when endotherapy fails
- Explore when rebleeding occurs in the elderly
- Explore an unstable patient
- Gastroduodenotomy, under-running of ulcer base for CDU and partial gastrectomy for gastric ulcer

### *Indications*

1. Failure of endoscopic haemostasis—prognostic factors are given below.
2. Rebleeding in the hospital (rebleeding is more common in gastric ulcer patients).
3. Bleeding requiring transfusion of more than 2000 ml blood in 24 hours (6 units).
4. Elderly patients with rebleeding.
5. Massive haemorrhage leading to shock or cardiovascular instability.
6. Recurrent haemorrhage requiring hospitalisation.

### *Types of Surgery*

1. ***Surgery for bleeding duodenal ulcer***

- Laparotomy and **anterior gastroduodenotomy.**
- Visualise the bleeding ulcer in the first part of duodenum.
- **Under-running** of the ulcer base by direct suture or 4 quadrant ligation of gastroduodenal artery by using nonabsorbable sutures (Fig. 53.37).
- **Gastroduodenotomy incision is converted into a pyloroplasty** followed by vagotomy which completes the treatment.

2. ***Surgery for bleeding gastric ulcer (benign)***

- Laparotomy, gastrotomy and visualise the bleeding ulcer.
- Under-running of the ulcer base. There are chances of rebleeding with this method.
- **Partial gastrectomy** is the best treatment provided general condition of the patient is good (Figs 53.38 and 53.39). Otherwise, local excision of the ulcer, vagotomy followed by GJ or pyloroplasty can also be done.

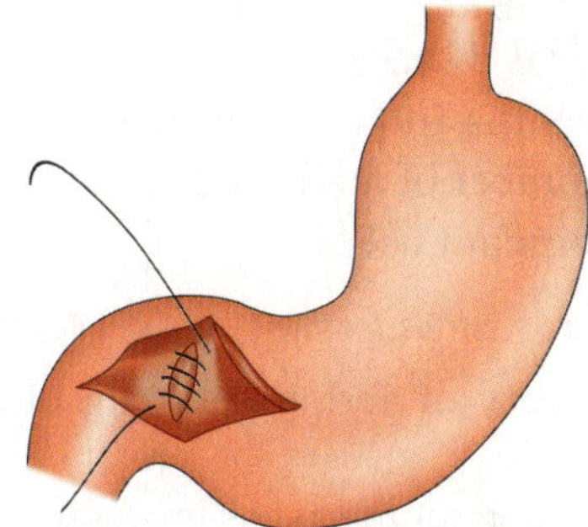

**Fig. 53.37:** Under-running of the duodenal ulcer

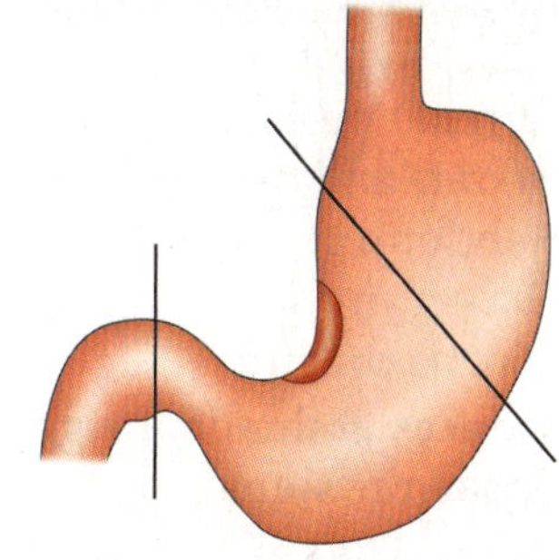

**Fig. 53.38:** Partial gastrectomy for gastric ulcer

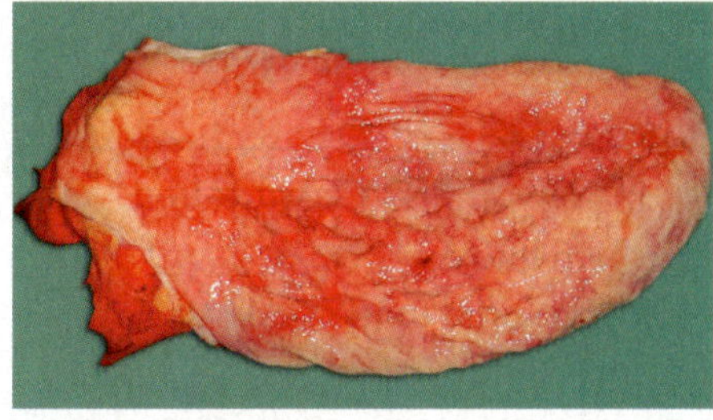

**Fig. 53.39:** Partial gastrectomy for bleeding gastric ulcer

- Haemostatic methods currently employed include thermotherapy (heater probe, multipolar or bipolar electrocoagulation) as well as injection of ethanol or epinephrine solutions.
- When the bleeding is controlled, long-term medical therapy includes antisecretory agents, usually in the form of a proton pump inhibitor, in addition to testing for *H. pylori* with treatment, if positive.
- If *H. pylori* is present, documentation of eradication should be performed after therapy.

## DIFFERENTIAL DIAGNOSIS OF HAEMATEMESIS (UPPER GI TRACT BLEEDING)

- 80% bleeding is from upper GI tract.
- Almost 20% is from lower GI tract (colon).
- 1% from small intestines.
- Bleeding proximal to ligament of Treitz.
- Haematemesis refers to vomiting of fresh red blood. Melaenemesis refers to vomiting of dark altered blood. However, both are included under upper GI tract bleeding. Small bowel, even though is a midgut structure, some of its lesions can produce haematemesis. Hence, they are also included under this heading.

### Causes (Fig. 53.40)

1. **Oesophageal causes**
   - Reflux oesophagitis
   - Mallory-Weiss syndrome
   - Oesophageal varices
   - Cancer of oesophagus, leiomyoma oesophagus.

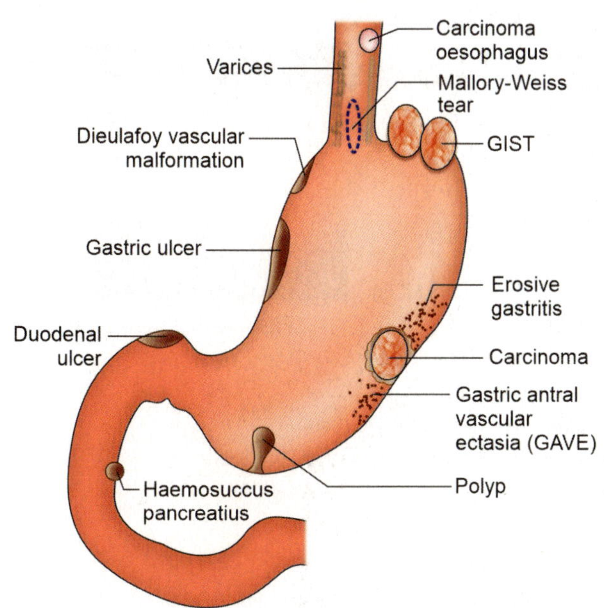


**Fig. 53.40:** Various causes of haematemesis

2. **Gastric causes**
   - Gastric ulcer
   - Gastric varices
   - Acute erosive gastritis
   - Gastric cancer
   - Stromal tumours—**GIST**
   - Lymphoma
   - Arteriovenous malformation
   - Gastric polyp
   - Dieulafoy vascular malformation
   - Gastric antral vascular ectasia (GAVE)
3. **Duodenal causes**
   - Duodenal ulcer
   - Arteriovenous malformation
   - Duodenal carcinoma
   - Aortoduodenal fistula diverticulae
   - Polyps
4. **Other rare causes**
   - Purpura
   - Haemophilia
   - Haemobilia
   - Pseudoaneurysms due to acute pancreatitis.

> *Pearls of Wisdom*
>
> Acute erosive gastritis, chronic peptic ulcer and oesophageal varices constitute almost 90% of the cases.

### Initial Assessment

Table 53.6 describes the initial assessment of upper GI tract bleeding. Two 16 gauge cannulae are secured for resuscitation in the emergency department. Patient should be stabilized first with Ringer lactate, blood transfusion and when he is stable, endoscopy is done.

### Investigations (Fig. 53.41)

- **Fibreoptic endoscopy** should be done on an emergency basis within 6 to 36 hours of admission. It can diagnose variceal bleeding, erosive gastritis, bleeding peptic ulcer, carcinoma stomach, etc.
- Only when endoscopy cannot yield any diagnosis, selective coeliac angiography should be done which can detect uncommon causes such as angiodysplasia of the stomach or bleeding from a rolling hernia, etc. Barium study is done to rule out intestinal causes in less urgent cases.
- **CT angiogram is the gold standard** investigation when haemobilia or haemosuccus pancreatitis is suspected (Figs 53.42 to 53.44).

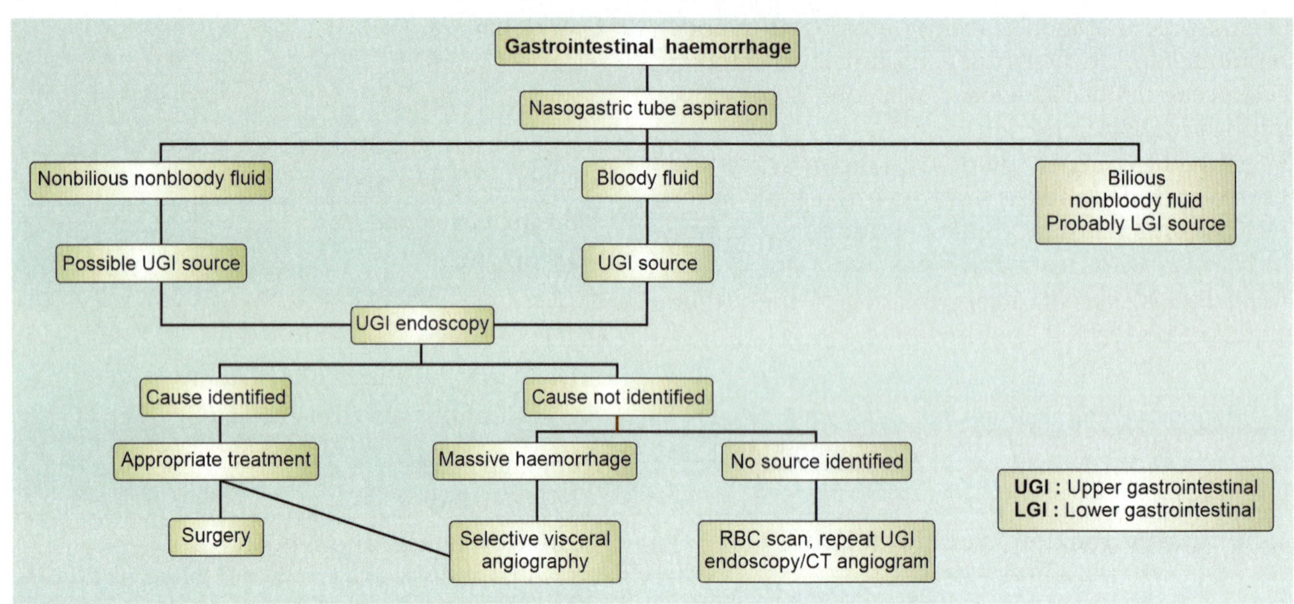


**Fig. 53.41:** Investigation algorithm of UGI bleeding (*Courtesy*: Dr Sibacis Bisoi, Assistant Professor, KMC, Manipal)

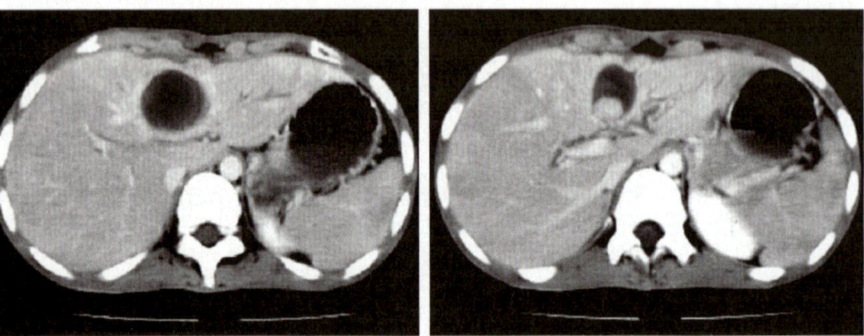

**Figs 53.42 and 53.43:** CT hepatic angiogram demonstrating extravasation of dye into a pseudoaneurysm of a branch of middle hepatic artery and thrombus—case of haemobilia

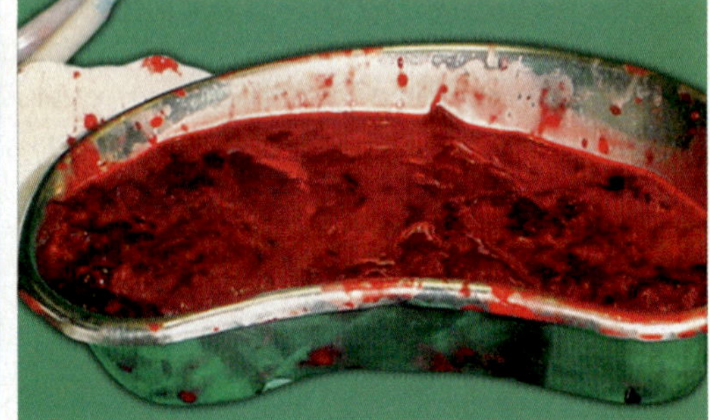

**Fig. 53.44:** Massive haematemesis in this patient of haemobilia

**TABLE 53.6:** Initial assessment

| History | Probable causes |
|---|---|
| 1. Abuse of drugs and alcohol<br>Previous abdominal pain<br>H/o jaundice, liver cell failure<br>Anaemia, loss of weight, loss of appetite<br>Violent vomiting—haematemesis | Acute erosive gastritis<br>Chronic peptic ulcer<br>Oesophageal varices<br>Carcinoma stomach<br>Mallory-Weiss syndrome |
| 2. General physical examination<br>• Testicular atrophy, gynaecomastia<br>• Palpable left supraclavicular node<br>• Arthritis—multiple joint involvement<br>• Purpuric spots (Fig. 53.45) | <br>• Cirrhosis of the liver<br>• Carcinoma stomach<br>• Acute erosive gastritis (use of NSAIDs)<br>• Bleeding tendencies |
| 3. Abdominal examination<br>• Palpable spleen, ascites<br>• Palpable stomach mass<br>• Tenderness in the epigastrium | <br>• Portal hypertension<br>• Carcinoma stomach<br>• Peptic ulcer disease |
| 4. Assessment of haemorrhage<br>Massive haemorrhage (more than 1,000 ml of blood)<br>Moderate haemorrhage (500–1000 ml of blood)<br>Mild haemorrhage (less than 500 ml of blood) | <br>Portal hypertension, acute erosive gastritis, chronic peptic ulcer<br>Chronic peptic ulcer<br>Other causes |

**Fig. 53.45:** Purpuric spots

## CAUSES OF UPPER GI TRACT BLEEDING (Figs 53.46 to 53.51)

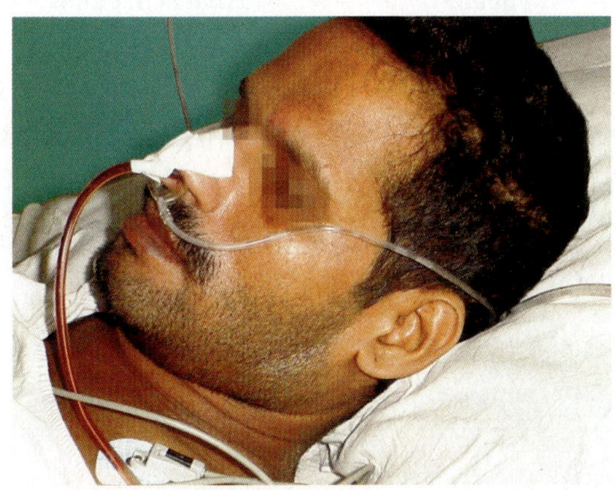

**Fig. 53.46:** Chronic duodenal ulcer with massive UGI bleeding. Diagnostic use of nasogastric tube is to detect active bleeding

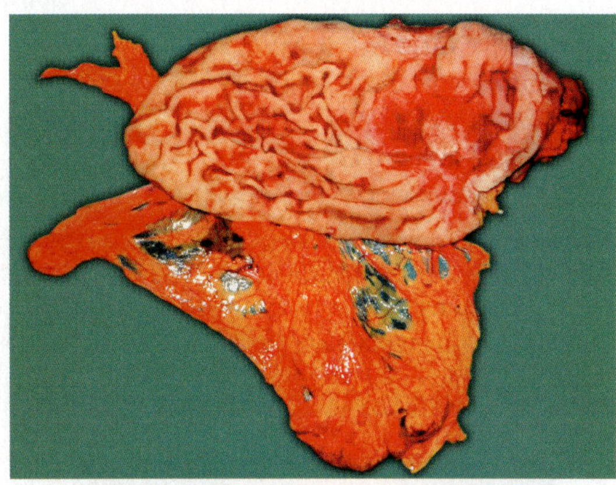

**Fig. 53.47:** Subtotal gastrectomy specimen showing bleeding gastric ulcer

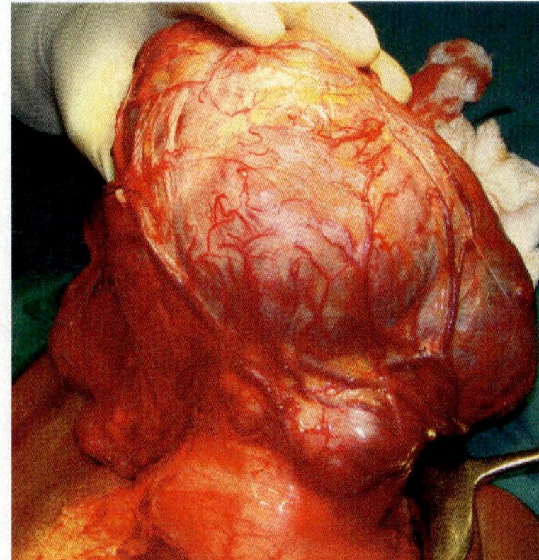

**Fig. 53.48:** Upper GI bleeding due to GIST of stomach

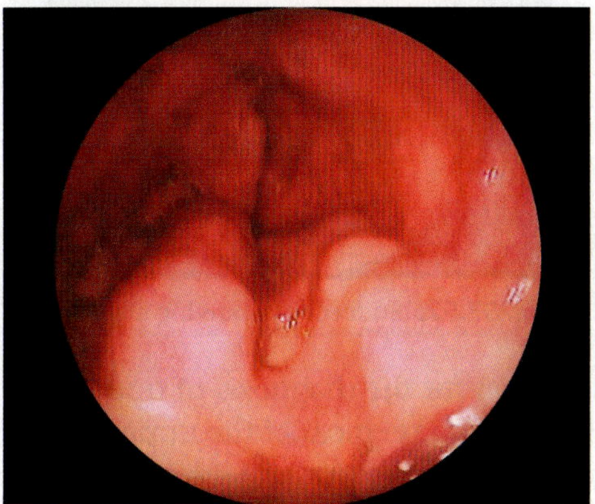

**Fig. 53.49:** Grade III oesophageal varices with bleeding

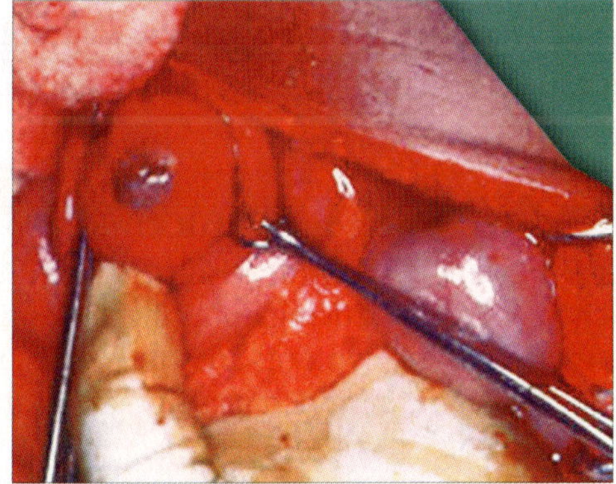

**Fig. 53.50:** Dieulafoy vascular malformation

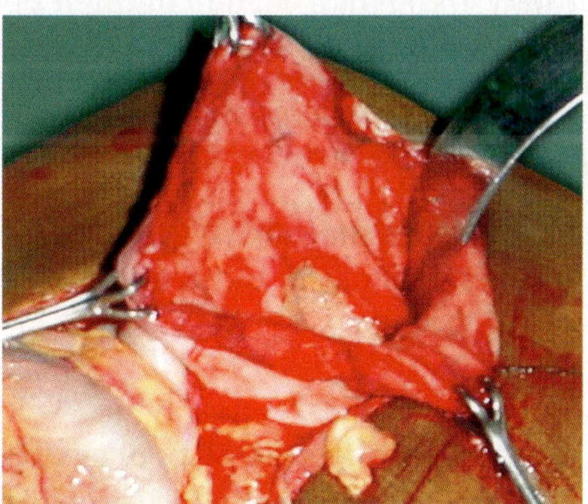

**Fig. 53.51:** Giant gastric ulcer with bleeding

### Treatment

Initial management is to treat the shock in the line discussed for peptic ulcer haemorrhage.

#### *Indications for Surgery*

1. Elderly patients with rebleed in the hospital
2. Rarity of blood groups
3. Spurting vessel in an endoscopy.

#### *Surgery*

- Surgical management of individual case has been discussed along with the concerned chapter. However, summary of the treatment is discussed in Table 53.7.
- Thus, upper GI bleeding can occur due to various causes. However, acute erosive gastritis, chronic peptic ulcer and oesophageal varices are the three important causes of bleeding. Endoscopy is the

**TABLE 53.7:** Surgery for haematemesis

| Causes | Conservative ⟶ Failure ⟶ | Surgical method |
|---|---|---|
| 1. Acute erosive gastritis | Yes | Rarely—gastrectomy |
| 2. Chronic duodenal ulcer | Yes | Vagotomy, under-running, pyloroplasty |
| 3. Chronic gastric ulcer | Yes | Partial gastrectomy |
| 4. Mallory-Weiss syndrome | Yes | Suturing of the tear |
| 5. Cancer of the stomach | Endoscopic snaring | Gastrectomy |
| 6. Duodenal polyp | No | Surgery, if endoscopic facility not available |
| 7. Haemobilia | Yes, therapeutic embolisation | Ligation of feeding vessel |
| 8. Variceal bleeding | Yes, sclerotherapy | Devascularisation |
| 9. Haemosuccus pancreatitis | Yes, therapeutic embolisation | Ligation of pseudoaneurysm |
| 10. Dieulafoy lesion | Yes, injection sclerotherapy | Wide excision |

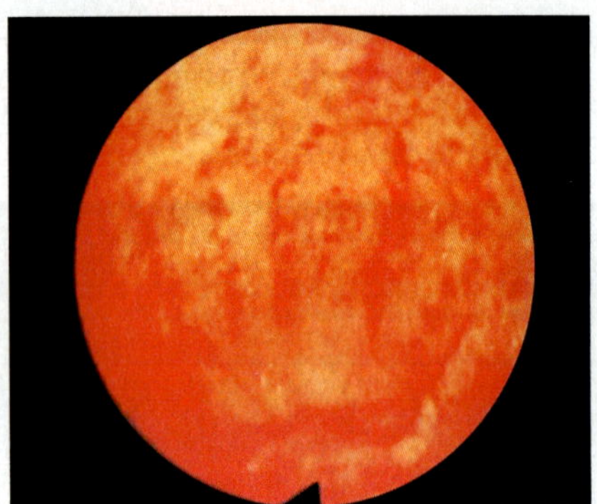

**Fig. 53.52:** Endoscopy showing erosions

investigation for the diagnosis of upper GI bleeding (Fig. 53.52). Today, most of the upper GI bleeding is managed either in the form of injection sclerotherapy, laser coagulation, or with powerful H2 blockers or proton pump inhibitors. In appropriate cases, surgery is definitely indicated. Some common conditions which give rise to haematemesis are discussed in the following pages.

## ACUTE PEPTIC ULCER

They are also called acute erosive gastritis/acute stress ulcers/acute steroidal ulcers and **acute gastric mucosal lesions (AGML)**.

### Aetiology

- Drugs—aspirin, analgin, steroids, phenylbutazone.
- Any stress or acute infection which results in sepsis.
- Following tetanus
- After burns, they are called **'Curling's ulcer'**.
- After head injury or neurosurgical operations, they are called **'Cushing's ulcer'**.
- Following **hypotension** and shock, there is **hypoperfusion,** which results in **mucosal ischaemia** and acute stress ulcers. Example: Myocardial infarction, trauma, sepsis.
- Excessive consumption of spirits and smoking.
- Respiratory failure can also produce acute erosions.

### Pathology

There is a diffuse mucosal damage and disruption of gastric mucosal barrier. Reflux of bile also may be a precipitating factor. This results in acute erosions when they are 1 to 2 mm or acute ulcers when they are 1 to 2 cm in size, shallow and well-demarcated. The entire stomach is involved by these ulcers.

### Clinical Features

- Dyspepsia due to minor bleeding.
- Haematemesis—sometimes massive, fresh bleeding can produce hypotension and shock.
- Acute abdominal pain due to acute erosions or perforation of an acute ulcer.
- In ICU: **Drop in blood pressure,** nasogastric aspirate of blood and/or melaena.

### Diagnosis

Emergency endoscopy to confirm diagnosis and to rule out other causes of upper GI tract bleeding.

### Treatment of Acute Peptic Ulcers with Bleeding

1. **Admission in intensive care unit (ICU)** (Key Box 53.15).
2. **Ryle's tube** to be introduced first and empty the stomach. It helps in reducing vomiting and sometimes aspiration of gastric contents into the lungs also. Ice cold water or saline stomach wash (vasoconstriction) reduces bleeding.
3. **Regular antacids** 20–30 ml, 2nd hourly, preferably cold antacids.
4. **Replacement of blood** specifically coagulation factors.

Key Box 53.15

**Very Important Measures in ICU**

- Correct coagulopathy
- Improve oxygenation
- Blood transfusion
- Control sepsis

5. **Injection Pantoprazole 20 mg IV**. Majority of cases respond to conservative line of treatment.
6. **Endotherapy:** If there is solitary bleeding site.
7. **Surgery:** With modern investigations and their therapeutic role in addition to good ICU care, availability of blood and nursing care, almost all cases of erosive gastritis can be managed without surgery. In spite of above treatment, if the condition deteriorates, a total gastrectomy or a subtotal gastrectomy may be necessary (very, very rare) as a life-saving measure.

## MALLORY-WEISS SYNDROME

### Aetiopathogenesis (Key Box 53.16)

- It occurs due to a tear in the gastric mucosa near the oesophagogastric (OG) junction.
- Also called partial thickness mucosal rupture.
- In Boerhaave syndrome, all layers are involved in a tear.

Key Box 53.16

**Conditions wherein Mallory-Weiss Tear is Seen**

- **S**pirit or alcohol
- **P**ancreatitis
- **I**nfarction—myocardial
- **R**enal failure
- **I**nfection—cholecystitis
- **T**umour—pregnancy

*Remember as* **SPIRIT**

### Clinical Features (Fig. 53.53)

- The patient is usually a middle-aged male who, after consumption of alcohol, vomits the food contents first. During the course of vomiting because of straining and retching, a tear develops near the oesophagocardiac junction. Hence, the **second vomitus contains blood**.
- Sometimes, the bleeding can be so massive to produce hypotension and shock. In 90% of cases, the bleeding stops spontaneously.

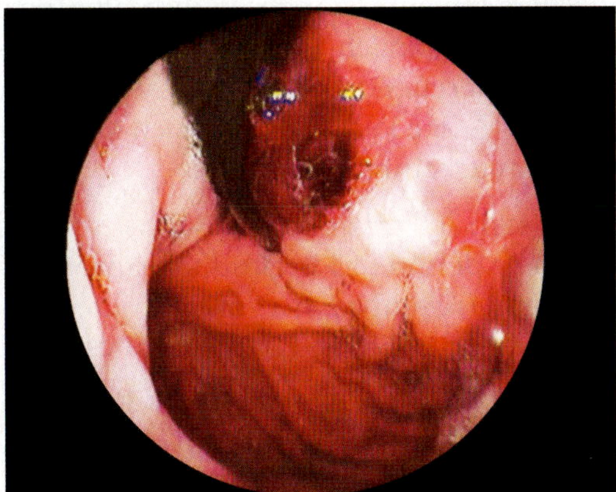

**Fig. 53.53:** Mallory-Weiss tear—with the endotherapy bleeding stopped (*Courtesy*: Dr Filipe Alvares, Gastroenterologist, KMC, Manipal)

### Treatment

- Urgent resuscitation of haemorrhagic shock.
- Endoscopy to confirm the diagnosis—tear is seen in the lesser curvature.
- Ryle's tube aspiration for 48–72 hours.
- Endotherapy—injection adrenaline 1:10,000 dilution is effective. If not, haemoclipping can be done.
- Multipolar electric coagulation
- When all other measures fail, **gastrotomy** (opening in the stomach) and under-running is necessary with 2–0 silk sutures.

## DIEULAFOY VASCULAR MALFORMATION

- In this condition, an unusually large artery runs in the submucosa which lies in close contact with mucous membrane (Fig. 53.54).
- Mucosal erosion precipitates the bleeding.
- In more than 80% cases, bleeding occurs within 6 to 8 cm from OG junction, at the lesser curvature.
- Endoscopy and endotherapy should be tried and if necessary, repeated also.
- Sudden, massive, painless, recurrent haematemesis with hypotension is the presenting feature.
- Angiography to confirm the bleeding lesion and gelfoam embolisation must be tried first.
- Failure to achieve control of the bleeding—**gastrotomy and wide excision** of the lesion should be done.

## GASTRIC ANTRAL VASCULAR ECTASIA (GAVE)

- It is an uncommon cause of chronic GI bleeding resulting in iron deficiency anaemia.
- It is also called **watermelon stomach** because of the presence of long red streaky area which are present in the stomach resembling a watermelon (Key Box 53.17).

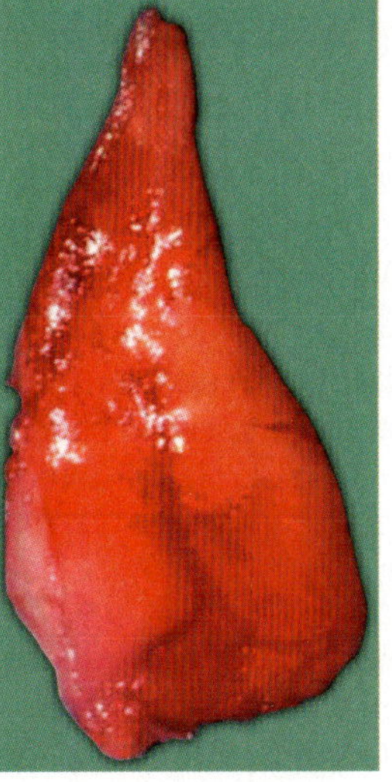

**Fig. 53.54:** Dieulafoy vascular malformation—excised

Key Box 53.17

**Watermelon Stomach (Gastric Antral Vascular Ectasia)**

- Women in their 50s are commonly affected
- Antrum is commonly involved
- TIPSS (*see* page 396) in patients with portal hypertension
- Ectasia of antral vessels gives rise to UGI bleeding
- Red parallel stripes on the mucosal fold are characteristic
- Mucosal fibromuscular hyperplasia and hyalinisation are present
- Endoscopy is the investigation of choice
- Liver disease in 25% patients—cirrhotic men
- Other diseases—autoimmune connective tissue disorder may be associated with this—also *Helicobacter pylori*
- No control of bleeding—antrectomy may be required

*Remember as* **WATERMELON**

### Subacute Complication of Peptic Ulcer

A small perforation of peptic ulcer which is sealed off by omentum may result in a residual abscess in one of the subphrenic spaces. It responds to conservative treatment. Otherwise, percutaneous drainage can be done with ultrasonographic guidance.

## CHRONIC COMPLICATIONS OF PEPTIC ULCER

### I. GASTRIC OUTLET OBSTRUCTION

**Earlier it was called pyloric stenosis. However, gastric outlet obstruction is a better word.** Chronic cicatrisation of a duodenal ulcer or juxtapyloric ulcer results in narrowing of pyloric antrum which is described as pyloric stenosis. In India, pyloric stenosis is more common in South Indian patients, who usually present with a long history of duodenal ulcer and a recent history of vomiting (Key Box 53.18).

Key Box 53.18

**Pyloric Stenosis**

- Pyloric stenosis in CDU—**Misnomer**
- Stenosis is very often found in the **first part of duodenum**
- In cases of pyloric channel ulcer, true pyloric stenosis occurs
- Metabolic changes, such as paradoxical aciduria (Fig. 53.55), are usually seen in patients with ulcer, **not in carcinoma** because of relative achlorhydria in the latter

### Symptoms

- Classical **hunger pain** of duodenal ulcer disappears. It may be replaced by a dull aching pain because of gastric distension. Colicky pain is due to hyperperistalsis of stomach.
- **Vomiting** is profuse, projectile, persistent, foul-smelling (because of stasis) and nonbilious.
- There may be **distension of upper abdomen** with epigastric fullness.

### Signs

1. **Visible gastric peristalsis (VGP):** Parenthesis "stomach that you see"—
   - It is a wave of contraction of the stomach which starts in the left hypochondrium, runs across the umbilicus and ends in the right hypochondrium. These contractions can be felt—**stomach that you feel**. Presence of VGP is diagnostic of pyloric stenosis (right to left peristalsis is seen in left-sided obstructive colonic tumours). **If VGP is not seen, it can be made prominent by:**
     - Asking the patient to drink at least 500–1000 ml of water (it is difficult. Try and see!).
     - Stimulating the abdomen by flicking movement.
2. **Succussion splash**
   - Should be done on 'fasting' stomach. This test should be done before asking the patient to drink water.
   - In pyloric stenosis, there is always residual fluid in the stomach, which gives a splashing sound that can be heard with/without stethoscope—**stomach that you hear**.

*Pearls of Wisdom*

Thus, the stomach which is seen, felt and heard is diagnostic of pyloric stenosis.

3. **Auscultopercussion test/auscultoscraping test** to find out the greater curvature of the stomach.

   **Procedure:** Keep the "bell" of stethoscope in the centre of epigastrium (ask the patient to hold the bell of stethoscope) and percuss radially. Percussion over the stomach gives a dull note because of presence of fluid. When the note changes, it indicates the greater curvature of stomach. Mark it on the abdomen (instead of percussion, scraping can be done with finger nail). A line joining 3 or 4 such marks outlines the greater curvature of stomach.

**Saline load test:** 700 ml of normal saline is infused into stomach over a period of 3 to 5 minutes through a nasogastric tube and is clamped. If a volume more than 350 ml can be aspirated after 30 minutes, it indicates obstruction.

### Electrolyte Changes in Gastric Outlet Obstruction

- Hypochloraemic alkalosis
- Hyponatraemia
- Hypokalaemia
- Paradoxical aciduria (Fig. 53.55).

Gastric outlet obstruction
↓
Vomiting
↓
Hypochloraemic alkalosis
↓
Excretion of HCl with sodium
↓
Hyponatraemia and dehydration
↓
Sodium retention, potassium and hydrogen excretion
↓
Hypokalaemia and paradoxical aciduria

**Fig. 53.55:** Pathogenesis of paradoxical aciduria

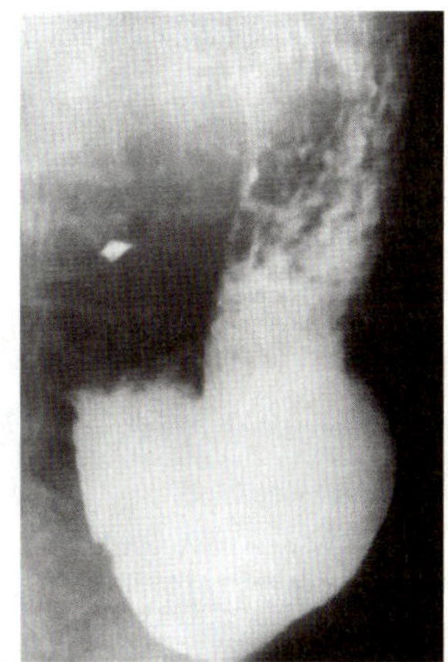

**Fig. 53.56:** Barium meal showing dilated J shaped stomach with mosaic appearance

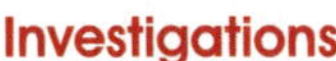

## Investigations

1. **Barium meal X-ray**
   - **Hugely dilated stomach (large and low stomach).**
   - Barium does not enter the duodenum. Barium mixed with food residue can give rise to ***mosaic appearance***. Delay in evacuation (on repeat X-ray) of barium into the duodenum is seen (Fig. 53.56).
2. **Gastroscopy**
   - The scope will not enter the duodenum. Stomach is full of foul-smelling food residue.
   - Gastroscopy is also done to rule out carcinoma of the stomach.
3. **Electrolyte study (*vide infra*)**

## Treatment (ABCDEF)

**A:** Aspiration with Ryle's tube—good stomach wash, twice a day is given to keep the stomach empty. Saline is used as it decreases oedema of the stomach wall. Stomach wash should be given for at least 3–5 days before surgery.

**B:** Blood is arranged for surgery. Blood may be required preoperatively to treat anaemia.

**C:** Charts: Adequate urine output is maintained by infusion of intravenous fluids.

**D:** Drug: Antibiotics for surgery.

**E:** Exploratory laparotomy: **Vagotomy followed by GJ is done.** Pyloroplasty should not be done because the duodenum is scarred, cicatrised, fibrosed and narrowed.

**F:** Fluids to correct electrolyte abnormalities. Pyloric stenosis patients can develop **"hyponatraemic, hypochloraemic, hypokalaemic alkalosis"**. Normal saline infusion is better initially than ringer lactate because ringer lactate can aggravate metabolic alkalosis.

- Postoperatively these patients recover very fast. Dehydration improves and nutritionally they show dramatic improvement. Even the gastric tone may return after a few years.

## Differential Diagnosis of Gastric Outlet Obstruction

There are two important causes for gastric outlet obstruction (Table 53.8). However, duodenum obstruction in the second part or third part by malignancies, annular pancreas or lymph nodal masses may give rise to persistent vomiting but usually it is bilious.

**TABLE 53.8:** Differential diagnosis of pyloric stenosis

| | **Cicatrised chronic duodenal ulcer** | **Carcinoma pyloric antrum** |
|---|---|---|
| 1. Age | 20–40 years | >40–50 years |
| 2. Duration of the symptoms | Long duration of abdominal pain and recent history of vomiting | Pain is usually absent, but vomiting is a feature<br>Symptoms are of short duration |
| 3. Appetite | Decreased because of vomiting | Severe loss of appetite |
| 4. Weight loss | Present | Significant |
| 5. Anaemia | Not a feature | Present |
| 6. Mass | Not palpable | Hard, irregular mass is palpable |

The palpable mass is the deciding clinical factor (sign). Other differences cannot truly differentiate between the two conditions. Rarely, carcinoma of the stomach is also seen in young patients at the age of 20. In congenital hypertrophic pyloric stenosis, the mass is palpable (*see* page 754).

### II. TEA-POT DEFORMITY OR HANDBAG STOMACH (Fig. 53.57)

- A long-standing lesser curve gastric ulcer causes shortening of the lesser curvature due to fibrosis. Such stomach resembles a tea-pot. As a result of this, the pylorus becomes nondependent. Hence, stasis occurs.
- **Treatment:** Partial gastrectomy followed by Billroth I anastomosis.

### III. HOURGLASS CONTRACTURE (Fig. 53.58)

- When a saddle-shaped ulcer in the lesser curvature gets cicatrised, it involves both surfaces of the stomach resulting in conversion of stomach into two compartments.
- Features of stasis such as fullness, distension and persistent vomiting are present.
- Females are affected more often.
- Weight loss is present. Appetite is decreased.
- It is treated by **Billroth I partial gastrectomy** with removal of 2nd pouch.

### IV. PENETRATION INTO PANCREAS

Posterior gastric ulcer can penetrate into pancreas, resulting in severe referred pain to the back resembling pancreatic pathology. However, this type of pain is relieved on lying down.

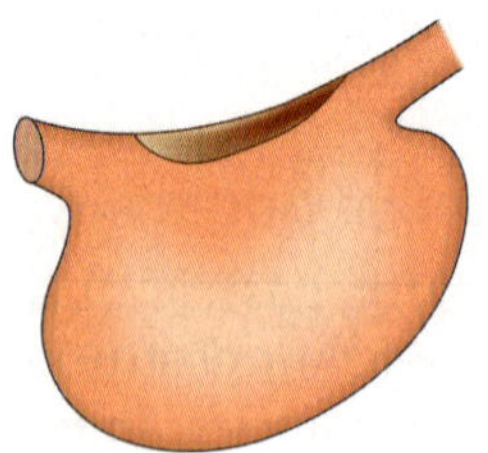

**Fig. 53.57:** Tea-pot deformity

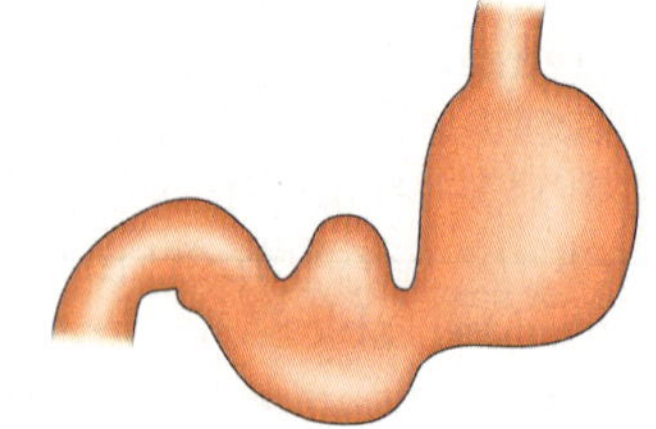

**Fig. 53.58:** Hourglass contracture of the stomach

> **SU28.9:** Describe and discuss the aetiology, the clinical features, investigations and principles of management of carcinoma stomach.

## CARCINOMA STOMACH

### Introduction

- Carcinoma stomach is more common (2 times) in men compared to women.
- Rare below 40. Average age is 63 years.
- Worldwide, it is the fourth most common cancer and second leading cancer of death.
- North Eastern part of India, the district of Aizawl in the state of Mizoram has recorded the highest incidence in the country as per NCRP 2013 (64.2/100,000 population). The highest incidence of gastric cancer in Mizoram has been attributed to smoking local cigarettes like maizol and Taibur-tobacco smoke infused water. This is followed by a Southern Indian state, Tamil Nadu, where the incidence is 12.2/100,000 population in men.
- Incidence of proximal gastric carcinoma is increased—may be due to obesity and in rich socioeconomic status patients (Key Box 53.19).
- Carcinoma distal stomach is more commonly associated with *H. pylori*.
- Proximal carcinomas are more advanced at the time of presentation than distal carcinomas.
- D2 gastrectomy is currently the recommended surgical choice for cases of resectable advanced disease.
- The 5-year overall survival for resectable GC is approximately 20 to 30% worldwide, but it is 70% in Japan and in other eastern countries.

**Key Box 53.19**

**Carcinoma Proximal Stomach (Cardia)**

- Incidence is increasing. Obesity and high socioeconomic group
- More aggressive
- Thin muscularis mucosa. Hence, submucosal invasion is seen early
- Diagnosis may also get delayed as endoscopy needs technical expertise
- Signet ring carcinoma is common here
- Surgical resection involves oesophageal anastomosis which is technically demanding. Leak rates are high
- Hence, prognosis is poor

**Sites:** Pyloric antrum is the commonest site. Refer Fig. 53.59 for sites and percentage of occurrence.

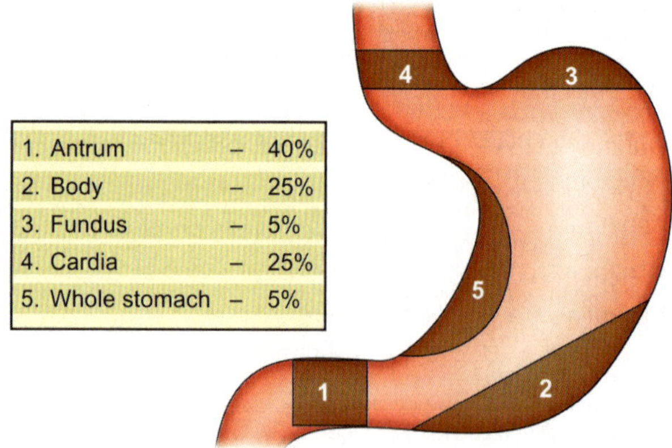


**Fig. 53.59:** Site and incidence of gastric cancer

## Risk Factors for Carcinoma Stomach

(Fig. 53.60 and Key Box 53.20)

### 1. Environmental and Dietary Factors

- The incidence is increased in persons who consume red meat, cabbage, spices, spirits, salt-fish (Key Box 53.20).
- Smoked salmon fish was responsible for increased incidence of carcinoma stomach in Japanese population. Probably, it is related to release of polycyclic hydrocarbons and aromatic amino acids. Smoking, spicy food and alcohol consumed over a period of many years produce chronic gastritis which may change into carcinoma of stomach.

**Pearls of Wisdom**

WHO recommends increased consumption of fruits and vegetables. Vitamin C is an antioxidant which is a protective agent. Ascorbic acid prevents conversion of nitrates to nitrites.

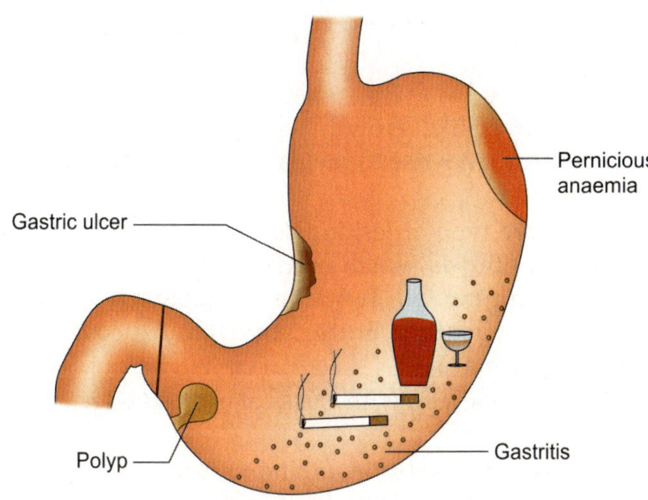


**Fig. 53.60:** Risk factors for carcinoma stomach

**Key Box 53.20**

**Food Products which may be Carcinogenic**

- Smoked food
- Spirits
- Smoking
- Salted food—salt based preservatives and lack of refrigeration, (pickles are rich in nitrates)
- Soil
- Diet low in carbohydrate
- Animal protein
- Rich fatty food
- High in complex carbohydrates
- *H. pylori* in contaminated water

### 2. Precancerous Conditions

a. **Atrophic gastritis:** This may be due to smoking, spicy food, continuous ingestion of drugs, reflux of bile into the stomach, etc.

b. **Pernicious anaemia:** Patients have increased risk (four to six times) of development of carcinoma when compared to general population. It causes atrophic gastritis and precipitates carcinoma of fundus of the stomach. Lesions are polypoidal and multicentric

c. Patients with **hypogammaglobulinaemia** (50-fold increase) are at high-risk.

d. ***H. pylori* infection** results in atrophic gastritis, followed by the intestinal type of gastric mucosa, metaplasia and then dysplasia. Eventually, it leads to **intestinal type of gastric cancer** (Figs 53.61 and 53.62). *H. pylori* can also cause proliferation of gastric cancer cells and decrease secretion of vitamin C. Cytotoxin associated gene A (Cag A) is associated with increased risk.
   - Also both **type A** and **type B** gastritis can predispose to carcinoma stomach. Type A—proximal stomach, type B—distal stomach. *It is an important modifiable risk factor.*

e. **Adenomatous polyps** which occur in the antrum have highest risk of malignant transformation (larger polyps, i.e. more than 2 cm—10 to 20% malignant transformation).
   - Polyp more than 2 cm, pedunculated polyp can be removed endoscopically. Higher chances of malignancy is seen in sessile polyps.

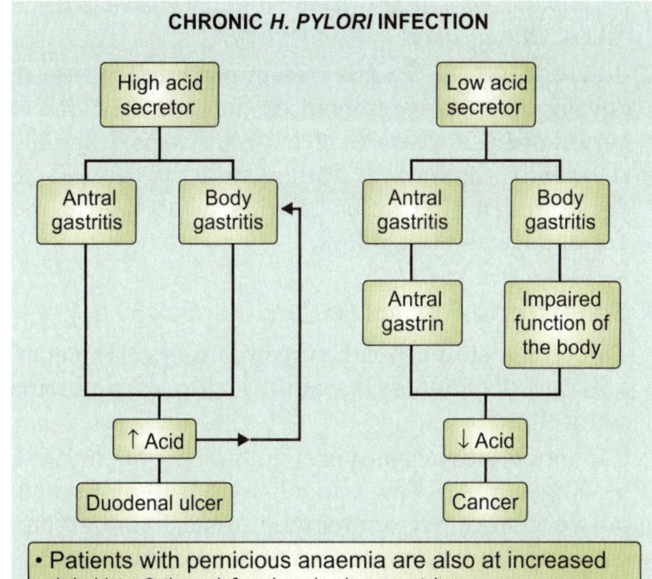


**Fig. 53.61:** *H. pylori* and pathogenesis of duodenal ulcer and carcinoma stomach

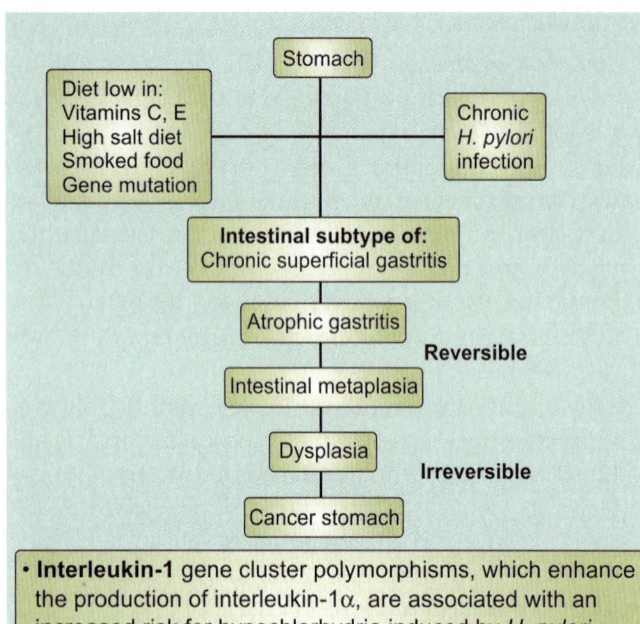


**Fig. 53.62:** Aetiopathogenesis of carcinoma stomach

f. **Menetrier's disease** is a protein-losing enteropathy, along with giant hypertrophy of gastric mucosal folds. It is a precancerous condition.

g. **Gastric ulcer (benign):** Incidence of malignancy is 2% (0.5 to 5%). Carcinoma arising in a gastric ulcer is called *"Ulcer Cancer of the Stomach"*.

h. **Previous GJ or gastric resection** predisposes to development of carcinoma of the stomach after a period of 15–20 years. Such a carcinoma is described as stump carcinoma. Pathogenesis is related to development of atrophic gastritis, achlorhydria and duodenogastric bile reflux.

### *3. Genetic and Familial Factors* (Key Box 53.21)

- Carcinoma stomach can run in families. However, only 10% of patients give family history of carcinoma stomach.
- Carcinoma stomach is more common in patients with blood group A. These patients have different mucopolysaccharide secretion in the stomach and greater susceptibility to ingested carcinogens. They develop diffuse type of carcinoma.
- Several genetic alterations have been identified such as activation of oncogenes, inactivation of tumour suppressor genes p53 and p16, reduction or loss in the cell adhesion molecule E-cadherin (met proto-oncogene).

Key Box 53.21

**Familial Gastric Cancer**

- Only 10% of patients give family history of carcinoma stomach
- Associated with mutation of E-cadherin gene
- Bonaparte (Napoleon) appears to have had this gene
- It is also called hereditary diffuse gastric cancer (HDGC)
- Diagnosis is made when carcinoma is detected below the age of 40 years
- E-cadherin mutation results in lifetime risk of gastric cancer by 60–90%.
- Hence prophylactic gastrectomy is recommended
- Familial diffuse gastric cancer (FGC)—at least 3 relatives in 2 generations are affected, one of them before 50 years of age.
- Hereditary nonpolyposis colon cancer carries—10% risk of gastric cancer.

- Mutation of E-cadherin gene causes hereditary diffuse gastric cancer. Defective DNA mismatch repair (MLH1 or MSH2 mutation) causes Lynch syndrome. They have increased risk of gastric and colon cancer.

## Gross Types

1. **Cauliflower**-like growth with friable tissue. This variety can give rise to melaena or bleeding causing anaemia.
2. **Infiltrative** type of lesion (diffuse) with dense submucosal fibrosis which converts the stomach into a small contracted, functionless stomach—**linitis plastica** or **leather bottle stomach.** Mucosa may appear normal.
3. **Ulcerative** variety, with classical everted edges with central slough.
4. **Ulcer cancer** refers to carcinoma arising in a pre-existing gastric ulcer. In this variety, complete destruction of the muscle coat is present.
5. **Colloid carcinoma:** In this condition, malignant cells are separated by colloid material. This is the type which is common in women and gives rise to Krukenberg's tumour—bilateral, bulky ovarian metastasis common in premenopausal women (signet ring carcinoma produces this).

## Pathology

- Ninety-five percent of all malignant gastric neoplasms are adenocarcinomas.
- The Lauren system separates gastric adenocarcinoma into intestinal or diffuse types based on histology (Key Box 53.22).
- Other histologic types include squamous cell carcinoma, adenoacanthoma, carcinoid tumours, GI stromal tumours, and lymphoma.

Key Box 53.22

**Lauren Classification System**

| Intestinal | Diffuse |
|---|---|
| Environmental | Familial, blood type A |
| Gastric atrophy, intestinal metaplasia | Does not arise in gastritis |
| Men > women | Women > men |
| Higher incidence with age | Younger age group |
| Gland formation present | Poorly differentiated, signet ring cells, no gland formation |
| Haematogenous spread | Transmural/lymphatic spread |
| Microsatellite instability *APC* gene mutations | Decreased E-cadherin |
| *p53*, *p16* inactivation | *p53*, *p16* inactivation |

## EARLY GASTRIC CANCER (Key Box 53.23)

- Early gastric cancer is defined as adenocarcinoma limited to the mucosa and submucosa of the stomach, regardless of lymph node status.
- The entity is common in Japan, where gastric cancer is the number one cause of cancer death, and where aggressive surveillance programs have been established.
- Approximately 10% of patients with early gastric cancer will have lymph node metastasis.
- Approximately 70% of early gastric cancers are well differentiated and 30% are poorly differentiated.
- The overall cure rate with adequate gastric resection and lymphadenectomy is 95%.
- In some Japanese centres, 50% of the gastric cancers treated are early gastric cancers.
- In the US, less than 20% of resected gastric adenocarcinomas are early gastric cancers.

Key Box 53.23

**Early Gastric Cancer (Japanese Classification)**

| | |
|---|---|
| **Type I** | Exophytic lesion extending into the gastric lumen |
| **Type II** | Superficial variant |
| **IIA** | Elevated lesions with a height no more than the thickness of the adjacent mucosa |
| **IIB** | Flat lesions |
| **IIC** | Depressed lesions with an eroded but not deeply ulcerated appearance |
| **Type III** | Excavated lesions that may extend into the muscularis propria without invasion of this layer by actual cancer cells |

## ADVANCED GASTRIC CANCER

It refers to involvement of muscularis mucosa and/or serosa with or without involvement of lymph nodes.

- The **Borrmann classification system** was developed in 1926 and remains useful today for the description of endoscopic findings (Fig. 53.63).

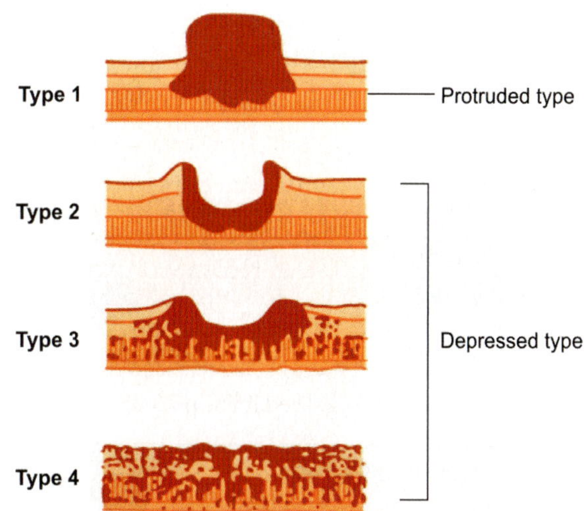


**Fig. 53.63:** Borrmann's classification (refer to advanced gastric cancer macroscopic type)

- The Borrmann system divides gastric carcinoma into five types depending on the lesion's **macroscopic** appearance.
  - **Type 1** represents polypoid or fungating lesions
  - **Type 2** ulcerating lesions surrounded by elevated borders
  - **Type 3** ulcerating lesions with infiltration into the gastric wall
  - **Type 4** diffusely infiltrating lesions
  - **Type 5** lesions that do not fit into any of the other categories.
- ***Linitis plastica*** is the term to describe type 4 carcinoma when it involves the entire stomach (Key Box 53.24 and Figs 53.64 to 53.66).

Key Box 53.24

**The Diffuse Form of Gastric Adenocarcinoma—Linitis Plastica**

- **Poorly differentiated**
- Lacks gland formation
- Composed of **signet ring** cells
- Consists of tiny clusters of small uniform cells
- Tends to spread submucosally
- Has less inflammatory infiltration
- **Metastases occur early**
- Intraperitoneal metastases are frequent
- Route of spread is generally by transmural extension and through lymphatic invasion
- Does not generally arise in the setting of prior gastritis
- **More common in women**
- Affects a slightly younger age group
- Association with blood type A and familial occurrences, suggesting a **genetic aetiology**
- The prognosis is less favourable for patients with diffuse-subtype histology.

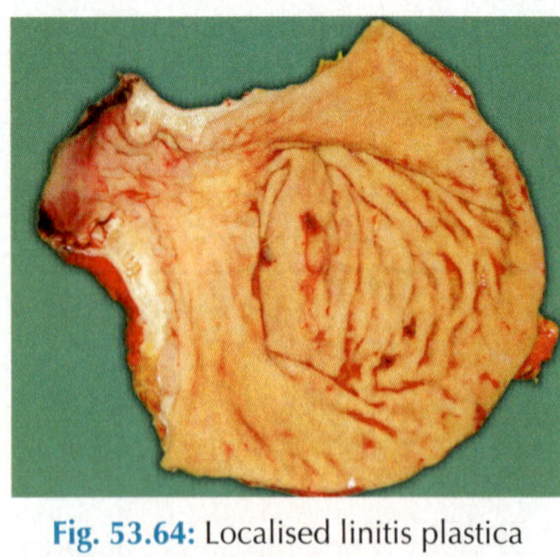

**Fig. 53.64:** Localised linitis plastica

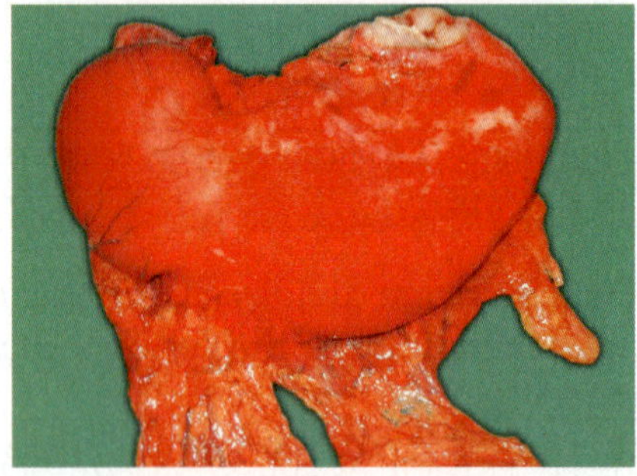

**Fig. 53.65:** Diffuse variety of carcinoma stomach

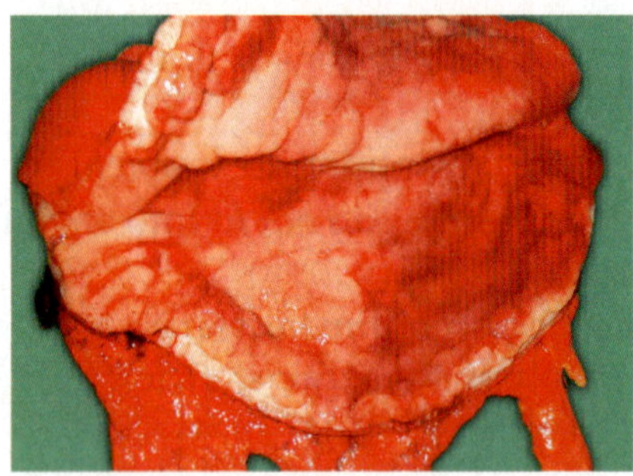

**Fig. 53.66:** Linitis plastica—opened specimen

- The original histologic classification system was developed by Borders in 1942.
- Borders classified gastric carcinomas according to the degree of cellular differentiation, independent of morphology, and ranged from 1 (well-differentiated) to 4 (anaplastic).

## WHO CLASSIFICATION: Five Main Categories

1. Adenocarcinoma 95%
   - Papillary, tubular
   - Mucinous
   - Signet ring
2. Adenosquamous cell carcinoma
3. Squamous cell carcinoma
4. Undifferentiated carcinoma
5. Unclassified carcinoma.

[1]If you remember **SOLID**, you will get solid marks.

## Clinical Features of Carcinoma Stomach (SOLID)[1]

- Very often patients would have vague symptoms—early satiety, flatulence, discomfort, pain in the upper abdomen.
- Early satiety is due to decreased distensibility of the stomach (Fig. 53.67).
- Anaemia is due to many factors (Key Box 53.25).

**S:** **S**ilent: Growth is silent but manifests as secondaries in the liver, ascites, Virchow's node, rectovesical deposits, (Blumer's shelf), umbilical nodule (Sister Mary Joseph's nodule), left axillary nodes (Irish nodes), palpable ovarian mass (Krukenberg tumour) (Figs 53.67 to 53.72).

**O:** **O**bstruction at pylorus (pyloric antrum) producing pyloric obstruction with features of vomiting with/without blood. Visible gastric peristalsis (VGP) (Fig. 53.69) can also be present. Obstruction at cardio-oesophageal junction produces dysphagia.

**L:** **L**ump in the abdomen which is hard and irregular. Clinically, stomach mass is differentiated from liver mass by features mentioned below.

1. Stomach moves with respiration.
2. Upper border of the stomach mass can be made out.
3. Anatomical location of the mass: Right hypochondrium in a pyloric mass, epigastrium and left hypochondrium in a mass arising from body of the stomach.
4. Knee elbow position: The mass falls forwards, unless fixed.
5. The mass may have intrinsic mobility.

**I:** **I**nsidious in onset: Anaemia, anorexia and asthenia of short duration.

**D:** **D**yspepsia in a man over the age of 40: Carcinoma stomach should be ruled out. Early gastric cancer presents as dyspepsia.

Nonmetastatic conditions such as thrombophlebitis (Trousseau's sign) and deep venous thrombosis can occur due to change in thrombotic and haemostatic mechanisms.

### Key Box 53.25

**Anaemia in Carcinoma Stomach**

- This is one of the common presentations. Often patients get investigated for anaemia by the physician only to discover carcinoma stomach.
- Achlorhydria results in poor conversion of ferrous to ferric which causes anaemia.
- 15% of patients may also develop haematemesis as in ulcerative lesions or proliferative lesions. GI blood loss also accounts for anaemia.
- Early satiety, loss of appetite and poor intake also contribute to anaemia (minor role).
- 40% of carcinoma stomach patients have anaemia.

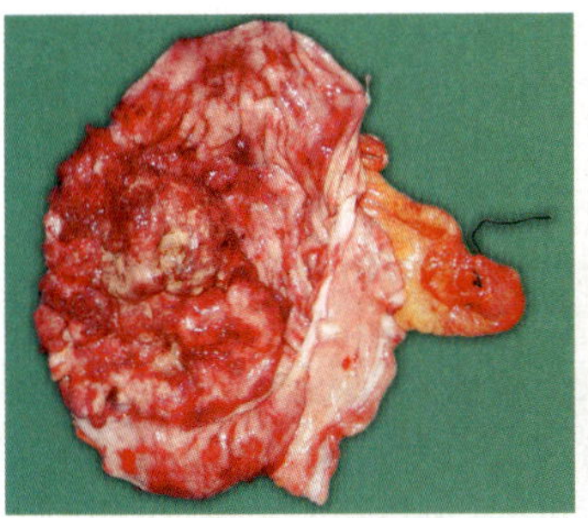

**Fig. 53.67:** Carcinoma stomach large ulcerative lesion with involvement of serosa

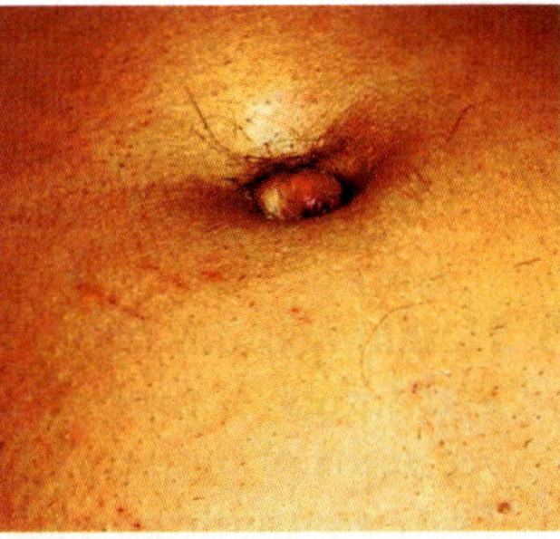

**Fig. 53.68:** Umbilical nodule—popularly called Sister Mary Joseph's nodule

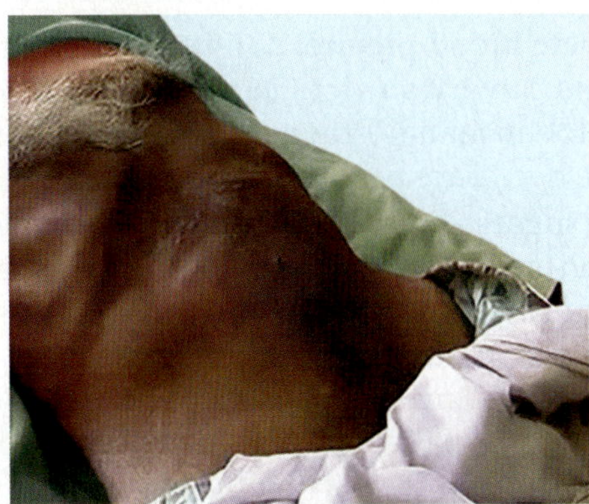

**Fig. 53.69:** VGP in a patient with carcinoma pyloric antrum

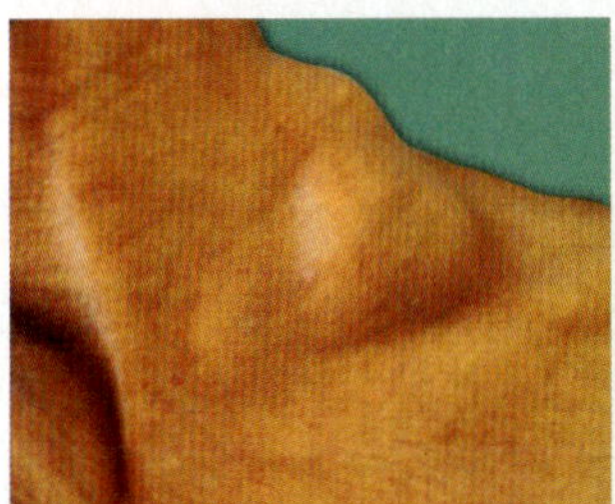

**Fig. 53.70:** Large supraclavicular nodes

**Fig. 53.71:** Krukenberg tumours

**Strong Suspicion of Carcinoma Stomach**

- New onset dyspepsia in men >50 years of age
- Unexplained anaemia
- Unintentional weight loss
- GI bleeding
- Iron deficiency anaemia
- Progressive dysphagia

**Clinical Signs of Inoperability**

- Ascites
- Secondaries in the liver
- Para-aortic lymph nodes
- Krukenberg tumours
- Sister Mary Joseph nodule
- Blummer shelf deposits
- Supraclavicular nodes—Virchow node
- Irish node

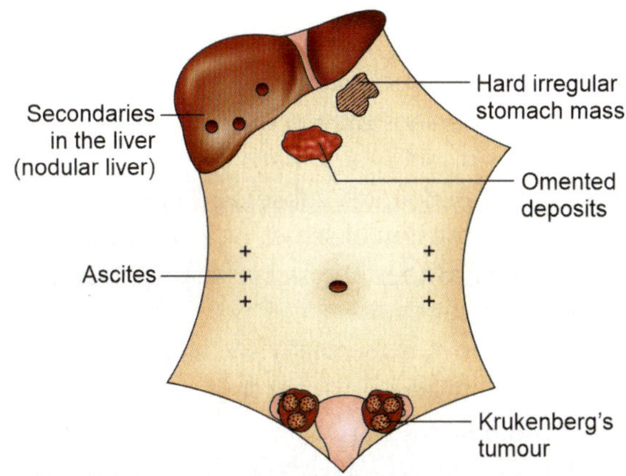


**Fig. 53.72:** Diagrammatic representation of secondaries in carcinoma stomach

**SISTER MARY JOSEPH NODULE**

- Sister Mary Joseph—head nurse to William Mayo
- Was first to notice that a 'nodule' in the umbilicus was often associated with advanced malignancy
- Presents as firm, red, nontender nodule
- Results from spread of tumour within the falciform ligament
- 90% of tumours are adenocarcinomas
- Commonest primaries are stomach and ovary
- Primary tumour is almost invariably inoperable

## Paraneoplastic Manifestations

- Sudden appearance of diffuse seborrhoeic keratoses (sign of Leser-Trélat) or acanthosis nigricans—velvety and darkly pigmented patches on skin folds.
- Hypercoagulable states (Trousseau's syndrome)
- Polyarteritis nodosa.

## Staging

Refer TNM staging. New clinical stage includes prognostic groups, cTNM, postneoadjuvant therapy pathologic stage groupings, ypTNM—new prognostic information change to anatomic boundary for staging carcinoma at oesophagogastric junction and changes to pathologic stage grouping. Refer NCCN guidelines for more details.

**TNM STAGING: AJCC 8th Edition**

| AJCC | TNM staging |
|---|---|
| **Primary tumour (T)** | |
| TX | Primary tumour cannot be assessed |
| T0 | No evidence of primary tumour |
| Tis | Carcinoma *in situ*. Intraepithelial tumour without invasion of the lamina propria |
| T1 | Tumour invades lamina propria, muscularis mucosa or submucosa |

*(Contd.)*

(Contd.)

| | |
|---|---|
| T1a | Tumour invades lamina propria or muscularis mucosa |
| T1b | Tumour invades submucosa |
| T2 | Tumour invades muscularis propria |
| T3 | Tumour penetrates subserosal connective tissue without invasion of serosa or adjacent structures |
| T4 | Tumour invades serosa (visceral peritoneum) or adjacent structures |
| T4a | Tumour invades serosa (visceral peritoneum) |
| T4b | Tumour invades adjacent structures |
| **Regional lymph nodes (N)** | |
| NX | Regional lymph nodes (S) cannot be assessed |
| N0 | No regional lymph node metastasis |
| N1 | Metastasis in 1–2 regional lymph nodes |
| N2 | Metastasis in 3–6 regional lymph nodes |
| N3 | Metastasis in 7 or more regional lymph nodes |
| N3a | Metastasis in 7 to 15 regional lymph nodes |
| N3b | Metastasis in 16 or more regional lymph nodes |
| **Distant metastasis (M)** | |
| M0 | No distant metastasis |
| M1 | Distant metastasis |
| **Histologic grade (G)** | |
| GX | Grade cannot be assessed |
| G1 | Well-differentiated |
| G2 | Moderately differentiated |
| G3 | Poorly differentiated |
| G4 | Undifferentiated |

## Spread

1. **Penetration of gastric serosa:** This is the most important prognostic indicator. When serosa is NOT penetrated, 50% survive for 5 years after resection. When serosa is penetrated, this figure drops to 20%. Once serosa is involved, adjacent organs such as liver, pancreas, spleen, omentum, transverse colon get involved. **Endoscopic ultrasound** is the best investigation to detect the involvement of layers in carcinoma of the stomach.
2. **Lymphatic spread:** More than 400 lymph nodes have been identified. Lymph node involvement is a poor prognostic indicator. 4 lymphatic zones have been described.
   - **Zone 1:** In the gastrocolic omentum along the right gastroepiploic vessels. This drains the pyloric antrum and lower half of greater curvature.
   - **Zone 2:** It lies in the gastrocolic omentum and gastrosplenic ligament along the left gastroepiploic vessels. This drains upper half of the greater curvature.
   - **Zone 3:** It lies in the lesser omentum draining proximal two-thirds of the stomach. From here, lymph drains into perioesophageal lymph nodes.
   - **Zone 4:** It is from distal portion of the lesser curve and pylorus along hepatic artery and right gastric artery into para-aortic nodes.
   - Lymph nodes have been given separate numbers. They are discussed under resections.
3. **Hematogenous spread:** Most common sites are liver and lungs. It produces extensive secondaries. They are signs of inoperability.
4. **Transcoelomic spread** results in ascites, Krukenberg tumour—bilateral bulky ovarian deposits and rectovesical deposits **(Blumer's shelf)**.

## Investigations

1. **Complete blood picture:** 20% of early gastric cancer patients have iron deficiency (microcytic, hypochromic) anaemia. Preoperative blood transfusion may be necessary before endoscopy.
2. **Blood** sugars, ECG and Echo, renal function, liver function are assessed and ECOG score is given so that whether these patients can undergo radical surgery/ preoperative–neoadjuvant chemotherapy/radiotherapy can be given or not. Preoperative optimization is done by normalizing blood sugar, renal function or cardiac function so as to get the best results.
3. **Flexible oesophagogastroduodenoscopy** (Figs 53.73 to 53.76)
   - Diagnosis of malignancy by ulcerated lesion with elevated edges, obliterated gastric rugae.

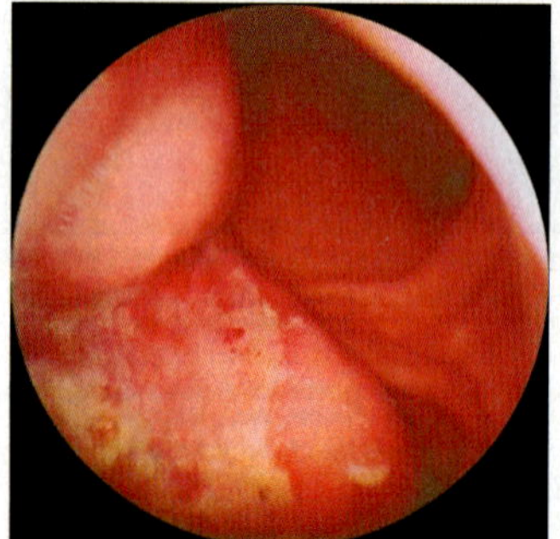

**Fig. 53.73:** Endoscopy showing superficial ulceration

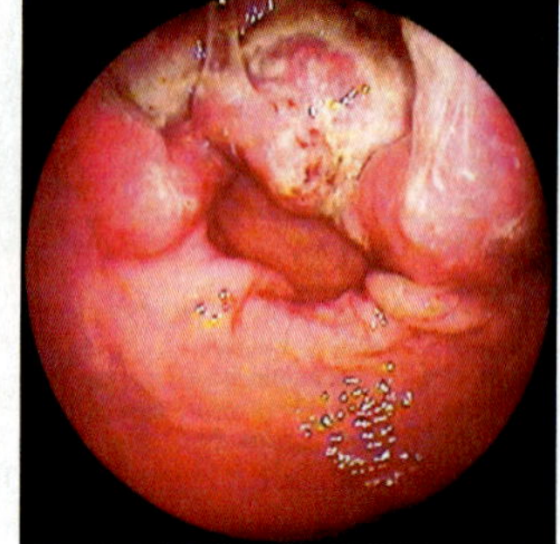

**Fig. 53.74:** Endoscopy showing ulceroproliferative growth

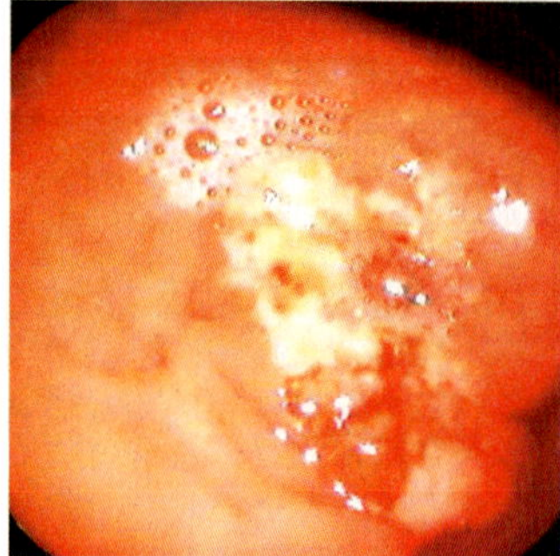

**Fig. 53.75:** Friable granular tissue—antral carcinoma

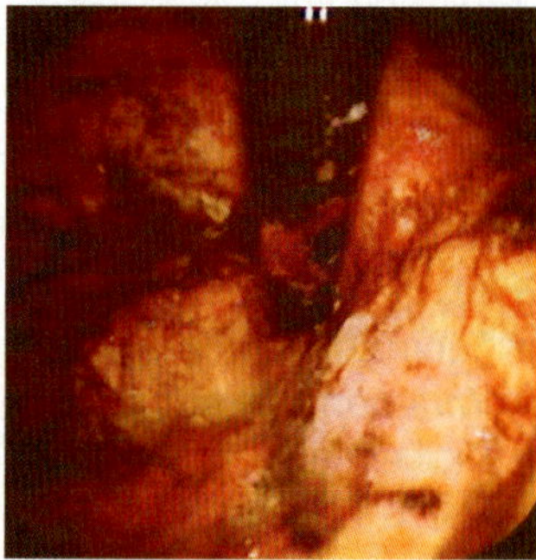

**Fig. 53.76:** Fundal carcinoma detected by J manoeuvre in endoscopy

- To know the extent of the lesion
- To confirm the diagnosis
- To take multiple biopsy—6 to 8 pieces
- Also, to aid brush cytology.

Biopsy is sent not only for histopathology but also for immune histochemistry. *Overexpression of HER-2 neu receptors is found in about 13 to 20% of gastric cancers.*

4. **Ultrasound of the abdomen**
   - To rule out secondaries in the liver.
   - To look for enlarged coeliac nodes.
   - Can detect ascites-guided fluid tap and cell cytology.
   - To detect Krukenberg tumour (pelvic CT).
   - Useful in detecting metastatic disease.
5. **CECT of the abdomen, pelvis and chest should be done** (Figs 53.77 and 53.78)
   - It is superior to ultrasound because it is objective and more specific.
   - Resectability—specially infiltration into pancreas, large fixed nodes at origin of left gastric artery, retroperitoneal structures are better appreciated.
   - However, detection of peritoneal disease sensitivity is only around 30–35%.

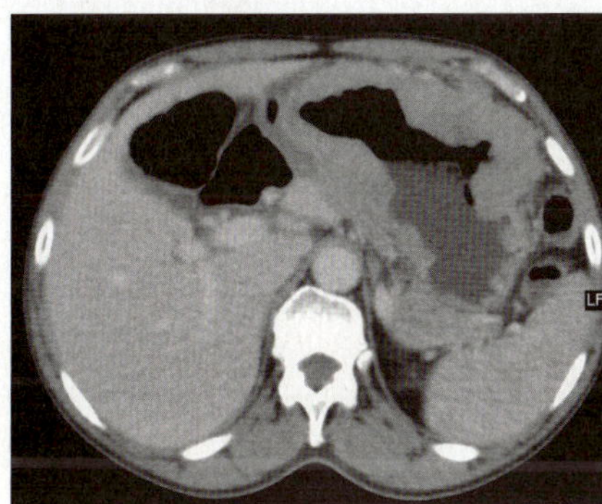

**Fig. 53.77:** CECT scan showing carcinoma body of the stomach—coronal section

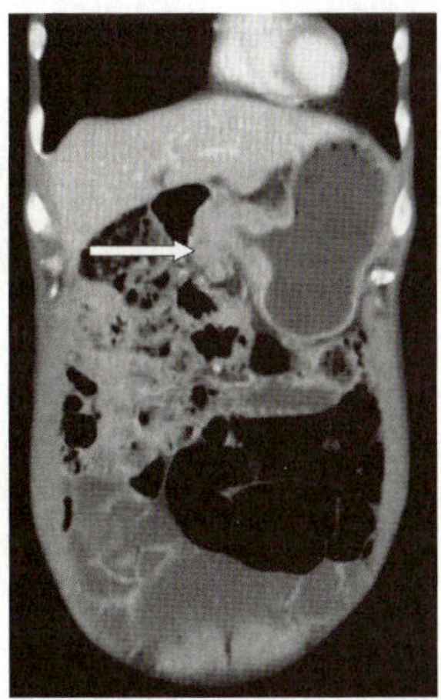

**Fig. 53.78:** Carcinoma pyloric antrum

6. **Endoscopic ultrasonography** can detect advanced tumours in 80% of patients. Overall staging accuracy is about 75%. However, it has significant limitations for staging mucosal disease. Flexible endoscope with 7.5 to 12 MHz transducer is used. Stomach is filled with water.

   5 alternating – hypoechoic and hyperechoic areas are recognised. Muscularis propria is 4th layer, involvement of this layer indicates T2. It can also detect 80 to 90% for nodal disease. If found, one can do nodal FNAC.
7. **Laparoscopy:** CT cannot detect liver or peritoneal metastasis (small <5 mm) and small lymph nodes. Laparoscopy is an ideal investigation. Almost 20 to 30% of so-called operable cases become inoperable. Laparoscopic peritoneal lavage for cytology is best test.
8. **Role of PET scan**
   - PET scanning is not routinely used in staging gastric cancer.
   - Gastric cancers have low avidity for 18F-fluoro-2-deoxyglucose.
   - In advanced cases, before doing a resection for controlling the locoregional disease, PET scan is done to rule out metastatic disease.
9. **CEA:** Carcinoembryonic antigen is elevated in about 60–70% patients. It indicates extensive spread of the disease. Also CA 19-9 (carbohydrate antigen) and alpha-fetoprotein can be done.
10. **Barium meal** has become obsolete (Fig. 53.79).

## Histopathology

It is an adenocarcinoma of the stomach. There are basically two types of gastric carcinomas as per **Lauren's classification**.

1. **Diffuse is more common in young, females and carries poor prognosis.** The leather-bottle stomach or linitis plastica is poorly differentiated with anaplastic cells. Signet-ring cell carcinoma and other poorly cohesive carcinomas are under diffuse variety as per WHO classification.

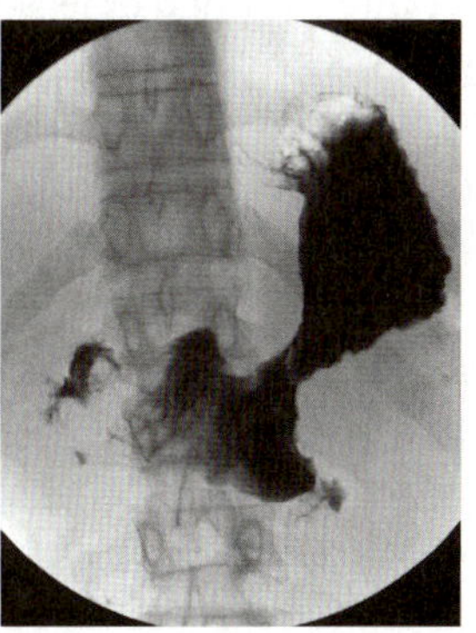

**Fig. 53.79:** Hourglass contracture of the stomach caused by carcinoma

2. **Intestinal is more common in elderly males.** It shows areas of intestinal metaplasia. It has better prognosis. Papillary adenocarcinoma, tubular adenocarcinoma and mucinous adenocarcinoma are subtypes as per WHO classification.
   - There are so many other varieties which are grouped under indeterminate type (WHO classification). Few of them are mixed, e.g. adenosquamous, carcinoma with lymphoid type, etc.
3. HER-2 neu receptors to be checked by immunohistochemistry.

## TREATMENT OF CARCINOMA STOMACH

- Surgical resection—gastrectomy, is the only potentially curative treatment for GC. Adjuvant and neoadjuvant perioperative chemotherapy and/or radiotherapy are now increasingly used in conjunction with surgery for locally advanced disease and in early stage of gastric cancer.
- Operable means cure is possible by doing radical surgery.
- Resectable means the growth can be removed.
- Inoperable means there are no chances of cure but growth may be resectable.

### Signs of Inoperability at Surgery

- Growth infiltrating into pancreas, engulfing pedicle of left gastric vessels to pancreas or posterior abdominal wall.
- Rectovesical deposits, due to peritoneal seedings which are felt during per rectal examination.
- Enlarged, fixed coeliac nodes, para-aortic nodes.
- Ascites, peritoneal deposits.

### Types of Resection

- Curative resection (R0) should be done whenever possible. Minimum 5 cm margin is required proximally. If serosa is involved, it qualifies for T3/T4 and not for curative resection
- Stage IA: Regionally confined disease should undergo primary surgical R-0 resection—radical subtotal gastrectomy.
- Stage T1a: Endoscopic resection for tumours less than 2 cm—curative.
- Stage II and III: Neoadjuvant therapy followed by radical resection. Curative but about 20%.
- Stage IV or inoperable patient with vomiting, if facilities are available, endoscopic stenting can be offered. Majority of these patients succumb to the disease by 3–6 months. Gastrojejunostomy is also another option provided some part of body of the stomach is healthy to consider anastomosis.
- Stage IV patient with bleeding, if fit for surgery: Palliative gastrectomy can be done to remove a fungating, ulcerative, bleeding mass. It gives better palliation.

### Terminology

- Japanese Research Society for gastric cancer advocates very aggressive resection including lymphadenectomy (Fig. 53.80). Hence, more details of lymph node stations are given in Table 53.9. However, the rest of the cancer research groups were not able to produce the same results as the Japanese.
- **D1** resection refers to the removal of primary group of nodes such as nodes along the lesser and greater curvature, and juxtapyloric nodes. If tumour and N1 nodes (group 1) resected = D1 gastrectomy. **This will become curative resection when lymph nodes are clinically not enlarged (N0) but they are removed** (Fig. 53.81).
- **D2** resection refers to the removal of lymph nodes such as left gastric, common hepatic, splenic, retropancreatic nodes, etc. If tumour and N2 nodes (group 2) resected = D2 gastrectomy.
  **This will become curative resection when lymph nodes are clinically enlarged (N1). So one step**

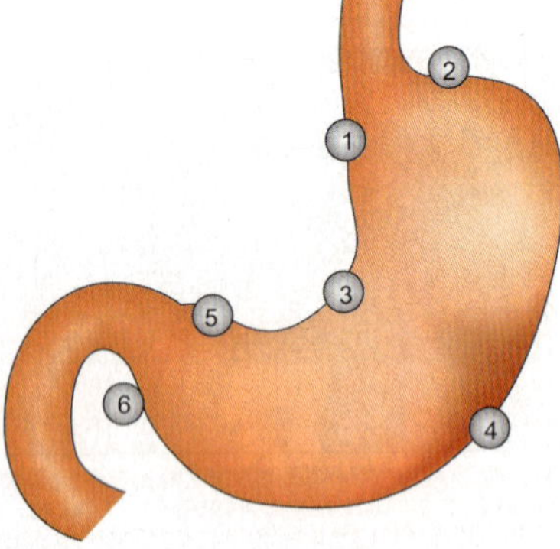


Fig. 53.80: Perigastric nodes: 1. Right pericardial, 2. left pericardial, 3. lesser curvature, 4. greater curvature, 5. suprapyloric, 6. infrapyloric

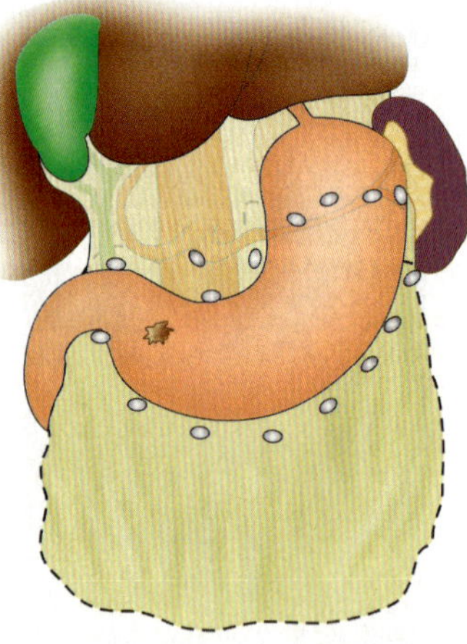

Fig. 53.81: Extent of D1 resection of tumour in distal one-third of stomach

**TABLE 53.9:** Grouping of regional lymph nodes

| Lymph node station (number) | Description | Location of primary tumour in the stomach | | |
|---|---|---|---|---|
| | | **Upper third** | **Middle third** | **Lower third** |
| 1 | Right paracardial | 1 | 1 | 2 |
| 2 | Left paracardial | 1 | 3 | M |
| 3 | Lesser curvature | 1 | 1 | 1 |
| 4 | Short gastric | 1 | 3 | M |
| 4 | Left gastroepiploic | 1 | 1 | 3 |
| 4 | Right gastroepiploic | 2 | 1 | 1 |
| 5 | Suprapyloric | 3 | 1 | 1 |
| 6 | Infrapyloric | 3 | 1 | 1 |
| 7 | Left gastric artery | 2 | 2 | 2 |
| 8 | Anterior common hepatic | 2 | 2 | 2 |
| 8 | Posterior common hepatic | 3 | 3 | 3 |
| **9** | **Coeliac artery** | 2 | 2 | 2 |
| **10** | **Splenic hilum** | 2 | 3 | M |
| 11 | Proximal splenic | 2 | 2 | 2 |
| 11 | Distal splenic | 2 | 3 | M |
| 12 | Hepatoduodenal | 3 | 2 | 2 |
| **13** | **Retropancreatic** | M | 3 | 3 |
| 14 | Superior mesenteric vein | M | 3 | 2 |
| 14 | Superior mesenteric artery | M | M | M |
| 15 | Middle colic (mesocolon) | M | M | M |
| 16 | Aortic hiatus (para-aortic) | 3 | M | M |
| 17 | Around lower oesophagus | – | – | – |
| 18 | Supradiaphragmatic | – | – | – |

Numbers 1–3: Group number M = Lymph nodes regarded as distant metastasis

**higher lymph nodes are cleared. Carcinoma stomach often causes local recurrence at the tumour site or in the locoregional lymph nodes. So aggressive approach of clearance of lymph nodes have been recommended** (Key Box 53.26 and Fig. 53.82).

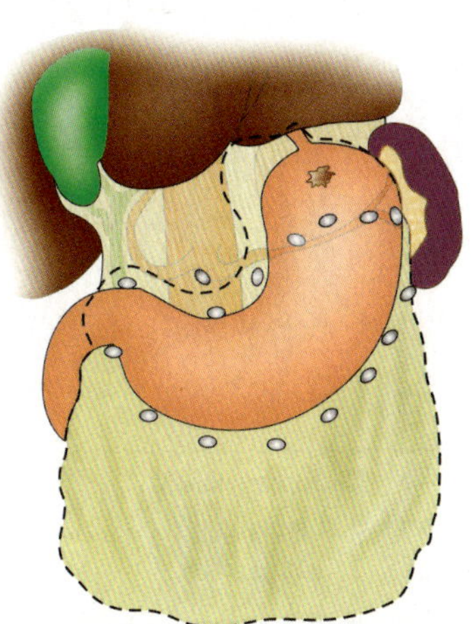

**Fig. 53.82:** D2 resection of tumours of the proximal third of stomach

- **D3** resection refers to D2 resection followed by the removal of lymph nodes such as para-aortic, porta hepatis nodes, behind the head of the pancreas, etc. (not done).

Key Box 53.26

**Pathological basis for D2 Dissection**

- Gastric cancer has a great propensity to spread through the rich plexus of lymphatics of the stomach to local or regional lymph nodes. Hence, the need to remove stomach and lymph nodes.
- **Gastric cancer, unlike breast cancer, remains for a long time as a locoregional disease.**
- It is striking too, that when gastric cancer recurs, it often does so locoregionally rather than more wide-spread dissemination.
- It is very rare for gastric cancer to recur 5 years after surgery, whereas for breast cancer, disseminated micrometastases continue to take their toll some 10–20 years after surgery.

### Curative Resections

A. Gastrectomy, and B. Endoscopic mucosal resections.

The term R status was first described by Hermanek in 1994 and is used to describe the tumour status after resection (Key Box 53.27). If no disease is identified in the lymph nodes, N0 nomenclature is used.

**A. *Gastrectomy:*** The extent of the gastrectomy (Figs 53.83 to 53.88) is site-dependent and focuses on complete removal of the gastric carcinoma with preferably a 5 cm margin from the gross edge of the tumour. Clearly, anatomic limitations influence this margin because in antral lesions close to or involving the pylorus, only a limited portion of the duodenum can be removed. In patients with a distal lesion, essentially a distal subtotal gastrectomy is performed regardless of T stage.

- **For proximal gastric cancers (fundic),** total gastrectomy is required.
- **For midbody or more extensive lesions**, total gastrectomy is required.
- **For more distal lesions,** a subtotal gastrectomy is the preferred approach.
- **Extended organ resection** is reserved for patients with apparently node-negative T4 lesions, in which complete resection requires resection of the invaded portions of the diaphragm, pancreas, spleen, adrenal gland or colon.
- These patients usually are pretreated with chemotherapy.

Key Box 53.27

**R-Resections**

- R0 describes a microscopically margin-negative resection, in which no gross or microscopic tumour remains in the tumour bed.
- R1 indicates removal of all macroscopic disease but microscopic margins are positive for tumour.
- R2 indicates gross residual disease. Since the extent of resection can influence survival, some authors include this R designation to complement the TNM system.
- Long-term survival can be expected only after a R0 resection; therefore, a significant effort should be made to avoid R1 or R2 resections.

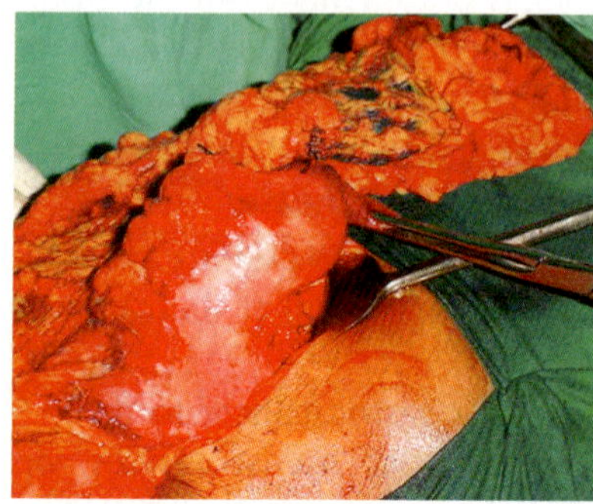

**Fig. 53.83:** Carcinoma stomach with involvement of serosa, endosonogram can detect this

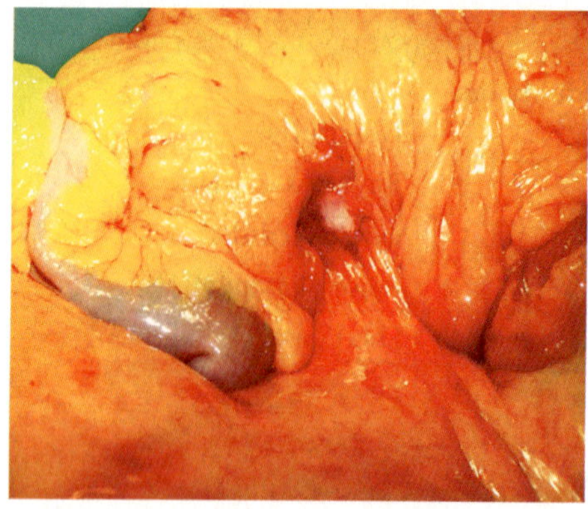

**Fig. 53.84:** Peritoneal metastasis from carcinoma stomach. Laparoscopy is the most ideal investigation to detect peritoneal metastasis

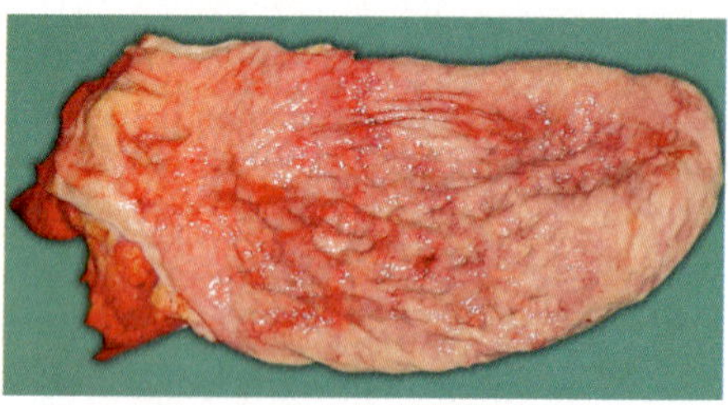

**Fig. 53.85:** Intestinal type—gland formation present, similar to adenocarcinoma colon—good prognosis

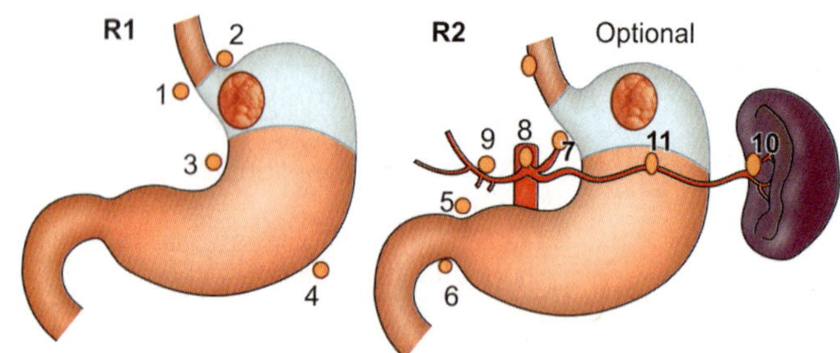


| | | |
|---|---|---|
| 1. Right cardiac | 5. Suprapyloric | 10. Splenic hilar |
| 2. Left cardiac | 6. Infrapyloric | 11. Splenic |
| 3. Lesser curvature | 7. Left gastric | |
| 4. Greater curvature (and short gastric) | 8. Hepatic | |
| | 9. Coeliac | |

**Fig. 53.86:** Proximal gastric cancer

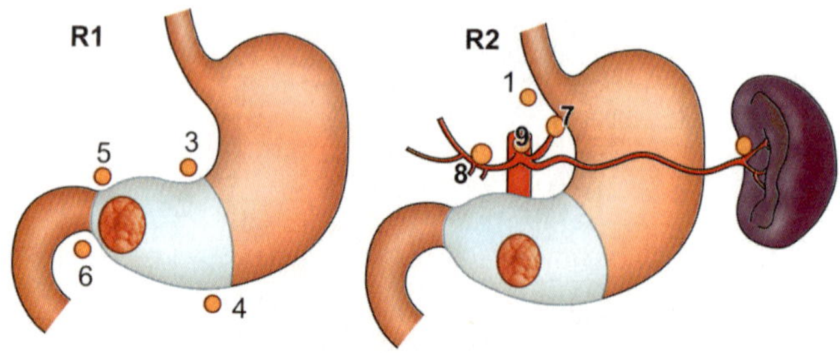


| | | |
|---|---|---|
| 1. Right paracardiac | 5. Suprapyloric | 8. Hepatic |
| 3. Lesser curvature | 6. Infrapyloric | 9. Coeliac |
| 4. Greater curvature | 7. Left gastric | |

**Fig. 53.87:** Distal gastric cancer

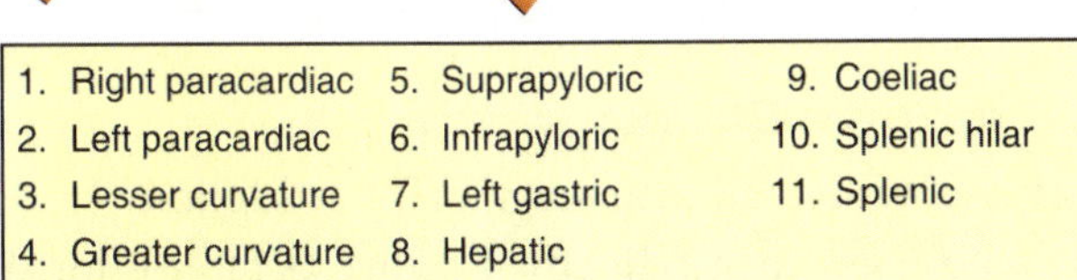

| | | |
|---|---|---|
| 1. Right paracardiac | 5. Suprapyloric | 9. Coeliac |
| 2. Left paracardiac | 6. Infrapyloric | 10. Splenic hilar |
| 3. Lesser curvature | 7. Left gastric | 11. Splenic |
| 4. Greater curvature | 8. Hepatic | |

**Fig. 53.88:** Mid-body gastric cancer

*Example:*

**Surgery: A standard D2 resection for gastric cancer involves:**

1. Removing part or whole of the stomach.
2. The N1 (groups 1–6) and N2 (groups 7–11) lymph nodes. Minimum of 15 lymph nodes need to be removed. More centers are recommending more lymph nodes removal.
3. The greater and lesser omentum and omental bursa.
4. The spleen and tail of the pancreas are removed, if infiltrated by the tumours of the proximal stomach in order to remove groups 10 and 11 lymph nodes. All attempts should be made to preserve these structures but remove lymph nodes.
5. The hepatoduodenal nodes—level 12—in antral tumours.
6. The splenic hilum and other nodes—level 10, 11, 12.

*Reconstruction*

- **Carcinoma of pyloric antrum and distal body of the stomach:** Radical subtotal gastrectomy—D2. Reconstruction is done by gastrojejunal anastomosis. Popularly called polya gastrectomy or Billroth II anastomosis (Figs 53.89 and 53.90).
- **Carcinoma of proximal stomach and diffuse carcinoma:** Radical oesophagogastrectomy (Figs 53.91 and 53.92): Removal of the entire stomach, lower end of oesophagus, with regional lymph nodes N2, followed by oesophagojejunal anastomosis.

**B.** ***Endoscopic/Endoluminal mucosal resection***

- This is indicated in early gastric cancer confined to mucosa. The cancer should be less than 2 cm and there should not be node enlargement. Small, high up lesions are ideal.
- Here, laparoscopic instrumentation is done under endoscopic guidance.
- Stomach is suitable for endoluminal surgery because it can be distended, and contents are sterile.
- Ideally cancer should be elevated variety and well differentiated.

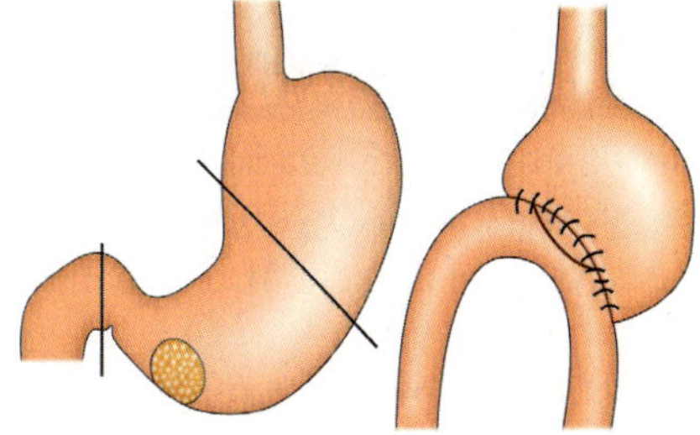

**Figs 53.89 and 53.90:** Radical subtotal gastrectomy with Billroth II anastomosis

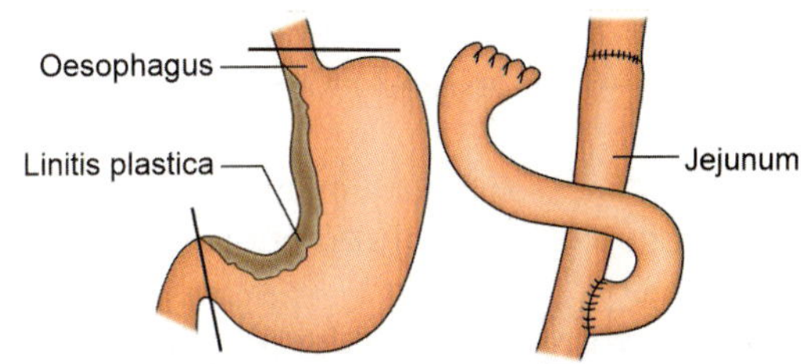


**Figs 53.91 and 53.92:** Radical total gastrectomy, with Roux-en-Y oesophagojejunostomy

- Normal saline is injected into submucosal plane and lesion gets elevated.
- It is excised with 1 cm margin up to muscularis propria at a deeper plane.

### *Palliative Resections*

1. Carcinoma pyloric antrum (inoperable): Palliative anterior GJ (Fig. 53.93) is done to relieve vomiting, by anastomosing a jejunal loop to the stomach in the prepyloric region. If posterior GJ is done, the growth may involve the GJ stoma early resulting in stomal obstruction. With anterior GJ, entero-enterostomy can be added to prevent bilious vomiting.
2. Palliative gastrectomy to get rid of ulcerated, necrotic or bleeding lesion.

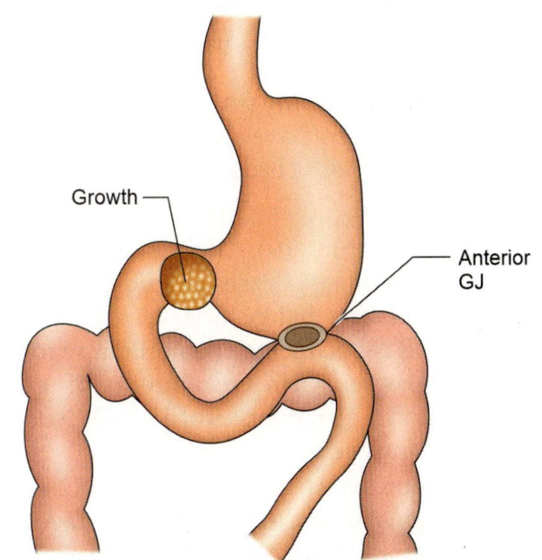


**Fig. 53.93:** Palliative anterior GJ

**KEY POINTS ON SURGERY FOR CARCINOMA STOMACH**

1. Carcinoma antrum and body—radical subtotal gastrectomy.
2. Carcinoma proximal stomach—radical total gastrectomy.
3. Inoperable carcinoma distal stomach—palliative anterior GJ.
4. Radical refers to removal of lymph nodes, fat, fascia greater and lesser omentum.
5. When level 1 to 6 (N1) nodes are removed along with stomach, it is D1 gastrectomy.
6. When level 7–11 (N2) lymph nodes are also removed along with 1–6 nodes and stomach, it is called D2 gastrectomy.
7. Early gastric cancer without lymph nodes can be treated with endoscopic mucosal resection or endoluminal gastric resection.
8. Palliative gastrectomy (subtotal) is worth considering in appropriate cases of obstruction/bleeding.

## Role of Chemotherapy

### *A. The Adjuvant Treatment*

***Postoperative chemotherapy:***

- Now, it is understood that gastric cancers partially respond to chemotherapy—in about 30% of cases given at advanced stage (results are better than cancer colon). Injection 5-FU (fluorouracil) 500 mg IV daily for five days, every 28 days. It can be given by IV infusion or IV bolus over 15 minutes.
- **Mechanism of action:** It is an antimetabolite and acts by interfering with DNA synthesis. Side effects are myelosuppression, mucositis, excessive lacrimation, nausea, vomiting, etc.
- Combination of 5-FU with adriamycin, mitomycin and cisplatin has also been tried. However, toxicity is more with these drugs. FAM (5-fluorouracil, adriamycin and mitomycin C) and ECF (epirubicin, cisplatin and 5-FU) are popular agents.
- Intraperitoneal mitomycin and mitomycin C—impregnated charcoal have also been used (target the recurrence site—gastric bed).

**Indications:**

1. R0 resection (free margins): Any tumour greater than T2 including selected T2 cases should be considered for adjuvant therapy that includes 1 cycle of 5-FU+/– leucovorin OR capecitabine chemotherapy followed by 5-FU+/– leucovorin OR capecitabine based chemoradiation 3–4 more cycles of 5-FU+/–leucovorin OR capecitabine chemotherapy.
2. R1 (microscopic margin positive) and R2 (grossly positive margins) regardless of the TMN stage should receive chemoradiation followed by further cycles of adjuvant chemotherapy.
3. If the patient has received preoperative chemotherapy/chemoradiation then:
   A. Adjuvant treatment is usually recommended beyond T2N0M0 which is usually 5-FU+/–leucovorin OR capecitabine based.
   B. If patient has received ONLY preoperative chemotherapy and the resection was R1/R2, then postoperative chemoradiation is advised.

### *B. Neoadjuvant Chemoradiation*

- Patients with a clinical stage of T2 or higher.
- It is advised in medically fit unresectable—locally advanced diseases which generally includes concurrent 5-FU/capecitabine-based chemotherapy.
- Chemotherapy alone may also be used as a neoadjuvant modality.
- Recommended radiotherapy dose is 45–50.4 Gy (at 1.8 Gy/fraction).
- *Trastuzumab (Herceptin) can be used in metastatic or locally advanced gastric adenocarcinomas which are* **overexpressing HER-2 neu receptors** in about 13 to 20% of gastric cancers.

## Role of Radiotherapy

External beam radiotherapy can also be used in metastatic cases as a part of palliation, especially when there is tumour bleed, gastric outlet obstruction due to the tumour pain. Dose for palliative radiotherapy is generally 30 Gy in 10 fractions over 2 weeks.

# OTHER TUMOURS OF THE STOMACH

## GASTROINTESTINAL STROMAL TUMOURS (GISTs)

- Previously named leiomyoma, leiomyosarcoma is called GIST today.
- In gastrointestinal tract, **stomach is the most common** site of GIST.
- **Bleeding** is the most common presentation. It occurs due to ulceration of mucosa which on endoscopy gives **appearance of cervix** (Figs 53.94A and B).
- Larger tumours can present with dysphagia, weight loss, anaemia and palpable mass (Fig. 53.95).
- ***The diagnosis of malignancy is by greater mitotic figures.***
- **If mucosa is not ulcerated, 'biopsy on a biopsy'** or 'well biopsy' is necessary.
- Immunohistochemistry is mandatory for diagnosis—**C Kit gene amplification: It is the tumour marker of GIST.**
- CT scan is a useful investigation (Fig. 53.96).
- Resection is the best treatment (Fig. 53.97).

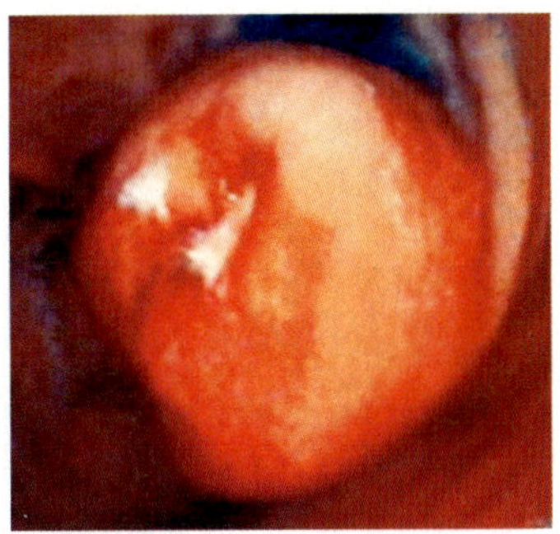

**Fig. 53.94A:** Bleeding ulcer of the stomach

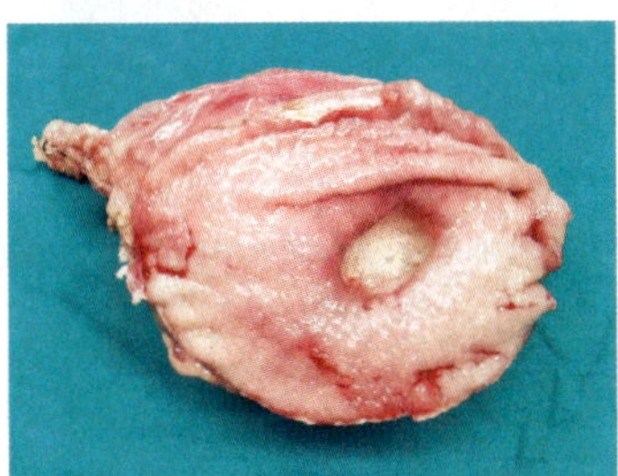

**Fig. 53.94B:** Wide excision specimen of GIST of the stomach showing ulcer crater. (*Courtesy*: Dr SS Prasad, Former Professor of Surgery, KMC, Manipal)

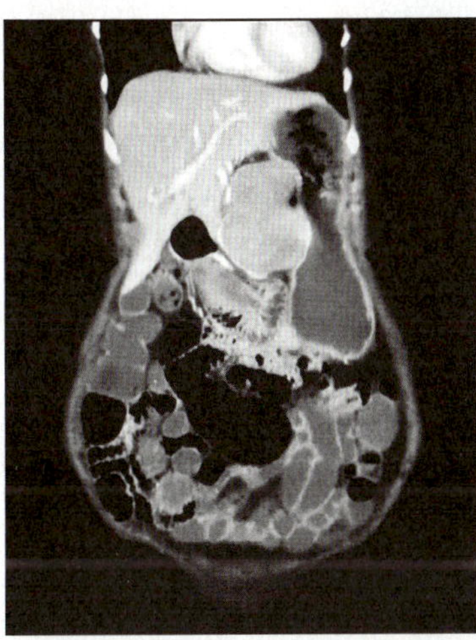

**Fig. 53.95:** Large GIST with air pocket. Torricelli-Bernoulli sign

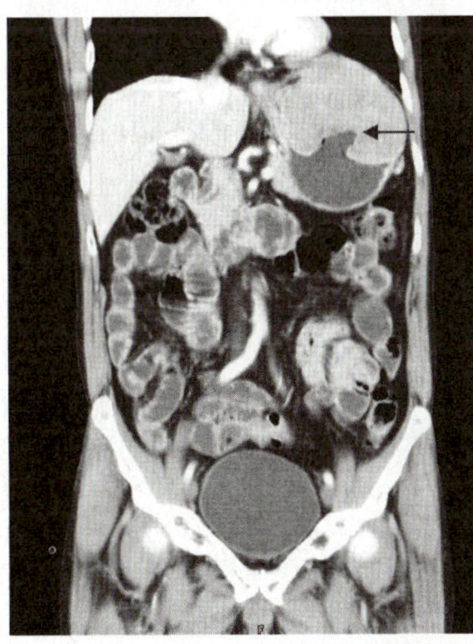

**Fig. 53.96:** CT GIST fundus

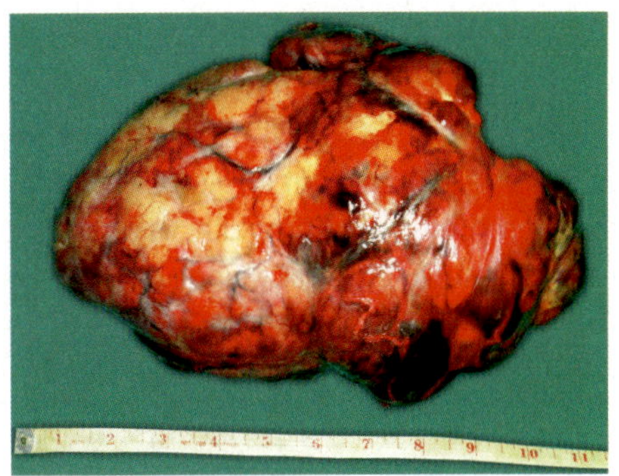

**Fig. 53.97:** GIST specimen

### Chemotherapy for GIST

Capsule Imatinib 100 mg 4 capsules—to a total of 400 mg per day is given till toxicity appears or metastasis or residual tumour regresses (investigated by CT scan).

## GASTRIC LYMPHOMA

- Incidence of primary gastric lymphoma is increasing.
- They are B cell derived from mucosa associated lymphoid tissue (**MALT**)—**MALTOMA**.
- Pain, weight loss, bleeding are common presentations.
- **6th decade** is the common age group.
- Endoscopic features are not specific but diffuse thickening with or without ulcerations may be seen.
- It is important to rule out **generalised process** by CT, ultrasound, bone marrow aspirate.
- Gastrectomy is the best treatment.
- Chemotherapy is better for systemic disease.

*Pearls of Wisdom*

Low-grade lymphoma associated with *H. pylori* infection may regress and totally disappear after eradication treatment for *H. pylori*.

## COMPLICATIONS OF VAGOTOMY AND GJ

Can be classified as complications of vagotomy, complications of GJ and complications of gastrectomy.

1. Stasis of food in the stomach resulting in nausea, loss of appetite, distension of upper abdomen, foul eructation, etc.
2. Denervation of gallbladder can cause gallstones.
3. Postvagotomy **diarrhoea**—can be very troublesome at times (Key Box 53.28).
4. Vagotomy produces hypoacidity which allows bacterial proliferation. Nitrates are reduced to nitrites which are carcinogenic. Such a malignancy which develops at GJ site is called **stump carcinoma**.

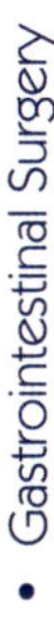

Key Box 53.28

**Causes of Diarrhoea**

- Vagotomy results in removal of parasympathetic influence on the function of foregut and midgut.
- Fast gastric emptying occurring due to GJ or gastrectomy.
- Hypoacidity resulting in bacterial proliferation causing enteritis.
- Bile salts also play a role.

## STOMAL OBSTRUCTION

It is due to oedema as in gastroduodenal anastomosis or nondependent drainage as in GJ. Sometimes, fat in the transverse mesocolon undergoes necrosis resulting in obstruction to the loops. Stomal obstruction also develops, if there is narrowing of the lumen. Treatment is conservative. Surgery may also be required later, after confirming obstruction by gastrografin studies.

## RETROGRADE JEJUNOGASTRIC INTUSSUSCEPTION (Fig. 53.98)

It develops if efferent and afferent loops are not sutured properly. It can appear at any time after surgery.

### Clinical Features

- Previous history of abdominal surgery (surgery done for peptic ulcer)
- Acute abdominal pain in upper abdomen
- Vomiting, sometimes blood stained
- **Palpable mass** in the upper abdomen.

### Investigation

Barium meal X-ray shows filling defect in the stomach (Fig. 53.99). Sometimes, following a barium meal, intussusception is reduced.

### Treatment

Reduction of the intussusception and suturing of intestinal loops properly. If the loops are gangrenous, resection may be necessary (Fig. 53.100).

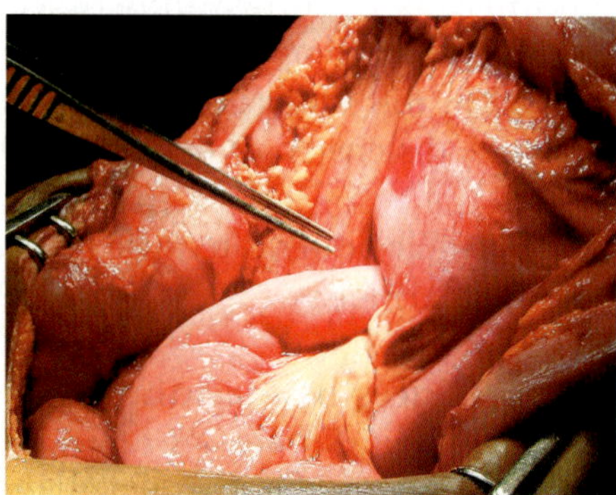

**Fig. 53.98:** Jejunogastric intussusception

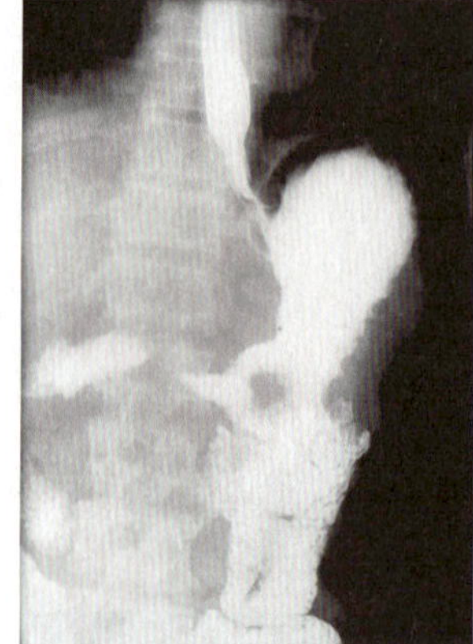

**Fig. 53.99:** Barium showing filling defect, in a patient who had undergone GJ

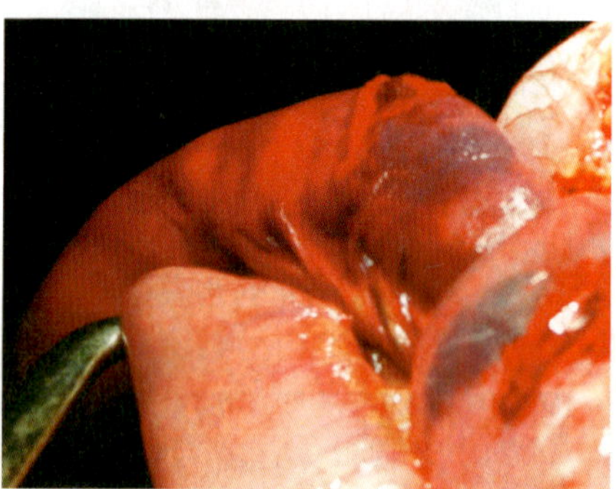

**Fig. 53.100:** Gangrene in jejunogastric intussusception

### Complication

Gangrene of intestine.

## GASTROJEJUNOCOLIC FISTULA

- It is a complication of GJ done for peptic ulcer, especially when vagotomy is not done or is incomplete.
- After a few years of GJ, a recurrent ulcer can develop at the stoma—GJ site.
- This recurrent ulcer slowly invades the adjacent structure such as the transverse colon resulting in gastrojejunocolic fistula.

### Clinical Features

- Previous history of vagotomy and GJ.
- Foul eructation and foul vomiting due to colonic contents entering the stomach which is loaded with faecal matter and foul contents.
- Intense diarrhoea due to severe jejunitis brought about by colonic bacteria entering the jejunum.
- Rapid deterioration in health—loss of weight, loss of appetite, dehydration and emaciation.

*Pearls of Wisdom*

Diarrhoea is not due to food entering the colon. Contents of the colon enter the stomach and then jejunum resulting in jejunitis causing diarrhoea.

### Diagnosis

Confirm by barium enema—barium entering the stomach (because of high pressure in the colon). Barium meal study should not be done (Fig. 53.101).

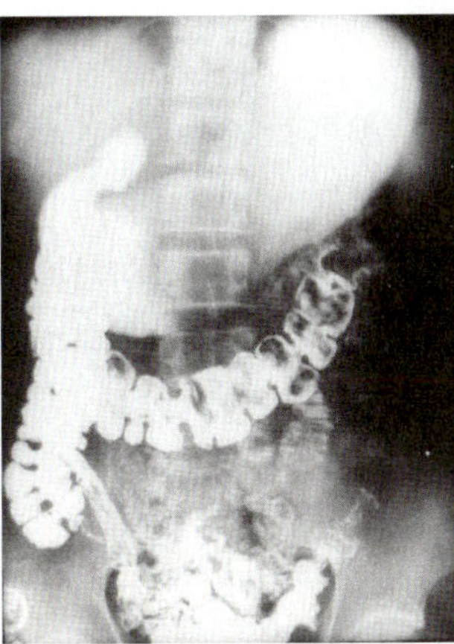

**Fig. 53.101:** Barium enema—barium entering into the stomach from colon (barium meal is not the investigation for gastrojejunocolic fistula)

### Treatment

- Triple resection (Figs 53.102 to 53.104).
- Preoperative preparation is necessary in the form of blood transfusion, stomach wash, nutritional supplementation and correction of dehydration.
- Resection of portions of stomach, intestine and colon followed by end-to-end anastomosis.

## STUMP CARCINOMA (Figs 53.105 to 53.107)

- It refers to carcinoma developing in the stomach after some surgery on the stomach. Classically, it happens after a gastrojejunostomy (GJ) Billroth II or after a pyloroplasty.
- It develops after 10 to 20 years of surgery.
- Reflux of bile, changes in the acidity due to vagotomy are a few factors that precipitate stump carcinoma. Metaplasia is due to enterogastric reflux and bacterial reduction of nitrates.
- Clinical features include sudden loss of appetite, loss of weight with or without mass abdomen.

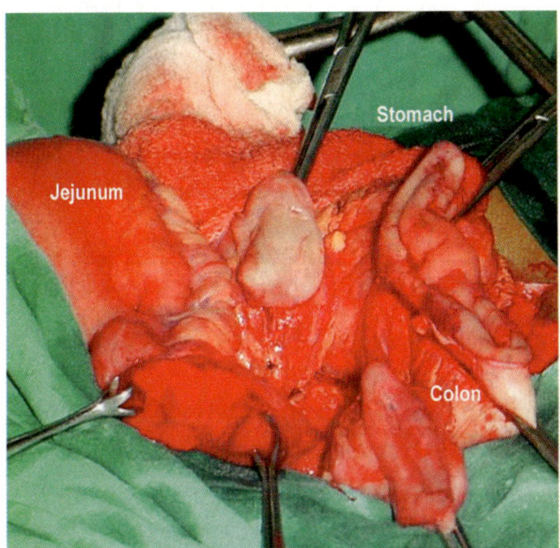


**Fig. 53.102:** Specimen of triple resection

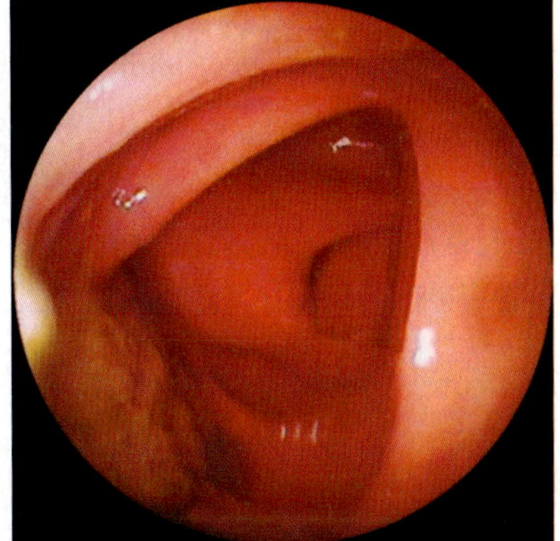

**Fig. 53.103:** Gastrojejunocolic fistula—gastroscopy shows faecal matter in the stomach, coming from colon (see the triangular folds of colon)

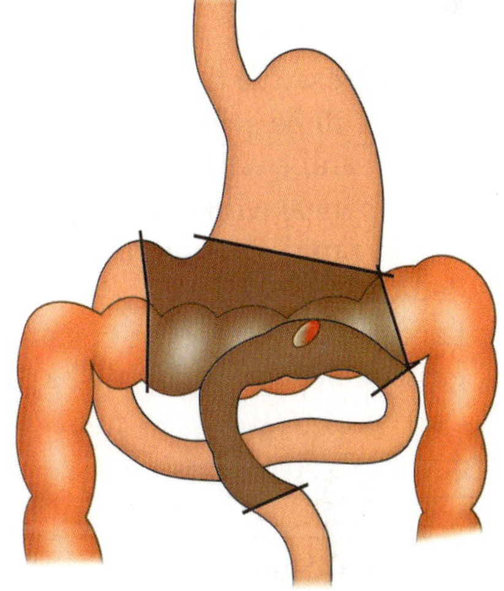

**Fig. 53.104:** Triple resection

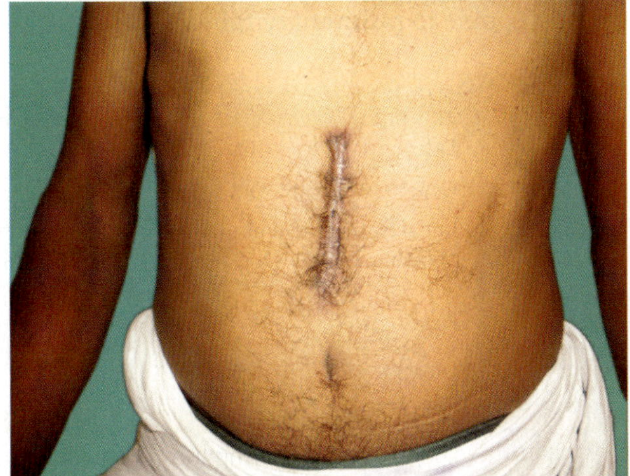

**Fig. 53.105:** GJ was done in this patient 20 years back. He came with stump carcinoma

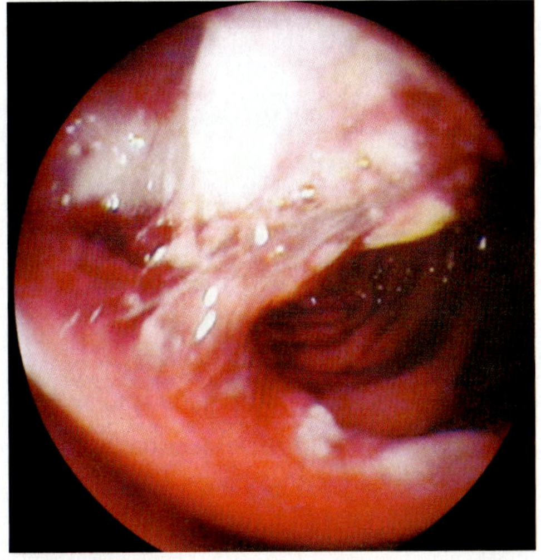

**Fig. 53.106:** Endoscopy showing stump carcinoma

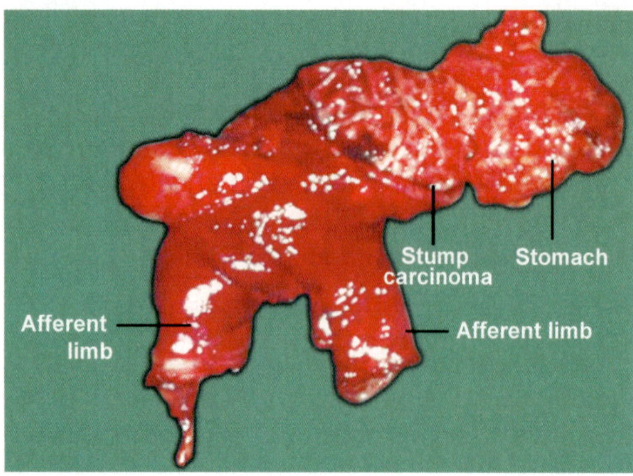


Fig. 53.107: Gastrectomy for stump carcinoma

- Diagnosis is by endoscopy (Fig. 53.106).
- Treated by resection. However, many cases are advanced and they are inoperable.

## GASTROILEOSTOMY (Fig. 53.108)

- It is an avoidable complication.
- Instead of the short loop—jejunum, ileum is anastomosed to the stomach.
- There will be severe uncontrolled diarrhoea, loss of weight and emaciation within a short period.
- Barium meal with fluoroscopy should be done which shows rapid flow of barium from stomach into the ileum.
- Laparotomy—undoing of gastroileostomy and fresh gastrojejunostomy should be done.

## POSTCIBAL SYNDROMES

This syndrome complex results due to rapid emptying of stomach contents to the distal intestines resulting in various physiological changes such as vasomotor symptoms, hypoglycaemia, etc. They are of two types. Their comparison is given in Table 53.10.

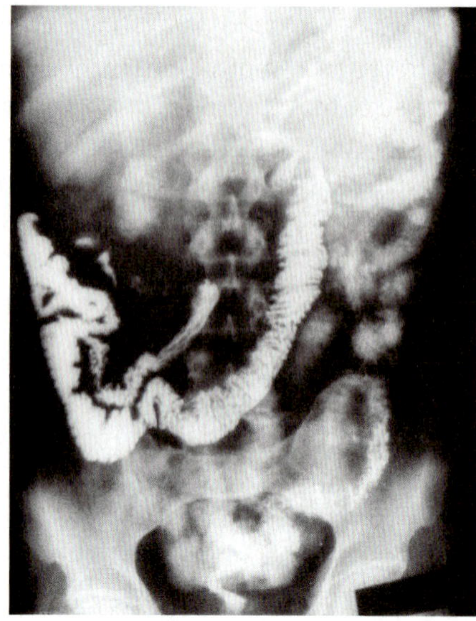

Fig. 53.108: Gastroileostomy—the biggest blunder a surgeon can do—it can be avoided by identifying the duodenojejunal flexure

*Pearls of Wisdom*

Alkaline reflux gastritis which develops after GJ should be differentiated from afferent loop syndrome (Table 53.11).

# COMPLICATIONS OF GASTRECTOMY

## NUTRITIONAL DISTURBANCES

- Vitamin $B_{12}$ and calcium deficiency.
- Megaloblastic anaemia occurs late due to gastric mucosal atrophy.
- **Iron deficiency anaemia**, common after gastrectomy when duodenum is bypassed because of deficient iron absorption.
- **Diarrhoea** is due to vagotomy causing intestinal hurry or due to dumping.
- Due to poor nutrition, there is **weight loss** and they are susceptible to **pulmonary tuberculosis**.

**TABLE 53.10:** Dumping syndrome—postcibal syndromes

| | Early | Late |
|---|---|---|
| Onset | Increased emptying immediately after meals | One to two hours afterwards |
| Causes | Rapid passage of food of high osmolarity from stomach into small intestine causes hypovolaemia. It is also due to loss of pyloric sphincter | Initial hyperglycaemia causes increased release of insulin which is followed by hypoglycaemia |
| Relief | Lying down | Glucose |
| Aggravating factors | More food, glucose, fullness | Exercise |
| Symptoms | Epigastric distension, sweating, diarrhoea | Tremors, fainting attacks (release of adrenaline) |
| Treatment | Small quantity, dry food. Over a period of time, symptoms settle down, less sugar content | Dietary adjustment of food |
| Incidence | More common (10%) | Less common (5%) |

**TABLE 53.11:** Comparison of chronic afferent limb syndrome and alkaline reflux gastritis

| | Chronic afferent limb syndrome | Alkaline reflux gastritis |
|---|---|---|
| Pain | After meals | Unrelated to meals |
| Vomitus | Bile<br>Relieves pain<br>Projectile | Bile and food<br>No changes in pain<br>Nonprojectile |
| Occult bleeding | Rare | Common |
| Cause | Limb obstruction—long loop | Enterogastric reflux (no obstruction) |
| Treatment | Avoid a long loop at surgery<br>Convert Billroth II to Billroth I<br>Roux-en-Y jejunostomy or jejunojejunostomy<br>(Braun modification of Billroth II) | High fat, amino acid regimen<br>Proton pump inhibitors<br>Ursodeoxycholic acid<br>Jejunojejunostomy, converting Billroth II to Billroth I can be done |

## DUODENAL FISTULA (Duodenal blow out)

It is the leakage of duodenal contents to the exterior. It commonly occurs after surgery.

### Causes

- After a partial gastrectomy/total gastrectomy, where the closure of duodenum was difficult.
- After closure of perforated duodenal ulcer, which gives way once again.
- Injuries to duodenum during right hemicolectomy, right nephrectomy, etc.

### Precipitating Factors

- Faulty technique of closure of duodenal stump.
- Severely inflamed duodenum due to an active ulcer.
- If there is a distal obstruction, it increases tension in duodenal loop and may result in fistula.
- Ischaemia of duodenal stump.

### Clinical Features

- Signs and symptoms develop usually after 4 to 5 days when oral fluids are commenced. These stimulate outpouring of biliary and pancreatic juices.
- Severe upper abdominal pain and guarding, rigidity, hypotension and shock-like features of biliary peritonitis develop, if there is no drainage tube.
- If drainage tube is kept in the first surgery, bile flows to the exterior. In such cases, signs of peritonitis are usually not present. However, severe electrolyte imbalance can occur (Fig. 53.109).

### Treatment

- Conservative treatment is successful in majority of the cases. Fistula heals in a few days, provided there is no distal obstruction. During this time hydration, electrolyte care is essential. Appropriate antibiotics are given.

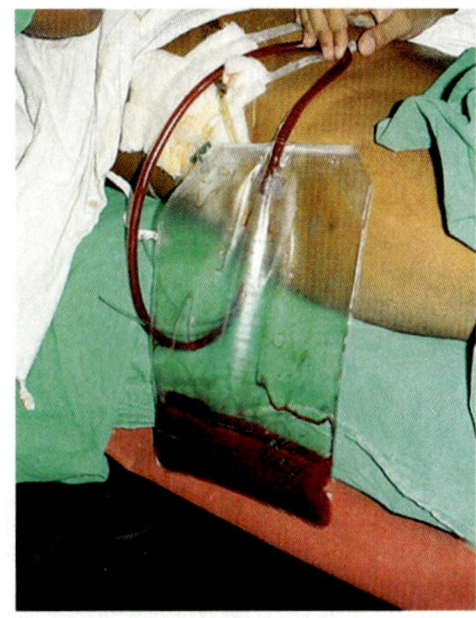

**Fig. 53.109:** Duodenal blow out following gastrectomy

- Surgical—if the fistula persists, laparotomy and closure of the fistula can be done by repairing with nonabsorbable sutures.

### Complications

- Biliary peritonitis
- Septicaemia, if bile is not drained outside.
- Excoriation of abdominal skin can be prevented by zinc oxide application.
- Fluid and electrolyte imbalance.

## RECURRENT ULCER

It can be true anastomotic ulcer (gastrojejunal, gastroduodenal or jejunal ulcer), or a gastric ulcer in the remnant, or recurrent ulcer following highly selective vagotomy (HSV).

### Incidence

- 3% after Billroth II gastrectomy
- 5 to 8% after vagotomy and GJ
- 40% after gastrojejunostomy
- 10 to 12% following HSV.

### Causes of Recurrent Ulcer (Fig. 53.110)

1. Incomplete vagotomy
2. GJ alone
3. Inadequate gastrectomy
4. Narrow stoma
5. Zollinger-Ellison syndrome
6. Hyperparathyroidism

### Symptoms

- Appears within 1 to 2 years after the operation.
- Severe persistent pain, 'boring' type, which gets worse within a few minutes of taking food. The pain is felt on the left side of the abdomen, near the umbilical region and it passes downwards.
- The pain is felt in the lower left chest following antecolic anastomosis. It is not relieved by antacids or milk unlike peptic ulcer. Bleeding may manifest as haematemesis, melaena or anaemia. Perforation can occur, resulting in peritonitis.

### Diagnosis

- Gastroscopy gives the correct diagnosis.
- Hypercalcaemia and hypergastrinaemia should be ruled out.

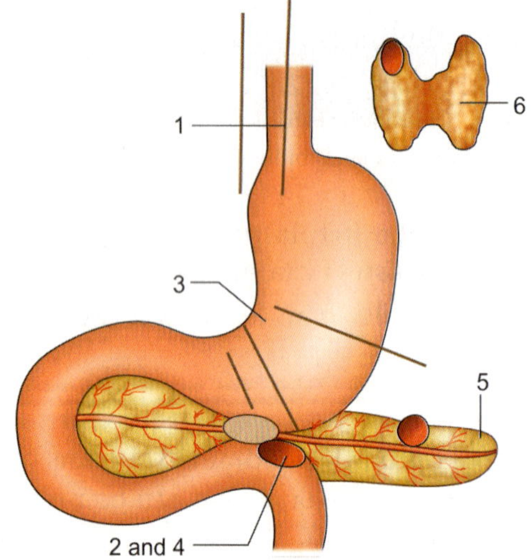


**Fig. 53.110:** Various causes of recurrent ulcer: 1. Incomplete vagotomy, 2. GJ alone, 3. Inadequate gastrectomy, 4. Narrow stoma, 5. Zollinger-Ellison syndrome, 6. Hyperparathyroidism

### Management (Table 53.12)

- Conservative treatment with $H_2$ receptor blockers is nearly always effective but relapse occurs, if they are stopped. Smoking should be stopped.
- However, definitive surgery is indicated in appropriate cases.

## ACUTE DILATATION OF STOMACH

### Aetiopathogenesis

1. Can occur after any operation, particularly splenectomy and pelvic procedures.
2. It can occur following fracture femur, application of plaster of Paris, etc. Malnutrition, excessive distension of the stomach due to ventilation, aerophagia are other precipitating factors.

There is a **sudden loss of sympathetic tone** resulting in massive dilatation of stomach. Improper Ryle's tube aspiration and permitting intake of oral fluids too early before paralytic ileus settles down are additional factors.

### Clinical Features

- History of surgery.
- **Hiccoughs**—due to irritation of under surface of the diaphragm, by the hugely distended stomach.
- Abdominal pain, vomiting, distension. Vomiting contains foul smelling dirty fluid and blood and is effortless.
- Features of shock. In untreated cases, can lead to cardiovascular collapse.
- **Effortless vomiting** of litres of dark watery fluid is characteristic of this condition.

### Treatment: Urgent resuscitation

- **Introduce a Ryle's tube and aspirate the stomach. It is the life-saving use of Ryle's tube** (Fig. 53.111).
- Rapid IV fluid replacement, with normal saline and dextrose saline. Both crystalloids and colloids may be necessary to treat the shock and electrolyte abnormalities.

**TABLE 53.12:** Management of recurrent ulcer

| Type of first surgery | | Corrective surgery |
|---|---|---|
| 1. GJ alone | ⟶ | Vagotomy |
| 2. Vagotomy + GJ (incomplete vagotomy) | ⟶ | Incomplete vagotomy is the cause. Usually posterior vagus is found and it has to be divided |
| 3. Vagotomy + GJ (complete vagotomy) | ⟶ | Stoma is not adequate. Partial gastrectomy is the ideal treatment |
| 4. Billroth partial gastrectomy | ⟶ | Vagotomy with or without revision gastrectomy |
| 5. HSV | ⟶ | Vagotomy + partial gastrectomy |

Fig. 53.111: Plain X-ray showing acute dilatation of the stomach. Ryle's tube insertion is a life-saving simple procedure in this condition

### Complications

- Pulmonary: In debilitated patients, aspiration may result in aspiration pneumonitis (Mendelson syndrome).
- It carries significant mortality.

## VOLVULUS OF THE STOMACH

- It is a rare condition in which stomach rotates in a horizontal (organoaxial) and vertical (mesentericoaxial) direction resulting in an acute abdomen.
- Organoaxial is more common.
- Many times, volvulus is intermittent.
- In general, initially the colon moves upwards and later greater curvature of the stomach.
- There is associated eventration of the diaphragm which also precipitates this condition (in children, congenital).
- In adults, diaphragmatic defects are more commonly traumatic or paraoesophageal herniation.
- Clinical features include epigastric pain, fullness and tenderness.

### Borchardt's Triad

1. Sudden, constant, severe upper abdominal pain
2. Recurrent retching with production of little vomitus
3. Inability to pass a nasogastric tube.

### Diagnosis

- Plain X-ray abdomen/chest: Gas-filled viscus.
- Barium meal can demonstrate twisted stomach.
- Upper GI scopy.

### Treatment

- Reduce the volvulus by dividing gastrocolic omentum.
- Fix the greater curvature of the stomach to the duodenojejunal flexure or perform a GJ without stoma.
- Repair of eventration.
- Fixing by tube gastrostomy can also be done.

## BEZOARS

- Bezoars are collections of **nondigestible materials,** usually of vegetable origin (phytobezoar) but also of hair (trichobezoar).
- **Trichobezoars** are concentrations of hair, generally found in long-haired girls or women who often deny eating their own hair (trichophagy) (Fig. 53.112).

### Causes

- **Phytobezoars** are most commonly found in patients who have undergone surgery of the stomach and have impaired gastric emptying.
- **Diabetics with autonomic neuropathy** patients are also at risk.

### Clinical Features and Diagnosis

- The symptoms of gastric bezoars include early satiety, weight loss, nausea, pain and vomiting due to **gastric outlet obstruction** with occasional gastric perforation and small bowel obstruction.
- **A large mass** may be palpable on physical examination and the diagnosis is confirmed by a barium examination or endoscopy.

### Treatment

- **Papain:** Enzymatic therapy to attempt dissolution of the bezoar.
  - Papain found in Adolph's Meat Tenderizer (AMT) is given in a dose of one teaspoon in 150 to 300 ml water several times daily.
  - The sodium concentration in AMT is high, so hypernatraemia may occur.
- **Cellulase** has been used with some success.

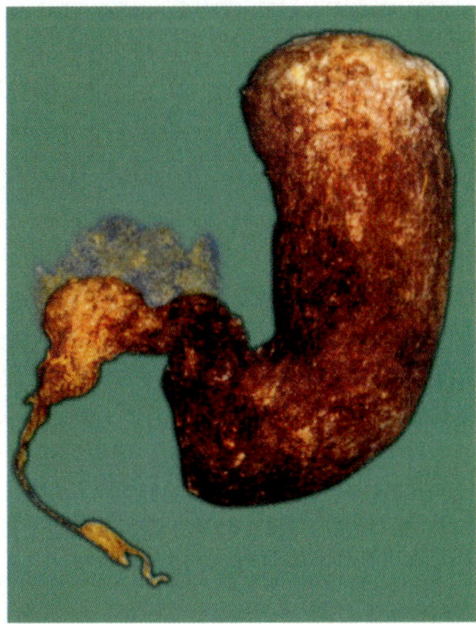

Fig. 53.112: Trichobezoar (*Courtesy*: Dr YV Krishna Rao, Professor of Surgery, Mamata Medical College and Hospital, Khammam, Andhra Pradesh)

- **Aggressive Ewald tube lavage or endoscopic fragmentation.**
- Failure of these therapies would necessitate surgical removal.

*Pearls of Wisdom*

Trichobezoars tend to form a cast of the stomach, with strands of hair having been observed as far distally as the transverse colon.

**SU28.8:** Describe and discuss the aetiology, clinical features, investigations and principles of management of congenital hypertrophic pyloric stenosis.

## IDIOPATHIC HYPERTROPHIC PYLORIC STENOSIS (IHPS)

### Aetiopathogenesis

- In this condition, there is **hypertrophy** involving the pyloric antral **circular muscle fibres**. Duodenum is normal (Fig. 53.113).
- The lumen is so much narrowed as to give rise to pyloric obstruction.
- Familial history can be obtained in a few patients.
- Prenatal incoordination of muscles, lack of nitric oxide relaxation of smooth muscles may be some factors responsible for IHPS.
- Risk factors in babies include birth by preterm birth, cesarean section, bottle feeding, and being first born male.

### Clinical Features

- **Incidence:** 1–2/1000 births. First born male child is affected very often. The child is normal at birth and the symptoms appear around 6–8 weeks.
- First symptom is **vomiting**. It is **projectile**, forcible, does not contain bile. A visible gastric peristalsis (VGP) can be seen especially when the mother feeds the child (Fig. 53.114).
- Loss of weight—dehydration.
- Constipation and oliguria are the features.
- *Per* abdomen—hypertrophied thickened pylorus can be felt as a mass in the right hypochondrium—'Olive like mass' (in adults with pyloric stenosis due to chronic duodenal ulcer, no mass is felt—Fig. 53.113).

Classic triad of IHPS is (projectile vomiting, palpable olive and visible peristalsis).

### Ultrasound

- Long axis view of pylorus demonstrates 'cervix' sign.
- Short axis view of pylorus demonstrates 'target' sign.

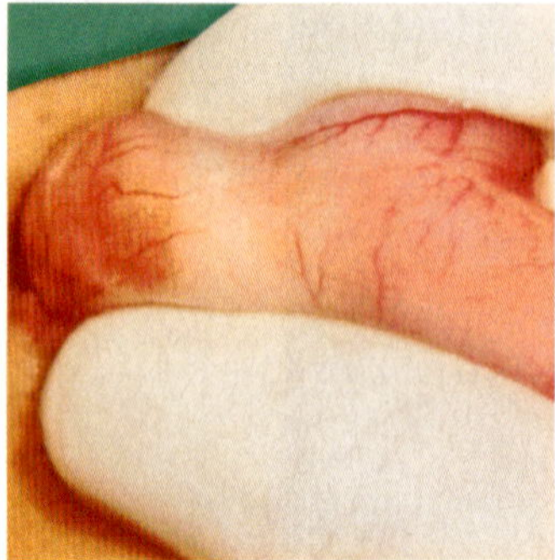

**Fig. 53.113:** Hypertrophied pylorus

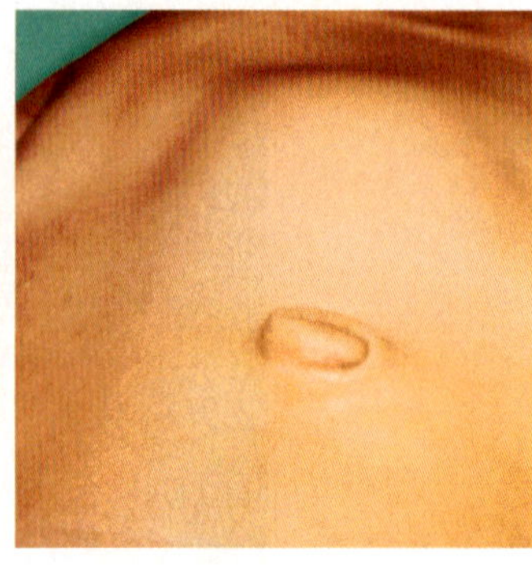

**Fig. 53.114:** Visible gastric peristalsis

- When muscle thickness is more than 7–15 mm size and pyloric canal length is 20–25 mm, it is diagnostic.

### Treatment

- Correction of dehydration and electrolyte disturbance by intravenous half normal saline must always precede surgery.
- **Ramstedt's pyloromyotomy** is the surgical treatment (Figs 53.115 to 53.118).
- Laparotomy is done and an incision is made through the serosa. It then cuts through the circular muscle fibres till all the muscle fibres are divided and the mucosa bulges out.
- Avoid injury to the mucosa. If mucosa is opened, it is sutured and reinforced by using omentum.

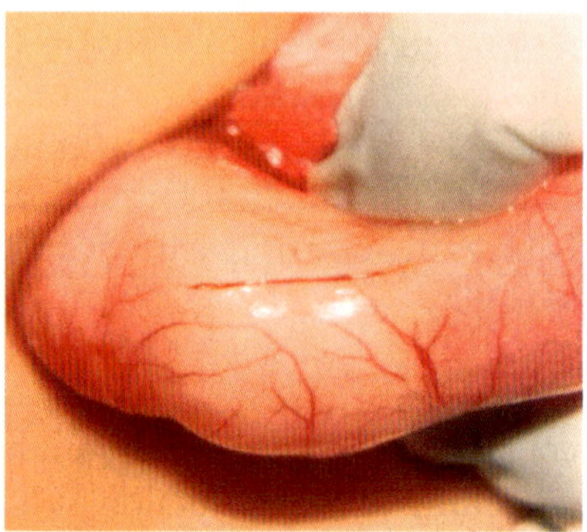

**Fig. 53.115:** Pyloromyotomy incision

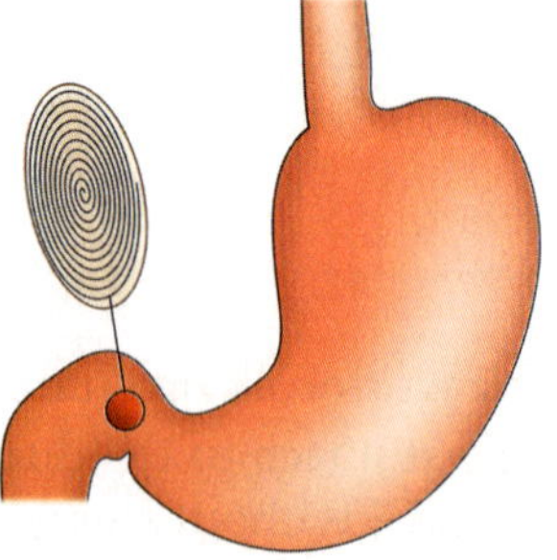

**Fig. 53.116:** Pyloric mass

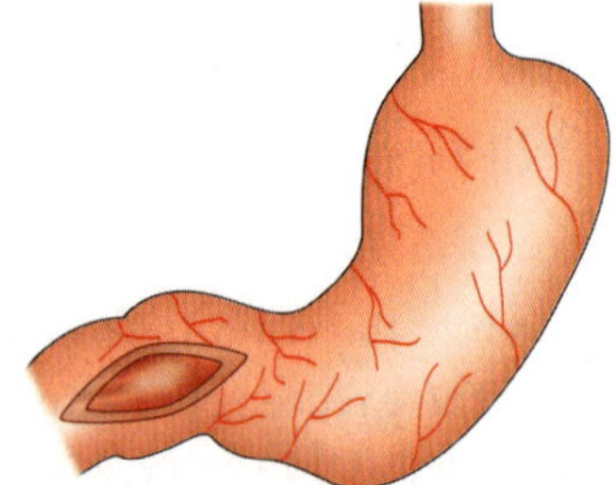

**Fig. 53.117:** Ramstedt's pyloromyotomy

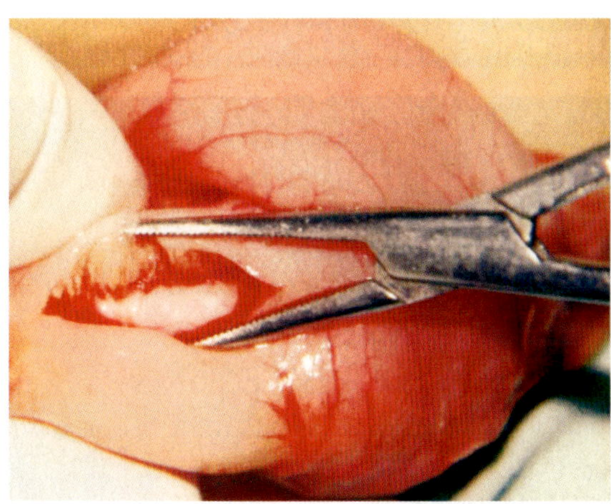

Fig. 53.118: Ramstedt's pyloromyotomy being done (*Courtesy*: Prof Vijaykumar, Head, Department of Paediatric Surgery, KMC, Manipal)

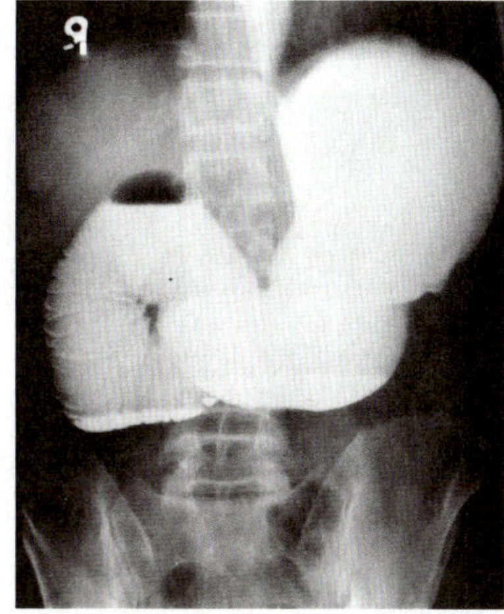

Fig. 53.119: Duodenal obstruction resulting in gross dilatation of duodenum—need for duodenojejunostomy than gastro-jejunostomy in these cases

## CHRONIC DUODENAL ILEUS

- It is also called superior mesenteric artery (SMA) syndrome, **Wilkie's disease or arteriomesenteric compression** (Figs 53.119 and 53.120). The third part of the duodenum is compressed between vertebral column and superior mesenteric vessels. Acute loss of fat and immobilisation with cast precipitates this disease. Hence, it is also called cast syndrome. Normal angle between superior mesenteric artery and aorta is 38–56°. Due to loss of fat or due to abnormal origin of the SMA, when the angle reduces to 6–25°, SMA syndrome occurs (for risk factor—*see* Key Box 53.29).
- In this condition, duodenum is dilated up to the 3rd part with obstruction to the 3rd or 4th part of duodenum (Fig. 53.119).
- Patients present with features of gastric outlet obstruction but vomitus contains bile—'Food Fear'.
- Abdominal pain is not severe as in intestinal obstruction but on careful questioning, history of true nature of spasmodic pain is obtained.
- This condition is often misdiagnosed.
- Barium meal demonstrates the obstruction—dilated stomach and duodenum.
- Duodenojejunostomy is the treatment of choice (Fig. 53.121).

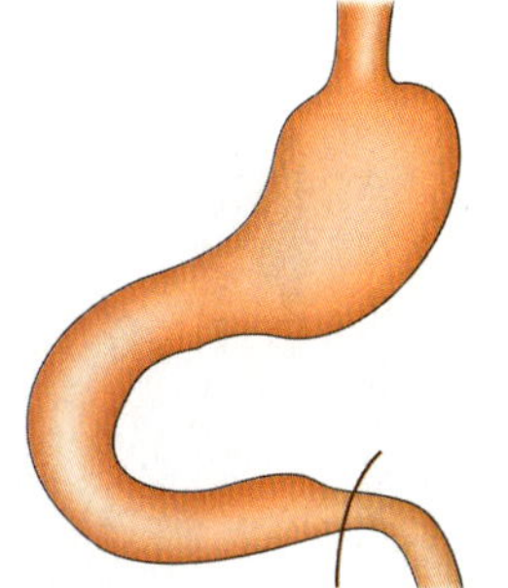

Fig. 53.120: Wilkie's disease—superior mesenteric artery syndrome

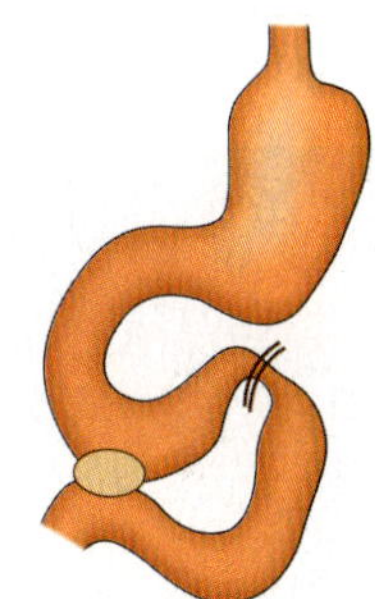

Fig. 53.121: Duodeno-jejunostomy

Key Box 53.29

**Risk Factors for SMA Syndrome**

- **A**sthenic and tall—thin and tall body build—aorto-mesenteric angle is narrow (congenital)
- **B**urns—prolonged bed rest → loss of weight
- **C**achexia, catabolic phases, cast application
- **D**uodenal insertion is high at ligament of Treitz
- **E**maciation, malnutrition
- **F**emales twice as susceptible
- **G**ut malrotation/poor motility of the gut
- **H**yperextension of spine. Lumbar lordosis

**ABCDEFGH** of SMA syndrome

### Differential Diagnosis

1. **Pyloric stenosis:** In this condition, vomitus does not contain bile. Barium meal X-ray shows distended stomach. Duodenum is not seen.
2. **Annular pancreas:** Rarely, it can present in adults with obstruction to the second part of the duodenum. Vomitus may contain bile. Barium meal X-ray shows dilatation of the first part and also the second part of the duodenum.
3. **Tuberculosis of lymph nodes** can compress the 3rd part of the duodenum and can mimic Wilkie's disease.

What is nutcracker syndrome?[1]

[1]Nutcracker syndrome is the entrapment of right renal vein between abdominal aorta and the SMA.

## IMAGES OF A 24-YEAR-OLD FEMALE WITH SMA SYNDROME (Figs 53.122 to 53.126)

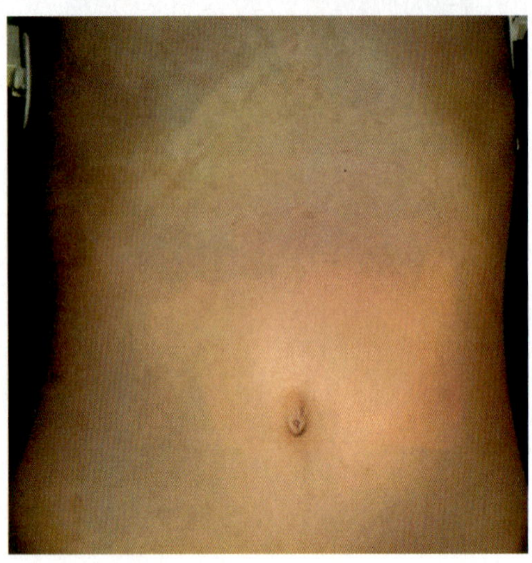

**Fig. 53.122:** A 24-year-old thin female patient presented with persistent bilious vomiting

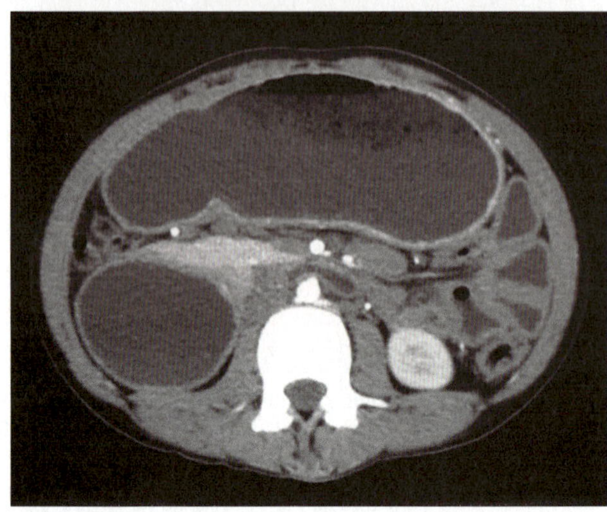

**Fig. 53.123:** CT scan revealed hugely dilated second part of the duodenum and stomach

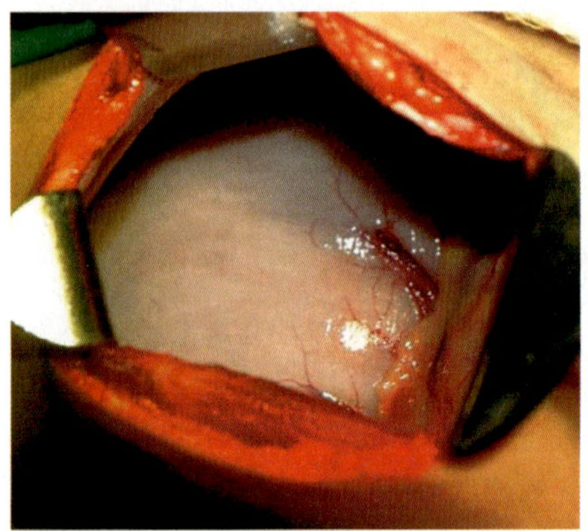

**Fig. 53.124:** At surgery, stomach was grossly distended with prominent vasculature

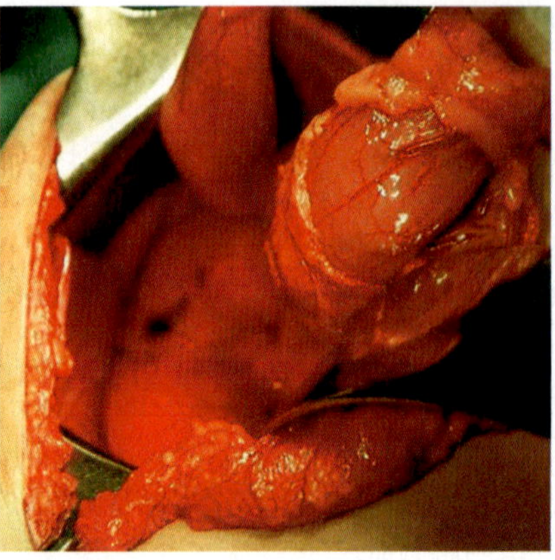

**Fig. 53.125:** You can see distended first and second part of the duodenum

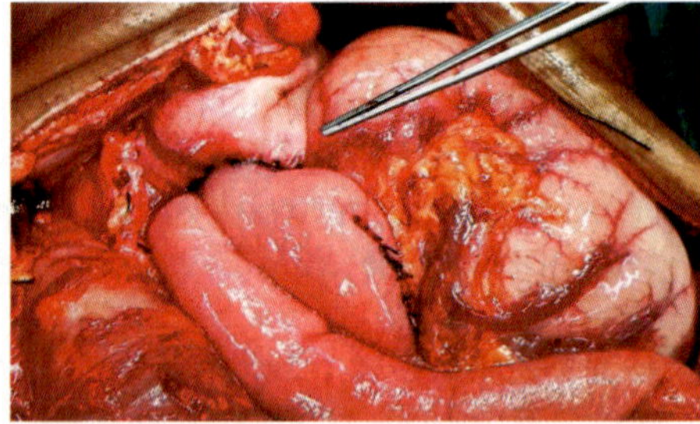

**Fig. 53.126:** Duodenojejunostomy is done in this patient (*Courtesy*: Dr SS Prasad, Dr Rajendra Benakatti, Dr Keerthan Kumar, Department of Surgery, KMC, Manipal)

## DUODENAL ANATOMY AND OBSTRUCTION

- There are many causes of duodenal obstruction in children.
- In adults, important causes are given in Table 53.13.

  **1st part:** Postbulbar ulcer with stenosis.

  **2nd part:** Two causes:

  1. Annular pancreas in adults
  2. Carcinoma head of pancreas

  **3rd part:** Three causes:

  1. Carcinoma head of pancreas
  2. Arteriomesenteric compression
  3. Tuberculosis/metastatic nodes causing compression of the 3rd part of duodenum. Most common cause of duodenal obstruction in adults is carcinoma pancreas.

  **4th part:** Carcinoma pancreas (Fig. 53.127).

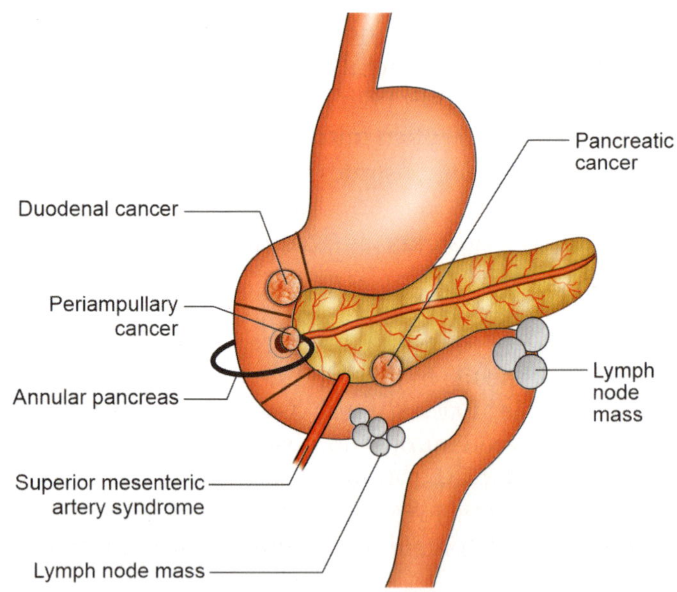



**Fig. 53.127:** Causes of duodenal obstruction

Section V • Gastrointestinal Surgery

**TABLE 53.13:** Anatomy of duodenum and surgical importance

| Parts | Development | Length | Relationships | Blood supply | Surgical importance |
|---|---|---|---|---|---|
| 1st part | Foregut | 2 inches | • Gallbladder<br>• Liver<br>• Bile duct<br>• Portal vein | • Superior pancreaticoduodenal<br>• Supraduodenal artery of Wilkie | • Perforation of 1st part (causes peritonitis)<br>• Injury to duodenum in laparoscopic cholecystectomy |
| 2nd part | • Foregut above ampulla of Vater<br>• Midgut below ampulla of Vater | 3 inches | Right lobe of liver transverse colon anteriorly and kidney, renal vessels posteriorly | | • Perforation of 2nd part manifests late because it is retroperitoneal<br>• Injury to duodenum in right hemicolectomy |
| 3rd part | Midgut | 4 inches | • Retroperitoneal fixed<br>• Anteriorly crossed by superior mesenteric vessels<br>• Posteriorly related to inferior vena cava | Inferior pancreaticoduodenal artery | Careful separation of mesenteric vessels from duodenum during pancreaticoduodenectomy |
| 4th part | Midgut | 1 inches | • Anteriorly by transverse colon<br>• Superiorly body of pancreas | Inferior pancreaticoduodenal artery | 4th part continues as duodenojejunal (DJ) flexure. It is an important landmark to identify first loop of jejunum during gastrojejunostomy |

## OBESITY, BARIATRIC AND METABOLIC SURGERY (Fig. 53.128)

### Introduction

Obesity is a chronic, complex disease that negatively affects one's health. It is characterized by excess fat in the body, which occurs when calorie consumption is significantly higher than calorie expenditure. Body mass index (BMI), which is measured in kg/m$^2$, is used to classify patient's weight. Morbid obesity (BMI >35 kg/m$^2$) may be associated with comorbidities, such as diabetes mellitus, hypertension, coronary artery disease, osteoarthritis, sleep apnoea, etc., which reduce life expectancy. Bariatric surgery is often performed to reduce excess body weight and is known as metabolic surgery when primarily carried out to manage associated comorbidities.

### Aetiology and Pathophysiology

The aetiology of obesity is multifactorial and occurs due to causes like a sedentary lifestyle, a familial tendency, environmental factors, psychosocial behaviour, a few medical conditions (e.g. Cushing's syndrome, hypothyroidism), and congenital diseases (e.g. Prader–Willi syndrome). An elevated BMI is associated with increased leptin levels. Obesity can affect any age and is becoming increasingly prevalent among children and adolescents. India has emerged as the third most obese nation after USA and China due to its socioeconomic changes. Obesity affects almost every organ of the body and causes many diseases that result in significant morbidity and mortality.

### Management of Obesity

Medically treatable causes for obesity should be evaluated by appropriate tests. If no cause is established, a trial of diet and exercise with behavioural changes should be prescribed. If this also fails, bariatric surgery should be considered after proper counselling. Patients with a BMI ≥35 kg/m$^2$ with comorbidities should be considered for surgery. Laparoscopic surgery is currently the standard of care, and robotic bariatric surgery is also sometimes adopted.

### Types of Bariatric Surgery

1. Restrictive procedure, e.g. laparoscopic adjustable gastric banding (LAGB) and laparoscopic sleeve gastrectomy (LSG)—this largely restricts food intake.
2. Restrictive procedures with some malabsorption: Roux-en-Y gastric bypass (RYGB), one anastomosis gastric bypass or mini gastric bypass (OAGB or MGB)—this restricts food intake and causes some malabsorption.
3. Malabsorptive procedures with some restriction: Biliopancreatic diversion (BPD), duodenal switch

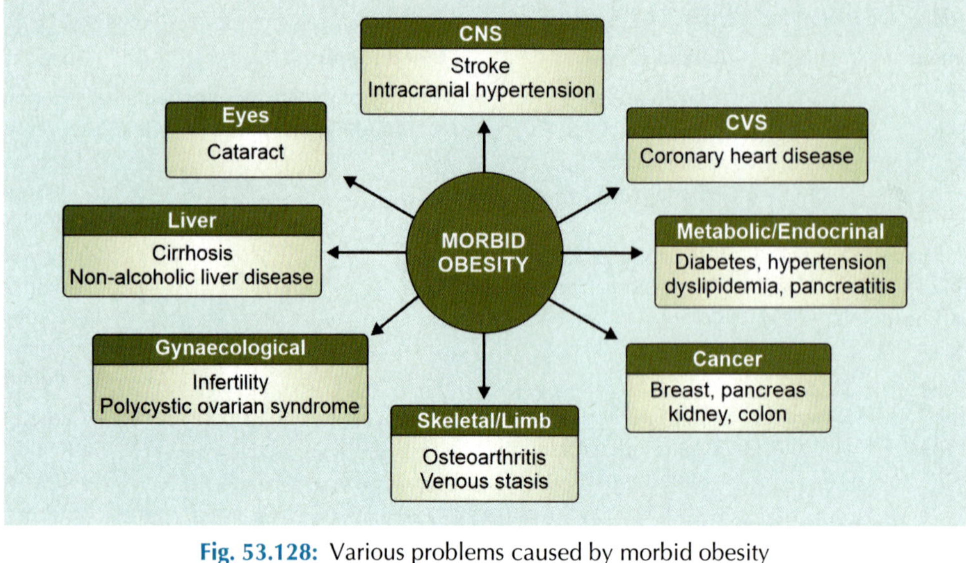


**Fig. 53.128:** Various problems caused by morbid obesity

(DS)—this causes severe malabsorption with less food restriction and is rarely performed in India.

## Indications for Bariatric Surgery

1. BMI >40 kg/m$^2$ or BMI >35 kg/m$^2$ with associated medical comorbidity.
2. Failed dietary therapy with above BMI levels.
3. Psychiatrically stable without substance abuse.
4. Knowledgeable about the operation to be performed and its sequelae.
5. Motivated individual.
6. Age >18 years and <70 years.

## Contraindications for Bariatric Surgery

I. **Medical:** Cirrhosis with portal hypertension, autoimmune connective tissue disorders, inflammatory bowel disease (IBD), chronic administration of steroids, poor fitness for general anaesthesia.

II. **Surgical:** Inability to ambulate, Prader–Willi syndrome (congenital obesity syndrome with severe hyperphagia, growth-hormone deficiency, hypogonadism, dysmorphic features, and cognitive impairment).

## Details of Surgery

1. **Laparoscopic RYGB** (Fig. 53.129): Gastric bypass, which was first described by Mason and Ito in 1969, incorporates a loop of jejunum anastomosed to a proximal gastric pouch. However, loop gastric bypass may result in bile reflux. To overcome this disadvantage, RYGB was developed, and it has now become one of the most commonly performed bariatric surgeries.
   - The roux limb should be at least 75 cm, and the biliopancreatic limb should be 100–150 cm.

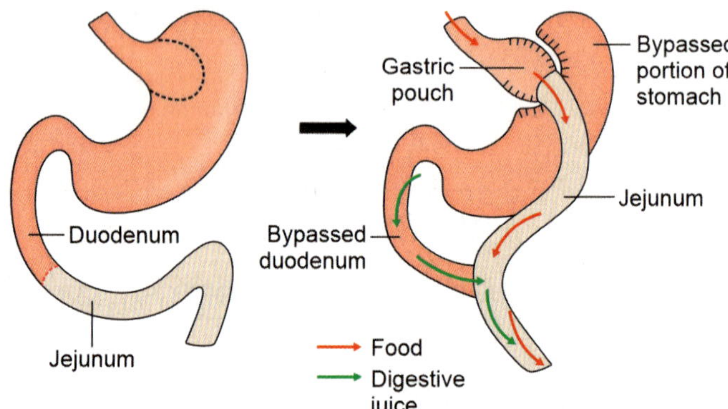


**Fig. 53.129:** Roux-en-Y gastric bypass (RYGB)

   - Enteroenterostomy (jejunum) is performed to prevent stenosis or obstruction.
   - All potential spaces for internal hernias should be closed using nonabsorbable sutures.
   - A small proximal gastric pouch (15–20 ml) should be constructed from the cardia of the stomach to prevent dilation and to minimize acid production.
   - The gastric pouch should be divided from the distal part of the stomach.
2. **Laparoscopic sleeve gastrectomy** (Fig. 53.130): It is widely practiced worldwide due to its simplicity. A narrow gastric sleeve is fashioned over a gastric calibration tube by stapling the stomach vertically, and the resected stomach is removed.
3. **One anastomosis gastric bypass or mini gastric bypass (OAGB or MGB)** (Fig. 53.131): This is a type of gastric bypass in which 150–200 cm of the jejunum is bypassed by anastomosing it to a long, narrow gastric pouch.

## Complications of Bariatric Surgery

a. **Staple line/anastomotic leaks:** These may be lethal, if not recognized early. The leak rate is high in the initial

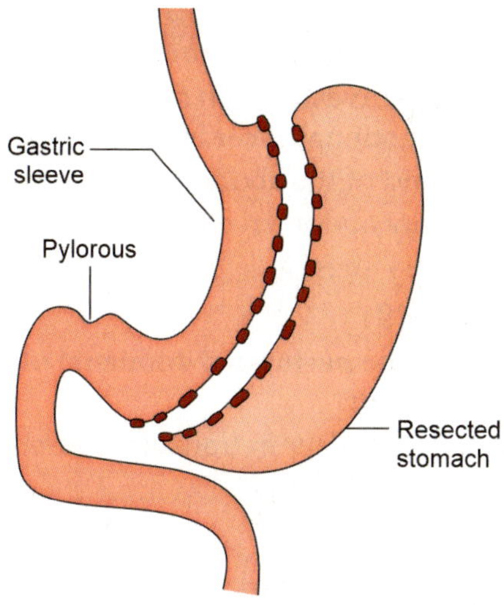


Fig. 53.130: Laparoscopic sleeve gastrectomy

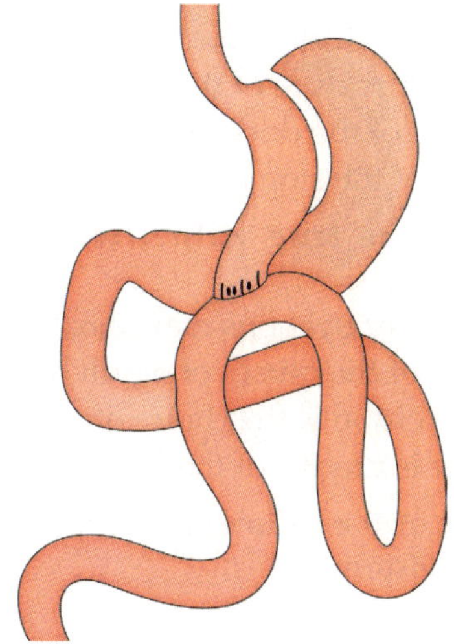

Fig. 53.131: One anastomosis gastric bypass or mini gastric bypass (OAGB or MGB)

period. More recent studies report anastomotic leak rates of 0.35–0.5%.

b. **DVT (deep vein thrombosis) and pulmonary embolism:** Obese individuals are prone to DVT. However, this has become uncommon with chemoprophylaxis and early mobilization.
c. **Nutritional deficiency:** Various nutritional deficiencies may occur due to severe food restriction and malabsorption, if the patient is not taking the required daily dose of additional nutritional supplements and adequate proteins.
d. **Bowel obstruction after Roux-en-Y gastric bypass (RYGB):** It occurs due to the potential for internal hernias, which commonly occurs after laparoscopic RYGB and is estimated to be between 3 and 4.5%. Two potential locations: (A) Petersen's space: It is the space caused by the herniation of intestinal loops through the defect between the small bowel limbs, the transverse mesocolon, and the retroperitoneum after RYGB. (B) Jejunojejunostomy mesenteric defect.
e. **Marginal ulcer:** It occurs in 2–10% of cases who undergo gastric bypass surgery. It may lead to perforation, stricture formation, or gastric pouch outlet obstruction, which will require endoscopic dilation, if it is not treated promptly.

## Recent Advances

Certain endoscopic procedures, such as gastric balloon and endoscopic sleeve gastroplasty, are being tried to limit food intake. The use of appetite suppressants or drugs that limit food absorption cannot be taken for long time without adverse effects. Research is now directed towards the role of altering gut microbiota to manage obesity.

## FURTHER READING

1. ASMBS Textbook of Bariatric Surgery.
2. www.theossi.com—Bariatric Surgery.

## MULTIPLE CHOICE QUESTIONS

1. **Regarding duodenum following are true, *except*:**
   A. Lined by mucus-secreting columnar epithelium
   B. Brunner's glands are present
   C. Duodenum can produce cholecystokinin
   D. Duodenum will not secrete secretin
2. **Following are true regarding blood supply of the stomach, *except*:**
   A. The fundus is supplied by left gastric artery
   B. Left gastric artery is a branch of coeliac axis
   C. Right gastroepiploic artery runs along greater curvature of the stomach
   D. Gastroduodenal artery is a branch of hepatic artery
3. **Duodenal ulcer commonly occurs in which part of duodenum?**
   A. First part B. Second part
   C. Third part D. Fourth part
4. **Following are true for *Helicobacter pylori* bacteria, *except*:**
   A. It is spiral shaped
   B. It hydrolyses urea
   C. It can produce cytotoxins
   D. Mostly, it is associated with type A gastritis
5. **Following are true for duodenal ulcer, *except*:**
   A. It occurs in the first part of the duodenum
   B. It may be associated with type B gastritis
   C. Smoking may precipitate development of ulcer
   D. It can erode branches of left gastric artery and result in massive bleeding
6. **Following are true for malignancy in a gastric ulcer, *except*:**
   A. It occurs rarely
   B. Occurs in the lesser curvature of the stomach
   C. It produces a notch in barium studies
   D. Converging rugosity is lost
7. **Most important cause of duodenal stump leakage after Billroth II gastrectomy is:**
   A. Efferent loop obstruction
   B. Oedema of the stump
   C. Kinking of the afferent loop
   D. Fat necrosis
8. **About truncal vagotomy which one of the following is not correct?**
   A. Decreases acid secretion
   B. Decreases parasympathetic activity
   C. Increases gallstones
   D. Increases constipation
9. **More accurate investigation for the diagnosis of the perforated duodenal ulcer is:**
   A. Ultrasound of the abdomen
   B. Plain X-ray abdomen erect position
   C. Plain X-ray chest
   D. CT imaging
10. **Treatment of the perforated duodenal ulcer include following, *except*:**
    A. Suturing the ulcer in transverse direction
    B. Truncal vagotomy
    C. Peritoneal toilet
    D. Omental patch
11. **The most common site of bleeding from peptic ulcer is:**
    A. Lesser curvature of the stomach
    B. Greater curvature of the stomach
    C. First part of the duodenum
    D. Fundus of the stomach
12. **Following are true with Dieulafoy's lesion, *except*:**
    A. It is an arteriovenous malformation
    B. It is one of the causes of occult bleeding
    C. Local excision is the choice of treatment
    D. The site is fundus of the stomach
13. **Which one of the following is the complication of gastrojejunostomy?**
    A. Gallstones
    B. Duodenal blow out
    C. Intussusception
    D. Diarrhoea
14. **Following are complications of vagotomy, *except*:**
    A. Diarrhoea
    B. Gallstones
    C. Achlorhydria
    D. Carcinoma stomach
15. **Hypochloraemic alkalosis in pyloric stenosis is treated by:**
    A. Normal saline
    B. Ringer lactate
    C. Isotonic saline with potassium
    D. Double strength saline
16. ***H. pylori* is an important factor for carcinoma stomach in which region?**
    A. Distal
    B. Proximal
    C. Body
    D. Gastro-oesophageal junction

**17. Which one of the following is not a risk factor for proximal carcinoma stomach?**
A. Chronic gastric ulcer
B. *H. pylori* induced gastritis
C. Pernicious anaemia
D. Obesity

**18. Which one of the following is not a feature of early gastric cancer?**
A. Confined to mucosa
B. Confined to mucosa and submucosa
C. Confined to mucosa with lymph nodes
D. Involving muscularis

**19. Following are features of gastrointestinal stromal tumours (GISTs) of the stomach, *except*:**
A. Stomach is the most common site of GIST
B. More than 5 cm size tumour is considered to have malignant potential
C. Wedge excision is the treatment of choice for small lesions
D. Always do lymphadenectomy with wedge excision

**20. Which one of the following features is false for gastrointestinal stromal tumour (GIST)?**
A. It is arising from mesenchymal tissue
B. Associated with tyrosine kinase C-kit oncogene
C. They are sensitive to tyrosine kinase antagonist imatinib
D. Lymph node spread is very common

**21. All are true for hormone ghrelin, *except*:**
A. Produced by gastric antrum
B. It is a hunger hormone
C. It stimulates growth hormone
D. It is produced by oxyntic glands

**22. About Roux-en-Y gastric bypass following are true, *except*:**
A. It is the most common procedure done now
B. It prevents bile reflux
C. It allows endoscopic examination of gastric fundus
D. Obilteration of Peterson's space is also a part of the procedure

**Answers**

| | | | | | | | | | |
|---|---|---|---|---|---|---|---|---|---|
| **1.** D | **2.** A | **3.** A | **4.** D | **5.** D | **6.** C | **7.** C | **8.** D | **9.** D | **10.** B |
| **11.** C | **12.** D | **13.** C | **14.** D | **15.** C | **16.** A | **17.** B | **18.** D | **19.** D | **20.** D |
| **21.** A | **22.** C | | | | | | | | |

Chapter 54

# Gallbladder and Pancreas

- Surgical anatomy
- Physiology
- Congenital anomalies
- Gallstones disease
- Acute cholecystitis
- Chronic cholecystitis
- Obstructive jaundice
- Stricture of CBD
- Choledochal cyst
- Caroli's disease
- Chronic pancreatitis
- Cholangiocarcinoma
- Congenital biliary atresia
- Carcinoma of gallbladder
- Carcinoma of pancreas
- Endocrine tumours
- Acute pancreatitis
- Pseudocyst
- Annular pancreas
- Ectopic pancreas
- Cystic fibrosis
- Pancreatic divisum
- Pancreatic fistula
- White bile
- Pancreatic ascites

## INTRODUCTION

- One may wonder why gallbladder and pancreas are discussed together!! Yes, biliary tract (gallbladder is an important part of that) ends after joining with pancreatic duct by opening into 2nd part of duodenum.
- Gallstones, when they block/pass through ampulla of Vater, produce acute pancreatitis.
- An important surgical condition—surgical jaundice or obstructive jaundice can be discussed better only if you know gallbladder and pancreas.
- Any surgery involving sphincter of Oddi in the form of sphincteroplasty/or removal (as in Whipple's pancreaticoduodenectomy), the gallbladder does not function and hence it needs to be removed.
- Embryologically, liver, biliary tree, ventral pancreas, gallbladder—all developed from a diverticulum on the ventral aspect of the foregut of the embryo.
- And gallbladder will be palpable in most of the cases of periampullary/carcinoma head of the pancreas.

> **SU28.1:** Describe the applied anatomy of biliary system. Describe the clinical features, investigations and principles of management of diseases of biliary system.

## SURGICAL ANATOMY OF THE GALLBLADDER AND BILE DUCTS

Gallbladder is a pear- or globular-shaped organ present in the right hypochondrium on the inferior surface of the liver, situated in the gallbladder fossa. It is about 8–12 cm long.

- **Fundus:** It is the dilated portion of the gallbladder adherent to undersurface of liver from which it can be separated easily.
- **Neck:** The narrow angulated distal portion of the neck is called ***Hartmann's pouch***—common site where stones occur and tend to stay for a long time (also called infundibulum of gallbladder) (Fig. 54.1).
- **Gallbladder** drains into the common bile duct (CBD) through ***cystic duct***, which is 3 cm long. It is lined by cuboidal epithelium. There are prominent mucosal folds within the cystic duct due to the presence of prominent circular muscle fibres underneath. Its lumen is usually 1–3 mm in diameter. Contraction of gallbladder produces a functional valve called ***valve of Heister*** which prevents the migration of stone into the CBD. The wall of cystic duct is surrounded by a sphincter structure called ***sphincter of Lutkens***. A spiral fold keeps cystic duct open for drainage of bile.

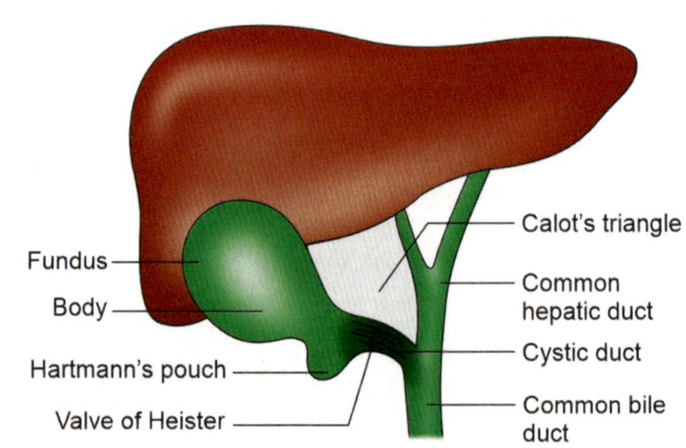


**Fig. 54.1:** Surgical anatomy of the gallbladder

### Cholecystohepatic Triangle or Calot's Triangle Boundaries

- **Lateral:** Cystic duct and gallbladder
- **Medial:** Common hepatic duct
- **Above:** Inferior surface of right lobe of the liver.

Calot's triangle is dissected free of all tissue except for the cystic duct and artery, and the base of the liver bed is exposed—**the critical view of safety—Strasberg et al** during cholecystectomy.

### Contents

- Right hepatic artery and its branch, the cystic artery
- Cystic lymph node of Lund.

### Blood Supply of Gallbladder

Cystic artery, a branch of right hepatic artery, arises behind the common bile duct. Soon, it branches out over the surface of gallbladder. ***Cystic artery is an end artery*** (Fig. 54.2). Multiple small veins from the surface of gallbladder join the liver surface. There is also a cystic vein, from the neck of gallbladder draining into portal vein directly. This explains early spread of gallbladder malignancy to the liver.

### Lymphatics

1. Subserosal and submucosal lymph nodes drain into *cystic lymph node of Lund* and from here they drain into nodes in the hilum of liver and coeliac nodes.
2. **Subserosal lymphatic vessels** of gallbladder are also connected to **subcapsular lymph channels** of liver, which accounts for frequent spread of carcinoma gallbladder to the liver.

### Anatomy of the Bile Ducts

- **Common hepatic duct (CHD)** is formed by the union of right and left hepatic ducts. It is 3 cm long, receives cystic duct and continues as common bile duct (CBD).
- **Common bile duct** is about 8 cm long. It has four parts: Supraduodenal, retroduodenal, infraduodenal and intraduodenal. Along with pancreatic duct, it forms ampulla of Vater. Controlled by sphincter of Oddi, it ends by an opening into the second part of duodenum (Fig. 54.3).

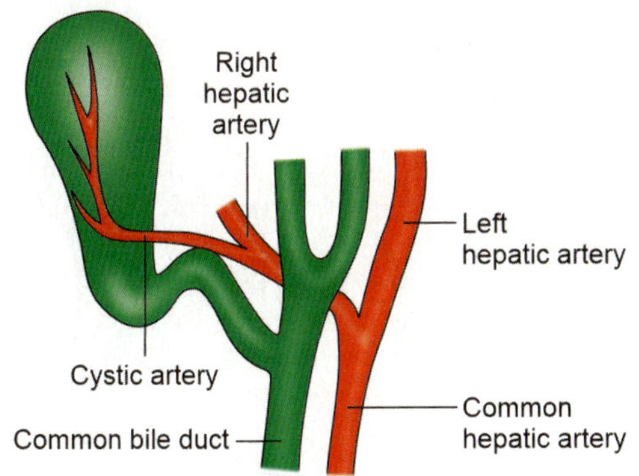


Fig. 54.2: Blood supply of the gallbladder

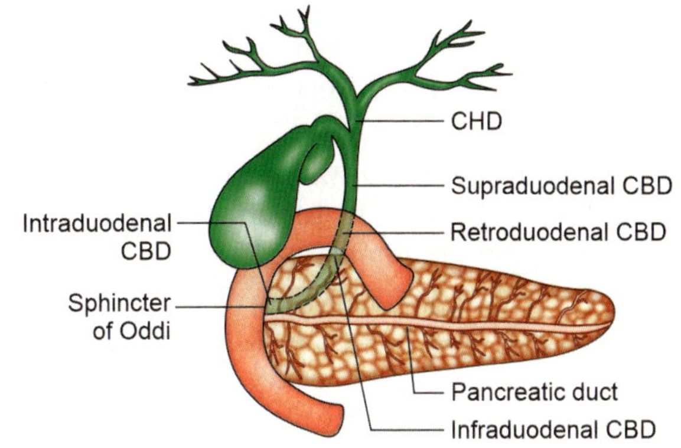


Fig. 54.3: Surgical anatomy of the bile ducts. Note how close gallbladder is to the duodenum (chances of injury in laparoscopic cholecystectomy)

## PHYSIOLOGY

### Functions of the Gallbladder

- **Reservoir for bile:** Bile excreted by the liver is stored in the gallbladder as total of about 500 to 1000 ml per day. At fasting, the tone of sphincter of Oddi is high. Food contents in the duodenum stimulates release of cholecystokinin, which causes gallbladder to contract.
- **Concentration:** Bile is 98% water. Due to active absorption of water, sodium chloride and bicarbonate, bile gets concentrated 5–10 times. Thus, a relative increase in bile salts, bile pigments, cholesterol and calcium occurs.
- **Mucus secretion:** It secretes about 20 ml mucus per day. Obstruction to the cystic duct causes mucocele of the gallbladder.

### Bile

- Secreted from hepatocytes.
- pH is more than 7.0.
- 500–1000 ml/day, 98% is water.
- Concentrated in gallbladder because of absorption of water. Capacity of gallbladder is 40–50 ml.
- Fatty food stimulation releases cholecystokinin, which stimulates gallbladder to contract and at the same time, sphincter of Oddi to relax.
- It also has inorganic ions (more than plasma) and hence, severe electrolyte imbalance is seen in biliary fistula.
- Cholesterol, synthesised in the liver, gives rise to bile acids—cholic and chenodeoxycholic acids. They are metabolised in the colon to deoxycholic acid and lithocholic acids.
- Main function of bile acids in the bile is to maintain cholesterol in solution.

## CONGENITAL ANOMALIES OF GALLBLADDER

**Absence of gallbladder:** Very rare; other variations include (Fig. 54.4):

A. **Floating gallbladder:** Results due to long mesentery. It is more vulnerable to torsion—a rare cause of recurrent upper abdominal pain. Such a gallbladder can be easily removed.

B. **Phrygian cap:** Cap which was worn by people of Phrygia (ancient Asian country, Mongolia). It is an anomaly connected with the fundus of the gallbladder.

C. **Double gallbladder:** The second one is always intrahepatic (rare).

D. **Absence of cystic duct:** Cholecystectomy becomes difficult. There are high chances of injury to the common bile duct.

E. **Low insertion of cystic duct:** Cystic duct opens into the common bile duct near the ampulla. This anomaly should be kept in mind when operating on cases of obstructive jaundice.

F. **An accessory or aberrant cholecystohepatic duct** is present in about 10% of the patients. It may be the cause of significant bile leakage after cholecystectomy. It is the segmental duct that joins biliary system outside the liver instead of within it.

G. Diverticulum of gallbladder

H. Cystic duct joining right hepatic duct

I. **Anomalies of blood supply**

1. Very, very tortuous hepatic artery: Caterpillar turn or Moynihan's hump. It runs in front of the origin of cystic duct.
2. Cystic artery is given anteriorly from right hepatic artery.

## BILIRUBIN METABOLISM

Quick summary of relevant bilirubin metabolism has been depicted in Fig. 54.5. For more details students can refer physiology books.

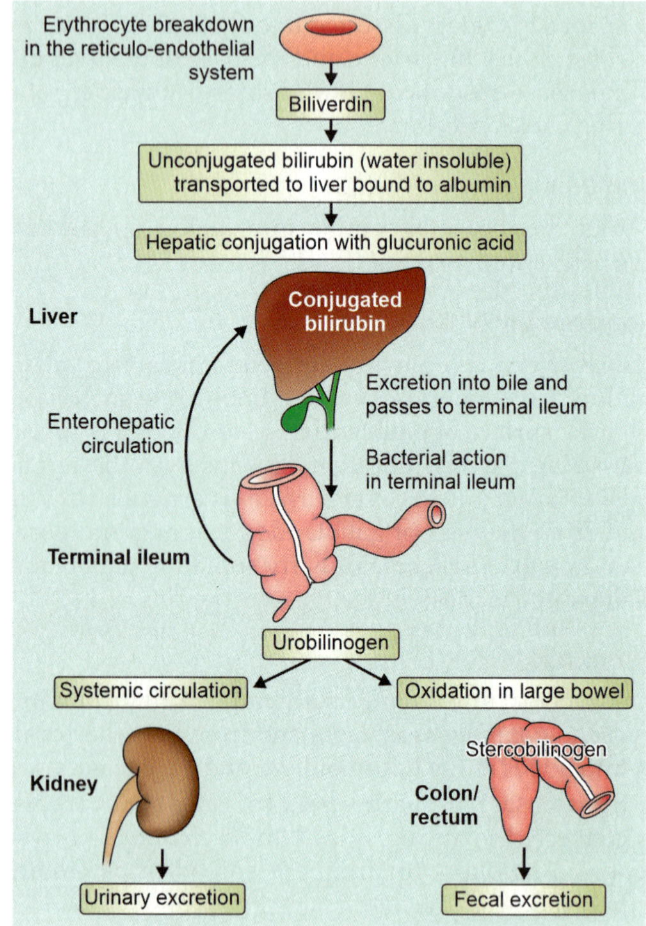


**Fig. 54.5:** Bilirubin metabolism

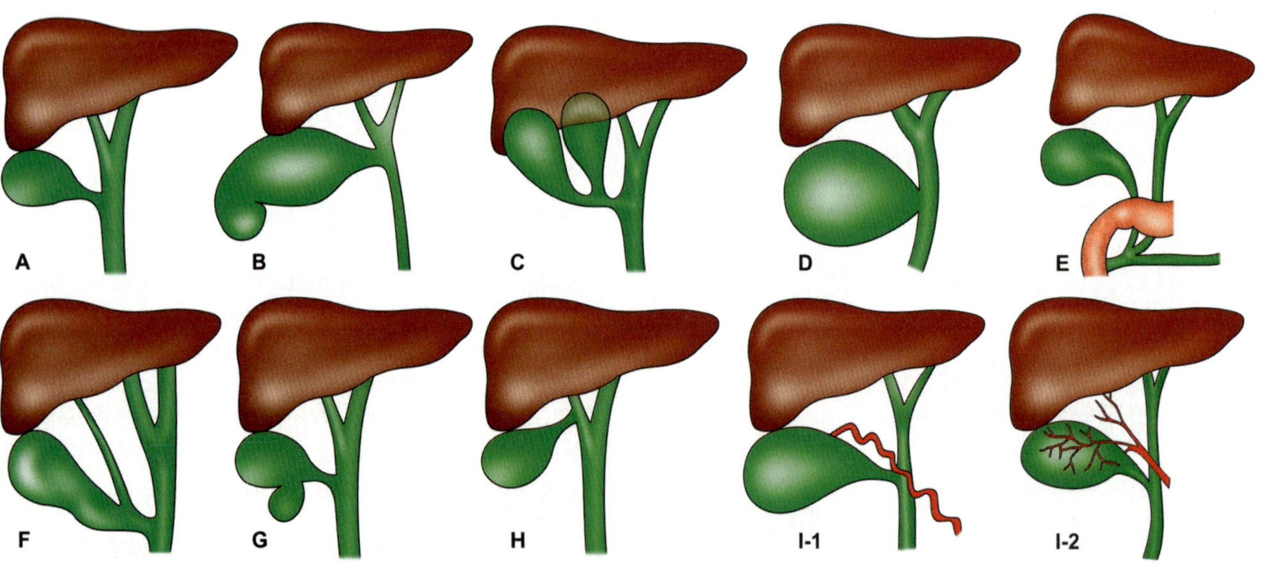


**Fig. 54.4:** Congenital anomalies of the gallbladder (*see* text A to I)

## GALLSTONE DISEASE (CHOLELITHIASIS)

### Aetiology

#### 1. Metabolic Causes

- Cholesterol is produced from the liver, which gives rise to bile acids. Cholesterol is insoluble and it must be transported within the bile salt micelles and phospholipid (lecithin) vesicles. Normal ratio of bile acids: cholesterol is 25:1 (Fig. 54.6).
- This ratio is necessary to maintain the cholesterol in liquid form by forming micelles. When the ratio drops down to 13:1 (which is called critical ratio), cholesterol crystals will nucleate and stones will form.
- Obesity, high calorie diet and medications which increase cholesterol secretion can result in stone formation.

#### 2. Infection

- It is the most common cause responsible for a gallstone in 80% of patients. Sources of infection are tonsils, tooth, bowel, etc.
- Organisms such as *E. coli, Proteus*, anaerobic organisms, streptococci, etc. reach the gallbladder wall through the bloodstream and form a focus/nidus around which cholesterol and bile salts get precipitated.
- Over a period of many years, this results in a mixed stone. They are usually multiple and occur in infected bile.

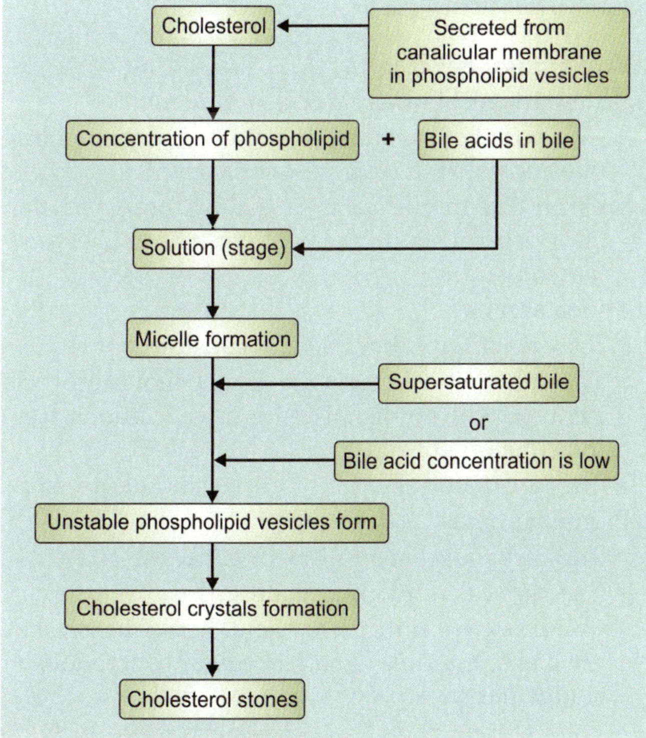


**Fig. 54.6:** Formation of cholesterol stones

**Pearls of Wisdom**

"A gallstone is a tomb stone erected in the memory of organisms within it". —Lord Moynihan

#### 3. Bile Stasis and Decreased Bile Acid Pool

- Pregnancy, oestrogens, following vagotomy and prolonged total parenteral nutrition are associated with bile stasis.
- They are prone to mixed stones as a result of bile stasis (Key Box 54.1).

**Key Box 54.1**

**Causes of Decreased Bile Acid Pool**

1. Cirrhosis of liver—pigment stones
2. Gastrectomy
3. Ileal resection
4. Malabsorption
5. Obesity
6. Hypercholesterolaemia

#### 4. Haemolytic Anaemia

- Examples: Hereditary spherocytosis, sickle cell anaemia.
- Bilirubin production is increased because of **increased breakdown of RBCs**. Since, the production is more, they cannot conjugate with glucuronic acid, which is produced at normal levels.
- Such **unconjugated bilirubin** combines with calcium and is excreted in the biliary tree resulting in calcium bilirubinate stones (pigment stones) not only in the gallbladder but also in the entire ductal system.

#### 5. Saint's Triad

Gallstones can occur along with two other conditions:
- Diverticulosis of colon
- Hiatus hernia

#### 6. Parasitic Infestation

- In Oriental countries, *Clonorchis sinensis* (Chinese liver fluke) infestations can cause stone in the biliary tree.
- *Ascaris lumbricoides* in the biliary tree may produce stones in the common bile duct.

#### 7. Due to Abnormal Mucus

It is produced in **congenital cystic fibrosis.** Gallstones occur in these children due to impairment of bile flow.

**Other Diseases Associated with Gallstone Disease**
- Diabetes mellitus
- Type IV hyperlipoproteinaemia
- Cirrhosis of liver
- Fistulae on treatment with total parenteral nutrition
- Gastric surgery

### 8. Risk Factors for Gallstone Disease (Fig. 54.7)

- Female sex
- Obesity
- Maturity onset diabetes
- Age >40 years.

### Types of Gallstones (Figs 54.8 to 54.10)

**1. Cholesterol stones**

- **Constitutes about 10% of the gallstones.**
- Occur in patients with increased cholesterol levels.
- Fatty women are commonly affected.
- It is single, solitary, occurs in aseptic bile. Sometimes they can be multiple. Precipitation of cholesterol gives rise to stone.
- Such stones can be silent for many years. They are radiolucent.
- Pigment can also get precipitated along with cholesterol.

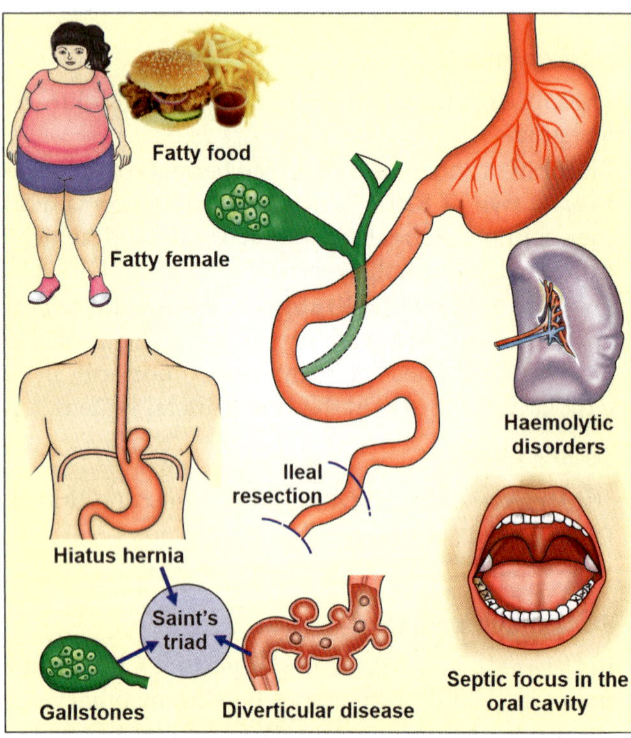


Fig. 54.7: A few risk factors for gallstone disease

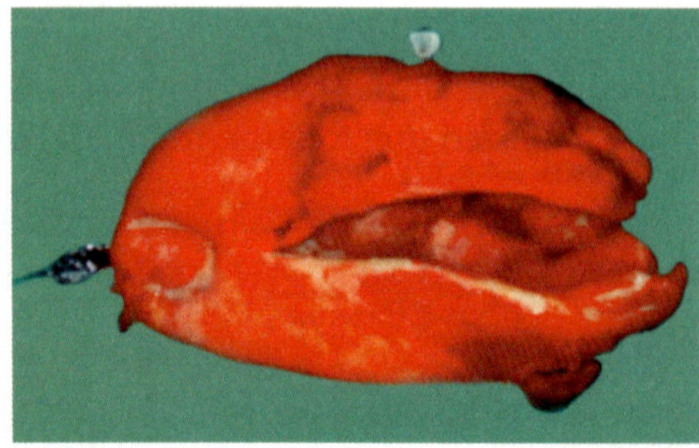

Fig. 54.8: Double GB with stones

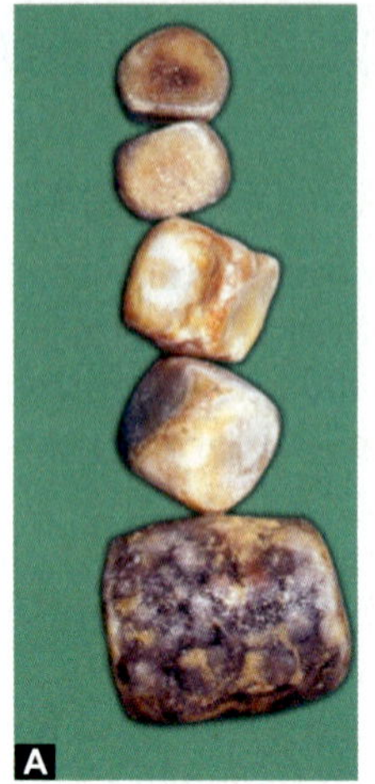


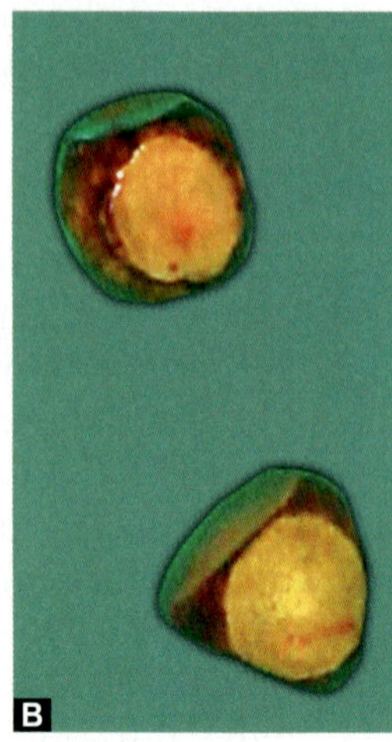


Fig. 54.9: Mixed stones—observe faceting—cause of gallstone colic

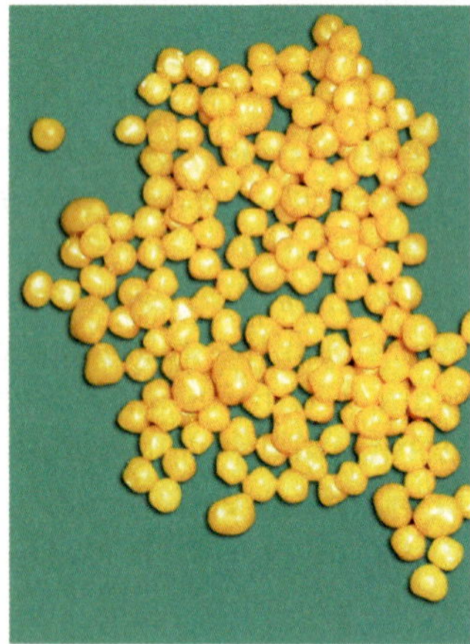

Fig. 54.10: Gallstones: Multiple small stones are responsible for obstructive jaundice by causing obstruction to CBD

**2. Brown pigment stones**

- **Rare in gallbladder, occurs in bile duct.**
- Composed of calcium bilirubinate, calcium palmitate and calcium stearate + cholesterol.
- Occur due to bile stasis caused by foreign bodies, endoprosthesis, *Clonorchis sinensis* and *Ascaris lumbricoides.*

**3. Mixed stones**

- They constitute about 80% of gallstones.
- They contain alternating layers of cholesterol and pigment with epithelial debris or vegetations, from infective organisms.
- They are multiple, small, faceted by mutual pressure.

**4. Pigment stones**

- They are found in 5 to 10% of patients.
- They are calcium bilirubinate stones.
- Commonly occur due to haemolysis. Hence, they are black, multiple, small, irregular concretions or sludge particles.
- For reasons not clear, **cirrhotic patients have increased incidence of black pigment stones.**

- Bacteria also have a major role to play in the formation of pigment stones. Patients with pigment stones have more sepsis than patients with cholesterol stones.

## Clinical Features (Complications of Gallstones)

Clinical presentation of these patients vary from **dyspepsia** to severe forms such as **pancreatitis and perforation of the gallbladder.** Complications are classified as in the gallbladder, in the CBD and in the intestines (Figs 54.11 and 54.12).

### In the Gallbladder

- Silent stones
- Flatulent dyspepsia
- Gallstone colic

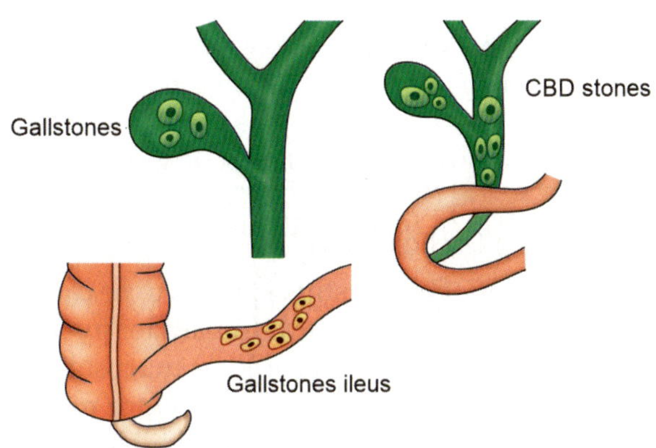


**Fig. 54.11:** Complications of gallstones

- Acute cholecystitis—Murphy's sign positive
- Chronic cholecystitis
- Mucocele—enlarged gallbladder without jaundice
- Empyema
- Perforation
- Carcinoma of the gallbladder
- Mirizzi's syndrome.

### In the Bile Duct

- Obstructive jaundice
- Cholangitis
- White bile
- Acute pancreatitis.

### In the Intestine

Acute intestinal obstruction (gallstone ileus).

## COMPLICATIONS IN THE GALLBLADDER

### Silent Stones

- This is usually a single, silent, cholesterol stone which is symptomless.
- It is accidentally discovered, may be by an ultrasound or plain X-ray abdomen (since calcium content is low in a cholesterol stone, it is very rarely visible in a plain X-ray).
- This stone rarely causes obstructive jaundice.
- Hence, it is left alone without treatment.

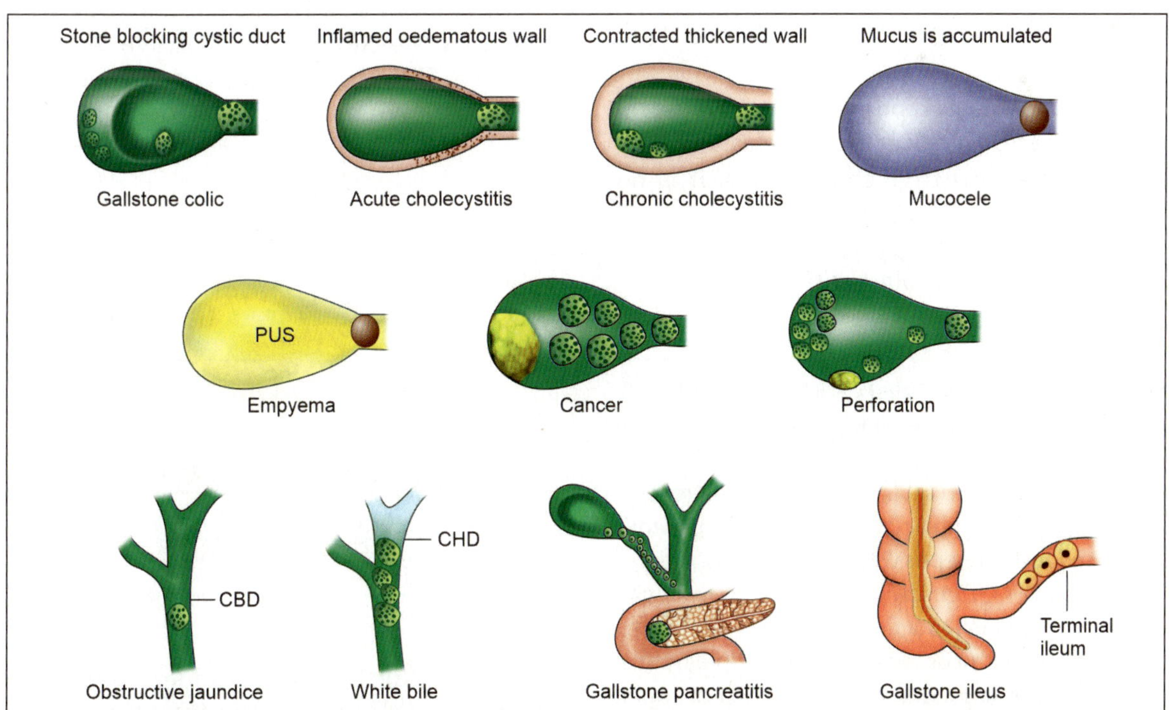


**Fig. 54.12:** Complications of gallstones. They are discussed in the subsequent pages

### Flatulent Dyspepsia

If an obese woman (fatty, fertile, flatulent, female in forties) complains of gaseous distention, intolerance to fatty food and discomfort in the abdomen, heartburn and belching, she probably has gallstones. These patients benefit from cholecystectomy.

### Gallstone Colic

- It usually occurs at night wherein a stone tends to block the cystic duct or neck of gallbladder in the supine position.
- It is a severe colicky upper abdominal pain felt in the right hypochondrium, may shoot to the back or between shoulder blades. The pain is continuous and lasts for a few hours. Pain may radiate to chest also.
  - The pain is due to spasm of gallbladder.
  - It is associated with vomiting due to reflex pylorospasm, restlessness and sweating.
  - There is tenderness in the right hypochondrium.
- Pain may last for a few minutes to a few hours.
- **Differential diagnoses include:**
  - Chronic duodenal ulcer
  - Reflux oesophagitis (some causes can present as precordial chest pain)
  - Pancreatitis
  - Myocardial infarction.

## ACUTE CHOLECYSTITIS

**Definition: Acute bacterial inflammation** of the gallbladder with or without stone.

### Types

- **Calculous:** Obstructive cholecystitis. It is the commonest variety. Calculi cause bile stasis.
- **Acalculous:** Nonobstructive cholecystitis. It is not uncommon and is seen in patients who are recovering from major illness (Key Box 54.2).
- **Acute emphysematous cholecystitis.**

Key Box 54.2

**Acalculous Cholecystitis–Percutaneous Cholecystostomy**

- In life-threatening situations with severe sepsis due to gallstones, percutaneous cholecystostomy seems to be a very good alternative to save the life of the patient.
- Indicated in acalculous cholecystitis in which the patient's condition is serious with sepsis with co-morbid conditions.
- Using ultrasound or CT guidance, a pigtail catheter can be inserted into the gallbladder, ideally transperitoneally.
- It is the treatment of choice for acalculous cholecystitis.
- 3–4 days later, when sepsis improves, laparoscopic/open cholecystectomy can be done.

### Bacteriology of Acute Cholecystitis

- Majority of the cases of calculous cholecystitis are due to organisms such as *E. coli*, streptococci, *Salmonella*, *Klebsiella*, etc.
- Typhoid fever can also cause **typhoid cholecystitis** around 2nd week of infection (Key Box 54.3).
- *Clostridial* infection of the gallbladder produces acute cholecystitis with toxaemia.

Key Box 54.3

**Typhoid Infection of the Gallbladder**

- *Salmonella typhi* or *S. typhimurium* are the organisms.
- Acute cholecystitis can occur in the 2nd week of typhoid fever.
- Long-lasting infections—chronic cholecystitis can occur.
- Bacilli can be present in the bile for a long time.
- Obstruction by a pre-existing stone or any other cause.
- Necrosis of GB, ulceration, perforation can be dangerous.
- Local tenderness, on the right side of abdomen, guarding can occur.
- Antibiotics against *Salmonella* must be given.

### Pathogenesis (Key Box 54.4)

- Acute calculous cholecystitis appears to be caused by obstruction to bile flow from gallbladder by stone or oedema formed as a result of local mucosal erosion and inflammation caused by stone. **Once mucosa is eroded, tissue planes are exposed to bile salts.** Toxic bile salts destroy cells by their detergent action leading to necrosis and perforation of gallbladder.
- At the same time, bacterial infection adds to the morbidity of acute cholecystitis. Positive bile cultures are found in 70% of cases of acute calculous cholecystitis.

Key Box 54.4

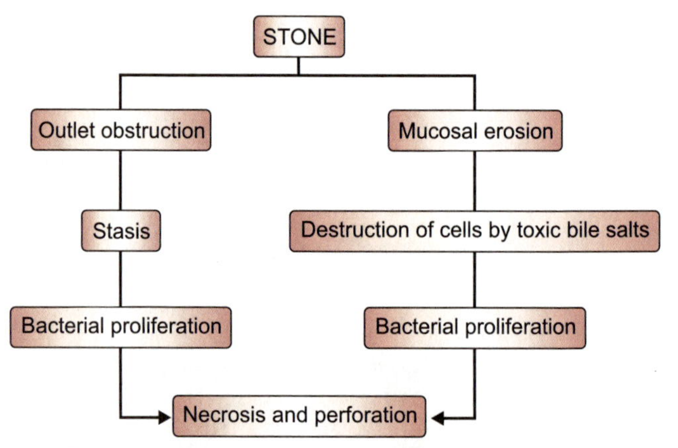


### Pathology

1. **Inflammation:** Entire gallbladder is inflamed, swollen and is friable. When the inflammatory exudate surrounding the gallbladder collects under the

diaphragm, it results in pain radiating to the right shoulder (C3, C4) due to phrenic nerve irritation. It may undergo complete resolution with antibiotic therapy but such recurrent attacks are common at a later date.

2. **Perforation:** Extensive ulcerations of gallbladder may result in perforation with biliary peritonitis and carries a very high mortality rate. **Perforation** can occur when the stone is impacted in the **Hartmann's pouch**.
3. **Obstruction** to the neck of gallbladder results in **mucocele** or **pyocele** (empyema). Empyema of the gallbladder can occur in diabetic patients and is associated with high grade fever, chills, rigors and even septicaemia.
4. **Gangrene** of gallbladder can occur, if the blood vessels get thrombosed. All these features are more in an obstructive variety.
   - If there is clostridial infection as can occur in diabetics because of extensive gas production in biliary tree and associated toxicity, perforation is likely even without a stone.
5. **Jaundice** as in hereditary spherocytosis (Fig. 54.13).

## Clinical Features

- A fatty, fertile, female is the typical victim who presents with severe upper abdominal pain. The pain is colicky in nature and more prolonged because of inflammation. Severe nausea and vomiting are present. In the initial phase, there is low grade fever, except in clostridial infection where there is high grade fever.
- Right shoulder pain is due to inflammatory exudate irritating under surface of the diaphragm (supplied by phrenic nerves C4–C5—shoulder region is supplied by supraclavicular nerves.

**Pearls of Wisdom**

You may be surprised to find a young boy, a girl or even a child with gallstones—suspect haemolytic anaemias.

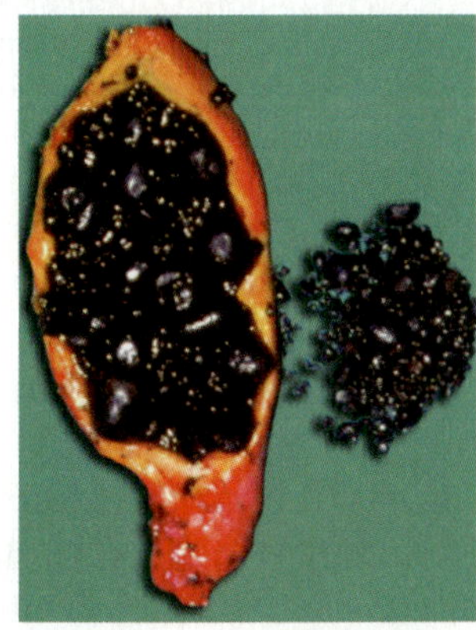

**Fig. 54.13:** Pigment stones—case of hereditary spherocytosis

## Signs

1. ***Murphy's sign***
   - Keep the fingers in the right hypochondrium and ask the patient to take a deep inspiration.
   - At the height of inspiration, there is a sudden catch in the inspiration.
   - It is due to inflamed gallbladder coming in contact with the abdominal wall under the fingers and producing pain. This is called **Murphy's sign positive**. It is a diagnostic sign of acute cholecystitis (Fig. 54.14).

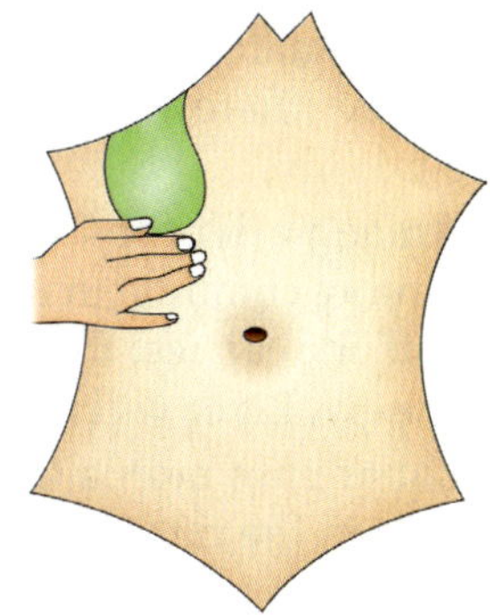

**Fig. 54.14:** Eliciting Murphy's sign

2. ***Boas' sign:*** An area of hyperaesthesia between 9th and 11th ribs posteriorly on the right side is a feature.
3. **Upper abdominal guarding, rigidity**.
4. **Vague mass** consisting of inflamed gallbladder, omentum, inflammatory exudate can be felt at times. Hence, even if a perforation occurs, generalised peritonitis is uncommon.

## Differential Diagnosis (DD) (Fig. 54.15)

1. **Perforated peptic ulcer:** Severe sudden pain, severe tenderness in the right hypochondrium, guarding and rigidity caused by perforated peptic ulcer, can mimic acute cholecystitis. Obliteration of liver dullness, coffee ground vomitus, generalised guarding and rigidity clinches the diagnosis of perforated duodenal ulcer.
2. **Acute pancreatitis:** A severe pain in upper abdomen, tenderness in the right hypochondrium

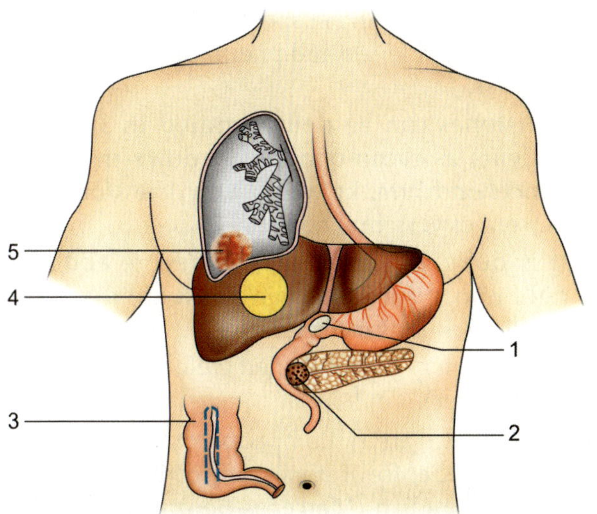


**Fig. 54.15:** Differential diagnosis of acute cholecystitis (*see* text)

and epigastrium mimic cholecystitis. One should remember that pain of pancreatitis is more severe and classically radiates to back.

3. **High retrocaecal appendicitis:** Especially when appendix is in the subhepatic position. Once inflammatory fluid spreads in the general peritoneal cavity, there will be more difficulty in diagnosing clinically.
4. **Amoebic liver abscess:** Can also mimic very closely. It is more common in male alcoholics. Liver is enlarged and one can feel the round lower border of liver very closely. Liver will be extremely tender.
5. **Lobar pneumonia (basal):** It can give rise to referred pain in the right hypochondrium with guarding and rigidity.

## Investigations

1. **Total WBC** count is always raised.
2. **Blood and urine sugar** estimation to rule out diabetes mellitus.
3. **Emergency ultrasonography** (Fig. 54.16)
   - To demonstrate stones, which cast **posterior acoustic shadow**.
   - Success rate is >95%.
   - It can demonstrate inflamed, thickened organ, in cases of acalculous cholecystitis.
   - More than 5–6 mm thickness of gallbladder suggests significant thickening.
   - Pericholecystic oedema may be present.
   - Demonstration of Murphy's sign, with the help of ultrasonography is possible which adds to the diagnosis.
   - Ultrasound can also measure gallbladder function by using ultrasonic dimensions of the gallbladder.
   - It can detect gallbladder polyps.
4. **Plain X-ray** abdomen erect position (Fig. 54.17). Not routinely done. If you suspect gallstone ileus, it may detect gas fluid levels and pneumobilia (Details later in page 986)
   - Gallstones can be demonstrated in 10% of the patients as radio-opaque shadows in the right hypochondrium. In lateral view, the stone is seen in front of vertebral bodies.
   - It is done for evaluation of severe abdominal right upper quadrant pain when the diagnosis of perforation is also considered.
   - Rarely, it may show calcified gallbladder (porcelain gallbladder).

   10% gallstones are radio-opaque, 90% gallstones are radiolucent. Centre of stones may contain radiolucent gas, either triradiate (**Mercedes-Benz sign**) or biradiate **(Seagull sign)**.

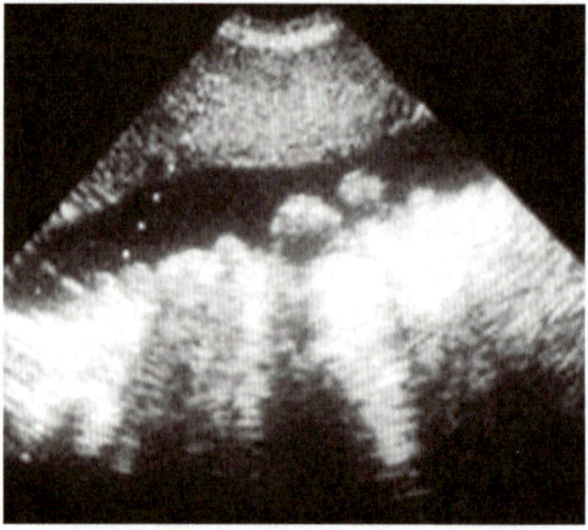

**Fig. 54.16:** Ultrasonography showing posterior acoustic shadows

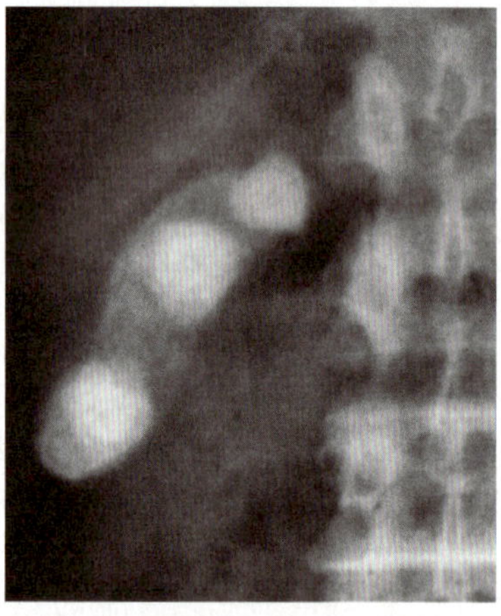

**Fig. 54.17:** Plain X-ray abdomen showing radio-opaque shadows

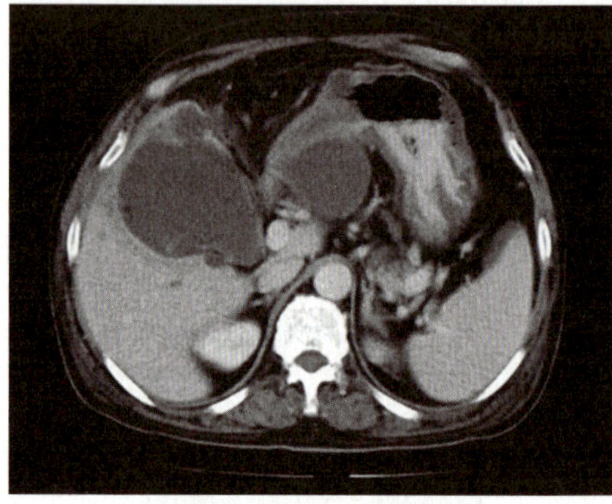

**Fig. 54.18:** Perforation of gallbladder

5. **CT scan** (Fig. 54.18)
   - It is done when ultrasound findings are not clear
   - It not only diagnoses gallstones, but also detects other complications such as perforation, stones in the CBD, etc.
   - Renal halo sign is due to fluid around.
   - Excellent investigation to diagnose gangrene in late cases of acute cholecystitis patients who present with septic shock.

## Treatment

### I. Conservative Treatment (60 to 70%) Followed by Cholecystectomy

Basically there are two types of cholecystectomy—one is early cholecystectomy and other is elective cholecystectomy.

Elective cholecystectomy is followed by many surgeons because many patients are elderly often diabetic or may be having cardiac comorbidity. Also inflammation would have resulted in so-called frozen or difficult 'Calot's triangle' dissection. During surgery, dissection may result in injuries to CBD, hepatic artery, portal vein, etc. Hence, these are managed conservatively till pain inflammation settles down. Principles of conservative treatment are given below.

1. **Admission**
2. **Aspiration** with Ryle's tube: Aspiration of HCl decreases the stimulus to the secretion of bile. Spasm of gallbladder may come down.
3. **Antispasmodics:** Injection tramadol 50 mg IV/IM is given and if necessary repeated.
4. **Antibiotics:** Broad spectrum antibiotics are given against gram +ve, gram –ve and anaerobic organisms. Cefazolin, cefuroxime or amikacin are the drugs of choice. The patient is kept nil orally for 2–3 days and during this time, IV fluids are given.

After 2–3 days, pain comes down, signs (tenderness) disappear and abdomen becomes soft. Ryle's tube is removed, clear oral fluid is given for 2–3 days followed by soft diet. After 6 weeks, the patient is advised to undergo elective cholecystectomy. Reason for conservative treatment is in majority of cases, inflammation will settle down.

### II. Early Laparoscopic Cholecystectomy—Lap Chole (Table 54.1)

- Patients in the first group need two admissions, cost is increased and return to work is also delayed.
- Hence, if a surgeon is experienced and the set up is good, one can proceed to early cholecystectomy from 2nd day to 7th day.
- It has been proved that even though gallbladder is inflamed, complications are no way more than elective cholecystectomy in the hands of experienced surgeon while performing laparoscopic cholecystectomy.
- Thus, if a firm preoperative diagnosis is established and some of the comorbid conditions are corrected (diabetes, hypertension, etc.), surgery can be done safely. This is called early cholecystectomy done within 48 to 72 hours.

### III. Emergency Cholecystostomy

- About 5% of cases of acute cholecystitis require emergency cholecystostomy.
- In these patients, high grade fever, sepsis, shock, high leukocyte count are the deciding factors.
- Acalculous cholecystitis and perforated gallbladder with peritonitis are definitely strong indications for emergency cholecystostomy.
- This is an attempt to decrease toxicity, fever and improve general condition.
- Either by open-laparoscopic method, a tube is inserted into gallbladder (Pig tail catheter/Malecot's) and the pus/necrotic tissue is drained out. Only an experienced surgeon can attempt cholecystectomy. Otherwise tube is inserted and fixed and brought outside.
- After 6–8 days later, cholecystectomy is done.

## Prognosis

- Overall death rate is 3–5%.
- Contributing factors for death are diabetes, age above 60 years, cardiovascular or pulmonary disease.
- Uncontrolled sepsis, intra-abdominal abscess (Table 54.1).

**TABLE 54.1:** Few important components of Tokyo guidelines in treating Acute Cholecystitis (AC)

| Grades of acute cholecystitis | ASA-PS scores | When to do cholecystectomy? | Comments |
|---|---|---|---|
| **Grade I (mild) AC** | **Patient can withstand surgery** | Early lap Chole within 24 to 72 hours | It is safe to do early cholecystectomy |
| | **Patient cannot withstand surgery** | Conservative treatment (antibiotics, nil oral, monitoring, pain relief) | |
| **Grade II (moderate) AC** | **Patient can withstand surgery** | Lap Chole within 3 to 4 days by skilled surgeon and high volume centre | It may be a difficult cholecystectomy. Calot's triangle may be masked. Care should be taken to avoid injury during surgery and a switch to open or subtotal cholecystectomy |
| **Grade III (severe) AC** | **Patient can withstand surgery** | **Early Lap-Chole can be performed by a specialist skilled surgeon and back up of ICU conservative treatment** | Intervention by percutaneous external drainage if severe sepsis and organ failure |
| | **Patient cannot withstand surgery** | Organ dysfunction restoration, delayed cholecystectomy | Culture of bile, recovery, ICU care |

*What is prophylactic cholecystectomy?*

It means removal of gallbladder with stones without symptoms. It is indicated in:

- Congenital haemolytic anaemia
- Patients undergoing bariatric surgery
- Porcelain gallbladder.

## CHRONIC CHOLECYSTITIS

- Recurrent attacks of cholecystitis will convert the gallbladder into a fibrosed, nonfunctioning, contracted, shrunken, small gallbladder. Gallbladder wall is grossly thickened. Stones are invariably present. Such patients present with classical fatty food intolerance. Murphy's sign is positive.
- They are diagnosed by ultrasound which reveals a small, contracted gallbladder. Oral cholecystography (OCG) used to be done to know the function of the gallbladder earlier.

### Treatment

Cholecystectomy (Fig. 54.19).

## CHOLECYSTOSES

### Definition

Uncommon group of conditions affecting gallbladder in which there are chronic inflammatory changes and hyperplasia of all tissue elements.

### Types

1. **Cholesterolosis** (strawberry gallbladder): Aggregations of cholesterol crystals in the mucosa/submucosa. Yellow specks of cholesterol crystals are seen when gallbladder is opened (xanthogranulomatous) (Key Box 54.5 and Fig. 54.20).

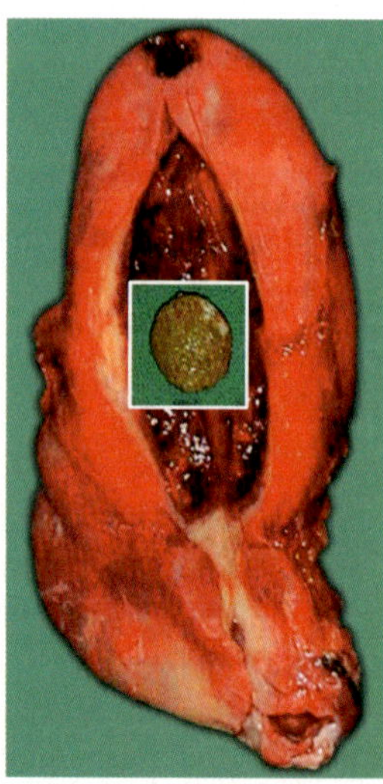

Fig. 54.19: Cholecystectomy specimen—observe thickened gallbladder wall

Key Box 54.5

**Xanthogranulomatous Cholecystitis**

- It is a pathological diagnosis.
- Gallbladder is chronically thickened, irregular with extension of yellow xanthogranulomatous inflammation to adjacent organs.
- It is thought to be due to bile penetrating gallbladder wall.

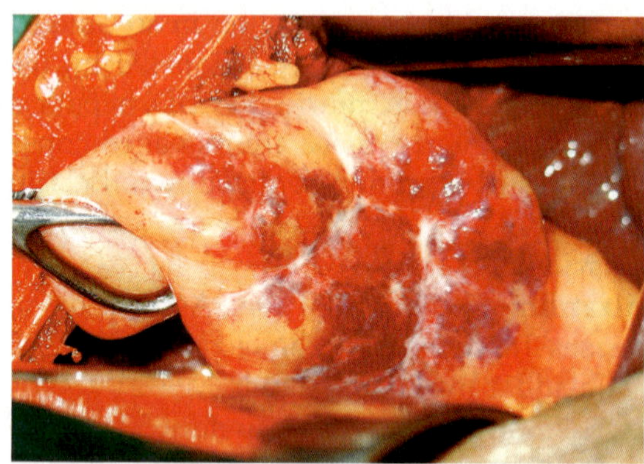

Fig. 54.20: Xanthogranulomatous cholecystitis at surgery

2. **Cholesterol polyposis** (gallbladder polyp): Polypoidal projections of mucosa in the gallbladder. ***Polyp longer than 1 cm or change in size requires surgery.***
3. **Cholecystitis glandularis proliferans:** Granulomatous thickening and hyperplasia of the gallbladder. All layers of gallbladder are thickened.
4. **Diverticulosis** of gallbladder.
5. Gallbladder wall with ***fistula***.

### Clinical Features

Dyspepsia, upper abdominal discomfort, Murphy's sign is positive.

### Management

Ultrasound to confirm the diagnosis followed by cholecystectomy.

## MUCOCELE (Figs 54.21 and 54.22)

- It occurs when there is a stone blocking the cystic duct and the bile is not infected.
- As a result of obstruction, all the bile within the gallbladder is absorbed and is replaced by the mucus secreted from gallbladder epithelium.
- Clinically, it results in a soft, fluctuant, globular mass in the right hypochondrium which moves with respiration. It needs cholecystectomy.

## EMPYEMA AND PERFORATION OF GALLBLADDER

- These are uncommon. Impacted stone, diabetes, virulent organisms precipitate pyocele and perforation.

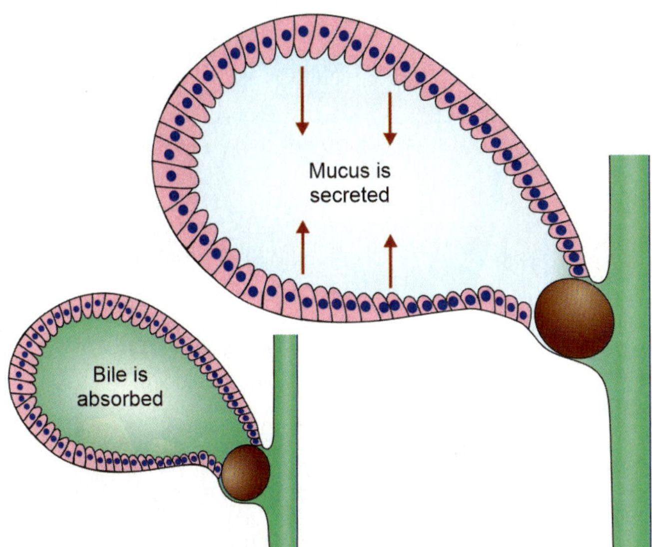


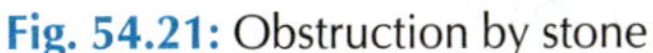

**Fig. 54.21:** Obstruction by stone

**Fig. 54.22:** Mucocele

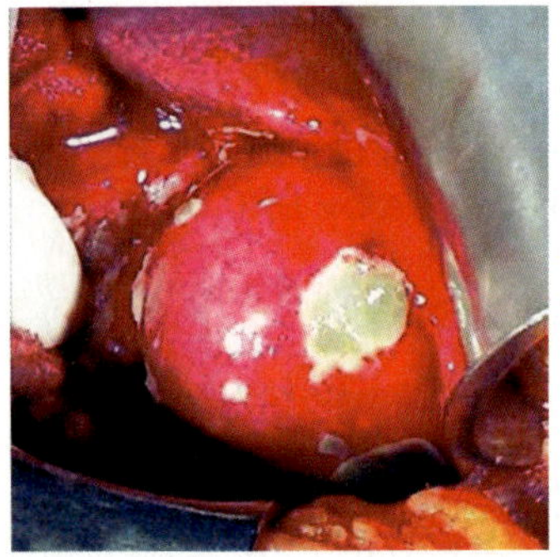

**Fig. 54.23C:** Gallbladder perforation at surgery

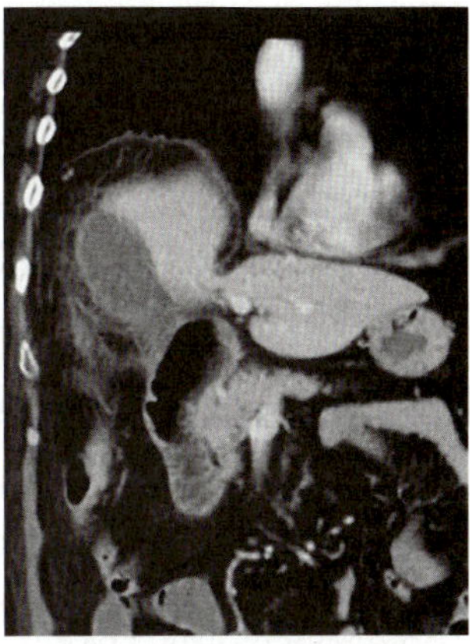

**Fig. 54.23D:** Acalculous cholecystitis—enlarged gallbladder with pericholecystitic oedema

- Patients present with high grade fever with chills and rigors, toxicity, high leucocyte count.
- Perforation can cause local abscess, if there are adhesions due to previous inflammation.
- Perforation into the general peritoneal cavity is rare but produces diffuse biliary peritonitis which has a high mortality rate.
- Urgent laparotomy, aggressive resuscitation, good antibiotic cover may help in reducing mortality. At laparotomy, removal of gallbladder is difficult. Hence, drainage of the pus and cholecystostomy with removal of gallstones can be done (Figs 54.23A to D).

**Three types** are (Fig. 54.24):

1. Localised perforation with pericholecystic abscess—managed by catheter drainage.
2. Free perforation into peritoneal cavity and peritonitis—urgent laparotomy drainage.
3. Hollow viscous perforation (duodenum).

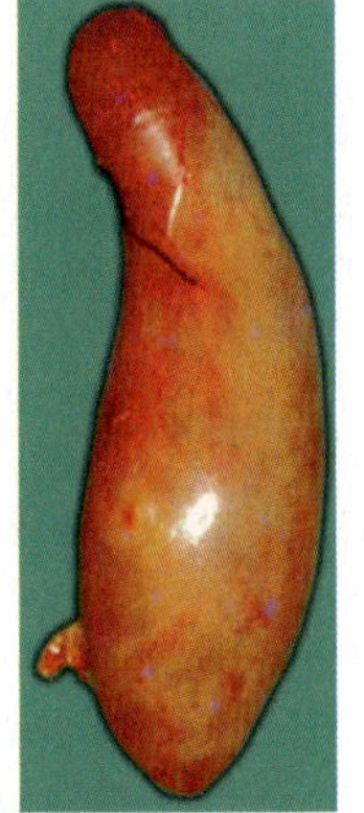

**Fig. 54.23A:** Empyema of gallbladder

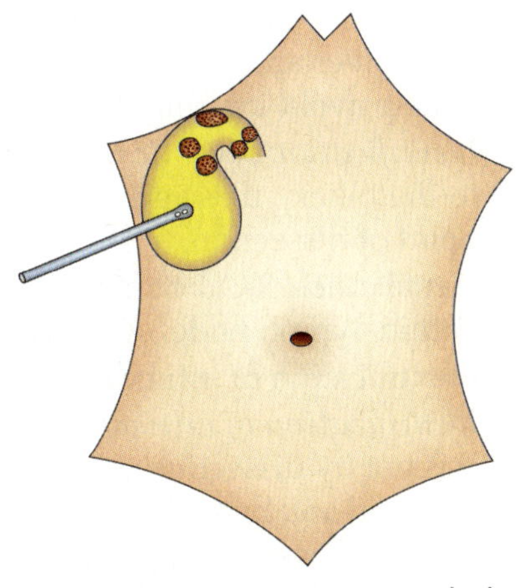

**Fig. 54.23B:** Percutaneous cholecystostomy for empyema of gallbladder

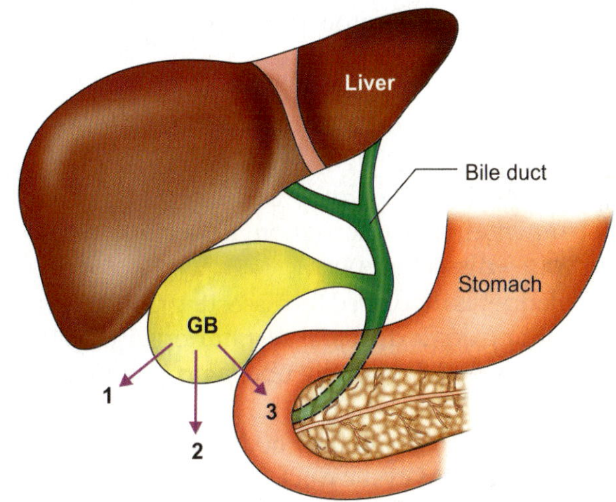


**Fig. 54.24:** Empyema of gallbladder—complications (*see* the text)

## CARCINOMA OF GALLBLADDER (see page 799)

Long-standing gallstones can bring about squamous metaplasia of gallbladder epithelium and can cause carcinoma of gallbladder. However, the incidence is very low. Hence, routine cholecystectomy is not advised for silent gallstones. Porcelain gallbladder is a precancerous condition.

**Porcelain Gallbladder**

- It occurs due to deposition of calcium carbonate in the gallbladder wall.
- Diagnosis can be made by plain X-ray of the abdomen.
- On ultrasound examination, calcification appears as hyperechoic semilunar structure with dense posterior acoustic shadowing.
- In case of difficulties, CECT can help to differentiate it from gallstones.
- Incidence of carcinoma gallbladder is around 1 to 5%.
- Prophylactic cholecystectomy is indicated.
- One should be ready to do hepatic resection, if required.

## MIRIZZI SYNDROME (Figs 54.25 and 54.26)

**Type I:** Compression of CBD without lumen narrowing.
**Type II:** Compression of CBD with lumen narrowing.
**Type III:** Compression causing CBD wall necrosis.
**Type IV:** Stone ulcerating into CBD resulting in cholecystocholedochal fistula. It is treated by ERCP.

## LAPAROSCOPIC CHOLECYSTECTOMY

It has become the most popular choice today. More than 95% of gallbladders can be removed through a laparoscope. Some principles and procedure of laparoscopic cholecystectomy are discussed below (Figs 54.27 and 54.32B).

### Procedure

- 1 cm incision is made below the umbilicus, through which a pneumoperitoneum is maintained by $CO_2$ insufflation.
- Following this, a laparoscope is introduced and a camera is attached. Three small, 1 cm incisions are made in epigastrium and ½ cm in the right hypochondrium. These are used for suction, instrumentation, cauterisation, dissection, retraction purpose—dissection port.
- Gallbladder is mobilised by dissecting Calot's triangle by isolating cystic duct and cystic artery. Retraction of Hartman's pouch laterally opens up Calot's triangle (Fig. 54.28).
- Thus, it gives a view of liver bed and two structures—cystic artery and cystic duct. It is called critical view of Strasberg (Fig. 54.29).
- Cystic duct and cystic artery are clipped and gallbladder is removed using gallbladder-holding forceps and is brought outside through the epigastric port (Figs 54.30 to 54.32).
- Bleeding from liver is controlled using lasers/cautery.

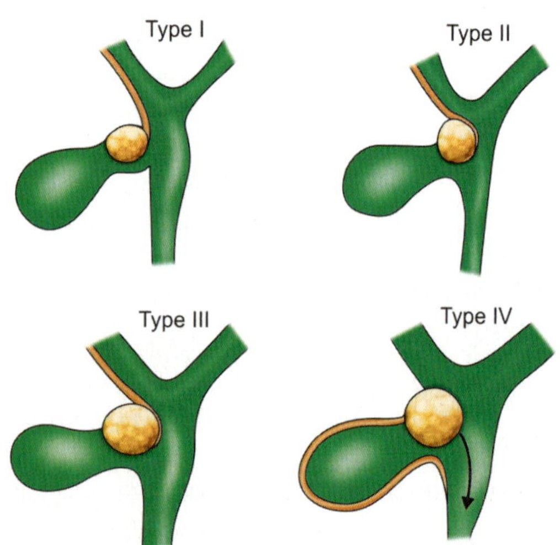


**Fig. 54.25:** Mirizzi syndrome

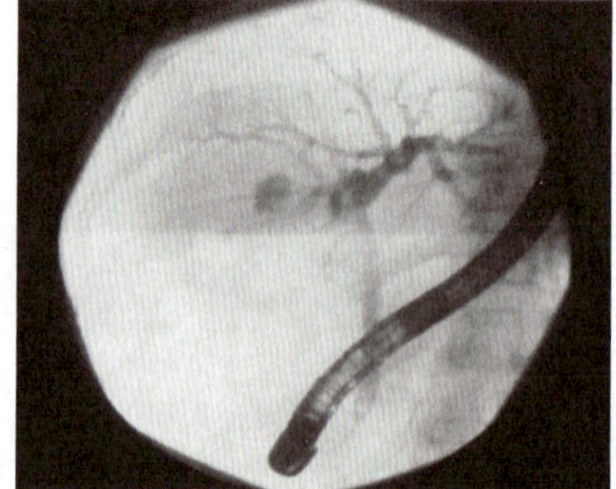

**Fig. 54.26:** ERCP showing Mirizzi syndrome

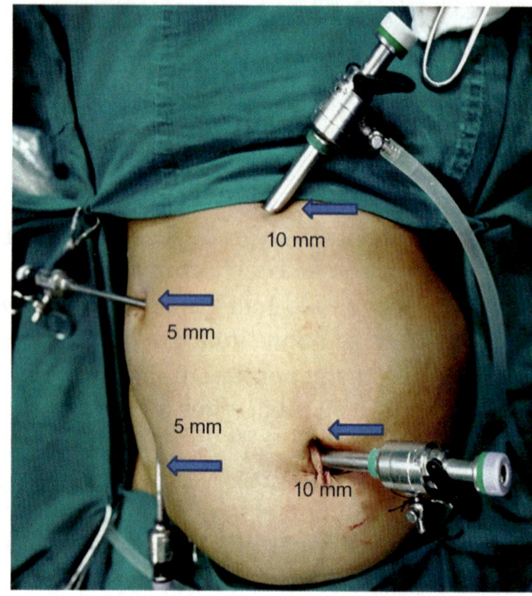


**Fig. 54.27:** Ports for laparoscopic cholecystectomy

- The procedure is done under general anaesthesia. It may take 1–3 hours depending upon the experience of the surgeon.

### Identification of Bile Ducts and Avoiding Injuries during Laparoscopic Cholecystectomy

- *Identification of Rouviere's sulcus:* This is an anatomical land mark—a fissure, 2–5 cm, between the right lobe of the liver and the caudate process. This can be used to help avoid injuring the common bile duct (CBD).
- *Identification of cystic lymph node:* Always lies lateral to the biliary tree and should form the medial end-point of dissection.
- Identification of Calot's triangle and identifying structures within–lymph node, cystic artery and cystic duct.
- Identification of infundibulum of the gallbladder.
- *Identification of critical view of Strasberg or safety:* It is got by dissecting the entire infundibulum of the liver bed and by freeing it of all fatty tissue, both in its dorsal and ventral aspects. We should see 2 structures entering into the gallbladder: Inferiorly cystic duct, superiorly cystic artery and liver is seen in between.

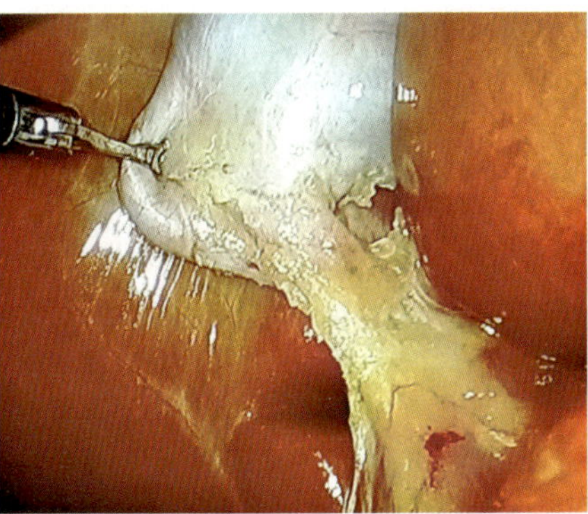

Fig. 54.28: First view of gallbladder once Hartman's pouch is retracted

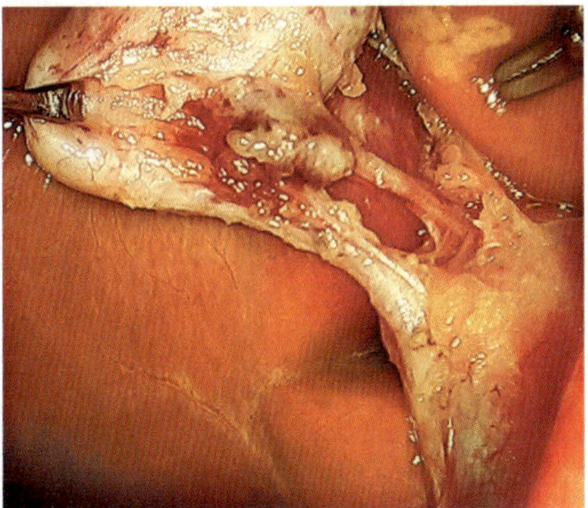

Fig. 54.29: Cystic artery and cystic ducts are seen—**critical view of safety** or **Strasberg** is achieved by dissecting the infundibulum off the liver bed, freeing it of all fatty tissue, both in its dorsal and ventral aspects

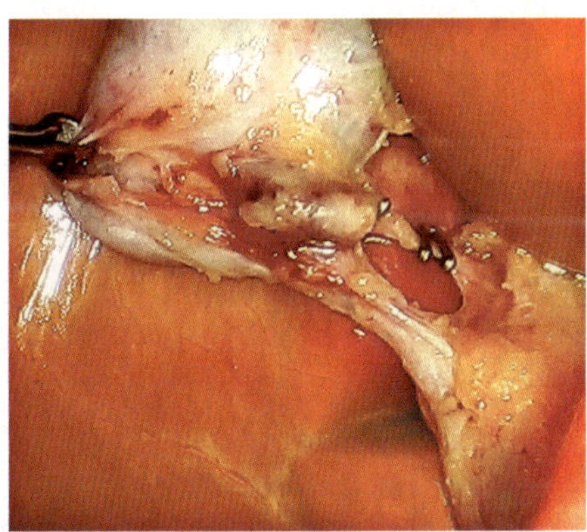

Fig. 54.30A: Cystic artery is ligated in 3 places

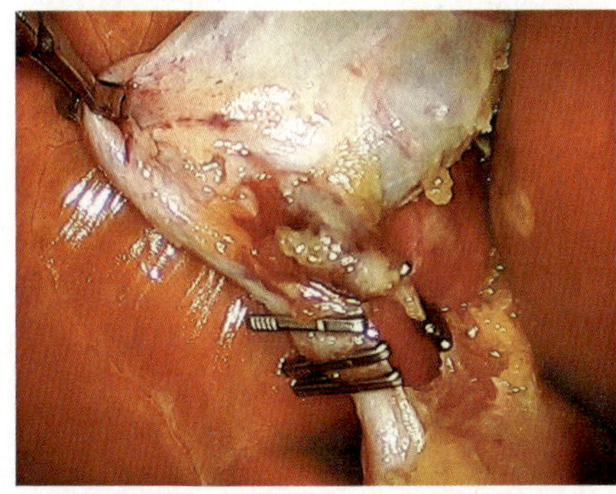

Fig. 54.30B: Cystic duct is clipped in 3 places

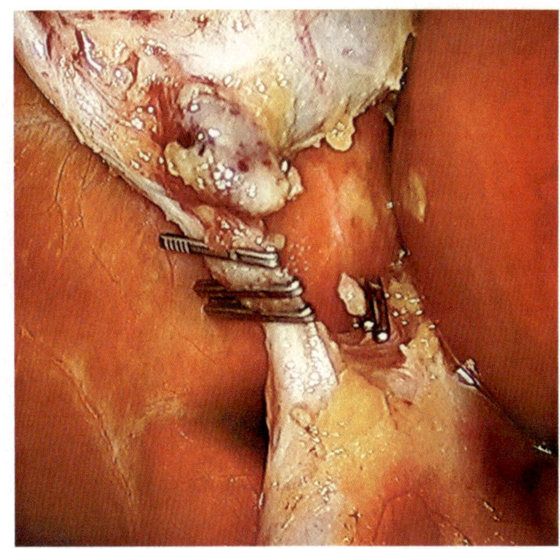

Fig. 54.31A: Cystic artery is divided

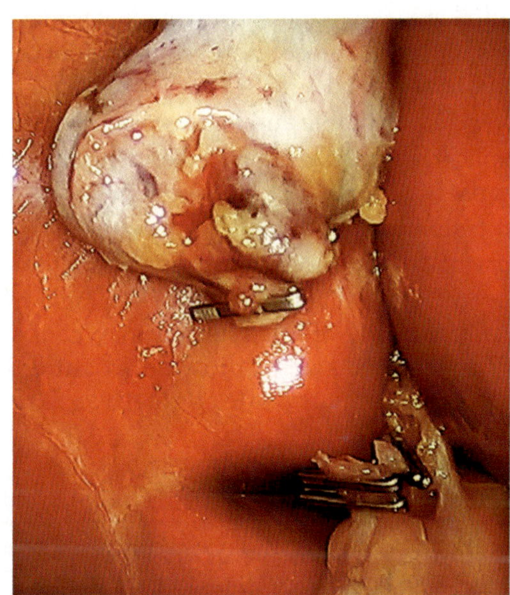

Fig. 54.31B: Both cystic artery and cystic duct are divided

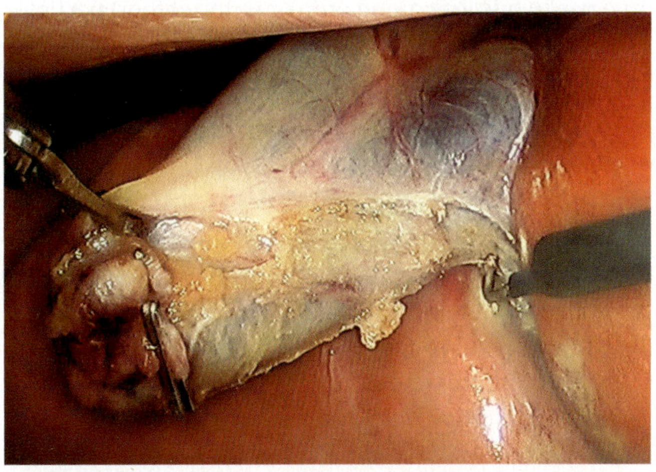

Fig. 54.32A: Gallbladder is dissected from liver bed

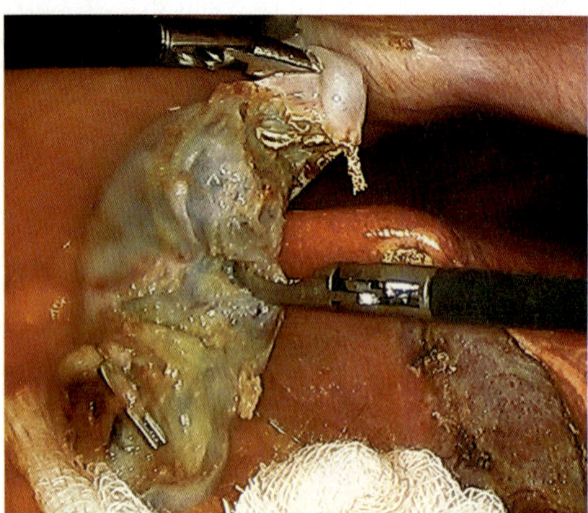

**Fig. 54.32B:** Gallbladder is completely dissected from the liver bed, placed in a bag and extracted

### Advantages

- Hospital stay is 1–2 days, recovery is very fast.
- Pain is minimal. Hence, mobilisation of the patient is much better and easy.
- It gives an acceptable and better cosmetic result.
- Complications such as adhesions and incisional hernia are rare.

  **Conversion to open when**
  - Very badly contracted, fibrosed gallbladder.
  - Very difficult gallbladder—Calot's triangle anatomy is not defined well. Dissection may cause injury to the bile ducts and can cause stricture. **Partial cholecystectomy is a safe alternative.**

## POSTOPERATIVE BILE LEAK FOLLOWING LAPAROSCOPIC CHOLECYSTECTOMY

Bile leak after laparoscopic cholecystectomy is uncommon but can occur in 0.3–2.7% of patients. It is defined as the persistent leakage of bile from the biliary tree. Injuries to CHD, CBD, accessory ducts; loosely applied clips or ligatures are the usual causes. Duodenal injury also will give rise to bile leak along with or without food particles.

***Diagnosis of bile leak***

- Look at the video recording
- Early ERCP and classify the injuries
- Classify (Examples are given below).

**Bile duct injury classification**

I. Strasberg A–minor leaks from cystic duct stump or minor biliary radicles to strasberg E–major duct transection–types

II. Hannover A1 to E 4
  - Plan the treatment
  - Resuscitation, stabilisation, investigations
  - Antibiotics
  - Drainage/surgery

**Treatment principles:**

If ultrasound-guided drainage is successful and adequate, then it is unusual for life-threatening peritonitis or sepsis to develop subsequently. Management is conservative with antibiotics and a daily assessment of drain output.

Drainage of 200 ml or less of bile per day, and reducing over a period of a few days, is likely to subside on its own. In some cases, this may be all that is necessary, and the bile leak will slowly reduce and stop.

Persistent drainage of 200 ml or more of bile per day over a period of a few days, elective ERC is performed. This may demonstrate the site of bile leak – placement of an (5–7 cm long) internal stent between the common bile duct and the duodenum.

**Exploration:** This is needed if patient condition is not stable, in sepsis, drainage of large collections, interloop collections, duodenal injuries, etc.

The best time for repair is at first surgery. Late cases wait for 6–8 weeks.

## MEDICAL TREATMENT OF GALLSTONES

It is indicated for **pure cholesterol** stones only.

### Patient Selection

- Patients with functioning gallbladder proven by OCG or scintigraphy.
- Young, thin, female patients.
- Tiny (<5 mm), translucent, floating stones.

### Drawbacks

- Recurrence of stones once treatment is stopped.
- Lifelong maintenance is needed.
- After dissolution of the stones, lithotripsy or extracorporeal shock wave lithotripsy should be done.

### Types of Medical Treatment

#### *1. Oral Dissolution Treatment*

- **Drugs used:** CDCA—chenodeoxycholic acid UDCA—ursodeoxycholic acid.
- **Mechanism of action:** They inhibit HMG-CoA, a rate limiting step in the synthesis of cholesterol, thereby increasing the bile salt pool. UDCA also acts by decreasing cholesterol absorption in GIT.

#### *2. Direct Contact Dissolution*

MTBE—methyl tert-butyl ether is the drug which is given through a catheter placed in gallbladder percutaneously.

***Drawbacks:*** Explosive and toxic, if it enters bile duct or duodenum.

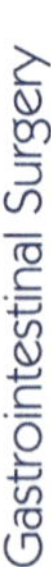

*Indications*

- High-risk patients with symptomatic stones, refusing surgery.
- The patient must have patent cystic duct (proven by OCG/scintigraphy).

*Side effects:* Haemorrhage and catheter displacement.

Thus, we have completed gallstones and their complications in the gallbladder. Now, we will study the anatomy of the pancreas. So that we can understand obstructive jaundice better.

> **SU24.2:** Describe the anatomy of the pancreas. Describe the clinical features, principles of investigation, prognosis and management of pancreatic exocrine tumours.

## SURGICAL ANATOMY OF THE PANCREAS

The pancreas is both endocrine and exocrine organ situated retroperitoneally behind the stomach. It is a soft and fleshy gland (pancreas—all flesh), extending from the duodenum on the right side to the spleen on the left side, the entire length being 6 inches (Fig. 54.33). It weighs approximately 80 g.

### Parts

- The *head* lies within the C-loop of duodenum. The uncinate process projects from the left inferior portion of the head over which course the superior mesenteric vessels. There are 5–6 small thin veins connecting this portion of the head with superior mesenteric veins. These veins have to be carefully divided during pancreaticoduodenectomy. Superior mesenteric vein continues above as portal vein after joining the splenic vein. During pancreaticoduodenectomy for periampullary carcinoma, infiltration into the portal vein should be ruled out before any major structure is divided. This is done by inserting a finger between the portal vein and head of pancreas, both from above and below.
- The *neck* is about 2 cm and is related posteriorly to superior mesenteric vessels.
- *Body and tail:* The head and neck continue as body which is placed transversely. It slopes upwards across the aorta and ends as tail of the pancreas, which is enclosed within lienorenal ligament along with splenic vessels. A large cystadenoma arising from the tail of the pancreas can move with respiration because of its contact with the spleen.

## BLOOD SUPPLY OF THE PANCREAS

### Arterial Supply (Fig. 54.33)

- Splenic artery is the chief artery supplying the neck, body and the tail. Arteria pancreatica magna refers to one large branch of splenic artery.

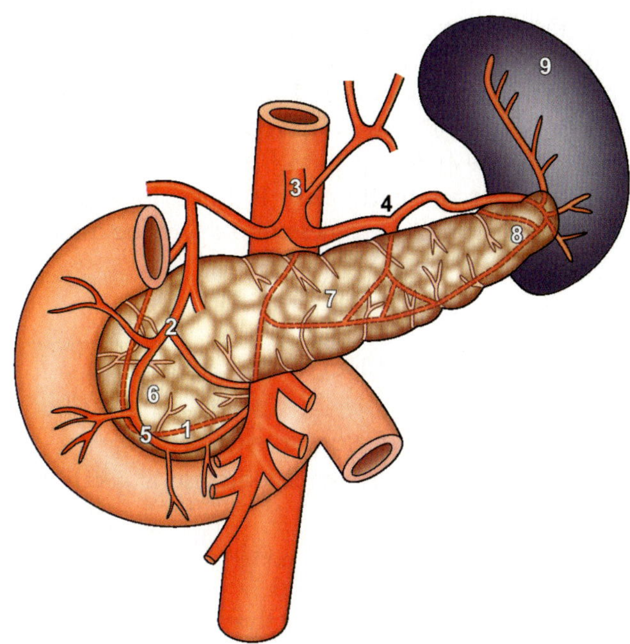


**Fig. 54.33:** Blood supply and parts of pancreas: 1. Uncinate process, 2. superior pancreaticoduodenal artery, 3. coeliac artery, 4. splenic artery, 5. inferior pancreaticoduodenal artery, 6. head of pancreas, 7. body of pancreas, 8. tail of pancreas, and 9. spleen

- Superior and inferior pancreaticoduodenal arteries supply not only head of pancreas but also the adjacent duodenum. Thus, during any surgery which involves excision of the head, the C-loop of the duodenum is also removed. Thus, pancreaticoduodenectomy becomes a major surgery.

### Venous Drainage

- Body, neck and tail drain into splenic vein by means of multiple small veins.
- The head is drained by superior pancreaticoduodenal vein which drains into portal vein and inferior pancreaticoduodenal vein drains into superior mesenteric vein.

### Islets of Langerhans (Endocrine)

- 75% : β cells
- 20% : α cells
- 4% : δ cells

### Pancreatic Duct

- The main pancreatic duct (duct of Wirsung), a tubular structure, drains entire pancreas from tail to the head. It joins the common bile duct and forms ampulla of Vater. This ampulla opens on the duodenal papilla (a nipple-like elevation) in the 2nd part of the duodenum. Normal diameter of pancreatic duct is 2–3 mm. When it is dilated more than 6–8 mm, as in chronic pancreatitis, longitudinal pancreaticojejunostomy can be done.

- Accessory pancreatic duct of Santorini drains the uncinate process and lower portion of the head and opens into the duodenum 2 cm above the opening of the main duct. The two ducts communicate with each other at many sites.
- The main pancreatic duct is lined by columnar epithelium which becomes cuboidal in the ductules.

### PANCREATIC JUICE

- Bicarbonate rich, protein rich, alkaline fluid
- 2.5 litres/day
- Rich in proteins—15 g of protein/day
- Thus acidic chyme in the duodenum is alkalinised by pancreatic juice.
- Protein is secreted by acinar cells, fluid and electrolytes by ductal cells.
- Secretions are stimulated by three phases:
  a. Cephalic phase is mediated by acetylcholine—10% of secretion
  b. Gastric phase—mediated by gastrin and vagus—15%
  c. Intestinal phase—75% release mediated by release of secretion from duodenal acidification and stimulated release of bile into 2nd part of duodenum following entry of fat and proteins.

## OBSTRUCTIVE JAUNDICE (SURGICAL JAUNDICE)

### Definition

- Jaundice that occurs due to obstruction to the outflow of bile is called obstructive jaundice.
- Since these cases have to be managed by surgical intervention, it is also called surgical jaundice.
- However, haemolytic jaundice cases are not obstructive but a few are managed by splenectomy, hence it is called as surgical jaundice.

### A CASE OF OBSTRUCTIVE JAUNDICE

**Definition:** Persistent progressive jaundice (may be with waxing and waning) with more than 50% of conjugated bilirubin or **jaundice associated clinically with yellow coloured skin and sclerae, nausea, pruritus, dark-coloured urine, and decolouring of the stool.** They constitute more than 90% of cases of obstructive jaundice treated surgically. The common causes of obstructive jaundice are stones in the common bile ducts, periampullary and carcinoma head of the pancreas. Palpable liver, palpable mass (cholangiocarcinoma, carcinoma head of pancreas) and palpable gallbladder (periampullary carcinoma) supports the diagnosis of malignancy. Charcot's triad page 779, Table 54.2 if present supports the diagnosis of stones in the CBD. Details have been given in the subsequent pages. Early diagnosis by imaging, endoscopy, ERCP, MRCP is possible.

### Aetiology (Fig. 54.34)

#### *I. Causes in the Lumen*

1. Stones in the common bile duct
2. Ova, cysts, ascaris worms
3. Hydatid cyst of the biliary tree
4. Stone in the pancreatic duct/CBD junction.

#### *II. Causes in the Wall*

1. Periampullary carcinoma
2. Bile duct stricture
3. Stenosis of sphincter of Oddi (papillary stenosis)
4. Klatskin's tumour—carcinoma of the bile duct where right and left ducts join
5. Choledochal cyst
6. Post-laparoscopic cholecystectomy.

#### *III. Causes from Outside* (due to Pressure)

1. Carcinoma head of pancreas
2. Chronic pancreatitis
3. Lymph nodes at the porta hepatis obstructing the biliary tree.

### Clinical Features

Firstly, differentiate choledocholithiasis from carcinoma pancreas (Table 54.2). Next, differentiate between ampullary and periampullary carcinoma pancreas (Table 54.3).

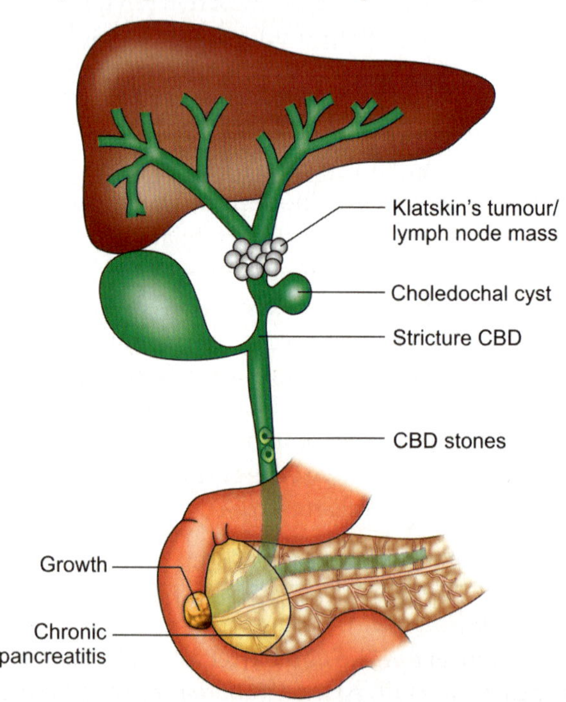


**Fig. 54.34:** Various causes of obstructive jaundice

**TABLE 54.2:** Differences between stone in the CBD and periampullary carcinoma (Ca)/Ca head of pancreas

| | Stone in the CBD | Carcinoma periampullary/head of pancreas |
|---|---|---|
| **1. Age** | 30–50 years | 50–70 years |
| **2. Sex** | More common in females | Equally common in both sexes |
| **3. Duration of symptoms** | Long duration | Short duration (1–3 months) |
| **4. Symptoms** | | |
| Pain | It is due to a stone blocking the CBD resulting in spasm of CBD. It is severe colicky pain like gallstone colic | There may be some discomfort in abdomen but colicky pain is not a feature. Pain is relatively rare in carcinoma head of the pancreas |
| Fever | As a result of obstruction, multiplication of organisms results in fever | When obstruction becomes severe, there is bile stasis Cholangitis, fever with chills and rigors can occur |
| Jaundice | Occurs due to obstruction. Once inflammation subsides, all these 3 symptoms are relieved partly but they recur after sometime. Hence, intermittent pain, intermittent fever, intermittent jaundice are classical of a stone in CBD— **Charcot's triad** | As a result of slow developing obstruction in periampullary region, jaundice is **persistent, progressive, painless, pruritic** In 5% of cases, growth may ulcerate into the duodenum. It can cause melaena and jaundice may temporarily sub-side. This happens in periampullary not in head of pancreas growth |
| Stools | Since the obstruction is never complete, clay-coloured stools are not commonly seen | Clay-coloured stools are common and when mixed with blood, it is called **silvery stools** or aluminium paint stools. This is called as Thomas' sign and it was first described by Heneage Ogilvie |
| Pruritus | May be present but mild | Severe—due to bile salts in the circulation |
| Loss of appetite | No | Significant |
| Loss of weight | No | Significant |
| **5. Signs** | | |
| Jaundice | Deep yellow | Sometimes, greenish yellow |
| Anaemia | Absent | It is usually present |
| **6. Per abdomen** | Liver can be enlarged due to back pressure. It is smooth, with round border, firm in consistency | Liver can be enlarged due to back pressure. In such cases, it has smooth surface. If it is nodular, with sharp border, hard in consistency, it is due to secondaries in the liver |
| **7. Gallbladder** | As a rule, gallbladder is not palpable | Gallbladder is palpable in 70–75% of cases |
| **8. Metastasis** | No | Left supraclavicular node, ascites, etc. may be seen |

**TABLE 54.3:** Differences between ampullary and periampullary carcinoma pancreas

| | Ampullary carcinoma | Periampullary carcinoma |
|---|---|---|
| Parts involved | Ampulla: (common channel), the intraduodenal portion of the bile duct and the intraduodenal portion of the pancreatic duct | Head of the pancreas, the distal common bile duct and the duodenum |
| Type of carcinoma | The intestinal type | Pancreatobiliary type |
| Incidence | Uncommon 6% | More common 20% |
| Ki-ras mutation | Around 35% | Around 90% |
| Prognosis | Good | Moderate |
| Clinical presentation | Ampullary tumours present with early jaundice, duodenal carcinoma presents with loss of weight, vomiting and cholangiocarcinoma with jaundice | Jaundice, fluctuant jaundice, loss of weight and appetite<br>Clay coloured stools |

## COURVOISIER'S LAW (Figs 54.35 and 54.36)

- In a jaundiced patient, if the gallbladder is palpably enlarged, it is not due to stones (Key Box 54.6). In case of stones, previous inflammation would have made gallbladder fibrotic and hence, will not be palpable.
- From clinical point of view, 90% of cases of obstructive jaundice are due to stones, periampullary carcinoma or carcinoma of the head of pancreas.

Key Box 54.6

**Clinical Features of Gallbladder Mass**

- Egg-shaped mass/pyriform shape
- Moves with respiration
- Tensely cystic, feels firm **(Murphy's point)**, located in the right hypochondrium
- Superficially placed
- Intra-abdominal, intraperitoneal

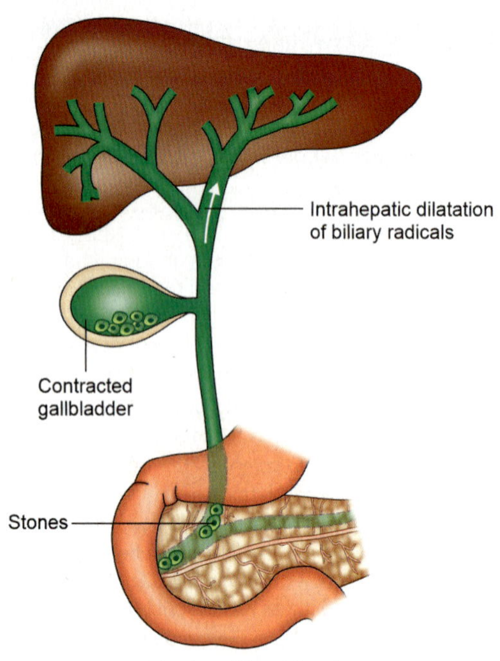


Fig. 54.35: Contracted thick gallbladder due to stones. Hence, not palpable

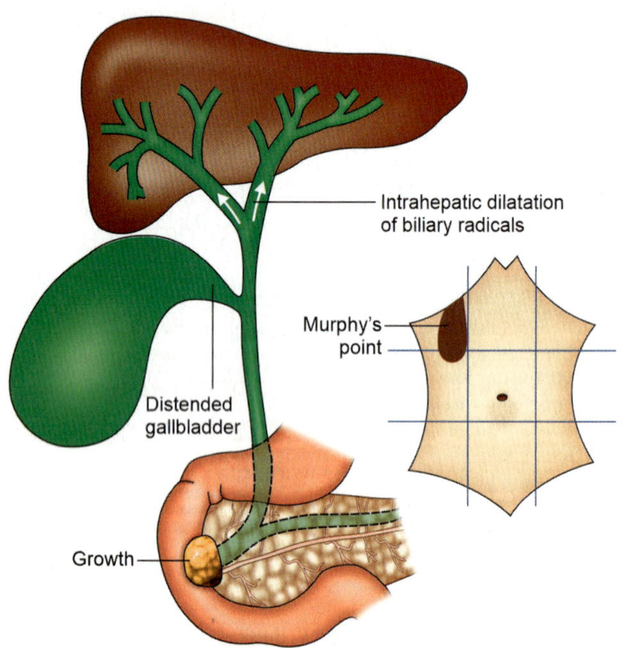


Fig. 54.36: Enlarged palpable gallbladder in cases of periampullary carcinoma

## Exceptions to Courvoisier's Law

1. Double impaction: One stone in the CBD and one stone in the cystic duct. Gallbladder may be palpable in such cases.
2. Periampullary carcinoma in a patient who has undergone cholecystectomy.
3. Primary oriental cholangiohepatitis causing stones in the CBD (gallbladder is normal in these cases). These stones are called primary CBD stones.

> **SU28.12.2:** Enumerate the causes, types, clinical features, investigations and management of a patient with cholelithiasis, and choledocholithiasis.

## CHOLEDOCHOLITHIASIS (see Table 54.1)

### Types of CBD Stones

I. **Primary stones:** These stones are formed in the CBD or within intrahepatic ducts. They are multiple, pigment stones or often mixed stones (Key Box 54.7). Various causes are:
   - Infections of biliary tree and infestation—parasites such as clonorchiasis.
   - Congenital—Caroli's disease or choledochal cyst.
   - Biliary dyskinesia—defective pathophysiology of biliary tree.
   - Other causes—diabetes, malnutrition.

II. **Secondary stones:** These stones originate from gallbladder and stay in CBD—usually supraduodenal portion—then get enlarged to attain large size over a period of time.
   These stones can give rise to cholangitis.

Key Box 54.7

**Primary CBD Stones**

- Only 4–12% of all CBD stones.
- These stones form primarily in common bile duct.
- Almost all primary CBD stones are pigment type (brown stones).
- Associated with bile duct stasis and infection (bacteria).
- Soft, easily crumble when manipulated.
- Associated with biliary stricture, papillary stenosis or sphincter of Oddi dysfunction.
- Mechanism; stasis—bacteria secrete bacterial glucuronidase which causes deconjugation of bilirubin diglucuronide, bilirubin gets precipitated as calcium salt.

### Natural History of CBD Stones (Key Box 54.8)

Key Box 54.8

**Natural History of CBD Stones**

| *Symptom* | | *% of patients* |
|---|---|---|
| Asymptomatic | — | 40% |
| Cholangitis | — | 20% |
| Jaundice | — | 20% |
| Biliary colic | — | 15% |
| Pancreatitis | — | 5% |

### Cholangitis

Bacterial infection of bile duct is called cholangitis.

#### *Predominant Organisms*

- *E. coli, Klebsiella, Pseudomonas,* enterococci, *Proteus.*
- Bacteroides and other anaerobes (*Clostridium perfringens*)

***Important causes***
- Choledocholithiasis
- Biliary stricture
- Neoplasm
- Less important causes are pseudocyst of pancreas, chronic pancreatitis stenosing sphincter of Oddi, biliary parasitic infections, etc.
- Post-ERCP, if stent cannot be passed as in obstructive jaundice cases.

### *Symptoms and Signs*

- Biliary colic, jaundice, chills and rigors are called Charcot's triad.
- Tenderness may be present in the upper abdomen.

### *Investigations*

- Leukocytosis, high bilirubin levels and alkaline phosphatase levels are diagnostic tests.
- Ultrasound, CT scans, ERCP are indicated to confirm/rule out the various causes.

### *Treatment*

- Intravenous antibiotics
- Emergency endoscopic sphincterotomy, extraction of stones in choledocholithiasis, endoscopic dilatation in cases of stenosis or stricture.
- Percutaneous transhepatic biliary drainage (PTBD) in high obstructions.
- Laparotomy—drainage of CBD—T-tube insertion.

### Reynolds' Pentad of Acute Obstructive Cholangitis

A few cases of CBD stones present with serious problems of cholangitis described as Reynold's pentad.

1. Persistent pain
2. Fever
3. Persistent jaundice
4. Shock
5. Altered mental status.

## INVESTIGATIONS IN OBSTRUCTIVE JAUNDICE

1. **Hb%** is low in malignancy.
2. **TC and DC** are increased in case of infections. High white cell counts suggest cholangitis and it becomes an indication for preoperative stenting in cases of carcinoma head/periampullary carcinoma. If cholangitis is due to CBD stones (more common), ERP followed by extraction of the stones with a stent is the initial definite treatment.
3. **PT and INR** may be increased in case of obstructive jaundice.
4. **Urine** for urobilinogen is negative in obstructive jaundice.
5. **Serum alkaline phosphatase:** Normal value 60–300 units/L. More than 500 units is suggestive of obstructive jaundice.
    - These are the enzymes which bring **hydrolysis** of phosphate esters in alkaline medium.
    - Sources of alkaline phosphatase include **liver, biliary tree**, bone, intestine, kidney.
    - Excretion is mainly through biliary tree (Key Box 54.9).

Key Box 54.9

**Alkaline Phosphatase**

- It is the product of epithelial cells of cholangioles—↑ levels are due to increased enzyme production.
- Intrahepatic cholestasis, cholangitis, and extrahepatic obstruction are the chief factors causing elevation.
- Focal lesions in the liver—single hepatic metastasis, liver abscess or a tumour can cause increased levels without jaundice.
- In cholangitis, bilirubin may be normal but alkaline phosphatase may be very high.
- 

| **Gross elevation** | **Mild elevation** |
|---|---|
| Obstructive jaundice, biliary cirrhosis, bone disease | Metastasis in the liver, hepatic abscess, hepatitis |

6. **Gamma-glutamyl transpeptidase (GGT):** It is the first enzyme to get elevated in obstructive jaundice. It persists for a longer period of time. It is not elevated in diseases of bones wherein ALP is elevated. However, it can be elevated in many malignancies including carcinoma prostate, carcinoma ovaries, etc.
7. **Abdominal ultrasound:** It is the **most useful, noninvasive, reliable and quick investigation for obstructive** jaundice. Dilated biliary radicles, both intrahepatic and extrahepatic, can be demonstrated (first clue in obstructive jaundice).
    - Gallstones can be diagnosed with their posterior acoustic shadow.
    - Mass lesion in the head region can be seen in cases of chronic pancreatitis or carcinoma head of the pancreas causing obstructive jaundice.
    - Ultrasound can detect multiple secondaries in the liver, thus, favouring the diagnosis of malignancy. However it is not an ideal investigation for CBD stones.
8. **Contrast enhanced CT (CECT) scan:** A head mass of even 2–3 cm in size and portal vein infiltration can be demonstrated by CT scan. Obliteration of fat plane between the mass and superior mesenteric vessels can be demonstrated by CT scan which decides the operability of periampullary carcinoma

or carcinoma head of the pancreas (Figs 54.37 to 54.40). It is a relative contraindication for surgery.

- CT scan cannot differentiate head mass of carcinoma from chronic pancreatitis. (PET scan may differentiate.)
- CT scan can also detect coeliac nodes, presence of which is a contraindication for radical resections (Key Box 54.10).
- Take precautions against contrast-induced nephropathy.

Key Box 54.10

**Investigation of Choice in Obstructive Jaundice**

- Gallstones: Ultrasound
- Suspected CBD stone: MRI
- Diagnostic and therapeutic for CBD stone: ERCP
- High bile duct stricture: MRCP
- Low-ampullary stenosis/strictures: ERCP
- Carcinoma head of pancreas/chronic pancreatitis: CT/ERCP

9. **Endoscopy** is useful to diagnose a periampullary carcinoma which may be seen as an ulcerative lesion in the second part of the duodenum. Biopsy can also be taken which shows adenocarcinoma (Fig. 54.41). Please note if a lesion is detected such as growth, no stenting/or intervention (ERCP) is done. However, when bilirubin levels are very high and to improve general condition of the patient, as in cholangitis, temporary stenting can be done.
   - In case of obstructive jaundice due to stones, smooth bulge can be seen in the second part of the duodenum. In carcinoma, ulcerated lesion can be seen.
10. **MRI:** When CBD stones are suspected, MRI is done. It is easy and no contrast is used. If stones are detected, one can proceed with ERCP and basketting of stones (Figs 54.42 and 54.43).
11. **Endoscopic retrograde cholangiopancreatography (ERCP)** (Figs 54.44 to 54.46).
   - With the help of a side viewing endoscope, ampulla of Vater is cannulated and a radio-opaque dye is injected.
   - It fills up the biliary and pancreatic system.

   ***Interpretation***

   - Stones appear as filling defects in the CBD or in the common hepatic duct (CHD) (Figs 54.44 to 54.46), which may be mobile (change position, if patient is moved).
   - A periampullary carcinoma gives rise to an irregular filling defect or there may be total cut off in the flow of dye. (Done for cholangitis due to carcinoma cases.)

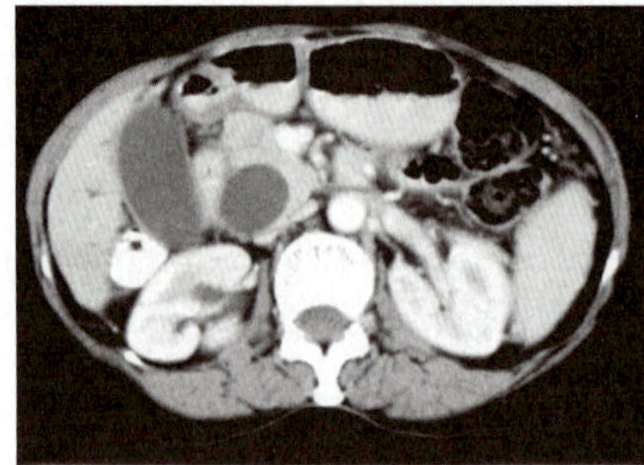

**Fig. 54.37:** CT scan showing hugely distended gallbladder and common bile duct—periampullary carcinoma. Growth was resectable. He underwent **Whipple's operation**

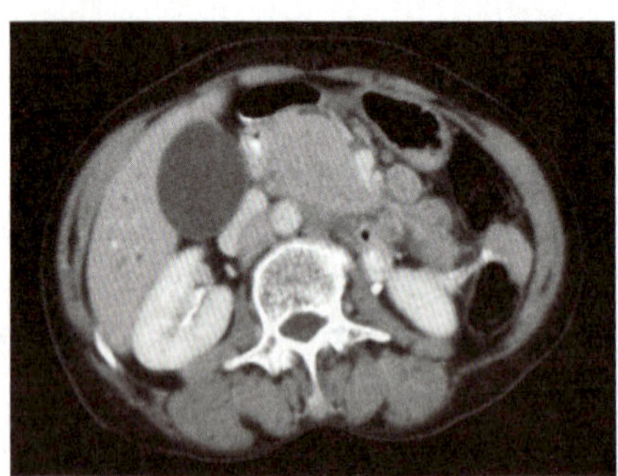

**Fig. 54.38:** Large 6 cm mass in the head of pancreas—patient not only had obstructive jaundice but also duodenal obstruction. He underwent **triple bypass**

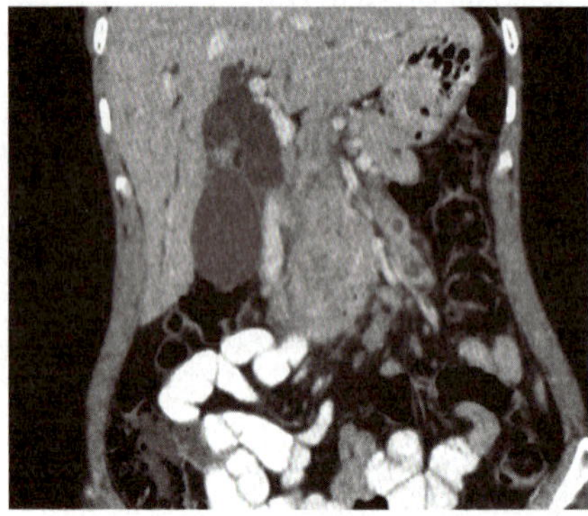

**Fig. 54.39:** 6 cm mass abutting mesenteric vessels and involving root of the mesentery. Such masses are usually nonresectable

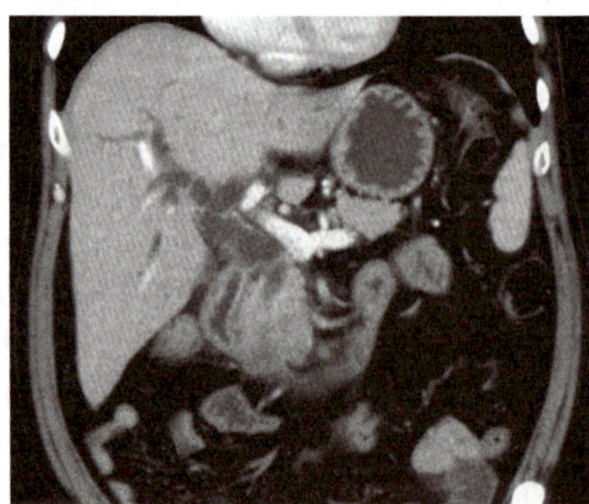

**Fig. 54.40:** Large head mass with obstructive jaundice with intrahepatic dilatation. When in doubt, diagnostic laparoscopy will help—to operate or palliate nonsurgically

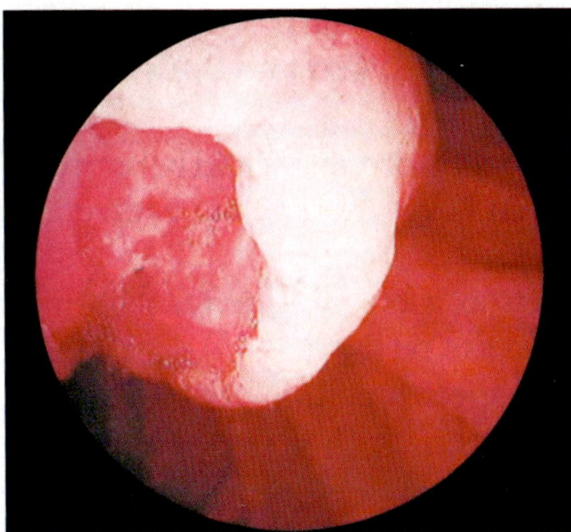

Fig. 54.41: Endoscopy showing growth in the periampullary region. These lesions are usually resectable

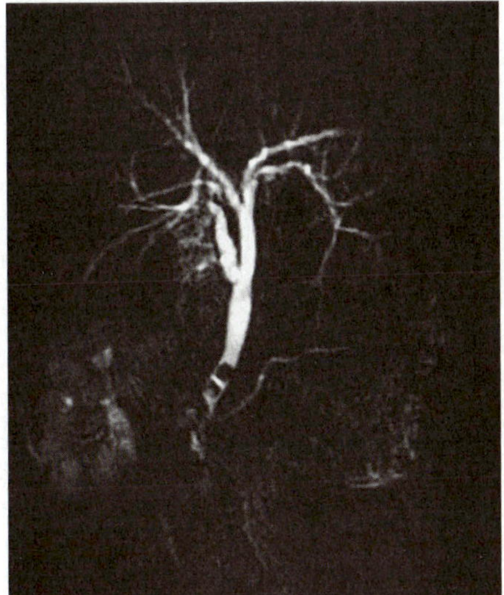

Fig. 54.42: MRI showing CBD stone

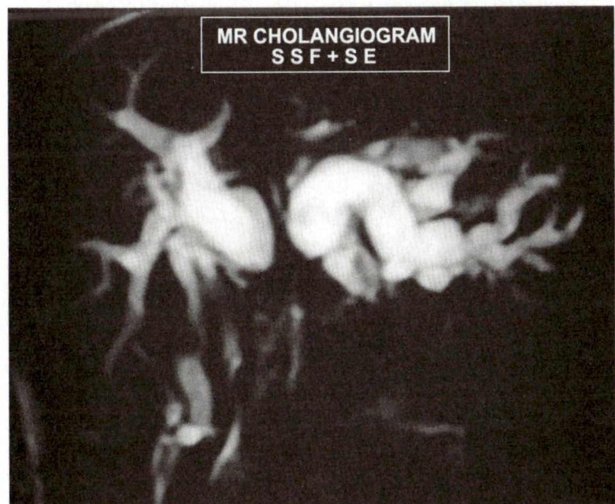


Fig. 54.43: MRC intrahepatic dilatation, another case of cholangiocarcinoma—biopsy is not possible with MRI. Brush cytology is possible while doing ERCP

- Chronic pancreatitis may show the dilated duct and stones in the pancreatic duct—***'chain of lakes' appearance***.

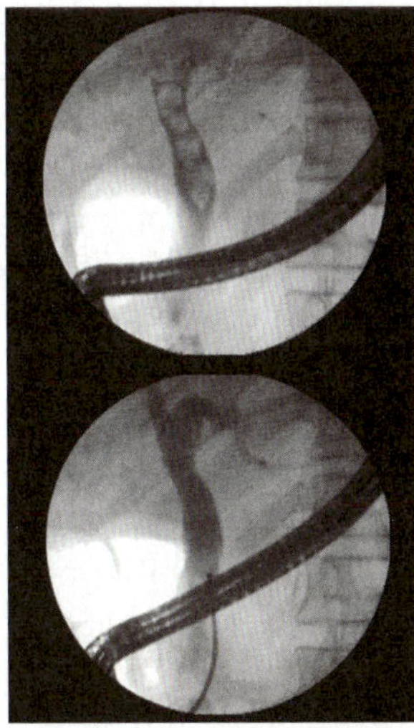

Fig. 54.44: ERCP showing stones in the CBD, stones are extracted and stent has been placed in the common bile duct

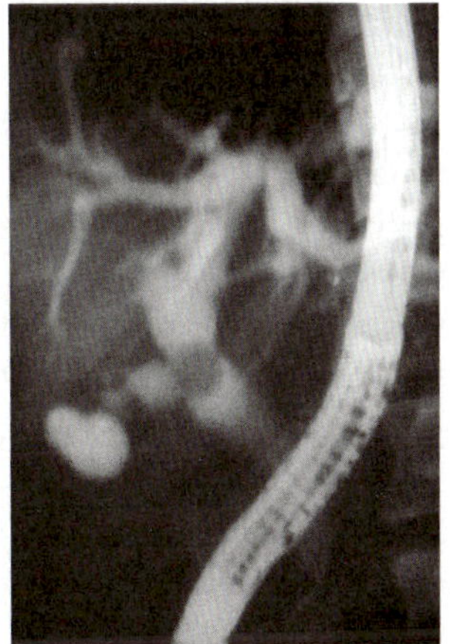

Fig. 54.45: ERCP showing stones in the CBD and contracted gallbladder

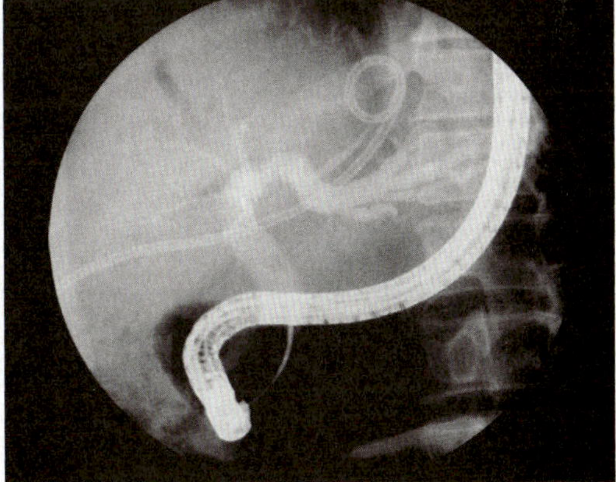

Fig. 54.46: ERCP basketting of stones followed by stent inserted into CBD

***Uses:*** If stones in the CBD are diagnosed, they can be treated in the following ways:

- Extraction by using a basket.
- Large stone can be crushed by using a lithotripter and can be extracted.

- Sphincterotomy (incision of sphincter of Oddi) can be done to facilitate extrusion of small stones.
- In patients with cholangitis with obstructive jaundice, stenting of common bile duct can be done to relieve obstruction. **Stent removal is necessary** at a later date.
- In selected patients with **biliary strictures**, stent is placed after ERCP to relieve obstructive jaundice (sometimes permanent in malignancies).
- In selected patients with **chronic pancreatitis**, pancreatic duct can be stented to relieve pain.

*Pearls of Wisdom*

ERCP and stenting is NOT indicated in operable cases of carcinoma periampullary/head of pancreas unless cholangitis is present.

***Complications:*** Severe infection of biliary tree (cholangitis) and acute pancreatitis can occur in 1–2% of the patients. Hence, prophylactic antibiotics are given before the procedure.

12. **Endosonogram:** Endoscopy aided ultrasound can detect missed stones in the CBD. It can also detect pancreatic head mass, lymph nodes. Endosono-guided FNAC can also be done (Fig. 54.47).
13. **Percutaneous transhepatic cholangiography (PTC):** Using an ultrasound image-intensifier, a dilated biliary radicle is identified within the liver and a fine needle (Chiba needle[1]) is introduced into it. The stylet is then removed and a radio-opaque dye injected. Chiba needle is 15 cm long and 0.7 mm in diameter (Figs 54.48A and B, Key Box 54.11).

***Precautions***

- Coagulation profile should be normal. Otherwise, vitamin K injection 10 mg is given IV or SC for 3 days.
- If there is a bleeding tendency, this procedure should not be done.
- Broad-spectrum antibiotics are given before the procedure.

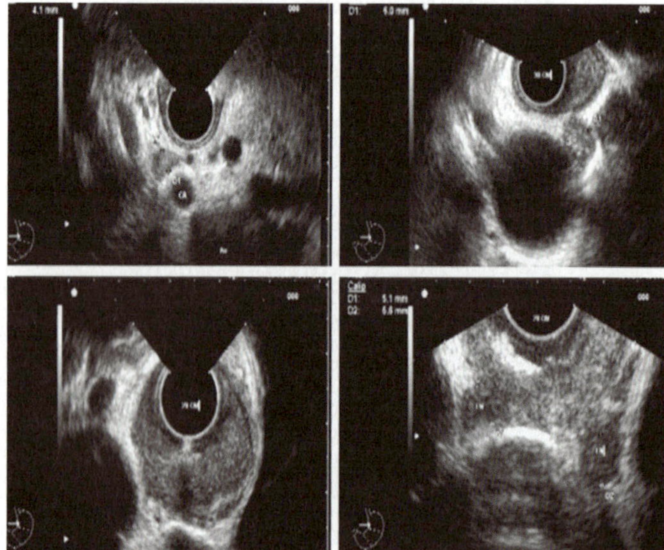

**Fig. 54.47:** Endosonography showing pancreatic tumour with celiac lymph nodes. (*Courtesy*: Dr Ganesh Pai, Head, Department of Medical Gastroenterology, KMC, Manipal)

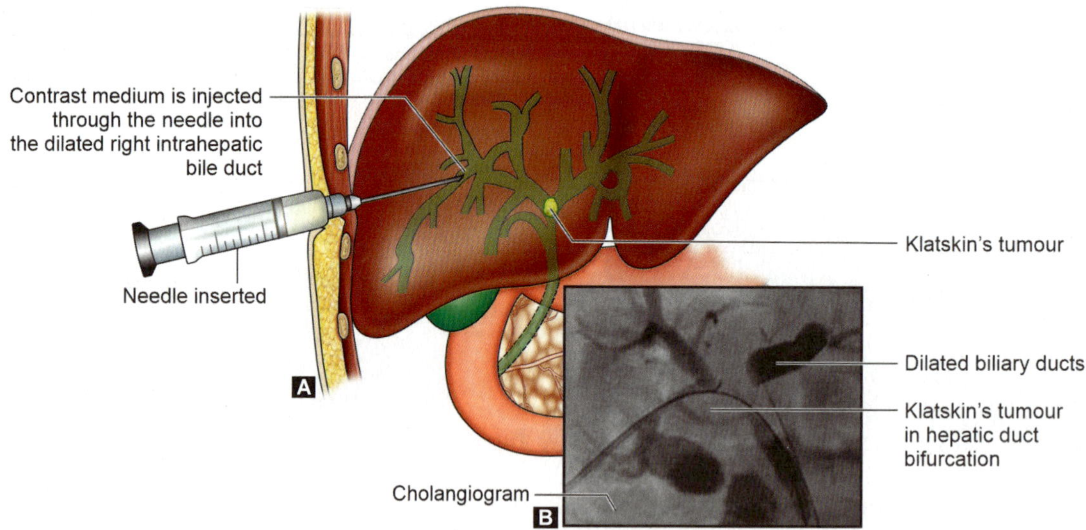


**Figs 54.48A and B:** (A) Percutaneous transhepatic cholangiography (PTC); (B) Dye had failed to fill-up the bifurcation of the common hepatic duct suggesting the obstruction (diagrammatic)

[1]Chiba: It is the name of a university in Japan.

Key Box 54.11

**Facts about PTC**

1. In the diagnosis of high strictures, PTC is better than ERCP.
2. It can also be used in ERCP failure cases.
3. In the diagnosis of Klatskin's tumour, PTC is extremely useful. It can also delineate the dilated proximal duct, which helps in planning for a biliary-enteric anastomosis.
4. Catheter can be kept in the bile ducts to provide external drainage as in strictures or in inoperable malignancies with obstructive jaundice (Fig. 54.48C).

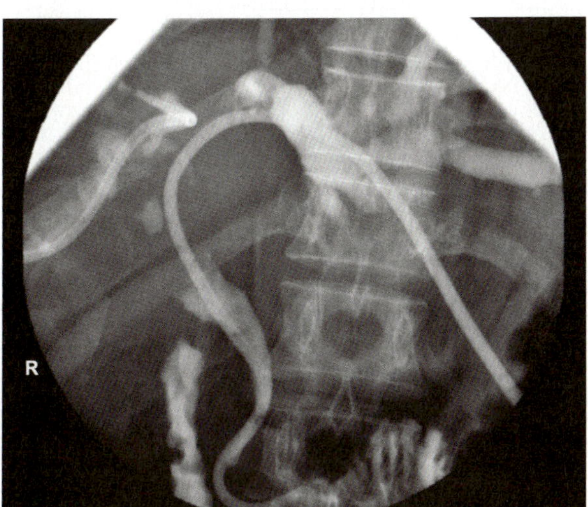


**Fig. 54.48C:** PTBD catheter inside CBD

*Complications*

- Infection, cholangitis, septicaemia
- Biliary leak can be significant producing abdominal pain and guarding. Hence, PTC should be done just prior to the surgery.
- Haemorrhage

**14. Diagnostic laparoscopy**

- It is used in many GI malignancies.
- It can be aided by laparoscopic ultrasound.
- It can complement the staging by CT, MRI, etc. It can improve prediction of resectability to about 98% accuracy.
- It is a simple but invasive investigation, requires 3 ports.
- Specially excellent to detect ***peritoneal metastasis*** (which cannot be picked by other tests) which is the sign of inoperability.

**15. CA 19–9:** Often head mass can be due to carcinoma/chronic pancreatitis. Biopsy is not mandatory. Clinical suspicion of a head mass may be treated with Whipple's pancreaticoduodenectomy. However, gross elevation of CA 19–9 (carbohydrate antigen) will suggest carcinoma.

### Summary of the Investigations in Cases of Obstructive Jaundice (Fig. 54.49)

- CBP, LFT is done first to know the type of jaundice and to know the general condition of the patient.
- If ultrasound detects IHBR and CBD stones, no other investigations are necessary. ERCP and basketing of the stones is done.
- If ultrasound shows doubtful stones, CECT is done.
- If periampullary carcinoma is suspected, side viewing endoscopy and biopsy is done followed by CECT to detect signs of operability.
- In high (at the porta hepatis or at confluence of left and right hepatic ducts) obstructions—MRI and CECT are done.

## TREATMENT OF OBSTRUCTIVE JAUNDICE

### Preoperative Preparation

In all malignancies, Kernofsky criteria or ECOG criteria (page no. 842) of performance status is calculated and discussion is done with patient and relatives regarding the plan of treatment—surgery, complications, chemotherapy, etc. Discussion of the disease and the performance status should be discussed in tumour board once staging is done and appropriate treatment is done.

1. Correction of fluid and electrolyte status, adequate hydration before surgery for 2–3 days is essential, especially when patients have vomiting or have developed sepsis.

   Adequate hydration is done to improve the urinary output.
2. Injection vitamin K, 10 mg, subcutaneously or intravenously for 3 days is given to correct the prothrombin time. If prothrombin time is not corrected with this treatment, **fresh frozen plasma** should be given.
3. Broad-spectrum antibiotics are given before, during and after surgery.
4. Adequate blood transfusion to correct anaemia.
5. Nutrition, especially in cases of low albumin.

### Treatment of CBD Stones

Once the diagnosis of CBD stones are confirmed by imaging, a few options are available depending upon expertise, facilities. They are given below.

1. ***Preoperative ERCP, sphincterotomy + extraction of stones followed by laparoscopic cholecystectomy:*** This method has become the choice today. Expertise and sophisticated equipment are necessary for this (Fig. 54.50).
2. ***Cholecystectomy*** is done first. This is followed by introduction of a cannula into the cystic duct and a radio-opaque dye is injected.

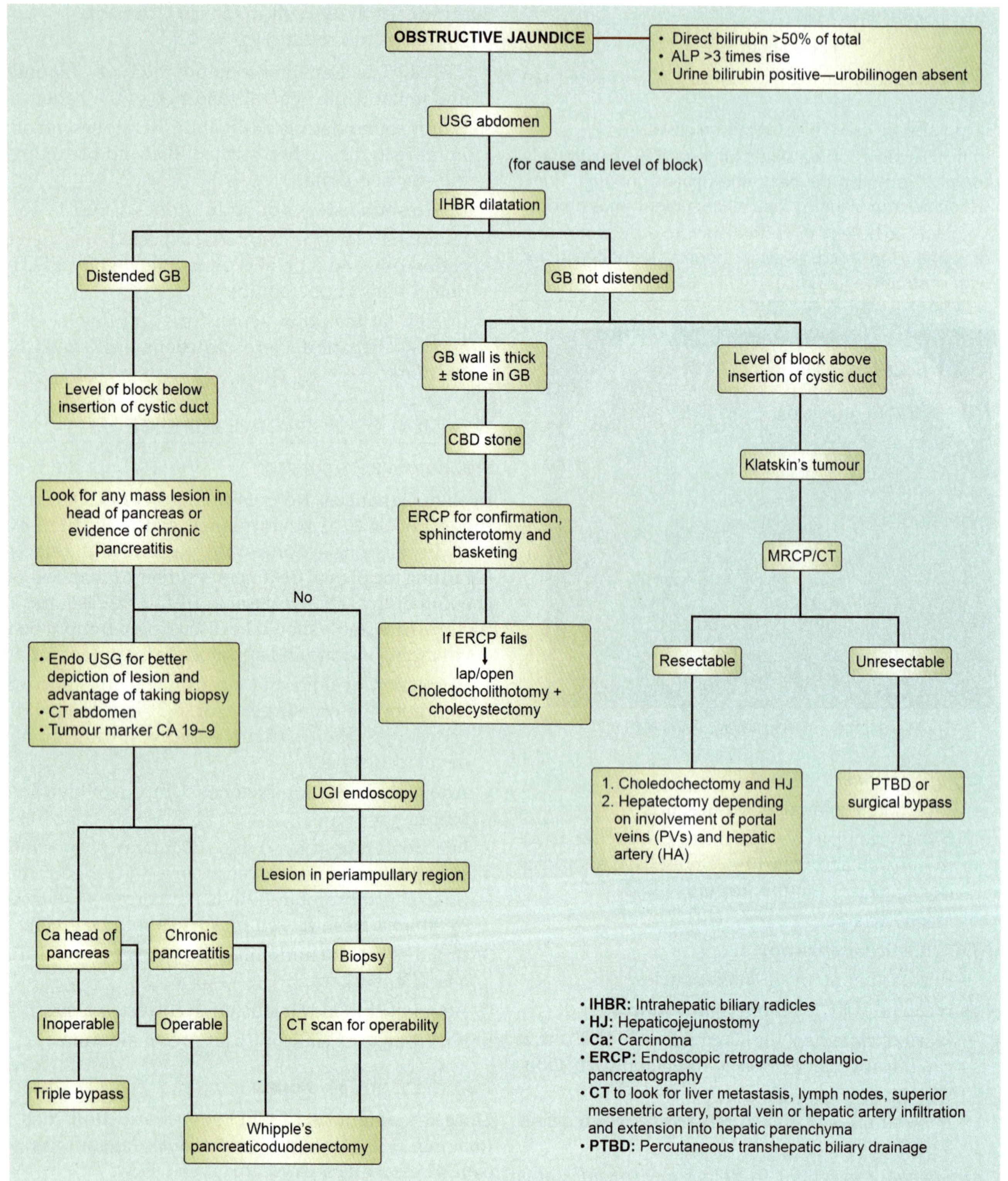


**Fig. 54.49:** Investigations and treatment of obstructive jaundice. (*Courtesy*: Dr Ankur Sharma, Assistant Professor, Department of Surgery, KMC, Manipal)

- This is called **OTC** (**O**n **T**able **C**holangiography). If the dye goes freely into the duodenum without filling defect, it is a normal OTC. If there are filling defects in the CBD, it is explored.
- **Precautions while doing OTC**
  - There should not be any air bubble in the syringe.
  - 5–10 ml of dye has to be injected.
  - Leakage of the dye should not occur.
  - OTC and CBD exploration can be done by laparoscopy only.

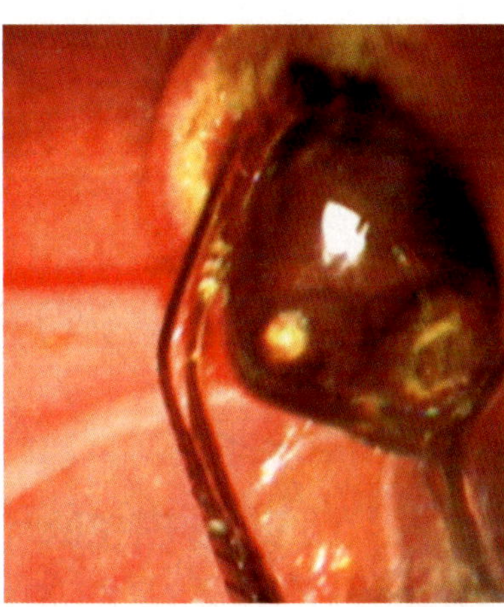

**Fig. 54.50:** Stone was removed through endoscopic papillotomy followed by basketing. There is a small risk of perforation and pancreatitis in these patients. Procedure is followed by a stent. (*Courtesy*: Dr Ganesh Pai, Prof and Head, Department of Medical Gastroenterology, KMC, Manipal)

3. ***Supraduodenal choledocholithotomy:*** Some patients come after Lap. cholecystotomy and failed ERCP and basketting. They are managed by open method. Supraduodenal CBD is explored through an incision over the anterior wall and the stones are removed. Operating choledochoscope is passed into the common hepatic duct and its branches and the stones, if present, are removed. Closure of the CBD is done after inserting 'T-tube'. After 8–10 days, a T-tube cholangiography is done and if the dye goes freely into duodenum and no filling defect is seen in the CBD, the T-tube is removed by gentle traction. By 10–12 days, the track is well formed. Hence, even if minor leak occurs, bile flows outside without causing peritonitis (Key Box 54.12, Figs 54.51A and B).

Key Box 54.12

**Indications for Exploration of CBD**

1. Ultrasound proven stones in CBD
2. OTC shows filling defect

4. ***Cholecystectomy + choledocholithotomy + choledochoduodenostomy:*** It can be done when CBD is dilated more than 1.5 cm in diameter and stoma should be at least 2–3 cm in size (Fig. 54.52). Indications are:
   - Recurrent stones in the CBD
   - Multiple intrahepatic stones (Caroli's disease)
   - Stricture of the lower CBD

   ***Advantages of choledochoduodenostomy***
   - Biliary leak is negligible
   - There is no worry, even if there are retained stones in the CBD.
   - It is a permanent solution for stenosis, stricture or multiple intrahepatic stones.

## TREATMENT OF PERIAMPULLARY CARCINOMA

### I. Surgical Treatment (Figs 54.53 to 54.58)

1. **Radical pancreaticoduodenectomy—'Whipple's operation'** (Figs 54.53 and 54.54).
   - In this operation, the growth along with 'C' loop of duodenum up to DJ flexure, proximal jejunum, head of the pancreas up to the neck are removed and partial gastrectomy is done. This is followed by:
     - Removal of lower CBD and gallbladder.
     - Pancreaticojejunal anastomosis (PJ), gastrojejunostomy (GJ) and choledochojejunostomy (CJ).

*Pearls of Wisdom*

Preoperative tissue diagnosis is NOT necessary with appropriate clinical and imaging findings, specially in head masses.

   - This is a major operation and carries 5–10% mortality due to pancreatic leakage or biliary leakage.

**'TUNNEL OF LOVE'**

During resectional surgery for pancreatic head and uncinate process tumours (Whipple's pancreaticoduodenectomy), after a preliminary search for metastases, a tunnel (the so-called tunnel of love) needs to be developed behind the neck of the pancreas and anterior to the underlying visceral vessels before concluding that the lesion can be resected. CBD is lifted gently by a tape and plane between CBD and portal vein is slowly developed by using a little finger from above. Another finger is inserted from below behind pancreas. Two should meet without any tissue.

   - Whipple's operation is indicated in cases of mobile growth with no metastasis and where the general condition of the patients is good.
   - Patients with cholangitis are treated with preoperative CBD stent followed 3–4 weeks later by Whipple's procedure.

2. **Pylorus-preserving pancreaticoduodenectomy (PPPD) or Traverso-Longmire procedure:** In this operation, pylorus is preserved. Thus, gastric motility is not disturbed (*see* Fig. 54.55).
3. **Triple bypass: Cholecystojejunostomy + enterostomy + gastrojejunostomy**
   - This is a palliative surgery in which distended gallbladder is anastomosed to a long loop of jejunum (40 cm) to relieve jaundice. To prevent food particles entering into the gallbladder, enteroenterostomy is done (*see* Fig. 54.50). Cholecystojejunostomy is easy to do compared to choledochojejunostomy which is superior bypass procedure.

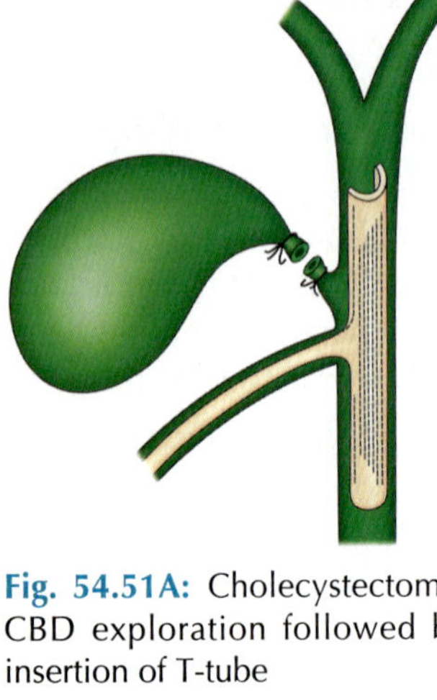

Fig. 54.51A: Cholecystectomy, CBD exploration followed by insertion of T-tube

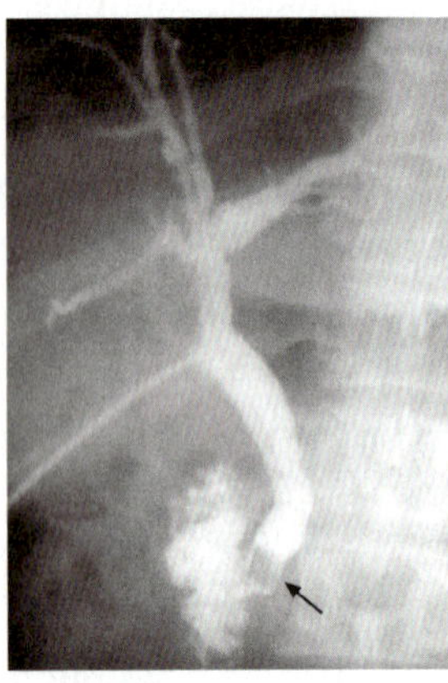

Fig. 54.51B: T-tube cholangiogram showing residual (retained) stone in the lower CBD—it was removed through endoscopic papillotomy and basketing

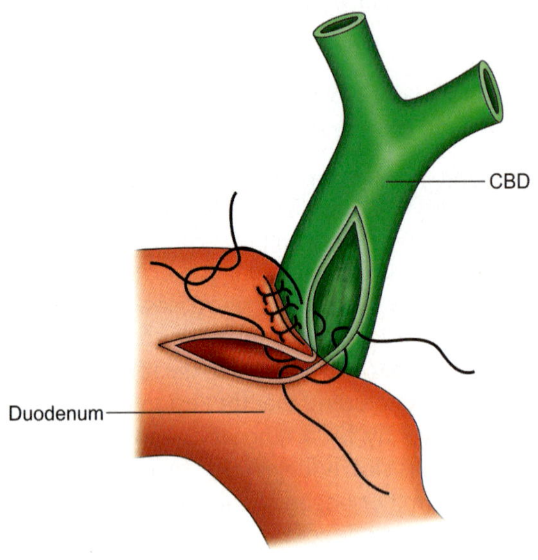


Fig. 54.52: Choledochoduodenostomy

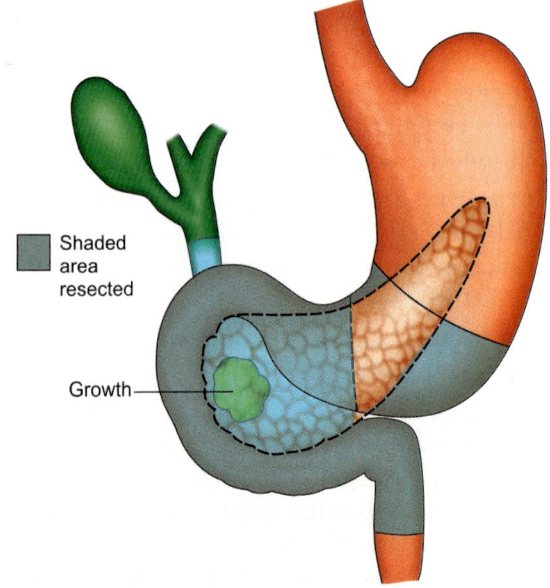


Fig. 54.53: Whipple's resection (diagrammatic)

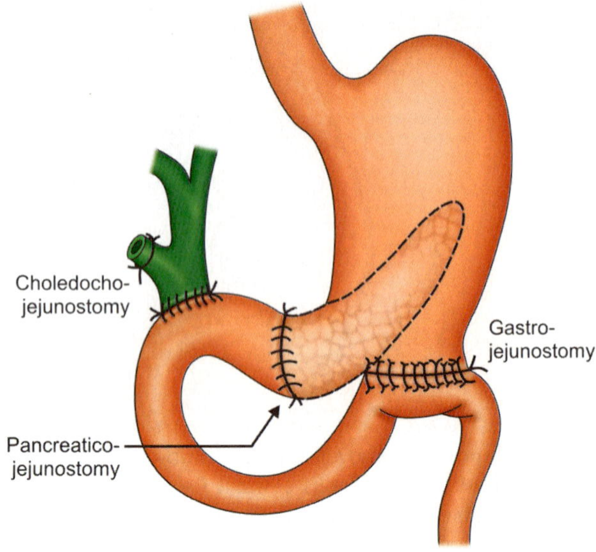


Fig. 54.54: Reconstruction following Whipple's operation

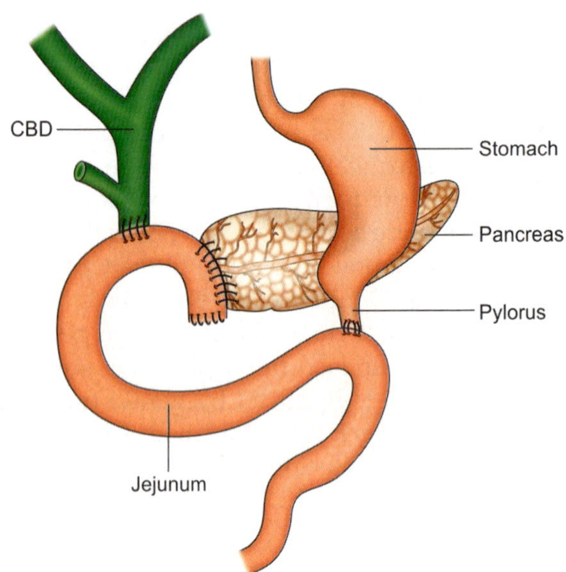


Fig. 54.55: Pylorus-preserving pancreaticoduodenectomy (PPPD)

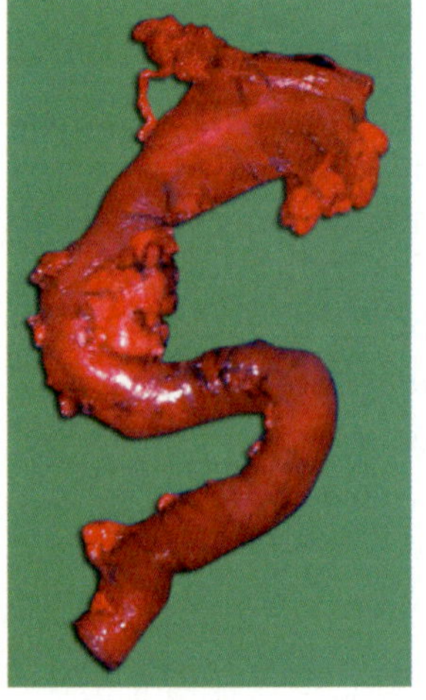

Fig. 54.56A: Whipple's resection specimen

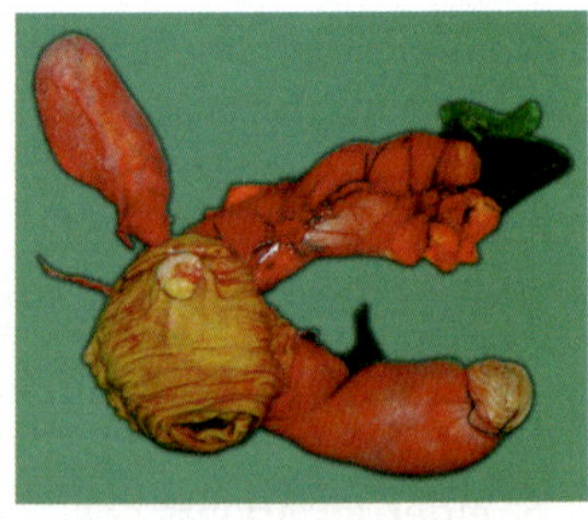

Fig. 54.56B: Whipple's specimen (*Courtesy*: Dr Satyanarayana N, Former Associate Professor, Yenepoya Medical College, Mangaluru)

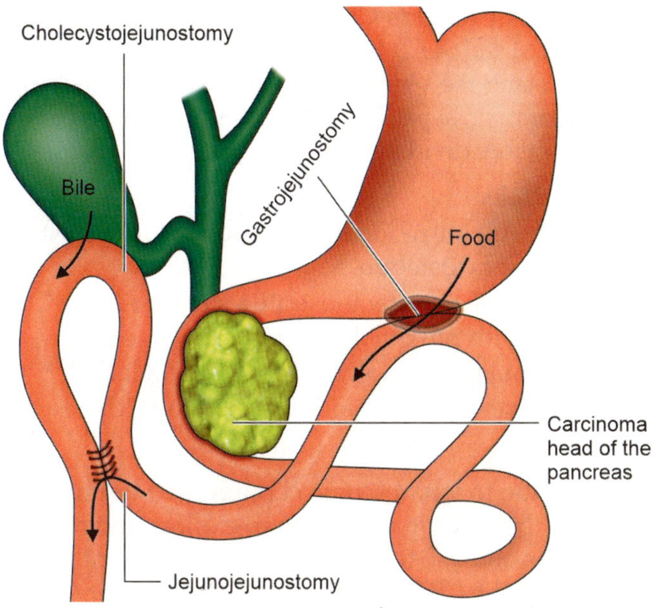


**Fig. 54.57:** Palliative triple bypass

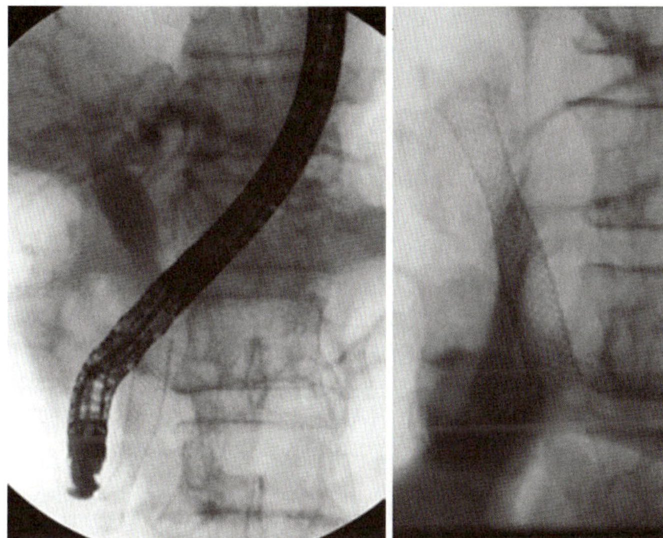

**Fig. 54.58:** Palliative stenting for carcinoma head of the pancreas

- Most of the patients develop duodenal obstruction caused by the growth in the postoperative period. Hence, a palliative GJ is done at the same time.
- In the absence of duodenal obstruction, if surgeon thinks that patient may live longer, beyond 6 months, GJ is indicated (for a possible duodenal obstruction occurring later).

### II. Nonsurgical Treatment

Very elderly patients (age criteria not clear) who are not fit candidates for surgery and patients who have metastasis can be treated by palliative stenting. However, results of a surgical bypass is superior to stenting. Also, the stent needs to be changed frequently.

## OTHER CAUSES OF OBSTRUCTIVE JAUNDICE

**SU28.12.4:** Classify biliary strictures. Enumerate the causes, clinical features, investigations and management of biliary strictures.

### STRICTURE OF THE CBD

- 80% of strictures occur following surgery on the biliary tree. They are called postoperative strictures. 20% are due to inflammatory pathology.
- It gives rise to slowly progressive, painless jaundice.
- Strictures account for 1–2% cases of obstructive jaundice.

#### Post Laparoscopic Cholecystectomy (Lap Chole)

The classification of bile duct injuries following Lap chole are classified as:

1. **Bismuth classification:** Five types of bile duct injuries are recognosed based on the distance from the hilar structure—bile duct bifurcation, the level of injury, the involvement of bile duct bifurcation, and individual right sectoral duct.
   - ***Bismuth classification of postoperative stricture:***
     **Type I:** Low common bile duct; stump >2 cm
     **Type II:** Middle common hepatic duct, stump <2 cm
     **Type III:** Hilar—confluence of right and left duct intact
     **Type IV:** Right and left ducts separated
     **Type V:** Involvement of the intrahepatic ducts.
2. **Strasberg classification:** It helps in differentiating small (bile leakage from the cystic duct or aberrant right sectoral branch) and serious injuries.
   Both these have been depicted in Fig. 54.59.

#### *Causes*

*1. Postoperative post-traumatic* (Fig. 54.60)

- ***Difficult cholecystectomy:*** When the gallbladder is fibrosed, densely stuck to the right hepatic duct or to the common bile duct or as in early cholecystectomy due to oedema around Calot's triangle, injury can occur to the right hepatic duct or to the CBD or CHD resulting in stricture.

*Pearls of Wisdom*

Difficult cholecystectomy, dangerous cholecystectomy and faulty dissection are the important factors for postoperative bile duct strictures.

- ***Dangerous cholecystectomy:*** Sudden bleeding from cystic artery can occur due to traction on the gallbladder or due to lack of gentleness in ligating cystic artery. Sudden application of an artery

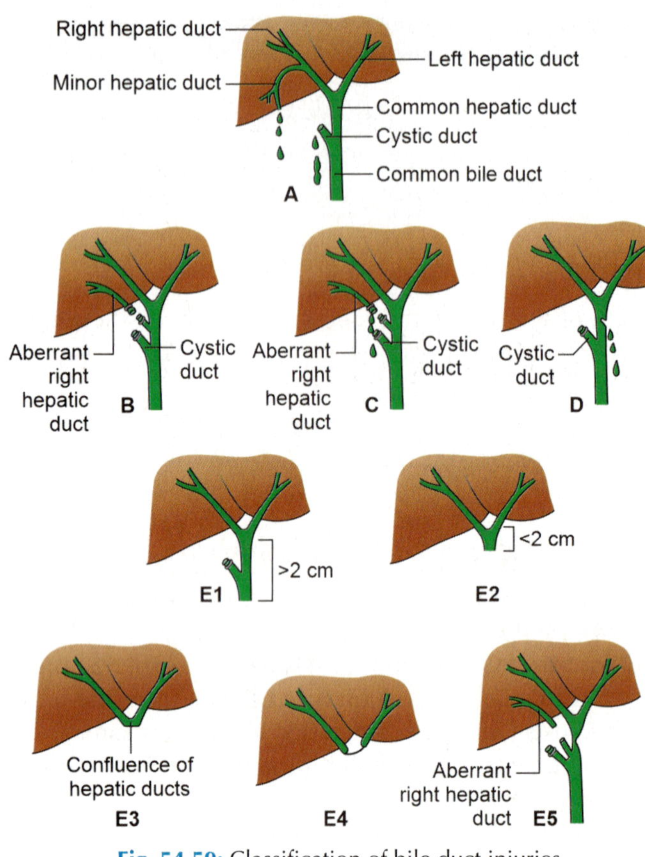


**Fig. 54.59:** Classification of bile duct injuries

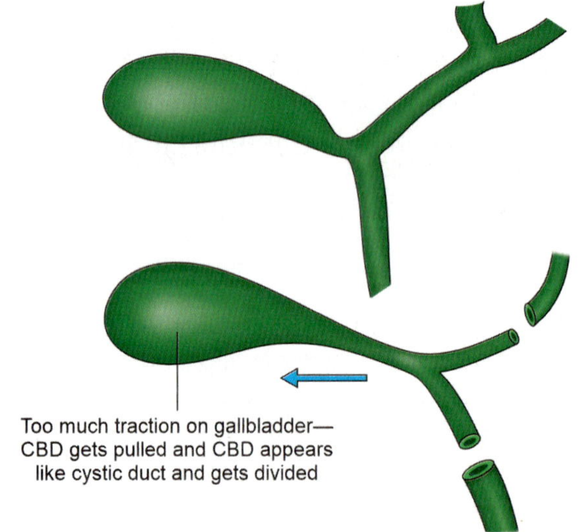


**Fig. 54.60:** Laparoscopy bile duct injury

forceps to control the bleeding may injure CBD. In such situations, packing the area, good suction and visualisation of the bleeding artery and ligation should be done. If the bleeding continues, the hepatic artery can be compressed between the finger and the thumb in the lesser omentum through the foramen of Winslow. This is called **Hogarth-Pringle manoeuvre**.

- ***Dissection at fault:*** Ignorance of anomalies such as short cystic duct or too much traction on the gallbladder distorts CBD and predisposes to injury (Figs 54.61 and 54.62). It is the duty of the surgeon to show his assistants the Y junction which is formed by the cystic duct, common hepatic duct above and common bile duct below before dividing any structures in this area.

### *Investigations*

- USG—to rule out residual stones in CBD, to demonstrate intrahepatic dilatation.
- ERCP or PTC may demonstrate a stricture in the CBD or CHD with proximal dilatation.
- T-tube cholangiography, if T-tube is in place.
- MRC is noninvasive and is better than PTC.

### *Treatment*

- If it is due to laparoscopic clipping without transection of the CBD, it is better to re-explore and remove the clips and a T-tube or an endoscopic stent can be placed in the CBD (Fig. 54.63).
- Late cases can be managed by choledochojejunostomy or hepaticojejunostomy by anastomosing a loop of jejunum to the dilated portion above the stricture. However, the general condition of the patient should be improved before surgery (Figs 54.64 to 54.68).

*Pearls of Wisdom*

Prevention is better than treatment. Try to prevent bile duct injuries during laparoscopic cholecystectomy.

### *2. Post-inflammatory*

Post-inflammatory strictures follow recurrent attacks of cholangitis due to:

- Stones in the CBD or CHD
- Parasites like *Ascaris lumbricoides* in the biliary tree or **Asiatic cholangiohepatitis** produced by Chinese liver fluke infestation (*Clonorchis sinensis*).
- Primary sclerosing cholangitis wherein the cause is not known.

### *3. Malignant strictures*

Malignant strictures are due to cholangiocarcinoma.

### *Clinical features*

- History of cholecystectomy in the past with or without profuse discharge of bile in the postoperative period.
- A slowly progressive, painless jaundice deepening day by day.
- Hepatomegaly due to back pressure.
- Recurrent cholangitis due to stasis of bile.

### *4. Sclerosing Cholangitis*

It is characterised by development of multiple strictures and dilatation of CBD with features of fibrous thickening of CBD.

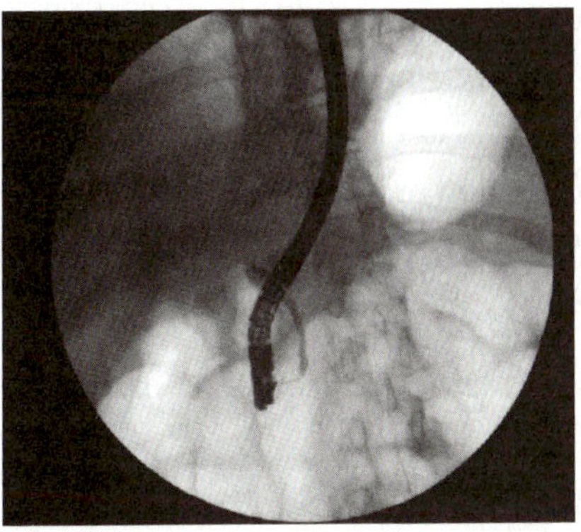

**Fig. 54.61:** ERCP showing complete transection of bile duct—type IV injury

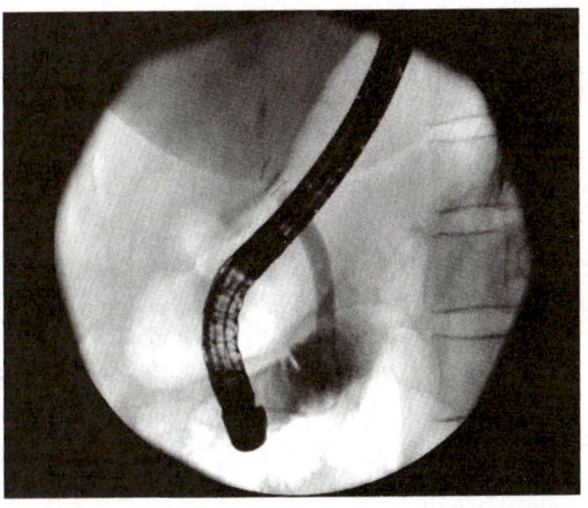

**Fig. 54.62:** CBD clipping—here, it was not transected. It was explored, clip removed and endoscopic stent was inserted

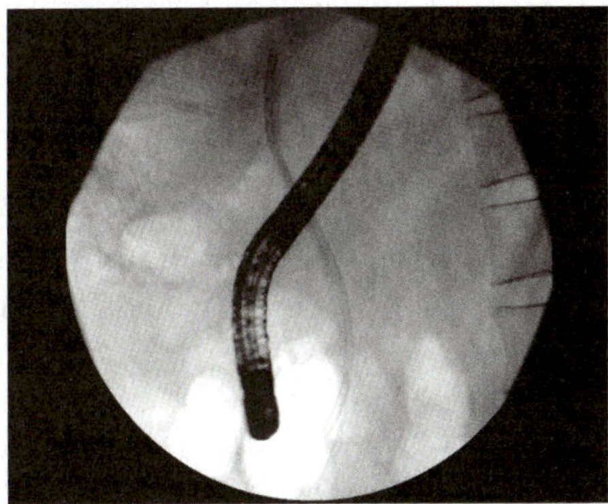

**Fig. 54.63:** Same patient as in Fig. 54.62. You can see the stent in the common hepatic duct. It was removed after 6 months

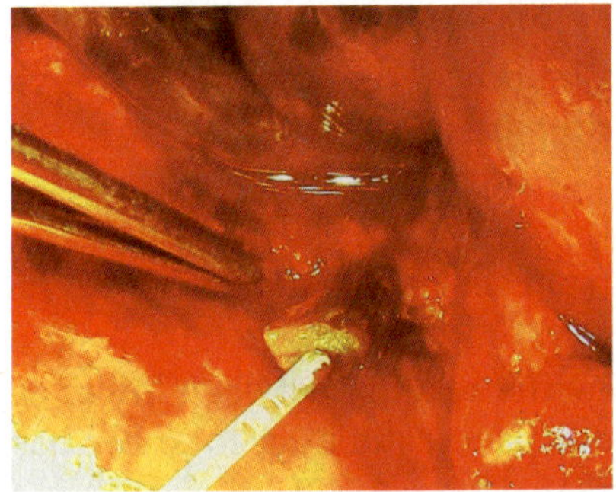

**Fig. 54.64:** Cut CHD—it was a difficult task to reach this area, it is trimmed for biliary enteric anastomosis

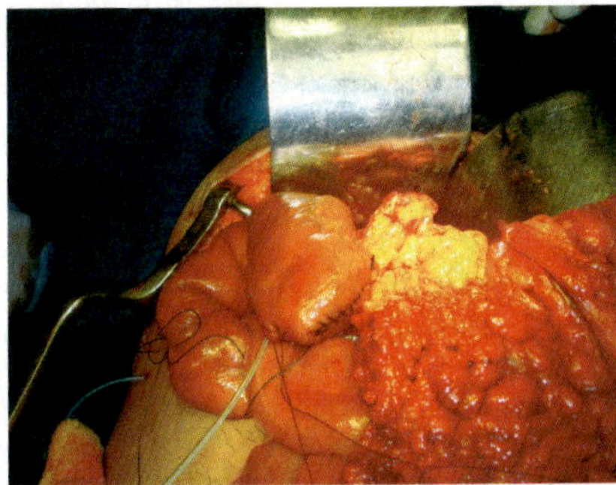

**Fig. 54.65:** Roux jejunal loop is prepared for hepaticojejunostomy

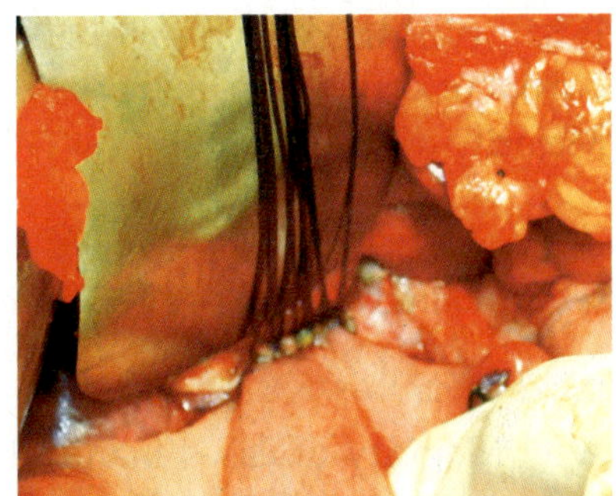

**Fig. 54.66:** Hepaticojejunostomy was done in another patient with type IV injury

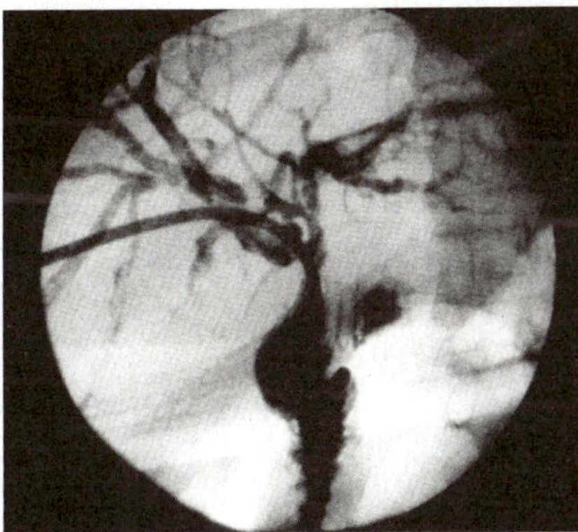

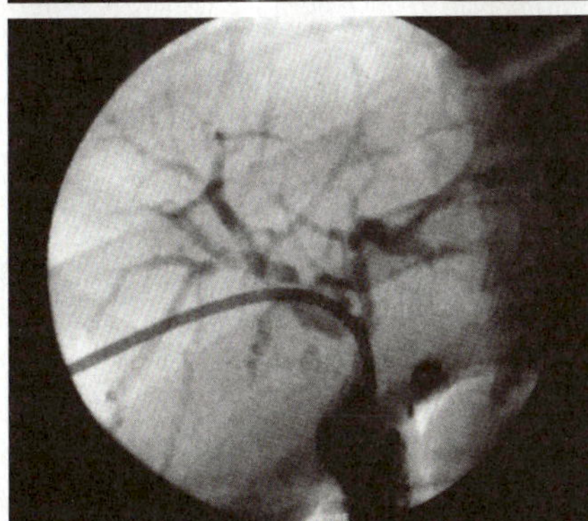

**Figs 54.67 and 54.68:** PTBD catheter was passed from above across strictured hepaticojejunostomy and dilatations were done in high strictures

### Types

- **Primary:** No cause is found. However, it can be associated with conditions given in Key Box 54.13.
- **Secondary:** It is due to stones or injuries.

Key Box 54.13

**Associated Conditions**

- Ulcerative colitis
- Crohn's disease
- Graves' disease
- Sjögren's syndrome

### Complications

Due to long-standing obstruction, biliary cirrhosis and cholangiocarcinoma can develop (Fig. 54.69).

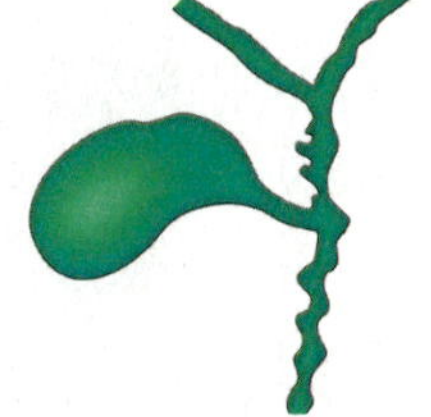

**Fig. 54.69:** Sclerosing cholangitis

### Diagnosis

- **Ultrasound** can demonstrate intrahepatic dilatation.
- **MRCP** is a noninvasive investigation which can demonstrate multiple strictures and dilatation.
- **ERCP** is the investigation of choice which can demonstrate the strictures in the CBD and dilatation

which is described as having a **beaded** appearance. However, the risk of suppurative cholangitis is present.

## Treatment

- It is difficult.
- Stenting is the choice although stents may have to be replaced or changed, if blockage occurs or if infection sets in.

> **SU28.12.3:** Describe the classification, aetiopathogenesis, clinical features, investigations and management for different types of choledochal cyst.

## CHOLEDOCHAL CYST

- It is a congenital cyst occurring in the CBD due to partial or complete weakness of the wall of the CBD.
- Majority of cases manifest by 1–2 years of age.

### Classification (Fig. 54.70 and Key Box 54.14)

***Recent advances: Type VI—cystic dilatation of cystic duct.***

### Clinical Features

- Age: Majority of cases manifest in children within 1–2 years of age. It can also present in adults.

Key Box 54.14

**Todani Classification**

| **Types** | |
|---|---|
| Type I: | Fusiform dilatation of CBD—commonest |
| Type II: | Lateral saccular diverticulum of the CBD |
| Type III: | Dilatation of intraduodenal segment of CBD (choledochocele) |
| Type IV: | Dilatation of CBD + intrahepatic biliary dilatation |
| Type V: | Multiple intrahepatic cysts—Caroli's disease |

- More common in **females**—4:1.
- **Abdominal distension** can be due to a large cyst. The cyst can be palpated per abdomen in the right hypochondrium.
- Slow progressive jaundice, recurrent attacks with abdominal pain and pyrexia.

### Investigations

1. **USG** will confirm presence of abnormal cyst. It is usually unilocular cyst.
2. **MRC:** It will define the relation between lower end of the bile duct and pancreatic duct to know basic anatomy (Fig. 54.71).

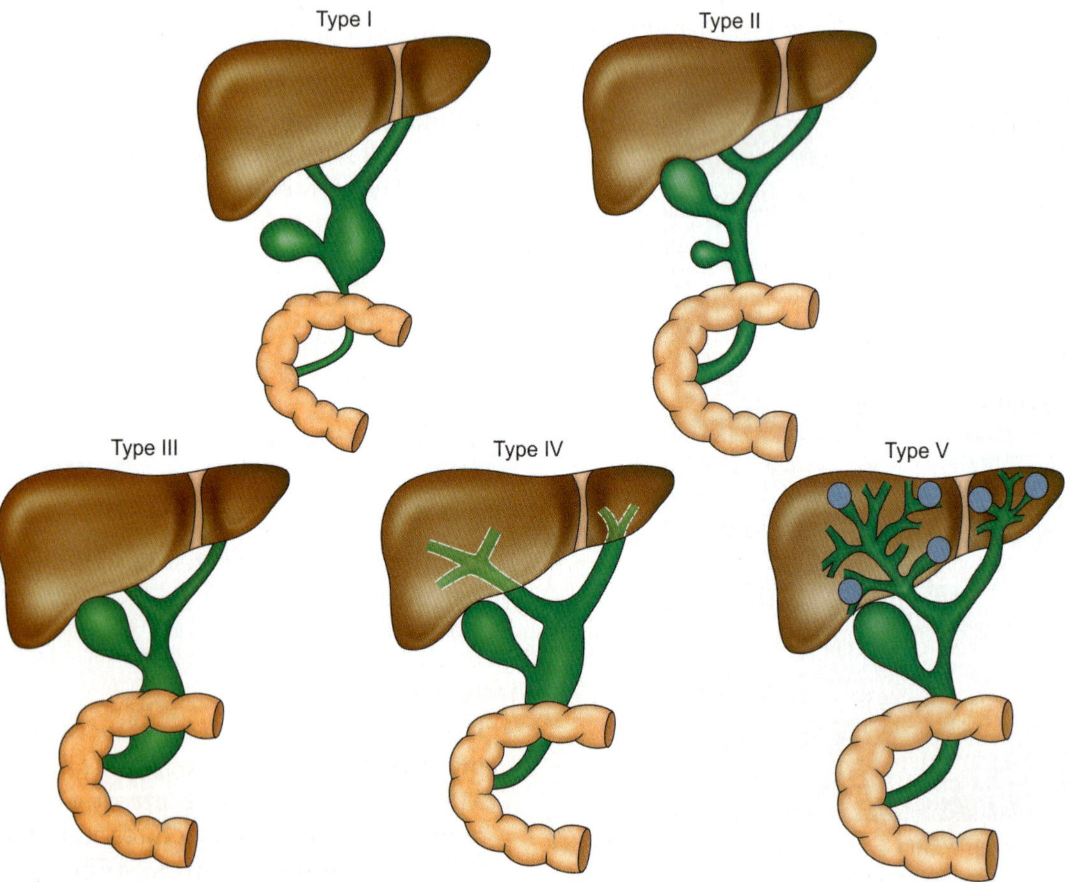


**Fig. 54.70:** Types of choledochal cysts

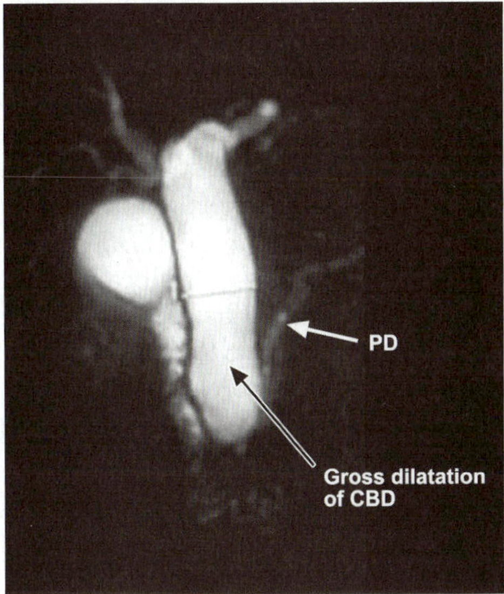


**Fig. 54.71:** MRC showing choledochal cyst

3. **CT** is also useful to know intrahepatic and extra-hepatic dilatation.
4. **ERCP** may be done, but it will not give any more information than MRC.

## Treatment

- **This anomaly is premalignant.** Change to carcinoma is a well-recognised complication and it carries poor prognosis. **Hence, excision of the cyst and reconstruction is the treatment of choice** (Figs 54.72 to 54.74).
  - **Type I:** Excision of the cyst followed by Roux-en-Y hepaticojejunostomy.
  - **Type II:** Excision of the diverticulum with suturing of CBD.
  - **Type III:** Endoscopic sphincterotomy is adequate (choledochocele).
  - **Type IV:** They are difficult to treat. Due to recurrent cholangitis, if total excision is not possible due to adhesions between the cyst and portal vein, **posterior wall of the cyst can be left behind**, after removal of mucosa. This is described as **Lilly's technique**.
  - **Type V** will be described later.

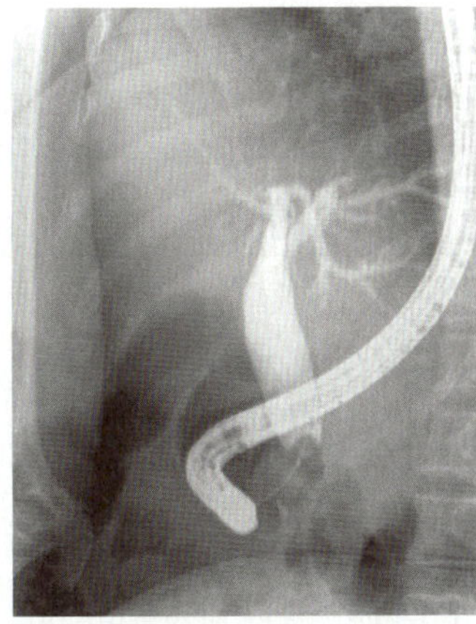

**Fig. 54.72:** ERCP showing choledochal cyst—type III treated by sphincterotomy

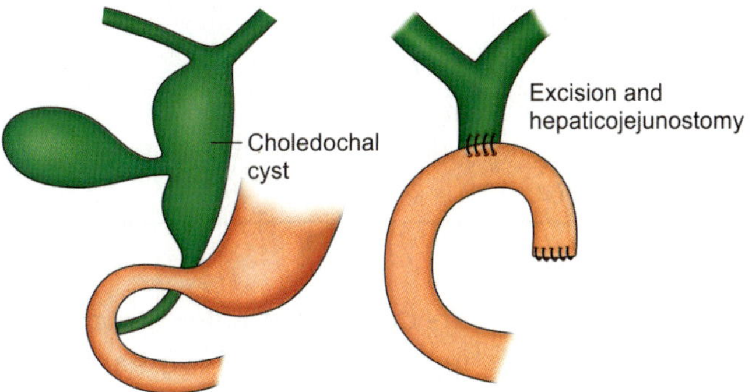


**Fig. 54.73:** Type I cyst

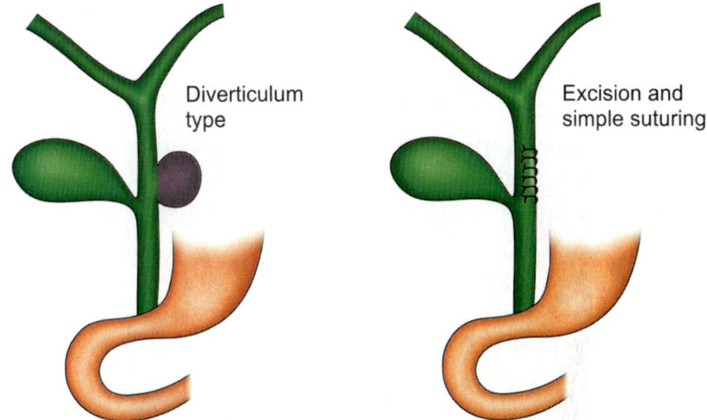


**Fig. 54.74:** Type II—excision and suturing

## Complications

1. **Recurrent cholangitis** with high-grade fever, resulting in biliary cirrhosis.
2. **Rupture of the cyst** resulting in biliary peritonitis.
3. **CBD stones**
4. **Carcinoma in the cyst** (25–30% of cases). It is a cholangiocarcinoma, common in types I and V.

## CAROLI'S DISEASE

- It is a hereditary condition wherein there is dilatation of intrahepatic ducts with stenotic segments in between.
- Multiple, irregular saccular dilatations are characteristic.
- It is also an example of ***type V choledochal cyst.***
  Two types:
  1. **Simple:** Presents later with abdominal pain and sepsis.
  2. **Periportal:** It occurs in childhood, presents as recurrent cholangitis.
- Diagnosed by ultrasound and CT scan. MRI and ERCP are other investigations (Fig. 54.75).
- Associated lesions are given in Key Box 54.15.

Key Box 54.15

**Associated Lesions**

- Congenital hepatic fibrosis
- Medullary sponge kidney
- Polycystic liver

## Complications

- Cholangitis: It occurs due to constant obstruction.
- Stones: Obstruction and stasis precipitate stone formation.
- Biliary cirrhosis
- Cholangiocarcinoma

## Treatment

Hepatectomy (Fig. 54.76), liver transplantation.

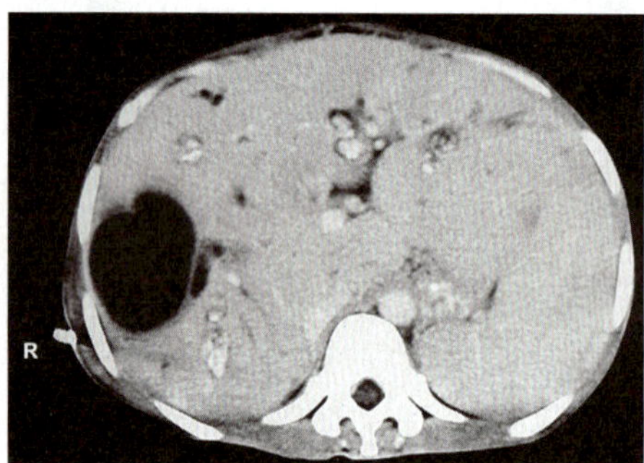


**Fig. 54.75:** Caroli's disease showing large cyst and intrahepatic dilatation

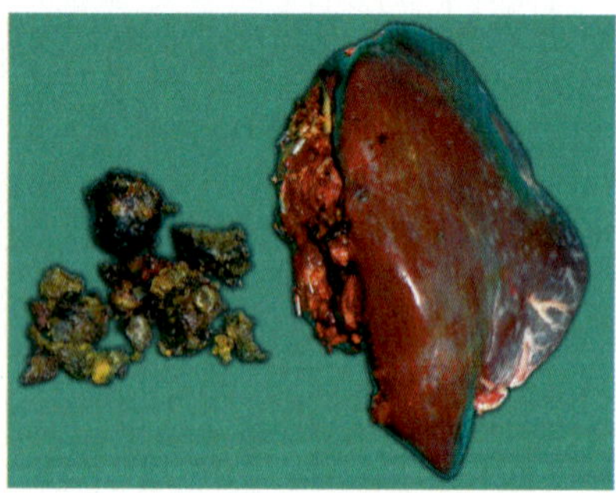

**Fig. 54.76:** Left lobectomy with extraction of stone—Caroli's disease. (*Courtesy*: Dr Nagaraj Palantkar, Consultant, Manipal Hospital, Bengaluru)

# CHRONIC PANCREATITIS

**SU24.1.3:** Describe the types, etiopathogenesis, clinical features, investigations and management of chronic pancreatitis. Also the various surgical modalities available for treatment of chronic pancreatitis.

## Definition

Diffuse inflammatory process of pancreas involving head, body and the tail resulting in permanent structural and functional damage to the pancreas.

## Causes

1. **Alcohol:** High alcohol consumption is the most frequent cause. Alcohol stimulates pancreatic secretion rich in protein. This forms plugs in the pancreatic duct and results in stasis of secretion and stone formation. Alcohol also causes spasm of sphincter of Oddi.
2. **Idiopathic:** It is common in Kerala, and was thought to be due to **consumption of tapioca** (Fig. 54.77). It is also called Kerala pancreatitis or **tropical pancreatitis**. It is now thought to be due to malnutrition. It is also called **fibrocalculous pancreatic diabetes**.
3. **Hereditary pancreatitis:** It is a genetic disorder transmitted as a Mendelian-dominant trait.
4. **Cystic fibrosis:** Generalised dysfunction of exocrine glands causes secretions to precipitate in the lumen.
5. **Hyperparathyroidism** favours precipitation of calcium intraductally. It can also activate pancreatic enzymes.
6. **Autoimmune pancreatitis:** Diffuse enlargement of pancreas and narrowing of pancreatic duct is seen. Autoantibodies may be present. IgG4 is increased.
   - Multiple joint pains, salivary gland infections may give clue to the diagnosis.

## Pathology

There is destruction of pancreas by ductal sclerosis, ductal strictures, glandular fibrosis and calcification, both intraductal and parenchymal (Key Box 54.16 and Fig. 54.78).

Key Box 54.16

**Chronic Pancreatitis Idiopathic Type**

- Common in **warm** climates (Kerala)
- Common in **young age**
- High incidence of **diabetes**
- High incidence of **stones** in the duct
- Increased chances of **parenchymal calcification**
- Increased chances of **pancreatic cancer**

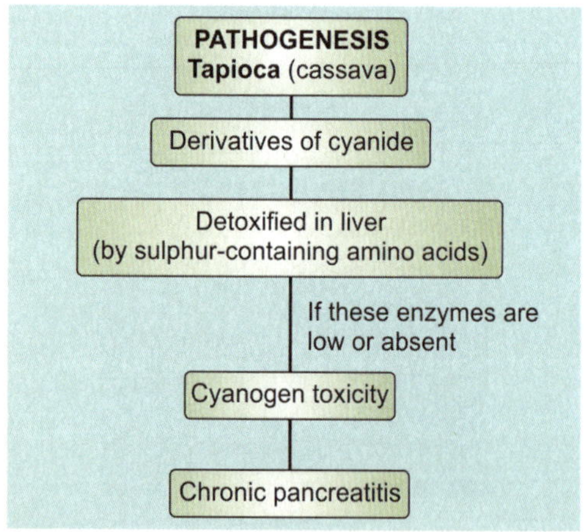


**Fig. 54.77:** Aetiopathogenesis of cassava pancreatitis

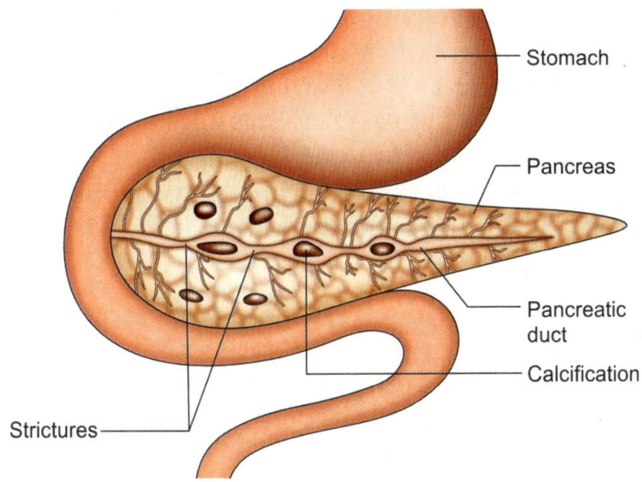


Fig. 54.78: Chronic pancreatitis showing pathological changes

### Clinical Features (you can remember as MOPED)

- **M**alabsorption occurs due to damage to exocrine glands resulting in steatorrhoea—10 to 15 stools per day, bulky, frothy, rich in fat, foul-smelling. Malabsorption indicates late disease and results in weight loss. Creatorrhoea refers to excessive loss of protein (Figs 54.79 and 54.80).
- **O**bstructive jaundice can occur due to oedema of the head of pancreas. Later, fibrous constriction of CBD due to fibrotic indurated mass in the head region can cause jaundice by compressing the CBD.
- **P**ain abdomen—upper abdominal pain radiating to the back in the region of L1 and L2 due to retroperitoneal inflammation (Key Box 54.17). Pain may be severe, sometimes radiating to both right and left sides. **The pain is due to multiple strictures in the pancreatic duct increasing the intraductal pressure.** It is relieved on stooping forward.
- **E**xploratory laparotomy—many cases are diagnosed at laparotomy where irregularity and hardness involving the entire pancreas are seen. Exploration is done for some other pathology.
- **D**iabetes—incidence of diabetes is about 10–20%. It should be suspected in diabetic patients with pain abdomen.

Key Box 54.17

**Pain in Chronic Pancreatitis**

- Parenchymal hypertension
- Perineural inflammation
- Ductal hypertension
- Pseudocyst formation
- Stenosis of bile duct

### Investigations

- **Plain X-ray** abdomen can demonstrate stones in the pancreatic duct or parenchymal calcification (Fig. 54.81).

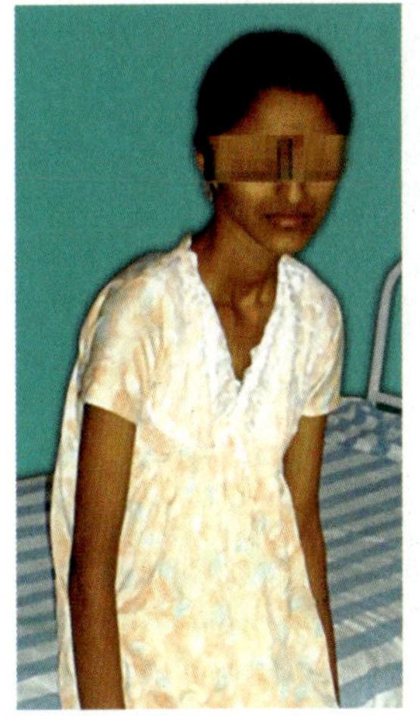
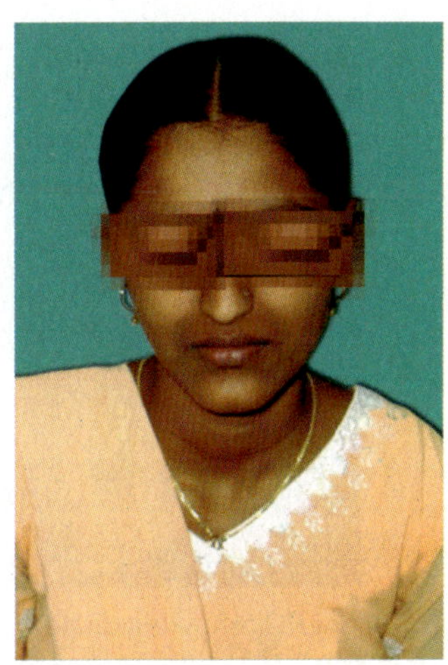

Figs 54.79 and 54.80: This 21-year-old girl was weighing 32 kg in 2006 when she underwent longitudinal pancreatico jejunostomy (LPJ) for failed medical treatment including stents. After 3 years, she has put on 22 kg weight

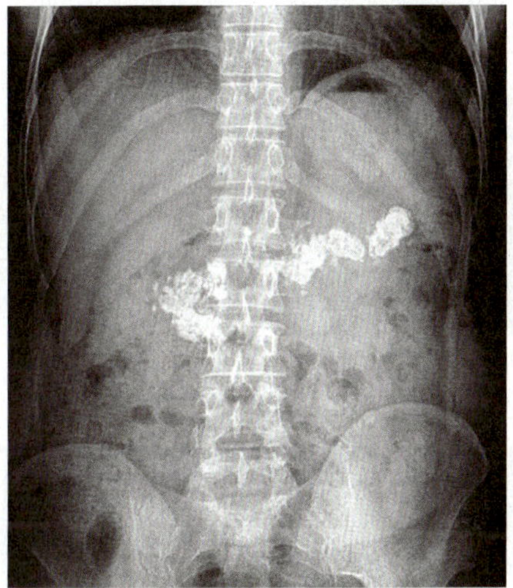

Fig. 54.81: Plain X-ray abdomen showing extensive calcification

- **USG** can detect the stones, stricture, dilatation and associated cysts.
- **ERCP** (Fig. 54.82)
  - Ductal distension, ductal stricture
  - Dilated pancreatic duct (diameter of the normal duct is 2 mm)
  - Demonstration of stones—appear as regular filling defect.
- **CT scan:** It can reveal ductal anatomy, head mass, size and configuration of pancreas (Figs 54.83 and 54.84).

### Complications

- Obstructive jaundice due to a mass lesion in the head region
- Carcinoma of pancreas
- Pseudocysts
- Steroids in autoimmune pancreatitis.

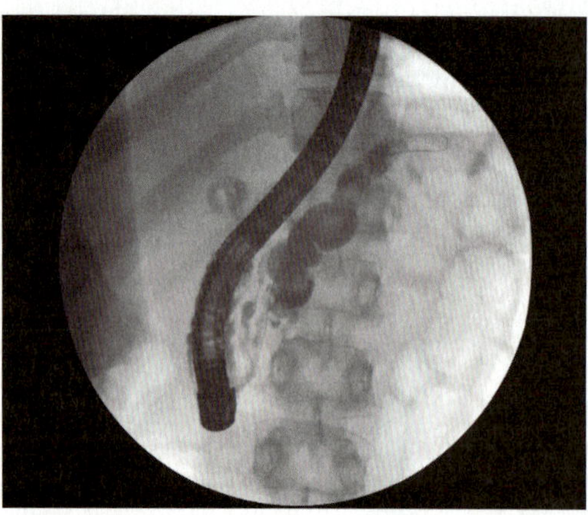

Fig. 54.82: ERCP showing dilated pancreatic duct—'chain of lakes' appearance

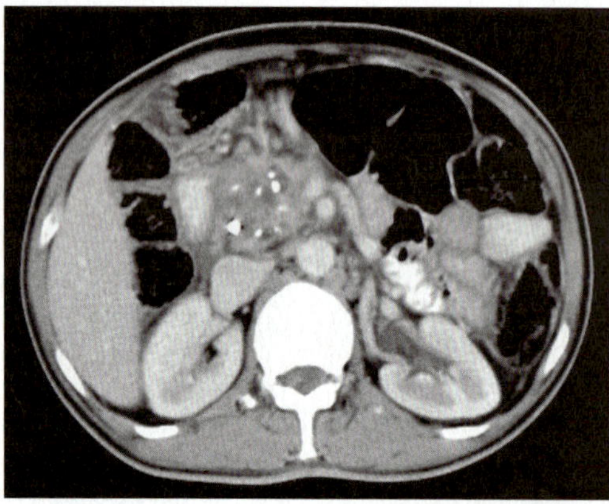

Fig. 54.83: CT scan showing chronic pancreatitis with head mass. This case should be treated with **head-coring** operation

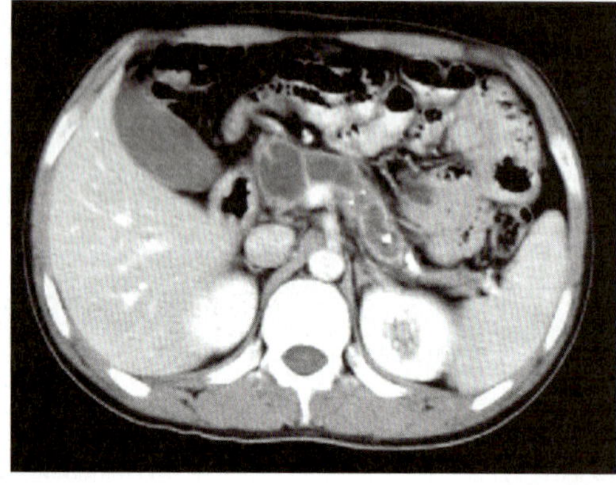

Fig. 54.84: CT shows dilated pancreatic duct of 10 mm in size with stones. ERCP is not required in such patients. This patient underwent LPJ

## Treatment

### I. Conservative

- Pain relief by analgesics, epidural analgesia, or splanchnic nerve block. Slow release opioid skin patches are useful.
- Supplement **pancreatic enzyme**—diet should be low in fat and **vitamin D** supplements should be given.
- Pancreatic enzymes not only help in treating exocrine insufficiency but they also denature CCK releasing peptide, thereby diminishing the release of CCK. Thus, pain is decreased. Six capsules of **pancreatin** are given.
- Control diabetes, stop alcohol consumption and tobacco smoking, antioxidants may help.

### II. Surgery

*Indications*

- Unrelieved pain
- Suspicion of carcinoma
- Complications:
  - Ascites
  - Cysts
  - Abscesses
  - GI bleeding—left-sided, portal hypertension, pseudoaneurysm
  - Obstructive jaundice
  - Duodenal obstruction.

*Types of Surgery* (Figs 54.85 to 54.91)

1. **Chronic pancreatitis involving tail of pancreas:** Distal pancreatectomy with removal of spleen.
2. **Diffuse chronic pancreatitis with dilated (large duct) pancreatic duct**
   - Duct is laid open widely, strictures are cut open, stones are removed and it is anastomosed to a loop of jejunum—longitudinal pancreaticojejunostomy (LPJ)—**Puestow's operation** (Roux-en-Y jejunal segment). The duct should be at least 6 mm in diameter. Sutures hold very nicely because of fibrosis of pancreas. Pain relief is obtained in about 80% of the cases. Pancreatic fistula is a complication of this surgery. Majority of the fistulae close spontaneously.
   - This is a bypass procedure which preserve endocrine and exocrine functions.
3. **Chronic pancreatitis with a head mass:** In this situation, doubt arises whether it is malignancy or not. Even trucut biopsy and frozen section are not foolproof. Hence, pancreaticoduodenectomy is advised, provided experience of the surgeon is good and the mortality rate is less than 5%.
4. **Chronic pancreatitis with bile duct obstruction:** If malignancy is ruled out, a bypass procedure is the treatment of choice.
   - Choledochojejunostomy is the ideal treatment.
   - Pancreaticoduodenal resection (Whipple) can also be done (as mentioned above).
5. **Chronic pancreatitis with duodenal obstruction:** Here also, resection of the head mass or gastrojejunostomy is the treatment of choice.

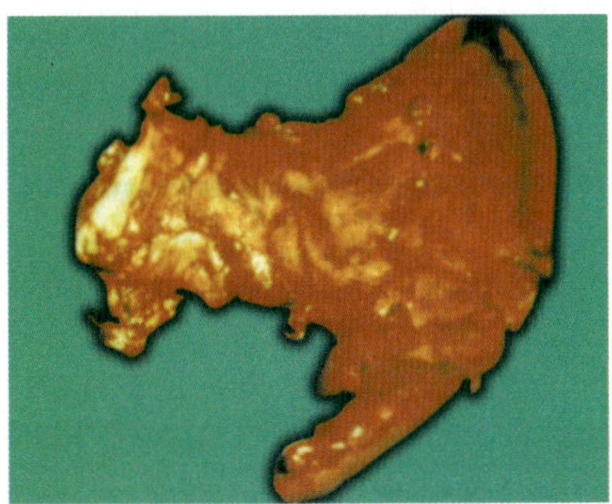

**Fig. 54.85:** Distal pancreatectomy. Chronic pancreatitis confined to tail of pancreas

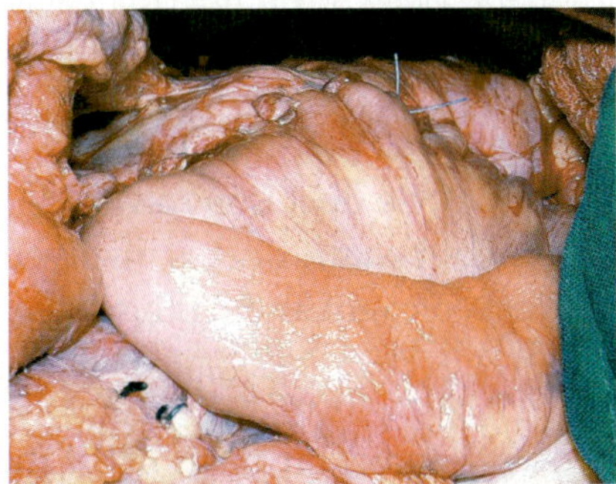

**Fig. 54.86:** Pancreaticojejunal anastomosis is being done

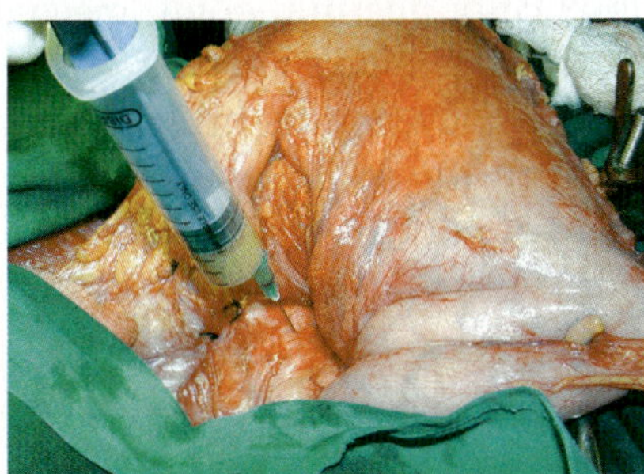

**Fig. 54.87:** Dilated duct is being aspirated to identify the duct followed by laying it open

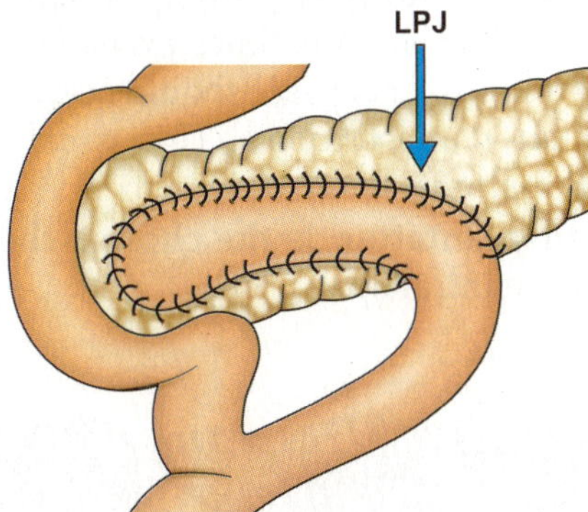


**Fig. 54.88:** Longitudinal pancreaticojejunostomy (diagrammatic)

6. **Chronic pancreatitis with ascites:** Treatment of choice is Puestow's operation (stenting may also relieve ascites).
7. **Resection:** A duodenum-preserving pancreatic head resection is called ***Hans Beger's procedure.*** Head-coring procedure is called ***Frey procedure*** (Figs 54.90 and 54.91 and Key Box 54.18).

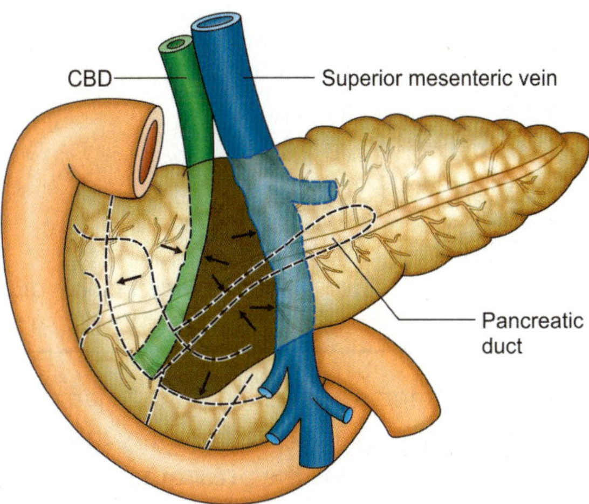


**Fig. 54.89:** The dark shaded area is called **pacemaker of chronic pancreatitis.** It should be removed in cases of head coring operation. It is a triangle between lower CBD, pancreatic duct and superior mesenteric vessels

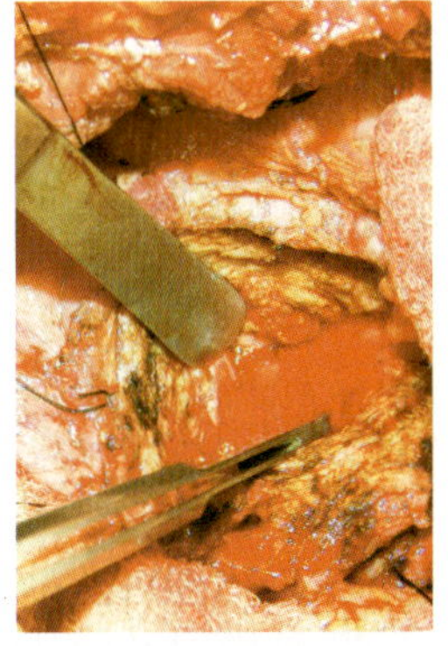

**Fig. 54.90:** Head coring is completed. You can watch thin rim of pancreatic tissue all around

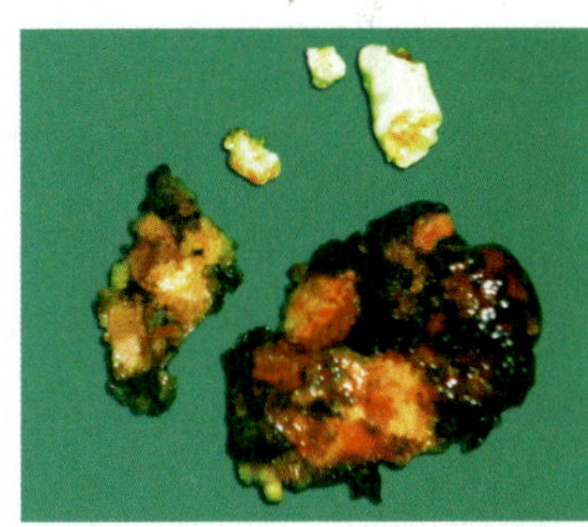

**Fig. 54.91:** Specimen of the portion of the head along with multiple stones

Key Box 54.18

**Head coring—Frey Procedure**

- **Pathologic key** to recurrent pancreatitis is localised to pancreatic head. It is called **pacemaker**.
- It is located in the **crucial triangle** (*see* Fig. 54.89) which has to be excised.
- Pain and recurrent pancreatitis will decrease after Frey procedure.
- Surgery can be done with minimum blood loss.
- Try **avoiding injury to lower CBD**—if necessary, CBD can be opened and a sound can be introduced.

## CHOLANGIOCARCINOMA—BILE DUCT CARCINOMA

**SU28.12.5:** Enumerate the types, etiopathogenesis, clinical features, investigations and management of cholangiocarcinoma.

- Patients with the **following diseases** have increased risk of developing cholangiocarcinoma (Key Box 54.19).

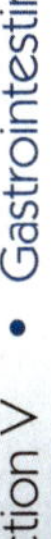

Key Box 54.19

**Risk Factors**

Cholangitis—primary sclerosing
Colitis—ulcerative
Clonorchiasis
Choledochal cyst
Caroli's disease
Chemical carcinogens like thorium, nitrosamines, diosmin
*Observe* **6 Cs**

- It is an uncommon cause of obstructive jaundice.
- Elderly males >60 years are commonly affected.
- **Obstructive jaundice** is the presenting feature.
- Tender hepatomegaly is present due to congestion and may be due to cholangitis.
- **Gallbladder is not palpable** in cases of cholangiocarcinoma unlike in periampullary carcinomas.
- Cholangiocarcinoma at the bifurcation of the hepatic duct is called **Klatskin's tumour**.

### Types

1. Perihilar is the most common, Klatskin's tumour comes under this.
2. Intrahepatic (10%)
3. Distal (CHD-CBD) 25%.

### Management

- Abdominal ultrasound, CT scan, ERCP will help in localising the site of obstruction (Figs 54.92 and 54.93). ERCP and stenting the CBD is indicated in inoperable cases. However, MRI is better.

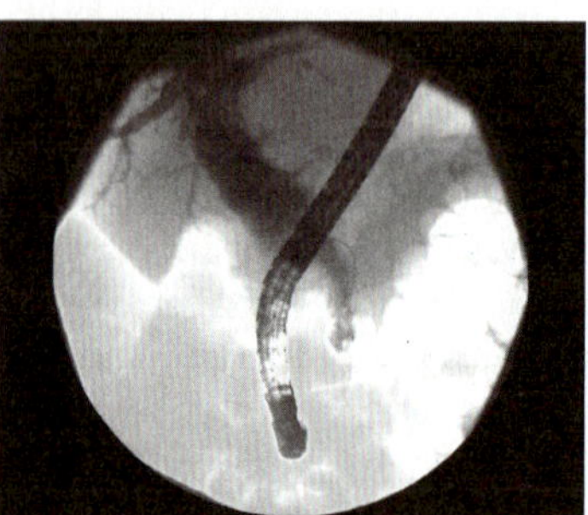

**Fig. 54.92:** ERCP showing cholangiocarcinoma

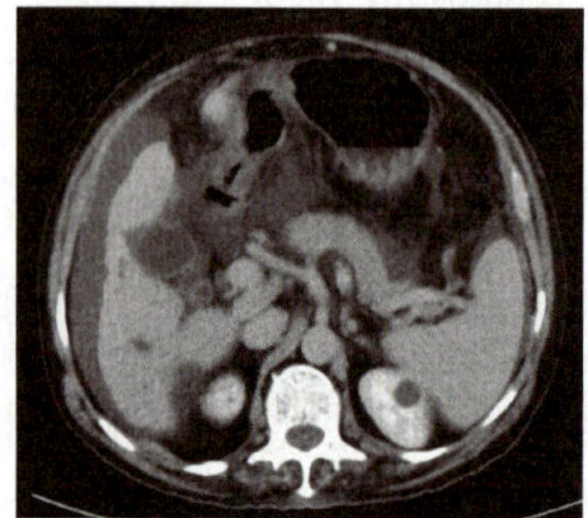

**Fig. 54.93:** CT scan showing extensive cholagiocarcinoma with ascites

- Treatment is difficult because most of the lesions are high up in the hilar region infiltrating the liver, portal vein, etc. Resection and hepaticojejunostomy or endoscopic stent placement are the treatment modalities available.
- Resection involves liver for hilar growth and for lower end growth.

## CONGENITAL BILIARY ATRESIA

### Aetiopathogenesis

A disease of unknown aetiology, though rare, is fatal. Viral aetiology and defective embryogenesis have been blamed for the development of biliary atresia.

### Types (Fig. 54.94)

- Type I: Common bile duct is involved.
- Type II: Common hepatic duct is involved.
- Type III: Atresia of right and left hepatic ducts.

### Clinical Features

- It presents as jaundice at birth or in the neonatal period.
- Due to absence of bile in the gut, meconium is not bile-stained. Hence, stools are pale.
- Gradually, due to backpressure, liver enlarges.
- Enlargement of the spleen may follow, if there is development of portal hypertension.
- Steatorrhoea, pruritus and clubbing are the other features.

### Treatment

- **Surgical drainage of bile** is the only available treatment provided patent bile duct or radicle is seen. Anastomosis of Roux-en-Y loop of jejunum to the dilated bile duct or sometimes excision of bile duct tissue up to the liver capsule should be done followed by Roux-en-Y anastomosis. This is called **Kasai's portoenterostomy**.
- **Liver transplantation** is the choice when there is atresia of the intrahepatic duct.

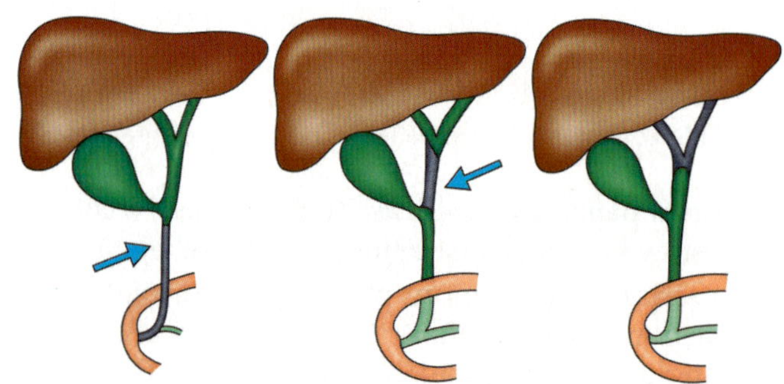

**Fig. 54.94:** Congenital biliary atresia—types I, II and III

### Complications

1. Recurrent cholangitis giving rise to hepatic fibrosis.
2. Biliary cirrhosis and portal hypertension.

## CARCINOMA OF GALLBLADDER

**Incidence:** It is common in North Eastern India. Occurs in elderly patients in their sixties/seventies.

### Aetiology

- **Gallstones:** 80–90% of gallbladder cancers are associated with gallstones. Calcification of gallbladder is associated with carcinoma gallbladder. Porcelain gallbladder is a precancerous condition. Incidence of malignancy may range from 1 to 5% of cases.
- **Chemicals:** High incidence of gallbladder and biliary cancer is noted in people who work in rubber industries.
- **Gallbladder polyp** (Fig. 54.95)
- **Dietary:** Adulterated mustard oil for cooking is found to precipitate carcinoma gallbladder.

### Pathology

- 85% of cases. It is usually adenocarcinoma. Undifferentiated carcinoma and squamous cell carcinoma may also occur. The tumour is most commonly nodular, infiltrates the entire gallbladder and adjacent tissues.
- Three types of adenocarcinomas have been identified: Nonpapillary adenocarcinoma, papillary adenocarcinoma and mucinous adenocarcinoma. Majority are nonpapillary adenocarcinoma.

### Clinical Features

- Significant weight loss, jaundice and mass in the right upper quadrant are common presentations. Clinically, it is palpable as a hard irregular mass.
- A few cases can present as chronic cholecystitis with a mass or acute cholecystitis. Ultrasonography may diagnose as stones and they are subjected to cholecystectomy. During surgery or postoperatively, the diagnosis gets confirmed.
- Obstructive jaundice, bleeding, ascites are late features.

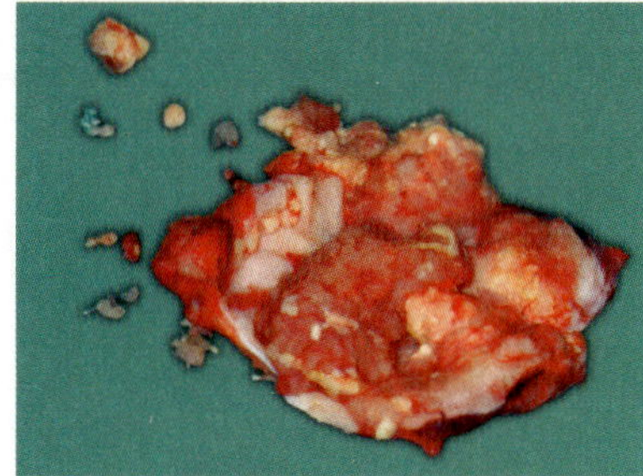

**Fig. 54.95:** You can see extensive carcinomatous polypoid lesions inside the gallbladder

### Staging

**TNM STAGING: Gallbladder cancer**

| Tumour (T) | | Metastases (M) |
|---|---|---|
| TX | Primary tumor cannot be assessed | M0 No distant spread |
| T0 | No evidence of primary tumor | M1 Distant spread |
| Tis | Carcinoma *in situ* | |
| T1 | Tumor invades lamina propria or muscular layer | |
| T1a | Tumour invades lamina propria | |
| T1b | Tumour invades muscular layer | |
| T2a | Tumour invades the perimuscular connective tissue on the peritoneal side without involving the serosa | |
| T2b | Tumour invades the perimuscular connective tissue on the peritoneal side without involving the liver | |
| T3 | Tumour perforates the serosa (visceral peritoneum) and/or directly invades the liver and/or one other adjacent organ or structure, such as the stomach, duodenum, colon, pancreas, omentum, or extrahepatic bile ducts | |
| T4 | Tumour invades main portal vein or hepatic artery or invades at least two extra-hepatic organs or structures | |
| **Nodes (N)** | | **Staging** |
| Nx | Regional lymph nodes cannot be assessed | Stage 0—Tis, N0, M0<br>Stage I—T1, N0, M0 |
| N0 | Regional lymph node metastasis | Stage IIA—T2a, N0, M0<br>Stage IIB—T2b, N0, M0 |
| N1 | Metastases to 1–3 lymph nodes | Stage IIIA—T3, N0, M0 |
| N2 | Metastases to >4 lymph nodes | Stage IIIB—T1 to T3, N1, M0<br>Stage IVA—T4, N0 or N1, M0<br>Stage IVB—Any T, N2, M0; Any T, any N, M1<br>*Note*: Stage I is Localised; Stages II to IV B are unresectable |

## Investigations

- CA 19–9 is elevated in 80% patients.
- Ultrasonography and endosonography are very useful investigations. Ultrasonography-guided FNAC can be done for histological diagnosis in suspected cases of gallbladder mass.
- CT scan is useful for staging—lymph nodes metastasis in the liver (Figs 54.96A and B).
- ERCP, if there is obstructive jaundice to localise the exact site and nature of obstruction.
- Diagnostic laparoscopy. If peritoneal metastasis is present, it is not worth resecting.
- MRCP can be done. It visualises bile duct better than CT scan.

## Treatment

- If gallbladder cancer is found at cholecystectomy and if **mucosa alone is involved**, then cholecystectomy is sufficient.
- If gallbladder wall is involved, then extended cholecystectomy is done (Fig. 54.97 and Key Box 54.20).
- Radiation has very small benefits.
- Chemotherapy also has been tried. 5-FU, mitomycin C, doxorubicin are the drugs used.

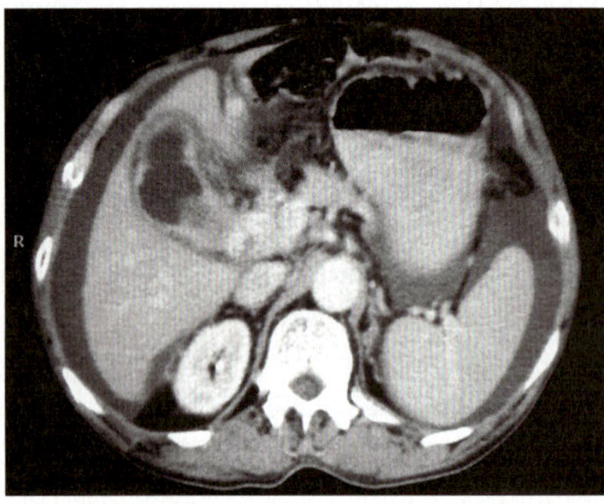


**Fig. 54.96A:** Advanced case of carcinoma gallbladder with ascites and liver infiltration

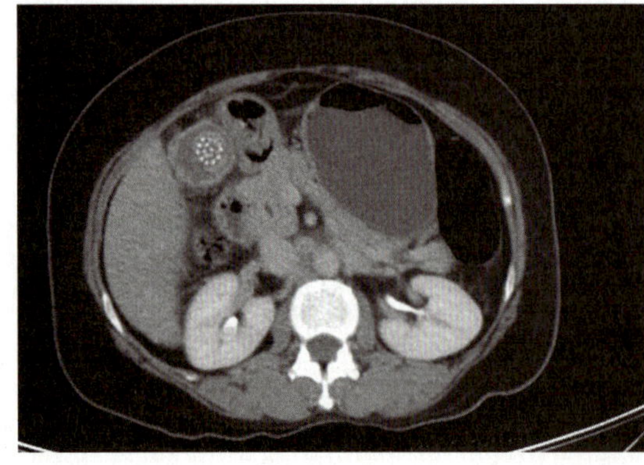

**Fig. 54.96B:** Gallstones with carcinoma gallbladder

### Key Box 54.20

**Extended Cholecystectomy**

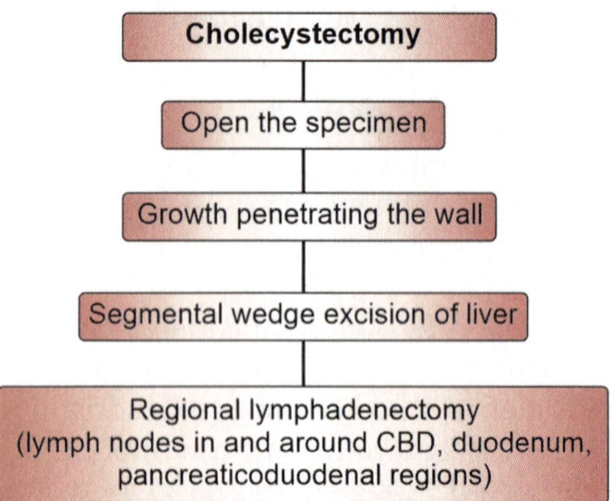


The usual blunder committed is doing cholecystectomy for a diagnosis of stone when it is actually a case of carcinoma gallbladder, inadequate surgery results in biliary fistula and hastens death

## Prognosis

In general, five-year survival is very poor (Key Box 54.21). Aggressive surgery and complete clearance give best result (Fig. 54.97).

### Key Box 54.21

**Gallbladder Cancer is the Worst, Why?**

- Biologically very aggressive cancer (unlike basal cell cancer, carcinoma colon, etc.)
- High incidence of lymphatic spread
- Easily spreads into liver by direct infiltration
- Spreads by blood, neural, intraperitoneal routes
- Intraductal extension into CBD causes obstructive jaundice
- Infiltration into stomach, colon, duodenum and liver can occur because of its location
- Radiation and chemotherapy is rarely of any benefit

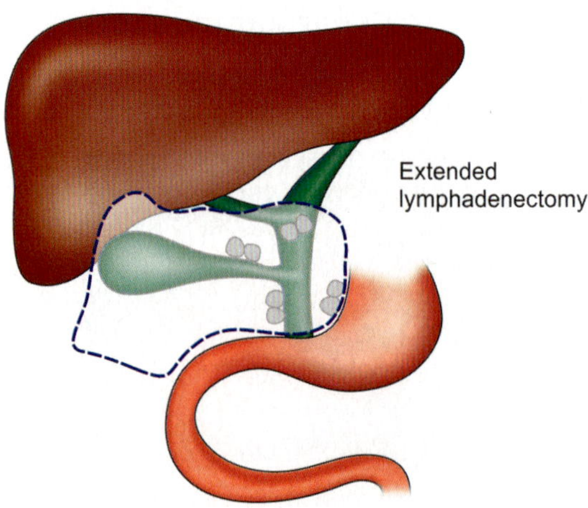


**Fig. 54.97:** Extended lymphadenectomy

### Rare or Uncommon Causes of Obstructive Jaundice (Table 54.4 and Fig. 54.98)

Parasites such as ascariasis, *Clonorchiasis sinensis* and biliary hydatid can give rise to obstructive jaundice.

Thus, we have discussed various causes of obstructive jaundice. Students should be able to differentiate between all these different causes and to offer an appropriate diagnosis in the examination. Each of these short topics can be asked as short notes in the theory paper and short cases.

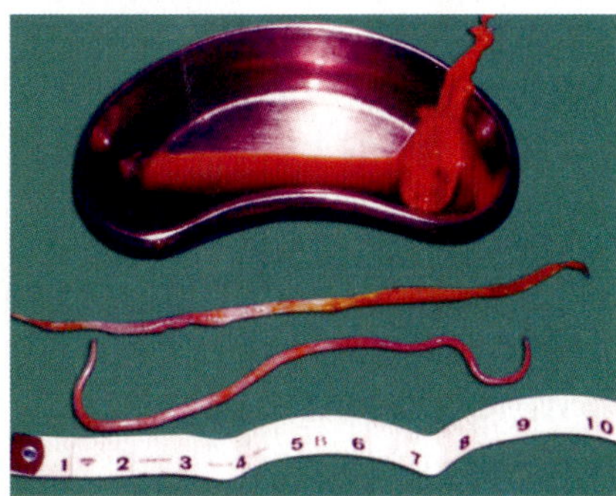

**Fig. 54.98:** Ascariasis of the biliary duct. (*Courtesy*: Dr CG Narasimhan, Consultant Surgeon, Mysuru)

## CARCINOMA OF PANCREAS

### Introduction

- 70% of the cases occur in the head of the pancreas including periampullary region.
- 30% occur in the body and the tail.
- 70% of cases are adenocarcinoma of duct cell origin.
- It is 4th leading cause of death due to cancer in males, after lung, colon, prostate.

### Aetiology

- **Chronic tropical pancreatitis** and hereditary pancreatitis are associated with pancreatic cancer—such malignancies can be multifocal.
- **Haemochromatosis** produces extensive calcification of pancreas. It is also a precancerous condition.
- **Diabetes:** Diabetic patients are 10 times more vulnerable to develop carcinoma of pancreas.
- **Other possible aetiological factors**
  - *Alcohol and smoking:* It is related to tobacco specific nitrosamines (including smokeless tobacco).
  - *Westernisation of diet:* Fatty food, rich in animal proteins can cause pancreatic cancer.
  - *Industrial carcinogens:* B11-naphthylamine, benzidine, gasoline are the possible agents.

### Pathology

- Periampullary refers to carcinoma arising from ampulla of Vater, the duodenal mucosa or the lower end of the common bile duct.
- Microscopically, the types are:
  1. **Mucus**–secreting carcinoma of ductal origin.
  2. **Nonmucus**–secreting carcinoma of acinar origin.
  3. **Anaplastic** carcinomas are poorly differentiated and tend to arise from the body of the pancreas.
  4. **Cystadenocarcinomas** are rare, slow-growing and tend to attain a large size.

### Clinical Features

- Periampullary and carcinoma head of pancreas present as obstructive jaundice (discussed already). Discussion here is on carcinoma body and tail of pancreas.
- Microscopically, the tumour shows malignant cells with a variable degree of differentiation, mitotic figures, etc. Not only it invades vessels and lymphatics, but also perineural spread occurs fast which explains backache (Key Box 54.22).

#### *Symptoms*

- Severe pain radiating to the back in the region of L1 and L2. It is due to infiltration of retroperitoneal nerve plexuses or pancreatic duct obstruction.

**TABLE 54.4:** Parasitic infestation of the biliary tract

| | Biliary ascariasis | Clonorchiasis | Biliary hydatid |
|---|---|---|---|
| 1. Causative organism | *Ascaris lumbricoides* (Fig. 54.98) | *Clonorchis sinensis* | *Echinococcus granulosus* |
| 2. Route of entry | Ampulla of Vater | Ampulla of Vater | Rupture of hydatid cyst of liver into biliary tree |
| 3. Complications | Stricture, suppurative cholangitis, liver abscess, empyema | Biliary pain, stone cholangitis, block, cirrhosis, bile duct carcinogenic | Obstructive jaundice, cholangitis |
| 4. Management | • Ultrasound, CT scan<br>• ERCP—worm can be extracted<br>• Open surgery<br>• Deworming | • Ultrasound, CT scan<br>• Cholecystectomy and T-tube drainage<br>• Choledochojejunostomy for a better drainage | • Ultrasound<br>• ERCP, sphincterotomy, stent<br>• Appropriate surgery |

Key Box 54.22

**Carcinoma of Pancreas—Pathology**

- More than 80% are **ductal adenocarcinomas**
- **Solid and scirrhous** tumours by nature
- Plenty of **neoplastic tubular** glands are seen
- **Desmoplastic** reaction is extensive (feels hard)
- Infiltrates locally—spreads along nerve sheaths, lymphatics and into blood vessels
- Being retroperitoneal in location, **manifests late**, **spreads fast and carries poor prognosis**

- Pain is so severe, often patient requests for narcotic analgesics.
- Gross weight loss in 3–6 months.
- Anorexia, asthenia and generalised weakness.
- Jaundice cannot occur in carcinoma body and tail of pancreas unless there are secondaries in liver or lymph nodes at porta hepatis.
- Symptoms of vomiting suggest duodenal obstruction.
- **Trousseau's sign**[1] (thrombophlebitis migrans):
  - Migrating thrombophlebitis of the legs can occur in visceral malignancies particularly from carcinoma of pancreas, rarely carcinoma stomach, colon, etc.
  - It is supposedly due to sluggish blood flow resulting in thrombus formation.
  - It is superficial and affects the leg veins, such as long saphenous vein.

*Pearls of Wisdom*

Sudden development of diabetes mellitus is an early manifestation of carcinoma pancreas in 25% of patients.

### Signs

- **Anaemia** may be present as in any other malignancy.
- **Jaundice** is not a feature. Left supraclavicular node may be palpable.
- **Per abdomen findings** (Table 54.5): Majority of these cases are advanced, fixed and are felt as a mass in the upper abdomen.

  **I. Characteristics of a pancreatic mass**
  - It is situated on the left side involving left hypochondrium, umbilical region and epigastrium.
  - It does not move with respiration because it is retroperitoneal.
  - It does not fall forwards in knee elbow position.
  - Can get above the swelling.
  - On percussion, it gives a resonant note because of anterior position of stomach.

  **II. Features of carcinoma**
  - It is common in elderly, male patients, smokers.
  - Hard, irregular, fixed lump.
  - Significant weight loss is present.

  **III. Evidence of metastasis:** Secondaries in the liver, ascites, rectovesical deposits.

[1]Trousseau's sign is also found in Buerger's disease.

**TABLE 54.5:** Differences between pancreatic mass and stomach mass

| Carcinoma body of the pancreas | Carcinoma stomach |
|---|---|
| Pain radiating to the back is the presenting feature | Vomiting, dyspepsia is present. Pain is not a feature |
| Haematemesis is not a feature | Haematemesis is a common feature |
| The mass does not move with respiration | Usually moves with respiration |
| Mobility is not a feature | Mobility is present |
| Knee elbow test—the mass does not fall forwards | Stomach mass falls forward (intraperitoneal), unless it is fixed |
| Retroperitoneal organ | Intraperitoneal |
| Percussion: Resonant note is obtained because of stomach anterior to it | Impaired note because of growth in the stomach |

### Differential Diagnosis

1. **Carcinoma stomach** infiltrating the pancreas
   - Such mass may not be mobile. It does not move with respiration because it is fixed to pancreas.
   - These patients will have vomiting first followed by backache at a later date.
2. **Carcinoma transverse colon**
   - Produces constipation and bleeding per rectum. Vertical mobility may be present.
   - Right to left peristalsis may be present.
3. **Para-aortic lymph node mass** may be due to: Intra-abdominal malignancies, lymphoma, testicular tumour, etc.

### Investigations

I. Investigations for periampullary carcinoma and carcinoma of head of pancreas (discussed before).

II. **Investigations for carcinoma of body and tail** (discussed here)

1. **USG:** First investigation of choice
   - Rules out calculous obstruction
   - Can detect a mass as small as 2 cm
   - Intraoperative ultrasound can be used to take a biopsy.

2. **Contrast-enhanced CT scan** (Figs 54.99 and 54.100)
    - Retroperitoneal invasion
    - Lymph node enlargement
    - Invasion of hepatic artery, superior mesenteric artery, ascites, liver metastasis—unresectable.
    - Infiltration of portal vein which makes it inoperable
    - In more than 70% of cases, pancreatic duct is dilated and in more than 60% of cases bile duct is dilated.
    - When both these ducts are dilated, it is most likely pancreatic cancer.
    - CT-guided aspiration biopsy is indicated for lesions to start neoadjuvant chemotherapy/RT (infiltrative lesions).
3. **ERCP** is indicated in the absence of a mass. Findings can be stenosis/obstruction.
4. **Carbohydrate antigen CA 19–9:** These are glycoproteins which are elaborated by malignancies. ***It is a tumour marker of pancreas to monitor carcinoma pancreas.*** Increased in 75% of patients with carcinoma pancreas and 10% of the patients in benign disease of pancreas, liver and bile ducts. Hence, it is not a diagnostic investigation. However, very high values suggest malignancy even when histology is inconclusive.

## Treatment

I. Periampullary carcinoma—Whipple's operation
II. Carcinoma of body and tail

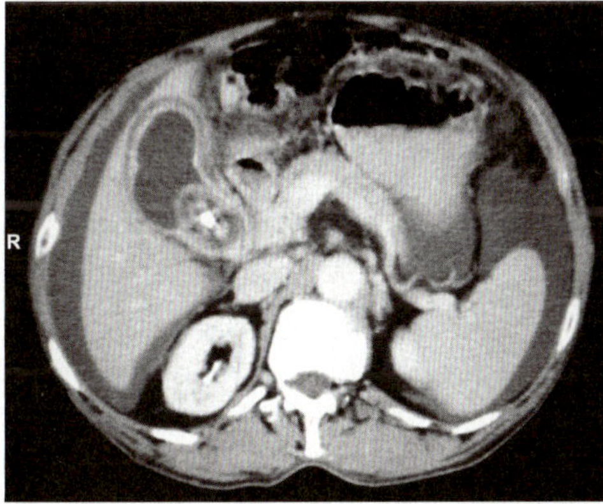


**Fig. 54.99:** Carcinoma body of the pancreas with para-aortic nodes and ascites

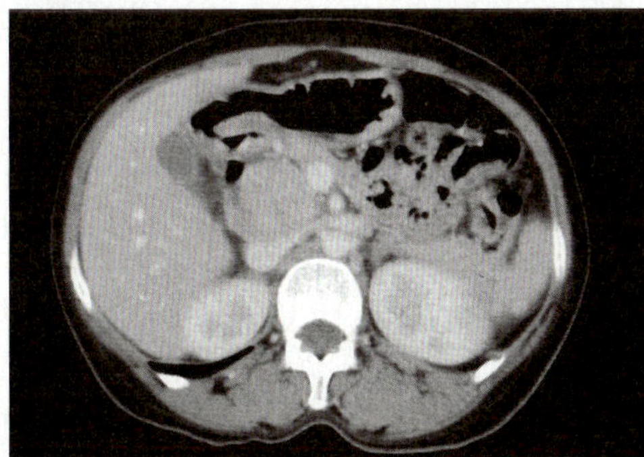

**Fig. 54.100:** Large mass in the head and body of pancreas

A. If the tumour is very small and diagnosed very early, they are ideally treated with **total pancreatectomy with removal of involved lymph nodes.**

B. Many cases are diagnosed late. They are inoperable either due to fixity to portal vein or due to metastasis. Hence, there is no role for curative surgery. For the confirmation of diagnosis, transabdominal USG-guided fine needle aspiration cytology can be done. Surgery is not indicated in such cases; only palliative treatment can be offered. Prognosis is very poor.
    - **Palliative radiotherapy:** 4000–6000 cGy units can be given. Response rate is 5–10%. It reduces size of the tumour and **some pain relief is obtained** (Table 54.6).
    - Palliative treatment is an important aspect of carcinoma pancreas even though such patients succumb to the disease within 3 to 6 months. Palliation is mainly to relieve pain.

## TRUE CYSTIC PANCREATIC NEOPLASMS (CPNS)

- These are uncommon tumours present predominantly in women (Key Box 54.23).
- Other rare tumours are cystadenocarcinoma, acinar cell cystadenocarcinoma, etc.
- These tumours can be confused with pseudocyst of the pancreas. Hence, they should be differentiated at surgery (Figs 54.101 and 54.102). Otherwise, gross blunders can take place (Table 54.7).
- Serous and mucinous are important. They are discussed in Table 54.8.

Key Box 54.23

**True Cystic Pancreatic Neoplasms (CPNS)**

**A. Serous cystadenoma: Benign**
- Common in women, located in head of pancreas. They account for 30% of all CPNs. They can be observed, if asymptomatic.

**B. Mucinous cystic neoplasms (MCNs)**
- More common in women
- More often found in body and tail
- More incidence than serous (40%)
- Considered premalignant
- Do not communicate with ductal system
- Lesions more than 2 cm need to be resected

**C. Intraductal papillary mucinous tumours (IPMTs)** (Figs 54.103 and 54.104)
- Slightly more common in males
- Communicates with duct
- Incidence is about 25%
- High malignant potential
- More common in head involving ampulla of Vater
- Treated by Whipple's resection

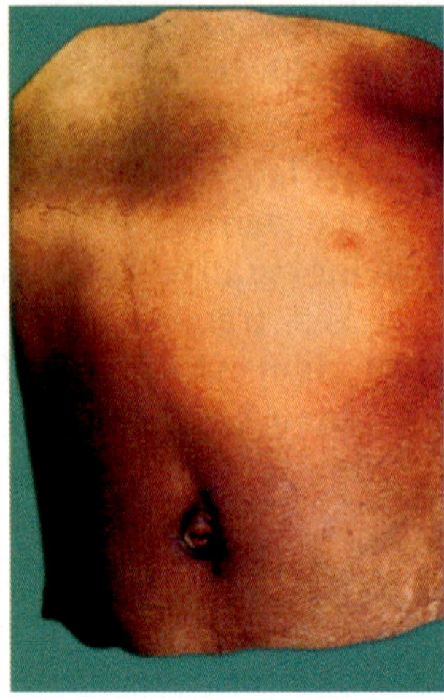

Fig. 54.101: Cystadenoma of the pancreas

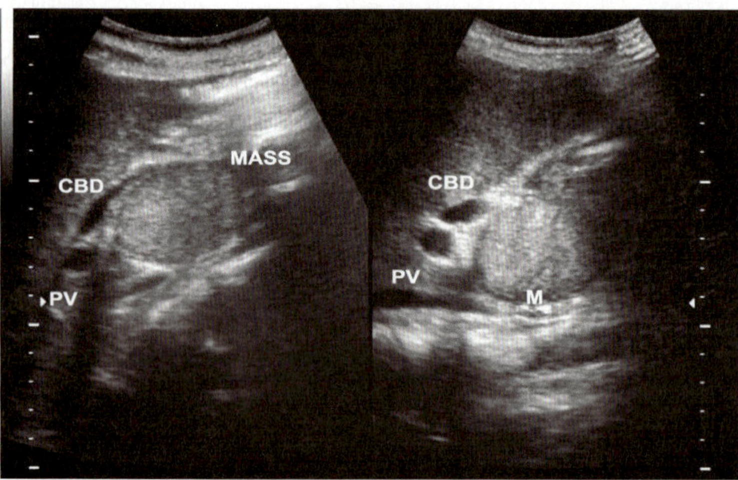


Fig. 54.102: Ultrasound showing cystic mass in the body of pancreas

**TABLE 54.6:** Palliation for carcinoma pancreas—3 chief symptoms

| Pain | Jaundice | Duodenal obstruction |
|---|---|---|
| • Sustained release oral narcotic drugs—morphine sulphate<br>• Celiac plexus nerve block (pain is due to invasion of retroperitoneal nerve trunks)<br>• Intraoperative celiac plexus block by injecting 50% alcohol directly into tissues along side of aorta<br>• Palliative RT and gemcitabine—survival improved by 1–2 months | • Stenting—recurrent obstruction and cholangitis chances are decreased<br>• Choledochojejunostomy, cholecysto-jejunostomy (if cystic duct enters CBD well above the growth)<br>• Surgical bypass has increased mortality and morbidity initially | • Occurs in 20% of patients<br>• Posterior dependent GJ is preferable—indicated in cases of symptoms such as vomiting |

**TABLE 54.7:** Differences between cystic neoplasm and pseudocyst

| | Cystic neoplasm | Pseudocyst |
|---|---|---|
| History of pancreatitis | Absent | Present |
| Imaging | May demonstrate *solid component* | Usually absent |
| ERCP | Mucin egress from bulging papilla in cases of IPMTs | No |
| Mucin content of fluid | Present | Absent |
| CEA in fluid | Increased in mucinous cystic neoplasms | Absent |
| CA 19–9 | Increased in malignant cystic neoplasms | Not elevated |
| Percutaneous wall biopsy | Epithelial lining can be present | No epithelial lining |

**TABLE 54.8:** Cystic neoplasms

| | Serous | Mucinous |
|---|---|---|
| Gender | No prediction | More common in women |
| Nature | Multiple cysts are present | More often multilocular |
| Cut surface | Microcystic adenomas with cut surface appearance of a sponge | Macrocystic adenomas with smooth lining with papillary projections |
| CT scan | CT may show cysts with calcification | Septal on CT scan is characteristic |
| Nature of fluid | Cystic spaces contain serous fluid | Cystic spaces contain mucus |
| Lining epithelium | Lining is by cuboidal epithelium | Lining is tall columnar and goblet cells |
| Malignant potential | No malignant potential | Most of them turn into cystadenocarcinoma |

Fig. 54.103: Intraductal papillary mucinous tumour (IPMT) at surgery. (*Courtesy*: Dr SS Prasad, Dr Sunilkrishna, Dr Rajendra Benakatti, Department of Surgery, KMC, Manipal)

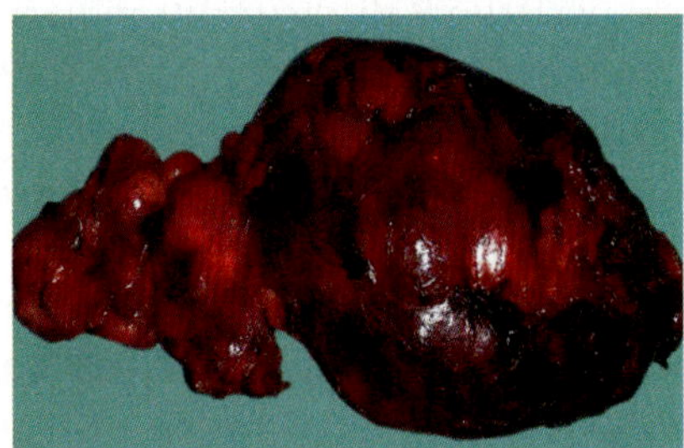

Fig. 54.104: Distal pancreatectomy specimen: Intraductal papillary mucinous tumour (IPMT) at surgery. (*Courtesy*: Dr SS Prasad, Dr Sunilkrishna, Dr Rajendra Benakatti, Department of Surgery, KMC, Manipal)

## ENDOCRINE TUMOURS OF THE PANCREAS

**SU24.3:** Describe the principles of investigation and management of pancreatic endocrine tumors.

These tumours are members of APUDOMA arising from APUD (**A**mine **P**recursor **U**ptake **D**ecarboxylation) cells. They are neuroectodermal in origin. Accordingly, following tumours can occur (Table 54.9A).

### Types

- **Sporadic:** Usually occurs as a single tumour.
- **Familial:** Occur with other adenomas as in multiple endocrine neoplasia syndrome—**MEN Type I:** Pituitary, parathyroid, pancreatic adenoma.

### INSULINOMA (β-CELL TUMOUR)

- Most common functioning islet cell tumour.
- Majority of the insulinomas occur in the tail and body of pancreas and majority of them are benign, one-third are malignant and one-third are multiple.
- It can be a single adenoma, can be due to diffuse hyperplasia or due to carcinoma.
- **Clinical features are that of hypoglycaemia** (Key Box 54.24 for other causes of hypoglycaemia).
- In early stages, it can mimic a duodenal ulcer. Due to hypoglycaemia, hunger pain develops and a tendency to ask for food is present.
- As it becomes severe, giddiness, dizziness, syncopal attacks, blurring of vision and diplopia can occur.
- Late stages—epilepsy, semiconsciousness and coma.

Key Box 54.24

**Persistent Hypoglycaemia—Causes**

- Insulinoma
- Hepatoma
- Hepatocellular damage
- Hypopituitarism
- Addison's disease
- Large mesenchymal tumour

### Whipple's Triad of Insulinoma

1. Attack of hypoglycaemia in morning hours, in the fasting state.
2. Symptoms are relieved on taking glucose.
3. Blood sugar in the fasting state is less than 45 mg% during the attack.

**Clinical Notes**

The author remembers a case of recurrent epilepsy getting admitted to the department of neurology. He was found to have hypoglycaemia and was diagnosed as insulinoma only during the 4th admission. A 3 cm benign insulinoma was enucleated from the pancreas. The patient is asymptomatic till date.

### Investigations

1. **Serum insulin** levels done by immunoassay method are found to be very high. Proinsulin levels and C-peptide level are also very high.

**TABLE 54.9A:** Summary of islet cells

| Islet cells | Active agent | Syndrome | Presentation |
|---|---|---|---|
| Alpha | Glucagon | Glucagonoma | Hyperglycaemia |
| Beta | Insulin | Insulinoma | Hypoglycaemia |
| Delta | Somatostatin | Somatostatinoma | — |
| G | Gastrin | Gastrinoma | Hyperacidity |

2. Persistent hypoglycaemia—blood sugar level of less than 50 mg/dl relieved by glucose is suggestive of insulinoma.
3. **USG and CT scan** of abdomen can demonstrate the tumour, if it is more than 2 cm. (Intraoperative ultrasound is a useful test.)
4. Selective angiography will demonstrate tumour blush as majority of them are very vascular.

### Treatment

- Enucleation is the treatment of choice.
- Resection of the tumour and if necessary distal pancreatectomy can also be done in selected patients.
- Diazoxide is given to suppress insulin release.
- For inoperable islet cell carcinoma, streptozocin is the best chemotherapeutic agents.

**Insulinoma—interesting most**

- The most common functioning islet cell tumour of pancreas
- Mostly are single (75%)
- Mostly multiple in 'MEN' syndromes
- Mostly benign (70%)
- Mostly occur in tail and body of pancreas
- Mostly present as bizarre behaviour confusing type due to hypoglycaemia
- Most useful diagnostic test—very high (disproportional) levels of insulin during fasting hypoglycaemia
- The most important test to localise the tumour before surgery is CT/MRI
- The most important test to localise at surgery is intra-operative ultrasound
- Mostly they can be enucleated when occur in the head
- Most insulinomas are small, less than 2 cm

## GASTRINOMA (ZOLLINGER-ELLISON SYNDROME)

Two types are recognised.

- **Type I (rare):** These have antral G cell hyperplasia, wherein gastrin is stored. Hypergastrinaemia with chronic peptic ulceration is a feature. Pancreas is normal.
- **Type II: May be due to an ulcerogenic,** non-β-islet cell tumour or sometimes diffuse hyperplasia of the islet cells. Tumour secretes gastrin and is usually found in the tail of the pancreas. 50% of them are malignant.
  - Intractable peptic ulceration, hypergastrinaemia with massive acid hypersecretion of up to 500 ml/hr can occur.
  - Diarrhoea, steatorrhoea and hypokalaemia occur due to acid irritating the small bowel activity (Key Box 54.25).

Key Box 54.25

**Gastrinoma should be Suspected in Following Situations**

1. **Unusual ulcer:** Peptic ulcer not responding to intensive medical treatment.
2. **Unusual recurrence:** Multiple recurrences in spite of the treatment.
3. **Unusual number:** Multiple ulcers scattered in the GIT.
4. **Unusual sites:** Ulcers present in the 2nd part of duodenum, an ulcer just distal to the ligament of Treitz.
5. **Unusual age:** Sudden development of an ulcer in a young boy or in a very elderly patient.

### Site

It commonly occurs in the gastrinoma triangle also called Passaro's triangle. Following three points form **Passaro's triangle**.

1. Junction of the cystic duct with the common bile duct (Fig. 54.105).
2. Junction between head and neck of pancreas.
3. Junction between second and third parts of the duodenum.

### Diagnosis

1. **Endoscopy** will show prominent mucosal folds and large amount of acid in the stomach.
2. **Serum gastrin** is increased above normal levels (normal value <150 ng/dl).
3. **CT scan and arteriography** may localise the tumour.

### Treatment

1. **Type I:** Partial gastrectomy to remove G cells-bearing area.
2. **Type II:** If the tumour is small, removal of the tumour can be done (enucleation).
3. If the **tumour is large,** Omeprazole 20 mg twice a day or Somatostatin derivatives have been used to control acidity. Total gastrectomy is the last resort, if gastrinoma is not found.

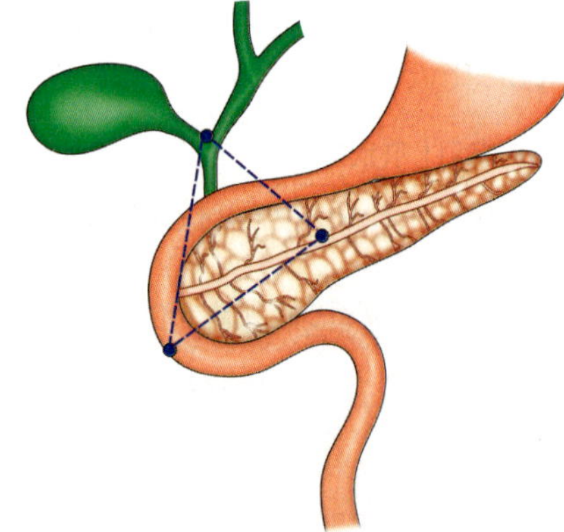

**Fig. 54.105:** Passaro's triangle of gastrinoma. (*Courtesy*: Dr Vidushi, Undergraduate student, KMC, Manipal)

## GLUCAGONOMA

- It arises from **alpha cells** producing glucagon. Around 90% are in the body and tail.
- Clinically, it presents with **extensive necrolytic migratory erythematous rashes**. Rashes occur due to low amino acid levels due to gluconeogenesis brought about by glucagon. Rashes involve legs and perineum.
- Age range is 20–70 years.
- This is common in women.
- **Mild diabetes**, weight loss, diarrhoea are the other features. Increased serum glucagon levels is diagnostic.
- Increased serum glucagon levels is diagnostic.
- Localisation is by elective arteriography and CT scan.
- **Treatment is enucleation.**

### Treatment Principles of Glucagonoma

- Correction of malnutrition by TPN (total parenteral nutrition).
- Treatment with somatostatin analogues.
- Enucleation is easy, if it is in the head.
- Considerable palliation, even if subtotal removal is achieved.
- Low dose heparin—before and after surgery—because of high-risk of DVT—pulmonary embolism.
- Streptozocin and dacarbazine are the most effective chemotherapeutic agents.

Thus, endocrine tumours of the pancreas are rare but when they occur, they can present with varying clinical manifestations which confuse a clinician. A high index of suspicion is necessary. They may be benign but can be fatal, if left untreated.

## ACUTE PANCREATITIS

**SU28.1:** Describe the clinical features, principles of investigation, prognosis and management of pancreatitis.

### Definition

It is defined as acute nonbacterial inflammatory condition caused by activation, interstitial liberation and autodigestion of pancreas presenting as acute abdominal pain.

- *Acute pancreatitis stings like a scorpion (produces severe pain).*
- *Acute pancreatitis drinks like a fish (produces dehydration).*
- *Acute pancreatitis eats like a wolf (pancreatic necrosis).*
- *Acute pancreatitis burrows like a rodent (produces fistula).*
- *Acute pancreatitis kills like a leopard (life-threatening).*

### Classifications

1. Marseille's classification
2. Modified Atlanta classification.

#### *1. Marseille's Classification*

1. Acute pancreatitis
2. Acute relapsing pancreatitis: In both these conditions, pancreas returns back to normal.
3. Chronic pancreatitis
4. Chronic relapsing pancreatitis: In both these conditions, there is always permanent damage to the pancreas.

#### *2. Modified Atlanta Classification*

The latest classification which is used is given in Tables 54.9B and C.

### Aetiology (Figs 54.106 to 54.108)

1. **Alcohol abuse (40 to 50%):** It is the **major cause of acute pancreatitis** in **our country** and is seen in about 50% of the cases. Alcohol stimulates pancreatic secretions rich in protein, forms protein plugs and results in obstruction to the pancreatic duct. Alcohol stimulates trypsinogen. It causes spasm of sphincter of Oddi. It also has **direct toxic effect on the pancreas**. Tobacco smoking contributes to its effects.
2. **Biliary tract disease:** Stone in the biliary tree (gallstone pancreatitis) is the major cause of acute pancreatitis in the Western world (40%). In our country, it may be responsible for pancreatitis in about 20–30% of patients.
3. **Collagen vascular disorders:** Autoimmune disease, such as polyarteritis nodosa, can be a causative factor in acute pancreatitis.
4. **Drugs:** Corticosteroids, tetracycline, oestrogens, azathioprine, valproic acid and diuretics can cause pancreatitis.
5. **Ductal:** Around 20%. Some of them are due to pancreatic divisum seen during ERCP. The opening of the minor papilla is inadequate for drainage of pancreatic juice. Ductal anomalies or APBDJ—abnormal pancreaticobiliary duct junction.
6. **Endoscopic procedures:** Sphincterotomy, cannulation of CBD or pancreatic duct, or basketing of stones from CBD can precipitate acute pancreatitis by duct disruption and enzyme extravasation.
7. **Familial or genetic** factors have been blamed for acute pancreatitis. Hereditary pancreatitis may be due to mutation of cationic trypsinogen gene. Symptoms begin in early childhood.
8. **Hyperparathyroidism** causing hypercalcaemia may stimulate pancreatic juices and can cause pancreatitis. It also facilitates precipitation of calcium in the ducts.

**TABLE 54.9B:** Pancreatic and peripancreatic collections

| Collection | Time after onset of pain (wk) | Pancreatitis subcategory | Location | Imaging features |
|---|---|---|---|---|
| APFC | ≤4 | IEP | Extrapancreatic | Homogeneous, fluid attenuation, conforms to retroperitoneal structures, no wall |
| ANC | ≤4 | Necrotizing pancreatitis | Intra- and/or extra-pancreatic | Inhomogeneous, nonliquefied components, no wall |
| Pseudocyst | >4 | IEP | Extrapancreatic | Homogeneous, fluid filled, circumscribed, encapsulated with wall |
| WON | >4 | Necrotizing pancreatitis | Intra- and/or extra-pancreatic | Inhomogeneous, nonliquefied components, encapsulated |

**TABLE 54.9C:** Modified Atlanta classification

| Acute Pancreatitis | | | |
|---|---|---|---|
| Two phases | Early<br>1st week | Late<br>After 1st week | |
| Severity | Mild<br>No organ failure | Moderate<br>Organ failure less than 48 h | Severe<br>Organ failure longer than 48 h |
| Two types | Oedematous | Necrotizing | |
| Complications | <4 Weeks: Acute peripancreatic collection<br>>4 Weeks: Pseudocyst | <4 Weeks: Acute necrotic collection<br>>4 Weeks: Walled-off necrosis | |

9. **Hyperlipidaemia** (>1000 mg/dl of triglycerides) can also cause pancreatitis. Dietary control can cure pancreatitis.
10. **Hypothermia** and **hypotension** can cause ischaemia to the pancreas resulting in acute pancreatitis.
11. **Injury to the pancreas** either postoperative or following penetrating injury can result in pancreatitis.
12. **Infection:** Viruses such as *Mumps* and *Coxsackie* can cause pancreatitis. Scorpion sting can also cause pancreatitic abnormality.

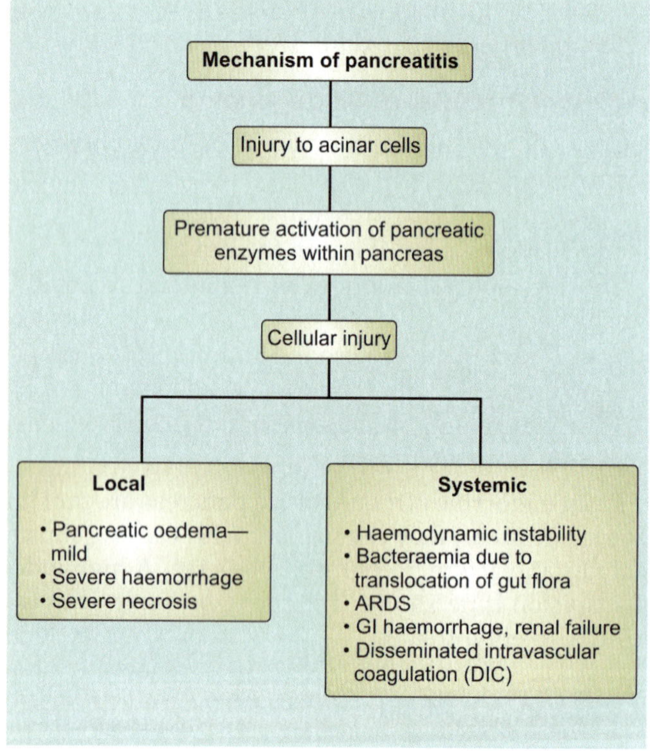


**Fig. 54.106:** Pathogenesis of tissue damage (*see* text)

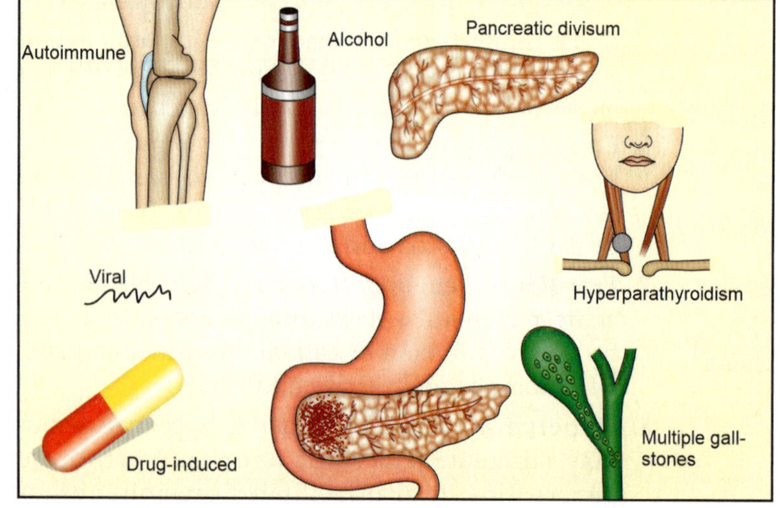


**Fig. 54.107:** A few causes of acute pancreatitis

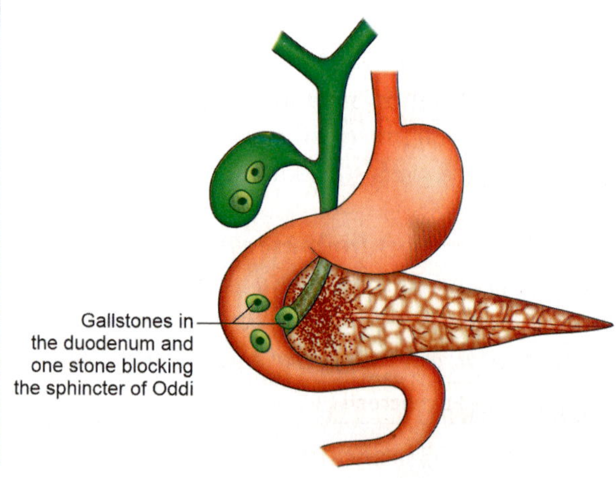


**Fig. 54.108:** Gallstone pancreatitis (diagrammatic)

13. **Postoperative pancreatitis**
    - It follows operations on CBD—open or laparoscopic. More common after T-tube insertions (now it is less).
    - Sphincteroplasty, ERCP, stone extractions
    - Pancreatic biopsy
    - Gastrectomy (distal/total)
    - Cardiac surgery. Here risk factors are perioperative administration of calcium, postoperative hypotension, preoperative renal failure.
14. **Idiopathic:** It is seen in about 15% of cases. Even though, classified as idiopathic (no cause is found), they are found to have sludge/gallstones undetected by ultrasound examination (Key Box 54.26).

Key Box 54.26

**Quick Reference to Common Causes of Pancreatitis**

- Pancreatitis in teens—suspect **hereditary or APBDJ**[1]
- Pancreatitis in women—suspect **gallstones**
- Pancreatitis in males—alcoholic pancreatitis
- Pancreatitis with **fleeting joint pains—autoimmune pancreatitis**
- Pancreatitis with bony lesions/cysts—**hyperparathyroidism**
- Pancreatitis with fever—viral

[1]Abnormal pancreaticobiliary duct junction

## Pathogenesis (Fig. 54.109)

- Autodigestion is the final common pathway leading to pancreatitis, a few theories have been explained as possible factors for autogenesis.
  1. **Obstruction/secretion:** Recurrent attacks of pancreatitis as in chronic cases can be due to multiple strictures, stasis, resulting in autodigestion.
  2. **Common channel theory:** In about 90% of cases, bile duct and pancreatic duct converge into ampulla of Vater. However, only in 10% of cases, they have common channel.
     Reflux of bile into pancreas has been blamed for 'gallstone pancreatitis'. However, strong evidence is lacking.
  3. **Duodenal reflux:** Activation of enzymes takes place in the duodenum through action of enterokinase. Hence, it is postulated that duodenal reflux is one of the causes of acute pancreatitis.
  4. **Back diffusion:** Back diffusion of pancreatic enzymes through the ductal epithelium is a possible factor, when damaged by alcohol/bile acids, etc.
  5. **Systemic sepsis:** Organ failure
     - ARDS, renal failure
     - Endotoxins originate from bacteria.
- Acute pancreatitis is an **autodigestion** following activation of trypsinogen. This is brought about by various agents mentioned above.

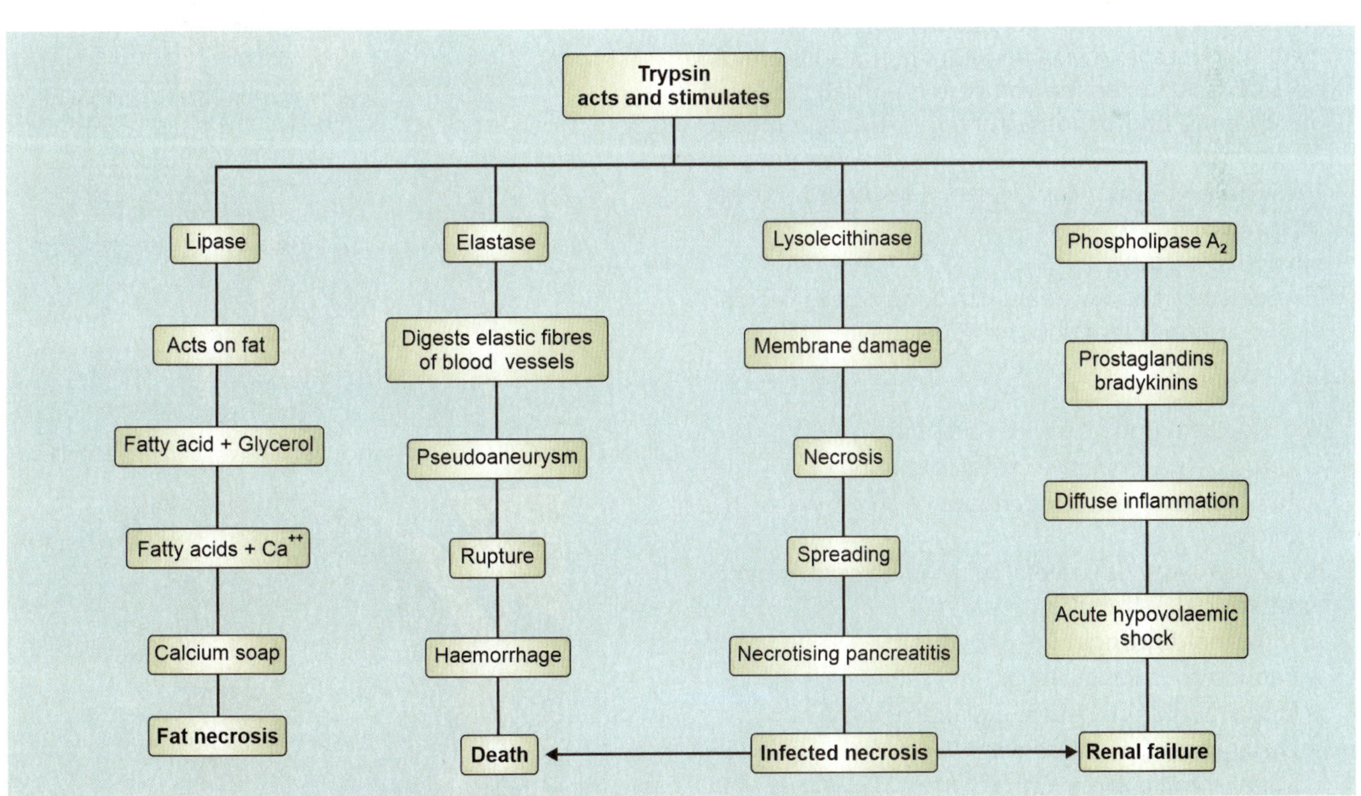


**Fig. 54.109:** Activation of trypsinogen to trypsin—pathogenesis of pancreatitis

- It may also be due to reflux of bile into the pancreas.
- Trypsinogen is converted into trypsin. It acts and stimulates:
  1. **Lipase:** Lipase splits the fat into fatty acids and glycerol. Fatty acids combine with calcium to form calcium soap. This is represented as fat necrosis seen in the omentum, subsynovial pockets of knee joint, etc. This also explains hypocalcaemia and tetany seen in acute pancreatitis.
  2. **Elastase:** It digests the elastic fibres of the blood vessels resulting in rupture and haemorrhage into the peritoneal cavity.
  3. **Lysolecithinase:** This is derived from the bile. It produces extensive tissue necrosis resulting in destruction of pancreas.
  4. **Prostaglandins, bradykinins, kallikrein, etc.:** These are the inflammatory mediators. They produce profound hypotension, shock and collapse, due to loss of fluid in the retroperitoneum (III space loss).
  5. **Extensive necrosis of pancreas:** It produces **MDF** (**m**yocardial **d**epressant **f**actor) which depresses ventricular contraction resulting in cardiac failure. Ultimate result is the development of **multiorgan failure**.

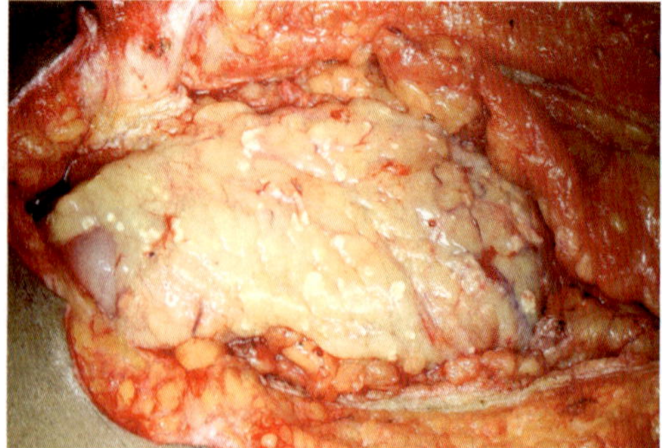

Fig. 54.110: Fat necrosis in the omentum

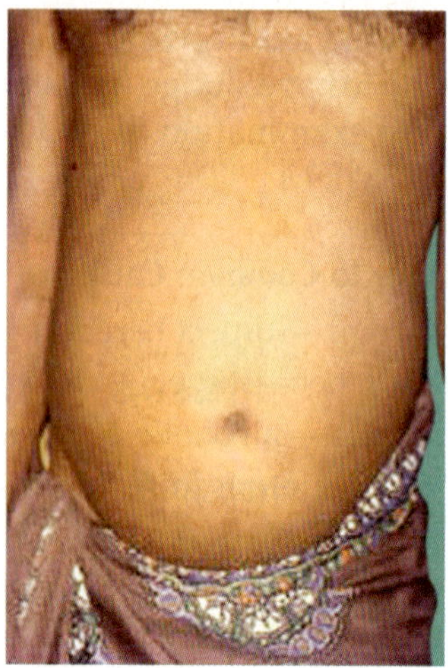

Fig. 54.111: Abdominal distension is due to paralytic ileus in the early stages. It can also be due to pancreatic ascites

## Clinical Features (Figs 54.110 to 54.113)

### *Symptoms*

- Severe upper abdominal epigastric pain radiating to the back increases over a period of hours—illimitable agony is a characteristic feature. It is partially relieved on stooping and bending forwards (Mohammedan Prayer sign). A meal or alcohol triggers the pain.
- Vomiting—frequent and effortless due to reflex pylorospasm.
- Fever—low grade.
- Haematemesis and melaena can occur due to necrosis of duodenum. It is a poor prognostic sign.

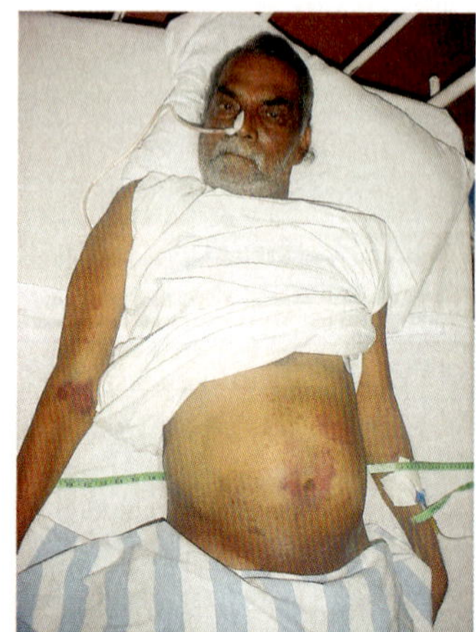

Fig. 54.112: Cullen's sign—discolouration around the umbilicus

### *Signs*

- **Febrile,** tachypnoeic patient in agony.
- **Cyanosis**—improper perfusion of lungs.
- **Faint jaundice** due to oedema of the head of the pancreas.
- **Features of shock**—feeble pulse, tachycardia, hypotension, cold extremities.
- **Abdominal findings**
  - Tenderness in epigastrium
  - Upper abdominal guarding and rigidity
  - Distension of the abdomen
  - Mass in epigastrium
  - Muscle guarding

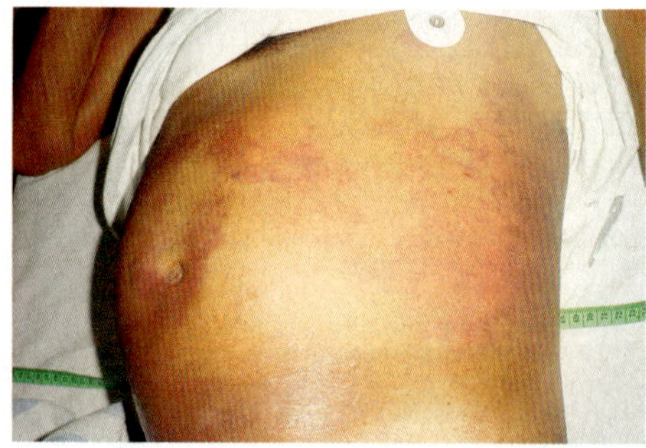

Fig. 54.113: Grey Turner's sign—discolouration in the flanks

- Abdominal distension due to either accumulation of blood or fluid in the peritoneal cavity or due to paralytic ileus.

- **Cullen's sign** (Fig. 54.112): Bluish ecchymotic discolouration seen around umbilicus (first described for ruptured ectopic pregnancy).
- **Grey Turner's sign** (Fig. 54.113)
  - Bluish discolouration in the flanks
  - Both these signs are due to peripancreatic and retroperitoneal haemorrhage and seepage of blood along fascial planes, into the anterior abdominal wall and spread through falciform ligament.
- **Evidence of respiratory signs:** Tachypnoea, dullness, effusion, crepitations, rhonchi (pulmonary oedema, ARDS).

### Systemic Complications

A. Disseminated intravascular coagulation as evidenced by:
  - Platelet count <100,000 cells/cumm
  - Fibrinogen <1 g/L
  - Fibrin split products >80 μg/dl

B. Metabolic disturbance (serum calcium <7.5 mg/dl)

### Local Complications

- Necrosis
- Abscess
- Pseudocyst

### Investigations

1. **Haemogram (CBP):** Hb% may be low due to haemorrhagic pancreatitis.
   Total count is raised above 15,000 cells/mm$^3$ due to inflammation.
2. **Blood for urea, creatinine** to rule out renal failure.
3. **Serum amylase** (widely used test) (Key Box 54.27).
   - Normal levels are 40–80 Somogyi units.
   - Values around 400 are suggestive and values more than 1000 Somogyi units are diagnostic of acute pancreatitis.
   - It is increased in the first 24–48 hours and returns to normal within 3–4 days (Key Box 54.27).
   - Persistent high level of amylase in acute pancreatitis indicates:
     - Unresolving inflammation
     - Recurrent attacks of pancreatitis
     - Complications—pseudocyst, pancreatic abscess
     - **Serum lipase levels—more specific** but difficult to measure. Lipase is only **secreted by pancreas.**

*Pearls of Wisdom*

Lipase levels tend to be higher in alcoholic pancreatitis and amylase levels are higher in gallstone pancreatitis.

Key Box 54.27

**Increased Amylase Levels—Seen in**

- Acute pancreatitis and its complications
- Parotitis
- Afferent loop obstruction
- Spasm of sphincter of Oddi
- Biliary peritonitis—duodenal injuries
- Mesenteric infarction
- Ruptured ectopic gestation

4. **Blood and urine sugar estimation:** Glycosuria is present in almost 100% of patients.
5. **Serum calcium levels:** Hypocalcaemia is seen, due to hypoalbuminaemia or fat necrosis.
6. Total proteins are usually low, especially albumin.
7. **Plain X-ray abdomen (erect position)** (Fig. 54.114)
   - **Calcification suggests chronic pancreatitis.**
   - To rule out perforation of peptic ulcer.
   - **Sentinel loop sign**—one dilated jejunal loop of intestine which is seen in the region of pancreas.
   - **Colon 'cut-off' sign** refers to mild distension of transverse colon with collapsed descending colon.
8. **Abdominal ultrasound**—can demonstrate oedematous pancreas, fluid in the abdomen or biliary tract disease.
9. **Contrast enhanced CT scan** of abdomen is done after 3–5 days in patients who fail to respond to conservative treatment. **If CT scan demonstrates infected necrosis, an urgent CT-guided FNAC is done and Gram stain is sent. If Gram stain is positive, it has to be treated urgently** (Figs 54.115 and 54.116).
   **Indications for CT scan in acute pancreatitis:**
   - Patients with severe pancreatitis
   - When the diagnosis is in doubt
   - Patients with organ failure
   - Patients with sepsis

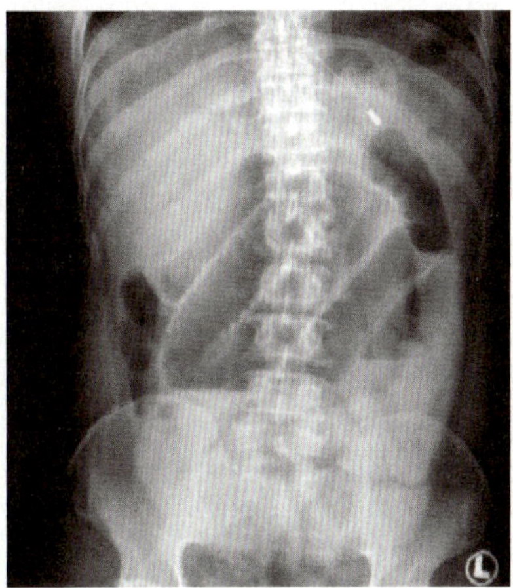


**Fig. 54.114:** Plain X-ray abdomen erect showing dilated jejunal loop due to paralytic ileus—sentinel loop sign

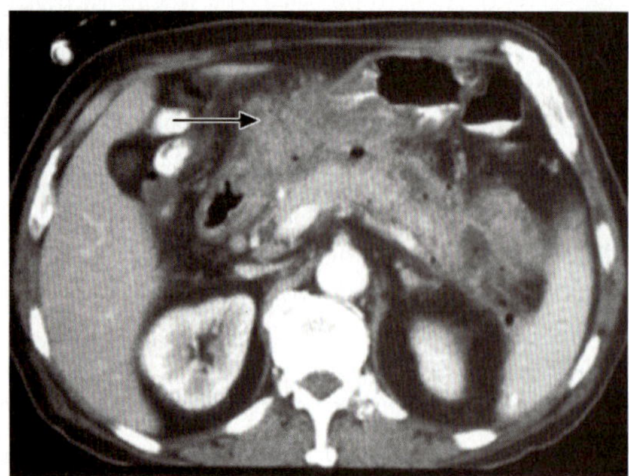

**Fig. 54.115: Contrast enhanced CT (CECT) scan** is the gold standard investigation in cases of acute pancreatitis. Useful between 4 to 7 days of acute pancreatitis. This photograph shows extensive necrosis. CT scan also helps in detecting pseudocysts, abscesses, presence of gallstones or any other unsuspected pathology in the abdomen. Modern thinking is to wait for 4–6 weeks for separation of necrosis before surgical necrosectomy

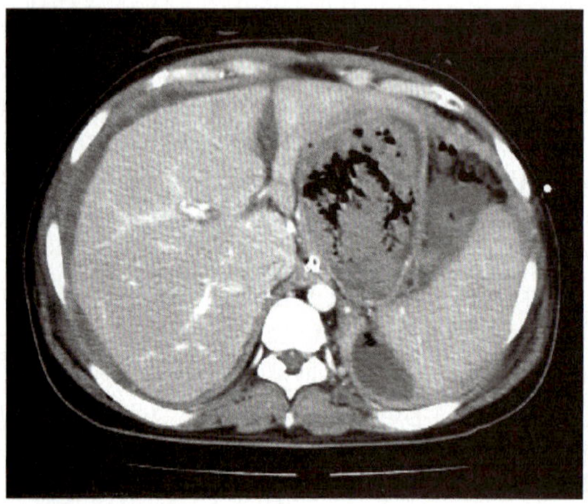

**Fig. 54.116:** CT scan showing infected necrosis with air pockets inside necrosis

- Localised complications such as pseudocyst, pseudoaneurysms
- Clinical deterioration.

## Prognostic Indicators/Criteria for Acute Pancreatitis

There are several scoring systems available, a few important ones have been given below. Atlanta's Criteria for Acute Pancreatitis is applied for organ failure. Ranson score is applied for severity prediction and Balthazar score is applied for CT severity index.

**Atlanta's criteria for acute pancreatitis**

*Organ failure as defined*

- Shock (systolic blood pressure <90 mmHg)
- Pulmonary insufficiency ($PaO_2$ <60 mmHg)
- Renal failure (creatinine level >2 mg/dl after fluid resuscitation)
- GI bleeding (>500 ml/24 hr)

**Balthazar-Ranson criteria for severity or computed tomography severity index (CTSI)**

| CT Grade | Score | Necrosis | Score | SI |
|---|---|---|---|---|
| A | 0 | None | 0 | 0 |
| B | 1 | One-third | 2 | 1 |
| C | 2 | One-half | 4 | 4 |
| D | 3 | >One-half | 6 | 7 |
| E | 4 | | | 20 |

A = normal

B = focal or diffuse enlargement of the pancreas

C = intrinsic pancreatic abnormalities associated with haziness and streaky densities representing inflammatory changes in the peripancreatic fat

D = single, ill-defined fluid collection

E = two or more multiple fluid collections

CTSI, 0–3, mortality 3% morbidity 8%

CTSI, 4–6, mortality 6%, morbidity 35%

CTSI, 7–10, mortality 17%, morbidity 92%

Severe pancreatitis is defined by the presence of any evidence of organ failure or a local complication.

## Management

- Almost always conservative. However, a few scoring systems have been followed (Table 54.10).

*Pearls of Wisdom*

Early aggressive fluid replacement is the key in the management of acute pancreatitis.

- Even though management principles of any acute abdomen includes 'nil per oral' so as to give rest to the part, in cases of pancreatitis it has been divided broadly into three categories. It is desirable to know the treatment followed for these categories. It has been given in Table 54.11 and Fig. 54.117.
- Those of you who find it difficult can remember at least a few fundamentals of managing acute pancreatitis. They are given in the form of simple headlines: **ABCDEF.**

**A: Aspiration** with Ryle's tube, to give rest to the pancreas in cases of vomiting (may be for one or two days).

**B: Blood transfusion** if Hb% is low, or albumin and amino acids if proteins are low.

**C: Charts**—increasing pulse, increasing temperature indicates pancreatic necrosis which requires different care.

**D: Drugs and fluids:** Drug of choice in acute necrotizing pancreatitis is injection imipenem. Dose is 1 g intravenous infusion twice or thrice daily. It is given to reduce further damage to pancreatic and peripancreatic tissues or to prevent progression to infected necrosis and multiorgan failure. Narcotic

**TABLE 54.10:** Prognostic indicators/severity predictors

| Ranson score | Glasgow Scale |
|---|---|
| **On admission**<br>Age >55 years<br>WBC count >16 × $10^9$/L<br>Blood glucose >10 mmol/L<br>LDH >350 units/L<br>AST >250 Sigma Frankel unit/unit | Age >55 years<br>WBC count >15 × $10^9$/L<br>Blood glucose >10 mmol/L<br>Serum urea >16 mmol/L<br>$PaO_2$ <60 mmHg |
| **After 48 hours**<br>Increase in blood urea nitrogen levels >5 mg%<br>Drop in haematocrit >10%<br>Arterial oxygen saturation ($PaO_2$ <60 mmHg)<br>Serum calcium <8 mg/dl<br>Base deficit >4 mmol/L<br>Fluid sequestration >6 L | **Within 48 hours**<br>Serum calcium <2 mmol/L<br>Serum albumin <32 g/L<br>LDH >600 units/L<br>AST/ALT >600 units/L<br>***Disease is classified as severe when three or more factors are present.*** |

**TABLE 54.11:** Management principles of acute pancreatitis

| | Acute oedematous (mild—80%) | Necrotising pancreatitis (sterile necrosis—10%) | Infected necrosis (very severe—5%) |
|---|---|---|---|
| **Admission IV fluids/ hypotension** | Acute ward with monitoring of vitals<br>**Early correction of hypotension,** hypovolaemia—crystalloids | Intensive care unit<br>IV fluids and inotropic* support may be required | Intensive care unit<br>May require inotropes and vasopressors for a long period |
| **Blood transfusion** | Rarely required | May be required | Definitely required |
| **Antibiotics** | No antibiotics | Early antibiotic prophylaxis is required | Broad spectrum antibiotics—imipenem, ciprofloxacin, metronidazole, etc. |
| **Oral/nutrition** | Oral fluids, soft diet by 3–4 days, once pain and ileus settle down | If pain is still present even after 4 days, nasojejunal feeding to be done | Enteral feeding/nasojejunal feeding. If calories are not sufficient, total parenteral nutrition is required |
| **Hypomagnesaemia/ hypocalcaemia** | Usually will not be a problem | Correction is required | Correction is required |
| **Oxygen** | By nasal cannula/face mask may be required | Early ARDS—ventilatory support | Ventilatory support may be required |
| **Role of surgery/ natural course** | Majority of patients will not require surgery. If gallstones are impacted at sphincter of Oddi, endoscopic basketing and laparoscopic cholecystectomy should be done | By 10–15 days, may resolve completely or may develop into pseudocyst or infected necrosis which require surgery | Ideal time to operate is after 4 weeks when necrosis is demarcated well.<br>Initial percutaneous CT guided or laparoscopic retroperitoneal aspiration (step up approach) followed by necrosectomy |

*Drug of choice in septic shock to treat hypotension and hypoperfusion is fluid boluses of crystalloids and norepinephrine

analgesics also can be given if pain is severe. Choice of fluid is Ringers' lactate. It is given at the rate of 125–150 ml/hr. Blood urea nitrogen (BUN) and creatinine should be used as markers to predict intravascular volume depletion and correction. Fluid resuscitation should be instituted early in cases of pancreatitis because of third space loss resulting in severe hypovolaemic shock. Hypovolaemia is due to endothelial cell damage and increased permeability.

**E:** Exploratory laparotomy (Key Box 54.28) is done when patient is **not improving** or when there is a complication of pancreatitis such as pancreatic fistula or necrosis. With the advent of wonderful imaging techniques, surgical intervention is rarely being done in the initial phase of acute pancreatitis. With conservative treatment, majority will return back to normal by 3–5 days. Those who develop complications are dealt with separately. Details are given later.

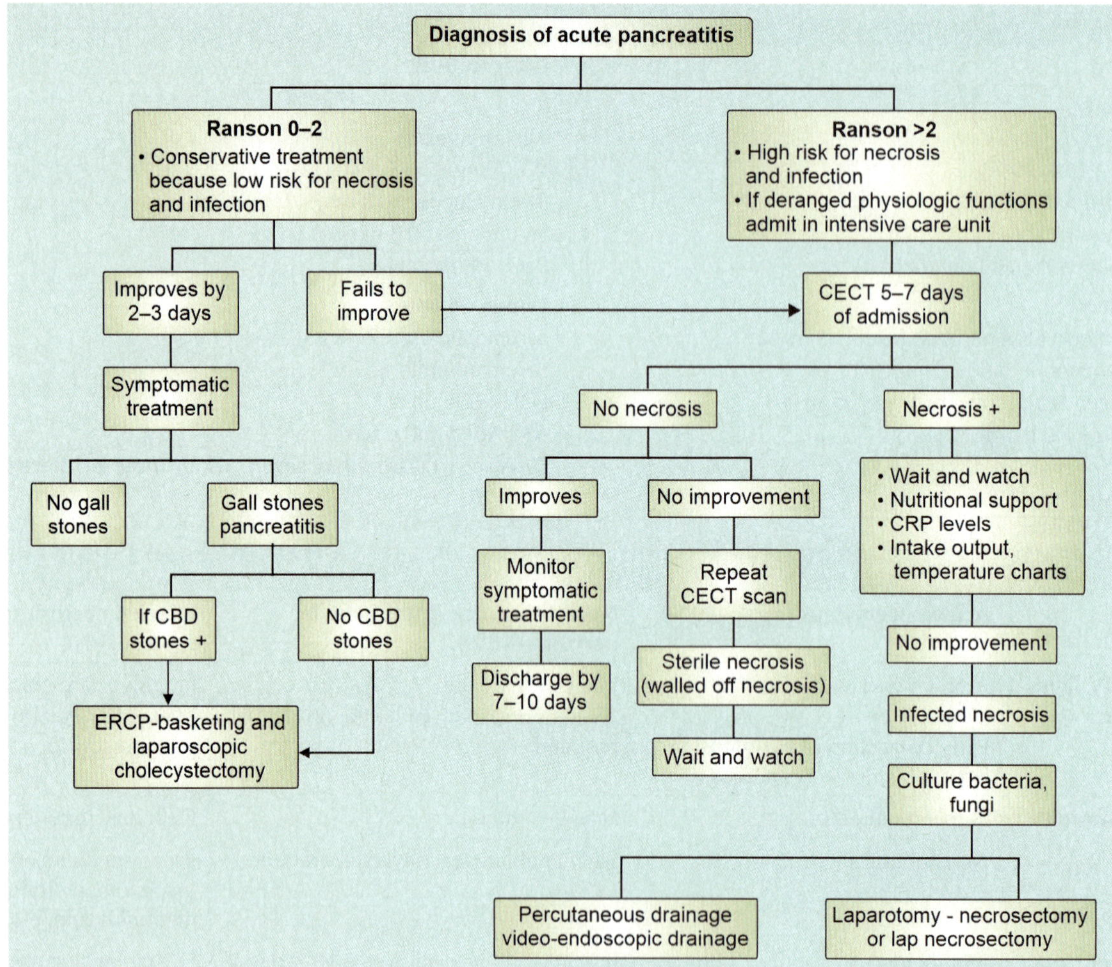


**Fig. 54.117:** Treatment of acute pancreatitis. (*Courtesy*: Dr SS Prasad, Dr L Ramachandra, Dr Kshama Hegde, Professor of Surgery, KMC, Manipal)

Key Box 54.28

### Indications for Surgery in Acute Pancreatitis

- Infected necrosis
- Pancreatic abscess
- Complications such as massive bleeding not responding to conservative treatment
- Cholangitis not responding to treatment

**F: Fluid** should be given early. Rapid infusion of 3–4 litres of Ringer lactate is used to treat hypovolaemic shock. Plasma or albumin may also be given.

- Factors predicting severe pancreatitis (Key Box 54.29).

Key Box 54.29

### Identification of Severe Pancreatitis

| | |
|---|---|
| Age | : >70 years |
| Obesity | : BMI >30 kg/m$^2$ |
| Pleural effusion | : Present |
| CT necrosis | : >50 |
| CT severity index | : CTSI |
| Persistent | : Organ failure |

*Pearls of Wisdom*

In cases of infected necrosis proved by CT-guided FNAC and Gram stain, necrosectomy should be done. Ideal time is 4–6 wks. First do percutaneous aspiration/drainage.

Details of the important aspects of treatment of acute pancreatitis are given in Fig. 54.117.

1. **Admission:** All patients with acute pancreatitis should be admitted and basic charts such as temperature, breathing, pulse, blood pressure, intake output abdominal girth are monitored. Those patients with frequent vomiting require nasogastric tube insertion for aspiration. Make a note of intake and output charts and accordingly fluid balance is maintained. Admission in ICU is recommended only in severe pancreatitis. Mild cases do not require oxygen supplementation. ARDS patients will require ventilator support and care in ICU early.
2. **Pain relief:** It is very important because pain is severe, deep and penetrates to the back. NSAIDs (non-steroidal anti-inflammatory drugs) such as paracetamol, ibuprofen are started. If the pain relief is not

sufficient, change over to powerful opioids, such as codeine. Still if pain persists, narcotic analgesics such as morphine or pethidine are recommended. Buprenorphine is better than pethidine because it is a long-acting analgesic and does not cause dependence. If pain is also due to stones in the CBD-gallstone pancreatitis, ERCP and extraction of stones is done.

3. **Fluid:** Fluid resuscitation in acute pancreatitis is an important step in resuscitation. Early aggressive hydration, defined as 250 to 500 ml/h of isotonic crystalloid solution (ideally lactated Ringer's solution), should be given to all patients during the first 12 to 24 h. However, if patient has cardiovascular, renal, or other related comorbid factors, then the fluid volume should be controlled or reduced. Once fluid replacement is adequate, there will be reduction in Hct and BUN levels over the first 24 h, particularly if they were high at the onset. In the same fashion, pulse rate, temperature, respiratory rate, blood pressure and urine output are monitored. Patients undergoing volume resuscitation should also undergo continuous pulse oximetry, receive supplemental oxygen as needed. Bedside ultrasound guided assessment of diameter of inferior vena cava also helps in assessing the fluid response. Passive leg raising is a simple bedside method to check for fluid response.
4. **Nutrition:** It is an important part of treatment in acute pancreatitis. If enteral or parenteral nutrition is given early in the treatment of acute pancreatitis, there is a lower risk of death than if no supplemental nutrition is given. Patients with mild pancreatitis can resume an oral diet as soon as their pain decreases say by 2 to 3 days after an attack of acute pancreatitis. Low-residue, low-fat, and soft diet are well tolerated and can be given. Idea is to decrease peristalsis activity because some degree of paralytic ileus exists even after 2 or 4 days. Early refeeding also seems to result in a shorter hospital stay.

***The enteral route is preferred over parenteral route because of following reasons:***
- Intestinal mucosal barrier is maintained.
- Prevents the intestinal atrophy, if patients are kept NPO for long period.
- Intestinal atrophy can promotes translocation of bacteria, thus sterile necrosis can turn to infective necrosis.
- Parenteral nutrition requires central IV catheters, thus the risk of infection of a catheter is present.
- Is less expensive.

A nasojejunal feeding tube is placed beyond the ligament of Treitz under radiological or endoscopic guidance. Reason being one can avoid stimulating the gastric phase of the digestive process. If one cannot insert nasojejunal tube, at least nasogastric feeding should be initiated. Whenever nasogastric tube is inserted, the GE junction sphincter does not function well and there is also paralytic ileus. So, to avoid aspiration, head end of the patient should be elevated to about 30 degrees (Fig. 54.118A).

5. **Antibiotics:** In mild cases of acute pancreatitis and in sterile necrosis, they are not indicated. However, if patient has some other pathology such as respiratory or urinary tract infection, antibiotics are given accordingly. In cases of infected necrosis, usual organisms are gram-negative such as *E. coli, Klebsiella*, and anaerobes. Thus, carbapenems, fluoroquinolones, and metronidazole are recommended.
6. **Role of surgery:** There is no role for surgery in mild pancreatitis cases. In cases of sterile necrosis, if they improve, no surgical line of treatment is required. Patients who develop infected necrosis (around 15–20 days) are carefully monitored and if they do not show improvement, percutaneous, retroperitoneal drainage of necrotic material, followed by pigtail catheter insertion is done. Same thing can also be done by **retroperitoneal videoendoscopic drainage**. If patients show complete relief, no surgery is required. **This is also called initial part of step-up approach treatment because around 3–4 weeks of time, necrotic pancreas is not very well demarcated.** However, if toxic features such as temperature, tachycardia, tachypnoea, hypotension, etc. are persisting and repeat CECT scans detect significant necrotic material, laparoscopic or open necrosectomy is done.

### Pancreatic Necrosectomy—Lap/Open Method

(Figs 54.118 to 54.123)

- Ideally done 4–6 weeks later when sepsis is still present.
- CT-guided FNAC/bacterial culture is a must.
- A midline laparotomy is done.
- Lesser sac is entered.
- Thorough debridement of the dead tissue is done.
- All fluid and tissue should be sent for aerobic and anaerobic culture.
- Blunt dissection rather than sharp dissection is done to minimise bleeding.
- Antibiotics of choice should be carbapenems and quinolones.
- Ileostomy should be done for retrocolic necrosis.
- Cholecystectomy should be done for gallstone pancreatitis cases.
- Perfect haemostasis should be achieved using manual compression, sutures and ligatures.

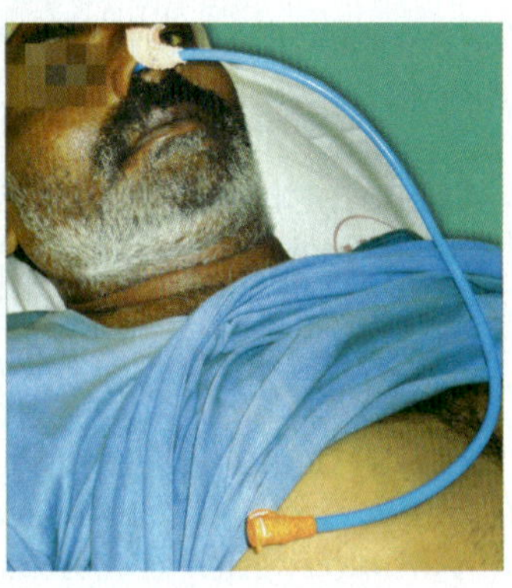

Fig. 54.118A: Acute necrotising pancreatitis. Patient had high temperature. Nasojejunal tube feeding is being done

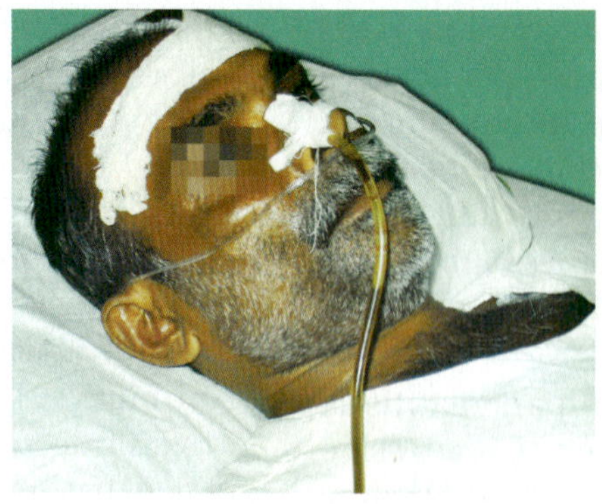

Fig. 54.118B: Acute necrotising pancreatitis with massive upper GI bleeding. Patient had high temperature, angiogram revealed pseudoaneurysm. He underwent therapeutic embolisation followed by necrosectomy

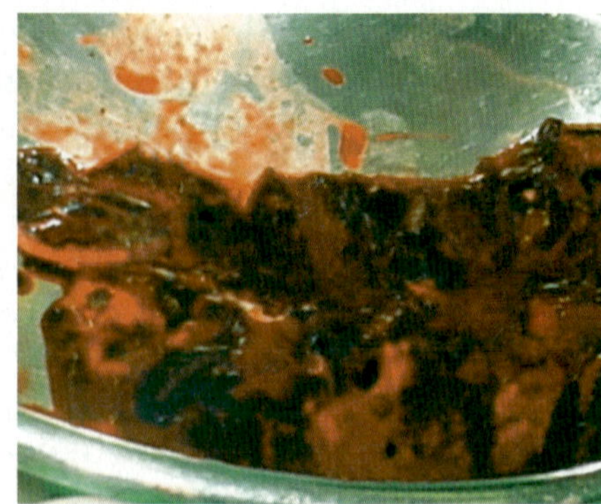

Fig. 54.119: Acute necrotising pancreatitis with massive upper GI bleeding. Patient had haematemesis of one litre of blood with clots

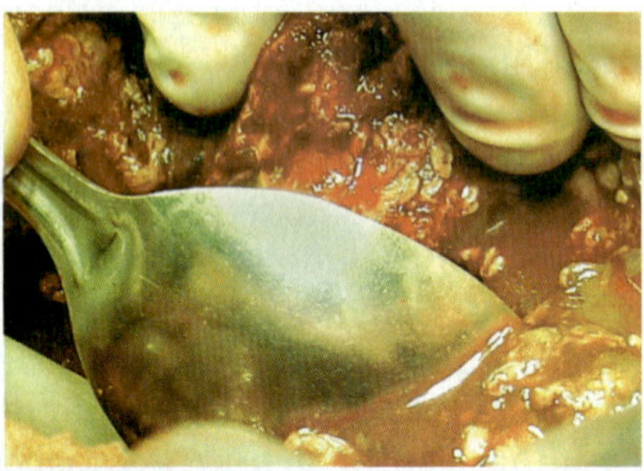

Fig. 54.120: You can see necrosectomy being done. It was done through lesser sac. Significant blood loss was present. Fingers are used to separate necrosis and it is removed with a spoon

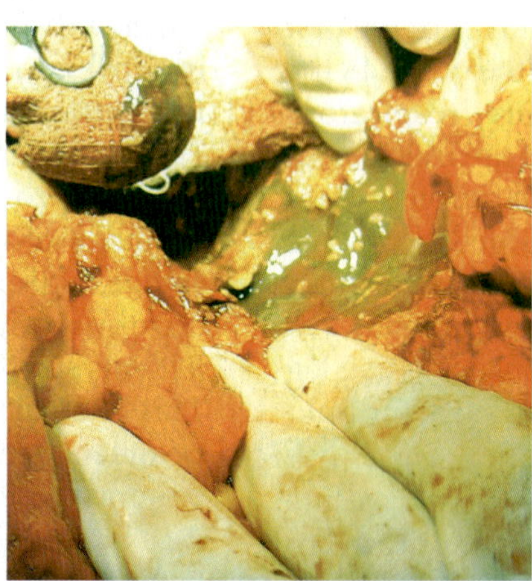

Fig. 54.121: After necrosectomy, pancreatic bed is washed with saline and tubes or sump drains are put so as to be able to irrigate in the postoperative period

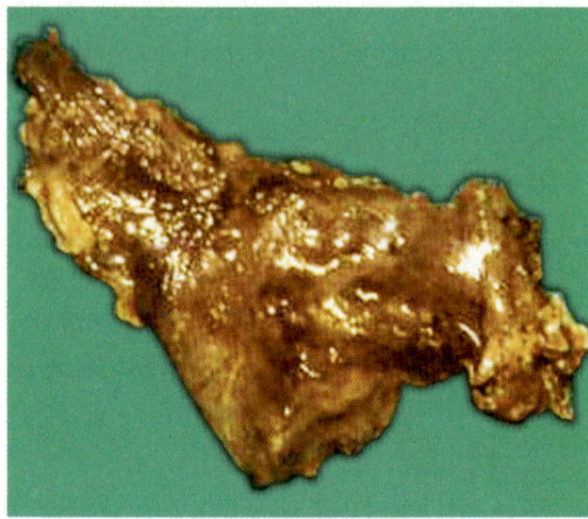

Fig. 54.122: Necrosectomy specimen

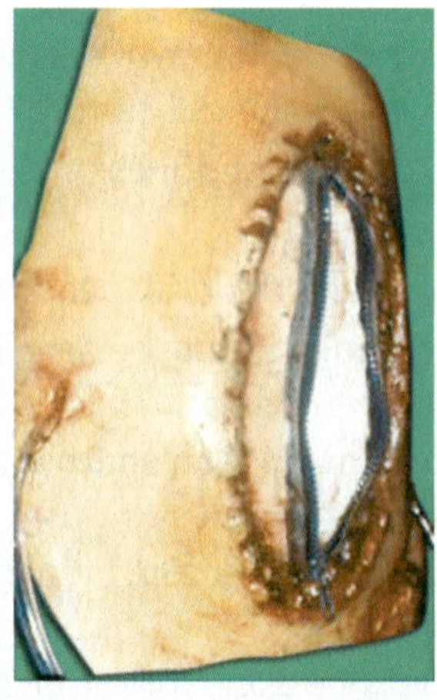

Fig. 54.123: After necrosectomy, it is better to perform zip laparotomy so that it can be opened any number of times for peritoneal toilet (*Courtesy*: Dr BH Ananda Rao, Prof and Head, Department of Surgery, Dr Siddhartha Bhandary and Dr Prashanth Shetty, Associate Professors, KMC, Manipal)

- In cases of early necrosectomy, lesser sac is packed, reoperation done after 48 hours—zipper closure of the abdomen is used.
- Continuous lavage of the lesser sac and retroperitoneum is done.
- Other alternate methods are closed packing.
- Today all these cases are done through minimally invasive methods.
- Endoscopic necrosectomy, retroperitoneoscopic necrosectomy is also done.

## Treatment of Gallstone Pancreatitis

If gallstone is obstructing the ampulla of Vater and causing pancreatitis, endoscopic sphincterotomy may be done within days. It has shown some benefit to the patients. After 2–3 weeks, once the jaundice subsides, cholecystectomy is recommended (Key Box 54.30).

Key Box 54.30

**Acute Pancreatitis**

- Lipase is a more reliable test because it is more pancreas-specific and remains elevated for long after onset of symptom
- However, amylase is widely used

It is not necessary to demonstrate CBD stone to prove the diagnosis of gallstone pancreatitis. Often stone has passed into duodenum

## Complications of Acute Pancreatitis (Table 54.12)

### *Systemic Complications*

1. **Shock**
   - Hypovolaemia and hypoperfusion are the major factors responsible for renal failure. Due to collection of large amount of fluid in the **third space**—peritoneal cavity, pleural cavity and extravascular space, shock occurs. Fluid replacement with blood or albumin should be done at appropriate time to treat the shock.
   - Electrolyte abnormalities should be corrected.
2. **Respiratory insufficiency:** Factors responsible for this are given in Key Box 54.31.

   Measurement of arterial blood gas values and administration of oxygen is enough in the initial stages. In late stages, pulmonary insufficiency needs to be treated with ventilatory support.
3. **Hypocalcaemia** needs to be treated with calcium IV. It is due to hypoalbuminaemia and due to calcium soap.
4. **Pleural effusion** is treated by pleural tap (ultrasound-guided), if it is symptomatic.
5. **ARDS, MODS:** Some mediators, such as phosphatase, damage alveolar membrane of lungs causing 'ARDS'. It manifests as respiratory failure.

**TABLE 54.12:** Complications of acute pancreatitis

| Local | General/systemic |
|---|---|
| ***Acute*** | ***Systemic*** |
| • Pancreatic necrosis (sterile)<br>• Pancreatic necrosis (infected)<br>• Pancreatic abscess<br>• Pancreatic ascites | • Pulmonary—ARDS<br>• Cardiac—shock, arrhythmias<br>• Renal—renal failure<br>• Gastro—ileus, intestinal colonic necrosis |
| ***Chronic*** | ***General*** |
| • Pancreatic pseudocyst<br>• Peritoneal fluid collection<br>• Pleural effusion<br>• Pseudoaneurysm<br>• Partial/splenic vein thrombosis | • Metabolic—hypercalcaemia, hypoglycaemia, hyperlipidaemia<br>• Haematological |

Key Box 54.31

**Respiratory Failure**

- Abdominal distension and elevation of diaphragm
- Intravascular coagulation in the lung
- Lecithin present in the pulmonary surfactant is altered due to lecithinase resulting in defective capillary alveolar exchange
- Defective ventilation caused due to pain
- Left-sided pleural effusion not responding to treatment

### *Local Complications*

1. **Pancreatic abscess** (Fig. 54.124)
   - It develops after 3–4 weeks of pancreatitis. Secondary infection in a pseudocyst results in pancreatic abscess. It usually points out on the left flank.
   - It has to be drained by CT-guided aspiration.
   - Laparoscopy may be necessary not only for the diagnosis but also as a therapeutic means for removal of necrotic pancreas.
   - Otherwise, open drainage of the abscess is required.
2. **Pseudocyst of pancreas** ***(vide infra)***
   - This complication is encountered after 2nd week following an attack of acute pancreatitis.
   - It is seen in about 20% of the patients.
3. **Perforation** of colon or stomach
4. **Pseudoaneurysm** resulting in massive upper gastrointestinal or lower gastrointestinal bleeding. Bleeding into the pancreatic duct is called **haemosuccus pancreaticus**.
   - This condition occurs due to enzymatic digestion of the blood vessels in the vicinity of pancreas. Thus splenic artery, gastroduodenal artery, etc. are commonly involved.
   - It has very high mortality. Prompt angiography followed by embolisation is the treatment.
   - Otherwise, laparotomy, ligation of pseudoaneurysm with or without intracystic ligation of the bleeders is the treatment (Figs 54.125 and 54.126).

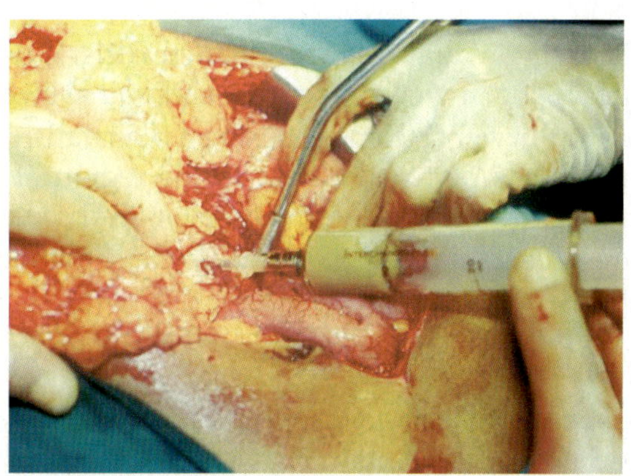

**Fig. 54.124:** Aspiration of pus from pancreatic abscess

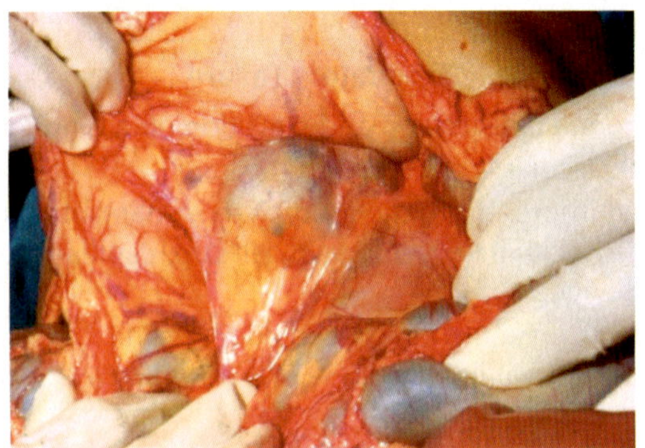

Fig. 54.125: Gastroduodenal pseudoaneurysm at surgery

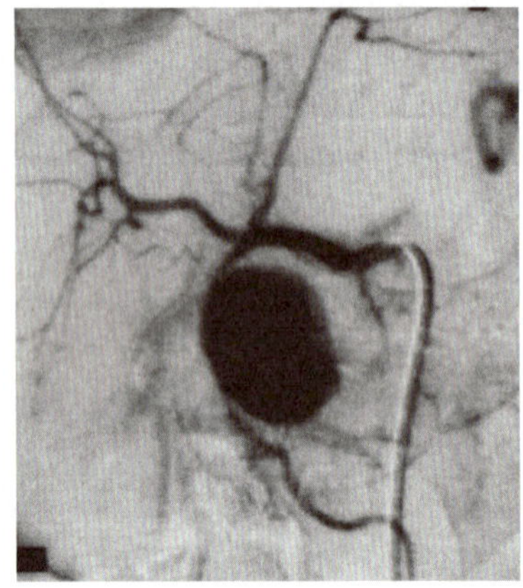

Fig. 54.126: Diagnosis by angiography

## PSEUDOCYST OF PANCREAS

### Definition

Collection of amylase-rich fluid in the lesser sac, due to pancreatic pathology. Fluid collection in the first 4 weeks is an acute fluid collection. After 4 weeks, it becomes an acute pseudocyst.

*Pearls of Wisdom*

It is called pseudocyst because it has no epithelial lining.

Fluid is enclosed by a wall of fibrous granulation tissue and is called a pseudocyst.

### Aetiology

1. Following an attack of **acute pancreatitis**, it usually appears after 4 weeks, as upper abdominal swelling.
2. **Blunt injury** of abdomen causing a ductal disruption wherein the pancreatic duct in the region of body is crushed against vertebral body results in a pseudocyst.
3. Some cause of **chronic pancreatitis** may be associated with pseudocyst.

### Locations of Pseudocyst

1. Between stomach and transverse colon
2. Between stomach and liver
3. Behind or below the transverse colon.

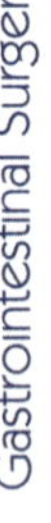


### D'egidio Classification of Pseudocyst

**Type I.** Acute postnecrotic pseudocyst that occurs after **an episode of acute pancreatitis** and is associated with **normal duct anatomy** and rarely communicate with pancreatic duct.

**Type II.** Post-necrotic pseudocyst that occurs after an **episode of acute on chronic** pancreatitis and have a diseased but **not strictured** pancreatic duct and **there is communication between the duct and pseudocyst.**

**Type III** (also called retention cyst) **occurs in chronic pancreatitis,** uniformly associated with a duct stricture and a communication between duct and pseudocyst.

### Clinical Features

1. Tensely cystic mass in the epigastrium, umbilical region or in left hypochondrium. Tensely cystic mass feels firm on palpation. Classically upper border of the mass is not felt.
2. Does not move with respiration because it is retroperitoneal in location.
3. It may have transverse mobility.
4. It does not fall forwards.
5. Percussion: It gives a **resonant note** because of stomach or intestine anterior to it.
6. **Transmitted pulsations** from aorta can be felt.
7. If a Ryle's tube is passed, it can be felt over the swelling. It is called **Baid sign**.
8. Depending upon the tension within the cyst, it can be tender or nontender.

### Investigations

1. **USG/CT:** It can detect size, location of cyst and wall thickness. Confirm that there is no neoplasm of the pancreas before doing cystogastrostomy (Fig. 54.127).

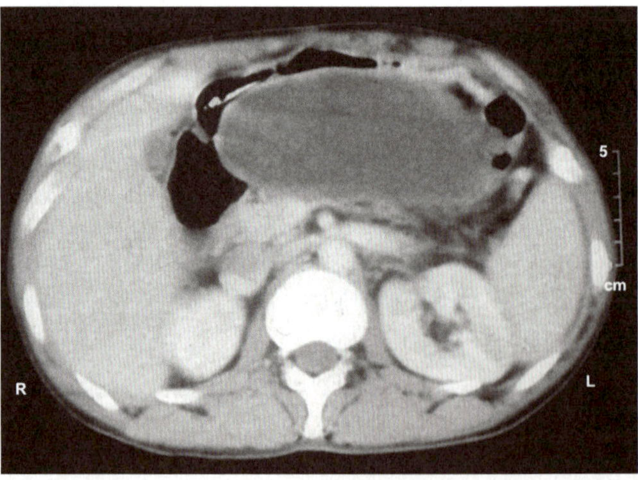


Fig. 54.127: CT scan: Classical pseudocyst pushing the stomach anteriorly—cystogastrostomy is ideal treatment

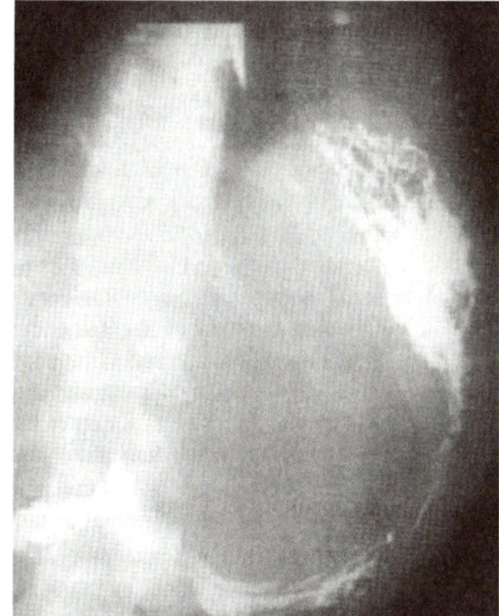

Fig. 54.128: Large pseudocyst behind the stomach demonstrated by barium meal

2. **Barium meal stomach:** In a lateral picture, the stomach is pushed anteriorly and increased vertebrogastric interval is seen (not done nowadays, Fig. 54.128).
3. **ERCP** may demonstrate communication of the cyst with the duct (routinely not done).

## Treatment (Fig. 54.129)

### *I. Conservative Line of Treatment*

- Majority of the pseudocysts following acute pancreatitis resolve spontaneously within 3–4 weeks.
- Hence, regular ultrasound examination is done to observe the pseudocyst.

### *II. Surgery*

Increase in size of cyst, severe pain, no response to conservative line of treatment are indications for surgery.

1. **Cystogastrostomy** (Figs 54.130 to 54.132)
   - ***Indications:*** Pseudocyst in relation to head and body of pancreas.
   - ***Timing:*** Surgery is done **after 6 weeks** because that is the time required for the wall to become fibrous.
   - ***Size*** of the cyst should be at least **6 cm**.
   - ***Procedure:*** Anterior gastrostomy is done and an incision in the posterior wall of stomach opens into the cyst cavity. The contents are drained, opening is enlarged and cut end of stomach in posterior wall is sutured to cut edge of cyst wall. After one week, the cyst collapses. For reasons not known, the food does not enter the cyst cavity. **Size of cystogastrostomy stoma is about 6 cm. This procedure can also be done by endoscopic method.**
2. **Distal pancreatectomy:** Cyst confined to the tail of the pancreas is treated with removal of the tail and the cyst.
3. **Cystojejunostomy:** By using Roux-en-Y loop can be done, **for large cysts** by suturing jejunal loop to the cyst in the most dependent area (Figs 54.133 to 54.135).

Pseudocyst
- Asymptomatic → Observe
- Symptomatic → ERP (MRP)
  - Communication → Endoscopic transpapillary stent → Surgical internal drainage ± resection
  - Stricture → Endoscopic internal drainage → Surgical internal drainage ± resection
  - Normal duct → Radiologic external percutaneous drainage
- Infected → Percutaneous drainage

Fig. 54.129: Management of pseudocyst

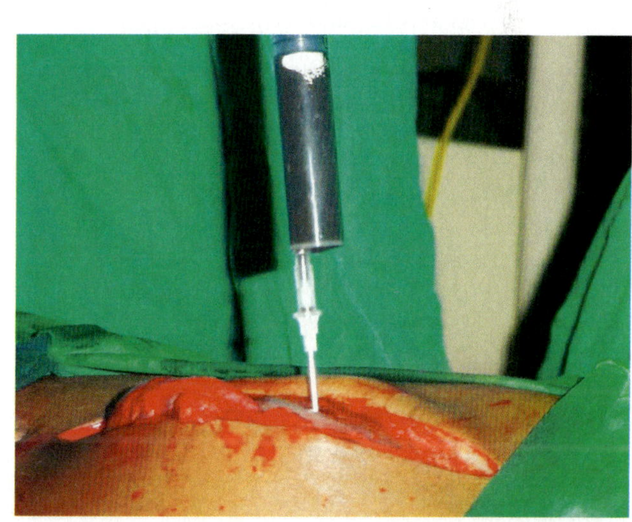

Fig. 54.130: Aspirated fluid is dark in colour, rich in enzymes—'engine oil' appearance

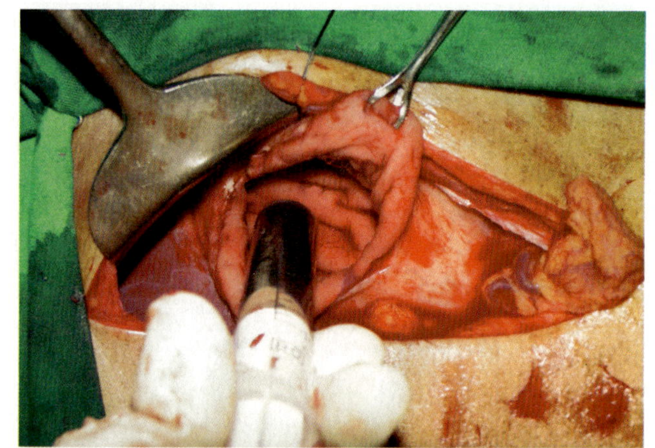

Fig. 54.131: Cystogastrostomy—anterior stomach wall is opened. Fluid is aspirated through the posterior stomach wall

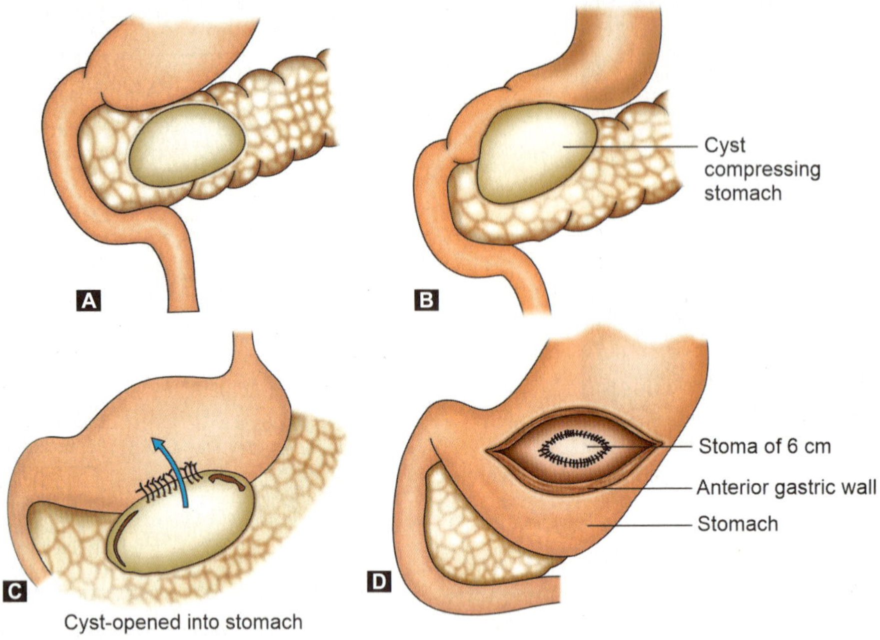


**Figs 54.132A to D:** Steps of cystogastrostomy. (*Courtesy*: Miss Vidushi, MBBS student, KMC, Manipal)

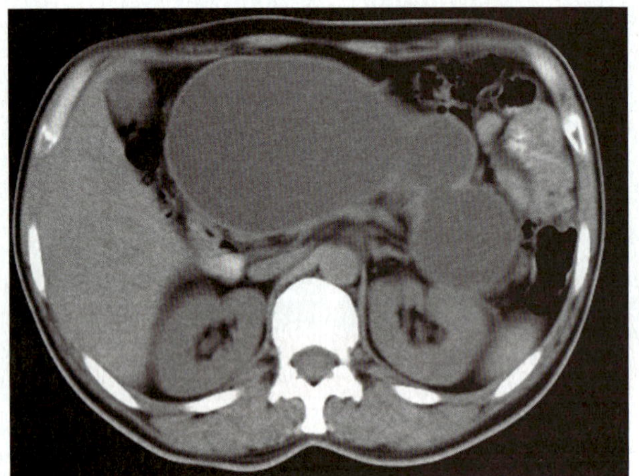

**Fig. 54.133:** CT scan showing large pseudocyst with multiple pockets. Cystojejunostomy is the ideal treatment

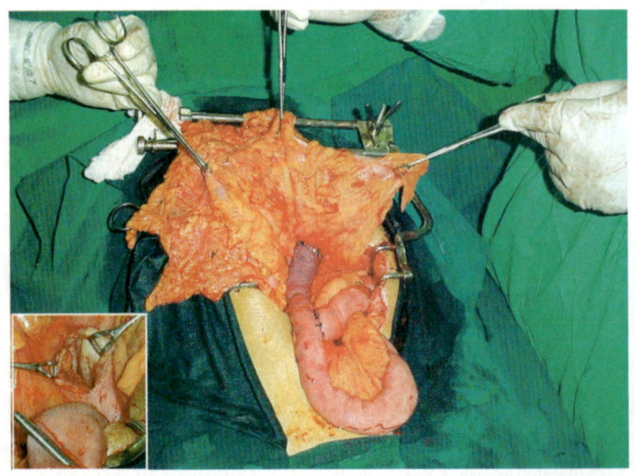

**Fig. 54.134:** Roux-en-Y cystojejunostomy at surgery, inset shows the opened cyst wall which is thick

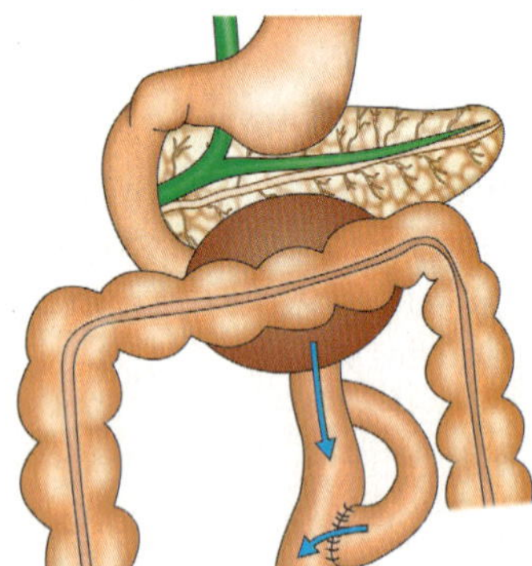

**Fig. 54.135:** Cystojejunostomy—diagrammatic representation

### III. Endoscopic Drainage

This is easy, less invasive and ideal in draining acute pseudocysts. This procedure can also be repeated. However, chances of introducing infection are present. Endoscopic method of draining the pseudocysts is also being done for chronic cysts (Fig. 54.136). Few important

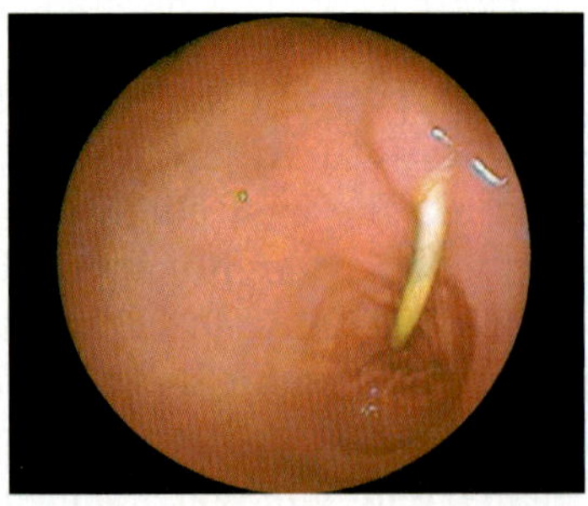

**Fig. 54.136:** Endoscopic cystogastrostomy—ideal to drain acute pseudocysts. After draining a nasobiliary catheter can be left in the cyst cavity. (*Courtesy*: Dr Filipe Alvares, Medical Gastroenterologist, KMC, Manipal)

points here are there should not be more than 3 mm gap between cyst and posterior gastric wall and at the site of incision in the posterior wall there should not be any varices.

## CONGENITAL ANOMALIES OF THE PANCREAS

### EMBRYOLOGICAL ANATOMY

- Pancreas is formed by fusion of ventral and dorsal buds. This will occur by 6 weeks. Malrotation of ventral bud causes annular pancreas.
- Ventral bud forms head and uncinate process.
- Ductal anomalies are given on page 822.

### ANNULAR PANCREAS

It is a rare anomaly which occurs due to persistence of a portion of the ventral pancreatic anlage which fails to rotate. As a result of this, second part of the duodenum is surrounded by a thin rim of pancreatic tissue. Hence the name, annular pancreas (Key Box 54.32).

Key Box 54.32

**Annular Pancreas**

- Persistent ventral 'anlage'
- Neonatal or adult age
- Barium meal—obstruction to second part of duodenum
- Plain X-ray—'double bubble'
- Duodenoduodenostomy is the treatment
- Never divide the annulus

#### Associated Anomalies

Intrinsic duodenal atresia or stenosis.

#### Clinical Features

- **Neonatal type:** It manifests early in life. It produces symptoms of acute intestinal obstruction with vomiting and inability to take food.
- **Adult type:** It manifests after the age of 20. Vomiting is bile-stained. Due to stasis in the pyloric antrum, features of duodenal ulcer may be present.

#### Investigations

- **Plain X-ray abdomen:** Double bubble appearance occurs due to dilated stomach and dilated proximal duodenum.
- **Barium meal:** X-ray can demonstrate obstruction to second part of duodenum.

#### Treatment

**Duodenoduodenostomy** is the treatment of choice. Otherwise, duodenojejunostomy can be done (Fig. 54.137).

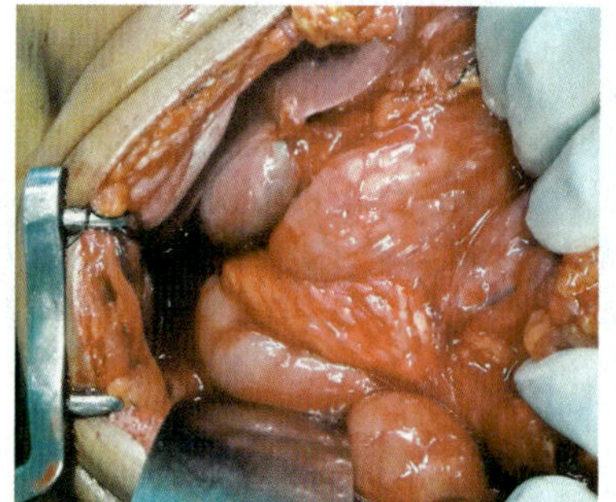

**Fig. 54.137:** Annular pancreas at surgery

*Pearls of Wisdom*

It is tempting to divide the thin pancreatic rim. This should not be done as it will result in a pancreatic fistula.

#### Differential Diagnosis

- Pyloric stenosis
- Wilkie's disease (chronic duodenal ileus).

### ECTOPIC PANCREAS

- This condition is not uncommon.
- Occasionally, at laparotomy for unrelated conditions, a soft to firm irregular tissue or nodule is found on the intestinal surface.
- Biopsy of this may come later as ectopic pancreas. Most of them are asymptomatic.
- It may be found in the submucosa of the stomach, duodenum, small intestines, Meckel's diverticulum or in the hilum of the spleen.

#### Complications

1. *In the stomach*: It may undergo cystic degeneration.
2. *In the intestine*: It can cause intussusception. Sometimes, it may be the source of gastrointestinal bleeding.
3. *In the Meckel's diverticulum*: Any of the complications mentioned above.

### CONGENITAL CYSTIC FIBROSIS

- It is inherited as an autosomal recessive disorder.
- It is a generalised dysfunction of exocrine glands resulting in defective mucus secretion.
- Malabsorption due to pancreatic insufficiency is a feature.
- Pulmonary disease due to bronchiolitis occurs later (Key Box 54.33).

Key Box 54.33

**Viscid Mucus—Conditions**

- Meconium ileus
- Cystic fibrosis of pancreas
- Respiratory tract infection
- Increased $Na^+$ loss in the sweat

### Pathology

The viscid mucin which is produced results in obstruction of the ducts and ductules. Stasis of pancreatic secretions, alveolar rupture due to increased pressure take place later. As a result of alveolar rupture, pancreatic enzymes leak outside resulting in pancreatitis.

### Clinical Features

1. **At birth:** Meconium ileus or meconium peritonitis is an important manifestation of cystic fibrosis of pancreas.
2. **In infants:**
   - Recurrent respiratory tract infection in the form of bronchiolitis and bronchiectasis results in cough with expectoration and dyspnoea.
   - Emaciation, steatorrhoea. Stools are pale and sticky.
3. **Older children:** Steatorrhoea, gross emaciation and wasting are the features. Due to poor nutritional status, cirrhosis of the liver with portal hypertension can be a feature.
4. **In adult:** Lucky survivors will suffer from gross wasting, diabetes, bronchiectasis, cirrhosis of the liver, sialoadenitis and choroiditis.

### Investigations

- Normal contents of the electrolytes in the sweat: $Na^+$—70 mmol/L, $Cl^-$—60 mmol/L, $K^+$— 20 mmol/L.
- In these patients, sodium excretion may be three to four times more than normal.

### Treatment (Only Symptomatic)

I. **Nutritional support**
   - Fat intake should be low, protein should be increased.
   - Pancreatic enzyme preparations (5 to 10 g) are given two to three times per day, to supplement pancreatic enzymes.

II. **Control infection:** Respiratory tract infection is treated with antibiotics, bronchodilators, mucolytic agents, etc.

III. **Role of surgery:** Indicated in meconium ileus to relieve intestinal obstruction.

## PANCREATIC DIVISUM AND DUCTAL ANOMALIES

- Pancreatic divisum is the most common congenital abnormality of the pancreas. It is found in 5–10% of patients.
- It is caused by failure of fusion of the dorsal and ventral portions of the developing pancreas. In the majority of patients, this anomaly is of no clinical importance.
- In a certain subset of patients, however, estimated to be approximately 5–20%, pancreatic divisum is a clinically important cause of abdominal pain, acute recurrent pancreatitis or chronic pancreatitis.
- **The frequency of pancreatic divisum in patients with pancreatitis in recent studies is approximately 10%** (Key Box 54.34).

Key Box 54.34

**Pancreatic Divisum**

- It is one of the uncommon causes of acute pancreatitis.
- In 10% of patients. Majority of pancreas drains through duct of Santorini through lesser papilla.
- Outflow obstruction—treated by sphincteroplasty of minor papilla.

### Pathophysiological Consequences

The cause of pancreatitis in this common anomaly is hypothesised to be caused by minor papillary insufficiency caused by papillary fibrosis and subsequent stenosis.

### Diagnosis

- The diagnosis is established by ERCP.
- MRCP is a noninvasive and accurate method of establishing the diagnosis. However, a negative MRCP does not exclude the diagnosis of divisum as the concordance with ERCP ranges from 50% to more than 70%.
- The accuracy of the MRCP may be improved by administration of secretin.

### Treatment

- In patients with minimal symptoms, treatment with pancreatic enzymes may reduce pancreatic secretion and hence, pain. Pain management referral may be necessary.
- Patients with acute pancreatitis are estimated to benefit from either surgical minor sphincteroplasty or endoscopic minor papillotomy.

A few anomalies of pancreatic duct are given below (Figs 54.138A to E).

A. Normal anatomy

B. Terminal end of accessory duct fibrosed

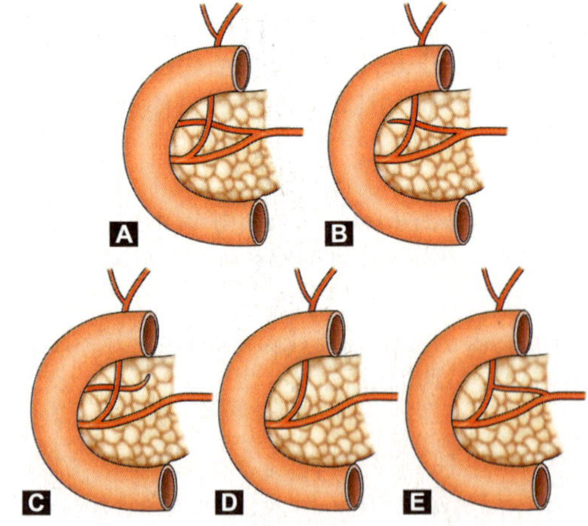


**Figs 54.138A to E:** Anomalies of pancreatic duct

C. Blind ending of accessory duct
D. Absent accessory duct
E. Blind end of accessory duct with main duct communication.

## MISCELLANEOUS

### PANCREATIC FISTULA

Most common after **pancreatic trauma** (Fig. 54.139).

#### Causes

1. **External fistulae** occur due to operative injury to the pancreas or due to a pancreatic anastomotic leak.
   - Injury to the tail of pancreas during splenectomy or adrenalectomy.
   - Injury to the head and body during radical gastrectomy.
   - Pancreaticojejunostomy for chronic pancreatitis or following Whipple's operation can also give rise to fistula in the postoperative period.
   - External drainage of an infected pseudocyst.
2. **Internal fistulae:** It can occur following a blunt injury abdomen wherein the neck of the pancreas is crushed against lumbar spine resulting in injury. Internal fistulae can communicate with pleural space resulting in a pancreaticopleural fistula.

#### Clinical Presentation

- In many cases, the patients present with a discharge of straw-coloured fluid from the drain site in the postoperative period.
- Internal fistula can manifest in a totally unexpected manner, sometimes, as a case of pleural effusion.

#### Investigations

- **Amylase** levels in the pleural fluid, peritoneal fluid and in the discharge will be high.
- Abdominal ultrasound is done to rule out a pseudocyst of the pancreas.

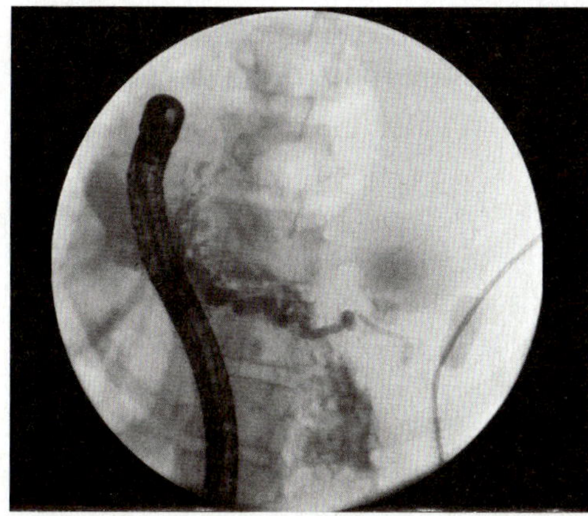

**Fig. 54.139:** Pancreatic fistula following acute pancreatitis

- **ERCP:** It can demonstrate leakage of the dye from the pancreatic duct into the surrounding area or along the fistulous tract and proximal obstruction, if any.
- **CT fistulogram** can define the exact site of communication to pancreas. It can define the length of the fistula also.
- **CT angiogram** is indicated in cases of bleeding associated with pancreatic fistula.

#### Treatment

1. **Conservative treatment:**
   - In majority of the cases following surgery, the fistulous discharge stops within one to three weeks of time. During this period, the skin is protected by application of zinc oxide cream. Electrolytes have to be checked frequently.
   - Injection octreotide in the dose of 50–100 mg, 8th hourly will help in decreasing fistula output by more than 80–90%.
2. **Stenting:** Endoscopy, ERCP followed by stenting can be tried. If successful, the fistula will often heal. It is very useful in blunt abdominal trauma and pancreatic ductal disruption.
3. **Surgical treatment:**
   - If the **fistula persists** in spite of conservative treatment, **fistulectomy** with removal of involved part of the pancreas and body or tail has to be done.
   - In very difficult cases (plastered abdomen) or in fistulas on the anterior abdominal side, **fistulo-gastrostomy** can also be done.
   - Pancreaticojejunostomy is another option.

#### Complications of Pancreatic Fistula

1. Secondary **infection**
2. **Massive bleeding:** It occurs due to digestion of elastin fibres of blood vessels resulting in pseudoaneurysms. Morbidity is high.
3. **Ramification** which means branching pattern of the fistula renders the surgery difficult.
4. **Bronchopancreatic fistula**—difficult to treat.

**Clinical Notes**

A patient was admitted to the hospital with acute breathlessness. He was found to have left-sided pleural effusion (massive). He had blunt injury abdomen 2 months back during which time laparotomy and closure of a proximal jejunal perforation had been done. There was no obvious sign of pancreatic injury. Aspiration of pleural fluid revealed high amylase. It was a case of pancreaticopleural fistula.

## WHITE BILE

- It is a misnomer (Fig. 54.140)
- In long-standing cases of obstruction to the CBD, the bile in the CBD gets absorbed and is replaced by mucus secreted from the CBD.
- It is not white but straw coloured.
- It is not bile but is mucus.

### Significance

- It indicates a long-standing obstruction.
- It has to be relieved as an urgent procedure.
- White bile is seen in:
  - Long-standing stricture of the CBD
  - Due to the stones in CBD
  - Rarely, seen in periampullary carcinoma.

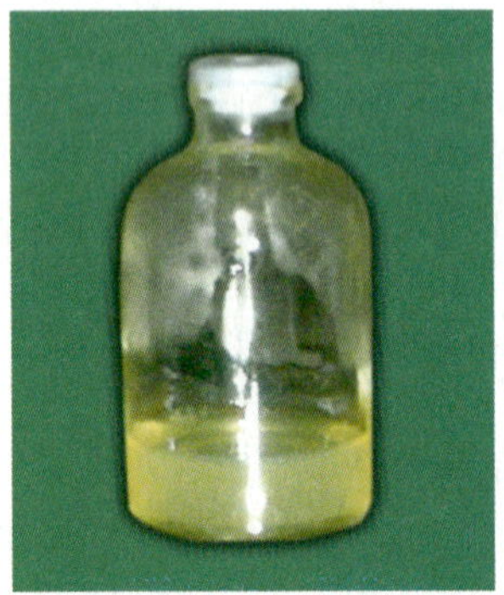

**Fig. 54.140:** White bile suggestive of severely impaired liver cell function

## PANCREATIC ASCITES

### Definition

- Accumulation of 'enzyme rich' pancreatic exudate in the peritoneal cavity is called pancreatic ascites.
- It is a protein-rich, noninfected fluid with protein levels greater than 25 g/L.

### Causes

- Acute pancreatitis mainly alcoholic
- Chronic pancreatitis
- Trauma to pancreas
- Ruptured pseudocyst

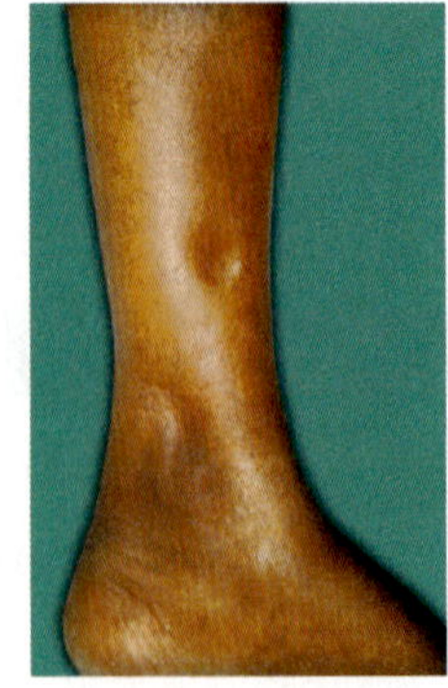

**Fig. 54.141:** Pedal oedema—severe hypoalbuminaemia

### Pathogenesis

- Disruption of ductal system of pancreas followed by spread of enzyme-rich fluid both anteriorly and posteriorly results in pancreatic ascites.
- Anterior rupture results in ascites.
- Posterior spread results in pleural effusion.

### Clinical Features

- History suggestive of pancreatitis, gross abdominal distention.
- Shifting dullness
- Breathlessness—due to pleural effusion.

### Investigations

- Serum amylase, may be elevated due to reabsorption across peritoneal membrane.
- Ultrasound/CT: It can detect fluid, pancreatic duct and guide aspiration.
- ERCP: May slow ductal communication.

### Treatment

- Repeated **tapping—**follow with **albumin infusion.** Most of the cases are associated with hypoalbuminaemia (Fig. 54.141).
- Octreotide to decrease pancreatic secretion.
- Total parenteral nutrition
- ERCP—pancreatic duct stenting
- Surgical: If there is no response by 2–3 weeks, resection (for tail lesion) or drainage for body lesion is indicated.

## MULTIPLE CHOICE QUESTIONS

1. **Which of the following statements is false for pseudocyst of pancreas?**
   A. It occurs in lesser sac
   B. Cystogastrostomy is usually the treatment of choice
   C. Better to operate after 2 weeks
   D. It has no epithelial lining
2. **Which of the following is not the cause for gallstone formation?**
   A. Saint's triad B. Haemolytic anaemia
   C. Infection D. Gastrojejunostomy
3. **Gallbladder carcinoma has following features, *except*:**
   A. It is squamous cell carcinoma
   B. It does cause jaundice often
   C. It does not respond to radiation
   D. Prognosis is very poor
4. **Most ideal and quick method for the diagnosis of gallstones is by:**
   A. Endosonogram B. MRI scan
   C. CT scan D. Ultrasound
5. **Following is not the feature of acute cholecystitis:**
   A. It causes pain in the right hypochondrium
   B. If it perforates, gas under diaphragm is detected by percussion
   C. Shoulder pain can occur
   D. Acalculous cholecystitis is due to hypotension
6. **Following is the most important sign of acute cholecystitis:**
   A. Pain in the right shoulder
   B. Intercostal oedema and tenderness
   C. Positive Murphy's sign
   D. Hyperaesthesia of the abdominal wall
7. **Cystic duct joins supraduodenal CBD in what percentage of the cases?**
   A. 80% B. 90%
   C. 70% D. 95%
8. **Porcelain gallbladder has following features, *except*:**
   A. It is calcification of the gallbladder
   B. Plain X-ray is not very useful to detect this
   C. CT scan will detect this
   D. It may be associated with carcinoma gallbladder
9. **Which one of the following is true for choledochal cyst?**
   A. Acquired dilatation
   B. Not premalignant
   C. Type I cyst is the most common variety
   D. Does not cause pancreatitis
10. **Which one of the features is true in gallstone ileus?**
    A. Obstruction is in terminal ileum
    B. Stone reaches ileum via ampulla of Vater
    C. Obstruction and features of perforation of gallbladder are found
    D. Cholecystectomy and extraction of the stones by enterotomy is done
11. **Following are true for acalculous cholecystitis, *except*:**
    A. It can be seen in septic shock due to hypotension
    B. Some features of cholecystoses may also be found
    C. *Salmonella typhi* can also give rise to acute acalculous cholecystitis
    D. Rare to get chronic cholecystitis in Salmonella cholecystitis
12. **Following are indications for common bile duct exploration, *except*:**
    A. Palpable stones in the CBD
    B. Dilated common bile duct
    C. Jaundice
    D. Thickened common bile duct
13. **Following are risk factors for cholangiocarcinoma, *except*:**
    A. Choledochal cyst
    B. Caroli's disease
    C. Primary sclerosing cholangitis
    D. Biliary stricture
14. **Which one of the following is true for carcinoma gallbladder?**
    A. It is common in males
    B. Disease occurs around 5th decade
    C. Gallstone disease does not predispose to carcinoma gallbladder
    D. Majority are adenocarcinoma
15. **Caterpillar hump is an anomaly of what structure?**
    A. Cystic artery B. Hepatic artery
    C. Coeliac artery D. Gastroduodenal artery
16. **Portal veins is formed at:**
    A. Posterior to head of pancreas
    B. Posterior to body of pancreas
    C. Anterior to neck of pancreas
    D. Posterior to neck of pancreas
17. **Following are true about anatomy of the pancreas, *except*:**
    A. 30% is by the head of pancreas
    B. 75% of islet cells are beta-cells producing insulin
    C. 80–90% pancreatic tissue is exocrine pancreatic tissue
    D. 5% of islet cells are A cells producing glucagon

**18. To avoid spillage of cells after FNAC of the pancreatic head mass which is the best investigation?**
A. Endoscopic biopsy
B. CT-guided biopsy
C. MRI-guided biopsy
D. Endosonographic biopsy

**19. Which one of the following is true for pancreatic divisum?**
A. Dorsal pancreatic duct become accessory duct
B. It does not cause pancreatitis
C. MRCP is not an ideal investigation for diagnosis
D. Endoscopic sphincterotomy has a definitive role

**20. Following are true for annular pancreas, *except*:**
A. It is more prevalent in children with Down syndrome
B. It surrounds 2nd part of duodenum
C. Duodenal obstruction causes vomiting in neonate
D. Gastrojejunostomy is the treatment of choice

**21. The use of ultrasound in the diagnosis of acute pancreatitis is mainly to:**
A. Rule out perforation
B. To look for oedematous pancreatitis
C. To rule out gallstones
D. To look for pancreatic stones

**22. Role of CT scan in acute pancreatitis include following, *except*:**
A. To detect gallstones
B. Diagnostic uncertainty
C. To detect necrotizing pancreatitis
D. To find out the localized complication

**23. Following are features of acute pancreatitis, *except*:**
A. Shock
B. Cullen's sign
C. Grey Turner's sign
D. Kehr sign

**24. Which one of the following is not routinely recommended in severe pancreatitis?**
A. Aggressive fluid resuscitation
B. Nasogastric feeding
C. ICU monitoring with oxygenation
D. Antibiotic prophylaxis

**25. Which one of the following is true for pancreatic necrosectomy?**
A. Usually done within 2–3 weeks of acute attack of pancreatitis
B. Gallstones, if present, should not be removed along with necrosectomy
C. Blunt dissection is the best technique
D. Feeding jejunostomy may not be useful

**26. Sudden rise in platelet counts in acute pancreatitis suggests:**
A. Pancreatic fistula
B. Bleeding
C. Portal vein thrombosis
D. Pancreatic necrosis

**27. Following are true about pseudocyst fluid, *except*:**
A. Ultrasound can easily detect pseudocyst
B. CEA levels are usually above 400 ng/ml
C. High amylase levels
D. Inflammatory cells in the aspirate

**28. Following are true for tropical pancreatitis, *except*:**
A. Starts in young age
B. High incidence of stone formation
C. High incidence of diabetes mellitus
D. Does not predispose to pancreatic cancer

**29. The best surgical treatment for chronic pancreatitis with dilated duct is:**
A. Frey's operation
B. Whipple's operation
C. Longitudinal pancreaticojejunostomy
D. Distal pancreatectomy

**30. Following are the risk factors for carcinoma pancreas, *except*:**
A. Cigarette smoking
B. Hereditary pancreatitis
C. Chronic pancreatitis
D. Female sex

**31. About porcelain gallbladder following is true:**
A. Requires conservative treatment
B. It cannot be detected by ultrasound
C. Prophylactic cholecystectomy is not indicated
D. It is a precancerous condition

**Answers**

| | | | | | | | | | |
|---|---|---|---|---|---|---|---|---|---|
| 1. C | 2. D | 3. A | 4. D | 5. B | 6. D | 7. A | 8. B | 9. C | 10. A |
| 11. D | 12. D | 13. D | 14. D | 15. B | 16. D | 17. D | 18. D | 19. D | 20. D |
| 21. C | 22. A | 23. D | 24. B | 25. C | 26. C | 27. B | 28. D | 29. C | 30. D |
| 31. D | | | | | | | | | |

Chapter

55

# Liver

- Surgical anatomy
- Physiology
- Pyogenic abscess
- Amoebic abscess
- Hydatid cyst
- Other cystic diseases
- Benign tumours
- Hepatoma
- Secondaries in the liver
- Portal hypertension
- Ascites in portal hypertension
- Portal gastropathy
- Portal biliopathy
- Budd-Chiari syndrome
- Role of octreotide in surgery
- Liver transplantation
- Haemobilia

### Introduction

Surgical anatomy of the liver is given here. However segmental anatomy and variations in vascular anatomy is given in page 838. This will help in understanding the concepts of liver resections.

## SURGICAL ANATOMY OF THE LIVER

- Liver is located in the right hypochondrium extending into epigastrium and left hypochondrium.
- It weighs about 1,500 g—three quarters of it is the right lobe and rest is the left lobe (Figs 55.1 and 55.2).

### Ligaments

- **Right triangular ligament** fixes the right lobe to the undersurface of the right dome of diaphragm. When this ligament is divided, right lobe can be mobilised and can be turned to left as during right hepatic lobectomy or to control bleeding from liver trauma.

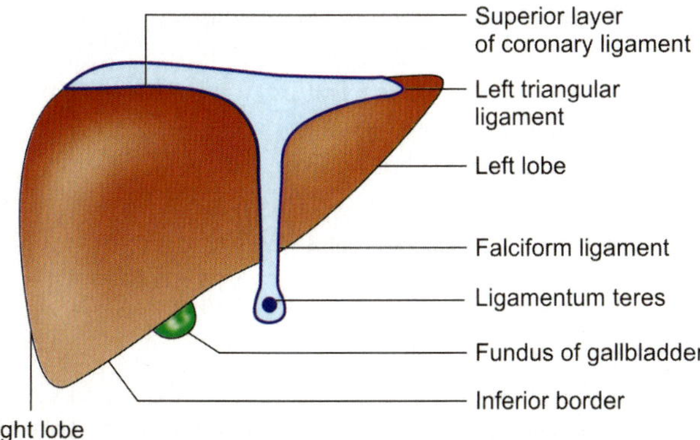


**Fig. 55.1:** Liver seen from the front

- **Left triangular ligament** fixes the left lobe to the diaphragm in a similar fashion. For a complete vagotomy, when this ligament is divided, left lobe can be easily retracted—vagotomy becomes easy. This ligament also needs to be divided to get access to retrohepatic inferior vena cava.
- **Falciform ligament:** It is the remnant of umbilical vein. It runs from umbilicus to the liver dividing the liver into right and left lobes, passing into the interlobar fissure. Division of superior leaves of falciform ligament helps in exposing suprahepatic inferior vena cava (IVC).

### Blood Supply

- 80% is derived from portal vein, 20% from hepatic artery.
- Right branch of hepatic artery supplies entire right lobe and left branch supplies the left lobe.
- Ligation of hepatic artery may not cause necrosis of liver in normal individuals. However, it can cause liver failure in cirrhotic patients (it was done in olden days to control secondaries in the liver), and in obstructive jaundice patients.

### Venous Drainage of the Liver

- Major venous drainage is through 3 hepatic veins: Right, middle and left. They join the inferior vena cava (IVC) immediately below the diaphragm. *Right hepatic vein has a small extrahepatic course.* On the other hand, middle and left hepatic veins usually join within liver parenchyma.
- In fact, these three veins keep the liver suspended.

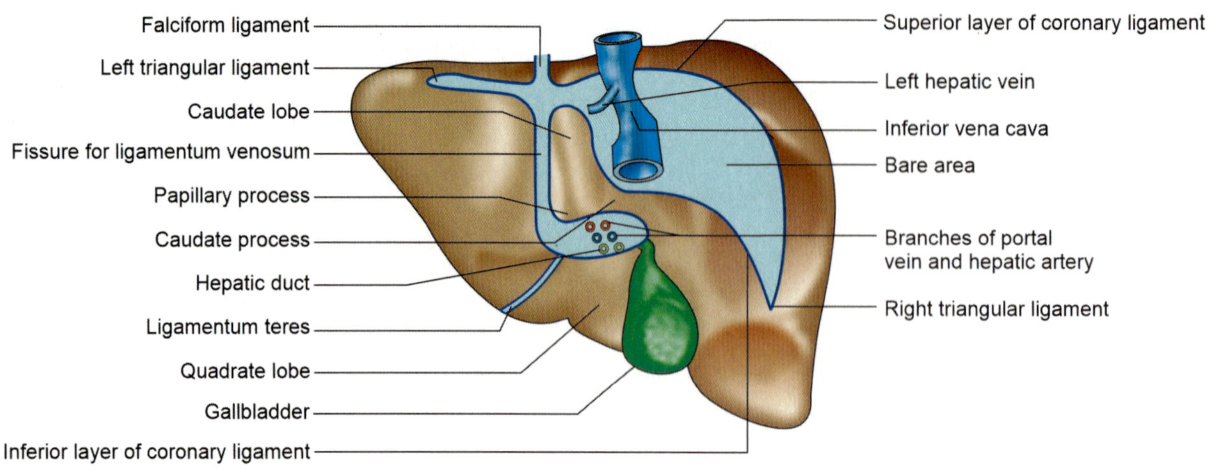


**Fig. 55.2:** Liver seen from behind and below

### Lymphatics

- Superficial lobules: Subcapsular course to diaphragm or to suspensory ligament or posterior mediastinum.
- Deep lobules: Along IVC or portal vein into porta hepatis.

### Hilum of the Liver

- This is also called **porta hepatis**. It has the most vital structures within it—hepatic artery, bile duct anteriorly and portal vein posteriorly.
- These structures are present within the free edge of lesser omentum—hepatoduodenal ligament.
- Within the hilum, these structures divide into right and left branches. Left bile duct has a **longer extrahepatic course** of approximately 2 cm. In CBD strictures, this can be used for **hepaticojejunostomy**.

### Regeneration

- Liver has an excellent **capacity for regeneration** after partial resection.
- A factor released from **pancreas** is supposed to be responsible for this.

### Hepatic Lobules

The ***functional unit*** of the liver is the hepatic lobule. Each hepatic lobule consists of sheets of liver cells, separated by hepatic sinusoids, venous channels which drain blood to central vein, a tributary of the hepatic vein from portal tracts that contain branches of the hepatic vein and portal vein.

## PHYSIOLOGY (Table 55.1)

**SU28.10.2:** Enumerate the types, etiopathogenesis, clinical features, investigations and principles in management of liver abscess. Also difference between the types of liver abscesses.

## PYOGENIC LIVER ABSCESS

### Causes (Fig. 55.3)

**I. Infection through the portal vein**

- Acute appendicitis
- Acute diverticulitis (sigmoid)

**TABLE 55.1:** Physiology of the liver

| Functioning of the liver | Significance |
|---|---|
| • Principal site of synthesis of all proteins **except globulins**, which are produced in reticuloendothelial systems | • Hypoalbuminaemia in chronic liver disease |
| • **Glucose metabolism, glycolysis and gluconeogenesis** | • Persistent hypoglycaemia is a feature of fulminant hepatic failure (FHF), also seen in hepatoma |
| • Synthesis of **clotting factors** | • Bleeding tendencies in chronic liver disease |
| • Maintaining **core body temperature** | • Hypothermia in FHF |
| • Bilirubin formation | • Congenital hyperbilirubinaemia and other |
| • Drug and hormone metabolism | • Hepatitis due to drugs such as rifampicin and other anti-tuberculous drugs |
| • Monitoring pH and correcting **lactic acidosis** | • Severely impaired in FHF |
| • Removal of endotoxins and foreign antigens | • Severely impaired in FHF |
| • Urea formation from protein catabolism | • After portacaval shunt, endotoxins bypass the liver, results in encephalopathy |

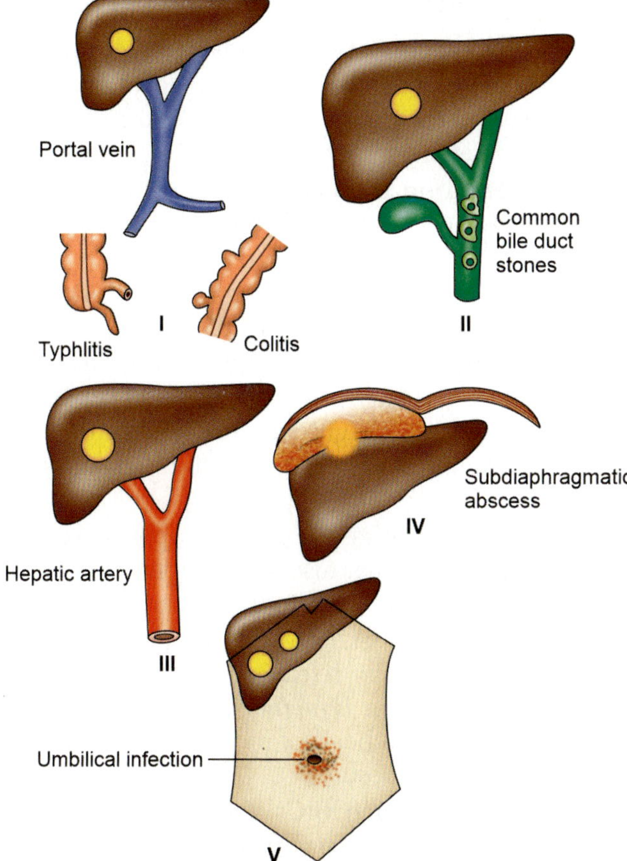


**Fig. 55.3:** Sources of pyogenic liver abscess

- Acute amoebic colitis
- Acute bacillary dysentery
- Ulcerative colitis

**II. Infection through the common bile duct (CBD)**
- Stricture of the CBD
- Periampullary carcinoma resulting in stasis of the bile, precipitating infection (cholangitis)
- Recurrent cholangitis due to stone in the CBD
- ERCP

**III. Infection through the hepatic artery**
- Septicaemia and pyaemia
- Actinomycosis of faciocervical region

**IV. Extension abscess**
- Subdiaphragmatic abscess
- Empyema thoracis
- Penetrating injuries

**V. Infection through umbilicus:** Neonatal umbilical sepsis giving rise to pyaemia.

### Certain Facts

- Majority of the infective bacteria are derived from gastrointestinal tract (Key Box 55.1).
- In majority of cases, it is **polymicrobial** infection.
- ***E. coli*** is the most common facultative organism.
- ***Bacteroides fragilis*** is the most common anaerobe.
- ***Candidal infection*** is increasing due to chemotherapy, especially for leukaemic patients.

Key Box 55.1

**Bacteriology**

| | |
|---|---|
| 1. Anaerobic bacteria | : 60% (Bacteroides fragilis) |
| 2. Enteric gram –ve bacteria | |
| ○ *Escherichia coli* | : 40% |
| ○ *Klebsiella pneumoniae* | : 10–20% |
| ○ Others | : 4–40% |
| 3. Gram +ve bacteria | |
| ○ *Staphylococcus aureus* | : 4–25% |

### Clinical Features

- Alcoholic males and debilitated men suffer more, probably because of poor immunity.
- Acute abscesses are usually multiple, chronic abscesses are single.
- Tender hepatomegaly, low grade or high grade pyrexia with abdominal discomfort are the main features.

### Investigations

- **Total WBC count** is raised.
- **Stool routine examination:** Amoebic cysts, culture and sensitivity for typhoid bacilli.
- **Abdominal ultrasound** and ultrasound-guided aspiration establishes the diagnosis.
- When in doubt, CT scan can be done (Figs 55.4 and 55.5), followed by FNAC which draws frank pus. Pus is sent for Gram's stain, culture and sensitivity. CT also helps in the diagnosis of ***associated conditions such as diverticulitis of the colon.***
- Further investigations are directed towards the associated conditions. **Examples:**
  - **Chest X-ray:** Air under the diaphragm (perforation of hollow viscus) or diagnosis of empyema thoracis.

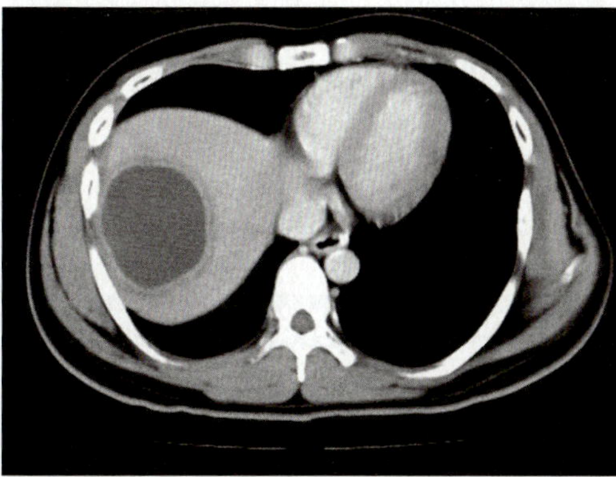

**Fig. 55.4:** CT scan showing hypodense lesion in the right lobe of liver suggestive of pyogenic liver abscess

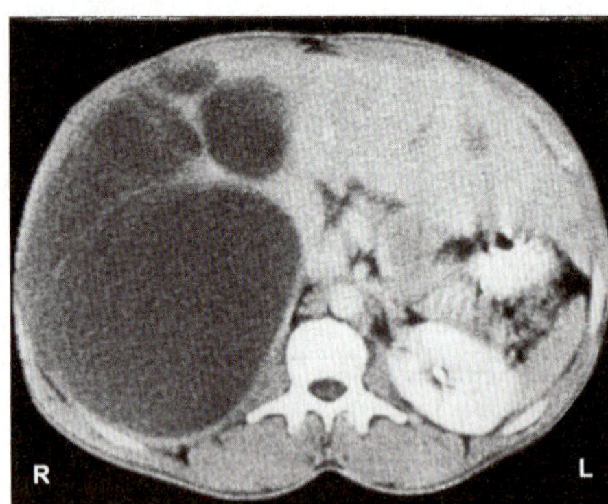


Fig. 55.5: CT scan showing multiple liver abscesses proved to be due to amoebiasis

### Treatment

1. **Conservative:** Multiple small abscesses may respond to antibiotics. However, they have to be given for 4 to 6 weeks.
2. **Percutaneous drainage** (Key Box 55.2):
   **Method**
   - Ultrasound or CT-guided aspiration and drainage by using a pigtail catheter.
   - Irrigation of abscess cavity with saline.
3. **Open (surgical) method** (Key Box 55.3): Laparotomy is required mainly to treat the primary causes, e.g. appendicectomy, drainage of appendicular abscess. If liver shows a significant abscess, it is drained. Alternately, a pigtail catheter is introduced into the abscess cavity and brought outside through a separate opening. It helps to drain for a longer period of time.
4. Laparoscopic drainage can also be done.

Key Box 55.2

**Percutaneous Drainage—Indications**

- Superficial abscesses
- Abscess with no intra-abdominal pathology
- Abscess of unknown aetiology

Key Box 55.3

**Open (Surgical) Method—Indications**

- Abscess with intra-abdominal pathology
- Ascites
- Deep-seated abscess
- Multiple abscesses

## AMOEBIC LIVER ABSCESS

It is also called **tropical abscess** (dysenteric abscess). It is the commonest extraintestinal manifestation of amoebiasis.

### Aetiopathogenesis

- This disease is caused by ***Entamoeba histolytica***.
- It is almost always a complication of amoebic dysentery. This can occur in the acute stage or in the chronic carrier stage.
  - **Infection from the caecum** (typhlitis) spreads through the tributary of **superior mesenteric vein.**
  - **From sigmoid colon**, through the tributary of **inferior mesenteric vein** (Fig. 55.6).
- The right branch of the portal vein is in direct line with the portal vein. Hence, by ***streamline phenomenon*** organisms reach the right lobe more often than the left lobe. The right lobe is also much bigger than the left lobe.
- In the right lobe, it is the posterosuperior surface which gets involved because it is extraperitoneal ***(bare area of liver)***. It has no peritoneal covering.
- After reaching the liver, the organism causes destruction of hepatocytes by releasing powerful ***cytolytic enzymes*** resulting in ***liquefaction necrosis***. It also causes aseptic thrombosis of blood vessels resulting in necrosis of liver tissue.
- At the same time, some RBCs[1] are also broken down. This causes ***anchovy sauce pus***, which is chocolate brown in colour, and is a mixture of broken down RBCs, hepatocytes, etc.
- **Green pus** is referred to pus mixed with bile, which is seen in a few patients.
- In majority of the cases, ***pus is sterile***. Secondary infection occurs in about 20 to 30% of the cases.
- Amoebae are rarely present in the pus but are present in the wall of the abscess cavity. The wall contains monocytes, plasma cells, lymphocytes and fibroblasts. Abscesses are multiple which fuse to form

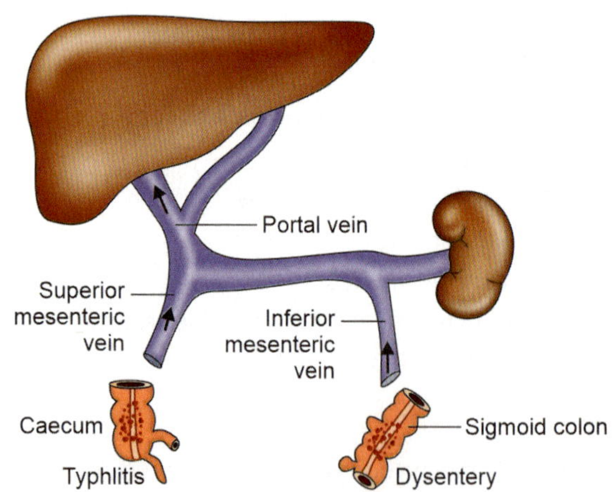


Fig. 55.6: Aetiopathogenesis of amoebic liver abscess

[1]Absence of WBC is an important feature. Hence, regeneration of abscess cavity is complete without scarring.

a single large abscess cavity in about 70% of the cases. Due to ***perihepatitis***, abscess gets fixed to the diaphragm resulting in immobility of the diaphragm. Liver abscess in the left lobe gets adhered to anterior abdominal wall.

- It is interesting to note that amoebic infection of gall-bladder and bile do not occur because of ***deleterious effect of bile on amoebae***.

### Clinical Features (Fig. 55.8A)

- **Male alcoholics** are commonly affected, in the age group of 20–40 years. It is eight times more common in men.
- Seen in patients with low socioeconomic status.
- Severe pain in the right hypochondrium is due to the enlarged liver. This stage is called stage of **amoebic hepatitis**. If USG is done, it may not demonstrate any abscesses but there may be many microabscesses. At this stage, there is low grade fever, weakness, anorexia, etc.
- High grade fever with chills and rigors develop if the stage proceeds to pyogenic liver abscess due to secondary bacterial infection of amoebic abscess.
- Thoracic symptoms such as nonproductive cough, pleurisy and right shoulder pain are common.

### Signs

- Anaemia, emaciation, toxic look and an earthy complexion are present.
- Jaundice may be present, if abscesses are multiple, due to compression of biliary radicles. However, it is rare (15%). It is of cholestatic variety.
- Liver is enlarged in the right hypochondrium, tender and soft (liver enlarges in upward direction) (Key Box 55.4).
- **Intercostal tenderness** differentiates it from acute cholecystitis. Intercostal oedema can also be present (Figs 55.7 and 55.8A).

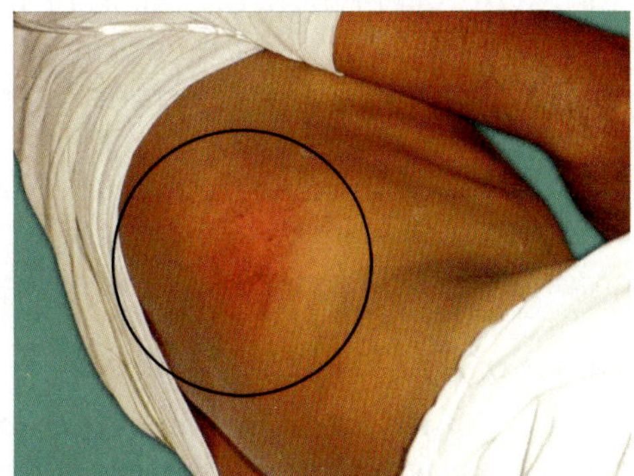

**Fig. 55.7:** Intercostal bulge and tenderness are important features of amoebic liver abscess of the liver—these signs are not seen in acute cholecystitis

> Key Box 55.4
>
> **Very Tender Liver**
>
> - Amoebic liver abscess
> - Hepatoma
> - Congestive cardiac failure

### Investigations

1. **Total WBC count** may be increased, if there is secondary infection.
2. **Stool examination** for ova and cysts of *Entamoeba histolytica* may be positive in 25% of cases.
3. **Serologic testing:** The indirect haemagglutination test is positive in 90–95% of patients with an amoebic abscess.
4. **Screening chest:** When the patient is asked to take a deep breath, right side of the diaphragm does not move due to inflammatory (**perihepatitis**) adhesions between liver and diaphragm. This is called **homolateral immobility of the diaphragm**. A small pleural effusion may also be present.
5. **Sigmoidoscopy** may demonstrate large, deep amoebic ulcers—**flask shaped**.
6. **Abdominal USG:** It is the investigation of choice.
   - To locate site of abscess and then to confirm diagnosis.
   - Ultrasound-guided needle aspiration can also be done and biopsy of abscess wall should be taken.
   - Multiple abscesses can be made out.
7. **CT scan** can demonstrate an abscess cavity as a low density zone surrounded by peripheral hypodense zone due to inflammatory reaction.

### Treatment

It can be classified into:

I. Conservative
II. Ultrasound-guided aspiration and pigtail drainage
III. Surgery—drainage.

### I. Conservative Line of Management

- It is indicated in ***amoebic hepatitis***. Tab. ***Metronidazole*** 400–800 mg 3 times a day is given for 14 days. The only recognisable side-effect is metallic taste.
- If the condition does not improve, injection ***Emetine*** 1 mg/kg body weight to a total of 60 mg/day deep IM for a maximum of 6 days is given.

### Side-effects and Precautions during Emetine Therapy

- Systolic BP should be at least 100 mmHg.
- ECG should be recorded before, during and after the therapy.
- Cardiotoxicity in the form of arrhythmias can occur.

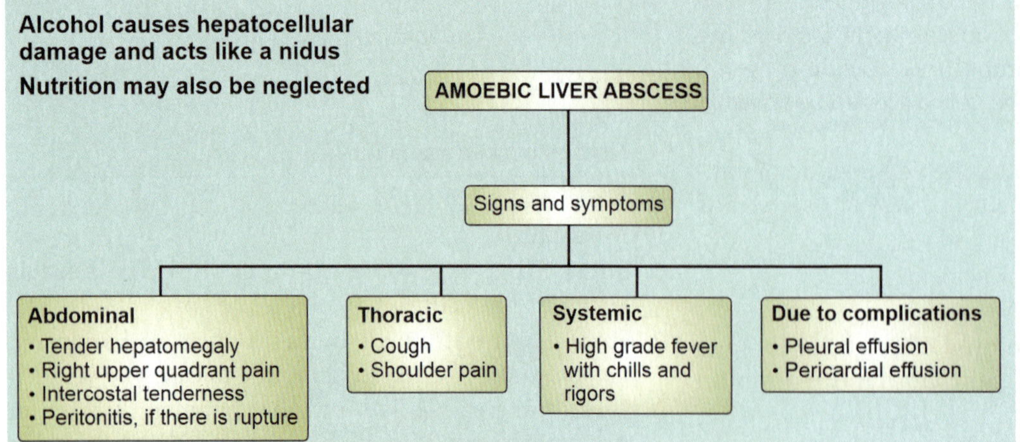


**Fig. 55.8A:** Clinical features of amoebic liver abscess

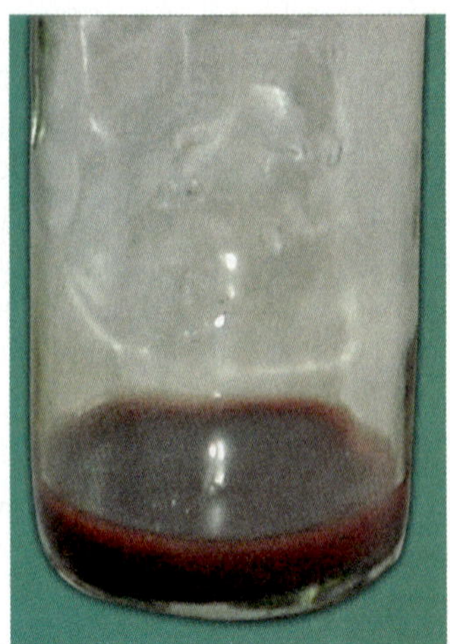

**Fig. 55.8B:** Anchovy sauce pus

- Absolute bed rest during treatment (because of these complications, it is not used nowadays).
- Adequate hydration, rest, analgesics to relieve the pain.

Improvement can be seen within one to two days in the form of disappearance of pain, fever and return of appetite.

### II. US-guided Needle Aspiration/Pigtail Catheter Drainage (Key Box 55.5)

- It is indicated in cases of ***amoebic liver abscess***.
- Before it is aspirated, coagulation profile should be normal and injection vitamin K 10 mg, IM should be given for at least 3 days.
- US-guided aspiration is also the treatment of choice where ***metronidazole is contraindicated***, e.g. 1st trimester of pregnancy.
- It can be easily done under local anaesthesia.
- Can be repeated, if pus recollects. Typically, it is anchovy sauce pus. Aspiration is followed by insertion of pigtail catheter.
- Before removal of the catheter do a repeat ultrasound to check for residual pus (Fig. 55.8B).

The clinical response to the aspiration may be observed as subsiding of fever (Figs 55.8B to 55.11).

Key Box 55.5

**Pigtail Catheter**

- They are the catheter used to drain clear fluids from cavities such as pleural fluid, ascites, bile, etc.
- Different sizes are available 8 to 12 French
- Radio-opaque polyurethane catheter
- Length—20 or 30 cm
- Large oval holes in pigtail for maximum drainage
- Thus, maximum efficiency is when 'transudate' pleural effusion is drained, as compared to empyema, haemothorax or anchovy sauce pus.

#### Complications

1. Bleeding—rare
2. Incomplete aspiration results in leakage of pus and bile into peritoneal cavity which may produce peritonitis. Hence, prophylactic antibiotics need to be given before and after the procedure along with metronidazole therapy.

### III. Surgery (Open Drainage) and Laparoscopic

#### *Indications*

1. Failure of US-guided needle aspiration.
2. Ruptured amoebic liver abscess with amoebic peritonitis.

#### *Procedure*

- Laparotomy is done first. Abscess cavity is identified. Contents are evacuated, a thorough peritoneal wash is given and a self-retaining **Malecot's catheter (any tube drain)** is introduced into the abscess cavity, brought outside and connected to a bag.
- With the advent of metronidazole, **amoebiasis cutis is rarely seen**. Hence, catheter can be safely placed inside the cavity and brought out. Malecot's catheter is now being replaced by other tube drains.
- Postoperatively for 3–5 days, necrotic liver tissue, anchovy sauce pus and blood drain outside.
- Once the drainage becomes minimal, Malecot's catheter is pulled out.
- Same procedure can be done by laparoscopic method.

#### *Complications of Amoebic Liver Abscess*

- **Amoebic peritonitis**, resulting in acute abdomen with shock. It has to be treated like any peritonitis—laparotomy, drainage of pus and drain the abscess cavity to outside (possibility of ***amoebiasis cutis*** is still present but rare).

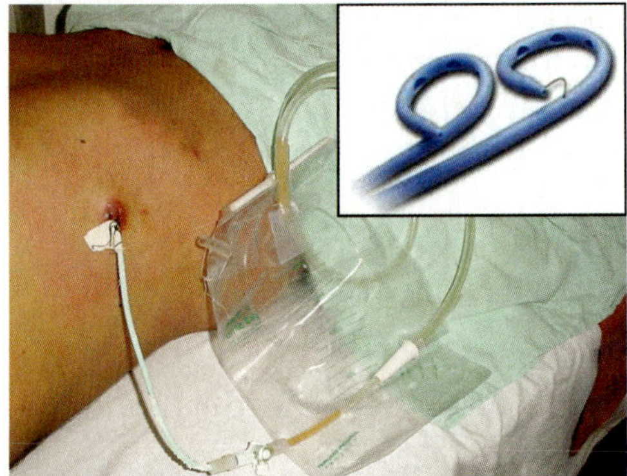

**Fig. 55.9:** Pigtail catheter drainage of amoebic liver abscess—it is a non-operative method of treatment

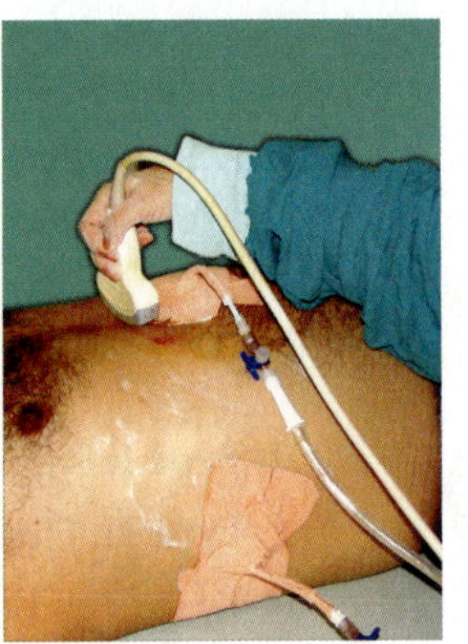

**Fig. 55.10:** Ultrasound is done to check residual abscess cavity

High temperature
Drainage done
Pulse rate
Normal temp.

**Fig. 55.11:** Temperature chart—once the drainage is done, temperature comes back to normal

**TABLE 55.2:** Differences between pyogenic abscess and amoebic liver abscess

| Pyogenic | Amoebic |
|---|---|
| Common sources are ascending cholangitis, instrumentation of common bile duct, ERCP, portal pyaemia, heamatogenous spread<br>Diabetes, immune compromised status | Source is from caecum/sigmoid colon: Organisms entry through the branches of superior and inferior mesenteric vein into the portal vein<br>Alcoholic men are commonly affected |
| Stage of hepatitis progressing to amoebic liver abscess<br>Usually multiple | Right lobe is more common especially bare area of the liver<br>Usually single |
| High grade fever, chills and rigors, jaundice, tender hepatomegaly and toxicity are common | Initially diarrhoea, blood and mucus in the stools. Then, high grade fever, chills and rigors, jaundice, tender hepatomegaly are common. Initially, systemic toxicity is not a feature |
| Diagnosis is by ultrasound and CECT scan. Other investigations such as MRCP or Chest X-ray depending upon the symptoms of the patient | Diagnosis is by ultrasound and CECT scan. Colonoscopy and biopsy of the ulcers in the sigmoid colon or in the caecum can be done. Stool can be sent for cyst and ova of *Entamoeba histolytica* |
| Treat the source–antibiotics (Broad spectrum antibiotics such as 2nd generation cephalosporins, metronidazole. If necessary, add Amikacin especially for gram-negative coverage depending upon the culture sensitivity pattern<br>Image guided percutaneous aspiration | Treat the source–antibiotics, image guided percutaneous aspiration. Injection metronidazole or tinidazole are the drugs used. If secondary infection is proved, other drugs are also added.<br>Amoebiasis cutis is rare. Hence, unilocular abscess can also be drained by percutaneous ultrasound guided aspiration. Rarely, open drainage may be required if there is a ruptured abscess with peritonitis. |

- Rupture into pleural space causing ***pleural effusion.***
- Rupture into the bronchus resulting in coughing out anchovy sauce (may be a natural cure)—***broncho-pleural fistula.***
- **Amoebic pericardial effusion** occurs due to rupture of left liver lobe abscess into pericardial space (Table 55.2).

**SU28.10.3:** Enumerate the etiology, pathogenesis, clinical features, investigations and various approaches in management of hydatid cyst of liver.

## HYDATID CYST OF THE LIVER

The disease is caused by *Echinococcus granulosus*, transmitted by dogs which are the chief mediators (host) and man is the intermediate host (Fig. 55.12). After swallowing the ova, they penetrate gastric mucosa[1], reach retroperitoneal structures, penetrate portal vein directly and then enter into liver. Having reached liver, the organisms grow and develop their own protective layer and form hydatid cyst.

### Layers of Hydatid Cyst (Fig. 55.13)

1. **The adventitia (pseudocyst)[2]:** This is the fibrous layer derived from the liver tissue. It is the reaction of liver to the parasite. It is adherent to the liver and cannot be separated—pericyst.
2. **The ectocyst (laminated membrane):** It is white and elastic and is produced by endocyst. It is this layer which gets peeled off at surgery.

[1]Reason why hydatid ova do not produce lesions in the intestine.
[2]It is the protective coat given by the host to the ghost.

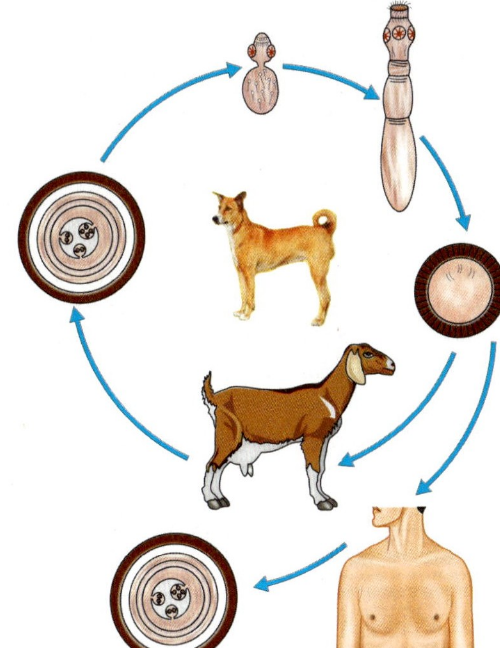
Fig. 55.12: Life cycle of hydatid cyst

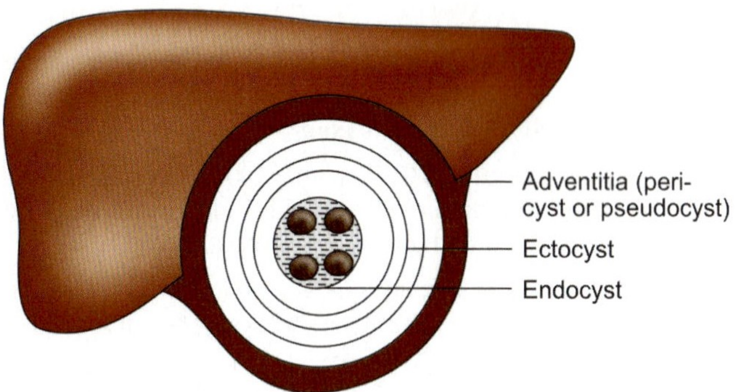

Fig. 55.13: Layers of hydatid cyst

3. **The endocyst:** This is called germinal epithelium and it is the innermost part of hydatid cyst. It secretes hydatid fluid inside and ectocyst outside. Within the hydatid fluid, the 'brood capsules' develop within which the scolices of *Echinococcus granulosus* develop.

### Clinical Features

- It can be silent—without any symptoms throughout life, accidentally discovered on routine examination.
- Dragging pain in the upper abdomen due to hepatomegaly.
- Liver is enlarged, has a smooth surface, round borders and is nontender.
- **Typical hydatid thrill** can be present on rare occasions. Hydatid thrill is demonstrated by 3-finger method. Keep 3 fingers over the liver, percuss over the middle finger and get the impulse by other 2 fingers (fluid thrill).
- Patient may present as an emergency with severe abdominal pain following minor trauma.
- May present as an emergency with features of anaphylatic shock without any obvious cause.

### Gharbi Classification

Five types have been identified:

**Type I:** Pure cyst—clear fluid

**Type II:** Fluid and detached germinative epithelium

**Type III:** Fluid collection with septa

**Type IV:** Heterogeneous cyst—hypo- or hyperechoic lesions

**Type V:** Calcified cyst and calcified wall.

### Investigations

1. **USG** can detect the cyst, localise the cyst and is used for aspiration purposes (details later—PAIR).
   WHO—Informal working group of Echinococcosis (WHO—IWGE) (USG classification)
   **Group 1:** Active group—cyst larger than 2 cm and often fertile
   **Group 2:** Transition group—cyst starting to degenerate because of host resistance or treatment; may contain viable protoscolices
   **Group 3:** Inactive group—degenerated partially or totally calcified cyst; unlikely to contain viable protoscolices.
2. **Plain X-ray abdomen** may demonstrate **speckled** calcification.
3. **CT scan** may be necessary in selected cases (Figs 55.14 and 55.15). The cyst which is superficial and has reached surface, should be operated upon.
4. **ERCP** if there is obstructive jaundice—in such cases, a wide sphincterotomy should be given so as to allow free drainage of the hydatid contents into the duodenum.
5. **Casoni's intradermal test:** Sensitivity and specificity of this test is low and hence, **no longer used**.
6. ELISA and immunoelectrophoresis may point towards the diagnosis.

### Treatment

It can be discussed under following headings.

#### *I. Conservative*

1. Calcified cysts are dead cysts. They are left alone.
2. Symptomless, small hydatid cyst can be left alone. Once symptomatic, or if the size is more than 5 cm, they may be treated.

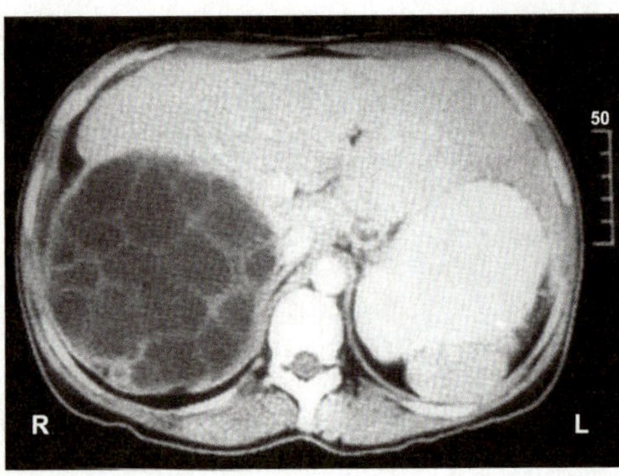


**Fig. 55.14:** CT scan of the liver showing classical cart wheel pattern—coronal section

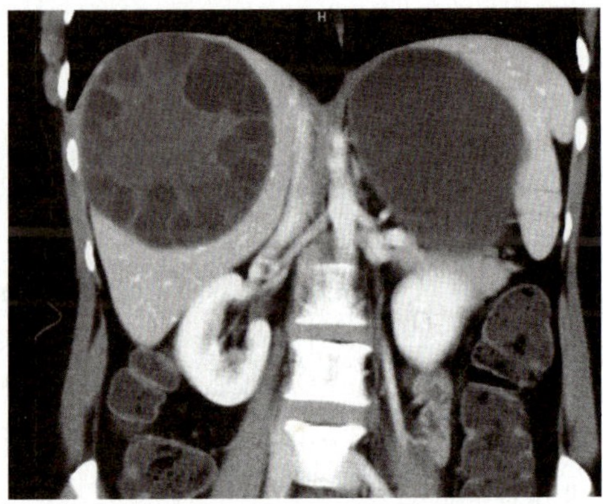

**Fig. 55.15:** CT scan of the liver showing classical cart wheel pattern—sagittal section

### *II. Medical Treatment* (Key Box 55.6)

- Albendazole 8 mg/kg or 400 mg BD is given for 21 days followed by drug holiday for 2 weeks.
  If no improvement occurs, maximum of 3 such cycles can be given.
- Watch for neutropenia.

**Key Box 55.6**

**Indications for Medical Treatment**

- Disseminated hydatid cyst
- Inaccessible for surgery (deep seated, multiple, recurrent)
- Patient unfit for surgery
- Contamination of peritoneal cavity at surgery

### *III. Surgery*

There are different types of surgeries for hydatid disease of the liver which have been summarised below. Indications are given in Key Box 55.7.

**Key Box 55.7**

**Indications for Surgery**

- Symptomatic cyst
- Asymptomatic patient with cyst >5 cm, noncalcified
- Infected cyst (Figs 55.20 and 55.21)

#### *Principles of Surgery*

1. **Laparotomy** and **isolation of the cyst** from peritoneal cavity by packs dipped in hypochlorite solution.
2. Aspirate the contents and inject **scolicidal agents** such as Savlon or hypertonic saline (Key Box 55.8).
3. Incise the cyst, **peel off the laminated membrane** by using sponge-holding forceps (Figs 55.16 to 55.19).
4. An attempt to remove adventitial layer may result in bleeding. It need not be removed.
5. At surgery, all laminated membrane, endocyst has to be removed. Perfect haemostasis must be achieved. Any bile leak to be sutured. Postoperative significant bile leak is managed by ERCP stenting.

**Key Box 55.8**

| Scolicidal agents | Side-effects |
|---|---|
| Hypertonic saline | Hypernatraemia |
| Chlorhexidine | Acidosis |
| Alcohol (80%) | Cholangitis |
| Sodium hypochlorite | Hypernatraemia |

#### *Precautions*

- Albendazole should be given before surgery.
- Avoid spillage into the peritoneal cavity to avoid peritoneal hydatid.
- **Injection hydrocortisone** 100 mg IV before, during and after surgery to avoid anaphylactic shock.

#### *Different Types of Surgical Procedures*

They have been summarised in Key Box 55.9. However, excision of the cyst leaving the adventitial layer is the most commonly performed surgery (Fig. 55.19).

**Key Box 55.9**

**Surgical Procedures**

- **Excision:** It is the most commonly performed operation.
- **Cystopericystectomy:** Here, the cyst is excised in a plane outside adventitial layer. It results in excessive bleeding but it removes the cyst completely.
- **Capitonnage:** If omentum is not available for closing the cavity, redundant cyst wall can be infolded into the cyst cavity and sutured.
- **Hepatic resection** in good centres when there are proper indications.

### *IV. Percutaneous Drainage*

- It is done after taking all necessary precautions/ equipment with all emergency drugs and with CT/ US guidance.
- It is also called **PAIR**—**P**uncture, **A**spiration, **I**njection and **R**easpiration.

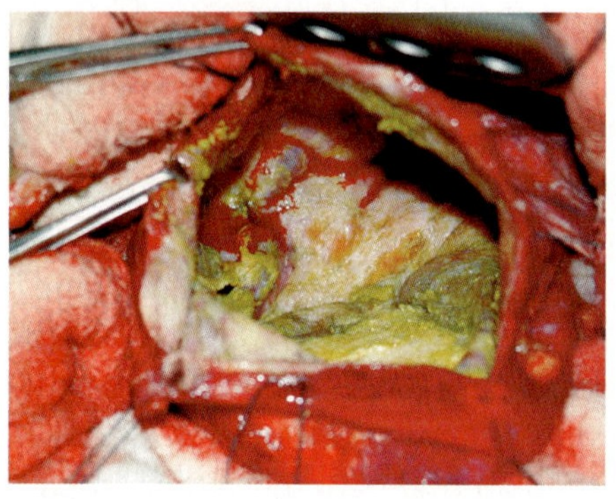
Fig. 55.16: Infected ruptured hydatid cyst—observe green colour due to biliary communication. In such cases, look for any bile leak and suture the opening of biliary duct branches

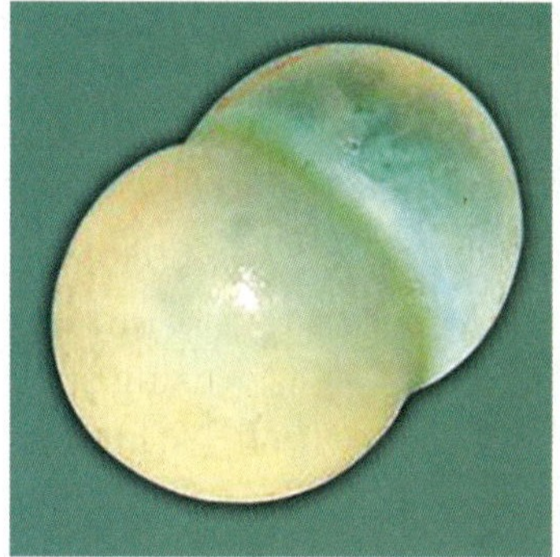
Fig. 55.17: Pearl-like daughter cysts (very precious!!)—Hydatid means dew drop in Latin and watery vesicle in Greek

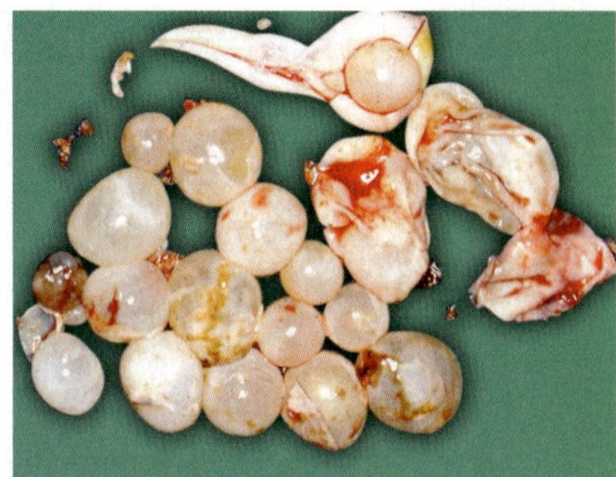
Fig. 55.18: Daughter cysts—it is important to clear all these to prevent recurrence. Please take care not to rupture them while removing

(*Courtesy:* Dr Geetha R, Dr Ankur Sharma, Dr Rajesh Nair, Department of Surgery, KMC, Manipal)

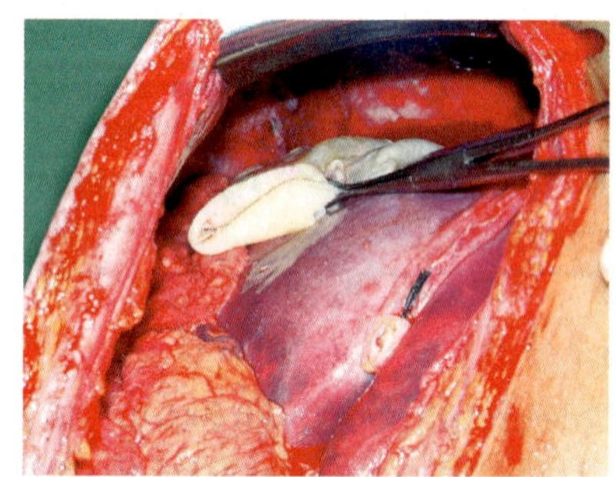
Fig. 55.19: Laminated membrane removed at surgery with sponge-holding forceps

## Indications (Figs 55.20A and B)

- Unilocular uncomplicated cyst
- Poor surgical candidate
- Previous multiple abdominal surgeries
- Relapse following surgery
- Management algorithm of hydatid cyst is given in Fig. 55.21.

## Contraindications to PAIR

- Multiple septal divisions, communicating cysts
- Dead or inactive cysts, laparoscopic approach for these procedures are being done.

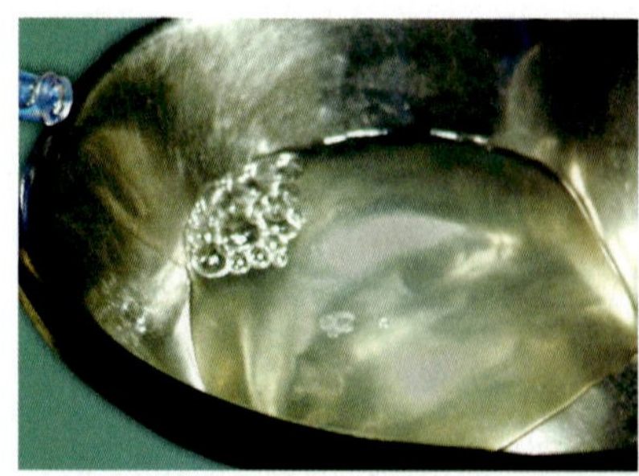
Fig. 55.20A: Clear fluid being aspirated as a part of PAIR treatment

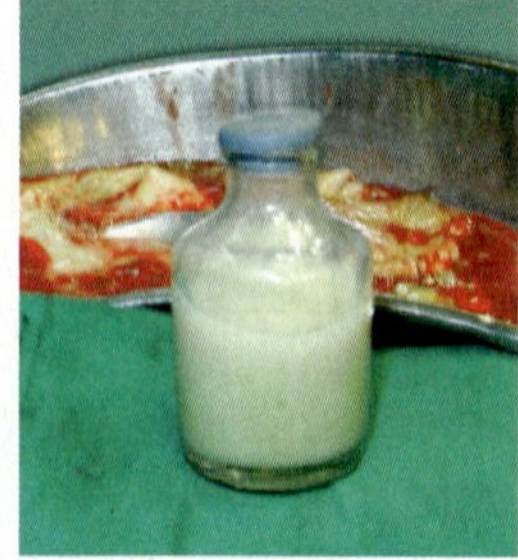
Fig. 55.20B: As the aspirated fluid was turbid, open drainage was done in this patient

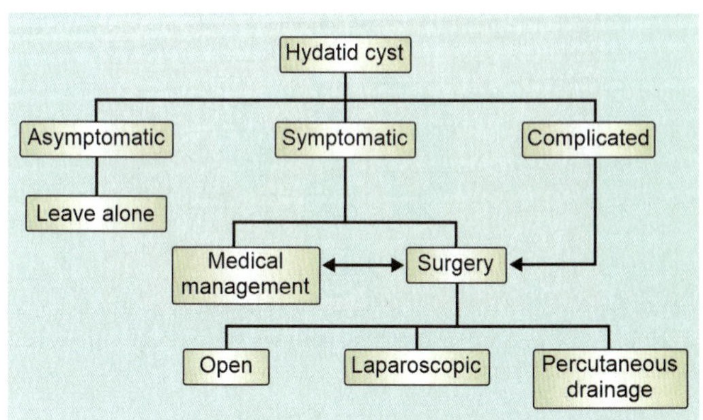

Fig. 55.21: Algorithm of management of hydatid cyst

Summary of the treatment of hydatid cyst of the liver is given in Fig. 55.21.

## Complications of Hydatid Cyst

1. **Rupture** of the cyst into the peritoneal cavity can occur due to trauma (rare) and may result in anaphylactic shock. It should be treated accordingly with injection hydrocortisone and laparotomy.
   Rupture can result in implantation of active cysts within peritoneal cavity and they grow within. Rupture through diaphragm can cause **empyema**. It can also rupture into biliary radicles and can cause obstructive jaundice.
2. **Jaundice** due to cysts within biliary tree or due to a large cyst compressing biliary ducts. ERCP followed by endoscopic removal of hydatid cysts from the common bile duct followed by sphincterotomy should be done.
3. **Suppuration** is rare due to the tough tunica adventitia.
4. **Calcification** of the cyst wall in long-standing cases (Fig. 55.22).

Other type of organism is ***Echinococcus multilocularis.*** This parasitic infestation is uncommon in our country but it is more severe (Key Box 55.10).

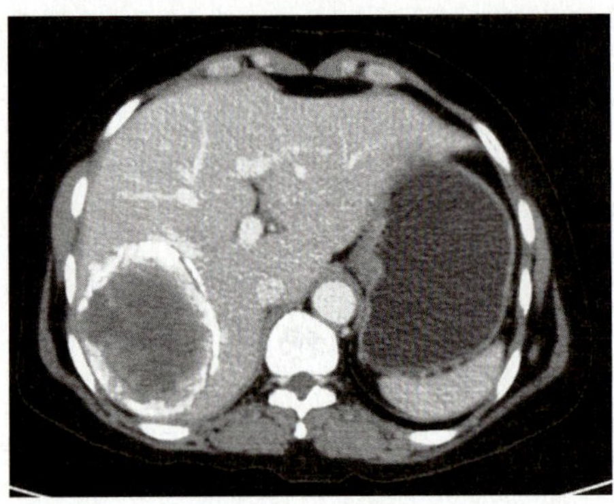

**Fig. 55.22:** CT of the liver—hydatid calcification

Key Box 55.10

***Echinococcus multilocularis***

- Alveolar echinococcosis
- It can cause **malignant hydatid disease** (misnomer). Difficult to treat. Hence, the name
- Needs resection
- It causes poorly demarcated honeycombed cystic specimen
- It infiltrates liver and invades vascular system

**SU28.10.5:** Enumerate the various benign neoplasms of the liver. The clinical presentation, investigations and principles of management of benign neoplasms of liver.

## OTHER CYSTIC DISEASES

### SIMPLE CYSTIC DISEASE

- When the cyst is thin walled, unilocular and regular, it is usually a simple cyst (Fig. 55.23).
- The host response is usually not present (unlike hydatid cyst).
- Incidentally discovered by ultrasound examination.
- Clinically, if they are big, liver will be palpable with smooth surface and round borders. It is nontender.

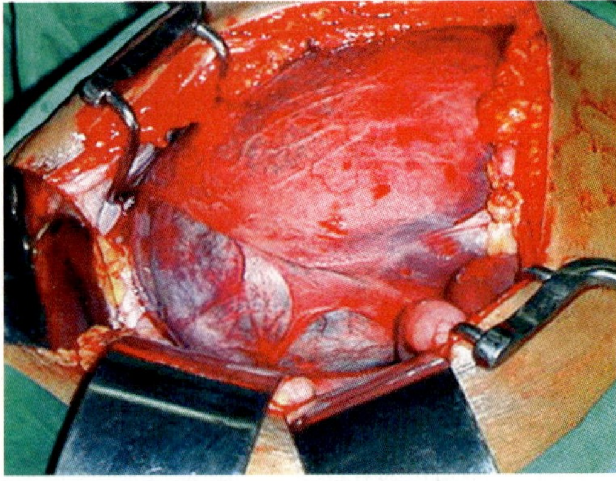

**Fig. 55.23:** Simple cyst at surgery. Observe the thin wall with slight bluish colour

- Asymptomatic cysts do not require any treatment.
- Ultrasound-guided aspiration, laparoscopic de-roofing and open surgical de-roofing are the methods of treating the cyst.
- Differential diagnosis includes hydatid cyst, polycystic disease.

### POLYCYSTIC LIVER DISEASE

- Congenital abnormality.
- Cysts occur within liver, pancreas and kidney (principally).
- Cysts are asymptomatic.
- Cysts do not produce liver cell failure (unlike polycystic kidneys).
- Cyst haemorrhage may be the presenting feature with right hypochondriac pain mimicking cholecystitis.
- CT scan and ultrasound are investigations.
- Cyst aspiration (PAIR like hydatid cyst), decompression may rarely be required in large painful lesions (laparoscopic).

*Observe* ***7 Cs of polycystic liver*** (Fig. 55.24).

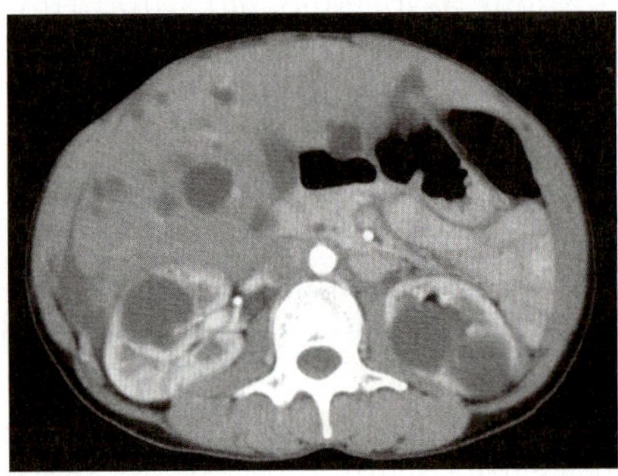

**Fig. 55.24:** CT scan showing polycystic liver and polycystic kidney

## BENIGN TUMOURS OF THE LIVER

- These are not uncommon tumours.
- They are more frequently diagnosed now with frequent use of ultrasound. Majority of them are asymptomatic and do not require specific treatment.
- Their removal should be attempted only by an experienced surgeon. Hepatic adenoma and focal nodular hyperplasia are compared in Table 55.3.
- They have a rare potential for malignant change.

### HAEMANGIOMA

- **Commonest benign tumour** of the liver.
- Majority (75%) occur in **women.**
- Most of them are **solitary**, **subcapsular**, occur in right lobe of liver.

| TABLE 55.3: Comparison of hepatic adenoma and focal nodular hyperplasia | |
|---|---|
| **Hepatic adenomas** | **Focal nodular hyperplasia** |
| Occur in young women | Occurs in young women |
| Occur due to oral contraceptive pills (OCPs) | Occurs due to oral contraceptive pills |
| Usually **solitary** | Can be **multiple** |
| Haemorrhage, rupture, necrosis can occur | Haemorrhage, rupture, necrosis do not occur |
| Can undergo malignant change | **Rarely, malignant** change can occur |
| If it is due to OCPs, it can regress after discontinuing OCPs. Otherwise, adenomas need to be resected | Generally does not regress |
| Kupffer cells are **not present** in hepatic adenomas | In addition to hepatocytes, it also contains Kupffer cells |

- It may be associated with **cavernous haemangioma** at some other sites such as head and neck region. Clinically, it is difficult to diagnose as it presents as hepatomegaly.
- **Kasabach-Merritt syndrome: Thrombocytopenia and consumptive coagulopathy.**
- Sometimes it may cause cardiovascular failure due to sequestration of blood.
- Ultrasound/CT scan can diagnose their location, number (single or multiple) or presence of any other complications associated with that (thrombosis, infection). MRI is a better investigation.
- Haemangioma **bigger than 8 cm** have **chances of rupture.**

## Treatment

1. **Transarterial embolisation (TAE)**
   - Indicated in large haemangiomas which are unresectable.
   - Large haemangiomas on the inferior surface of the liver are ideally suitable for the treatment (Figs 55.25 to 55.27).
   - Embolic materials
     (A) Temporary: Gel foam
     (B) Permanent: Steel coils, polyvinyl alcohol, isobutyl cyanoacrylate.
   - Polyvinyl alcohol particles 300–500 μm in size are used often.
2. They can be resected or can be enucleated.

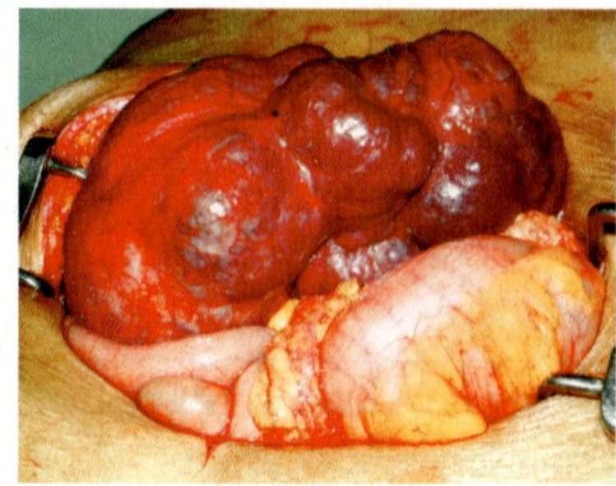

Fig. 55.25: Haemangioma arising from the inferior surface of the liver, is exposed at surgery

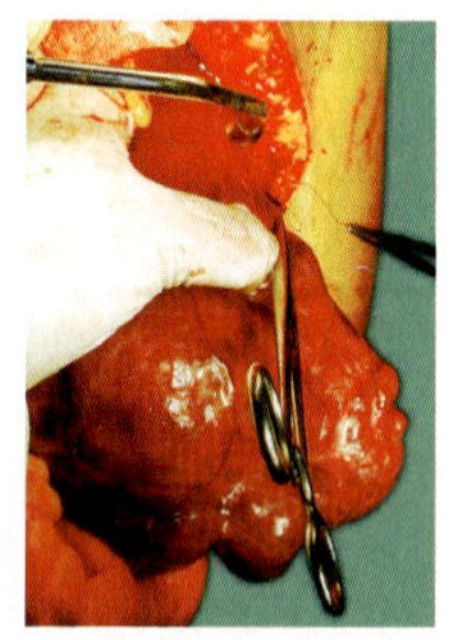

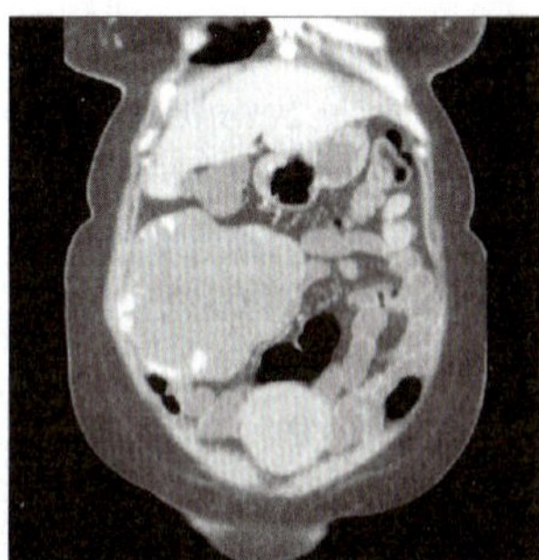

Figs 55.26 and 55.27: As it had a very narrow strip of the liver tissue, it was easily excised

**Caution:** Before putting a needle into the space occupying lesion in the liver, make sure it is **NOT a haemangioma**.

## Differential Diagnosis

Hepatoma, liver cysts, liver abscess.

Other benign tumours are **hepatic adenomas** and **focal nodular hyperplasia**.

# PRIMARY LIVER CANCER—HEPATOMA OR HEPATOCELLULAR CARCINOMA (HCC)

- Before discussion on HCC, one has to have a knowledge about segmental anatomy of the liver, which forms the basis of hepatic resection.
- Even though the details about hepatic resection may not be required for undergraduate students, it is desirable to know about the segmental anatomy to have a better understanding about hepatic resection.

**SU28.10.1:** Describe the segmental anatomy of liver and the variations in vascular anatomy of liver (Table 55.4).

## SEGMENTAL ANATOMY OF THE LIVER

- The liver is divided into two lobes by the main portal fissure, which is also called **Cantlie's line**. This line extends from the gallbladder fossa to the left side of

| TABLE 55.4: Variations in the vascular anatomy of the liver | |
|---|---|
| **Normal** | **Variations** |
| Common hepatic artery (CHA) usually originates from the celiac trunk | CHA can arise from superior mesenteric artery (SMA) or the left gastric artery (LGA) |
| In the porta hepatis, main hepatic artery is located. It divided into right and left hepatic artery | In about 40% of cases it is the only artery without any branches |
| Normal hepatic artery | Accessory hepatic artery can be present ranging from 4 to 40% of patients |
| Portal vein divides into right and left branches | Number of branches may vary. Segment 4 may receive as many as 7 branches sometimes |

IVC and is inclined at an angle of 75° to the horizontal plane. The main portal fissure is a constant feature. Each lobe is equal in size.

- The **right portal fissure** divides the right lobe into an anteromedial and posterolateral sector. The right hepatic vein courses along this fissure. This fissure is inclined at an angle of 40° with the horizontal.
- The left portal fissure divides the left lobe into an anterior and posterior sector, and it is in this fissure that the left hepatic vein courses.
- The liver is further divided into segments, which represents the smallest anatomic unit of the organ. In the right lobe, each of the two sectors is divided into two segments: The anteromedial sector and posterolateral sector. The anteromedial sector is divided into segment V anteriorly and segment VIII posteriorly, while the posterolateral sector is divided into segment VI anteriorly and segment VII posteriorly.
- In the left lobe, the anterior sector is divided into segment IV (or quadrate lobe) and the segment III. The posterior sector is comprised of only one segment, segment II. The Spigelian lobe or segment I is considered as an ***autonomous*** segment. It is also labelled ***caudate lobe***.
- Each segment has its own identifiable portal vein, hepatic arterial supply, bile duct and hepatic veins. All these segments can be removed individually. However, segment I receives tributaries from both the right and left branches of portal vein and hepatic artery. ***However, hepatic venous drainage is independent and may terminate directly into IVC*** (Fig. 55.28).

## Introduction

Hepatocellular carcinoma is uncommon in United States but more in Asians. It arises from hepatocytes. When it arises from biliary epithelial cells, it is intrahepatic cholangiocarcinoma. In neonates, it is hepatoblastoma as it resembles foetal liver.

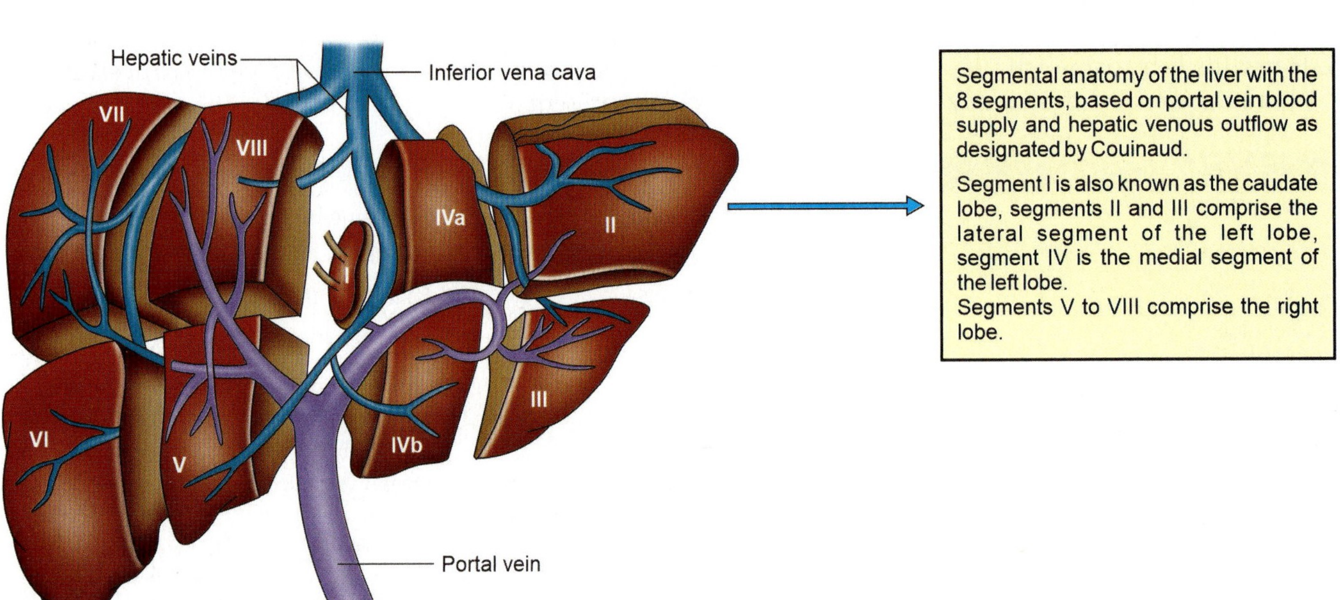


Segmental anatomy of the liver with the 8 segments, based on portal vein blood supply and hepatic venous outflow as designated by Couinaud.

Segment I is also known as the caudate lobe, segments II and III comprise the lateral segment of the left lobe, segment IV is the medial segment of the left lobe.
Segments V to VIII comprise the right lobe.

**Fig. 55.28:** Segmental anatomy of the liver

**SU28.10.6:** Describe in detail the aetiopathogenesis, premalignant conditions, clinical features, investigations, staging and treatment options available for treatment of hepatocellular carcinoma. Also types of hepatic resections.

## Aetiology of HCC

1. **Hepatitis B virus (HBV):** High titres of hepatitis B surface antigen (HBsAg) was found in 50 to 60% of patients with HCC. Its incidence is higher in chronic carriers and it is increased, if patients consume alcohol, aflatoxin and tobacco.
2. **Hepatitis C virus (HCV):** HCV infection induces cirrhosis and increases the incidence of development of HCC.
3. **Hepatitis D:** It is another viral infection also called **delta hepatitis**. This virus requires hepatitis B virus (HBV) for replication. It can cause dangerous hepatitis—HCC.
4. **Cirrhosis:** It is a definite premalignant condition. A palpable hard liver in a cirrhotic patient suggests development of HCC. **It is the single most common risk factor for HCC.**
5. **Aflatoxin consumption** (a fungus found in infected butter yellow, bread) is responsible for increased incidence of HCC as in Mozambique.
6. **Oral contraceptive pills** are known to cause adenoma and there is a rare chance of adenoma turning into HCC.
7. **Other risk factors:** Heavy alcohol consumption, cigarette smoking, diabetes mellitus, haemochromatosis are the other factors responsible for HCC. ***Wilson's disease is rarely associated with increased risk of HCC.***
8. Hereditary tyrosinaemia is a metabolic disorder characterised by deficiency of enzyme fumaryl acetoacetate resulting in, accumulation of toxic tyrosine metabolites—can progress to HCC.
9. **Other causes:** Type I glycogen storage disease and familial polyposis coli, alpha-1 antitrypsin deficiency, Budd-Chiari syndrome. It is 4 times more common in Asians and two times in Hispanics. Less common in Caucasians.

**Pathology:** It is a highly vascular tumour and fatal if left untreated. Few types and histological features are given below:

| ***Histologic variants of HCC*** | ***Pathology:*** Histology types |
|---|---|
| 1. Fibrolamellar<br>2. Mixed hepatocellular cholangiocarcinoma cellular<br>3. Clear cell variant<br>4. Giant cell variant<br>5. Childhood HCC<br>6. Carcinosarcoma<br><br>*Refer to Table 55.5 | • It is a highly vascular tumour with indistinct margin<br>• **Hanging type:** It is attached to the liver by a small stalk—easily resected<br>• **Pushing type:** A tumour pushing the blood vessels. It is also resectable<br>• **Infiltrative type:** Difficult to resect because of infiltration into surrounding structures.<br>• Hence, in cirrhotic patients, resection is not advisable |

## Clinical Features

- **Age group:** Highest incidence is found after 50 years of age. It is rarely seen in children also.
- **Sex:** ***Male alcoholics*** are commonly affected.

*Pearls of Wisdom*

Thus, almost 80% of the cases are due to underlying chronic hepatitis B and C virus infection.

- A *slow growing* mass in the right hypochondrium. It is the enlarged liver with an irregular surface and is hard in consistency. Evidence of cirrhosis may be present.

**TABLE 55.5:** Comparison of HCC and fibrolamellar carcinoma

| | **Hepatocellular carcinoma** | **Fibrolamellar carcinoma** |
|---|---|---|
| 1. Age (years) | 50–60 | 20–30 |
| 2. Sex | More common in males | Equal in both sexes |
| 3. Aetiology | Cirrhosis | Does not arise in a cirrhotic liver |
| 4. Involvement of lobe | Right lobe | Left lobe |
| 5. Gross pathology | Solitary or nodular, central necrosis is common | Solitary or nodular, central necrosis is not common |
| 6. Microscopy | Basic structure is trabecular pattern with acidophilic cytoplasm and large nuclei | Deeply eosinophilic hepatocytes, fibrous stroma is arranged in the form of thin hyalinised bands in layers<br>Hence the name, **fibrolamellar** |
| 7. Resectability rate | Less | More |
| 8. Prognosis | Not good | Good |

- It can be a ***rapidly growing*** neoplasm, highly vascular and clinically palpable as a soft to firm pulsatile mass with or without a bruit.
- Rapid development of ***anorexia, asthaenia, anaemia and loss of weight***.
- Jaundice is not common unless the tumour arises in a cirrhotic liver in hepatocellular failure.
- Worsening of portal hypertension.
- **Low grade pyrexia** is common. It is due to tumour necrosis.
- Liver being an important organ of metabolism, **hypoglycaemia** is found in 10% of the patients.
- Ascites
- **Triad of abdominal pain, weight loss and abdominal mass** is the most common clinical presentation.

### Spread of Hepatoma

1. **Direct infiltration** of the neighbouring structures such as diaphragm results in hiccoughs due to irritation of phrenic nerve.
2. **Lymphatic spread:** Lymph nodes at the hilum (porta hepatis) are involved first. Later, mediastinal nodes and left supraclavicular nodes (Virchow's node) are involved.
3. **Blood spread** causes massive malignant pleural effusion by dislodgement of tumour emboli into inferior vena cava because of spread through the hepatic veins. Vertebral involvement follows soon.
4. **Haemoperitoneum** due to spread involving peritoneal surface or due to rupture of an enlarging hepatoma may occur.

### Investigations

1. **CBP:** Hb% is usually low.
2. **Liver function tests** may show hepatocellular failure in the form of high bilirubin, low albumin and high globulin levels.
3. **Chest X-ray/CT chest** to look for pulmonary metastasis pulmonary metastasis.
4. **Abdominal USG:** Findings:
   - Diffuse distortion of hepatic parenchyma and a well-circumscribed hyperechogenic mass suggests HCC.
   - **Mosaic pattern** of the tumour with thin halo and lateral shadows, **nodule in nodule pattern** with separating fibrous septa and **posterior echo enhancement**.
   - **Tumour thrombi** in portal vein, hepatic vein or IVC.
5. **Contrast enhanced CT of the abdomen**[1]: It appears as a hypodense mass with internal mosaic architecture in the early phase and hypodense lesion with enhanced fibrous capsule in late phase. Guided FNAC can be done to confirm the diagnosis. A small fear of tumour embolisation *via* portal venous radicles exists and is a complication. Enhancement in arterial phase and washout in delayed portovenous phase is diagnostic of HCC (Figs 55.29 and 55.30).

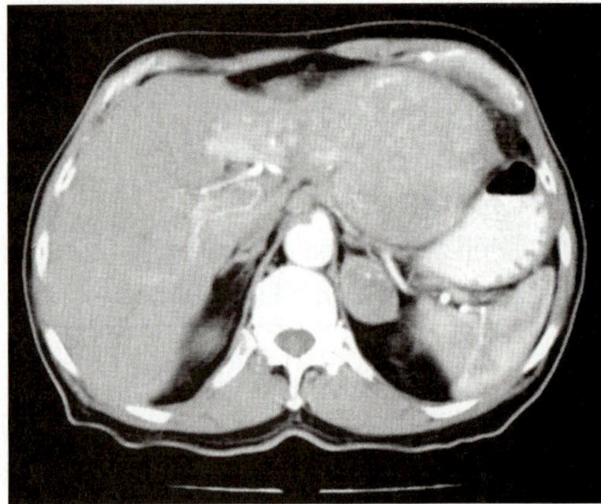

**Fig. 55.29:** CT scan showing a large hypodense mass lesion in the left lobe

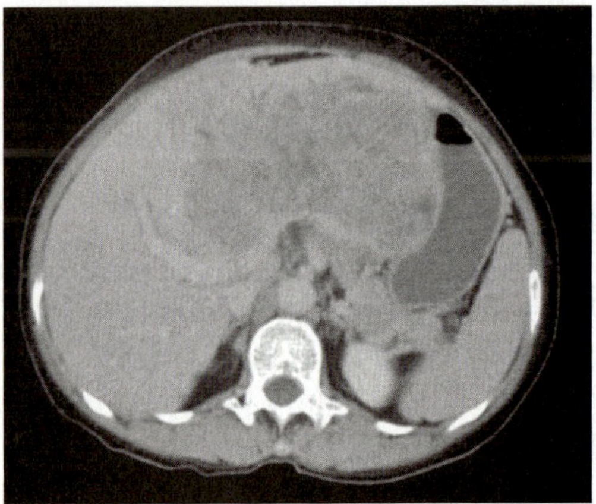

**Fig. 55.30:** CT scan showing a large hepatoma displacing the portal vein branches

6. **Alpha-fetoprotein**
   - It is a foetal antigen which disappears after birth. Hence, it is not measurable in normal persons.
   - Values above 20 ng/ml are suggestive of hepatoma.
   - Levels above 400 ng/ml in a cirrhotic patients with hypervascular mass larger than 2 cm in diameter is diagnostic.
   - α-fetoprotein levels indicate size of the tumour, invasion and even recurrence.
   - In patients who are not operated, levels reflect response to treatment (Key Box 55.11).
   - Values around 200 ng/ml is also seen with regenerating nodules.
   - 20 to 40% HCCs do not secrete LFP.

[1]Triple phase—precontrast, early vascular or arterial, portal phase and delayed phase—multislice spiral CT is the gold standard investigation for liver tumours. If clinical, radiological and biochemical features strongly suggest HCC, there is no need to prove histopathological diagnosis by FNAC.

Key Box 55.11

**Increased α-Fetoprotein Levels**

1. **Hepatoma—hepatoblastoma**
2. Carcinoma stomach
3. Carcinoma pancreas
4. Embryonal cell carcinoma of testis

**Not increased in fibrolamellar carcinoma**

7. **Selective angiography:** It is done only if hepatic resection is planned. It can demonstrate a highly vascular tumour (tumour blush due to neovascularisation) or involvement of portal vein thrombus in the IVC. Hence, venous phase must be recorded. It can define arterial supply also.
8. **MRI:** It appears as a high intensity lesion (adenomatous hyperplasia as a low intensity lesion).

   MRI is much more sensitive for diagnosis of 1–2 cm HCC.
9. **Liver biopsy for HCC:**
   - It is done only in unresectable cases or metastatic disease before starting other treatment such as chemotherapy, etc.
   - The images from contrast CT scan and MRI and raised levels of α-fetoprotein—almost always suggest HCC. Hence, biopsy is not done.
   - Also chances of haemoperitoneum and peritoneal implantation of tumour cells present.
   - Core-biopsy has increased risks of all the complications mentioned above.
   - With normal INR, fine needle aspiration can be done in selected cases (clinical trials) with minimal risk.

## Differential Diagnosis (Key Box 55.12)

- Secondaries in the liver—nodular surface and usually both lobes are enlarged.
- Polycystic disease of the liver.
- Hydatid cyst of the liver—smooth surface, round borders.

  Refer TNM staging of liver cancer.

Key Box 55.12

**Differential Diagnosis**

- Fibrolamellar carcinoma
- Secondaries in the liver
- Haemangioma
- Focal nodular hyperplasia
- Polycystic liver

**TNM STAGING: AJCC 8th edition–hepatocellular carcinoma**

**Primary tumour (T)**

**T1a** Solitary tumour ≤2 cm with/without vascular invasion

**T1b** Solitary tumour >2 cm without vascular invasion

**T2** Solitary tumour >2 cm with vascular invasion or multifocal tumours, note >5 cm

**T3** Multiple tumours at least one of which is >5 cm

**T4** Single tumour or multifocal tumours of any size involving a major branch of the portal vein or hepatic vein or tumour(s) with direct invasion of adjacent organs other than the gallbladder or with perforation of visceral peritoneum

**Regional lymph nodes (N)**

**Nx** Regional lymph nodes cannot be assessed

**N0** No regional lymph node metastasis

**N1** Regional lymph node metastasis

**Distant metastasis (M)**

**M0** No distant metastasis

**M1** Distant metastasis

| **Stage** | | | |
|---|---|---|---|
| **Stage IA** | T1a | N0 | M0 |
| **Stage IB** | T1b | N0 | M0 |
| **Stage II** | T2 | N0 | M0 |
| **Stage IIIA** | T3 | N0 | M0 |
| **Stage IIIB** | T4 | N0 | M0 |
| **Stage IVA** | Any T | N1 | M0 |
| **Stage IVB** | Any T | Any N | M1 |

## Prognosis

Prognosis of HCC depends upon not only about stage of the disease but also about whether patient can withstand/tolerate surgery or not? As most of the patients have active hepatitis/cirrhosis, resection may carry very high mortality. Hence, the Eastern Cooperative Oncology Group (ECOG) have adopted a performance status which is called ECOG performance status as given below.

**ECOG**

0. Fully active, able to carry on all pre-disease performance without restriction.
1. Restricted in physically strenuous activity but ambulatory and able to carry out work of a light or sedentary nature, e.g. light house work, office work.
2. Ambulatory and capable of all self-care but unable to carry out any work activities. Up and about more than 50% of waking hours.
3. Capable of only limited self-care, confined to bed or chair more than 50% of waking hours.
4. Completely disabled. Cannot carry on any self-care. Totally confined to bed or chair.
5. Dead

## CHILD-TURCOTTE-PUGH (CTP) SCORE

Classification of hepatocellular function in cirrhosis

| Points | 1 point each | 2 points each | 3 points each |
|---|---|---|---|
| Bilirubin mg/dl | <2 | 2–3 | >3 |
| Albumin (g/L) | >35 | 25–35 | <25 |
| Ascites | None | Easily controlled | Poorly controlled |
| Encephalopathy | None | Grade I–II | Grades III–IV |
| INR | <1.7 | 1.7–2.2 | >2.2 |
| A—5–6 points<br>C—10–15 points | | B—7–9 points | |

INR: International normalised ratio.

### Treatment of Hepatocellular Carcinoma

It can be classified under following headings.

1. **Resection** is the best possible treatment for hepatocellular carcinoma. Up to 3 segments of the liver can be resected. Rest of the liver will be enough to maintain life provided remaining liver is healthy/ noncirrhotic (Flowcharts 55.1, 55.2 and Table 55.6).
   - Functional liver remnant (FLR) should be >20% of standardised total liver volume after resection.
   - The remnant liver should have vascular inflow, venous outflow, biliary drainage.
   - Two contiguous liver segments must be left behind (Figs 55.31 to 55.34).
2. **Systemic chemotherapy** using intravenous doxorubicin has been tried with some success in the postoperative period. Intra-arterial 5-FU has also been tried.
3. **Transcatheter arterial embolisation (TAE):** By introducing gel foam into the branches of hepatic artery some amount of tumour necrosis occurs. This arterial embolisation is combined with chemotherapeutic agents such as doxorubicin, results are better because the tumour has prolonged exposure to the drug. This is called **transarterial chemoembolisation**

**Flowchart 55.1:** Various segments for liver resection

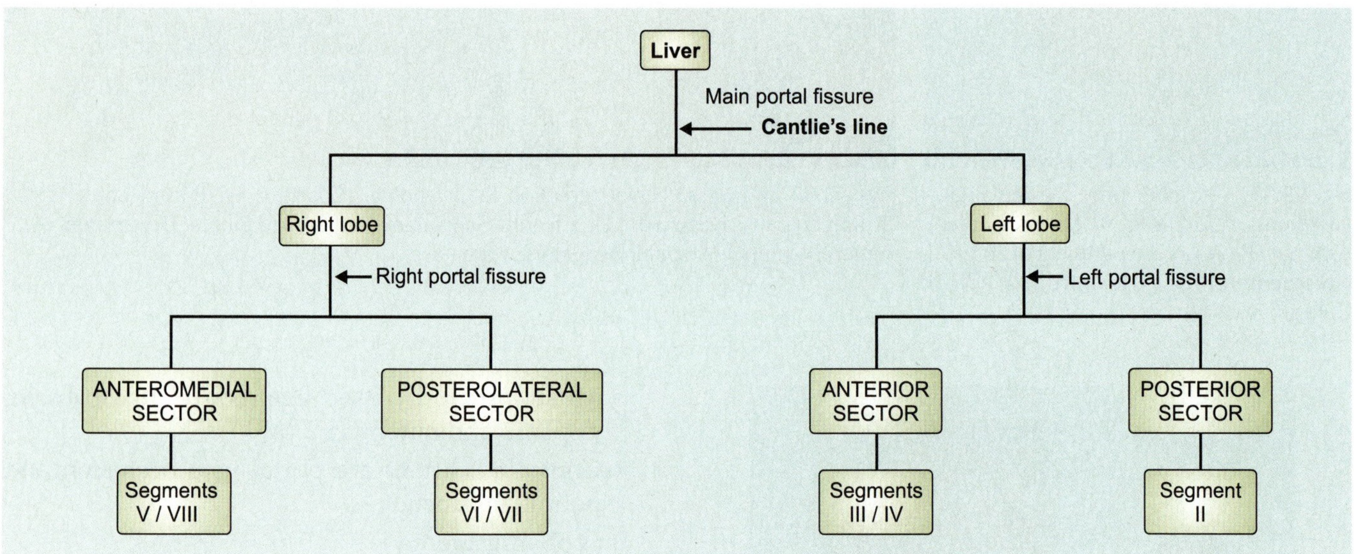


**Flowchart 55.2:** Treatment of HCC

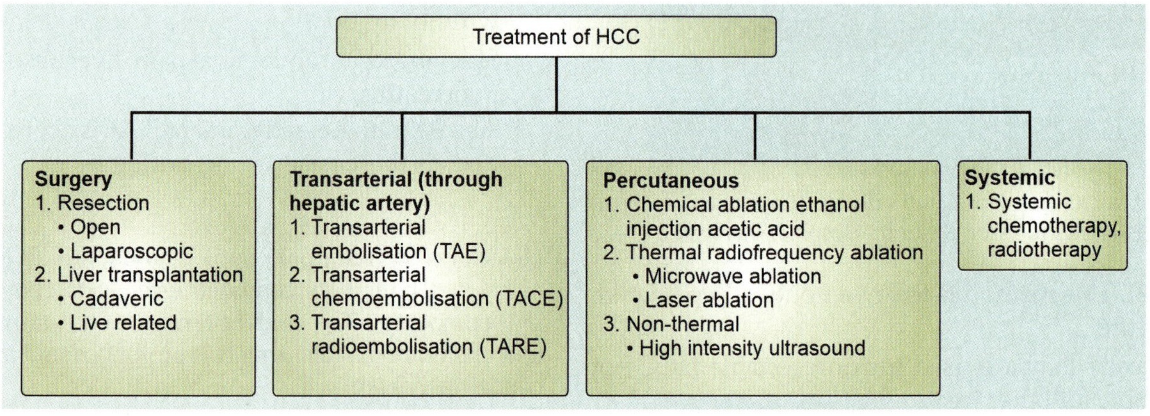

**TABLE 55.6:** Types of hepatic resections

| Hepatic resection | Nomenclature |
|---|---|
| 1. Resection along the main portal fissure, separating right and left lobes of the liver | • Right or left lobectomy |
| 2. Resection of entire right lobe and the medial segment of left lobe | • Right extended lobectomy or trisegmentectomy |
| 3. Removal of segments II and III | • Left lateral segmentectomy |
| 4. Removal of a single segment | • Unisegmentectomy |
| 5. Removal of 2 or more segments | • Plurisegmentectomy |
| 6. Removal of segments VI and VII | • Right lateral sectorectomy |
| 7. Removal of a small portion of liver, entirely within a single segment or transferring segmental plane | • Wedge resection |

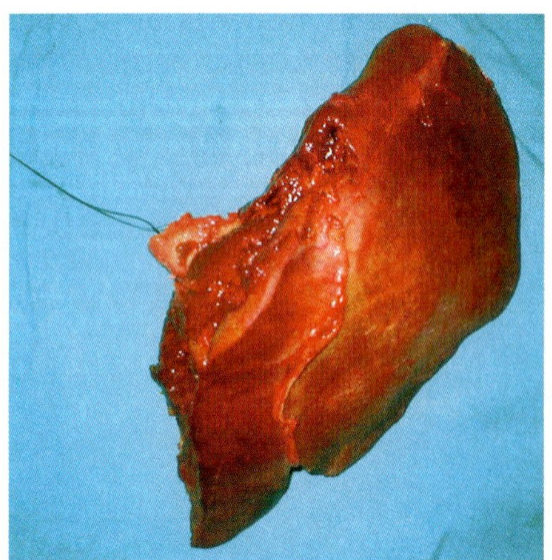

**Fig. 55.31:** Left lobectomy for cholangiocarcinoma. (*Courtesy*: Dr Ramesh Rajan, Associate Professor, Department of Surgical Gastroenterology, Trivandrum Medical College, Kerala)

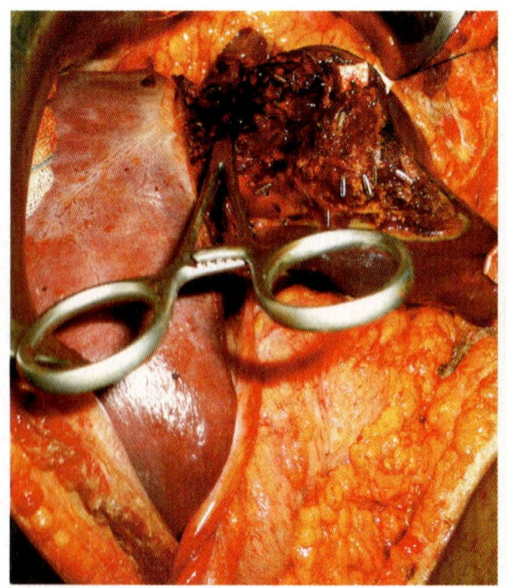

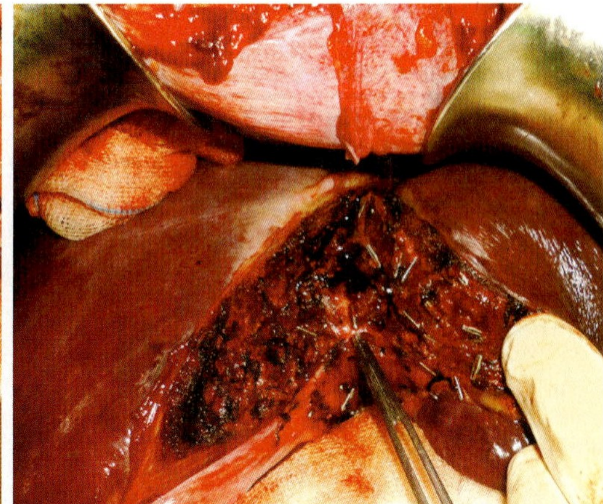

**Figs 55.32 and 55.33:** Liver resection for adenoma. (*Courtesy*: Dr Prasad Babu TLVD, Dr Ramcharan Thyagarajan, Dr Srikanth Gadiyaram, Prof Sadiq S Sikora, Department of GI Surgery, Manipal Hospital, Bengaluru, Karnataka)

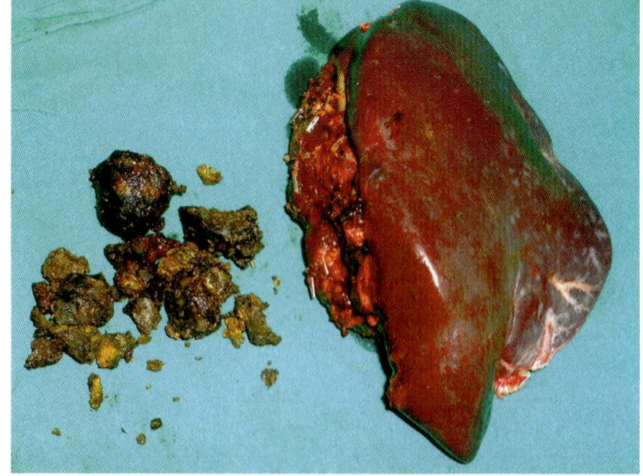

**Fig. 55.34:** Liver resection for Caroli's disease (*Courtesy*: Dr Nagaraj Palankar, Assistant Professor, Kasturba Hospital, Manipal)

**(TACE)**. This method is followed only as a palliative procedure.

- Basically they are used for unresectable HCC not suitable for other treatments.
- Most commonly used agents are doxorubicin, cisplatin and mitomycin.
- Contraindications are portal vein occlusion and poor liver function.

**Embolising agents:**

- Gel foam
- Chemotherapeutic agent (like doxorubicin) with or without lipiodol
- Side-effects are abdominal pain, liver abscess, acute pancreatitis, etc.
- As a definitive curative intent, TAE is not recommended, as there is no strong evidence.

*Pearls of Wisdom*

Lipiodol is derived from poppy seed oil. It is an iodinated ester. It is highly concentrated ester, gets concentrated by hepatocytes. The contact time between tumour cells and chemotherapeutic agents is prolonged and it leads to cancer cell death.

4. **Transarterial radioembolisation (TARE)**
- It is another option for unresectable HCC.
- It is called internal radiation.
- Most commonly used radioactive material is Yttrium-90 ($^{90}Y$).
- It emits β-radiation.
- It is delivered through feeding vessels of the tumour.
- Thus, any tumour, any size, any nodule can be irradiated.
- Survival is prolonged with this treatment.
- Can be used in cirrhotic patients of poor liver function.
- It is indicated in advanced disease, portal vein thrombosis.
- Thus, later resection or transplant can be option.

5. **Percutaneous ethanol ablation (PEA):** It is cheaper and is a palliative treatment. Tumour less than 3 cm and nodules not more than 3 are candidates. It reduces the tumour size and decreases pain.
   - Tumour necrosis occurs as a result of cellular dehydration denaturation of proteins and occlusion of small tumour vessels.
   - It requires 4–6 sessions under ultrasound guidance with 2–10 ml alcohol injection.
   - Injections are given on an outpatient basis. Easy to give because of the soft consistency of the tumour.

6. **Radiofrequency ablation (RFA)**
   - It is now being tried for inoperable tumours or patients who are not ideal candidates for surgery, as per Milan's criteria.
     **Indications:** Tumour deep in parenchyma, away from hilum and less than 3 cm.
   - Electrical energy (500 kHz) is delivered through a 18G needle inserted under US or CT guidance through the skin into the tumour. In the following few months, the tumour is destroyed and the cells are killed.
   - The route of insertion of this needle can be percutaneous, laparoscopic or by open route.
   - There should not be any evidence of extrahepatic disease preoperatively or intraoperatively.
   - **Mode of actions:** Cytodestruction of the tumour. In one sitting 6–7 cm of necrosis zone can be achieved for a 5 cm tumour.
   - In most cases a tumour can be adequately treated in one session. The procedure can also be repeated. It is done under general anaesthesia.
   - It is better to avoid RFA when the tumour is in the hilar plate wherein portal vein and the hepatic arterial branches enter the liver. Damage to these structures and bile duct can occur.
   - Thus, RFA is considered for small HCCs, CP grade A cirrhotic patients who are not candidates for resection and it is to be considered as bridging procedure before transplantation.

7. **Injection octreotide**, an analogue of somatostatin, has been used in advanced cases. It has shown promising results in decreasing the size of the tumour. It also reduces the pain and discomfort. This is combined with chemotherapy such as gemcitabine and carboplatin. However, the treatment is costly and results are temporary.

8. **Sorafenib** is the drug of choice in advanced HCC and with good liver function.
   - It is a multi-tyrosine kinase inhibitor.
   - It promotes apoptosis and inhibits angiogenesis.
   - These agents because of their mode of action, inhibit cell proliferation and thus control growth and improve survival. It also inhibits vascular endothelial growth factors (VEGF).
   - Thus, it is indicated in management of advanced HCC with good systemic function.
   - **Side effects:** Fatigue, skin rashes, hand-foot syndrome, hypertension, hair loss, itching.

## LIVER RESECTIONS

It should be the first choice in HCC, provided there is no extrahepatic disease or vascular invasion. After getting a negative margin, adequate functioning liver tissue should be present.

### Incision

- Aim of the incision is to get adequate exposure.
- A transverse abdominal incision in the right upper quadrant with a vertical extension to xiphoid process gives excellent exposure to the liver.

### Mobilisation of the Liver

- The key point is division of ligaments which are attached to it or which support the liver and suspend the liver.
- The falciform ligament is divided and followed along anterior surface of the liver.
- The left triangular ligament is divided by gentle pull on the left lobe of liver towards right side.
- The right triangular ligament is divided between diaphragm and right lobe of the liver by traction and countertraction.
- Lesser omentum is divided. Thus, separating the liver from stomach.
- Small multiple veins from the inferior surface of the liver join inferior vena cava. These should be divided.
- Lastly, hepatic veins are dissected and divided above renal veins.

### Hilar Dissection

- Cholecystectomy is done by ligating cystic artery and cystic duct. The CBD is then exposed at the free edge of lesser omentum. A sling is applied around CBD to isolate it and gently traction is applied.
- This visualises the common hepatic artery.
- By dissection of common hepatic artery, its right and left branches are dissected out.
- Slings are applied to these arteries, portal vein is exposed. This facilitates freeing of portal vein by dividing lymphatic tissues joining portal vein.
- The congenital anomalies such as aberrant right hepatic artery and accessory left hepatic artery also should be looked for.
- CBD, CHD, left and right hepatic ducts are exposed at the hilum.

### Division of the Parenchyma

- This requires ligation of artery or branch by 4/0 prolene, transfixation of the bile duct by 4/0 PDS and transfixation of portal vein with 4/0 prolene.
- Once the demarcation appears on the liver, parenchyma is divided by using diathermy.
- Cavitron ultrasonic surgical aspirator (CUSA) is the commonly used dissector for dividing liver parenchyma.
- Vessels and bile duct branches which are exposed are clipped or diathermised.
- Continue dissection till you reach hepatic veins/ branches. They are ligated or divided.

### Segmental and Local Resection

- Since each segment (*see* segmental anatomy) carries its own arterial supply, venous drainage and bile drainage, resection can be done with 1 cm margin.
- In a few cases, hilar dissection may not be necessary.

### Complications

- Intraoperative bleeding
- Biliary leakage
- Hepatic decompensation
- Ascites due to portal HTN, severing of lymphatics
- Infection

> **SU28.10.7:** Enumerate the clinical features, investigations and management of various types of secondaries in the liver.

## A CASE OF SECONDARIES IN THE LIVER

*Refer to Digital Content.*

## PORTAL HYPERTENSION

*Refer to Digital Content.*

## MISCELLANEOUS

*Refer to Digital Content.*

## MULTIPLE CHOICE QUESTIONS

1. **Which of the following statements is false about hepatic encephalopathy?**
   A. It is caused by ammonia
   B. Precipitated by sedatives
   C. Not precipitated by bleeding into gastrointestinal tract
   D. Precipitated by diuretics
2. **About hepatorenal syndrome following are true, *except*:**
   A. It can occur in sepsis
   B. Most of them have advanced liver disease
   C. It is associated with profuse intrarenal vasodilatation
   D. Orthotopic liver transplantation can reverse hepatorenal syndrome
3. **Which of the following is not the cause for overproduction of bilirubin?**
   A. Total parenteral nutrition
   B. Haemolytic anaemias
   C. Blood transfusion
   D. Gilbert's syndrome
4. **Triad of Sandblom includes the following, *except*:**
   A. Colicky abdominal pain
   B. Obstructive jaundice
   C. Haematemesis or melaena
   D. Sepsis
5. **The following are indications for percutaneous method for drainage of pyogenic liver abscess, *except*:**
   A. Superficial abscesses
   B. Abscess with no intra-abdominal pathology
   C. Abscesses of unknown aetiology
   D. Multiple abscesses
6. **Very tender liver is a feature of the following, *except*:**
   A. Secondaries in the liver
   B. Amoebic liver abscess
   C. Hepatoma
   D. Congestive cardiac failure
7. **A differentiating feature of amoebic liver abscess from acute cholecystitis is:**
   A. Intercostal tenderness
   B. Abdominal tenderness
   C. Guarding
   D. Fever
8. **The drug of choice for the treatment of amoebic liver abscess is:**
   A. Penicillin
   B. Gentamicin
   C. Metronidazole
   D. Cotrimoxazole
9. **The following are scolicidal agents, *except*:**
   A. Hypertonic saline
   B. Chlorhexidine
   C. Sodium hypochlorite
   D. Hydroxyethyl starch
10. **Indications for PAIR in the treatment of hydatid cyst includes:**
    A. Relapse following surgery
    B. Multiple septal divisions
    C. Communicating cysts
    D. Dead or inactive cysts
11. **The following feature is true about *Echinococcus multilocularis*, *except*:**
    A. Alveolar echinococcosis
    B. Causes malignancy
    C. Poorly demarcated honeycombed cystic lesion
    D. Infiltrates liver and invades vascular system
12. **A 65-year-old patient presents with the following: Serum bilirubin: 4 mg%, serum albumin: 1.8 mg%, INR: 2. He has gross ascites and is drowsy. What Child-Pugh Class does he belong to?**
    A. A B. B
    C. C D. D
13. **The following are features of polycystic liver disease, *except*:**
    A. They are usually asymptomatic
    B. The cysts do not produce liver cell failure
    C. They are acquired
    D. Cysts also occur in kidneys and pancreas
14. **Which of the following is the commonest benign tumour of the liver?**
    A. Haemangioma
    B. Adenoma
    C. Focal nodular hyperplasia
    D. Hepatoma
15. **For purposes of hepatic resection, the liver can be divided into ______ number of segments.**
    A. 2 B. 4
    C. 6 D. 8
16. **The main portal fissure is also called:**
    A. Cantlie's line
    B. Murphy's line
    C. Spigelian line
    D. Macewen's line

**17. The following conditions are associated with increased risk of hepatocellular carcinoma, *except*:**
A. Hepatitis B carrier state
B. Cirrhosis
C. Malignant hydatid cyst
D. Aflatoxin consumption

**18. Up to ______ segments of the liver can be resected safely without the danger of hepatic failure provided rest of the liver is normal.**
A. 2 B. 3
C. 4 D. 5

**19. Transcatheter arterial embolisation is a good option in the treatment of hepatocellular carcinoma in following situation:**
A. Serum bilirubin >3 mg%
B. Tumour thrombus in the main portal trunk
C. Early hepatocellular carcinoma
D. Inoperable tumours

**20. Which of the following is true criteria for secondaries in the liver?**
A. Single lobe enlargement
B. Rounded border
C. Soft in consistency
D. Nodular liver

**21. Commonest gastrointestinal tract primary in a nodular liver secondaries is from:**
A. Stomach B. Pancreas
C. Gallbladder D. Duodenum

**22. Portal hypertension is defined as a portal venous pressure exceeding _____ mmHg.**
A. 5 B. 10
C. 15 D. 20

**23. Portal vein normally carries _______ % of blood supply to liver.**
A. 25 B. 50
C. 75 D. 100

**24. Causes of bulky secondaries include the following, *except*:**
A. Malignant melanoma
B. Carcinoid tumours
C. Colloid carcinoma rectum
D. Testicular tumours

**25. Which of the following is true about the use of vasopressin in variceal bleeding?**
A. 20 units is diluted in 200 ml of saline and given over 20 min
B. Causes coronary vasodilatation
C. Is a powerful inotrope
D. Is a splanchnic vasodilator and reduces pressure in the splanchnic vessels

**26. Gastric transection of Tanner is an operation performed for:**
A. Carcinoma stomach
B. Carcinoma pancreas
C. Portal hypertension
D. Hepatocellular carcinoma

**27. About sorafenib following are true, *except*:**
A. It is tyrosine kinase inhibitor
B. It has anti-angiogenesis property
C. Vascular endothelial growth factor is inhibited by sorafenib
D. It is not a drug for hepatocellular carcinoma

**Answers**

| | | | | | | | | | |
|---|---|---|---|---|---|---|---|---|---|
| 1. D | 2. C | 3. A | 4. D | 5. D | 6. A | 7. A | 8. C | 9. D | 10. A |
| 11. B | 12. C | 13. C | 14. A | 15. D | 16. A | 17. C | 18. B | 19. D | 20. D |
| 21. A | 22. C | 23. C | 24. D | 25. A | 26. C | 27. D | | | |

Chapter

56

# Spleen

- Surgical anatomy
- Functions of the spleen
- Congenital abnormalities
- Rupture of the spleen
- Complications of splenectomy
- Idiopathic thrombocytopaenic purpura
- Hereditary spherocytosis
- Acquired autoimmune haemolytic anaemia
- Thalassaemia
- Sickle cell anaemia
- Splenectomy for other conditions
- Splenic artery aneurysm
- Hairy cell leukaemia
- Overwhelming postsplenectomy infection
- Interesting 'most common' for spleen

## INTRODUCTION

Diseases of the spleen and causes of enlargement of the spleen are a great concern for physicians. Dozens of differential diagnoses of splenomegaly are being taught in medicine. However, a surgeon's role in the treatment of an enlarged spleen is minimal. However, it is he **who does this 'magic' of removing** the spleen within minutes and saves the life of a patient with a ruptured spleen. A surgeon plays a major role by **treating hypersplenism with splenectomy**. In this chapter, only topics related to surgeon's interest are dealt with. Other topics are mentioned briefly.

## SURGICAL ANATOMY (Fig. 56.1)

**SU28.11:** Describe the applied anatomy of spleen.

The spleen is an anatomically small organ, hidden underneath the **9**th to **11**th ribs (dull note on percussion) measuring 1 × 3 × 5 inches and weighing about 7 oz (80–300 g). It lies in intimate contact with the under-surface of the diaphragm. This explains why a splenic abscess can rupture through the diaphragm causing empyema. When blood collects due to splenic injury, it irritates the diaphragm causing referred pain to the shoulder tip (**Kehr's sign**).

The **anterior border** is **notched** and is in contact with the stomach. It is enclosed by the **gastrocolic omentum**. The surgical importance of this is that when traction is applied on the stomach during vagotomy, a splenic capsular tear can occur, resulting in bleeding. The **two leaves** of gastrocolic omentum pass backwards in front of the kidney forming the **lienorenal ligament** (Fig. 56.2). This ligament is responsible for some part of the posterior fixation of the spleen. When this ligament is divided, the spleen can be brought to the surface of the wound during splenectomy.

The inferior part of the **hilum** of the spleen is (just) in contact with the **tail of the pancreas**. Often, during an emergency splenectomy, the tail of pancreas can get injured, resulting in a pancreatic fistula (Figs 56.2 and 56.3).

### Splenic Parenchyma

- It is **highly vascular**.
- Splenic pulp has red pulp and white pulp.
- **Red pulp** is a honeycombed vascular space which is made up of cords of reticular cells and sinuses.
- **White pulp consists of lymphatic tissue** and lymphoid follicles containing lymphocytes, plasma cells and macrophages.

### Blood Supply

- **Arterial supply:** Splenic artery is a branch of celiac artery. At the hilum of the spleen, it divides into 4–5 trabecular arteries and then branches into central arteries. Central arteries pass through white pulp and give radial branches to periphery including distal red pulp. Anatomical knowledge of these branches helps when performing partial splenectomy for ruptured spleen. (The blood flow rate through spleen is about 300 ml/min.)

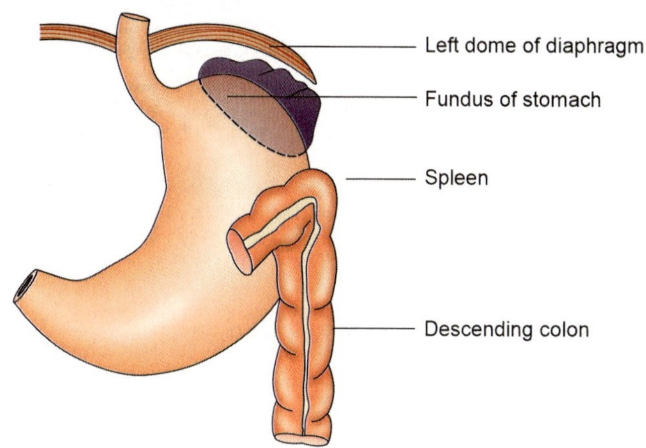


**Fig. 56.1:** Location of the spleen in relation to the fundus of the stomach and the diaphragm

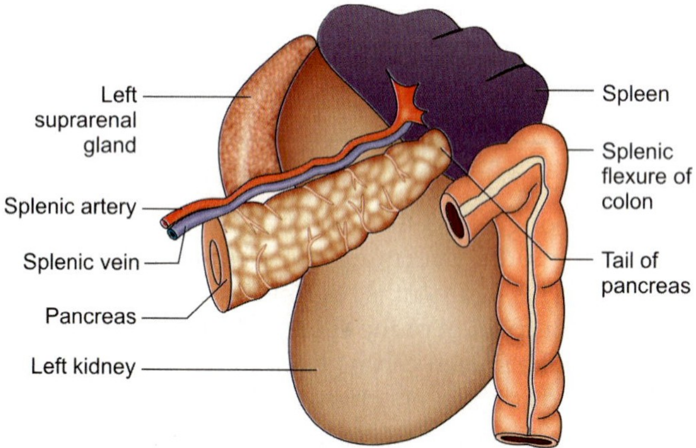


**Fig. 56.2:** Visceral relations of the spleen



**Fig. 56.3:** Peritoneal ligaments attached to the spleen and common sites of accessory spleen

- Spleen has 3–7 segments and each has its own vascular supply. Splenic artery divides into larger superior artery and smaller inferior artery. ***Lacerations of the spleen parallel to segmental vessels*** result in minimal haemorrhage. Lacerations perpendicular to the segments result in significant haemorrhage.
- In children, splenic capsule is thick and more tolerant to damage. Hence majority of the children with blunt abdominal trauma to the spleen are managed by conservative/non-operative treatment.
- **Venous drainage:** Four to five branches of the vein join and form the splenic vein. This forms the portal vein by joining with superior mesenteric vein behind the 2nd part of the duodenum.

### Lymphatic Drainage

The lymph drains into hilar nodes, then into retro-pancreatic nodes and finally into celiac nodes. Since it has intimate contact with the fundus of the stomach and tail of the pancreas, spleen also used to be removed (nowadays not done) along with the stomach and tail of the pancreas during radical gastrectomy and distal pancreatectomy.

## FUNCTIONS OF THE SPLEEN

1. **Destruction:** The process of removal of abnormal aged, damaged red blood cells is called *culling*. *Culling*, the Greek word, implies sorting a collection of two groups: One that will be kept and the other that will be rejected. For example, spherocytes, in hereditary, spherocytosis are broken down in spleen. This happens in red pulp.
2. **Production:** Production of lymphocytes, monocytes and plasma cells. Lymphopoiesis continues throughout life. Lymphocytes take part in immune response of the body.
3. **Antibody production:** Spleen synthesises antibodies in its white pulp. It removes antibody-coated bacteria and antibody-coated blood cells via blood and lymph node circulation.
4. **Immune response:** White pulp is composed of Malpighian corpuscles. They are composed of B lymphocytes and T lymphocytes—which are in periarteriolar lymphoid sheaths (PALS). Thus white pulp plays a major role in active immune response through humoral and all mediated pathways.
5. **Reservoir of platelets:** It is a storehouse of platelets, which are released into circulation in an emergency situation. Thus when spleen is enlarged, 80% of the platelets are sequestrated resulting in thrombocytopenia.

*Pearls of Wisdom*

Splenomegaly typically involves expansion of red pulp.

6. **Immune function:** It is the major site for synthesis of tuftsin, a peptide that stimulates phagocytic activity of leucocytes. Opsonins are antibodies produced by spleen against bacteria and fungi.

7. **Removal:** Heinz bodies, Howell-Jolly bodies, etc. are removed from RBCs. These cells are non-deformable intracellular substances.
8. **Erythrocyte production:** During foetal development, white and red blood cells production occur till 5th month of gestation. In adults, in case of myelofibrosis, erythopoiesis can occur.

## CONGENITAL ABNORMALITIES

1. **Accessory spleens: Splenunculi:** They are found in about 10–20% of the population.
   - They can be found near the hilum of spleen, tail of pancreas, splenic ligaments or in the mesocolon.
   - In diseases of the spleen (haemolytic anaemia, thrombocytopenic purpura), all these accessory spleens have to be removed along with spleen.
2. **Splenic agenesis** is rare.
3. **Polysplenia** is rare. It occurs due to failure of splenic fusion.
4. **Wandering spleen** is due to loose ligaments. It is more vulnerable for torsion.
5. **Hamartoma:** Rare, small masses of 1 cm in diameter. It may be in lymphoid tissue also (Hamartoma = misfire).

## RUPTURE OF THE SPLEEN

> **SU28.1.1:** Describe the clinical features, investigations and principles of management of splenic injuries.

### CAUSES

- **Blunt injury abdomen**
  - Injury to the left side of chest, left lower rib fractures, due to fall from a tree, road traffic accidents can be associated with splenic rupture.
  - Retroperitoneal haemorrhage, fracture spine and renal injuries may be associated with splenic injury.
- **Penetrating injuries** to the abdomen may cause **rupture of spleen**.
- **Spontaneous** rupture of the spleen is seen in malaria and infectious mononucleosis, rarely in sarcoidosis, haemolytic anaemia and leukaemia.
- **Iatrogenic:** Splenic capsule may be torn during surgical procedures such as vagotomy or gastrectomy due to traction on the stomach.

### TYPES OF INJURIES

Most of these injuries are diagnosed by CT scan today (CT classification is given).

1. **Subcapsular haematoma:** A capsular tear or parenchymal tear results in subcapsular haematoma.
2. **Clean (incised wounds):** This can happen in sharp injuries, Staal injuries (not common) or operative injuries.
3. **Lacerated wounds:** Often they are multiple as in blunt injuries abdomen.
4. **Hilar injuries** with **pedicle avulsion** are the most serious injuries. Need urgent laparotomy and ligation of bleeders and splenectomy. Otherwise, death will occur.
5. **Splenic injury** with other organs. Tail of pancreas, diaphragm, left kidney, left colon.

### Splenic Injury CT Scan Grading (Fig. 56.4)

**Grade I:** Nonexpanding subcapsular haematoma <10% surface area
Nonbleeding capsular laceration with <2 cm deep parenchymal involvement.

**Grade II:** Nonexpanding subcapsular haematoma 10–50% surface area.
Nonexpanding intraparenchymal haematoma <2 cm diameter
Bleeding capsular tear or parenchymal laceration 1–3 cm deep

**Grade III:** Expanding subcapsular haematoma or intraparenchymal.
Bleeding subcapsular haematoma or subcapsular haematoma >50% surface area
Intraparenchymal haematoma >2 cm
Parenchymal laceration >3 cm deep

**Grade IV:** Ruptured intraparenchymal haematoma with active bleeding.
Laceration involving segmental or renal vessel >25% spleen volume devascularised.

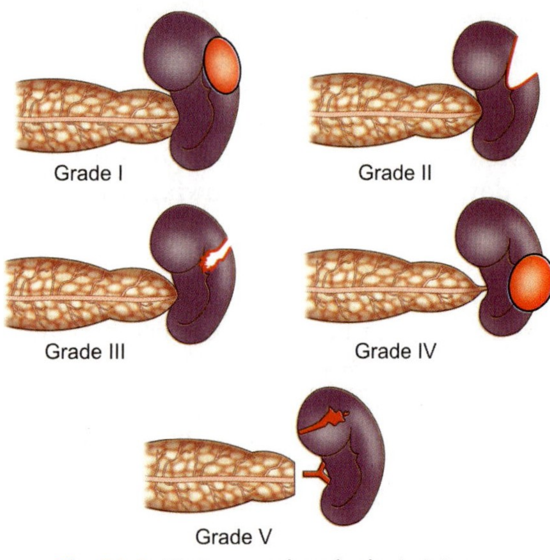

**Fig. 56.4:** Various grades of splenic injury

**Grade V:** Completely shattered or avulsed spleen. Hilar laceration which devascularises entire spleen.

## CLINICAL PRESENTATION

It can be divided into three groups:

1. **Tearing of splenic vessels:** Avulsion of splenic pedicle can result in severe haemorrhage and shock. Death can occur within a few minutes. Even in the best of the situations, death cannot be prevented often.
2. **A slow developing haemorrhagic shock** followed by recovery. Examination reveals evidence of intraperitoneal bleeding. This can occur due to a capsular tear or injury to the splenic parenchyma. Its clinical features are as follows:
   - Anaemia—pallor
   - Pulse—tachycardia, more than 100/min
   - BP—low/hypotension
   - Cold, clammy extremities
   - Abdominal distension
   - Paralytic ileus develops slowly
   - Guarding and rigidity
   - **Kehr's sign** is positive. Irritation of undersurface of the diaphragm by the blood causes irritation of phrenic nerve (C3, 4). Thus, this pain is referred to shoulder region (supraclavicular nerve C4).

> *Pearls of Wisdom*
>
> Kehr's sign can be elicited by elevation of the foot end of bed for about 10 minutes.

   - **Ballance's sign:** Blood in the vicinity of spleen is fresh blood which is coagulated and blood in the periphery is not coagulated. Hence, there will not be shifting dullness on the left side of the abdomen but can be present on the right side.
   - **Saegesser's splenic point of tenderness:** An area of tenderness on the left side between sternomastoid and scalenus medius (rare sign).
3. **Initial features of haemorrhagic shock, recovery and sudden haemorrhagic shock** after a few hours to a few days. It is due to the following reasons:
   - Greater omentum seals off a tear which gets reopened after some time. Time period is called **"latent period of Baudet"**.
   - A subcapsular haematoma which had developed, ruptures after some time.
   - Associated injury to the tail of pancreas causes release of enzymes which digests the tissues at a later date. This variety is called "delayed type of shock" or delayed rupture of spleen.

> *Pearls of Wisdom*
>
> In polytrauma, if a hypotensive patient responds to intravenous fluids, it is a hypovolaemic shock. Head injury is rarely a cause of hypovolaemic shock.

## COMPLICATIONS OF SPLENIC INJURIES

1. Haemorrhagic shock—if not treated—multiorgan failure results.
2. Disseminated intravascular coagulation due to massive bleeding and blood transfusion.
3. Injuries to the tail of pancreas—manifesting later as pancreatic ascites, pancreatic fistula or pseudocyst of pancreas.
4. Splenic artery pseudoaneurysm.
5. Splenic arteriovenous fistula.

## INVESTIGATIONS

1. **Hb%** estimation, PCV (packed cell volume) estimation (however, in appropriate cases, it should be repeated at frequent intervals to detect continuing haemorrhage).
2. **Four quadrant tap/aspiration** by using a fine needle (23 gauge) demonstrates blood either fresh or old. However, diagnostic peritoneal lavage **(DPL)** is more reliable (*vide infra*).
3. **Emergency USG** can (FAST refer page 1141) reveal a splenic tear, a subcapsular haematoma and can rule out other injuries. It is the most important investigation in suspected cases of splenic injury.
4. CT scan is more reliable. It should be used in cases of doubtful diagnosis and stable patients.[1] It also rules out hollow viscus perforation, pancreatic injuries, etc. (Fig. 56.5).
5. **Diagnostic peritoneal lavage (DPL):** It is indicated in blunt injury abdomen where there are **equivocal signs** or **doubtful signs** of peritonitis.
   - **Indications:**
     - Unconscious patient with polytrauma with signs of abdominal injury.
     - Unexplained shock
     - Associated spinal cord injury
   - **Procedure** (Fig. 56.6):
     - A 1 cm incision is made in the subumbilical region under local anaesthesia (LA) after emptying the bladder. The peritoneum is opened and a 12 or 14 Fr peritoneal dialysis catheter is introduced into the peritoneal cavity.
     - The skin is closed and 1000 ml normal saline is allowed to flow over 30 minutes.

[1]Deaths have been reported in CT scan room, in unstable patients with haemoperitoneum.

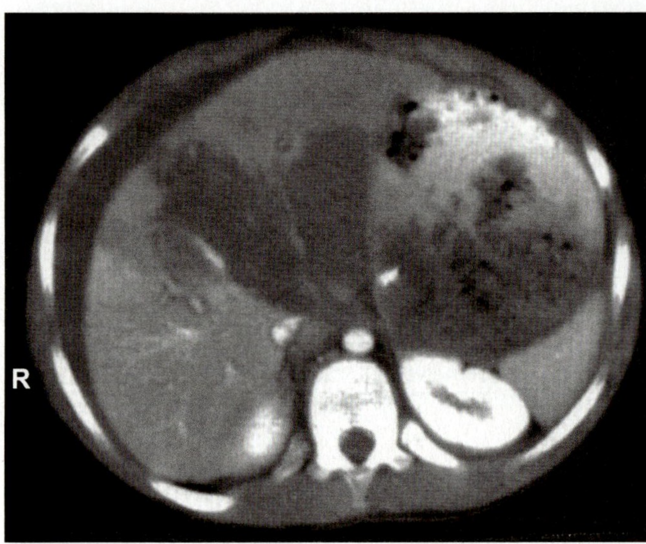


Fig. 56.5: CECT showing splenic and liver injuries

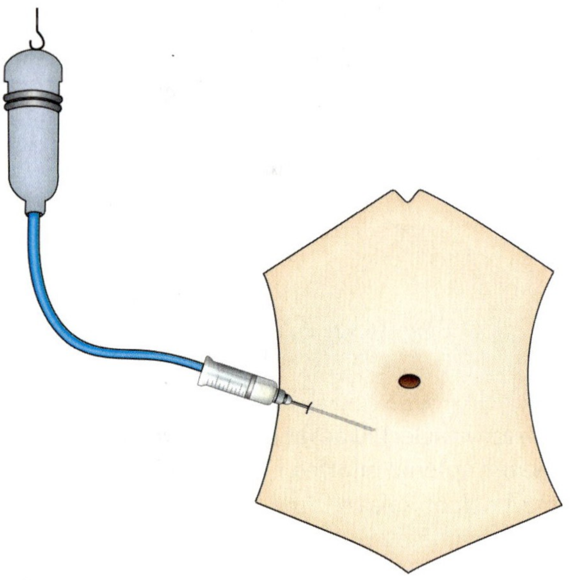

Fig. 56.6: Diagnostic peritoneal lavage

- The patient is turned to the right and left sides and fluid is allowed to flow out.

- **DPL is positive when:**
  1. Fresh blood of more than 20 ml is removed immediately after inserting dialysis catheter and it does not clot.
  2. RBC count 1,00,000/mm$^3$ or WBC >500/mm$^3$.
  3. Amylase level of over 175 units/dl.
  4. Bile, food or any other fresh contents.
  5. Gram stain is positive in the contents of lavage.
- Diagnostic accuracy is around 95%. DPL is useful to rule out intestinal injury in addition to intraperitoneal bleeding.

> *Pearls of Wisdom*
>
> DPL is more sensitive for mesenteric injury than CT scan. However, in early diagnosis of hollow viscus injuries, DPL is superior to CT scan. However, with the availability of ultrasound and CT scans, this investigation is rarely performed today.

6. **Plain X-ray abdomen**[1] erect **should not be done in an emergency situation** when patients are in shock. In suspected cases of perforation of hollow viscous (polytrauma) and only in stable patients, it can be done.

## TREATMENT (Key Box 56.1 and Fig. 56.7)

### 1. Emergency Splenectomy

- Haemodynamic instability is the main indication for emergency splenectomy. Blood pressure less than 90 mmHg and heart rate more than 130 per minute is a clear indication for surgery.

  When there is active bleeding with hypotension due to large lacerations, emergency splenectomy is the treatment of choice since it is quick, easy to perform and can be life-saving. The splenic artery is ligated first at the upper border of pancreas followed by splenic vein. In desperate situations, the spleen is mobilised by incising the lienorenal ligament, a large arterial clamp is applied at the splenic hilum and splenectomy is done (Fig. 56.8).

Key Box 56.1

**Treatment—4 Headings**

- Emergency splenectomy – Massive bleeding and unstable
- Splenorrhaphy – Stable
- Partial splenectomy – Stable
- Nonoperative – Stable patient

### 2. Partial Splenectomy (Fig. 56.9)

- It can be done because the splenic artery gives an **upper polar branch and a lower polar branch** which again divides into 2 branches. Hence, when one of the branches of splenic artery is ligated, the bleeding stops and a partial splenectomy can be done comfortably.
- After splenectomy, the spleen can be cut into multiple pieces and can be implanted within the greater omentum. The spleen survives because of neovascularisation and functions like a spleen in the production of antibodies. This can be done in children.

[1]Please do not make an unstable patient stand for the sake of X-ray. He may collapse due to hypotension.

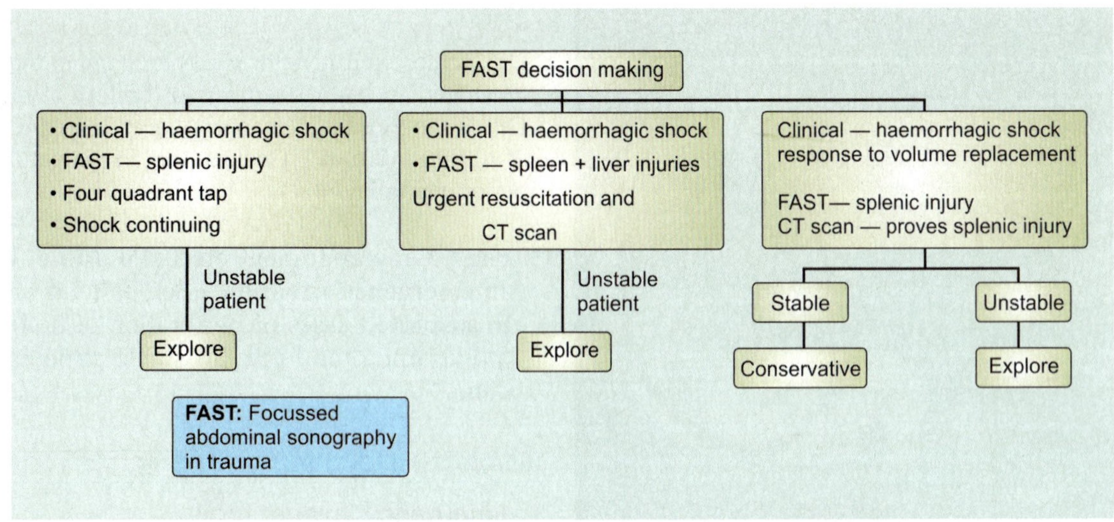


**Fig. 56.7:** Management of splenic rupture

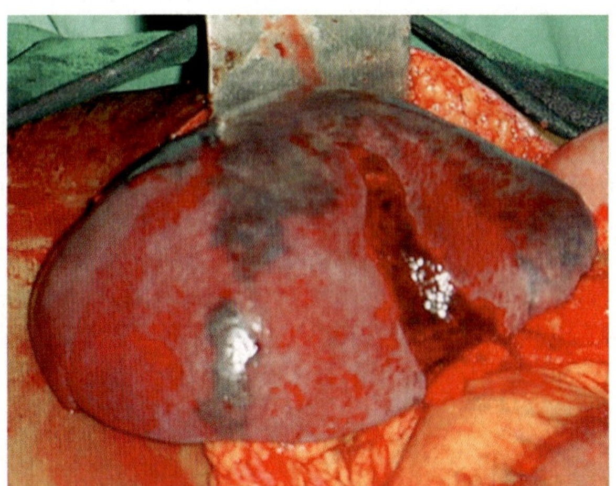

**Fig. 56.8:** Large laceration of the spleen

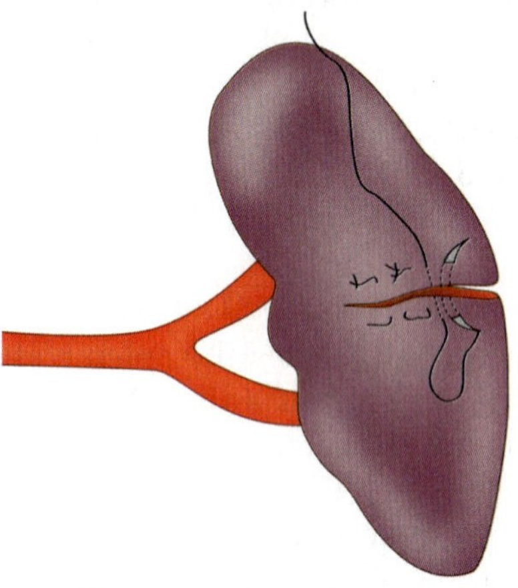

**Fig. 56.9:** Splenorrhaphy

### 3. Splenorrhaphy (Fig. 56.10)

- It is a method of preservation of spleen when the general condition of the patient is reasonably good.
- In this, a small tear is sutured by using chromic catgut and can be wrapped using greater omentum.

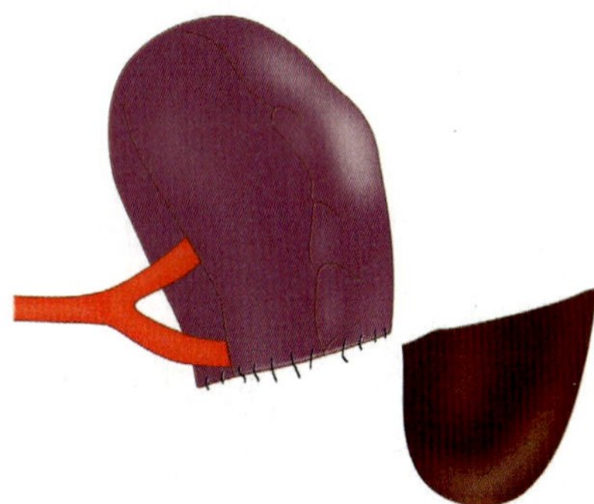

**Fig. 56.10:** Partial splenectomy

### 4. Nonoperative or Conservative Treatment

- It is safe in selected adult and paediatric patients with isolated splenic injuries.
- Small risk of delayed rupture should be explained to the patient (Key Box 56.2).

Key Box 56.2

**Nonoperative Treatment Patient Selection**

1. Haemodynamically stable patients after initial evaluation.
2. No other associated organ injuries which require laparotomy.
3. No extra-abdominal injuries which may preclude assessment of abdomen.
4. Facilities for emergency resuscitation, ultrasonography, CT scan should be available.
5. Patient must be willing for hospitalisation and close observation.
6. Regular monitoring by duty doctors, expert nursing staff who maintain hourly vital charts.

- Patients are admitted in intensive care unit. Serial monitoring of haemoglobin, total WBC counts are done. Abdominal girth and blood pressure are monitored. If there is any doubt of hypotension, exploration is done.

- While managing following patients, utmost care should be given with the non-operative treatment.
  1. Older patients above the age of 50
  2. Grade 3 and 4 injury
  3. More than 500 ml of blood detected by the CT scan
  4. Other solid organ injury (liver)
  5. Systemic vascular abnormalities, such as pseudoaneurysm or AV fistula, etc.

*Pearls of Wisdom*

If any vascular abnormalities are detected by CT scan, embolisation should be attempted first. In majority of the cases, bleeding will stop. If bleeding continues, they should be taken for splenectomy.

## EARLY: COMPLICATIONS OF SPLENECTOMY

1. **Pancreatic injury (0–6%):** Treated by drain placement and measuring drain amylase. Usually, it is a minor discharge, generally settles over a few days.
2. **Vascular injury (2–3%):** Slippage of ligature (splenic artery), hilar dissection, capsular tear during retraction. Needs to be identified and sutured or coagulated or clamped.
3. **Injury to bowel:** Colon, stomach. These can be avoided with careful dissection techniques. During ligation of short gastric arteries too close to the stomach side, injury to the stomach can occur. It is repaired in two layers. Colonic injury can occur during dissection to separate the lower pole. It is also repaired in the similar manner.
4. **Diaphragmatic injury:** This can happen when adhesions are present between spleen and diaphragm due to perisplenitis or recurrent infarctions. Simple suturing is enough, if recognised.
5. **Splenosis:** This refers to multiple small implants of splenic tissue on the peritoneal surface following traumatic rupture of spleen. They can give rise to adhesions.
6. **Pulmonary:** These are common complications. Generally get unnoticed. It can range from minor cough to atelectasis to pneumonia and pleural effusion. Basal atelectasis is one of the common causes of postoperative fever.
7. **Paralytic ileus:** Treated by drip and suction.
8. **Haematemesis** can occur due to congestion of the gastric mucosa as a result of ligation of the short gastric vessels.
9. **Subphrenic abscess:** Not common. If it occurs, percutaneous drainage and antibiotics (Fig. 56.11).
10. **Wound problems:** Haematomas, seromas and wound infection.
11. **Thrombocytosis and thrombotic complications:** Sometimes it can be dangerous. They can present as abdominal pain and vomiting which is confused for incision pain, gastritis, etc. Ultrasound examination is a must. One of our patients had portal vein thrombosis which was managed by anticoagulants. Platelet count after splenectomy was 8 lakh/mm$^3$.

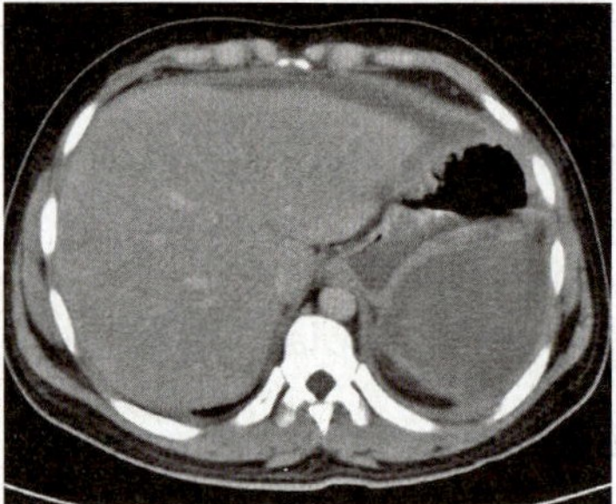

**Fig. 56.11:** Post-splenectomy large collection

## INDICATIONS FOR SPLENECTOMY

**I. Always indicated**

a. Primary splenic tumour
b. Hereditary spherocytosis

**II. Usually indicated**

a. Primary hypersplenism
b. Chronic ITP
c. Splenic vein thrombosis
d. Splenic abscess

**III. Sometimes indicated**

a. Splenic injury
b. Autoimmune haemolytic disease
c. Elliptocytosis haemolysis
d. Nonspherocytic congenital haemolytic anaemia
e. Hodgkin's disease with anaemia
f. Thrombotic thrombocytopenic purpura
g. Idiopathic myelofibrosis
h. Splenic artery aneurysm
i. Wiskott-Aldrich syndrome (Key Box 56.3)
j. Gaucher's disease.

Key Box 56.3

**Wiskott-Aldrich Syndrome**

- X-linked disorder predominantly presents as features of thrombocytopenia such as epistaxis, bloody diarrhoea, petechiae in young age
- Combined 'B' and 'T' cell immunodeficiency causes eczema
- More incidence of malignancies
- Spleen destroys platelets count as low as 20,000 or 40,000 cells/microlitre
- The best treatment is human leukocytic antigen (HLA) matched sibling bone marrow transplantation
- Otherwise—splenectomy and antibiotics are the treatment of choice

**IV. Rarely indicated**

a. Chronic leukaemia
b. Thalassaemia major
c. Sickle cell anaemia
d. Felty's syndrome
e. Hairy cell leukaemia.

## HAEMATOLOGICAL INDICATIONS FOR SPLENECTOMY

### IDIOPATHIC THROMBOCYTOPENIC PURPURA (ITP)

- This condition occurs due to development of autoantibodies against patient's own platelets (Key Box 56.4).
- Normal levels of platelets are between 1,50,000 and 4,00,000 cells per $mm^3$.
- The spleen is probably responsible for sequestration of platelets and for production of antibodies.

Key Box 56.4

**Other Causes of Purpura**

- ↓ Production: Cytotoxic drugs, aplastic anaemia.
- ↑ Consumption of platelets: DIC as in septicaemia.
- ↑ Destruction: SLE, infectious mononucleosis.
- ↑ Capillary fragility: Steroid-induced or Henoch-Schönlein purpura.

#### Types

**Type 1:** Acute—children: Follows an acute infection and resolves spontaneously in about two months.

**Type 2:** Chronic—adults: Longer than six months. No cause is identified.

#### Clinical Features

- Condition is common in females, F : M :: 3 : 1.
- **Purpuric patches** (ecchymosis refers to skin discolouration due to extravasation of blood) are found on the buttocks and petechial haemorrhages (spots) are found on the limbs. These are **dependent areas** having high intravascular pressure (Figs 56.12 to 56.14).
- All types of haemorrhages are common and can be mild or moderate (Key Box 56.5).

Key Box 56.5

**Common Types of Haemorrhages**

- Epistaxis
- Menorrhagia
- Haematemesis
- Bleeding gums
- Haemarthrosis
- Haematuria

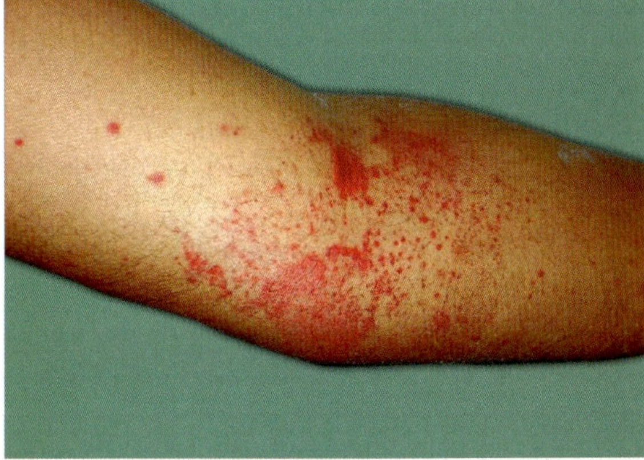

**Fig. 56.12:** Purpuric spots in the forearm

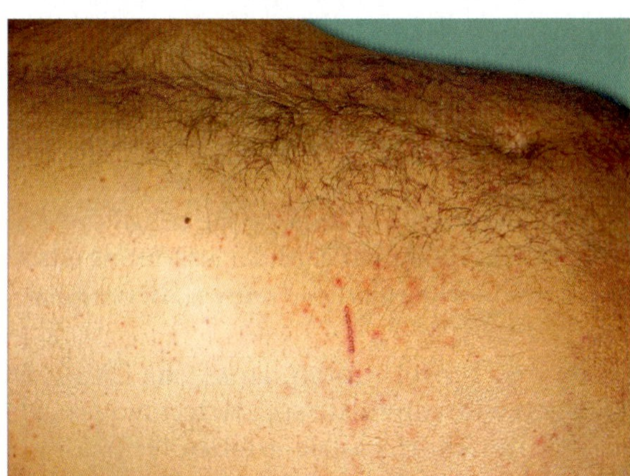

**Fig. 56.13:** Purpuric spots on the abdomen

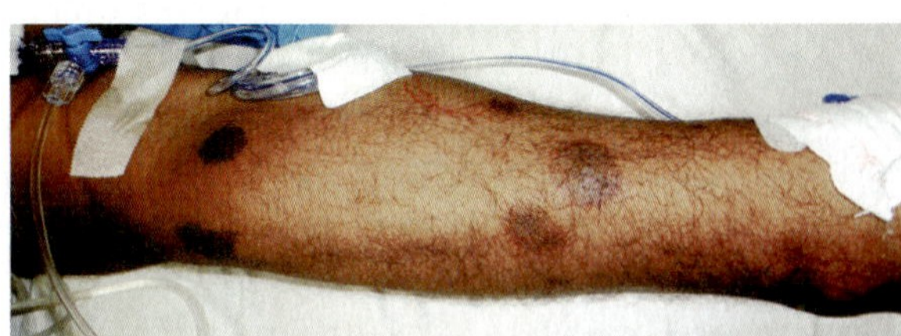

**Fig. 56.14:** Severe sepsis with thrombocytopenia

- Intracranial haemorrhage is found in 1–2% of patients but it may be the cause of death.
- In 25% of cases, the spleen is just palpable (small size).
- **Hess tourniquet test:** More than 20 petechiae in a circle of 3 cm diameter in cubital fossa suggests purpura.

*Pearls of Wisdom*

If the spleen is big, it is not ITP.

#### Investigations

- Bleeding time is prolonged in purpura. Clotting and prothrombin times are normal.
- Platelet count is reduced.
- Bone marrow biopsy: Precursors of platelets (megakaryocytes) are increased.

### Treatment

#### *In Children*

- Spontaneous regression occurs in majority of cases.
- Short course of corticosteroids is beneficial. Tablet prednisolone in the dose of 10 mg/day over a period of 6 weeks is given.

#### *In Adults*

**Splenectomy** is indicated in the following situations:

- ***When ITP has presented for more than 6–9 months.***
- ***When ITP has relapsed in spite of steroids,*** the patient is given a trial of prednisolone, 1 mg/kg/day. Platelet count rises within 7 days of starting steroids after which splenectomy can be done (Key Box 56.6).
- Also indicated, if a patient has two relapses on steroid therapy or if the platelet count is low.

Key Box 56.6

**Surgery in ITP**

- Can be done even when platelets are as low as 10,000 cells/mm$^3$.
- **Diathermy** is used to open layers of the abdomen.
- **Ligate splenic artery first** at the upper border of pancreas after opening lesser sac.
- **Splenectomy is not difficult. Accessory spleen** (15–30%), if present, should be **removed**.
- Platelet transfusion may be required postoperatively, if there is bleeding.
- **Two-thirds** of patients will be **cured** by surgery.
- 15% will show improvement.
- Remaining will not benefit.

### Results

70–80% of patients respond permanently and do not require any further treatment. Counts rise above 1,00,000/mm$^3$ in 7 days. Even if counts are not raised, recurrent bleeding rarely occurs.

### Haemolytic Anaemia

This type of anaemia results from an increased red cell destruction which occurs in the spleen. The lifespan of red blood cells is also shortened. Hence, irrespective of the cause of haemolytic anaemia, these cases can benefit from splenectomy. **Anaemia, jaundice** and **splenomegaly** are the triad of haemolytic anaemia.

#### *Causes of Haemolytic Anaemia*

1. Hereditary spherocytosis
2. Acquired autoimmune haemolytic anaemia
3. Thalassaemia
4. Sickle cell disease

## HEREDITARY SPHEROCYTOSIS

This hereditary disorder is transmitted by either parent as Mendelian autosomal dominant. The disease is characterised by a **defect in cell wall protein of the red cell, namely spectrin,** which increases reflux of sodium into the cell. This causes the biconcave red cell to swell and become spherical. Hence, the name spherocytosis.

### Consequences of Spherocytes in Circulation

1. The spherocyte is already weak. Adding onto this, there is a greater loss of membrane phospholipid which results in a delicate fragile spherocyte.
2. Because of the altered shape, **oxygen and energy requirements of RBCs increase which cannot be met by the spleen**. In the spleen, they are destroyed and release excessive haemoglobin which is converted into bilirubin.
   - The amount of bilirubin produced is increased and most of it is unconjugated. It gets attached to albumin as it is **lipid soluble** and, therefore, cannot be excreted in the urine. Hence, this type of jaundice is also known as acholuric jaundice.

*Pearls of Wisdom*

Most of this bilirubin is excreted in the biliary tree resulting in pigment stones in the biliary tree.

### Clinical Features (Figs 56.15 to 56.18)

- Commonly seen in young children but can manifest in adults also.
- Seen equally in both sexes.
- History of recurrent attacks of jaundice can be elicited from childhood.
- Jaundice is mild, never deep, not associated with itching or bradycardia.
- **Pallor** is an important feature due to destruction of the red cells.
- **Acute haemolytic crisis:** It is precipitated by an acute infection or stress. Abdominal pain, nausea, vomiting, pyrexia and pallor are the features. The condition can be confused for an abdominal emergency. In severe cases, anaemia, thrombocytopenia, leukopaenia can occur.
- **Spleen is moderately enlarged.** The liver is also palpable in a few cases.
- In adults, **gallstone colic** and obstructive jaundice due to **CBD** stone can also complicate the disease process. Incidence of gallstone disease is around 50%. **It is common after the age of 10.**
- Leg ulcers may occur as a result of anaemia.

*Pearls of Wisdom*

Young, pale, jaundiced, fatigued child with gallstones—think of hereditary spherocytosis.

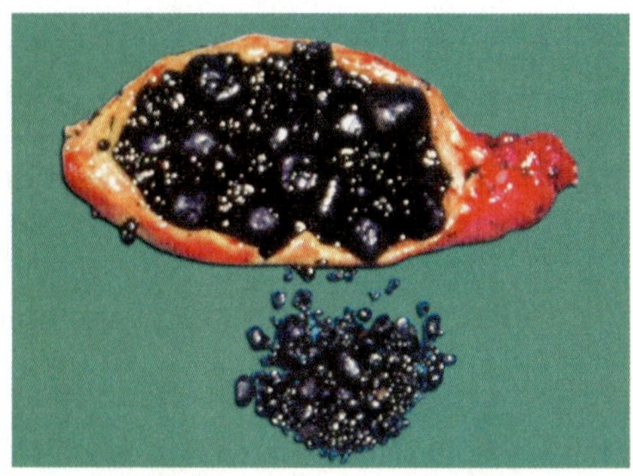

Fig. 56.15: Pigment stones

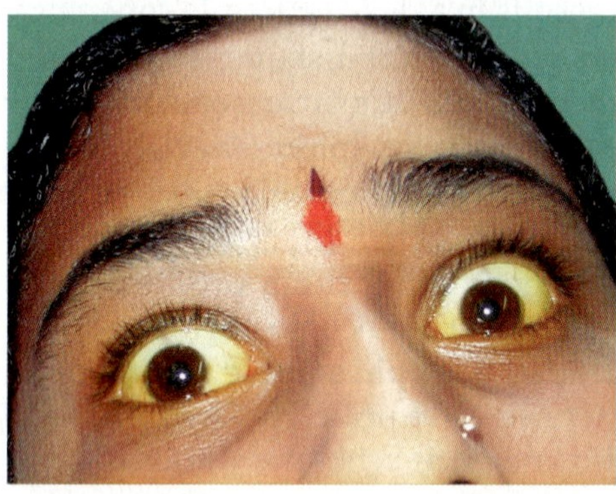

Fig. 56.16: Case of hereditary spherocytosis with faint jaundice in a 22-year-old girl

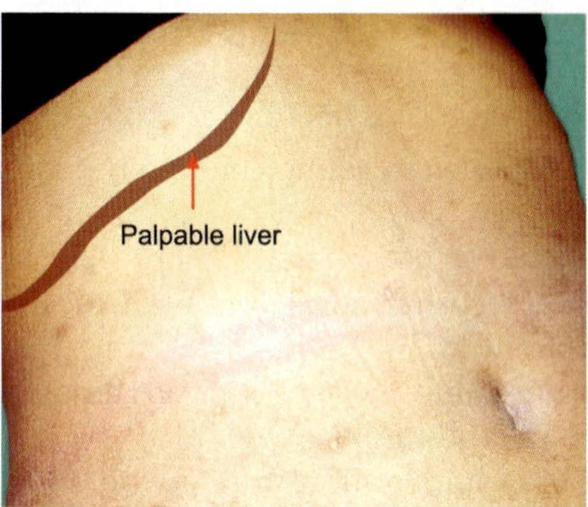


Fig. 56.17: She also had 2 cm enlarged liver and gallstones

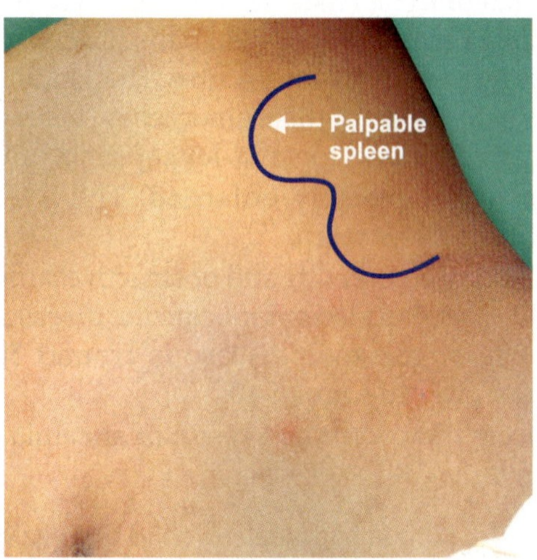


Fig. 56.18: Splenomegaly—its size was 5 cm

### Investigations

1. **Peripheral smear: Spherocytes** are present.
2. **Reticulocyte count is increased (15–25%):** These are immature red cells which are discharged by the bone marrow due to loss of red cells.
3. **Coombs' test is negative:** Serum bilirubin is mildly elevated and most of it is unconjugated.
4. **Fragility test:** Normal red cell haemolysis occurs in **0.47%** saline solution. Here, it occurs at **0.6%** or even in weaker solution.
5. **Ultrasound** abdomen is done to rule out gallstones.

### Treatment

**Splenectomy is the treatment** including removal of accessory spleen.

- Ideally, it should be done from the age of 6 to 10 years. Why after 6 years? The incidence of post-splenectomy sepsis is more when splenectomy is done within 6 years of age. Why before 10 years? After 10 years of age, the incidence of gallstone increases.

**Splenectomy** helps in the following ways (Figs 56.16 to 56.18)

1. By decreasing erythrocyte destruction, anaemia improves, thus avoiding blood transfusions.
2. Erythrocytes achieve normal lifespan. Hence, jaundice also disappears.
3. Leg ulcers heal quickly.
   - If gallstones are also found in these cases, laparoscopic splenectomy and cholecystectomy can be done in the same sitting.

*Pearls of Wisdom*

Hereditary elliptocytosis is also a genetic disorder wherein RBCs are oval in shape. It also responds to splenectomy.

## ACQUIRED AUTOIMMUNE HAEMOLYTIC ANAEMIA

Due to an autoimmune reaction, the red cell surface is damaged and it gets destroyed in the splenic red pulp. Antibodies develop against red cell antigens. In 50% of cases, the cause is not known. The following are the probable causes:

- SLE, lymphoma, chronic lymphocytic leukaemia
- Drugs: Methyldopa, mefenamic acid
- Exposure to chemicals or infections.

### Clinical Features

- More common in females after 50 years of age.
- Splenomegaly, moderate in size.
- Gallstones are found in around 25% of the cases.

### Investigations

- Anaemia is present.

- Spherocytes may be present because of damage to the red cell surface.
- Coombs' test is positive.

### Treatment

- It is a self-limiting disorder. Reassurance plays an important role.
- **Corticosteroids:** A short course of prednisolone 60 mg/day is given.
- Splenectomy is done when steroid response is not satisfactory. ***80% of patients respond to splenectomy.***

## THALASSAEMIA

It is also called Cooley's anaemia, Mediterranean anaemia, Heinz body haemolytic anaemia.

### Aetiopathogenesis

- It is a hereditary disorder, transmitted as a **dominant trait.** It is characterised by a defect in haemoglobin peptide chain synthesis. Depending on type of peptide chain involvement, it is classified into α, β and γ. However, β-thalassaemia is more common. There is a decrease in haemoglobin and red cells will be destroyed prematurely due to intracellular precipitates **(Heinz bodies)**.
- When it is a heterozygous disorder, it is called beta-thalassaemia minor and when homozygous, it is called beta-thalassaemia major (Cooley's anaemia). **The abnormal gene is inherited from either or both the parents**.

### Clinical Features

- Severe anaemia resulting in weakness, lethargy, leg ulcers, etc.
- Splenomegaly is mild to moderate in size. Sometimes, it is massive resulting in abdominal discomfort or may cause abdominal distension.
- Jaundice due to haemolysis. Liver can also be enlarged.
- To compensate for anaemia, bone marrow hyperplasia occurs resulting in bossing of skull and prominent malar bones. Thalassaemia major usually manifests in the first year of life.

### Complications

1. **Haemosiderosis** (deposition of iron in tissues) of pancreas results in chronic pancreatitis and diabetes.
2. **Hepatic cirrhosis** due to liver haemosiderosis.
3. **Aplastic crisis** with severe life-threatening infections.
4. **Gallstones** occur in about 20% of cases.

### Investigations

- Peripheral smear demonstrates microcytic hypochromic anaemia. Red cells are small, thin and are resistant to osmotic lysis.
- Haemoglobin electrophoresis reveals reduction or absent levels of haemoglobin A (HbA). There is a compensatory increase in foetal haemoglobin (HbF).

### Treatment

- **Blood transfusion:** Multiple repeated transfusions may be necessary.
- **Surgical:** Splenectomy is indicated in a few cases who require multiple transfusions and patients with gross splenomegaly.

## SICKLE CELL ANAEMIA OR SICKLE CELL DISEASE

This is a hereditary haemolytic disorder in which haemoglobin A is replaced by haemoglobin S (HbS). This results in crescent-shaped erythrocytes. This HbS molecule crystallises, if there is hypoxia, strenuous work or due to dehydration. As a result of this, red cells are distorted and elongated. Therefore, blood viscosity is increased, causing obstruction in the splenic circulation (Key Box 56.7).

Key Box 56.7

**Functional Abnormalities in Sickle Cell Anaemia**

- Spleen sometimes acts as a large reservoir for red cells and the sickle cells are destroyed.
- Antibody production is decreased.
- Spleen's ability to filter *Streptococcus pneumoniae* is reduced.

### Effect of HbS Blockage

- Splenic microinfarcts
- Splenomegaly or **autosplenectomy** due to repeated infarcts (Fig. 56.19).

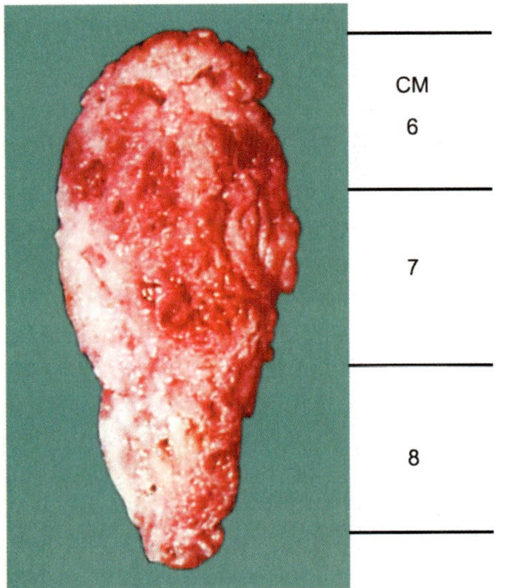


**Fig. 56.19:** Sickle cell anaemia—Nugget spleen (3 cm size). An example for autosplenectomy

### Clinical Features

- The disease is very common in Africans. Most of the patients in India have high HbF levels which protect HbS. Hence, symptoms are not seen in the first few weeks.
- Abdominal pain is due to recurrent infarcts or due to gallstone in a few patients.
- Skin ulcers occur due to anaemia or hypoxia.

*Pearls of Wisdom*

Microinfarction of carpal and tarsal bones resulting in bony pains is described as hand-foot syndrome.

### Investigations

- Peripheral smear demonstrates sickle cell.
- Haemoglobin electrophoresis to identify the type of haemoglobin.

### Treatment

- Folic acid supplements
- Splenectomy has a doubtful value. It is indicated only when excessive numbers of RBCs are sequestrated causing anaemia (Table 56.1 for comparison).

### Complications

- Infarct of cerebrum resulting in hemiplegia.
- Mesenteric infarction resulting in gangrene of the bowel.
- Pulmonary infarction resulting in chest pain.

## SPLENECTOMY FOR OTHER CONDITIONS

### HYPERSPLENISM

It is defined as pancytopaenia in the presence of normal or hypercellular bone marrow. Following are the causes of hypersplenism:

It usually involves red pulp expansion. It must be remembered that in cirrhosis of the liver, 15% of patients develop hypersplenism. Anaemia and thrombocytopenia are mild. Rarely requires splenectomy (a few causes are given below):

- **Tropical splenomegaly** due to malaria, kala-azar or schistosomiasis, etc. Since these diseases are endemic in tropical countries, it is called tropical splenomegaly. Gross enlargement of the spleen and hypersplenism are indications for splenectomy in such cases.
- **Myeloproliferative disorders:** Splenectomy reduces need for transfusion and may relieve abdominal discomfort.
- **Portal hypertension:** Maximum benefit is in segmental portal hypertension with oesophagogastric varices (Fig. 56.20).
- **Genetic:** Gaucher's diseases.
- **Neoplastic infiltration.**
- **Inflammatory disease:** Sarcoidosis, lupus erythematosus.
- Chronic infections, such as tuberculosis, brucellosis and malaria.
- **Chronic** haemolytic diseases—spherocytosis, thalassaemia, glucose-6-phosphate dehydrogenase deficiency, elliptocytosis.

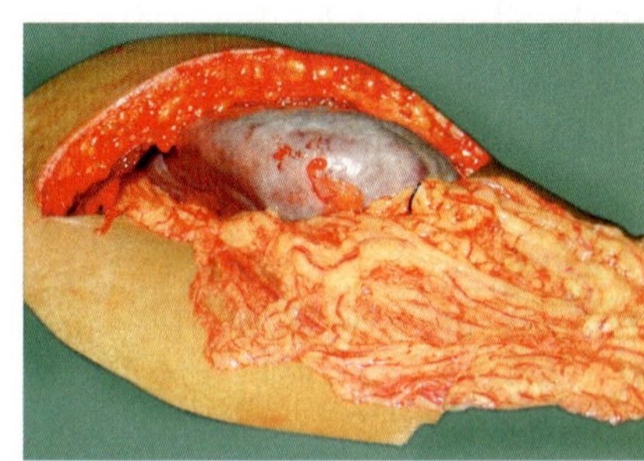

**Fig. 56.20:** Splenectomy done for left-sided portal hypertension due to splenic vein thrombosis

**TABLE 56.1:** Summary of haemolytic anaemias

| | Aetiology | Shape of RBC | Spleen | Investigation | Treatment |
|---|---|---|---|---|---|
| 1. Hereditary spherocytosis | Increase in red cell permeability to sodium | Spherocyte | Large | Reticulocyte count | Splenectomy very beneficial |
| 2. Autoimmune haemolytic anaemia | SLE, drugs | Spherocyte | Medium size | Coombs' test is positive | Steroids: Splenectomy in steroid failure cases |
| 3. Thalassaemia (Cooley's anaemia) | Reduction of β-chain of haemoglobin | Small, thin and no shape | Moderate size | Resistance to osmotic lysis Electrophoresis HbA | Splenectomy for bulky spleen and in patients requiring frequent blood transfusion |
| 4. Sickle cell | HbA is replaced by HbS | Sickle shape | Mild and later not palpable | Electrophoresis HbS | If hypersplenism +, splenectomy |

## CYSTS OF THE SPLEEN (Figs 56.21 to 56.23)

- ***Parasitic cyst*** is rare. Typically, it is caused by echinococcal disease **(hydatid disease)**.
- ***Traumatic cysts*** are due to a haematoma giving rise to liquefaction. These are false cysts of the spleen.
- ***Congenital cysts*** can be due to a dermoid cyst, haemangioma or lymphangioma.
- ***Better*** save the spleen by deroofing cyst wall.

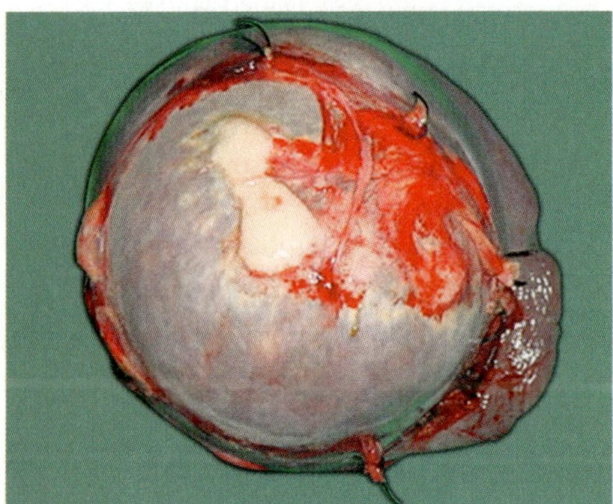

**Fig. 56.21:** Simple cyst of the spleen resulting in compression of the spleen—appearance like that of a ***globe***

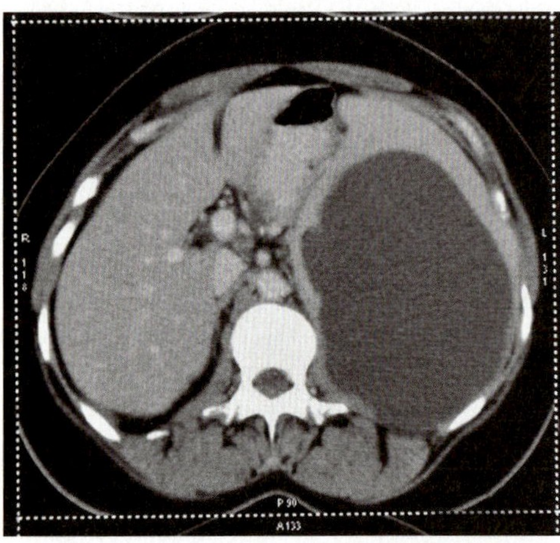

**Fig. 56.22:** Splenic cyst coronal view

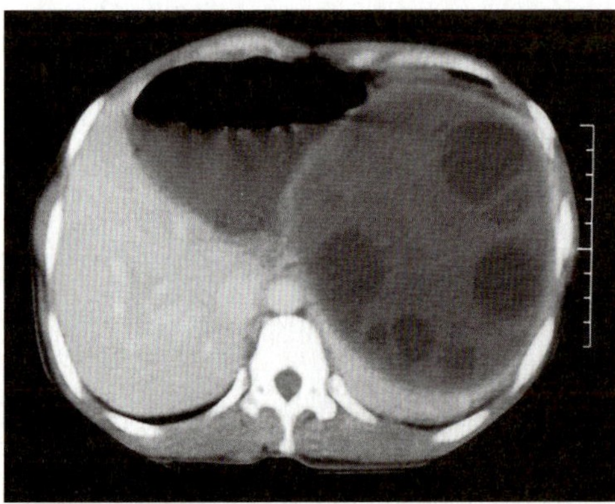

**Fig. 56.23:** Splenic hydatid cyst (*Courtesy*: Prof Dr Anandravi BN, Dr Balakrishna, Dr Dinesh, Dr Ravi, KR Hospital, Mysuru)

## TUMOURS OF THE SPLEEN/NEOPLASMS

- Among neoplasms, **lymphoma** is the commonest cause of ***enlargement*** of spleen. Spleen used to be removed as a part of a staging laparotomy. Now, it is very rarely removed. Patients with **large spleen** of chronic myeloid leukaemia, Gaucher's disease and hairy cell leukaemia (details later) will also benefit from splenectomy.
- **Fibrosarcoma** and **angiosarcoma** are rare malignant tumours.
- **Haemangioma** is the ***most common benign tumour*** of the spleen. It may turn into haemangiosarcoma.
- **Spleen** is removed in oesophagogastrectomy or upper carcinoma stomach—only when it is directly infiltrated. Sometimes it happens in carcinoma tail of pancreas/splenic carcinoma.

## OTHER INDICATIONS FOR SPLENECTOMY (Figs 56.24 and 56.25)

- **Splenic abscess** can occur due to infected septic emboli from otitis, typhoid fever or due to thrombosis of splenic vein causing infarction followed later by infection (Key Box 56.8). **Tubercular abscess** of the spleen is rare. It is usually affected secondary to abdominal or pulmonary tuberculosis.
- **Felty's syndrome** refers to splenomegaly, neutropenia with rheumatoid arthritis. After splenectomy, leg

Key Box 56.8

**Causes of Splenic Abscess**

**S**almonella infection
**P**aratyphi infection
**L**abour—puerperal sepsis
**E**ar infection—otitis
**N**ecrosis of pancreas
**I**nfection of bone—osteomyelitis
**C**hronic disease—tuberculosis

*Remember as* **SPLENIC**

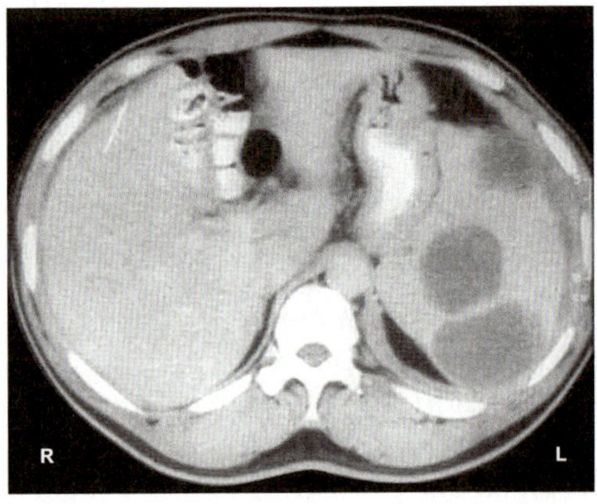


**Fig. 56.24:** CT scan showing multiple splenic abscesses

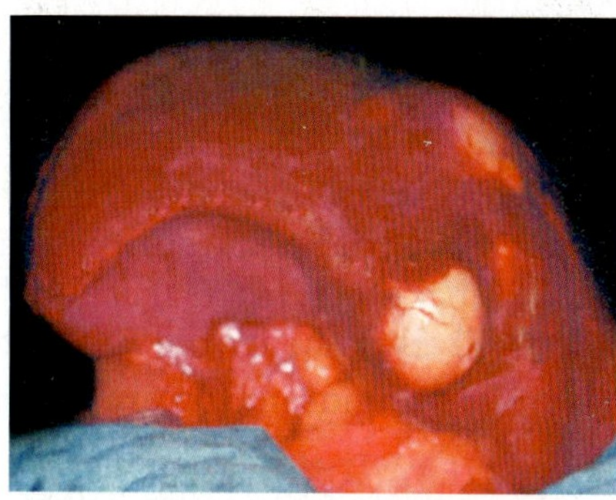

**Fig. 56.25A:** Same patient as in Fig. 56.24 with multiple abscesses in the spleen

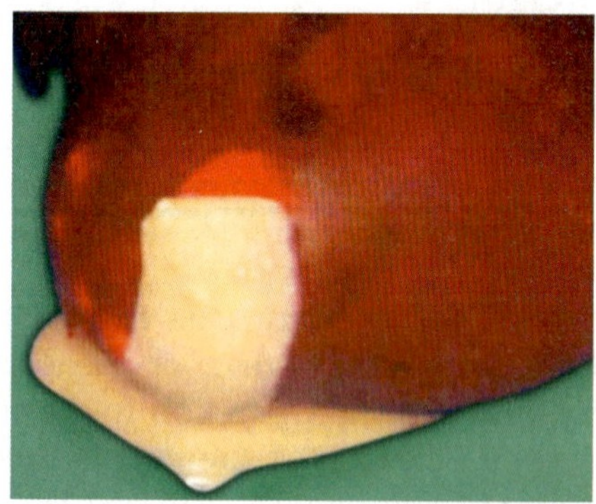

**Fig. 56.25B:** Incision of the abscess after splenectomy

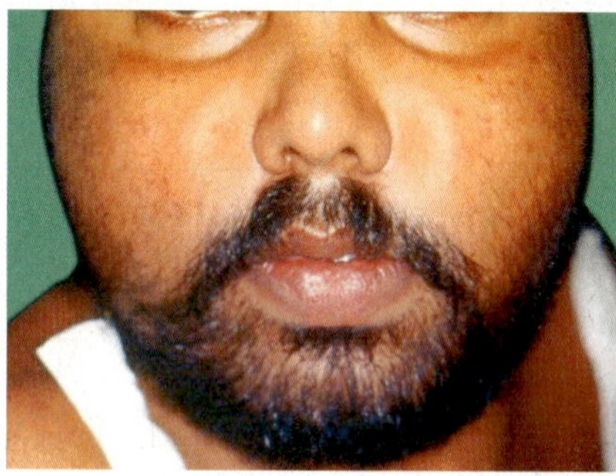

**Fig. 56.26:** Felty's syndrome. The patient had received steroids for one year. See the cushingoid facies

ulcers heal quickly and neutropenia also improves. The patient may respond to steroids better and the incidence of recurrent infection becomes less (Fig. 56.26).

## SPLENIC ARTERY ANEURYSM

It is an uncommon condition. More common in women, and some of them occur during *pregnancy*.

### Causes

- **Atherosclerosis:** Commonly seen in elderly patients.
- **Congenital:** Young patients. These patients may present for the first time during pregnancy with enlargement or rupture.
- **Acute pancreatitis:** Inflammatory process may give rise to pseudoaneurysm, especially because of pancreatic necrosis. This is the reason why CECT scan is done after 5 to 7 days of acute pancreatitis when patients are not improving.

### Clinical Features

- Pain and vomiting—haematemesis
- Thrill or bruit
- Calcification in a routine X-ray
- Rupture and features of haemorrhagic shock.

### Investigations (Figs 56.27 to 56.29)

- Ultrasound/CT scan
- Angiography

### Treatment

- **Non-operative:** Embolisation of splenic artery (Fig. 56.30).
- **Operative:** Ligation of splenic artery at the upper border of pancreas after opening lesser sac followed by splenectomy.
- **Rupture:** Carries high mortality rate.

#### Clinical Notes

A 49-year-old female came with chief complaints of pain abdomen since 10 years, aggravated since 10 days. Pain was in the left hypochondriac region, epigastrium and radiating to the back. She was a known case of chronic calcific pancreatitis and was treated many times. CT scan revealed chronic calcific pancreatitis with splenic artery pseudoaneurysm (2.5–3 cm). Angiogram revealed a pseudoaneurysm arising from main branch of splenic artery. Coiling of the pseudoaneurysm was done using 3 nester coils—one 5.0 cm × 3 cm and two 5 cm × 4 cm. After embolisation, the pseudoaneurysm decreased in size. Danger lies in rupture of pseudoaneurysm and massive bleeding.

## HAIRY CELL LEUKAEMIA (HCL) (Fig. 56.31)

- The cells on a blood smear have an irregular outline due to the presence of filament-like cytoplasmic projections. Hence, the name **hairy cells**.
- HCL is a clonal proliferation of abnormal B cells (very rarely T cells).

### Clinical Features

- Anaemia
- Recurrent infection
- Massive enlargement of spleen.

### Investigations

- Blood counts are low. White cell count may be raised with circulating hairy cells.
- Bone marrow has increased cellularity with characteristic infiltration by **hairy cells**.

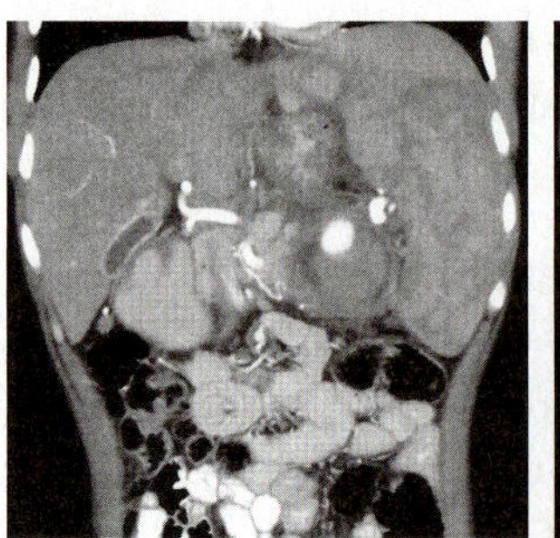
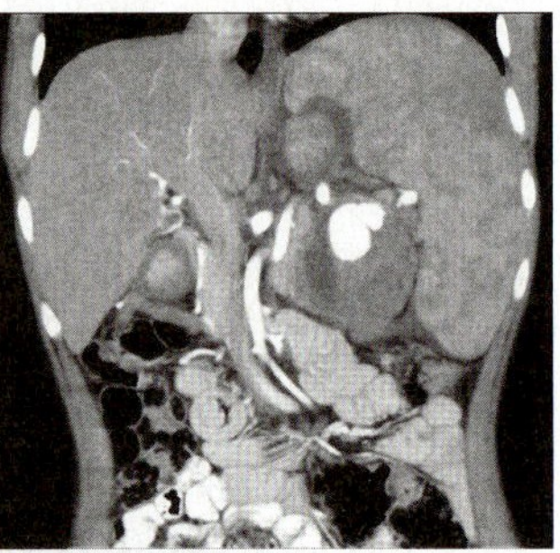
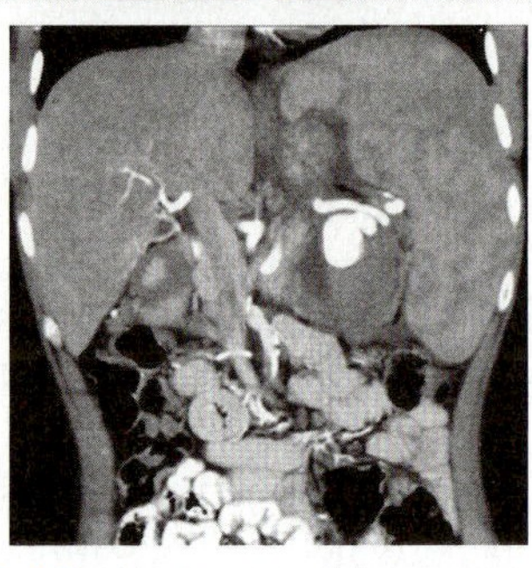

**Figs 56.27 to 56.29:** A 28-year-old man presented with pain abdomen. CT scan showed splenic artery aneurysm with haematoma and thrombus suggestive of ruptured splenic artery aneurysm. He also had splenomegaly and features of portal hypertension. He was alcoholic. He might have had pancreatitis and developed splenic artery aneurysm (*Courtesy*: Prof Sampath Kumar, Dr Basavaraj Patil, Dr Dinesh, Dr Pawan kumar Addala, Department of Surgery, KMC, Manipal)

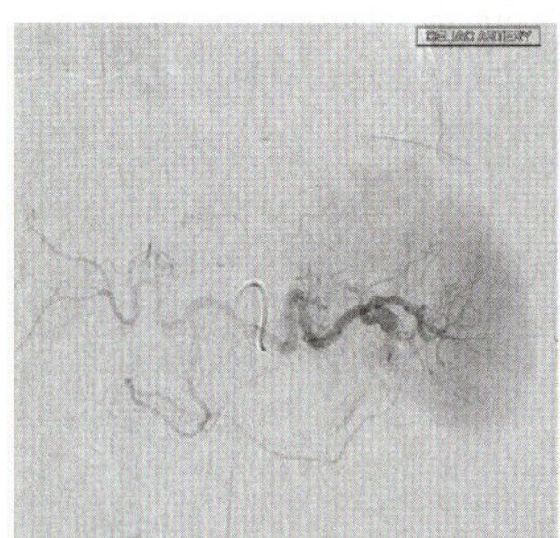
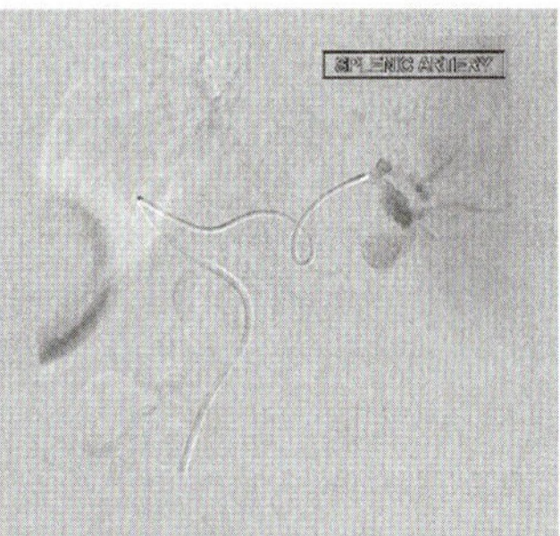
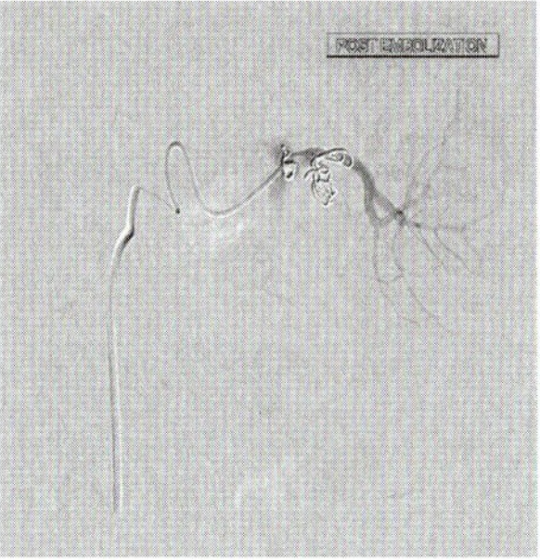

**Fig. 56.30:** Splenic artery embolisation. You can see reduction in the size of pseudoaneurysm in the last picture (*Courtesy*: Dr Rajgopal V, Dr Sunil Krishna, Dr Chitra Bhatt, KMC, Manipal)

### Treatment

- Drug: 2-Chloradenosine acetate (2-CDA) has been beneficial. It can induce remission.
- Splenectomy is indicated in cases of diagnostic difficulties and in very large spleens.

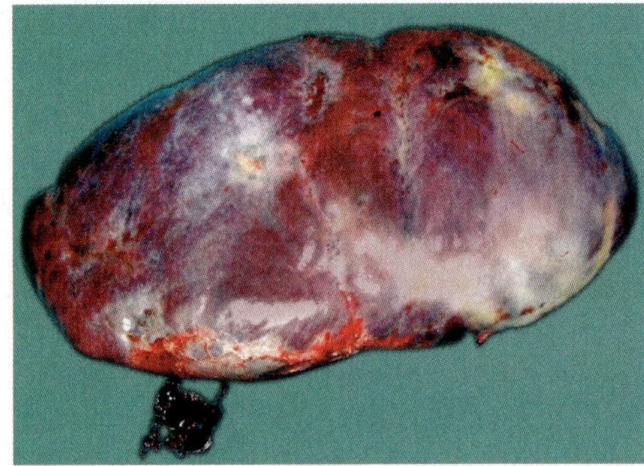

**Fig. 56.31:** Patient had pyrexia of unknown origin with pancytopaenia. Spleen was enlarged. Splenectomy was done and the biopsy report was non-Hodgkin's lymphoma

## OVERWHELMING POST-SPLENECTOMY INFECTION (OPSI)

**SU26.11:** Describe the post-splenectomy sepsis—prophylaxis.

### Definition

It is a generalized non-specific flu-like prodrome followed by rapid deterioration to serious full-blown fulminant septic shock within 24–48 hours of the onset. It is also called as post-splenectomy sepsis.

### Introduction

It is a medical emergency and if it not treated, cardiovascular collapse and death can occur. OPSI has high mortality rates. Fever, body ache, myalgia, chills are a few features of OPSI. Once symptoms start, symptoms deteriorate and the patient progresses to coma, acidosis, respiratory distress, septic shock. Within 24 to 48 hours, disseminated intravascular coagulation (DIC) can occur. Mortality rates can be very high (40 to 50%). Spleen is the most commonly injured organ in blunt abdominal trauma.

### Bacteriology and Pathogenesis

- The bacteria covered with a polysaccharide capsule are called as encapsulated bacteria. *Streptococcus pneumoniae, Klebsiella, Hemophilus influenzae, Neisseria meningitidis*, and *Pseudomonas aeruginosa* are examples.
- Normally, encapsulated pathogens are opsonized with antibodies. After that, phagocytosis takes place in the spleen by specialized macrophages. Thus, patients are more prone to develop serious infection and sepsis after splenectomy.

### Factors Precipitating OPSI

- Loss of splenic phagocytic function
- Low levels of serum immunoglobulin levels

- Low activity- suppression of lymphocyte sensitivity
- Loss of functioning of opsonin.

### Prevention

- Educating patients including children and parents is also an important part of prevention of OPSI.
- In all elective cases, vaccination should be given against *S. pneumoniae, Hemophilus influenzae* type b, *Neisseria meningitidis* and influenza at least 2 weeks before surgery and annually.
- Daily antibiotics for at least 2 years after splenectomy should be given, more so in children. In emergency cases, vaccines should be given as soon as possible.
- Any infections should be treated as emergency with by antibiotics.

### Treatment

- Early diagnosis
- Vancomycin/Ceftriaxone
- Early goal directed therapy to treat shock.

Following are the recommendations; to avoid OPSI (Key Box 56.9).

**Key Box 56.9**

**Penetrating Wounds**

- Represents mainly stab and gunshot wounds
- Immediately pack the wound
- Intercostal chest tube
- Thoracotomy mandatory

### *I. Elective Splenectomy*

- All children who undergo splenectomy before 5 years of age, should receive daily dose of penicillin until 10 years.
- *Haemophilus influenzae* type B vaccination for all irrespective of age and pneumococcal vaccine to be given (repeated once in 5 years).
- Meningococcal protection for only those who travel to high-risk areas.

**Pearls of Wisdom**

Vaccination should be given at least 2 weeks before elective splenectomy.

### *II. After Emergency Splenectomy*

- Vaccines should be given as early as possible. However, protection is **not always** guaranteed.
- Daily dose of oral prophylaxis with penicillin, erythromycin or amoxycillin to all children till 10 years who undergo splenectomy before the age of 5.

### Benefits of Splenectomy

Benefits of splenectomy in Fig. 56.32.

**INTERESTING 'MOST COMMON' FOR SPLEEN**

- Haemangioma is the most common benign tumour of the spleen.
- Lymphoma is the most common cause of enlargement of spleen (in India, malaria is the cause).
- It is the most common solid organ injured in blunt abdominal trauma.
- Most common cause for splenic rupture is blunt abdominal trauma.
- Most significant benefit of doing a splenectomy for hypersplenism for segmental left-sided portal hypertension.
- Most commonly performed investigation for suspected splenic trauma is abdominal ultrasound.
- Most common malignancy affecting spleen is lymphoma.
- Most common complication of splenectomy is pulmonary complication.
- Most common neoplasm of spleen—lymphoma.
- Most common primary tumour of spleen—haemangioma.
- Most common primary malignant tumour of the spleen—haemangiosarcoma.
- Most common infection after splenectomy is by *Streptococcus pneumoniae.*
- Most common indication for splenectomy—splenic trauma.
- Most common indication for splenectomy in elective setting—ITP.

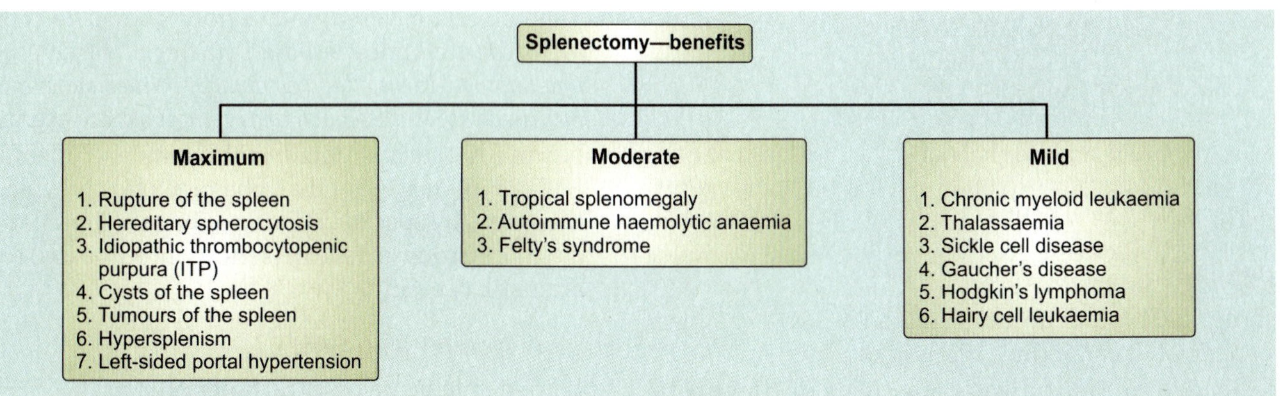


**Fig. 56.32:** Benefits of splenectomy

## MULTIPLE CHOICE QUESTIONS

**1. In splenic injury, Kehr's sign refers to:**
A. Absence of shifting dullness on the left side of abdomen
B. Tenderness on the left side between sternocleidomastoid and scalenus medius muscle
C. Tender left iliac fossa
D. Shoulder pain due to irritation of the undersurface of the diaphragm

**2. Spontaneous rupture of the spleen is seen in the following, *except*:**
A. Idiopathic thrombocytopenic purpura
B. Malaria
C. Infectious mononucleosis
D. Leukaemia

**3. Diagnostic peritoneal lavage is said to be positive in all of the following, *except*:**
A. Fresh blood >20 ml is aspirated after inserting dialysis catheter
B. Gram stain is positive in the contents of the lavage
C. RBC count >100,000 cells/cu mm
D. Amylase level of 75 units/dl

**4. The following is not true about nonoperative treatment in splenic trauma, *except*:**
A. Hemodynamically stable patient
B. Hollow viscus injury
C. Close monitoring is available
D. Hospitalisation is required

**5. Big spleen is not a feature of:**
A. Malaria
B. Idiopathic thrombocytopenic purpura
C. Portal hypertension
D. Leukaemia

**6. The following is true about purpura:**
A. Bleeding time is prolonged
B. Clotting time is prolonged
C. Prothrombin time is prolonged
D. Activated partial thromboplastin time is prolonged

**7. Which of the following vaccinations has to be given after splenectomy to prevent overwhelming post-splenectomy infection?**
A. Measles vaccine B. Pneumococcal vaccine
C. Hepatitis vaccine D. Varicella vaccine

**8. The following is true about splenectomy in idiopathic thrombocytopenic purpura (ITP):**
A. Is required in all cases of ITP
B. Must be done when platelet count is >100,000 cells/cu mm
C. Accessory spleens, if present must be left behind
D. Two-thirds of patients will be cured by surgery

**9. The following is true about splenectomy for hereditary spherocytosis:**
A. Splenectomy should be done as a last resort
B. Splenectomy must be done either before 6 years or after ten years of age
C. Accessory spleen, if present must be left behind
D. Jaundice disappears after splenectomy

**10. The most common benign tumour of the spleen is:**
A. Haemangioma B. Lymphoma
C. Tuberculoma D. Lipoma

### Answers

**1.** D **2.** A **3.** D **4.** B **5.** B **6.** A **7.** B **8.** D **9.** D **10.** A

Chapter 57

# Peritoneum, Peritoneal Cavity, Mesentery and Retroperitoneum



**SU28.3.1:** Describe applied anatomy and physiology of peritoneum.

### Introduction

Peritoneal cavity is the largest cavity in the body accommodating various viscera. It is divided into ***greater*** and ***lesser sac*** (omental bursa) which communicate through the ***foramen of Winslow*** or epiploic foramen. The peritoneum lining inner side of the parietes is called ***parietal peritoneum***. It is ***very sensitive*** and is innervated by both somatic and visceral afferent nerves. This explains the ***sharp, localised, cutting*** pain of peritonitis. Diaphragm and central part of the peritoneum is supplied by phrenic nerve (C4) and partly by intercostal nerves. Rest of the peritoneum is supplied by intercostal nerves and lumbar nerves.

***Lesser omentum:*** It is also called hepatoduodenal ligament. It extends from the duodenum to the liver. This has two layers and within these layers are the common bile duct, hepatic artery and hepatic portal vein.

## PERITONEUM

### Applied Anatomy: Lining of Peritoneum

**The peritoneum is lined** by simple squamous epithelium of mesodermal origin called mesothelium with surface area 1.0 to 1.7 $m^2$ and a thin layer of fibroelastic tissue. It is parietal peritoneum. A large peritoneal defect heals within a few hours because of these mesenchymal cells (flattened polyhedral cells—mesothelium). Applying this principle, some surgeons do not close the peritoneal layer after laparotomy. When parietal peritoneum is reflected into viscera, it is called visceral peritoneum.

It covers viscera and is supplied by autonomic nervous system. Hence, it is not sensitive. Thus, gastrojejunostomy (for gastric outlet obstruction) can be done under local anaesthesia but distension and traction to the bowel causes pain. During herniorrhaphy under spinal anaesthesia, handling of bowel or traction on the bowel can produce uncomfortable upper abdominal pain.

- *In men, peritoneal cavity is completely sealed, hence cannot get infected.*
- *In women, it is communicated to exterior through fallopian tubes. Hence, infection can occur.*

### Applied Physiology: Fluid

Peritoneal surface is a semipermeable membrane with an area comparable to that of cutaneous body surface. Nearly 1 $m^2$ of the total 1.7 $m^2$ area participates in fluid exchange with extracellular fluid space at the rate of 500 ml or more per hour.

It normally contains less than 50 ml fluid. When it is insulted by infection, a large amount of fluid can collect in this space giving rise to severe fluid and electrolyte imbalance. This is described as ***III space loss,*** e.g. ***peritonitis, pancreatitis***. Peritoneal fluid helps in smooth gliding of intestines. Absorption of fluid and secretion of fluid are some important functions of peritoneum (Key Box 57.1).

### Absorption and Exudation

This takes place through capillaries and lymphatics present in between the two layers of peritoneum.

Key Box 57.1

**Normal Peritoneal Fluid—Transudate**

- Specific gravity below 1.016
- Protein concentration less than 3 g/dl
- White blood cell count less than 3000 cells/L
- Complement mediated bacterial activity
- Lack of fibrinogen related clot formation

This principle is applied in **dialysis**. The direction of circulation is towards subdiaphragmatic lymphatics.

### Protective Function

It secretes prostaglandins, interferons and free radicals which help in some protection against peritonitis.

**Circulation of peritoneal fluid and its surgical importance:**

- Stomata are nothing but intercellular pores over the peritoneum covering inferior surface of the diaphragm. They communicate with lymphatic pools in the diaphragm.
- During expiration, diaphragm relaxes, pores open and peritioneal fluid is drawn into stomata.
- During inspiration, diaphragm contracts, the fluid particle enter into lymphatic pools in the diaphragm and through mediastinal lymphatics propelled into thoracic duct.
- Movement of the fluid is in the cephaloid direction.
- Thus in cases of severe intraperitoneal sepsis, it is no wonder that sepsis can spread so rapidly.

**Fitz-Hugh-Curtis Syndrome**

- It is exclusively seen in women/adolescent girls secondary to pelvic inflammatory disease.
- Caused by gonococci and chlamydial infections.
- Severe perihepatitis, irritation of diaphragm, peritonitis are features.
- Tetracycline, doxycyclines, metronidazole are a few drugs, to treat this disease.

## INTRA-ABDOMINAL SEPSIS

### Introduction

Intra-abdominal sepsis is one of the most challenging situations in surgery occurs due to peritonitis. The mortality ranges from 4 to 40% in Britain. It depends upon several factors which include severity of infection, experience of the surgeon, patient's condition, comorbidity and bacterial load. They require intensive care unit with strict monitoring. An attempt has been made here to discuss common causes of sepsis and peritonitis and its management.

### Types of Intra-abdominal Sepsis

- **Complicated:** Infection process proceeds beyond the organ into peritoneum causing localised or generalised peritonitis, e.g. perforated duodenal ulcer.
- **Uncomplicated:** Infection involves only one organ and does not spread into peritoneum, e.g. appendicitis **in early cases.**
- **Infectious:** Primary, secondary and tertiary peritonitis.
- **Sterile.**

**SU28.3.2:** Describe the causes, clinical features, investigations, management and complications of localised and generalised peritonitis.

## ACUTE PERITONITIS

### Definition

Inflammation of the peritoneum is called peritonitis.

#### I. *Primary Peritonitis*

- Spontaneous peritonitis of childhood
- Spontaneous peritonitis of adults
- Tuberculous peritonitis
- Peritonitis associated with dialysis

#### II. *Secondary Peritonitis*

This term refers to peritonitis from an intra-abdominal source and is the most common form of peritonitis. The following are the causes for secondary peritonitis (Fig. 57.1):

1. **Perforation of a hollow viscus**
   - Perforated duodenal ulcer, gastric ulcer
   - Perforated enteric ulcer, tubercular ulcer
   - Perforated Meckel's diverticulum
   - Perforated colonic ulcer
   - Ruptured appendicitis

   Fluid which is spilled into the peritoneal cavity (*Example:* Blood and bile) can travel along paracolic gutter and manifest as pain in the right iliac fossa, causing guarding and rigidity. This has been called **Valentino syndrome** (*see* later on page 870).
2. **Direct spread: Post-inflammatory**
   - Acute cholecystitis—gangrenous
   - Acute appendicitis
   - Gangrene of the intestine
   - Acute necrotising pancreatitis
3. **Penetrating injuries to the abdomen,** where the organisms gain entry from outside.
4. **Postoperative peritonitis** is due to the introduction of infection during surgery which might be due to:
   - Postoperative leaks
   - Foreign body (mop) in the abdomen

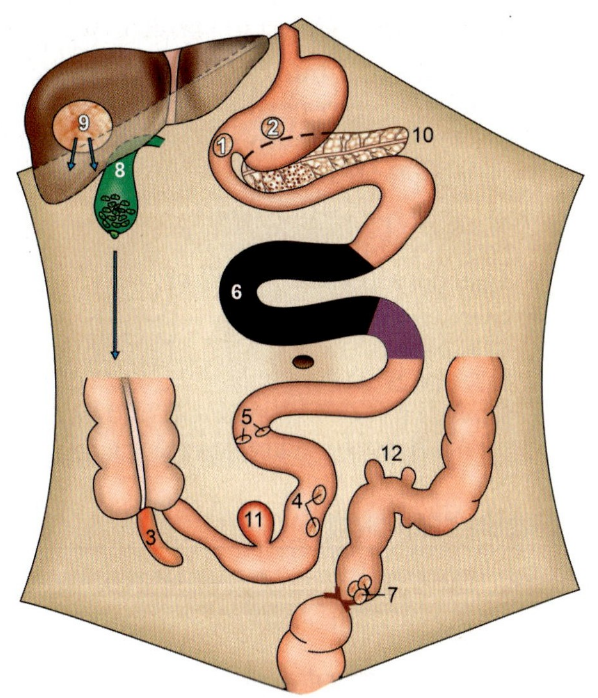


| Common causes of perforation |
|---|
| 1. Perforated duodenal ulcer |
| 2. Perforated gastric ulcer |
| 3. Perforated appendicitis |
| 4. Perforated enteric ulcers |
| 5. Perforated tubercular ulcers |
| 6. Gangrene intestine |
| 7. Perforated carcinoma left colon |

| Uncommon causes of peritonitis |
|---|
| 8. Ruptured amoebic liver abscess |
| 9. Perforated gallbladder |
| 10. Necrotising pancreatitis |
| 11. Perforated Meckel's diverticulum |
| 12. Sigmoid diverticular perforation |

**Fig. 57.1:** Common causes of generalised peritonitis

5. **Parturition peritonitis:** It refers to peritonitis after pregnancy and delivery.
6. **Blunt injuries to the abdomen**

## Classification of Peritonitis

- **Primary peritonitis:** Diffuse bacterial infection caused by single organism without loss of integrity of the GI tract.
- **Secondary peritonitis:** Loss of integrity of the GI tract, multiple organism.
- **Tertiary peritonitis:** It occurs due to recurrent infection after 48 hours—after adequate control of secondary peritonitis. A prolonged systemic inflammation is responsible leading to a higher chance of systemic inflammatory response syndrome, sepsis, severe sepsis, or septic shock. Mortality ranges between 30 and 60%.

## Scoring Systems

Many scoring systems are available. A few important ones are given below. They can predict survival or outcome. They are as follows:

A. **The Manheim Peritonitis Index (MPI) score:** It is a reliable scoring system depending upon several factors as given below.

   Presence of organ failure, time more than 24 hours, presence of malignancy, origin of sepsis, faecal peritonitis, generalised peritonitis.

B. **SOFA score:** Sequential Organ Failure Asssessment Score. The score is based on six different scores, one each for respiratory, cardiovascular, hepatic, coagulation, renal and neurological systems. Factors taken into consideration are: $PaO_2/FiO_2$ (mmHg), Glasgow Coma Scale, mean arterial pressure or administration of vasopressors required, bilirubin (mg/dl) [µmol/L], platelets × $10^3$/ml, creatinine (mg/dl) [µmol/L] (or urine output).

C. **APACHE II score (Acute Physiology Age Chronic Health Evaluation–Knaus et al., 1985):**
   - $AaDO_2$ Alveoloarterial (Aa) Difference (D) of Oxygen ($O_2$) partial pressure difference or $PaO_2$ (depending on $FiO_2$)
   - Temperature (rectal)
   - Mean arterial pressure
   - pH arterial
   - Heart rate
   - Respiratory rate
   - Sodium (serum)
   - Potassium (serum)
   - Creatinine
   - Hematocrit
   - White blood cell count
   - Glasgow Coma Scale

   - These were measured during the first 24 hours after admission.
   - The score is not recalculated during the stay; it is by definition an admission score.

## Pathophysiology

- **Sepsis and septic shock:** Life-threatening organ dysfunction caused by dysregulated host response to infection requiring vasopressor to maintain mean arterial pressure of 65 mmHg or greater and serum lactate greater than 2 mmol/L in the absence of hypovlaemia is described as septic shock.

- Once sepsis or SIRS sets in, it results in loss of large quantity of fluids resulting in hypoperfusion. At the same time, aerobes and anaerobes act synergistically and release inflammatory mediators including toxins. Also translocation of bacteria can occur even after control of sepsis due to more oxygen delivery after control of disease. Plasma lactate or increases resulting in acidosis. Net result is development of shock and **multiorgan failure**.

## Pathogenesis (Fig. 57.2 and Flowchart 57.1)

Due to any one of the reasons mentioned above, infection sets in and the causative organisms multiply in the peritoneal cavity.

- **Gram-negative organisms:** *Escherichia coli (E. coli), Proteus, Klebsiella*. They are present in the small and large bowel. They are the commonest organisms producing peritonitis (Key Box 57.2).
- **Enterococci:** *Streptococcus faecalis* needs bile to grow. It is present in the urinary tract, genital tract and also in the intestines. However, both aerobic and anaerobic streptococci are the second most common organisms producing peritonitis. They are the chief organisms in puerperal sepsis.
- **Bacteroides:** They are anaerobic organisms, present mainly in the lower intestine.
- **Bacteria from outside alimentary canal:** Gonococci, pneumococci, tubercular organisms, etc.
- These organisms proliferate in the peritoneal cavity resulting in peritonitis. A large amount of fluid gets secreted into the peritoneal cavity resulting in 3rd space loss which leads to severe **hypovolaemic shock**. This fluid is rich in proteins, bacteria and toxins. Due to powerful endotoxins released by gram-negative bacteria, endotoxic shock or septic shock (*refer* to shock), ensues.
- The fluid is rich in fibrinogen which forms fibrin and helps in localisation of infection (Fig. 57.3).
- Peritoneum loses its shiny surface, becomes reddish and oedematous and is covered with thick fibrinous exudate.

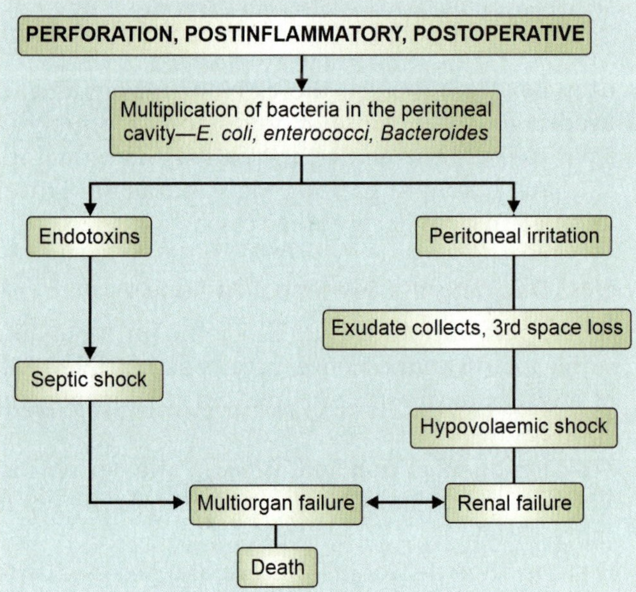


**Fig. 57.2:** Pathophysiology of peritonitis

**Flowchart 57.1:** Pathogenesis of peritonitis

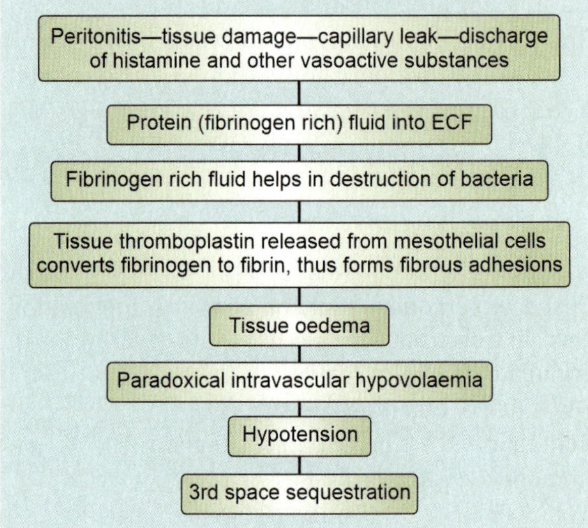


Key Box 57.2

### Organ-specific Organisms

- **Gastric perforations:** Sterile with minimum gram-positive organisms.
- Ileal perforation, appendicitis—aerobic bacteria in 30% patients, anaerobic in 10% patients. Predominant aerobic bacteria include gram-negative *E.coli*, streptococci, *Proteus* and *Klebsiella*.
- **Colonic-rectum:** Faecal spillage produces a load of $10^{12}$ or more—gram-negative and anaerobic bacteria per gram of stools.

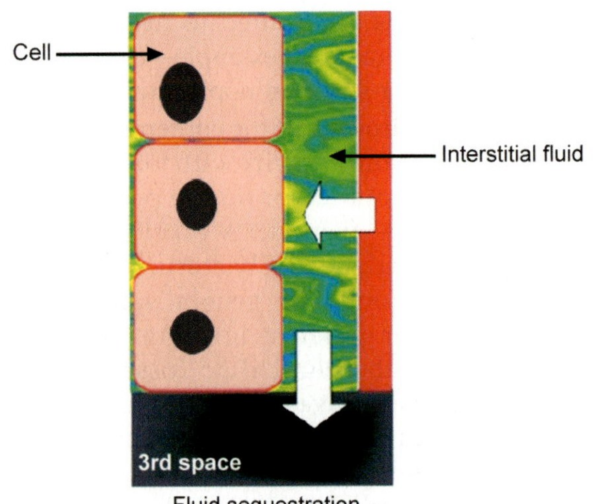

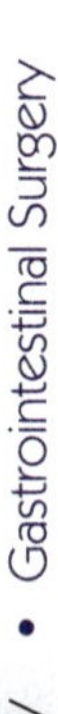


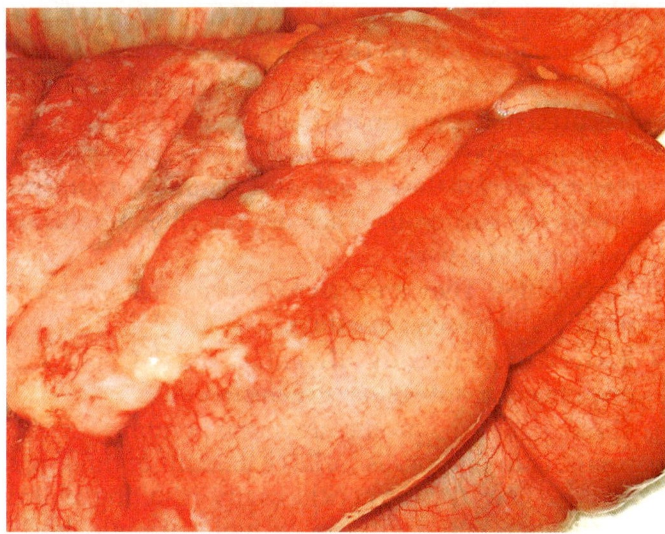

**Fig. 57.3:** Fibrin plaques: Early cases of peritonitis with fibrin plaques all over the peritoneal cavity

**Key Box 57.3**

**Valentino Syndrome—Valentino Appendix**

- **Rudolph Valentino** was an Italian actor who lived in early 20th century.
- On August 15, 1926, he was admitted with the diagnosis of appendicitis and gastric ulcers, with peritonitis.
- He underwent appendicectomy.
- Continued to have peritonitis.
- He developed pleural effusion and sepsis.
- Dies after a few days of surgery.
- In retrospect what he had was duodenal ulcer perforation.
- It is also called **Valentino syndrome** because in any inflammation of the upper abdominal viscera, contents can travel down the right paracolic gutter into the right iliac fossa resulting in pain and tenderness mimicking acute appendicitis.

- **Omentum:** It is a fatty apron with rich blood supply. A mobile double-layered peritoneal fold acts like a policeman to seal the area of infection or perforation. *Examples:* Perforated duodenal ulcer, acute appendicitis, acute diverticulitis, etc. Probably it also serves to supply collateral blood supply to the ischaemic viscera. In addition, it has immunological functions such as supply of phagocytes which destroy unopsonised bacteria.

## Types of Peritonitis

A. **Local peritonitis:** If a perforation is small and if it is sealed off immediately by omentum, it will give rise to local peritonitis. *Examples:* Small gastric ulcer perforation, diverticular perforation, gallbladder perforation. Anatomical factors also play a role in local peritonitis. *Examples*: Retrocaecal appendicitis with perforation. It is behind the caecum and in retroperitoneum. Signs are confined to right iliac fossa only. In posterior gastric perforations or acute pancreatitis, signs are limited to upper abdomen. Pelvic peritonitis is another example—occur following septic abortions or salpingo-oophoritis.

B. **Generalised peritonitis:** If the contents of the viscus leak into the peritoneal cavity with force, as it occurs in intestinal perforation or due to perforation of a free lying organ—example: Meckel's diverticular perforation. Virulence of bacteria is more as in colonic perforations with generalised peritonitis. Duodenal ulcer perforation can manifest as severe pain in the right iliac fossa mimicking appendicitis. **Many have been mistakenly operated for appendicitis because the right paracolic gutter is broad and contents travel down into right iliac fossa.** This has been referred to as **Valentino syndrome** (Key Box 57.3). Before the days of ultrasound, it used to be not uncommon to do appendectomy in a patient who had acute pancreatitis. Inflammatory exudate gravitating along right paracolic gutter resulted in pain in right iliac fossa.

## Factors Deciding the Severity of Peritonitis

- **Clean perforation:** Upper GI-gastric juice remains sterile for 6–8 hours. Hence, in early stages, there will be mild chemical peritonitis and early treatment gives good results.
- **Distal gut perforation and infected bile peritonitis:** Very dangerous and severe, causing sepsis and septic shock early.
- Postoperative peritonitis that usually occurs due to anastomotic leak is also dangerous.
- A perforation sealed off early by omentum causes mild peritonitis. Retrocaecal appendicitis produces minimal local peritonitis.
- On the other hand, perforated Meckel's diverticulitis produces diffuse peritonitis soon (Key Box 57.4).
- A few causes of peritonitis are shown in Figs 57.4 to 57.14.

**Key Box 57.4**

**Factors Affecting Diffuse Peritonitis**

- Speed of peritoneal contamination, e.g. perforation of Meckel's diverticulum
- Stimulation by purgatives
- Virulence of organisms
- Perforation in a closed loop obstruction
- Immunocompromised status
- Young children. Omentum is thin and small

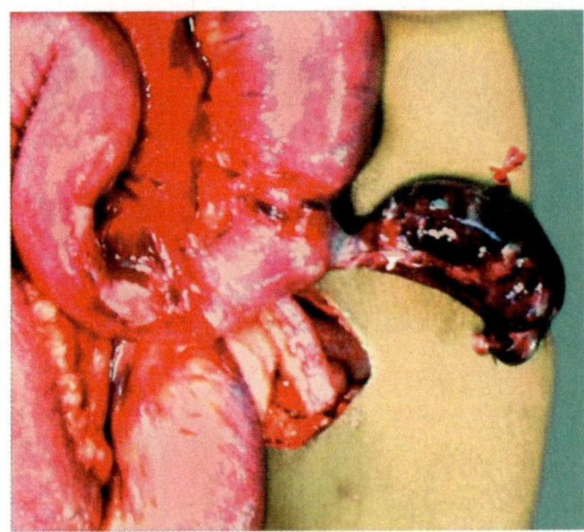

Fig. 57.4: Meckel's diverticulitis

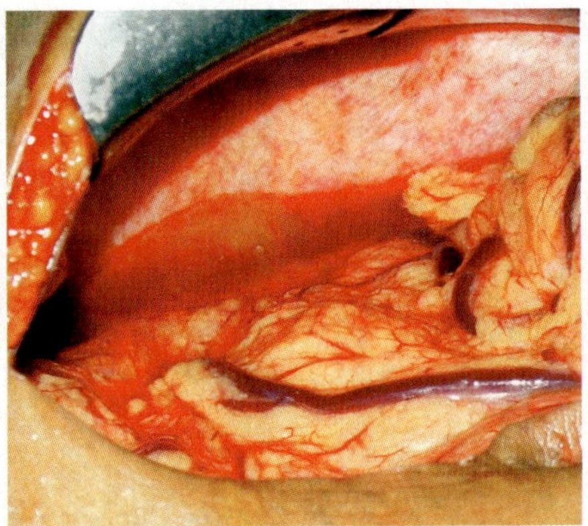

Fig. 57.5: Peritonitis due to ileal perforation consequent to tuberculosis. Usually it is an ulcerative variety

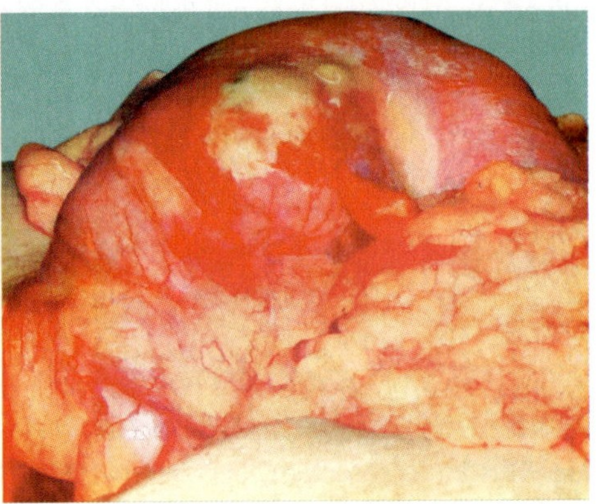

Fig. 57.6: Transverse colon injury due to steering wheel—simple closure in early cases without much peritonitis. Otherwise resection/closure with or without diversion ileostomy may be required

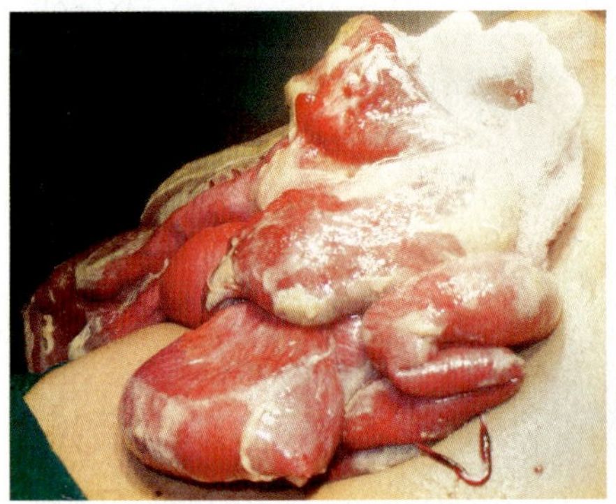

Fig. 57.7: Enteric perforation which is 4 days old—very friable edges. Re-leak after suturing is common

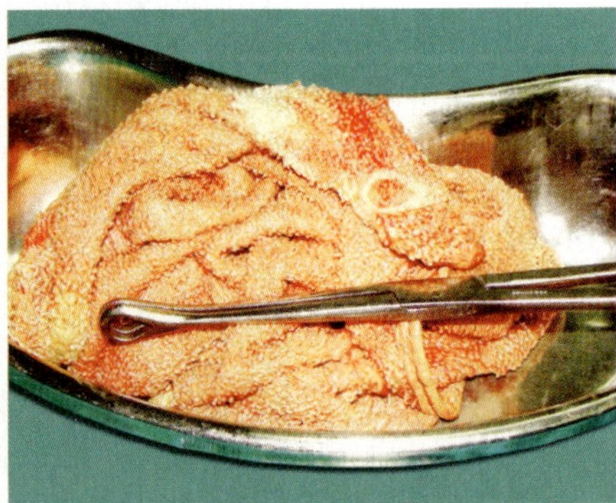

Fig. 57.8: Postoperative peritonitis due to a mop left behind following caesarean section. Always count the mops and instruments before closure of the abdomen. It is a good practice

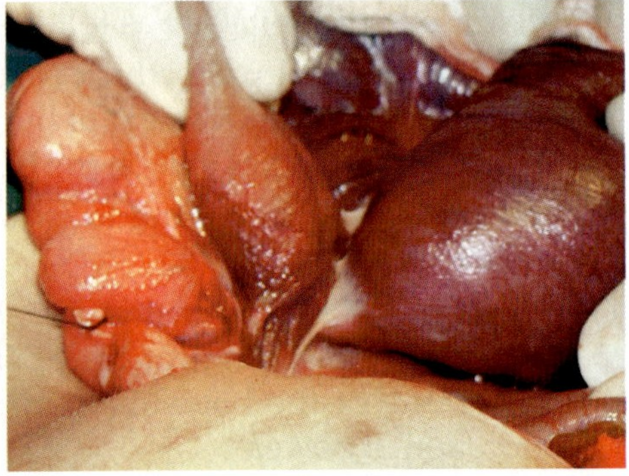

Fig. 57.9: Fibrous band causing gangrene of the terminal ileal loop resulting in peritonitis. The patient had pelvic peritonitis due to tuberculous salpingitis. That resulted in bands

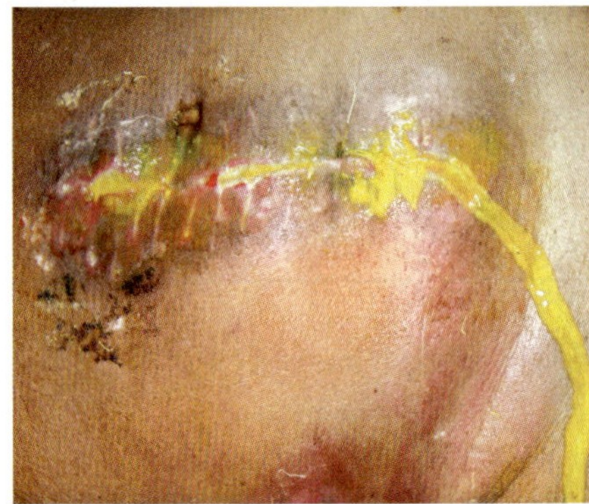

Fig. 57.10: Faecal peritonitis and faecal fistula due to anastomotic leak following right hemicolectomy. Ischaemia and tension at the suture line are the two common causes for the leak

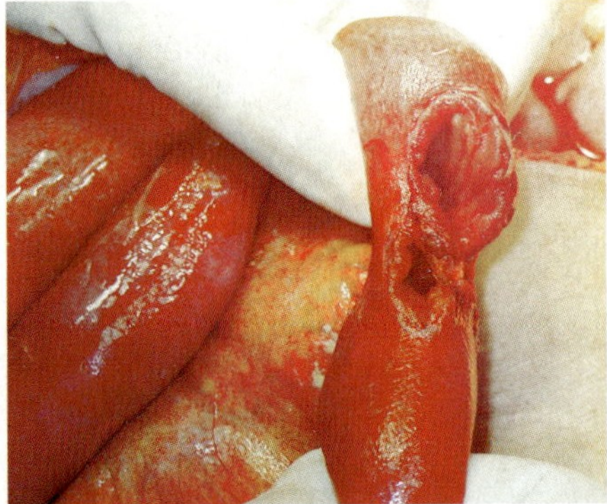

Fig. 57.11: Proximal jejunal transection following blunt abdominal trauma. It is one of the common sites affected in blunt abdominal trauma

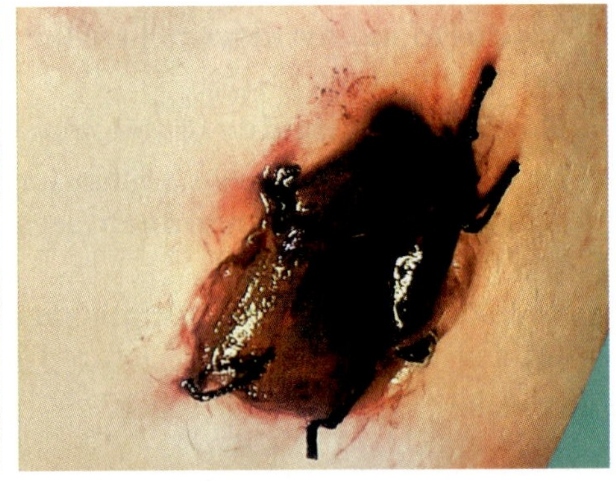

Fig. 57.12: Colostomy gangrene—the intra-abdominal segment was also gangrenous. It is important to always check for the vascularity of the colostomy site before closing abdominal incision

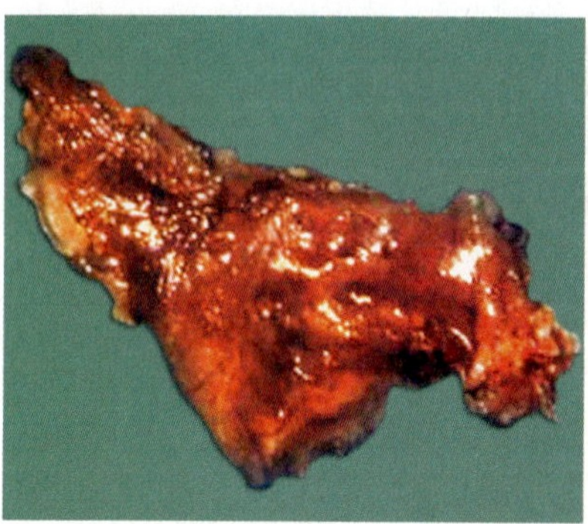

**Fig. 57.13:** Necrosectomy specimen—acute pancreatitis

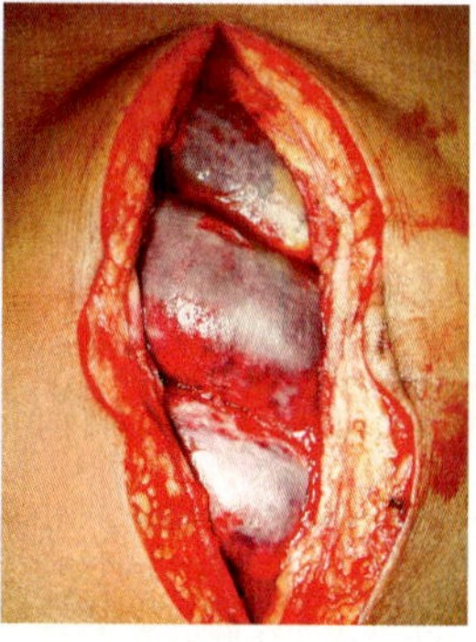

**Fig. 57.14:** Mesenteric ischaemia giving rise to gangrene

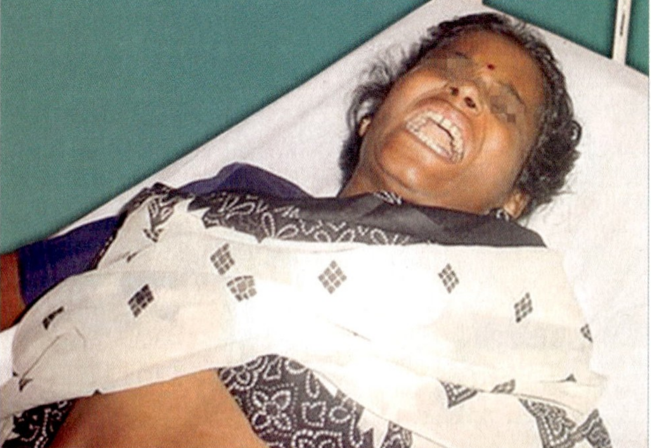

**Fig. 57.15:** Rebound tenderness is the diagnostic sign of peritonitis

## Clinical Features

It depends upon whether it is localised peritonitis or generalised. In cases of retrocaecal appendicitis, the abdominal signs may be minimal but guarding and rigidity of the back muscles is characteristic. Features of generalised peritonitis are as follows:

- **Severe abdominal pain** which is cutting in nature, becomes worse on movement of the abdominal wall. Hence, the patient lies still on the bed.
- **Persistent vomiting** is due to irritation of parietal peritoneum.
- **The pulse rate is increased.** An increase in the pulse rate may be an early indication of peritonitis, in cases of gangrene of the bowel or peritonitis following perforation of bowel.
- **High-grade fever with chills and rigors** indicates a septicaemic process.
- **Cough tenderness** indicates parietal peritoneal inflammation. Abdominal tenderness is elicited in all quadrants of the abdomen **(Dunphy's sign)**.
- **Rebound tenderness (Blumberg's sign):** Abdomen is pressed for a few seconds. The patient experiences pain. Sudden release of pressure causes severe pain. It is due to sudden movement of the sensitive parietal peritoneum (Fig. 57.15).
- **Guarding** and **rigidity** of abdominal wall.
- Bowel sounds are absent. Distension of the abdomen occurs within a few hours due to accumulation of fluid and paralytic ileus.
- **End-stage disease:** Hippocratic facies (Key Box 57.5 and Fig. 57.16).

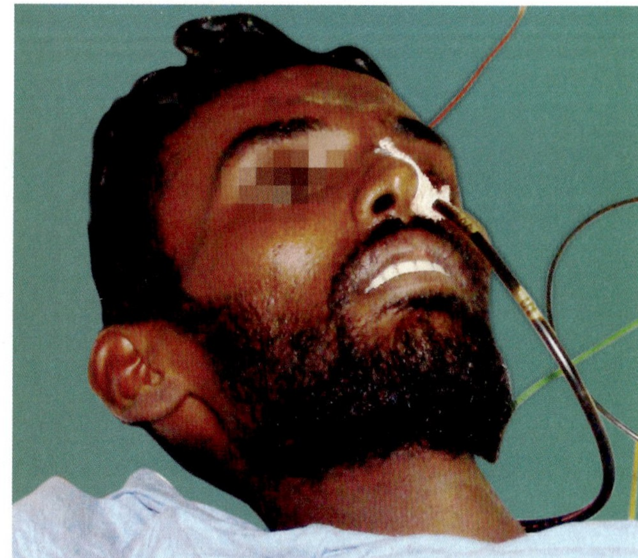

**Fig. 57.16:** Hippocratic facies: sunken eyes, drawn in cheeks, dehydrated, blood in the Ryle's tube

Key Box 57.5

**Hippocratic Facies**

- Hollow, bright eyes
- Pale and pinched face
- Cold perspiration in the head and brows
- Blue lips
- Dry, cracked tongue

## Investigations

1. **Complete blood picture** shows **high total count** with predominant neutrophil count.
2. **Blood** examination for **sugar** is done to rule out diabetes mellitus. Empyema gallbladder with or without perforation can present as septic shock. Often, they are diabetic.
3. **Plain X-ray abdomen, chest and upright**
   - **Gas under the diaphragm**—perforation (Figs 57.17 to 57.19).
   - **Ground glass appearance**—a smooth homogenous appearance due to accumulation of fluid (Fig. 57.20).

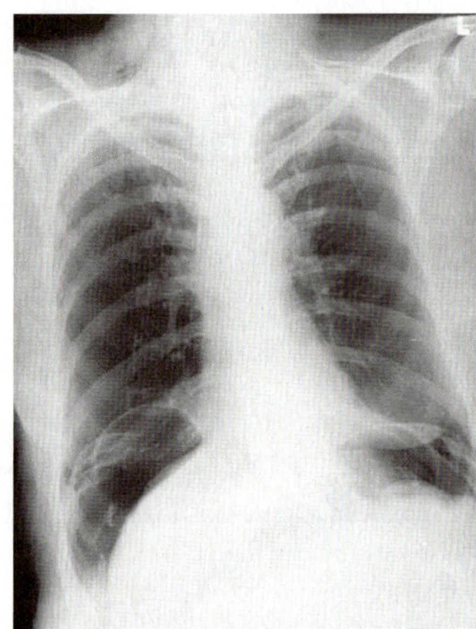

Fig. 57.17: Chest X-ray showing free gas under diaphragm

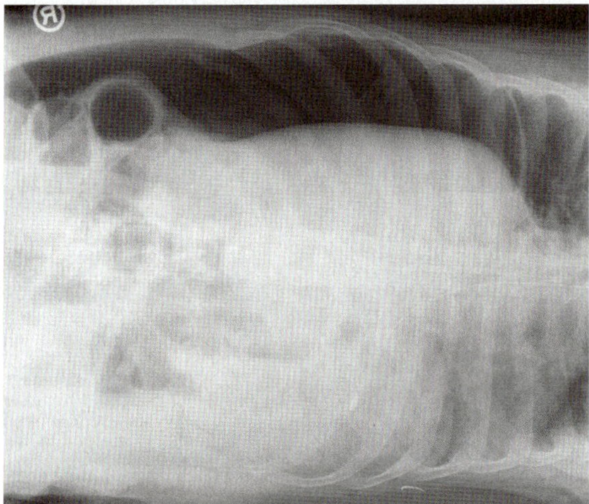

Fig. 57.18: Lateral decubitus X-ray showing free gas in the peritoneal cavity. (This position of the patient is used when patient is in shock or no able to stand)

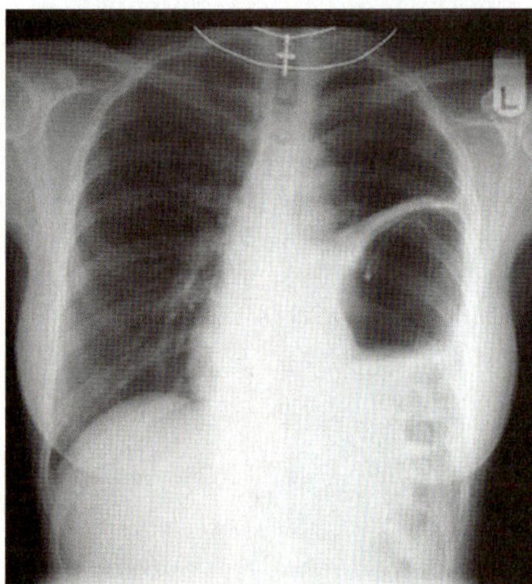

Fig. 57.19: Diaphragm is elevated—fundic air bubble is in the chest—traumatic diaphragmatic hernia

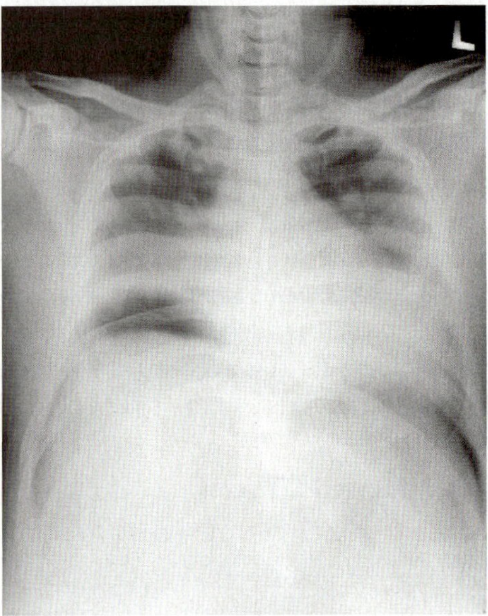

Fig. 57.20: Subphrenic abscess—mild pleural effusion on both sides

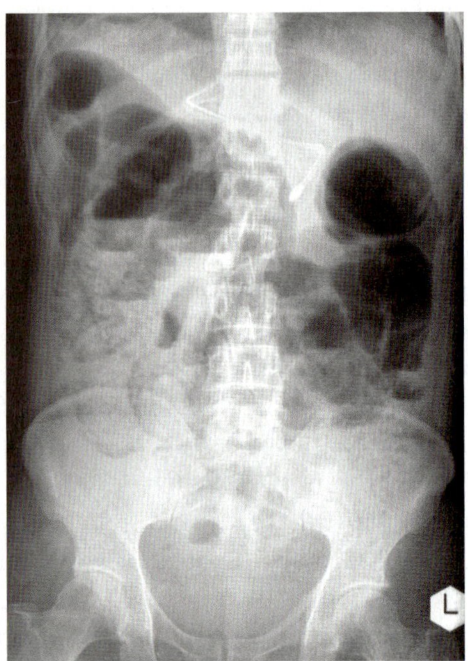

Fig. 57.21: Gas in the bowel wall (pneumatosis) indicates gangrene of the bowel

- Air in the bowel wall—gangrene (Fig. 57.21).
- Obliteration of psoas shadow and preperitoneal fat planes.

4. **Abdominal USG** to detect **fluid in the abdomen**. Following are different fluids which may give clue to the diagnosis:
   - Frank pus—peritonitis of more than 48 hours old
   - Bile—green coloured—duodenum, stomach, gallbladder perforation
   - Faeculent—dark green coloured thick aspirate with faecal odour—ileal perforations, postoperative anastomotic leaks

- Serous—exudative—early acute pancreatitis, tuberculous peritonitis
- Haemorrhagic—haemorrhagic pancreatitis
- Food particles—hollow viscus perforation

Thus ultrasound has so many advantages even though it may not point at the specific site. However, probe tenderness with fluid in the right iliac fossa may suggest acute appendicular perforation. It may not be possible to aspirate very thick contents such as anchovy sauce pus from ruptured amoebic liver abscess but ultrasound will provide clue about the liver abscess.

5. **Contrast-enhanced CT scan**
   - When the signs and symptoms are equivocal, CT is the ideal investigation.
   - CT can diagnose hollow viscus perforation, especially when there is no gas under the diaphragm.
   - CT can detect ischaemic changes due to gangrene of the bowel-gas in the bowel wall-pneumatosis (Figs 57.22 and 57.23).
   - CECT has higher sensitivity and specificity but it has radiation exposure of almost 200 chest X-rays.
   - CT can diagnose unsuspected and unexpected lesions in the abdomen including diverticular perforations, internal herniation and gangrene, acute pancreatitis, etc.
   - Adequate hydration and normal renal function (as indicated by normal creatinine values) are important before a contrast-enhanced CT scan.
6. **Abdominal tap**
   - Aspiration of blood indicates haemoperitoneum or gangrene of the bowel.
   - Aspiration of bile indicates biliary peritonitis due to perforation of duodenal ulcer, gallbladder or intestine.
   - **Aspiration of frank pus** indicates peritonitis due to gram-negative bacteria. Foul-smelling pus is due to anaerobic bacteria producing free fatty acids and their esters. Always send the fluid for culture sensitivity (Fig. 57.24).
   - Amylase estimation should be done to rule out pancreatitis.
7. **MRI:** It is costly, may not be available all the time. Indicated in pregnant patients with abdominal pain and ultrasound is inconclusive.
8. **Diagnostic laparoscopy** can be used in suspected cases of peritonitis (Key Box 57.6).

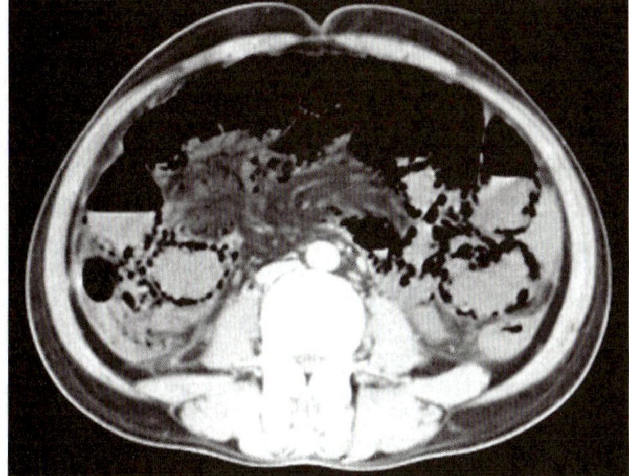

**Fig. 57.22:** CT showing air in the bowel wall—case of superior mesenteric ischaemia

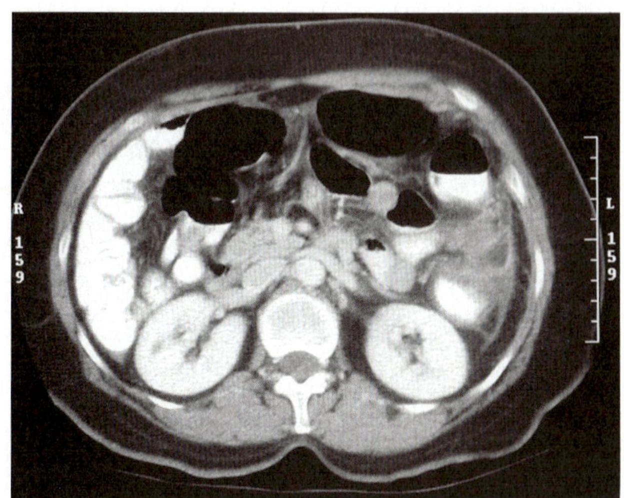


**Fig. 57.23:** CT showing hypodense lesion in the left iliac fossa—a case of sigmoid diverticular perforation

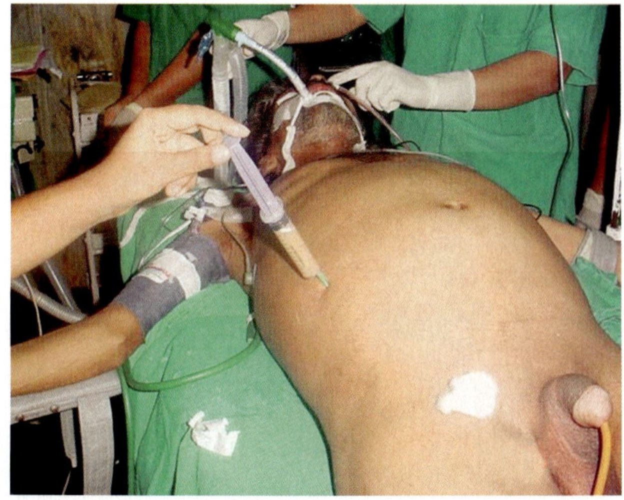

**Fig. 57.24:** Diagnostic tap showing pus following rupture of empyema of gallbladder

Key Box 57.6

**Diagnostic Laparoscopy**

- It can be used to reconfirm peritonitis.
- It can diagnose pancreatitis (laparotomy may be avoided).
- It can also treat primary cause, e.g. laparoscopic closure of duodenal ulcer perforation.
- Peritoneal toilet can be given.
- It can rule out other causes.
- In blunt injury, **it can detect diaphragmatic injury**—herniation of bowel, etc.

*Pearls of Wisdom*

When in doubt, do laparoscopy: It can reveal 'hidden' pathology.

## Treatment

1. **Aspiration:** Nasogastric aspiration with Ryle's tube helps in decreasing gastrointestinal secretion. Thus it reduces abdominal distension. It also prevents vomiting and gives rest to the gut. Indirectly, it reduces 'bacterial load' contaminating peritoneum.
2. **Bowel care and blood:** Purgatives should not be given as it may result in perforation. Blood is arranged for surgery.
3. **Charts:** Temperature, pulse rate, respiratory rate, intake-output charts are maintained.
4. **Drugs** are given against gram-positive, gram-negative and anaerobic organisms (Key Boxes 57.7 and 57.8).

Key Box 57.7

**Selection of Antibiotics**

- 2nd or 3rd generation cephalosporins should be started as early as possible.
- Once culture and sensitivity reports are available (after surgery), antibiotics can be changed.
- Antibiotics should also cover aerobes and anaerobes.
- Should not have serious toxicity, especially amikacin which has nephrotoxicity. Hence, use them carefully (check creatinine).

Key Box 57.8

**Early Aggressive Resuscitation**

- **Restore** intravascular volume. **Crystalloids:** Ringer lactate or isotonic saline stay in the intravascular space for a short period, larger volumes required.
  **Colloids:** Longer duration of action, smaller volumes are sufficient and can be used in cardiac patients. Not the choice.
- **Restore** oxygenation by face mask or mechanical ventilation, as necessary.
- **Restore perfusion:** Dopamine/dobutamine/noradrenaline.
- **Restore** normality by 'war' against sepsis—**ANTIBIOTICS** and surgical removal of **SEPSIS**.

5. **Exploratory laparotomy** and appropriate surgery is done followed by thorough peritoneal toilet/wash with normal saline.
6. **Fluids:** IV fluids are given before, during and after surgery. Central venous cannulation and measurement of central venous pressure (CVP) is indicated in unstable patients to guide fluid therapy. If not possible, an ***emergency cut down*** (venesection)—cephalic or basilic vein, is done followed by fluid infusion. Preoperatively, the aim is to maintain at least 30 ml/hr of urine output.
   - Ringer lactate solution is an ideal replacement.

**PRINCIPLES OF SURGERY FOR PERITONITIS**

**Exploratory laparotomy**
- Generous incision
- Extendable

**Exudative secretions drained out**
- Drain the fluids, send for culture and sensitivity
- Thorough peritoneal wash

**Explore the diseased region**
- Gently by separating loops and in between loops

**Establish the diagnosis**
- Identify site of perforation, gangrene, etc.

**Eradicate cause of sepsis**
- Resection anastomosis
- Suturing, appendicectomy, etc.

You explore the abdomen; Establish the diagnosis; Eradicate the cause and Eliminate the exudate

### Principles of Surgery for Peritonitis

(Key Box 57.9, Figs 57.25 to 57.29)

1. Adequate **incision** is used—upper/mid/lower midline.
2. As soon as the peritoneal cavity is opened, purulent fluid comes out. The fluid is collected and sent for **culture** and **sensitivity**. Greenish fluid indicates a hollow viscus perforation. All the fluid is drained, the source of peritonitis is identified and appropriate surgical procedure is done. **Examples are:**

Key Box 57.9

**Principles of Surgery**

- Incision
- Establish the diagnosis
- Exploration
- Pus culture and sensitivity
- Treat the cause—control of sepsis
- Peritoneal toilet
- Drain
- Closure
- Debridement of dead and necrotic tissues
- Devices (Infected) removal
- Drainage of pus
- Decompress abdominal cavity
- Damage control surgery are few principles for quick recall

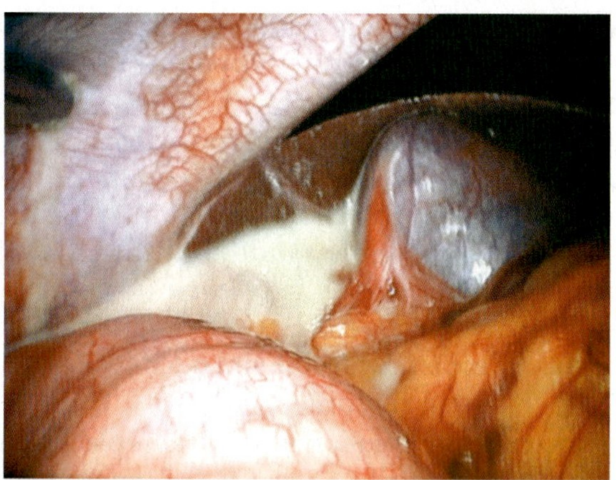

Fig. 57.25: Laparoscopy showing pus

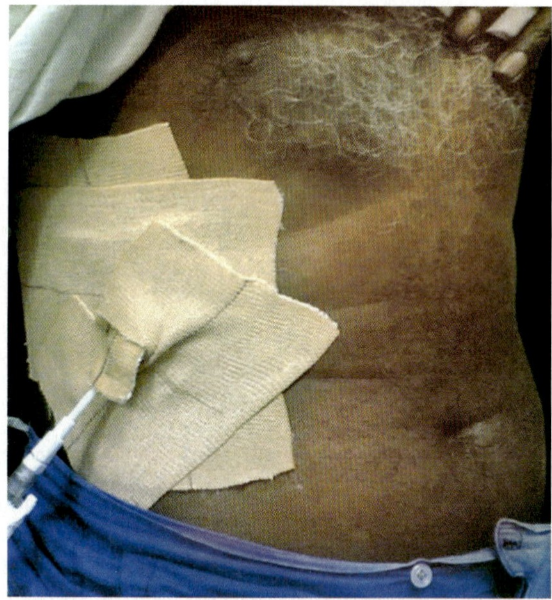

Fig. 57.26: A late case of duodenal ulcer perforation who presented with peritonitis with sympathetic pleural effusion. Laparotomy, closure of perforation and feeding jejunostomy were done. Drains in the subhepatic space and right pleural cavity were placed. Patient had stormy postoperative period with biliary fistula, which was closed after 6 weeks

- Appendicectomy for appendicitis.
- Closure of perforation for perforated peptic ulcer.
- Closure or resection for ileal perforation.
- Resection of the bowel for gangrene.

**Control of sepsis:** This is the most important step of treatment of peritonitis. Removal of septic focus is a primary aim—examples: Appendicectomy, perforation closure (duodenal ulcer) or resection (intestinal or colonic perforation) or cholecystostomy in difficult perforated gallbladder diseases. However, all the septic foci in the abdomen have to be removed—necrotic material, pus pockets and food particles. Thorough irrigation with warm saline cleans up subhepatic spaces, pelvic spaces and interloop collections. Primary anastomosis in presence of sepsis may result in leak and postoperative peritonitis. It is better to do colostomy or ileostomy in such cases. Incision can be partially closed leaving the skin open—sutures can be tied after 2 days in the ward.

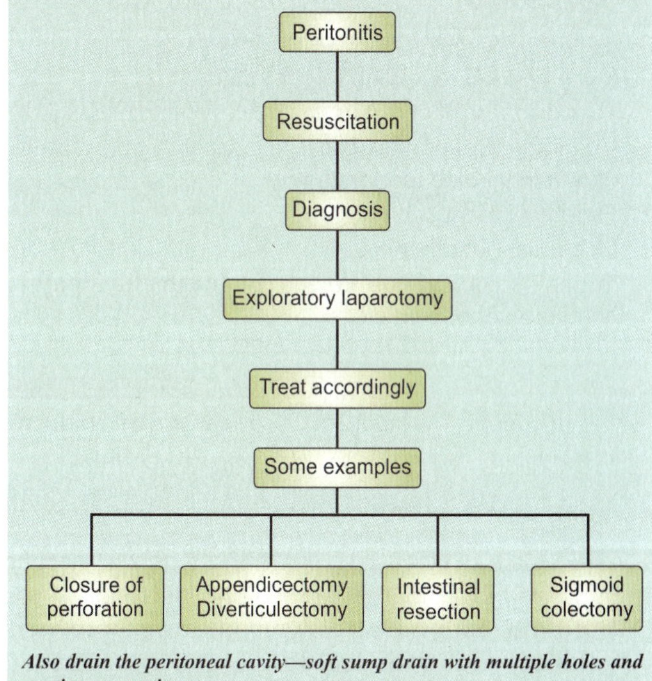


Fig. 57.27: Principles of management of peritonitis—identifying the source of sepsis and elimination is the key to success

3. It is better to use **nonabsorbable suture** material such as silk for intestinal anastomosis or for closure of perforation. In the presence of infection, absorbable sutures, such as catgut, get absorbed very fast.
4. A thorough **peritoneal wash/lavage** is given by using warm saline (up to 3–5 litres) to avoid intraperitoneal abscesses. Antiseptic agent such as betadine solution should be avoided because they can cause adhesions (Key Box 57.10).
5. Peritoneal cavity is drained to the exterior by using **tube drains**. These are kept in the subhepatic space and in the pelvic cavity.

Key Box 57.10

**Peritoneal Lavage**

- Used in diffuse peritonitis.
- 3–5 litres of isotonic crystalloid solution is used.
- Avoid antibiotic solution or povidone iodine solutions—they may induce more adhesions.
- Aminoglycoside lavage may cause respiratory depression due to neuromuscular blocking action of these drugs. Mops must be used to dry the peritoneal cavity. If fluid is left over, it may dilute the opsonins and thus decrease phagocytosis.

6. The wound is irrigated with **antiseptic agents**.
7. **Tension sutures** are put depending upon the severity of the peritonitis to prevent burst abdomen.
8. **Laparostomy (*vide infra*):** This method of exposing the peritoneal cavity can be done in selected cases, if abdominal compartment syndrome is suspected.

### Nonoperative Treatment of Peritonitis

1. Too sick a patient to tolerate the surgical procedure.
2. Sealed perforation.
3. Localised peritonitis—may resolve with treatment.

- In very sick patients, image guided drianage of septic focus can be done by pig tail insertion.

**Refer Chapter 11, nutrition in surgical patients**
- Sepsis is a catabolic event.
- Cytokines and TNF, insulin resistance play a role.
- Glucose is an essential part of nutrition and should amount to at least 500 kcal per day.
- Glucose gets converted to carbon dioxide and when in excess, can increase respiratory load.
- To reduce this, 50% daily energy requirements can be provided using lipids.
- Proteins should also be provided, bearing in mind, the increased protein catabolism in sepsis.

### Laparostomy

This refers to leaving peritoneal cavity exposed to outside without approximation of the anterior abdominal wall. Some situations arise, especially in emergency cases, where this is required. Hence, it is important to know how to deal with this situation (Figs 57.28 and 57.29).

#### *Indications of Laparostomy*

When a second look procedure is contemplated, e.g. acute pancreatitis, mesenteric ischaemia.

#### *Types*

1. **Open laparostomy:** Abdominal fascia and peritoneum are not sutured.

   ***Advantages:*** Abdominal compartment syndrome can be prevented. Details are given later.

   ***Disadvantages:*** Significant fluid loss and secondary infection.

2. **Closed laparostomy or mesh laparostomy:** Here the fascial layer is closed by using marlex mesh or prolene mesh or even a zip to protect exposed viscera.

   ***Advantages:*** One can minimise infection.

   ***Disadvantages:*** Abdominal compartment syndrome and perforation of bowel can occur.

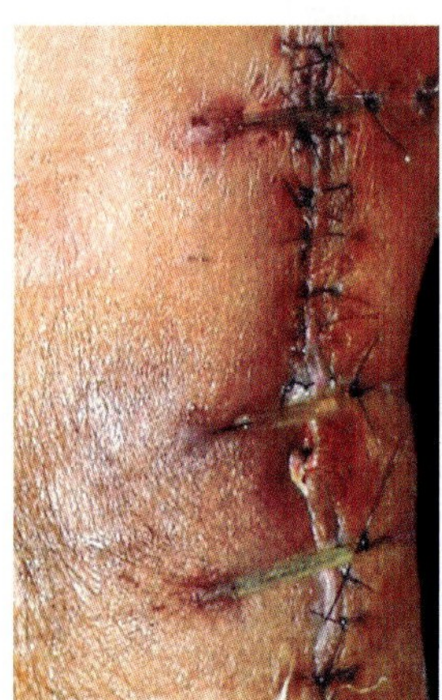

**Fig. 57.28:** Tension sutures

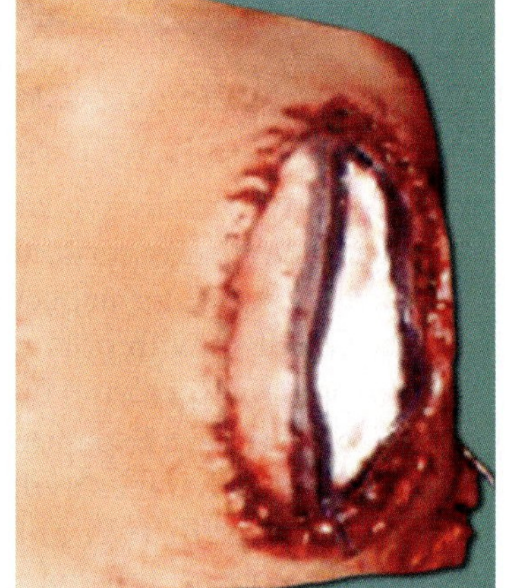

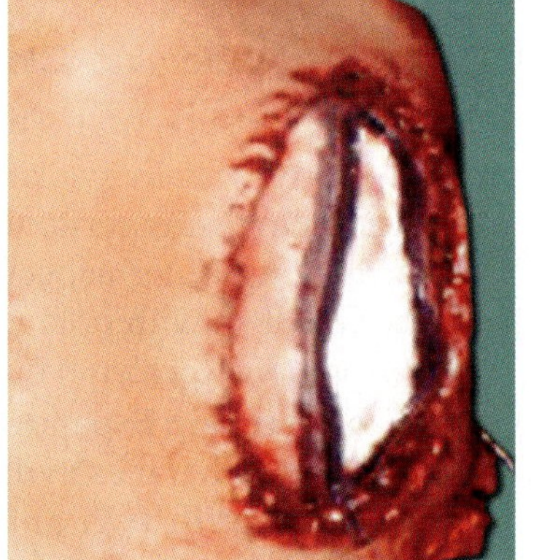

**Fig. 57.29:** Zip closure of peritoneum

## ABDOMINAL COMPARTMENT SYNDROME

### Introduction

The phrase "abdominal compartment syndrome" was coined in 1984 when Irving Kron, described the measurement of intra-abdominal pressure as a means of developing criteria for abdominal decompression to improve organ function.

### Definition

- Abdominal compartment syndrome (ACS) is defined as a sustained increase in IAP more than 20 mmHg with or without an abdominal perfusion pressure (APP) < 60 mmHg) that is associated with new organ dysfunction/failure (Fig. 57.30).
- Intra-abdominal pressure (IAP) is the pressure concealed within the abdominal cavity. Normal IAP is 0–5 mmHg showing phasic variation with respiration.
- Intra-abdominal pressure is measured to detect abdominal compartment syndrome and to decide on the requirement of a decompression so as to improve organ function.

### Final Effects

The adverse physiological effects of intra-abdominal hypertension (IAH) affect almost every organ system

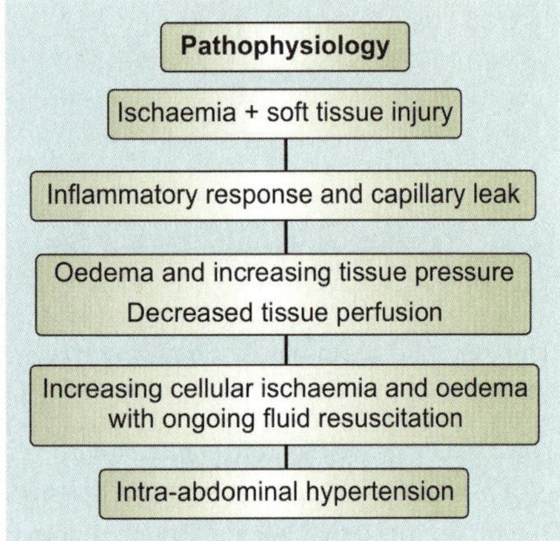


**Fig. 57.30:** Pathophysiology of abdominal compartment syndrome

resulting in ACS. The major systems affected, in decreasing frequency of incidence and morbidity are: Pulmonary, cardiovascular, renal, splanchnic, central nervous system. Thus, the end result can be:

- Intractable hypoxia, hypercarbia, ARDS
- Cardiac insufficiency and cardiac arrest
- Oliguria, anuria, acute renal failure
- Cerebral oedema and anoxia.

### Grading of IAP (Burch)

| | | |
|---|---|---|
| **Grade I** | : | IAP 12–15 mmHg |
| **Grade II** | : | IAP 16–20 mmHg |
| **Grade III** | : | IAP 21–25 mmHg |
| **Grade IV** | : | IAP >25 mmHg |

### Risk Factors

#### A. Diminished abdominal wall compliance

- Acute respiratory failure with elevated intrathoracic pressure.
- Abdominal surgery with primary fascial or tight closure. Example: Reduction of massive hernia (Figs 57.31 and 57.32).
- Major trauma/burns
- Prone positioning, head of bed >30°
- High BMI, central obesity

#### B. Increased intraluminal contents

- Gastroparesis
- Acute gastric dilatation

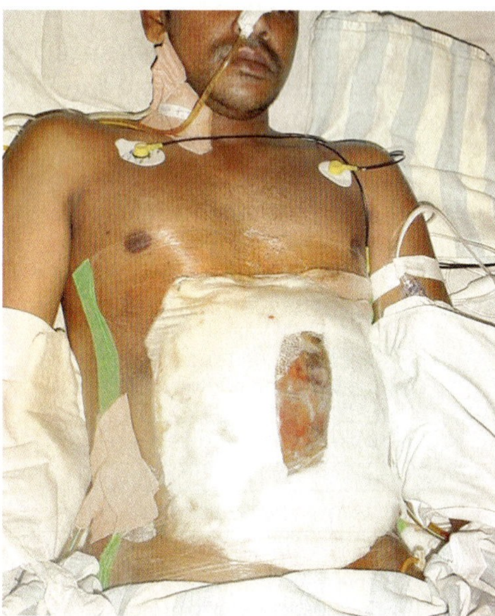

**Fig. 57.31:** This boy had abdominal compartment syndrome after reduction of intestinal contents from left thoracic cavity (a case of left diaphragmatic hernia) and we could not close the abdomen. It was covered with a thin plastic sheet—you can see the intestine. It took two months for granulation tissue to cover the defect. Eventually, he recovered with an incisional hernia. Bogota bag or vac are the other alternative methods of closure

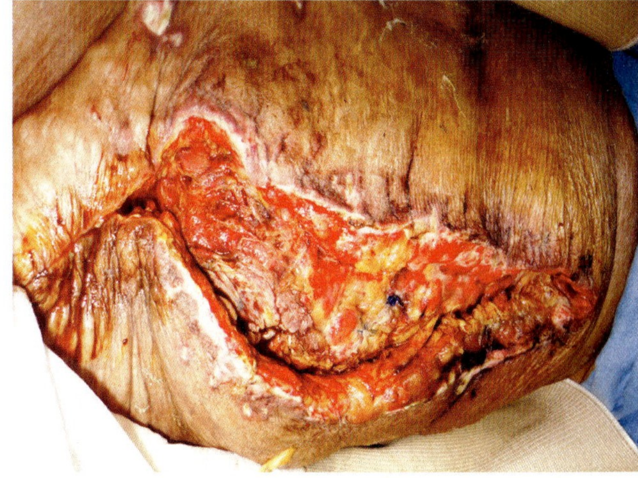

**Fig. 57.32:** Loss of abdominal layers following reduction of a massive ventral hernia

- Ileus
- Colonic pseudo-obstruction

#### C. Increased abdominal contents

- Haemoperitoneum/pneumoperitoneum
- Ascites/liver dysfunction
- Laparoscopy

### IAP Measurement—Principles

- Expressed in mmHg (1 mmHg = 1.36 cm $H_2O$).
- Measured at end expiration
- Performed in supine position
- Zeroed at mid-axillary line at the level of iliac crest.
- Performed with an instillation volume of no greater than 25 ml of saline (for bladder technique).
- Measured 30–60 sec after to allow bladder detrusor muscle relaxation (for bladder technique).

### Medical Treatment

- Close monitoring of patient's vitals
- Blood transfusion when required
- Nutritional supplements—intravenous/TPN

### Surgery

#### I. *Temporary Abdominal Closure*

- Towel clip closure, only skin closure.
- Mesh—commercially available meshes with absorbable surface facing intraperitoneum and non-absorbable surface facing outer aspect of the wound are used. Example: Mesh with polygalactin (vicryl) inside and polypropylene (prolene) outside can be used.
- **PTFE mesh repair:** Expanded polytetrafluoroethylene (ePTFE) is another mesh which is used. It is a surgical biomaterial with two antimicrobial preservative agents—chlorhexidine diacetate and silver carbonate. It also enhances tissue ingrowth.

- **Bogota bag: A Bogota bag** is a sterile plastic bag used for closure of abdominal wounds.[1] It is generally a sterilised, 3-litre genitourinary irrigation bag that is sutured to the skin or fascia of the anterior abdominal wall. The Bogota bag acts as a hermetic barrier that avoids evisceration and loss of fluids. Another advantage to the Bogota bag is that the abdominal contents can be visually inspected which is particularly useful in cases of ischaemic bowel. Thus, it is useful in resections following mesenteric ischaemia. In our country, we can use urosac bag (which can be split open) or even a thin plastic sheet can be used like a Bogota bag (*see* Fig. 57.31).

**Clinical Notes**

A young boy of 18 years, who suddenly had breathlessness was found to have diaphragmatic hernia. After reduction and closure, patient developed ACS. Reopening of abdomen was done and peritoneum was not closed but a 'cover' was given by using 'urosac' bag which was split open. Wound was allowed to heal by granulation tissue.

- **Vacuum-assisted closure (VAC):** It has been extensively used in the management of leg ulcers specially diabetic ulcers. It has been used in a few cases of severe pancreatitis. Here it is called open abdomen negative pressure therapy system. It removes debris, inflammatory exudates.

### II. *Definitive Abdominal Closure*

- Primary closure. It is done layer by layer. Non-absorbable suture is usually selected.
- Synthetic mesh
- Biologic mesh
- Component separation

*Pearls of Wisdom*

No doubt, drainage of the septic focus is the most important step in controlling sepsis.

## COMPLICATIONS OF PERITONITIS

1. **Severe hypovolaemic shock** giving rise to renal failure. It can be prevented by adequate hydration of the patients and careful usage of antibiotics such as gentamicin.
2. **Septic shock, multiorgan failure** and death occur in late cases of peritonitis.
3. **Subacute intestinal obstruction** due to postoperative adhesions. They are easily separable adhesions.
4. **Subphrenic abscess**
5. **Pelvic abscess**

**SU28.4.1:** Etiopathogenesis of intraperitoneal abscess.
Pelvic abscess and subphrenic abscess are two major groups. Intraperitoneal abscesses including interloop collections can occur in acute appendicitis or following acute Meckel's diverticulitis, etc. More details are given later.

## SUBPHRENIC ABSCESS

### Introduction

- As a result of peritonitis, residual abscess can collect in the intraperitoneal cavity. Pus that collects under the diaphragm is described as subphrenic abscess. Subphrenic abscess is the commonest intra-abdominal abscess.
- Gastrointestinal perforations, postoperative leaks, penetrations, trauma and puerperal sepsis are the common causes of subphrenic abscess.
- Blood clots, bacteria laden fibrin and neutrophils contribute to an abscess. To understand the etiopathogenesis of subphrenic abscess and treatment, we need to study anatomy of subphrenic spaces first.

### Surgical Anatomy

There are five subphrenic spaces between the diaphragm and the liver bounded by various peritoneal folds. Four are intraperitoneal and one is extraperitoneal. The spaces, boundaries and the common causes of pus in these spaces are described in Table 57.1 and Figs 57.33 to 57.35.

### Aetiopathogenesis (Fig. 57.36)

- The causative organisms of peritonitis are *Escherichia coli*, enterococci, *Klebsiella*, *Enterobacter*, *Proteus*, *Bacteroides*, etc.
- The high incidence of subdiaphragmatic abscess is due to constant circulation of fluid from below upwards because of the following reasons:
  1. Upward movement of diaphragm during expiration
  2. Decreased intra-abdominal pressure
  3. Capillary action.

**Subphrenic abscess is common on the right side because of the following reasons:**

1. Right paracolic gutter is wide and deep and colophrenic ligament is absent.
2. Left paracolic gutter is narrow and colophrenic ligament is present on the left side.
3. Majority of diseases affect right side (perforation, liver abscess, appendicitis, gallbladder disorders, etc.) (Fig. 57.36).

**TABLE 57.1:** Subphrenic spaces, boundaries and common causes of involvement

| Spaces | Boundaries | Common causes |
|---|---|---|
| 1. Right anterior intraperitoneal space | It lies between right lobe of the liver and diaphragm<br>Posteriorly—anterior layer of the coronary ligament and right triangular ligament. On the left side is the falciform ligament | Perforated duodenal ulcer, gastric ulcer, cholecystitis |
| 2. Right posterior intra-peritoneal space (Rutherford Morrison's hepatorenal pouch) | It lies below the right lobe of the liver<br>Inferiorly—hepatic flexure and transverse colon<br>Medially—second part of the duodenum<br>Laterally—abdominal wall. This is the biggest intra-peritoneal space | Appendicitis, cholecystitis<br>Perforated duodenal ulcer<br>Upper abdominal surgery |
| 3. Left anterior intraperitoneal space | Above—diaphragm. Posteriorly—left triangular ligament, left lobe of the liver, lesser omentum, anterior surface of the stomach. Right side—falciform ligament<br>Left side—spleen | Surgery on stomach—gastrectomy<br>Distal pancreatectomy. Left hemicolectomy |
| 4. Left posterior intraperitoneal space (lesser sac) | In front—by lesser omentum and posterior surface of the stomach. Behind—pancreas, suprarenal, left kidney<br>On the right side—foramen of Winslow through which it communicates with the greater sac | Pseudopancreatic cyst<br>Perforated gastric ulcer |
| 5. Midline extraperitoneal space (bare area of the liver) | Above—upper layer of coronary ligament<br>Below—lower layer of coronary ligament<br>Left—inferior vena cava | Amoebic hepatitis<br>Pyogenic liver abscess |

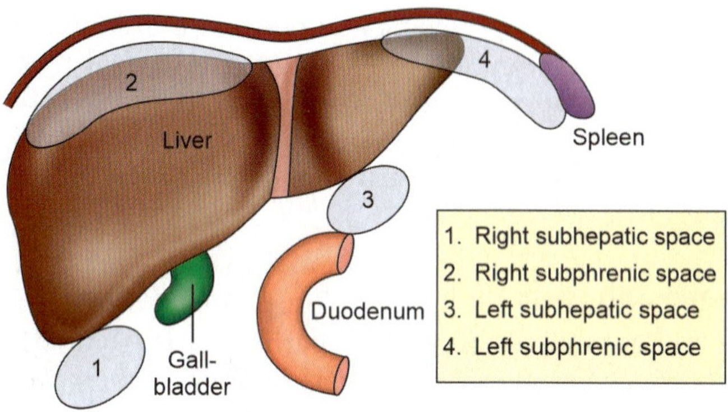


**Fig. 57.33:** Subphrenic spaces in sagittal section

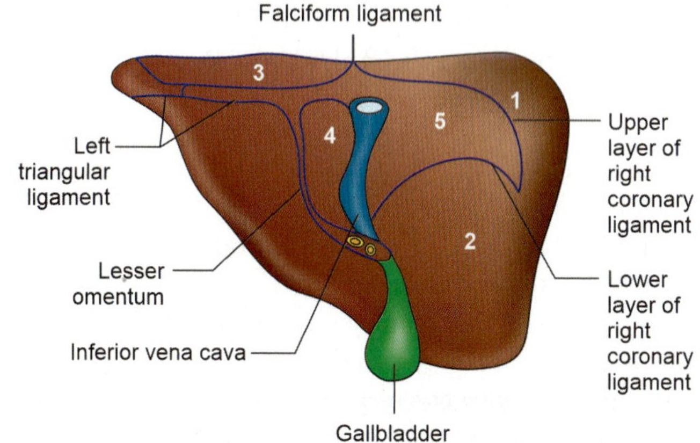


**Fig. 57.34:** Subphrenic spaces (Table 57.1 for numbers)

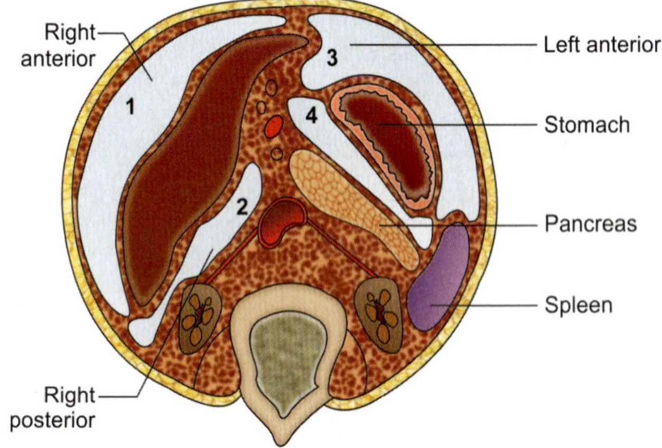


**Fig. 57.35:** Cross-section showing subphrenic spaces: 1. Right anterior intraperitoneal space, 2. right posterior intraperitoneal space, 3. left anterior intraperitoneal space, 4. left posterior intraperitoneal space (lesser sac)

## Clinical Features

- A patient who is recovering from peritonitis complains of *fever with sweating*. Initially, fever is low grade, continuous. Later, there is high-grade fever with chills and rigors.
- **Deterioration of health** occurs very fast with wasting and anorexia.
- **Shoulder pain** is due to irritation of undersurface of the diaphragm by the pus (sensory fibres of the phrenic nerve are irritated—C3, C4).

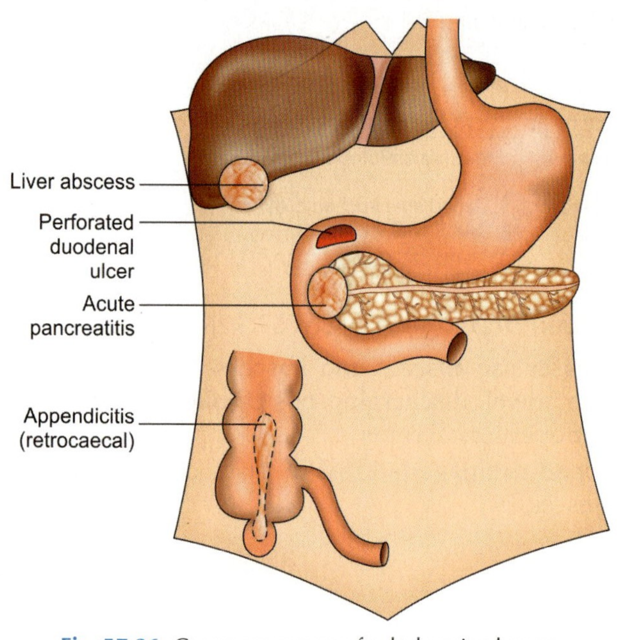


Fig. 57.36: Common causes of subphrenic abscess

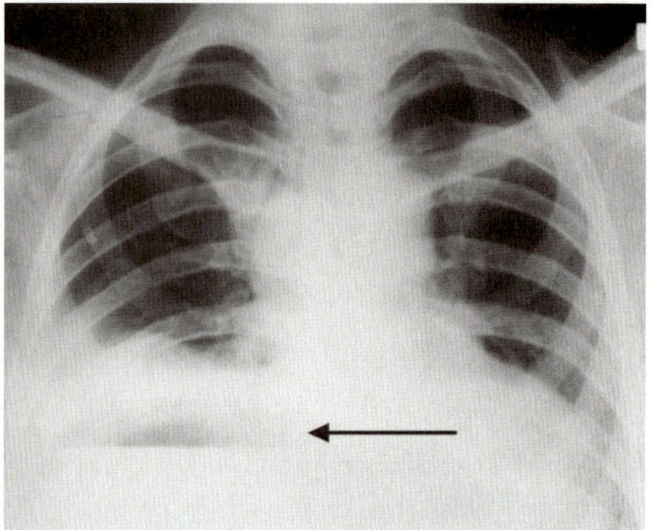

Fig. 57.37: Plain X-ray—gas and fluid level under diaphragm: PA view and lateral view

- Postoperatively, the patient is not doing well—prolonged ileus.
- Anorexia, wasting, hiccup, dry cough.

*Pearls of Wisdom*

A postoperative patient who has pyrexia, prolonged ileus, poor appetite and progressive deterioration of health has subphrenic abscess.

- **Tenderness** is present in the epigastrium on deep palpation.
- Common causes of postoperative fever are absent, e.g. thrombophlebitis, urinary tract infection.

*Pearls of Wisdom*

Pus nowhere, pus somewhere, pus under the diaphragm—Harold Barnard.

## Investigations

1. **Total count** with neutrophil count.
2. **Plain X-ray abdomen** (erect)—may show gas and fluid level under the diaphragm (Fig. 57.37).
3. **Ultrasonography** confirms the site of abscess, number of abscesses, loculations, etc.

   Abscess is characterised by hypoechogenic cavity surrounded by sharp distinct echogenic wall. It can be therapeutic to insert catheter for drainage.
4. **CT scan** demonstrates well defined, low density mass, the rim of which is enhanced after intravenous injection of contrast medium. The mass tends to be round because of centripetal expansion—high sensitivity >95% (Fig. 57.38).

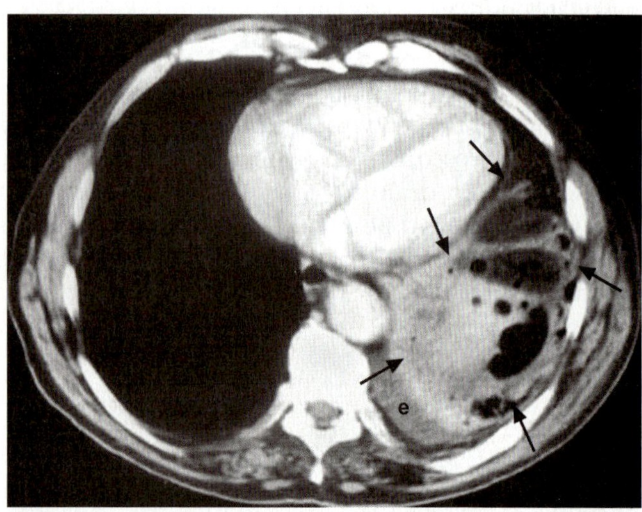


Fig. 57.38: CT scan showing left subphrenic abscess with air foci suggesting infected necrosis following acute pancreatitis—a pigtail catheter is inserted (also *see* Fig. 57.39)

## Treatment (Flowchart 57.2)

Today with the availability of sophisticated imaging facilities, percutaneous drainage has become the choice of therapy rather than surgery. Both have been described in next column. Always antibiotics are given to treat intra-abdominal sepsis in addition to drainage of pus—Image guided aspiration/laparosocpic or open method.

### I. *Percutaneous Drainage*

It can be done with the help of ultrasound or CT scan, provided the abscess cavity is unilocular, and the track is safe.

**Flowchart 57.2:** Goals of the treatment

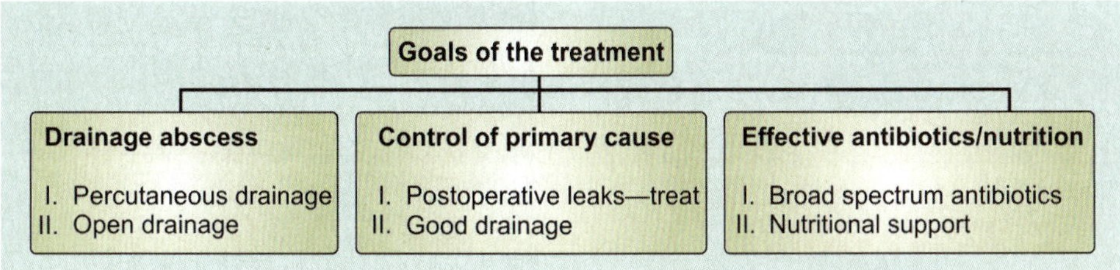


*Types*

A. ***Pigtail catheter*** (using Seldinger's technique): It is a small tube used to drain bile, urine, pancreatic fluid or abscess (Fig. 57.39).

B. ***Trocar catheter:*** 12–16 F trocar is used.

C. ***Sump catheter:*** It has a double lumen which permits irrigation as well as drainage and allows a good suction (Key Box 57.11).

**Pearls of Wisdom**

More than 90% of subphrenic abscesses are managed by percutaneous drainage successfully.

### II. *Laparoscopic Drainage*

With imaging, majority of subphrenic abscesses are treated by laparoscopic method. It is not only minimally invasive, but can drain all cavities, open loculi and a thorough lavage can be given. If any foreign body is present, it can be removed. However, if adhesions are present, damage to intestine can occur.

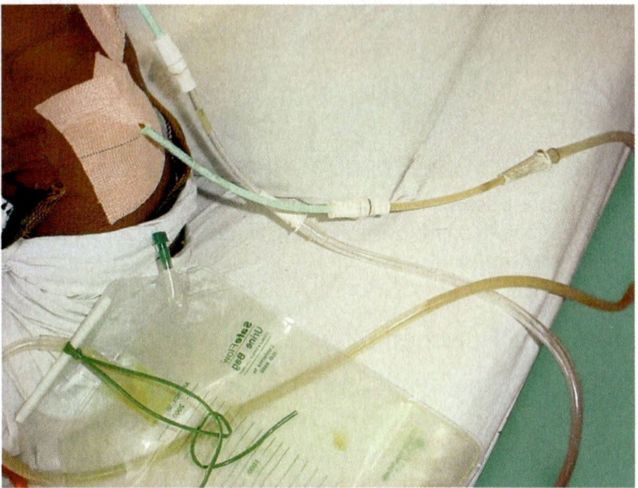

**Fig. 57.39:** Pigtail catheter drainage of left subphrenic abscess following gastric ulcer perforation

**Key Box 57.11**

**Indications for Removal of Catheter**

- Drainage less than 10 ml/day
- No fever, no pain
- WBC counts return to normal

### III. *Open Drainage* (Key Box 57.12)

- Lesser sac abscess and abscesses connected with the bowel, discharging pus or bile, are drained by intraperitoneal route.
- Open drainage is ideal in cases of multiloculated abscesses.

**Key Box 57.12**

**Indications for Open Drainage**

1. Multiloculated abscess
2. Persistent fistula discharging pus—communication with bowel
3. Thick viscid content
4. Failure of percutaneous aspirations
5. Abscess very close to IVC/diaphragm
6. Abscess with foreign body (MOP)

## PELVIC ABSCESS

This refers to accumulation of pus in the rectovesical pouch or pouch of Douglas (rectouterine pouch).

### Causes

- **Any peritonitis,** commonly following perforation due to ***acute appendicitis*** or following salpingo-oophoritis can result in pelvic abscess. The rectovesical pouch is the most dependent part in the body. Hence, the septic emboli accumulated in peritoneal space give rise to pelvic abscess.
- **Anastomotic leakage** is also an important cause.
- Perforated duodenal ulcer, perforated ileal ulcers are the other common causes.

### Clinical Features

- History of surgery/peritonitis
- Postoperative ***high-grade fever***
- History of **discharge of mucus per rectum** for the first time in a patient who is **recovering from peritonitis** suggests pelvic abscess. It occurs due to irritation of the rectum. Increased frequency of micturition occurs due to irritation of bladder.
- Deep tenderness in the suprapubic region.

- Continuing infection even after surgery—leak from an anastomotic line.
- Inadequate peritoneal toilet at the time of first surgery
- Inappropriate antibiotics.

### Diagnosis

- Confirmed by **per-rectal examination**. A **tender boggy** swelling is felt in the anterior wall of rectum. **Ultrasound** can define an abscess and can detect the size of the abscess.
- **CT scan** is very useful in defining pelvic abscess, its extent and to detect presence of a foreign body (Fig. 57.40).

### Treatment (Fig. 57.41)

- Under general anaesthesia, a proctoscope is introduced and a nick is made in the anterior wall of the rectum to open into the abscess cavity. Pus is drained with a sinus forceps through the rectum. There is no peritoneal contamination. The cavity collapses after a few days. Postoperatively, the patient is given broad-spectrum antibiotics.
- In females, pus can be drained through posterior fornix.

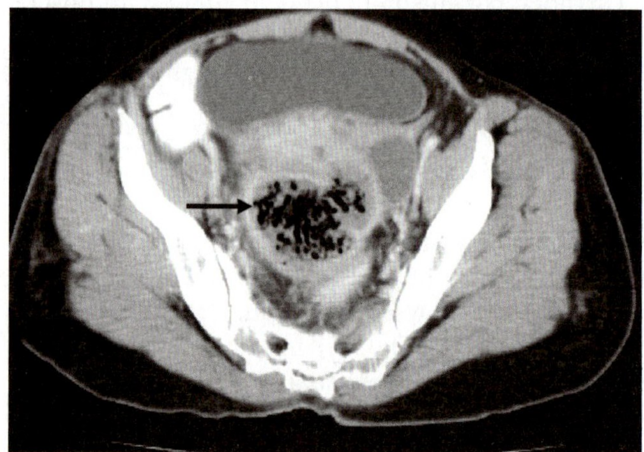

**Fig. 57.40:** CT scan showing gauze pieces—she had persistent foul-smelling vaginal discharge

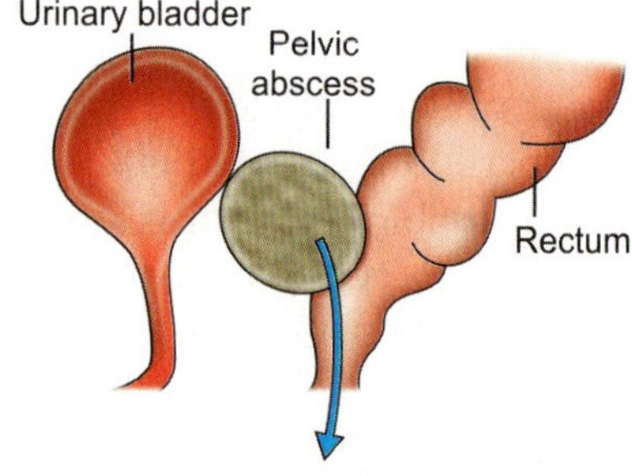


**Fig. 57.41:** Drainage of pelvic abscess through the rectum

**Clinical Notes**

A 36-year-old lady underwent vaginal hysterectomy for dysfunctional uterine bleeding. To control the bleeders, several gauze pieces were used without a proper count. After 2 weeks, purulent discharge per vagina, fever, ill health were reported. Ultrasound done showed a pelvic abscess. CT scan done in our hospital showed foreign body with air trap suggesting gauze pieces. Her abdomen was explored, abscess drained and the gauze pieces were removed.

## SPECIAL TYPES OF PERITONITIS

**SU28.3.3:** Summarize the tubercular peritonitis (*see* Page 905), spontaneous bacterial peritonitis, pneumococcal peritonitis, familial mediterranean fever (periodic peritonitis).

## PNEUMOCOCCAL PERITONITIS

- Primary variety is more common. Girls of 3–6 years of age are usually affected. Infection spreads from female genital tract through vagina.
- Malnourishment precipitates pneumococcal peritonitis.
- In boys, blood spread can occur following upper respiratory tract infection.

### Clinical Features

- High grade fever with features of toxaemia.
- Bloody diarrhoea and frequency of micturition are indicative of pelvic peritoneal inflammation.
- Other features of peritonitis are present.

### Diagnosis

Aspiration of peritoneal fluid demonstrates high WBC count—30,000/mm$^3$. More than 90% are polymorphs.

### Treatment

Laparotomy and drainage of pus (odourless and sticky initially and creamy or purulent in the later stages), followed by appropriate antibiotics.

## PRIMARY STREPTOCOCCAL PERITONITIS

- Infants and children less than 4 years are commonly affected.
- Peritoneal exudate is cloudy and contains flakes of fibrin.
- Symptoms of gastroenteritis—greenish watery stools are present.
- Source of infection is tonsillitis, pharyngitis, etc.
- Treated with injection crystalline penicillin.

## PARTURITION PERITONITIS

- This occurs after delivery, if proper aseptic precautions are not taken. The incidence has come down in the recent years. Attempted abortions by using instruments

**TABLE 57.2:** Summary of various types of peritonitis

| Type | Age | Route | Exudate |
|---|---|---|---|
| Pneumococcal | 3–6 years | Vagina | Odourless, sticky, turbid pus with high-grade fever |
| β-haemolytic streptococci | Children | Vagina | Cloudy and fibrin flakes + |
| Parturition | 20–40 years | Vagina | Thick pus + |
| Tuberculous | 20–40 years | Pulmonary tuberculosis | Straw-coloured fluid + tubercles + |
| Perforation peritonitis | 20–40 years | Hollow viscus | Foul-smelling exudate + |

Key Box 57.13

**Abortion Peritonitis**

- Instrumentation
- Puerperal sepsis
- Offensive lochia
- Pelvic peritonitis
- Infertility

which are not sterile results in peritonitis. Most of the time, peritonitis is confined to pelvis with paralytic ileus, mucous diarrhoea and offensive lochia (Key Box 57.13). Late cases develop generalised peritonitis, intra-abdominal abscess, intestinal obstruction and infertility. Table 57.2 gives summary of various types of peritonitis.

- Other name for this type of peritonitis is abortion peritonitis.

## SPONTANEOUS BACTERIAL PERITONITIS (SBP)

As the name suggests, in this condition, there is no demonstrable intra-abdominal disease responsible for peritonitis, such as perforation, abscess, gangrene, etc.

### Types

1. **In infants:** It is more common in female children. Spread is by haematogenous route. The causative organisms are *Streptococcus pneumoniae.* It may follow respiratory tract or urinary tract infection (Key Box 57.14).
2. **In adults:** Male alcoholic patients are commonly affected followed by patients with chronic liver disease. Causative organisms are *E. coli, S. faecalis,* etc.

Key Box 57.14

**Risk Factors**

**CHILDREN**

- Malnutrition
- Malignancy
- Chemotherapy
- Splenectomy

*Low protein in the ascites prevents opsonisation of bacteria*

**ADULTS**

- Cirrhosis → *Usually associated with SBP*
- Nephrotic syndrome
- Chronic renal failure

- **Portal hypertension** increases **permeability of gut wall**, thus increasing bacterial migration. These bacteria which colonise in the small bowel reach systemic circulation **because of shunting of blood around liver** sinusoids. **Portal lymph also gets contaminated** giving rise to increased ascitic fluid. So, this is translocation of bacteria.
- It is interesting to note that it is rare for anaerobic microorganism to produce SBP. Due to high volume of oxygen in the intestinal wall, they cannot translocate.

### Clinical Features

- **Dull aching** pain in the abdomen with low-grade fever.
- **Rebound tenderness** is present, bowel sounds are absent or sluggish—abdominal distension.
- Cirrhotic patients may develop ***coma*** with onset of primary bacterial peritonitis.
- **Septic shock** is a late feature with a high mortality rate.

### Investigations

- Leucocytosis, ↓albumin, ↑prothrombin time suggests sepsis.
- **Peritoneal tap and Gram staining** of the fluid.
- The diagnosis of SBP is made when ascitic fluid contains more than 250 neutrophils/$mm^3$. Ascitic fluid also has low protein.
- Ascitic fluid culture is usually monomicrobial.
- **Laparoscopy** may help to rule out intra-abdominal emergencies, such as perforations, etc.
- **Ultrasound** can detect nature of the liver and amount of fluid in the abdomen.
- **CT scan** when in doubt about the diagnosis.

### Treatment

- Conservative treatment is followed, provided secondary bacterial peritonitis is ruled out.
- Broad-spectrum antibiotics, such as aminoglycosides with 3rd generation cephalosporins are the ideal choice. Metronidazole can also be added.
- Instillation of antibiotic solution into ascitic fluid to achieve a quick and high concentration.
- If laparotomy is done, peritoneal wash or toilet is given.

## PERIODIC PERITONITIS

- Also called familial Mediterranean fever.
- It is of unknown aetiology.
- It affects children, young adults and females.
- Presents as abdominal pain, tenderness, pyrexia and increased total WBC count.
- When in doubt, laparotomy should be done.

**Some Salient Features (*Observe* 11Ps)**

- **Pyrin**—a protein product from the gene—MEFVgene mutation causes this
- **Pain** abdomen and tender abdomen
- **Pyrexia**
- **Pain** in the thorax
- **Period** of 2–3 days, it occurs and slowly remission occurs
- **Patients** are usually ***children***
- **Principally** occurs in ***Arabs, Armenians*** and ***Jews***
- **Primarily** runs in families
- **Peritoneal** inflammation is present
- **Polymorph** leucocyte count is increased
- **Prevent** recurrence—colchicine therapy

## POSTOPERATIVE PERITONITIS

### Introduction

It should be suspected following surgery on intestines or biliary tract, when a patient who is recovering from paralytic ileus starts deteriorating or when paralytic ileus does not return back to normal.

### Aetiology (Figs 57.42 and 57.43)

- Leakage from anastomotic line—most common
- Iatrogenic visceral trauma
- Foreign bodies
- Suture line leakage

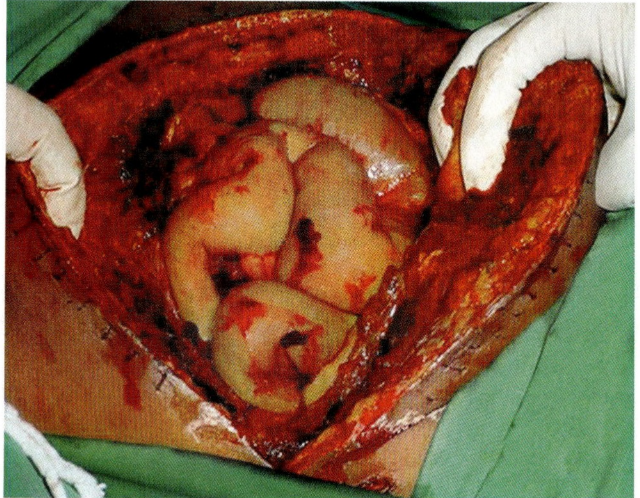

**Fig. 57.42:** Postoperative peritonitis due to post-cholecystectomy leak

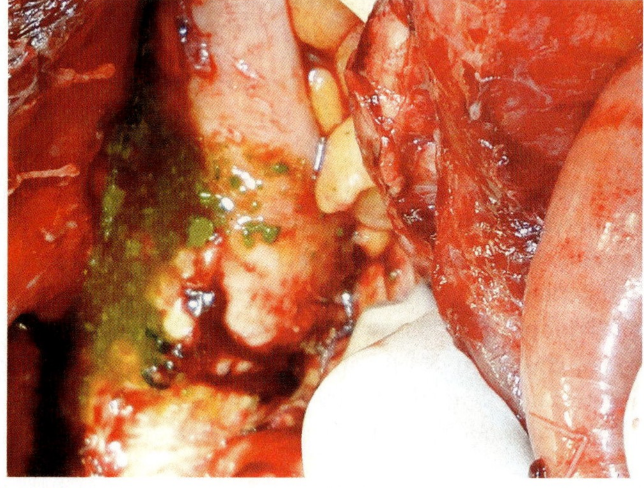

**Fig. 57.43:** Postoperative peritonitis due to anastomotic leak with faecal peritonitis

**1. Foreign bodies responsible for postoperative peritonitis**

| *Macroscopic* | *Microscopic* |
|---|---|
| • Gossypiboma | • Barium |
| • Textiloma | • Cloth piece |
| • Surgical drains | • Faecal matter |
| • Suture materials | • Necrotic tissue |
| • Surgical clips | • Talcum powder |
| • Implants | |
| • Instruments | |

**2. Presentation of foreign body**

| | |
|---|---|
| • Abdominal pain | • Intestinal obstruction |
| • Mass abdomen | • Fistula and sinus |
| • Granuloma, fever | • Extrusion—sometimes the foreign body may be visible to the exterior |

### Causes of Delay in the Diagnosis

- Presence of fever is attributed to other sources of infection such as urinary tract infection, thrombophlebitis, etc.
- Presence of pain and tenderness is attributed to recent laparotomy scar.
- Steroid therapy masks the local signs and symptoms.
- Administration of antibiotics would have reduced the severity of peritonitis (masking effect) only to manifest as septicaemia some time later.

### Bacteriology

**Common organisms in postoperative peritonitis**

| | |
|---|---|
| A. Gram –ve bacilli | *E. coli* |
| *Klebsiella* | *Proteus* |
| *Pseudomonas* | |
| B. Anaerobes | Bacteroides |
| *Clostridium* | Peptostreptococci |
| Fusobacteria | |
| C. Gram +ve cocci | Enterococci |
| Staphylococci | Streptococci |

## How to Suspect Postoperative Peritonitis

- Patient who is recovering from initial surgery, complains of abdominal pain and distension. He is not well. Has fever (Fig. 57.44).
- Tenderness is a feature.
- Deterioration after 3–5 days of operation (the time when anastomotic dehiscence takes place).
- Delay in recovery from paralytic ileus—abdominal distension.
- Evidence of toxaemia—tachycardia, tachypnoea.
- Free drainage of bile and faecal matter or pus from the drain site or the main wound.
- Oliguria may be an early indicator of postoperative sepsis.
- Guarding, rigidity may be present but minimal.

## Treatment of Postoperative Peritonitis (Fig. 57.45)

**I. Anastomotic leak:** Majority of the cases are due to anastomotic leak.

- Wait and watch policy is done, if contents are coming out freely and patient is haemodynamically stable, no tachycardia, no tachypnoea, no hypotension.
- Send few important investigations and inflammatory markers such as total WBC, CRP (C-Reactive proteins) and lactate levels. If these are elevated and patient is not improving further testing to be done.
- CECT of abdomen is done to rule out fistula tract/ communication/foreign bodies, etc.

  **Examples:** If a leak is detected from duodenal ulcer perforation closure site, re-suture it. Then add feeding jejunostomy and drain peritoneal cavity.
- If right hemicolectomy has leaked, explore, trim the edges, suture healthy tissue and do a protective proximal ileostomy.

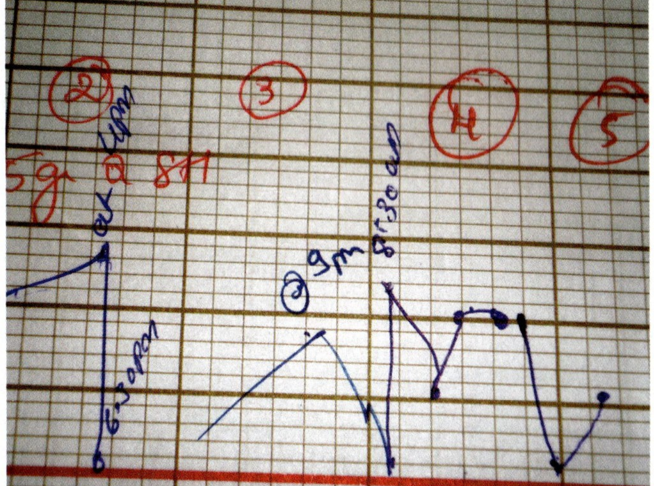

Fig. 57.44: Postoperative peritonitis due to anastomotic leak with faecal peritonitis—look at the temperature chart

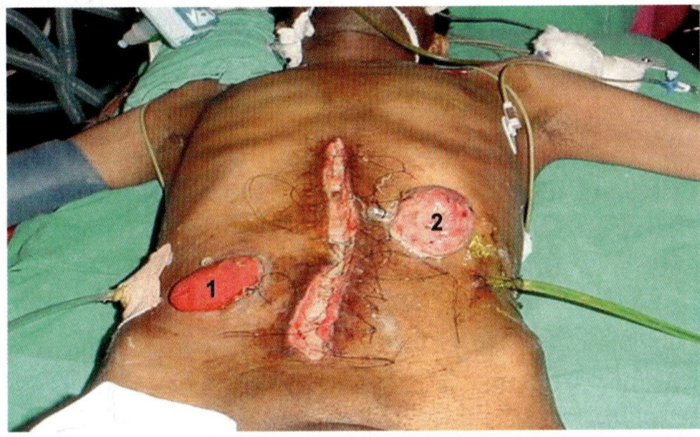


Fig. 57.45: Postoperative peritonitis due to leak following right hemicolectomy for carcinoma caecum. There were 2 sites of leak: 1. Ileocolic anastomotic site, 2. proximal jejunum. Both were exteriorized. You can see the wound left open with loose skin sutures—they will be tied after 3–4 days. This is to prevent wound infection (almost inevitable)

- If a colocolic anastomosis has leaked, redo the anastomosis, with or without proximal stoma.

*Pearls of Wisdom*

1. While doing an ileocolic or colocolic anastomosis for 2nd time, check for adequate vascularity of both ends of the bowel. Suture, if bowel is pink and mesentery shows pulsations. The suturing must be gentile but tight. It should not be too tight.
2. A proximal diversion ileostomy or colostomy is better.
3. Improve nutrition by total parenteral nutrition.

**II. Prevention of gossypiboma (mop)**

- Double counting
- Sponges with radio-opaque markers
- Avoid using packs—fascial closure
- Intraoperative radiology
- High degree of suspicion (*see* clinical notes)

**III. Specific treatment** (Key Box 57.15)

Key Box 57.15

**Treatment**

- Danger lies in delay, not in reoperation
- Leak or abscess cavity is confirmed by abdominal ultrasound/CT scan.
- Exploration (preparation similar to a routine laparotomy)
- Resection or resuturing, ileostomy, colostomy
- Drainage of abscess cavity
- Refashioning of colostomy, if it is retracted
- Appropriate antibiotics
- Delayed closure of skin
- Peritoneal lavage
- Once abscess is drained or leakage is prevented, recovery is wonderful.

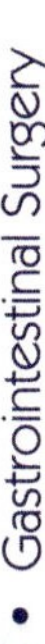

### Poor Prognostic Factors in Postoperative Peritonitis

- Increasing age
- Organ(s) failure
- Colonic perforation
- Multiple abscess
- Lesser sac abscess
- Malnutrition
- Postoperative pneumonia
- **Anergy:** It (immunologic tolerance) refers to the failure to mount a full immune response against a target.

## BILIARY PERITONITIS

- Leakage of bile into the peritoneal cavity results in biliary peritonitis.
- It will be more obvious and can be detected early, if a drainage tube has been kept.

### Causes

1. **Surgery on the gallbladder**
    - Leakage from the cystic duct
    - Injury to the right hepatic duct
    - Leak from accessory cholecystohepatic duct
2. **Surgery on the CBD**
    - Retained stones in the lower CBD (postoperative)
    - Loose sutures over CBD
    - T-tube not anchored properly
3. **Surgery on the duodenum**
    - Sphincteroplasty
    - Partial gastrectomy
    - Perforation of sutured duodenal ulcer
4. **Injury to the duodenum**
    - During nephrectomy, hemicolectomy
    - Blunt injury
5. **Instrumentation:** ERCP, stenting or following duodenal polypectomy.
6. **Diseases of the gallbladder:** Perforation or gangrene of the gallbladder.

### Clinical Features (Fig. 57.46)

- In majority of the cases, the local signs are confined to one quadrant of the abdomen in the form of guarding and rigidity.
- There may be excoriation of the skin due to drainage of bile to the exterior.
- However, when the anastomosis gives way, generalised peritonitis can occur.
- In untreated cases, septicaemic shock can develop.
- Untreated patients have high mortality rates.

### Treatment

**Basic principle** is in cases of post cholecystectomy, if the drain is in place, leaks are less than 200 ml per day and patient is not in sepsis, one can wait and watch. The fistula will heal over 1–2 weeks time. However, any fistula output more than 200 ml per day and with or without toxic features/sepsis/deterioration, better to get ERCP followed by stenting of the biliary duct. Septic focus inside abdomen, has to be drained out.

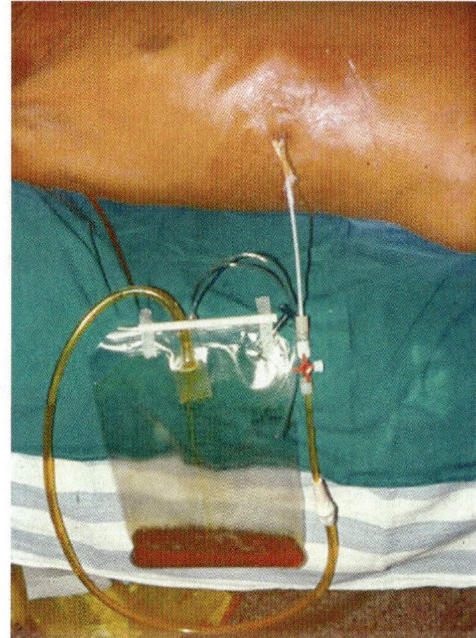

**Fig. 57.46:** Post-cholecystectomy bile leak due to injury to the common bile duct. Majority of such leaks can be managed conservatively. If the leak continues, get an ERCP done and treat the cause accordingly

Feeding jejunostomy is a very useful procedure in all cases of reperforation of sutured duodenal ulcers or difficult duodenal ulcer closures.

It should be remembered that feeding jejunostomy is temporary and is kept till it is assured that there is no leak from the operated site. If there is no peritonitis, the patient has passed flatus and stools, jejunostomy tube is removed.

Feeding jejunostomy should be done carefully with proper placement of catheter within the small bowel, fixing it firmly both inside and outside the abdominal wall and fixing to the bowel wall.

#### Complications of feeding jejunostomy

- Bile leak from the entry point.
- Tube blockage, if it is not flushed properly after feeding.
- Bleeding, displacement and intussusception.

## GRANULOMATOUS PERITONITIS

- Talc, gauze, starch, etc. are causative factors.
- It occurs many weeks after surgery.
- Low-grade fever, weight loss, distension, crampy abdominal pain are the features.

- Laparoscopy is the key investigation. One can visualise granuloma and biopsy can be taken. Also, fluid can be aspirated and sent for histopathology. High concentrations of lymphocytes are present in both.
- Symptomatic treatment—sinus, fistula needs to be treated.
- Intravenous prednisolone followed by oral prednisolone for 2–3 weeks is given.

### Prevention

- Cleaning the gloves by wiping before handling bowel, prevents many cases of granulomatous peritonitis.
- In the initial surgery, all the foreign bodies including ova, cysts of parasites, ascariasis and ingested food particles have to be removed.

## TUMOURS OF THE PERITONEUM

- **Primary:** Mesothelioma is the tumour to be remembered. It is more common from the pleura. In the abdomen, pelvic peritoneum is the common site.
- **Secondary** tumours are—pseudomyxoma peritonei and carcinoma peritonei.

## PSEUDOMYXOMA PERITONEI

- In this condition, peritoneal cavity is filled with mucoid substance (jelly-like) brownish or yellowish.
- **Mucinous adenocarcinoma of the ovary** is the cause.
- Primary tumour is **very slow growing** and metastasis is exceptional.
- Ruptured mucinous adenocarcinoma appendix and/or ovarian adenocarcinoma are the causes.
- Once rupture takes place, peritoneal cavity is studded with jelly-like mucous-secreting tumours which appear as large loculated cystic masses.
- From the appendix (Key Box 57.16), it can be benign-mucinoma of appendix to mucinous adenocarcinomas.

### Clinical Features

- Age group: 40–50 years. Equal incidence in both sexes.
- The patients can present with slow, painless and progressive abdominal distension. No shifting dullness.
- A few patients present with features of intestinal obstruction.

Key Box 57.16

**Sites**

- Appendix—common site
- Ovary—common site
- Intestines—not uncommon sites
- Uterus, urachus—rare sites

- Recurrence can occur because the tumour is locally malignant.

### Investigations

CECT of abdomen/pelvis is done to get details about any previous pathology in the appendix or ovary.

### Treatment

- Remove as much as possible **(debulking)**. This is described as cytoreduction.
- Appendicectomy, omentectomy, peritonectomy.
- Reject the involved organs (adjacent to tumours) may be colon, small bowel, etc.
- Hyperthermic intraperitoneal chemotherapy (HIPEC) (Key Boxes 57.17 and 57.18).

Key Box 57.17

**Treatment of Pseudomyxoma Peritonei**

- Remove as much as possible-cytoreduction.
- Resect the adjacent involved tissues.
- Kill cancer cells by hyperthermia-intraperitoneal chemotherapy.
- Doxorubicin, mitomycin, oxaliplatin are the common drugs.
- Technique of HIPEC is called coliseum technique.

Key Box 57.18

**Hyperthermic Intraperitoneal Chemotherapy (HIPEC)**

- Advantage of HIPEC is high concentration of drugs locally and low levels in the systemic circulation.
- Also these drugs from the peritoneal cavity get into portal veins, act on metastasis, if present in the liver.
- Hyperthermia kills the malignant cells locally at the temperature around 41 to 43°C.
- Hyperthermia added by cytoxic drugs results in increased cytotoxicity.

**Two methods are available for HIPEC**

1. Open method: It is called coliseum technique by Sugarbaker.
   - A Tenchkhoff catheter with 4 closed suction drains is used. They are passed through abdominal wall.
   - 30 to 90 minutes perfusion is done.
2. Closed technique: Laparotomy is done and skin edges are closed. It is much more rapidly acting.

**Drugs used:**

- These are the primary drugs used to treat original cancer.
- Carrier solutions are 1.5% dextrose isotonic solution which is used for peritoneal dialysis, most commonly used.
- Mitomycin C 15 mg/m$^2$ for appendicular carcinoma, Doxorubicin 15 mg/m$^2$ for colonic carcinoma and ovarian carcinoma are used.

## CARCINOMA PERITONEI

This name is applied to an advanced stage of intra-abdominal malignancy involving the entire peritoneal cavity.

Carcinomas of the stomach, colon, pancreas, breast and ovary are the common causes.

### Features at Laparotomy

- Multiple firm to hard nodules on the visceral and parietal peritoneum.
- Dense adhesions between the intestinal loops and other viscera.
- Plaques on the intestinal surface
- Widespread secondaries in the liver
- Entire omentum will be studded with hard nodules. It is called omentum cake.
- Ascites: Straw-coloured or haemorrhagic
- Greater omentum being the **policeman** and a great drain pipe of the abdomen with rich lymphatics, is studded with nodules.
- Low protein ascites is more vulnerable for risk of developing peritonitis. **Incidence of peritonitis in malignant ascites cases is low because of increased immunoglobulin levels in malignant ascites and increased opsonic activity.**

### Differential Diagnosis

- The most common differential diagnosis is tuberculosis (peritoneal). These nodules are firm and greyish.
- Acute pancreatitis with fat necrosis: This is due to calcium soap. They are yellow and soft.
- Ruptured hydatid cyst
- Lymphomatous nodules
- Ruptured GIST (not common, Fig. 57.47)

### Treatment

1. Radioactive gold ($^{198}Au$) instillation into peritoneal cavity.
2. Tamoxifen is useful for ascites due to carcinoma of the breast.

## THE OMENTUM

Surgically important diseases in the omentum are:

1. **Tuberculous peritonitis:** Here omentum is involved. It becomes nodular because it is studded with tubercles. Classically seen in children who are brought with abdominal distension. On palpation, omentum is felt as granular mass in the upper abdomen which moves with respiration. Laparoscopy, biopsy and antitubercular treatment is given in Fig. 57.48.

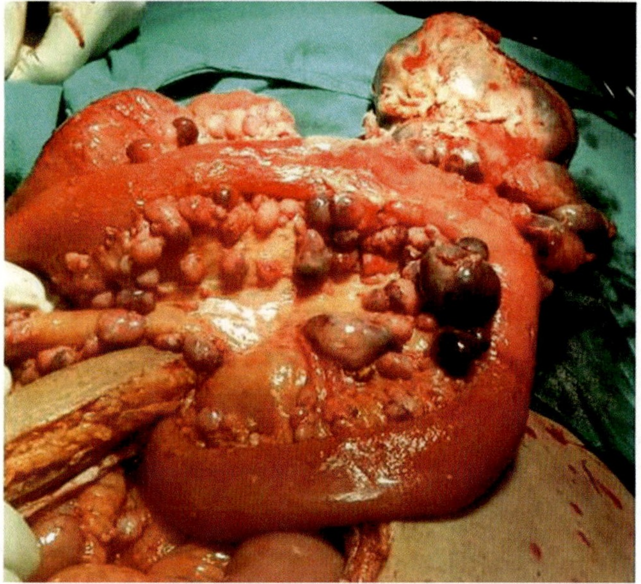

**Fig. 57.47:** Disseminated perforated GIST of small intestines. (*Courtesy:* Dr Jyothi, Head, Department of Surgery, GIMS, Gadag, Karnataka)

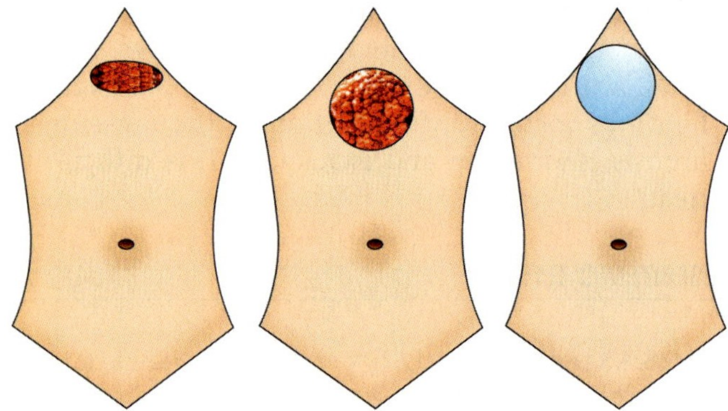

**Fig. 57.48:** Rolled up omentum in tuberculosis

**Fig. 57.49:** Omental cake in metastasis

**Fig. 57.50:** Omental cyst (lymphatic)

2. **Metastasis:** Carcinoma stomach, colon, pancreas commonly result in metastasis and they give rise to omental cake (Fig. 57.49).
3. **Tumour (cyst):** Omentum is the site of omental cyst which is a lymphatic cyst (Fig. 57.50). It is a slow-growing, painless swelling in the upper abdomen. On examination, the patient is a child or an adult, with a smooth, firm mass in epigastrium which moves with respiration. Excision of the lymphatic cyst is the treatment. Massive cyst can be confused for ascites.
4. **Torsion:** It is a rare surgical emergency wherein torsion of omentum occurs due to old **adhesions** or it is primary due to lengthy mobile omentum. It produces symptoms/signs similar to that of appendicitis. Laparotomy and excision of gangrenous omentum have to be done.

5. **Non-Hodgkin's lymphoma** can affect ometum and can give rise to granularity.
**Complications:** Haemorrhage into the cyst.

## MESENTERY

- **Anatomy:** Given on page 900.
- Mesenteric tear has been discussed on page 901.
- Mesenteric lymphadenitis has been discussed on page 907.

### MISTY MESENTERY

- It means increase in the mesenteric fat and it is a finding in the multi-detector CT scan.
- **A few pathological conditions which may give rise to this entity are:** Acute pancreatitis, retroperitoneal haemorrhage, malignancies.
- Once the source is treated, the findings may reduce or may disappear.
- Hence, follow-up CT scans are required.
- **Weber-Christian disease:** Lipodystrophy and mesenteric lipogranuloma are the features. In this condition, it should be called mesenteric panniculitis. Findings include inflammation of the mesentery, fibrosis, shortening and ischaemia. It is difficult to treat.

### MESENTERIC CYST

> **SU28.4.3 and SU28.4.4:** Define and classify mesenteric cyst. Pathology, clinical features, differential diagnosis, investigations and management of mesenteric cyst.

These are congenital cysts, enterogenous or chylolymphatic. It manifests in young children or during adolescence. Typically, the cyst is located in the umbilical region which moves at right angles to the direction of mesentery (Fig. 57.51).

#### Types of Mesenteric Cysts

(Figs 57.52 to 57.54, Key Box 57.19)

A. **Chylolymphatic cyst** is a lymphatic cyst arising from mesentery of ileum. It is a thin-walled cyst with clear fluid or chyle. It has a separate blood supply. Hence, enucleation is the treatment without sacrificing the bowel.

B. **Enterogenous cyst** is a duplication cyst from the intestine or due to diverticulum of the mesenteric border of the intestine. It is thick walled and contains mucus. This cyst is treated by excision of cyst with bowel segment because both share the same blood supply.

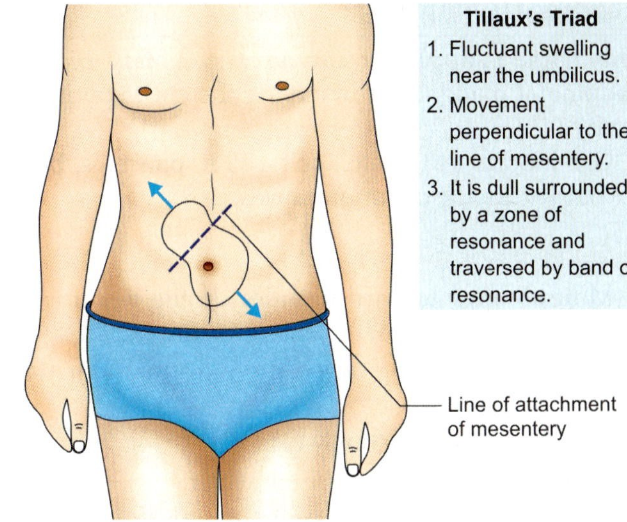


**Fig. 57.51:** Mesenteric cyst and its movements at right angles to the direction of mesentery (diagrammatic)

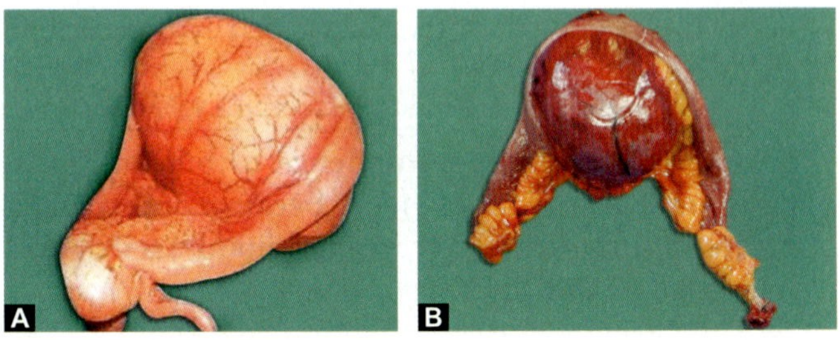


**Figs 57.52A and B:** (A) Mesenteric cyst excised in toto; (B) Enterogenous cyst. (*Courtesy:* Dr Jayan, Professor of Surgery, Calicut)

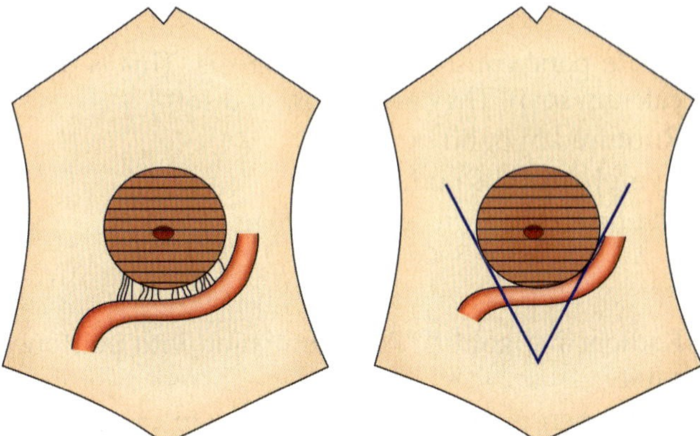

**Fig. 57.53:** Chylolymphatic cyst—it can be excised with-out resection of the bowel

**Fig. 57.54:** Enterogenous cyst—it requires excision of intestine along with the cyst

**Key Box 57.19**

**Mesenteric Cyst—Types**

- Chylolymphatic cyst
- Enterogenous cyst
- Urogenital remnant
- Teratomatous dermoid cyst

### Complications

- Torsion of the cyst resulting in acute abdominal pain.
- Rupture of the cyst due to trauma
- Haemorrhage into the cyst

## RETROPERITONEUM

### ANATOMY

**Retroperitoneal space:** The retroperitoneal space lies between the peritoneum and the posterior parietal wall of the abdominal cavity and extends from the diaphragm to the pelvic floor.

- **Superiorly**—12th thoracic vertebra and lateral lumbocostal arch.
- **Inferiorly**—base of the sacrum, iliac crest, and iliolumbar ligament.
- **Anteriorly**—posterior parietal peritoneum.
- **Posteriorly**—fascia overlying the quadratus lumborum and psoas major muscles.

### Important Anatomical Organs (Fig. 57.55)

1. **Urinary:** Adrenal glands, kidneys, ureter, bladder
2. **Circulatory:** Aorta, inferior vena cava
3. **Digestive:** Oesophagus (thoracic part), rectum (part of middle third and lower third is extraperitoneal).
4. The head, neck, and body of the pancreas, the duodenum, except for the proximal first segment, ascending and descending portions of the colon.

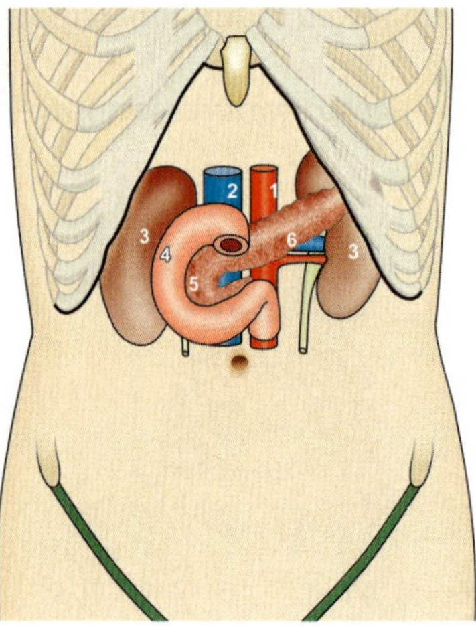

**Posterior abdominal wall includes the following structures**

1. Abdominal aorta
2. Inferior vena cava
3. Right and left kidneys with ureters
4. Duodenum on the right side
5. Head of pancreas in the concavity of duodenum
6. Body and tail of pancreas across the posterior abdominal wall towards the left kidney

**Fig. 57.55:** Anatomical organs in the retroperitoneal space

### IDIOPATHIC RETROPERITONEAL FIBROSIS—ORMOND'S DISEASE

> **SU28.4.6:** Describe etiology, clinical features, differential diagnosis and management of retroperitoneal fibrosis.

- This is one of a group of fibromatosis (other being Dupuytren's contracture and Peyronie's disease).
- Other types of fibrosis such as mediastinal fibrosis, sclerosing cholangitis may also be associated features.
- Riedel's thyroiditis may be associated with this condition.
- As collagen encases ureters, they present with ureteric obstructions, requiring ureteric stenting.
- Steroid therapy is the treatment of choice.
- Tamoxifen may help.
- It can present with lower back pain, renal failure, hypertension, deep vein thrombosis and other obstructive features.

  *See* Key Box 57.20 and Clinical Notes.

**Key Box 57.20**

**Idiopathic Retroperitoneal Fibrosis—Causes**

**I**diopathic—Ormond's disease
**D**rugs—chemotherapy, methysergide, β-adrenoreceptor antagonists
**I**rritation—blood, urine, bowel contents
**O**thers—autoimmune
**P**eritoneal disease—secondaries
**A**ortic aneurysm—inflammatory type
**T**rauma
**H**ereditary/familial
**I**nflammation—chronic
**C**arcinoid
*Remember as* **IDIOPATHIC**

**Clinical Notes**

- One day I was urgently called to assist the urosurgeon who had opened the abdomen for ureterolysis. Following was the clinical picture.
- A 76-year-old lady was admitted under urology for the diagnosis of renal failure. An ultrasound abdomen showed bilateral hydronephrosis. She was diagnosed to have idiopathic retroperitoneal fibrosis and posted for ureterolysis. To my surprise, when I explored, the patient had carcinoma colon in three places (synchronous), carcinoma caecum infiltrating right ureter, carcinoma sigmoid colon infiltrating left ureter and carcinoma transverse colon. She underwent total colectomy with ileorectal anastomosis. Ureteric reimplantations were done into bladder. She lived for 3 years and then succumbed due to liver metastasis.

### RETROPERITONEAL CYST

- Very often, it is a painless, smooth, firm enlargement.
- May have minor degree of mobility.
- These cysts are either lymphatic cysts or derived from the remnant of Wolffian duct. A few of them are teratomatous dermoids.

- Benign retroperitoneal cysts are usually mesothelial or mesonephric in origin; rarely, rupture of the biliary tree can result in bile-filled cysts.
- **Gross:** These cysts are not connected to the kidney or adrenal; usually filled with clear or straw-coloured fluid.
- **Histology:** These cystic structures may be lined by mesothelial, enteric (glandular), or columnar epithelium.
- They can be unilocular or multilocular.
- CT scan is required to differentiate it from hydronephrosis.
- Excision is the treatment.

## RETROPERITONEAL ABSCESS

### Causes

1. Renal source: Pyonephric abscess
2. Tuberculosis of spine (Pott's spine)
3. Haematoma: Fracture spine/pelvis
4. Acute pancreatitis (on right side)
5. Retrocaecal appendicitis (on right side)
6. Sigmoid diverticulitis.

### Diagnosis

- Ultrasound or CT scan-guided aspiration.
- Culture of the pus and antibiotic sensitivity.

### Treatment

Aspiration, appropriate antibiotics and open drainage.

## PSOAS ABSCESS

Three types have been recognised:

1. **Primary psoas abscess:** It is caused by haematogenous spread of *Staphylococcus aureus*. Source may be occult—tonsils, middle ear, etc. More common in children and young adults. Poor nutrition, may be a contributing factor—it is **monomicrobial**.
2. **Secondary psoas abscess:** Secondary to intestinal perforation, e.g. Crohn's disease. It is **polymicrobial.** Other causes are diverticular perforation, acute pancreatitis, etc.

   *Clinical features*

   Fever, flank pain, and flexion of the hip joint are triad of psoas abscess. Pain on extension confirms the diagnosis.

   *Management*

   - CT scan is the diagnostic test. Gas bubbles are diagnostic of an abscess.
   - Treatment include percutaneous catheter drainage, treatment of the source of infection with antibiotics.
   - If necrotic tissue does not drain well or if patient is not improving, open drainage should be done.
3. **Tuberculous spine:** Lower thoracic (T10) and upper lumbar spine are commonly affected (Fig. 57.56).

### Clinical Features

- Pain in the back (localised to lesion) or referred pain, if there is a collapse.
- Evening pyrexia
- Protective muscular spasm, especially of sacrospinalis.
- Collapse of the anterior portion of vertebral body results in angular deformity—gibbus.

### Route of Psoas Abscess

- Pus enters psoas sheath and tracks downwards and causes mass in the iliac fossa.
- From here, it traverses beneath inguinal ligament.
- If untreated, it collects in the subcutaneous plane.

### Investigations

- **Chest X-ray, ESR, sputum AFB**
- **Spine X-ray**—AP and lateral view. The earliest sign is a decrease in the intervertebral space.
- **MRI** can detect spine lesion, cold abscess
- **CT/MR-guided aspiration of pus**/biopsy to prove histological diagnosis.

### Treatment

- Cold abscess—aspiration followed by antituberculous treatment.
- Unstable/collapse spine—costotransversectomy—lateral thoracotomy.

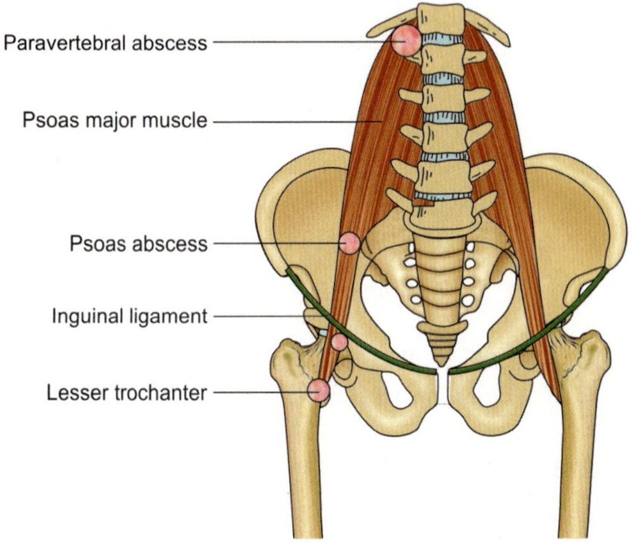


**Fig. 57.56:** Various sites of tubercular cold abscess arising from tuberculosis of the spine

## RETROPERITONEAL TUMOUR

**SU28.4.7:** Describe classification, clinical features, investigation to make diagnosis and management of retroperitoneal tumours.

### Definition

- The term retroperitoneal tumour (**RPT**) is usually confined to primary tumours arising in other tissues in this region, e.g. muscle, fat, lymph nodes, nerves (Tables 57.3 to 57.5). (**Jean Lobstein**, French pathologist and surgeon in 1829—coined the term **retroperitoneal tumour**).
- Other tissues refer to—tumours of retroperitoneal organs such as kidneys, ureters, pancreas and adrenals are conventionally not included in retroperitoneal tumours.

**TABLE 57.3:** Tumours of mesodermal origin (75%)

| | |
|---|---|
| Fatty tissue origin | *Lipoma/liposarcoma* |
| Smooth muscle origin | *Leiomyoma/leiomyosarcoma* |
| Connective tissue origin | *Fibroma/fibrosarcoma* |
| Lymphatic origin | *Lymphangioma/lymphangiosarcoma* |
| Mesenchymal origin | *Myxoma/myxosarcoma* |
| Vascular origin | *Haemangioma/haemangiosarcoma/ haemangiopericytoma* |
| Unknown origin | *Xanthogranuloma* |

**TABLE 57.4:** Tumours of notochordal or embryonic rests origin

| | |
|---|---|
| Embryonic origin | *Benign or malignant teratomas* |
| Notochordal origin | *Chordomas* |

**TABLE 57.5:** Tumours of neurogenic origin (25%)

| | |
|---|---|
| Germ cell origin | *Benign or malignant teratomas* |
| Sympathetic origin | *Chordomas* |
| Adrenochromaffin origin | *Cortical carcinoma/pheocromocytoma* |

### Introduction

- Uncommon (0.2–0.6% of all tumours)
- **Malignant** in 80–85% of cases (of these, 35% are sarcomas).
- **Sex:** No differences
- **Age:** Most occur between the sixth and seventh decade of life.
- Because of their location, these lesions usually demonstrate **indolent growth** and present as relatively large lesions.
- Their proximity to vital structures (especially vascular) makes **resection difficult**.

### Aetiology

1. Idiopathic: The actual cause is not known.
2. History of radiation: Accidental or given for lymphoma.
3. Exposure to vinyl chloride/thorium dioxide
4. **Familial disorders:** Gardner's syndrome, familial neuroblastoma, neurofibromatosis, Li-Fraumeni syndrome.

### Symptoms of RPT

- **Abdominal mass (80%):** Slow growing painless mass is the most common presentation. Typically confined to one side rather than centre (Key Box 57.21).
- **Nausea, vomiting** and weight loss in about 20 to 30% of patients.
- **Compressive symptoms:** Abdominal pain, constipation, recent haemorrhoids, haematochezia can occur. Back pain and sciatica (30%) are common and are confused for spine pathology.

  Unilateral lower extremity oedema and pressure symptoms including secondary varicosities are common.

  Acute urine retention, dysuria and increased frequency can occur due to compression on urinary bladder.
- **Paraneoplastic syndrome**, such as intermittent hypoglycaemia, can occur in liposarcoma/fibrosarcoma and catecholamine excess in paragangliomas.

Key Box 57.21

**When to Suspect Retroperitoneal Sarcoma**

- Recent finding of large abdominal mass
- Recent lower limb swelling
- Recent varicosities
- Recent varicocele
- Recent haemorrhoids
- Recent loss of weight

### Signs of RPT

- Usually large abdominal mass, firm to hard, irregular.
- Nonmobile or restricted mobility
- Not moving with respiration
- Does not fall forward (knee elbow position)
- Resonant tone on percussion—due to bowel anteriorly.
- Transmitted pulsations may be felt.

### TNM Staging

- Tumour differentiation: Score 1, 2 and 3
- Mitotic count: Score 1, 2 and 3
- Necrosis score: Score 0, 1 and 2

| Tumour (T) Category | | T Criteria | | |
|---|---|---|---|---|
| TX | | Primary tumour cannot be assessed | | |
| T0 | | No evidence of primary tumour | | |
| T1 | | Tumour <5 cm in greatest dimension | | |
| T2 | | Tumour 5 to 10 cm in greatest dimension | | |
| T3 | | Tumour >10 to 15 cm in greatest dimension | | |
| T4 | | Tumour >15 cm in greatest dimension | | |
| **Stage** | **Grade** | **Tumour** | **Nodes** | **Metastasis** |
| IA | G1, GX | T1 | N0 | M0 |
| IB | G1, GX | T2, T3, T4 | N0 | M0 |
| II | G2, G3 | T1 | N0 | M0 |
| IIIA | G2, G3 | T2 | N0 | M0 |
| IIIB | G2, G3 | T3, T4 | N0 | M0 |
| IV | G any | T any | N1 | M0 |
| IV | G any | T any | N any | M1 |

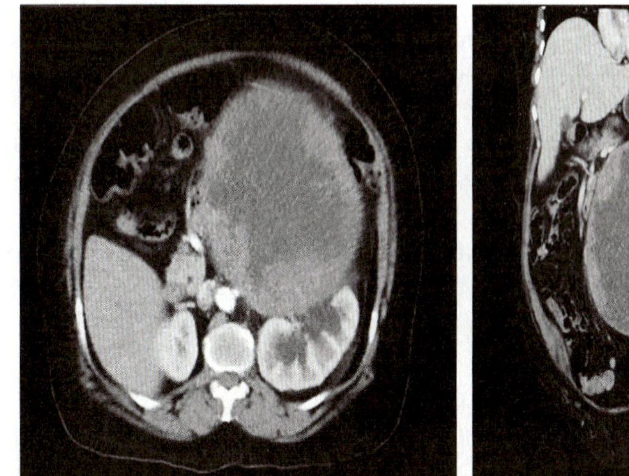
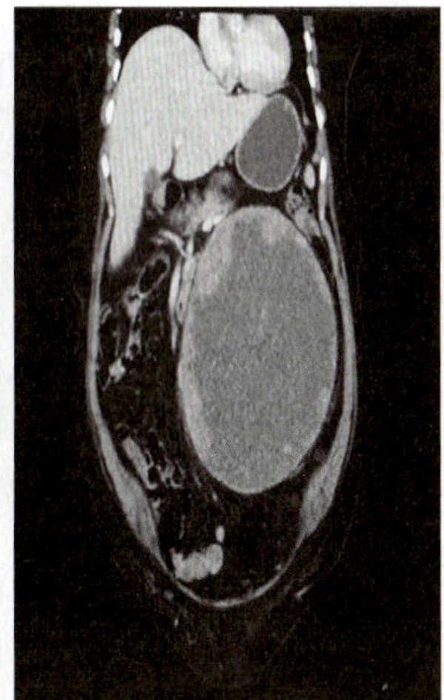
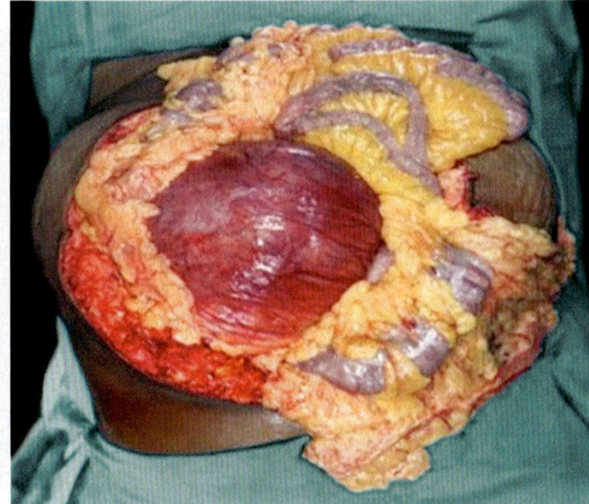

Fig. 57.57: A large well-defined peripheral nodular enhancing mass lesion with central non-enhancing areas (necrotic areas) and few peripheral chunks of calcification is noted arising from the retroperitoneum. Observe the change in the axis of the left kidney also.

## Differential Diagnosis

- Lymphoma
- Germ cell tumours
- GIST
- Metastatic testicular cancers

## Investigations

Preoperative planning to assess the extent of the disease is essential because successful surgery is defined by complete excision of the mass with adequate margins of normal tissue.

1. **CBP**
2. **LFT:** Increased alkaline phosphate may indicate secondaries.
3. **RFT:** Compressive uropathy with high urea and creatinine.
4. **Tumour markers:** AFP, beta-HCG—germ cell tumour.
5. **LDH in lymphoma/GCT:** LDH levels indicate tumour burden and growth rate.
6. **CT scan** (Key Box 57.22)
   - Delineate the anatomic limits of the lesion (Fig. 57.57).
   - Vascular involvement—vena cava, aorta, renal vessels.
   - Assess the integrity and function of adjacent organs—renal function is one of the important advantages of CT scan.
   - Visceral metastases +/–. If present, it is inoperable but resection after giving neoadjuvant therapy is still worth trying.
   - Para-aortic, iliac, mesenteric lymphadenopathy.
   - Axial skeleton and renal involvement (Key Box 57.22).

Key Box 57.22

**CT Scan: Typical Findings**

- **Lipoma:** Homogenous fatty density
- **Malignant fibrous histiocytoma:** Calcifications
- **Neurofibroma:** Homogenous low density
- **Teratoma:** Mixed components
- **Paraganglioma:** Para-aortic location
- **Neuroblastoma:** Calcified tumour, usually in children
- **Leiomyosarcoma:** Large areas of necrosis
- **Liposarcoma:** Heterogenous fatty density
- **Hemangiopericytoma:** Hypervascularity

7. **CT-guided core biopsy or laparoscopy and biospy:** Reserved for cases in which a diagnosis will change therapy, such as the need for neoadjuvant chemotherapy for:
   - GIST—imatinib mesylate
   - Germ cell tumours
   - Lymphomas
   - Metastatic testicular tumours.

## Treatment

Surgery is the main modality and the most effective modality of the treatment. It can be curative, if R-0 resection is achieved. Chemotherapy, radiotherapy are complementary to surgery. A few cases are also managed by neoadjuvant therapy.

### I. *Surgery*

**Principles:** Extirpative surgery is the principal and most effective form of therapy for primary retroperitoneal tumours. **Tumour histology, tumour size, or patient age are** *not significant factors in survival* in multiple-variable analysis. Therefore, carefully planned and skillfully executed surgical therapy is critical for any chance at long-term success.

**Adjuvant therapy:** This includes radiotherapy and chemotherapy.

High local recurrence rate and eventual mortality from this disease has prompted the exploration of adjuvant therapeutic modalities. **Postoperative radiation increases toxicity to surrounding structures.**

**A. Radiotherapy**

Radiotherapy: Two types:

1. EBRT—external beam radiotherapy
2. Brachytherapy for retroperitoneal leiomyosarcoma.

*Advantages*

- The viscera are often displaced by the tumour volume and a lack of surgical adhesions further reduces dose to the bowel.

**TEN COMMANDMENTS OF ROLE OF A SURGEON IN SARCOMA**

1. Biopsy site should be excised en bloc with the definitive surgical specimen (If biopsy is done)
2. Circumferential mobilization from all around
3. Do not ligate any major structure—renal pedicle, middle colic artery until and unless operability is decided. In doubtful cases, look into root of mesentery
4. Tumour must be removed in toto–avoid spillage.
5. Dissection should be through grossly normal tissue planes uncontaminated by tumour. R-0 RESECTION
6. Surgical clips should be placed to mark the periphery of the surgical field
7. En bloc resection of the sarcoma and contiguous organs that are macroscopically involved by tumour, multivisceral resection
8. No attempt is made to resect organs that merely lay adjacent to the tumour and are not involved.
9. If surgical margins are positive on final pathology, surgical re-resection should be considered unless bone, nerve, major blood vessels are involved.
10. Margins should be documented by both the surgeon and the pathologist.

**Enneking classification**

In his classification scheme, the four types of surgical margins were termed intralesional, marginal, wide, and radical (compartmental). The basis of the classification was the relationship of the margin to the tumor and its pseudocapsule. (Refer also page 291 in chapter 33)

- Effective radiation dose is lower in the preoperative setting.

**B. Chemotherapy**

- Doxorubicin is the foundation for chemotherapy in advanced sarcoma.
- **MAID regimen:** Mesna, adriamycin (doxorubicin), ifosfamide, and dacarbazine have been successful in neoadjuvant programmes for sarcomas of the extremities compared with historical controls.

## DIFFERENTIAL DIAGNOSIS OF RETROPERITONEAL SARCOMA

These are pathological variants. It is difficult to consider them as a diagnosis on clinical grounds. However, more common ones have to be considered first such as liposarcoma. Patients with von Recklinghausen's disease may have neural tumours. A few differential diagnosis are given below.

### Liposarcoma

Most common of primary RPT, 20% from retroperitoneum. More often about 30 to 40% of them arise from peri-nephric fat tissue.

- **Histological types**
  1. Well-differentiated liposarcoma (low grade)
  2. Myxoid/round cell liposarcoma (50%—most common)
  3. Pleomorphic liposarcoma (10–15%—high grade)
  4. Dedifferentiated liposarcoma—the rate of metastasis depends on the degree of tumour differentiation, with nearly 90% of poorly differentiated tumours metastasizing.
- **Pathology:** The key feature of a liposarcoma is the lipoblast, which is essentially an immature fat cell. **LIPOBLASTS** have multiple fat vacuoles which compress the nucleus, creating a scalloped appearance.

## Leiomyosarcoma

- 50% from retroperitoneum—Female: Male—2:1
- Site of origin (soft tissue, vascular or superficial), although many of the soft tissue lesions are believed to originate from smaller blood vessels (Figs 57.58 to 57.60).

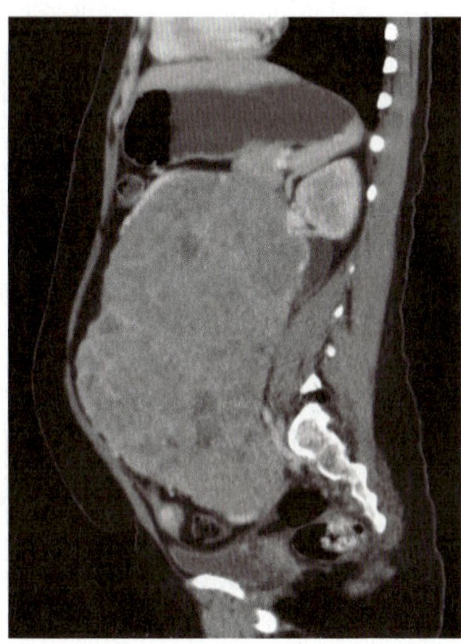

**Fig. 57.58:** CECT scan showing a large soft tissue tumour with areas of necrosis

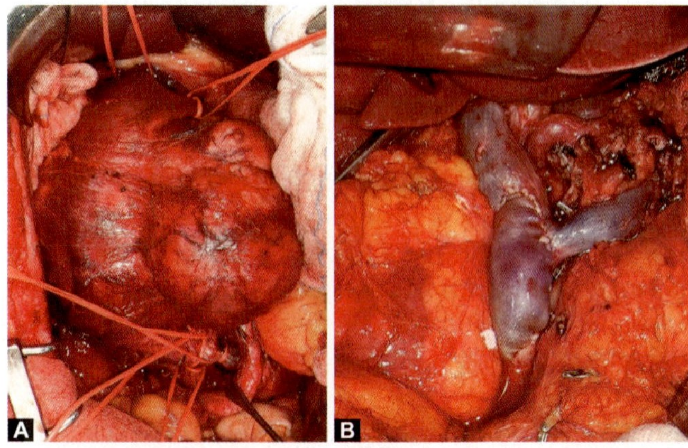

**Figs 57.59A and B:** (A) Shows tumour which is at surgery found to be arising from inferior vena cava; (B) Inferior vena cava is seen after complete excision of the tumour

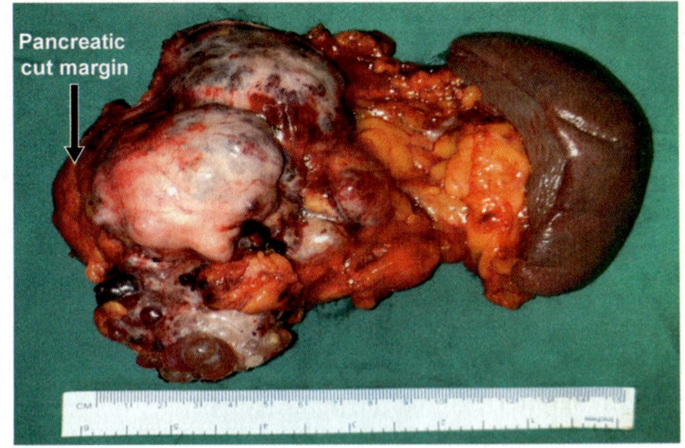


**Fig. 57.60:** Large pancreatic tumour from body of pancreas is excised along with spleen.

- Immunohistochemistry stain for smooth muscle myosin, vimentin, and actin and less often for desmin. (*Leiomyomas stain positive for desmin, which separates them from their malignant counterpart.*)
- They stain negative for S-100.

## Undifferentiated Pleomorphic Sarcoma—(Previously known as Malignant Fibrous Histiocytoma (MFH)

- Less common in the retroperitoneum.
- In the majority of cases, undifferentiated pleomorphic sarcoma affects the extremities. They are high grade tumours. Stage 3 or 4.
- It has an aggressive biological behaviour and a poor prognosis.
- Most undifferentiated pleomorphic sarcomas.
- They frequently metastasize (30–50% at diagnosis)
- Local recurrence is common despite adequate and aggressive treatment.
- The overall 5-year survival is between 25–70%.

## Retroperitoneal Teratoma

- These are the tumours arising from totipotential cells. Thus, they can have ectoderm, mesoderm or endoderm elements.
- 10% of all primary RPT.
- Rare in adults because of its congenital nature.
- Solid teratoma malignant (likely).
- Malignant mature cystic teratomas (0.2 to 2% of cases) have the potential to metastasise to sites such as the retroperitoneal lymph nodes and lung parenchyma.

## Rhabdomyosarcoma

- 6% in retroperitoneum
- More common in children
- Sporadic—most common
  - Genetic risk factor—10–33%: Li-Fraumeni syndrome, neurofibromatosis.

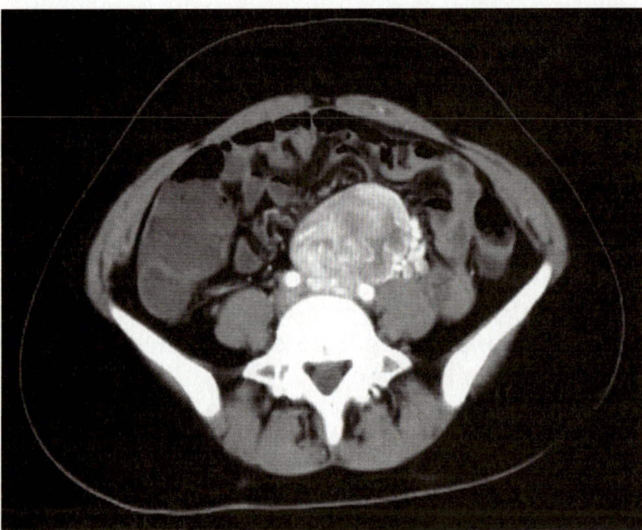

**Fig. 57.61:** Paraganglioma retroperitoneum. Arterial phase-Brilliant enhancement

## Schwannoma

- Majority has mutations in *NF2* gene.
- Majority are sporadic tumours.
- A minority (10%) are associated with syndromes, such as neurofibromatosis type 2, schwannomatosis and multiple meningiomas.
- Hallmark of schwannoma is alternating areas of cellular (Antoni A) and hypocellular (Antoni B) areas.

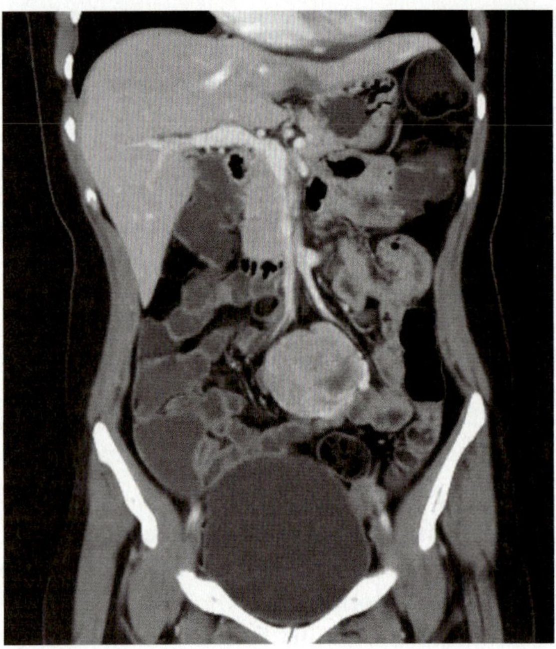

**Fig. 57.62:** Paraganglioma: Iliac artery + iliac vein seen. Left iliac vein compressed. Leash of vessels supplying tumour are also seen.

- Retroperitoneal tumours are larger and often show degenerative changes, such as cystic change, haemorrhage and calcifications.
- Immunohistochemistry: Diffuse S-100+ is characteristic (Figs 57.61 and 57.62).

## MULTIPLE CHOICE QUESTIONS

1. **One need not close peritoneal layer after laparotomy because:**
   A. The peritoneum can get stuck to the bowel
   B. Flattened mesothelial cells heal within a few hours
   C. The peritoneum tears when closure is attempted
   D. It is very painful postoperatively
2. **Peritoneum can be used for dialysis because:**
   A. It is close to kidney
   B. It is faster than haemodialysis
   C. Capillaries and lymphatics between two layers of peritoneum help in absorption and exudation
   D. It covers entire abdomen
3. **Which of the following is an example of primary peritonitis?**
   A. Tuberculous peritonitis
   B. Perforation peritonitis
   C. Postoperative peritonitis
   D. Parturition peritonitis
4. **Which of the following organisms are most commonly involved in secondary peritonitis?**
   A. Enterococci
   B. Streptococci
   C. Staphylococci
   D. Pneumococci
5. **The following are the typical features of acute generalised peritonitis, *except*:**
   A. Abdominal pain
   B. Persistent vomiting
   C. Bradycardia
   D. High-grade fever with chills
6. **Abdominal tap is done in peritonitis for all of the following roles, *except*:**
   A. Aspiration of blood to indicate haemoperitoneum
   B. Aspiration of pus indicating infection with gram-negative bacteria
   C. Aspiration of bile indicating biliary peritonitis
   D. Aspiration of urine indicating ureterocele
7. **The following suture material is best suited for closure of bowel perforation:**
   A. Silk B. Polypropylene
   C. Nylon D. Polyglactin
8. **History of mucus discharge per rectum for the first time in a patient who is recovering from peritonitis suggests:**
   A. Anal prolapse B. Pelvic abscess
   C. Proctitis D. Colitis
9. **What forms the anterior relationship of Rutherford Morrison's space?**
   A. Liver B. Kidney
   C. Diaphragm D. Duodenum
10. **Subphrenic abscess is common on the right side because of the following reasons, *except*:**
    A. Majority of the diseases affect right side
    B. Right lung is larger because of the anatomical position of the liver
    C. Left paracolic gutter is narrow and colophrenic ligament is present on the left side
    D. Right paracolic gutter is large and colophrenic ligament is absent on the right side
11. **Indications for open drainage of subphrenic abscess include the following, *except*:**
    A. Persistent fistula discharging pus
    B. Thick viscid pus
    C. Abscess very close to IVC/diaphragm
    D. Single loculus
12. **Intra-abdominal pressure exceeds ________ cm $H_2O$ in abdominal compartment syndrome.**
    A. 15 B. 25
    C. 35 D. 45
13. **Following are features of tuberculous peritonitis, *except*:**
    A. Tubercles over peritoneal surface
    B. Encysted form
    C. Can be a miliary form
    D. Transudate
14. **The best form of treatment for 10 cm size retroperitoneal sarcoma is**
    A. Neoadjuvant Imatinib
    B. Neoadjuvant chemotherapy
    C. Neoadjuvant radiotherapy
    D. Wide excision
15. **The following catheters are commonly used for percutaneous drainage of subphrenic abscess:**
    A. Pigtail catheter
    B. Trocar catheter
    C. Sump catheter
    D. Foley's catheter
16. **More reliable sign of peritonitis is:**
    A. Cough tenderness
    B. Tenderness on pressure
    C. Rebound tenderness
    D. Guarding

**17. Presence of sunken eyes, pale and pinched face, dry cracked tongue, cold perspiration and cyanosis are all typical features of:**

A. Hippocratic facies
B. Gargoyle facies
C. Marshall hall facies
D. Mask like facies

**18. Following are risk factors for spontaneous bacterial peritonitis, *except*:**

A. Cirrhosis
B. Nephrotic syndrome
C. Chronic renal failure
D. Carcinoma stomach

**19. which of the following is true for pneumococcal peritonitis?**

A. Common in young boys
B. Age is around 15 years
C. Peritoneal fluid is transudate
D. It is typically odourless

**20. Following are about pseudomyxoma peritonei, *except*:**

A. Common in women
B. Ovary is the main source
C. Surgery cannot cure the disease
D. Chemotherapy is also used

## Answers

| | | | | | | | | | |
|---|---|---|---|---|---|---|---|---|---|
| 1. B | 2. C | 3. A | 4. A | 5. C | 6. D | 7. D | 8. B | 9. D | 10. B |
| 11. D | 12. C | 13. D | 14. D | 15. A | 16. C | 17. A | 18. D | 19. D | 20. B |

Chapter 58

# Small Intestine

- Embryology and development
- Anatomy
- Physiological functions
- Abdominal tuberculosis
- Tuberculous peritonitis
- Tuberculous mesenteric lymphadenitis
- Intestinal tuberculosis
- Inflammatory bowel diseases
- Ileostomy
- Crohn's disease
- Surgical complications of enteric fever
- Intestinal amoebiasis
- Radiation enteropathy
- Peutz-Jeghers syndrome
- Adenocarcinoma
- GIST
- Neuroendocrine tumours
- Short gut syndrome
- Intestinal fistulae
- Small intestinal diverticula

### Introduction

Truly speaking small intestines extends from pylorus to ileocecal junction. However, for all practical purposes, it is discussed as starting from duodenojejunal flexure till caecum. Small intestines play an important role not only in the transfer of food contents distally but in the digestion, absorption and secretion of the contents. Being the central portion of the gastrointestinal (GI) tract with long length, many diseases affect the intestine. Surgically important topics such as intestinal tuberculosis, inflammatory bowel diseases and few tumours are discussed in this chapter.

## EMBRYOLOGY AND DEVELOPMENT

**SU28.13:** Appreciate anatomy and physiology of the small intestine.

- Small intestine develops from midgut.
- This midgut loop has cranial and caudal limbs.
- As the elongation starts from 5th week of foetal life, cranial limb develops into distal duodenum, jejunum and proximal ileum.
- Distal ileum and proximal two-thirds of transverse colon are developed from caudal limb.
- Midgut also rotates 270°. Thus, proximal jejunum will go to left side and ileum will go to right side.
- Anomalies can occur during rotation resulting in malrotation.
- Vitellointestinal (VI) duct joins the junction of cranial and caudal intestines which is about 2 feet away from ileocaecal junction.
- When VI duct is not obliterated, various anomalies occur. One of them is Meckel's diverticulum.
- Caecum which is present in the right hypochondrium descends into the right iliac fossa region.

## ANATOMY

- Small intestine consists of proximal 2/5 jejunum and distal 3/5 ileum. It is about 6 metres in length.
- Small intestine starts at duodenojejunal flexure just to the **left of the inferior mesenteric vein.**
  **Surgical importance:** To identify the first (short) loop of jejunum for gastrojejunostomy.
- Small intestine ends at ileocaecal junction. In cases of intestinal obstruction, trace up to ileocaecal junction. If caecum is distended, it is a case of large bowel obstruction. If caecum is collapsed, it is a case of small bowel obstruction.
- Jejunum resides in the left side of the peritoneal cavity and ileum on the right side.
- Differences between jejunum and ileum have been given in Key Box 58.1.

### Blood Supply (Fig. 58.1)

- Superior mesenteric artery is the **artery of the midgut** which supplies the entire midgut (entire small

Key Box 58.1

**Differences between Jejunum and Ileum**

| | Jejunum | Ileum |
|---|---|---|
| **Length** | 2/5 | 3/5 |
| **Diameter** | Wider (2–4 cm) | Less (2–3 cm) |
| **Wall** | Thick and double (mucous membrane can be felt) | Thin |
| **Colour** | Deep red | Pale pink |
| **Peyer's patch** | Very, very less | More |
| **Blood supply** | Long and a few vasa recta (1 or 2) | Short and numerous (5 or 6) |
| **Mesentery** | Transparent, less fat | More fat |

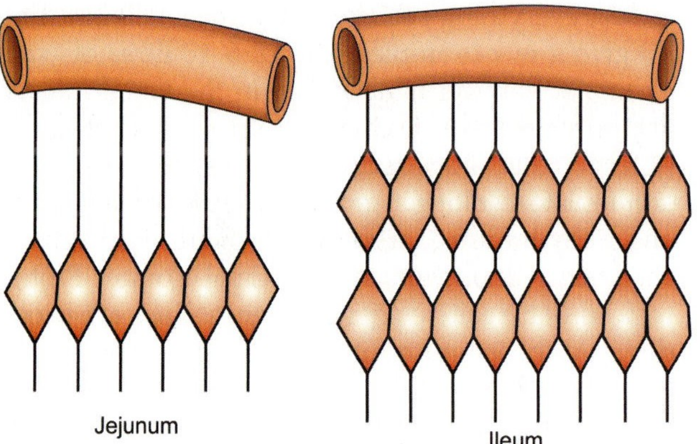


**Fig. 58.1:** Blood supply—jejunum and ileum

intestine). Jejunal arteries are end-arteries. Occlusion of SMA at the origin results in massive gangrene and the condition is fatal.

- Mesenteric border of the intestine gets more blood supply when compared to anti-mesenteric border. Hence, in cases of diminished blood supply, anti-mesenteric border becomes ischaemic first.
- Venous drainage is through superior mesenteric vein. Superior mesenteric venous occlusion is also fatal left untreated.

Details with pictures of these have been given in page 991 under Mesenteric vascular Occlusion in Chapter 60.

## Mesentery

- It is a fan-shaped fold of peritoneum which attaches jejunum and ileum to posterior abdominal wall.
- Blood vessels and lymphatics course in between the folds of peritoneum.
- It extends from the left of duodenojejunal flexure (left of L2) vertebra to the right sacroiliac joint, thus fixing the ileocaecal junction there.

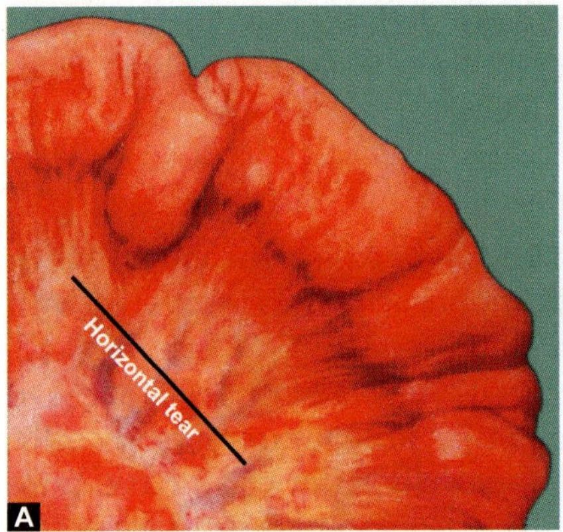


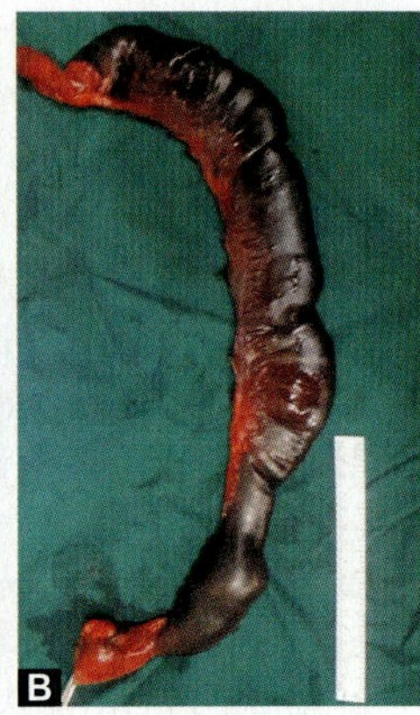


**Figs 58.2A and B:** (A) Observe blood supply of the mesentery and it is natural that a horizontal tear causes more gangrene; (B) Large mesenteric horizontal tear resulting in gangrene

- The importance of direction of the mesentery is appreciated in the following examples:
  A. **Mesenteric cyst** moves at right angles to the direction of the mesentery (*see* page 890).
  B. **Mesenteric lymph nodes** can be clinically palpable as a nodular or a smooth mass (*see* page 907).
  C. **Horizontal tear** in the mesentery causes more gangrene of the bowel than vertical tear (Figs 58.2A and B).
- **Structures crossed by mesentery:** Duodenum, aorta, inferior vena cava, right ureter, right psoas major and right gonadal vein.

## Innervation

- **Parasympathetic:** These are derived from vagus. It is secretomotor, thus helping in secretion and motility of small intestines. Nerve fibres traverse through coeliac ganglion. Afferent fibres do not carry pain impulses.
- **Sympathetic:** These fibres arise from three sets of splanchnic nerves. Their ganglion cells are located in a plexus around base of superior mesenteric artery. Pain is mediated through sympathetic system.

## Lymphatics

- From mucosa, lymphatics pass through the wall of the bowel to regional lymph nodes, then into lymph nodes at base of superior mesenteric artery.
- Then, it flows into cisterna chyli and then into thoracic duct and empty into venous system at confluence of left internal jugular and subclavian veins. Extravasation of few tumour emboli outside this confluence results in enlargement of supraclavicular lymph nodes. They are about 4 to 6 in number and are called **Virchow's nodes. This clinical sign is described as Troisier's sign**[1].

[1]Virchow's nodes are named after Rudolf Virchow (1821–1902), the German pathologist who first described the nodes and their association with gastric cancer in 1848.

- Peyer's patches are major deposits of lymphatic tissue in the distal bowel. Tuberculosis and typhoid fever affect the Peyer's patches.

## Microscopic Anatomy

- Basic unit of small bowel mucosa is the villus, which is a finger-like projection. Each villus is covered with tall columnar epithelium.
- Goblet cells, Paneth cells and endocrine cells are seen in the crypts. Goblet cells are mature mucous cells. Endocrine cells (enterochromaffin cells) have cytoplasmic granules which secrete 5-hydroxytryptamine, neurotensin, glucagon and motilin. Importantly, mucosal cell-mediated immunity is brought by mucosal T lymphocytes. Paneth cells are secretory cells located in the crypts of Lieberkühn. They play an important role in host defence and immunity by producing antimicrobial peptides, proteins and other components.

## PHYSIOLOGICAL FUNCTIONS

- **Motility:** Two types of muscle contractions occur—one which does not propagate—it exposes the food contents to the absorptive surface for a longer time by causing segmentation allowing better absorption of the food. Another type is peristaltic which propagates the food contents. Control of peristalsis is done by myenteric plexus. Time taken by the solid food contents to reach from mouth to colon is about 24 hours (Key Box 58.2).

Key Box 58.2

**Functions of the Small Intestine (SI)**

- Digestion and absorption
- Synthesis of lipoproteins
- Secretion of regulatory peptides
  - Secretin
  - Cholecystokinin
  - Somatostatin
  - VIP
- Immune function: Production of immunoglobulins (IgA). The **B** cells and **T** cells help in phagocytosis and secretion of cytokines.

- **Absorption and digestion:** Except calcium and iron, almost everything is absorbed in the small intestines. To give a few examples: Out of 6–10 litres of water, almost 80% water is absorbed in the small intestine and only 10–20% is discharged into colon. Thus in cases of terminal ileal obstruction, about 8–10 litres of fluid accumulate resulting in gross distension of the abdomen and dehydration. Carbohydrates and fat are mainly absorbed in duodenum and proximal jejunum. Proteins require pancreatic enzymes. Hence, they are broken down in the jejunum into amino acids and peptides. Conjugated bile acids are absorbed in the terminal ileum wherein enterohepatic circulation takes place and again they are secreted in the bile. Thus in ileal resections or diseases like Crohn's disease, more amount of bile acids enter colon resulting in diarrhoea due to increased secretion of water and electrolytes (Table 58.1).

**TABLE 58.1:** Absorption and digestion

| | Amount (normal) | Absorption | Process | Any other |
|---|---|---|---|---|
| Water | 8 to 10 litres/day enters into small intestine (SI) | Almost 90–95% only 500 ml enters the colon | Simple diffusion | Also along with water, there is active transport of sodium, glucose or amino acids |
| $Na^+$ | 130–140 mEq/μl | Active transport through basolateral membranes | $Na^+$ absorbed, $H^+$ secreted into lumen | $H^+$ combines with $HCO_3^-$ and forms carbonic acid |
| Calcium | 9–11 mg% | Proximal jejunum and duodenum | Enhanced by vitamin D and PTH | |
| Iron | Ferritin levels—12 to 300 nanogram per ml of blood for males and 12 to 150 nanogram per ml for females | Absorbed as **heme** in the duodenum | Absorbed as ferritin or transported to plasma bound to transferrin | Helps in erythropoiesis |
| Vitamins | The normal range for vitamin $B_{12}$ in the blood is between 200 and 900 nanograms per millilitre (ng/ml) | Most of vitamins are absorbed in proximal jejunum except vitamin $B_{12}$ which is absorbed in the terminal ileum | Vitamin $B_{12}$ will bind to (or complex with) intrinsic factor and gets absorbed | Resection of terminal ileum or diseases affecting terminal ileum such as Crohn's disease and tuberculosis affects this vitamin $B_{12}$ absorption |

## ABDOMINAL TUBERCULOSIS (TB)

### Introduction

Abdominal tuberculosis is a common extrapulmonary manifestation of tuberculosis. Disease is caused by *Mycobacterium tuberculosis*. Approximately 15–25% of cases with abdominal TB have concomitant pulmonary TB. Tuberculosis (TB) is a life-threatening disease which can virtually affect any organ system. Incidence in the West has also increased due to immigrant population and increased incidence of HIV infections. In India, extrapulmonary TB is also showing re-emergence due to incomplete treatment and occurrence of multi-drug-resistant strains. Initial few pages will give you classification, pathophysiology and investigations of abdominal tuberculosis, followed by details about each type of tuberculosis.

### Definition

The term abdominal tuberculosis includes tuberculous infection of gastrointestinal tract, mesenteric lymph nodes, peritoneum, omentum and solid organs related to gastrointestinal tract such as liver and spleen.

### Classification (Key Box 58.3)

Key Box 58.3

**Various Forms of Abdominal TB**

- **I. Peritoneal tuberculosis:** Acute, chronic
  - A. Chronic forms
    1. Ascitic type (wet)
       - Generalised
       - Localised
    2. Fibrous type (dry)
       - Adhesive, plastic
       - Miliary nodule type
  - B. Tuberculosis of peritoneal folds
    1. Mesenteric adenitis
    2. Mesenteric cysts/abscesses
    3. Bowel adhesion
- **II. Gastrointestinal**
  1. Ulcerative
  2. Hyperplastic
  3. Sclerotic/plastic
- **III. TB of solid viscera**
  1. Liver
  2. Spleen

### Routes of Spread of Infection and Pathogenesis

1. Intestinal tuberculosis is caused by *Mycobacterium tuberculosis* from **swallowed sputum** (pulmonary tuberculosis) or milk (milk-borne infection—*Mycobacterium bovis*). From intestinal tuberculosis, mesenteric nodes get involved and later, the peritoneum can get involved.
2. **Blood spread:** Infection from pulmonary tuberculosis can spread through blood during bacteraemic phase. Untreated patients can develop liver, spleen involvement in the form of multiple tubercles.
3. **Lymphatic spread** from tuberculosis of intestines.
4. **Genitourinary tuberculosis:** From here, cephalad spread occurs and thus, peritoneum gets affected.

### Pathology and Pathogenesis

The spread from ingestion of infected sputum or ingested unpasteurized milk is the main cause for intestinal tuberculosis. It is submucosal tubercle which later ulcerates into mucosa followed by spread else where. This happens within 2 to 4 weeks of infection (Fig. 58.3).

### Investigations

It is important to realise that there are so many investigations for abdominal tuberculosis. **Although it is essential to have a theoretical knowledge about all these investigations, all of them need not be done during clinical management.**

To give an example: If chest X-ray and sputum AFB are positive, and patient has inetstinal tuberculosis symptoms, one should start ATT (need not do costly investigations such as CT scan or even diagnostic laparoscopy, etc.). Investigations done by the clinician should be complementary to each other.

1. **Complete blood picture (CBP)** which includes Hb%, TC, DC and ESR. Haemoglobin may be low indicating anaemia. Anaemia has to be corrected before surgery.
2. **ESR** will help in equivocal cases. High ESR values may direct to investigate in more details. More importantly, decreasing ESR in patients on anti-tuberculous treatment will reflect positive response of the treatment.
3. **Sputum AFB (acid-fast bacilli):** Demonstrated by Zeihl-Neelsen method. Many patients, with abdominal tuberculosis will not have pulmonary tuberculosis. However, if sputum is present, it must be tested for AFB.
4. **Chest X-ray** may suggest tuberculosis in the form of cavity, calcification, etc. In such patients, bronchoscopy washings or biopsy may clinch the diagnosis.
5. **Mantoux test** is nonspecific but a strong ulcerated Mantoux test result suggests tuberculosis.
6. **Ultrasound**, being a noninvasive investigation, is an imaging of choice.
   - Ascites can be demonstrated and the aspirated fluid is sent for analysis.

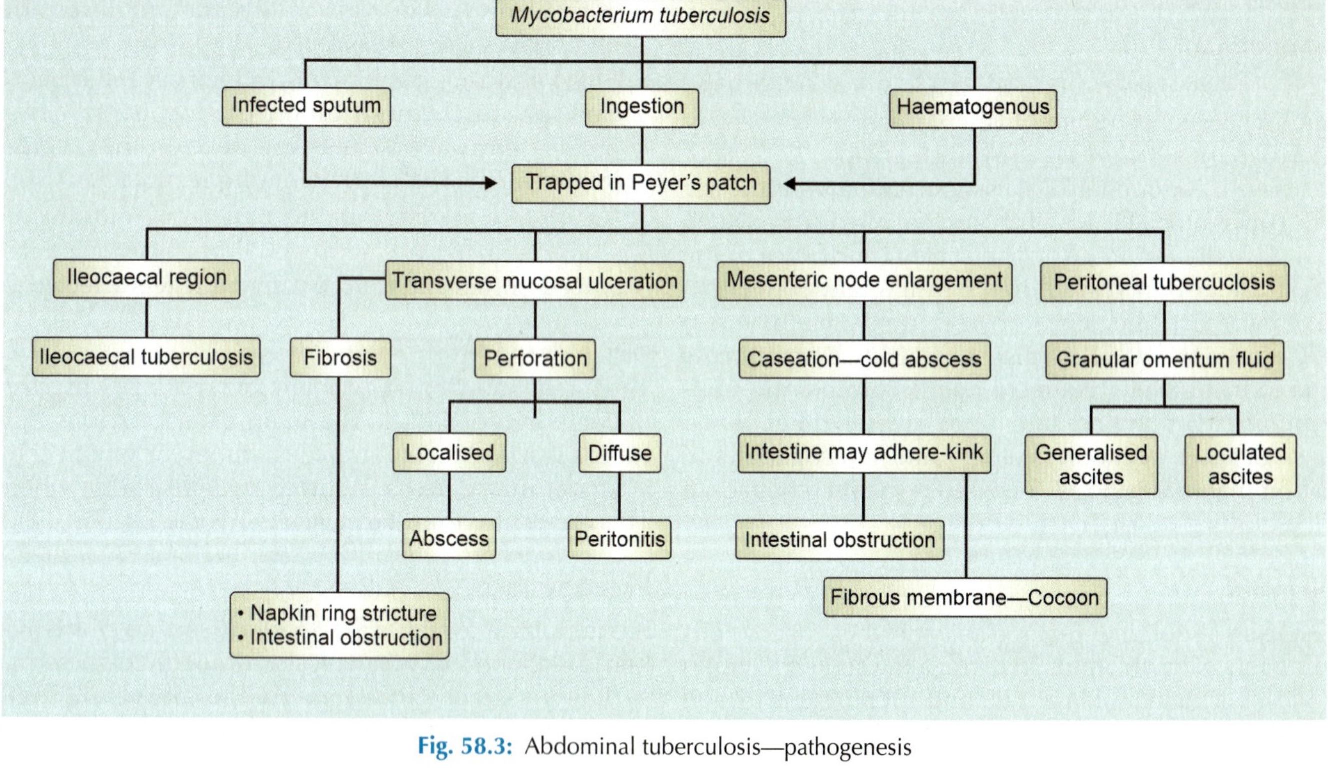


**Fig. 58.3:** Abdominal tuberculosis—pathogenesis

- Focal ascites between loops of bowel—**Club sandwich sign** may be seen.
- Enlargement of mesenteric lymph nodes (common) and retroperitoneal nodes (uncommon) can be detected.
- Dilated loops and sometimes peritoneal tubercles are seen as echo-poor shadows.
- Thickening of omentum, mesentery, peritoneum can be found out. (However, CECT is a better investigation to detect these).
- **Pseudokidney sign:** Pulled caecum identified in the right hypochondrium.
- Hepatosplenomegaly may be present.

7. **Ascitic fluid analysis:** Ultrasound-guided fluid is aspirated and about 20–40 ml is sent for analysis (Key Box 58.4).
8. **CECT: Contrast enhanced CT scan of the abdomen:** CT scan is objective. All the findings which can be detected by ultrasound can be confirmed by CT scan. Addition of the contrast is definitely more superior in detecting strictures, dilatations, perforations, and more importantly loculated ascites and intra-abdominal collections. CT-guided biopsy can be done. If distension or matting of loops and adhesions are present, it is not safe.
9. **Barium studies:** These are not done routinely. If diagnosis is possible by the various investigations mentioned above, there is no necessity to do them. In fact, it can harm the patient by precipitating obstruction and barium peritonitis, if there is a perforation. Few findings in barium studies can be:
   - Small bowel enema—enteroclysis: Dilatation and narrowed segments in partial obstruction, narrowing of terminal ileum (**Fleischner's sign**), fibrotic terminal ileum opening into the contracted caecum (**Stierlin's sign**).
   - Barium enema: Pulled up caecum, normal acute ileocaecal angle becomes obtuse or sometimes straightening of the ileocaecal angle.

Key Box 58.4

**Ascitic Fluid Analysis (Straw-Coloured Fluid)**

- Specific gravity is increased—2020 or more
- Glucose <30 mg%
- AFB is rarely demonstrated <3% of cases
- Increased white cell count (>500/cells/cumm), predominantly lymphocytic
- Increased total protein (>2.5 g/dl)
- Serum/ascitic fluid albumin gradient (SAAG*) <1.1 g% units
- LDH >90 units/L
- Decreased pH
- Increased adenosine deaminase
- Bacterial isolation and culture is possible in 20–45% of patients.

*__SAAG__ = Serum albumin level—ascitic fluid albumin level

10. **Endoscopy: Upper gastroduodenoscopy** may detect tubercles in the stomach or duodenum—rare.
    - **Push enteroscopy also called small bowel enteroscopy:** Ulcers in the proximal jejunum can be detected and biopsy can be taken—chances of perforation are high.
    - **Colonoscopy** can detect nodular lesions, ulcerations in the colon—caecum and terminal ileum (last 10 cm of ileum should be entered and biopsy should be taken).
11. **Laparoscopy:** This is a diagnostic investigation as it gives the tissue diagnosis (Figs 58.4 and 58.5). One can also evaluate all possible viscera, peritoneum, omentum and pelvic organs. **Biopsy is possible under direct vision.** Findings can be: Straw-coloured peritoneal fluid, abscesses secondary to perforation, rolled up omentum, tubercles on the peritoneal surface, matting of the loops of bowel, adhesions, bands, strictures and dilatations. Other findings which can be appreciated are: Shortened mesentery, caseation of lymph nodes (pseudomesenteric cyst), pulled up caecum and hepatosplenomegaly. Laparoscopy can also be therapeutic, if a stricture is identified, the diseased loop is isolated, brought out and resection and anastomosis/stricturoplasty done (Key Box 58.5).
    - Adhesiolysis can also be done.

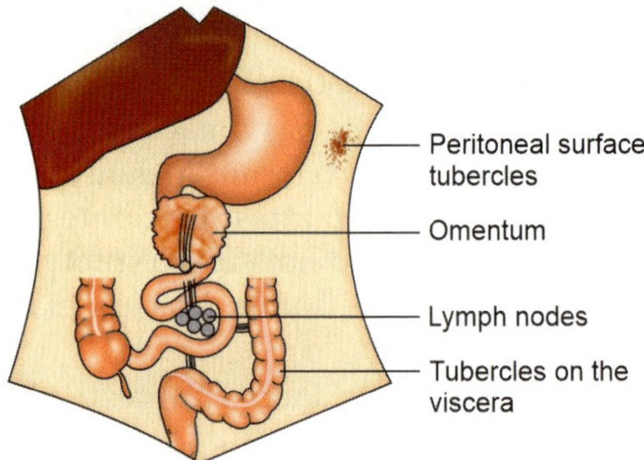


**Fig. 58.4:** Various sites from where laparoscopic biopsy can be taken in suspected case of abdominal tuberculosis. Biopsy from peritoneal surface and omentum is safe. Otherwise lymph node biopsy can be done

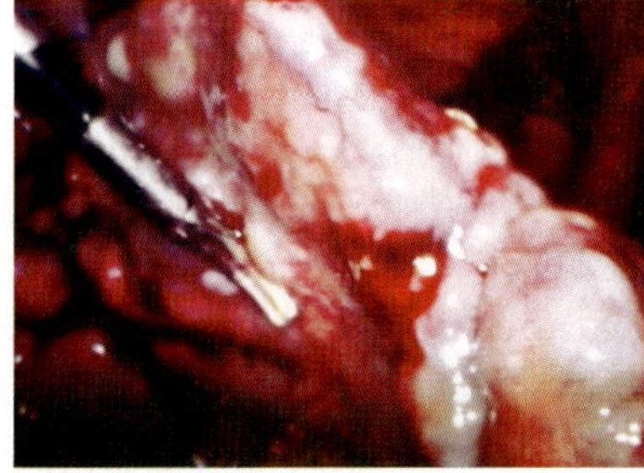

**Fig. 58.5:** Extensive abdominal tuberculosis. Laparoscopic biopsy being done

Nucleic acid amplification testing (NAAT)—CBNAAT (cartridge based NAAT)/Xpert MTB/RIF helps in both diagnosis of TB and about rifampicin resistance. It should be done in all patients.

Key Box 58.5

**Laparoscopy—Important Findings**

- **L**ymph nodes enlargement
- **A**dhesions, matting
- **P**eritoneal nodules
- **A**scites—aspiration—AFB staining
- **R**olled up omentum
- **O**bstruction, stricture

*You can remember as* **LAPARO**

12. **Polymerase chain reaction (PCR):**
    - It is a technique used in medical and biological research labs.
    - One can do functional analysis of genes; useful in the diagnosis of hereditary diseases.
    - Helps in detection and diagnosis of infectious diseases, such as tuberculosis.
    - Laparoscopically biopsied tissue can be sent for PCR. It can detect 1–2 organisms or 8 fg of mycobacterial DNA.
    - Positive PCR indicates infection but it need not be active infection. Hence, it is inferior to tissue diagnosis.
    - PCR has 97% sensitivity and 99% specificity.

*Pearls of Wisdom*

One can get a diagnosis of tuberculosis from sputum AFB being positive, from tissue diagnosis by endoscopy or CT guided biopsy of solid lesions such as lymph nodes or liver or spleen.

## TUBERCULOUS PERITONITIS

**SU28.3.3:** Summarize the tubercular peritonitis.

In most of the cases, tuberculous peritonitis results from reactivation of latent primary peritoneal focus (Key Box 58.6).

It can be of two types: Acute and chronic. Basically, it produces the following pathological changes:

1. Intense exudation which causes ascitic form
2. Exudation with minimal fibroblastic reaction—loculated form
3. Extensive fibroblastic reaction—plastic form
4. Fibroblastic with secondary infection—purulent form.

Key Box 58.6

**Tuberculous Peritonitis**

- Cirrhosis
- HIV infection
- Diabetes mellitus
- Underlying malignancy
- Dialysis
- CAPD

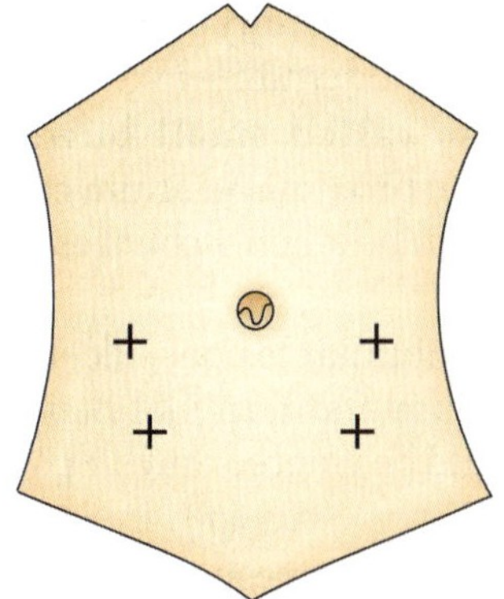
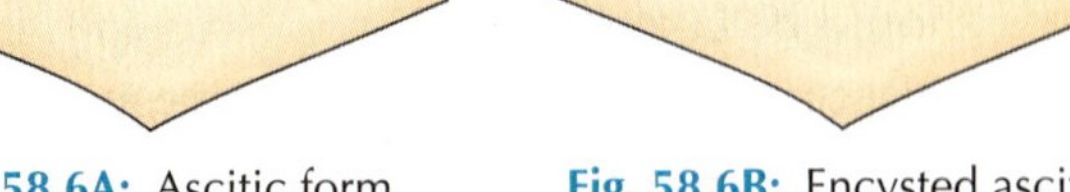
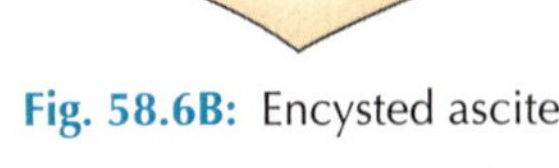

**Fig. 58.6A:** Ascitic form **Fig. 58.6B:** Encysted ascites

## Types

1. **Ascitic form** (Fig. 58.6A) (generalised variety)
   - It is common in children and young adults. The child is brought to the hospital with abdominal distension.
   - Omentum can be felt as a rolled up transverse mass, which is nodular due to extensive fibrosis. Abdomen has a doughy feel with fluid giving rise to shifting dullness.
   - Aspiration of peritoneal fluid reveals exudate, which is rich in lymphocytes. Other causes of increase in proteins in ascitic fluid is given in Key Box 58.7
   - Peritoneal cavity contains pale-straw-coloured fluid and the peritoneal surface is studded with tubercles.
   - Umbilical hernia or congenital hydrocele appears in children due to increased intra-abdominal pressure.
   - Tuberculous peritonitis can be associated with infections of pleural space and pericardial space (effusion). It is called **polyserositis** syndrome.

Key Box 58.7

**Causes of Exudative Ascites—Increase in Protein**

**P**ancreatic ascites
**R**are cause: Meig's syndrome
**O**cclusion: Budd-Chiari syndrome
**T**ubercular peritonitis
**E**xcess of chylomicrons
**I**nfective: Peritonitis
**N**eoplasm of peritoneum (carcinoma peritonei)

*Remember as* **PROTEIN**

2. **Loculated or encysted form** (Fig. 58.6B and 58.7)
   - In this variety, ascitic fluid is present in one quadrant of the abdomen which is sealed off by matted intestinal coils surrounded by omentum. It gives rise to localised swelling. These patients have no shifting dullness. Doughy feel of abdomen, tense cyst which feels firm on palpation, surrounded by tympanitic note of intestines clinches the diagnosis.
   - It commonly presents in adults.

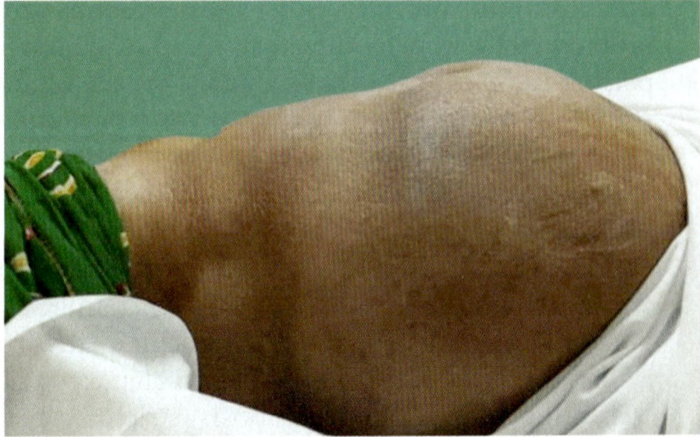

**Fig. 58.7:** A 50 years lady with lower abdominal distension

   - **Differential diagnosis:** Pseudocyst of the pancreas, mesenteric cyst, retroperitoneal cyst.

3. **Fibrous peritonitis (plastic)** (Fig. 58.8)
   - In this variety, **there is no ascites** but there is extensive fibrosis which results in **dense adhesions** between the coils of intestines. Intestines are matted, distended and not able to empty properly due to adhesions and bands. It is associated with **strictures**.
   - This gives rise to blind loop with **steatorrhoea** and **emaciation**.
   - Usually, it presents with **intestinal obstruction** at a later date due to fibrous band which needs to be divided to relieve the obstruction. In some occasions, it is not possible to enter the peritoneal cavity, due to dense adhesions.
   - It is **not uncommon** to create openings in the bowel (accidental enterotomy) at laparotomy and end with a helpless situation wherein one will not be able to close the perforation. The net result is fistula formation.
4. **Fibroblastic variety with secondary infection** (Fig. 58.9)
   - Seen in females as a complication of genitourinary tuberculosis (tuberculous salpingitis).
   - The spread occurs through the female genital tract and there is always secondary infection.

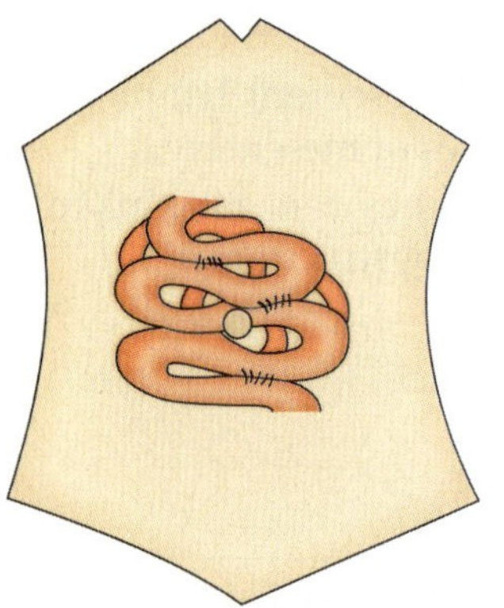
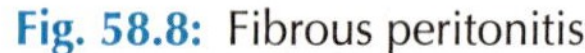

Fig. 58.8: Fibrous peritonitis

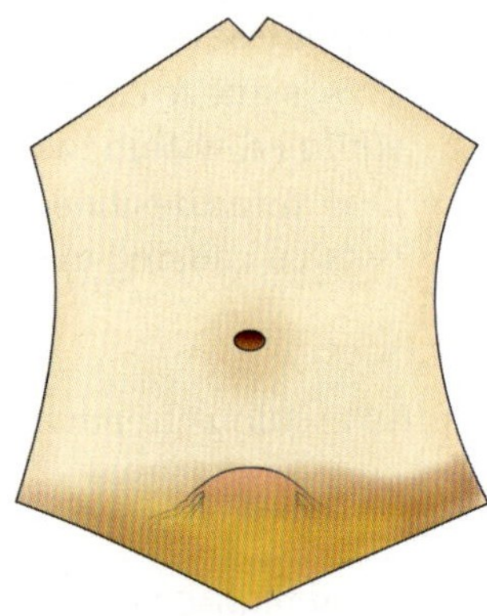

Fig. 58.9: Purulent type

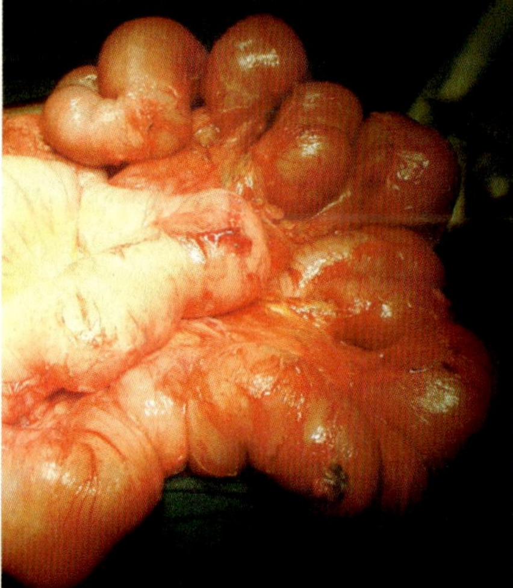

Fig. 58.10: Fibrous bands

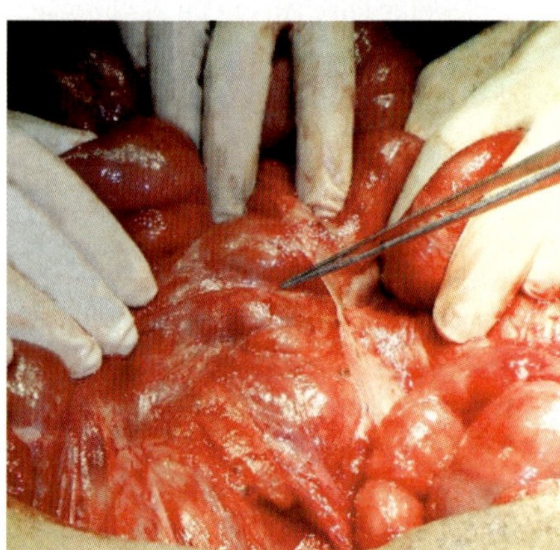

Fig. 58.11: Adhesive form

- It presents as pelvic peritonitis–pain, fever, lower abdominal distension, guarding and rigidity. Diagnostic laparoscopy: The peritoneal cavity is seen studded with tubercles, cold abscesses and pus.
- Laparotomy, drainage of pus, followed by anti-tuberculous treatment is the choice of therapy.
- It carries poor prognosis because of complications such as toxaemia and faecal fistula formation.
- *See* also Figs 58.10 to 58.13.

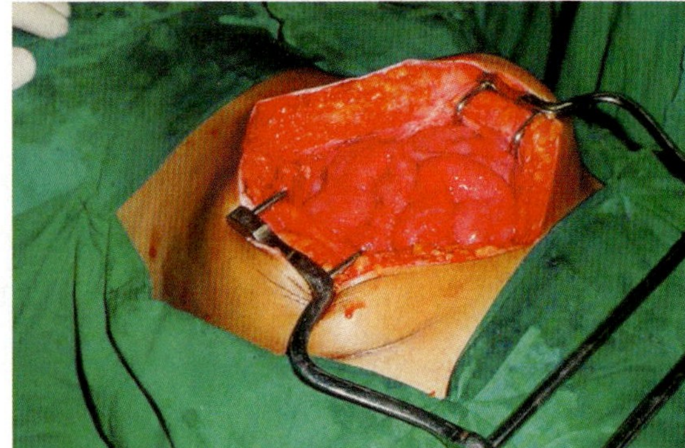

Fig. 58.12: Tubercles on the peritoneal surface

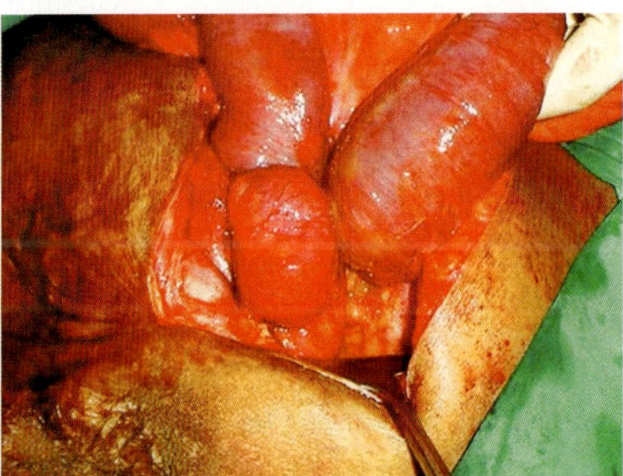

Fig. 58.13: Tuberculous peritonitis

## TUBERCULOUS MESENTERIC LYMPHADENITIS

### Clinical Presentation

1. **As a calcified lesion** (Fig. 58.14) along the line of mesentery, which extends from L2 vertebra, at the left of vertebral column to the right sacroiliac joint. In 50% of cases, there is no active infection but in the remaining, there is infection. If the symptoms are that of tuberculosis, antituberculous treatment should be given. The shadows caused by lymph nodes are round to oval, mottled and may be regular or irregular.
2. **Acute mesenteric lymphadenitis** (Fig. 58.15)
   - Common in children, clinically mimics acute appendicitis.
   - Pain in the right iliac fossa, vomiting, fever, rigidity can be present.
   - On palpation, tender mass of swollen lymph nodes can be felt in the right iliac fossa.
   - Laparotomy, appendicectomy and biopsy of the lymph node is the procedure of choice.
3. **Chronic lymphadenitis** (Fig. 58.16) in children presents as **failure to thrive**. Fever, loss of weight, loss of appetite, emaciation and pallor are present. Abdomen is protuberant. On deep palpation, nodes can be felt in the right iliac fossa. These nodes have to be differentiated from nodes that enlarge due to lymphoma.

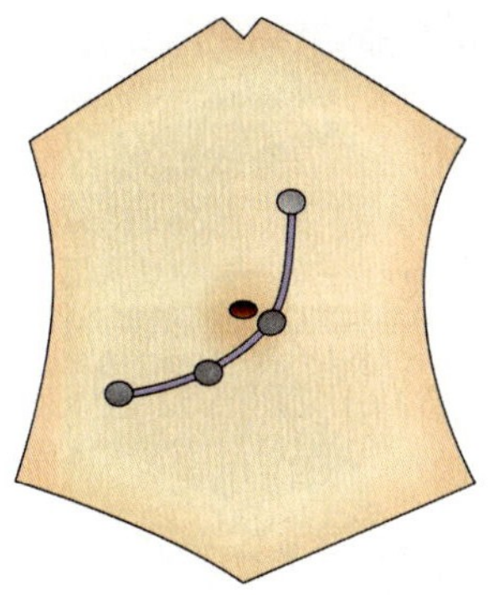

**Fig. 58.14:** Mesenteric lymph nodes

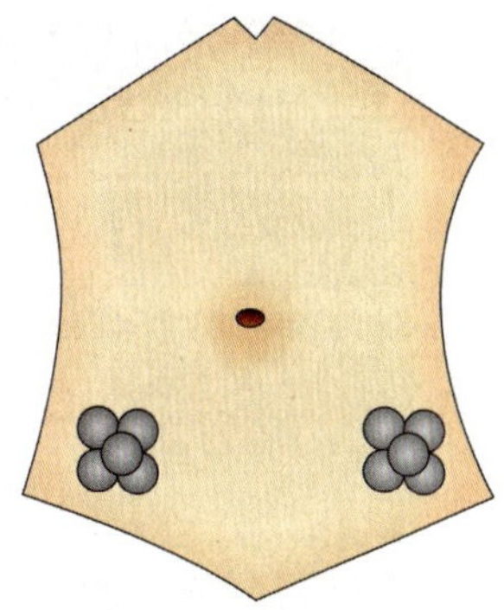

**Fig. 58.15:** Acute lymphadenitis

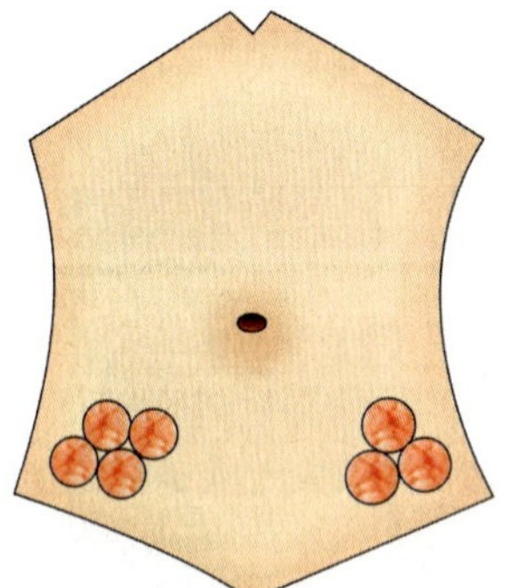

**Fig. 58.16:** Chronic lymphadenitis

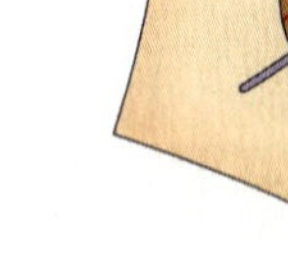

**Fig. 58.17:** Pseudomesenteric cyst

4. **Pseudomesenteric cyst** (Fig. 58.17)
   - This is due to caseation of mesenteric lymph nodes confined within two leaves of mesentery.
   - Due to adhesions, intestines can get kinked or twisted causing intestinal obstruction.

### Treatment

Antituberculous treatment.

## INTESTINAL TUBERCULOSIS

**Ileocaecal region is commonly involved** in tuberculosis because of the following reasons:

- Abundant Peyer's patches
- Alkaline media
- Bacterial contact time is more
- Minimal digestive activity
- Maximum absorption in the area
- Stasis due to valve—**ileocecal valve, Tulp's valve, Tulpius valve** or **Bauhin's valve.**

### Types (Table 58.2 for comparison)

1. Ulcerative variety
2. Hyperplastic variety
3. Mixed (sometimes)

**TABLE 58.2:** Comparison of two forms of intestinal tuberculosis (TB)

| | **Ulcerative variety** | **Hyperplastic variety** |
|---|---|---|
| 1. Aetiology | Secondary to pulmonary TB. Occurs due to swallowing of TB bacilli (*Mycobacterium tuberculosis*) | It is a primary intestinal TB, due to *M. bovis.* Milk-borne infection or due to *Mycobacterium tuberculosis*—low grade infection |
| 2. Site | Terminal ileum | Ileocaecal region |
| 3. Virulence of the organism | More virulent | Less virulent |
| 4. Resistance of body | **Very poor** | Good |
| 5. Pathology | Multiple ulcerations in the terminal ileum with/without involvement of lymph nodes. **Ulcers are transverse**. Serosa is reddened and oedematous | It is **low grade, chronic continuous inflammation** involving ileocaecal region resulting in cicatrising **granuloma** in right iliac fossa (mass in right iliac fossa) |
| 6. Clinical features | Symptoms of **pulmonary TB,** blood and mucus in stool resulting in gross emaciation and cachexia. Diarrhoea is also a feature | Abdominal pain and diarrhoea may be the initial symptoms for a long time and later fever, weight loss and subacute intestinal obstruction occur |
| 7. Complications | • **Acute** TB, ulcer perforation—Treatment is laparotomy and resection of bowel. If 2 ends of resected bowel are healthy, vascular and not edematous, anastomosis is done. Otherwise, anastomosis and covering (proximal) ileostomy is done which needs to be closed after 4 to 6 weeks later<br>• **Chronic:** Healing of ulcer results in **stricture** of terminal ileum and **subacute intestinal obstruction** | Nodular, mobile, **firm mass** in the right iliac fossa which later produces subacute **intestinal obstruction.** Plain X-ray abdomen shows multiple gas and fluid levels suggestive of intestinal obstruction (Fig. 58.24) |
| 8. Barium meal follow through (Figs 58.24 and 58.25) | Demonstrates a stricture, or multiple strictures. In the initial stages, ileum is not seen due to hypermotility | **Barium enema** can demonstrate (i) contracted caecum, (ii) pulled up caecum (subhepatic), (iii) luminal obstruction, and (iv) obtuse ileocaecal angle |
| 9. Chest X-ray and sputum AFB | Positive | Negative |
| 10. **Colonoscopy and biopsy** (Fig. 58.27) | To confirm the diagnosis | To confirm the diagnosis |

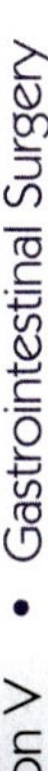

### Clinical Features (Figs 58.18 to 58.20)

- Few features of intestinal tuberculosis such as vague ill health, noisy abdomen, loose stools, evening rise in temperature, not putting on weight are common.
- **Abdominal pain:** It is the most common symptom (90%) of patients. It can be a dull, vague pain or colicky pain (stricture) which increases after taking food or relieved by vomiting. Often patient modifies his diet and eats less and more liquids to avoid pain, thus slowly loses weight. Severe colicky abdominal pain vomiting and distension indicate intestinal obstruction.
- **Diarrhoea:** Watery, small quantity, abnormally foul smelling. It may alternate with constipation. Frequency of stools will be much more in Crohn's disease compared to intestinal tuberculosis.
- **Abdominal distension:** It is due to ascites and sub-acute intestinal obstruction.
- Fever with night sweats, weight loss is very common. Anorexia, tiredness, pallor may be the presenting features. Tuberculosis accounts for 5–9% of all small intestinal perforations in India, and is the second commonest cause of intestinal perforation after typhoid fever.

**Fever with Night Sweats**

- Normal for body temperature to increase at night
- Activation of immune system
- Decrease in cortisol and adrenaline levels at night
- Attention of the patient

### Signs

- Typically patients are **malnourished and pale**.
- **Visible intestinal peristalsis** may be seen.
- **Distended bowel loops** can be palpated.
- **Doughy abdomen** in case of peritoneal involvement.
- **Rolled up omentum in the epigastrium,** mass in the right iliac fossa due to hyperplastic caecum or in the lumbar region due to pulled up caecum, can be the features. Details about the mass is given in the Table 58.2. (*Refer* Figs 58.21 to 58.23).

### Investigations (Refer Table 58.2)

Once intestinal tuberculosis is suspected, the basic investigations such as complete blood picture, chest X-ray, ultrasound and CECT of abdomen are done (Details have been discussed earlier in this chapter). Again to repeat, no barium studies to be done when there is suspicion of obstruction. Final histopathological diagnosis is established by colonoscopy enter terminal ileum and take multiple biopsies (at least 6). The tissue samples are not only sent for histopathology but also for CB-NAAT.

A. **The caseation necrosis** in granulomas is the histologic hallmark of TB.

   **In intestinal tuberculosis,** the granulomas are multiple, larger (more than 200 μm) and coalescent in mucosa and submucosa—**Langhan type of giant cells.** CB-NAAT has to be done in all cases to look for rifampicin resistance. Few investigations and pictures are given below (Figs 58.24 to 58.27).

B. **The yield of organisms on smear and culture is low. Staining for acid-fast bacilli is positive in less than 3% of cases. A positive culture is seen in only 20% of cases.**

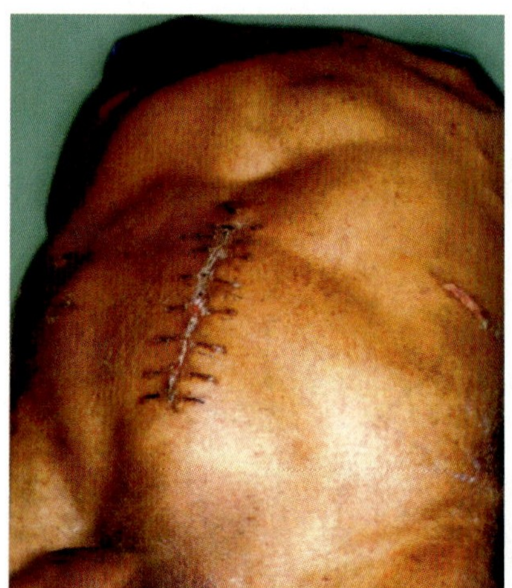

**Fig. 58.18:** Step ladder peristalsis is seen in a patient who underwent appendectomy for pain in the right iliac fossa. A diagnosis of appendicitis was made and appendicectomy was done. Postoperatively, he had step ladder peristalsis. Initial surgeon had missed the diagnosis

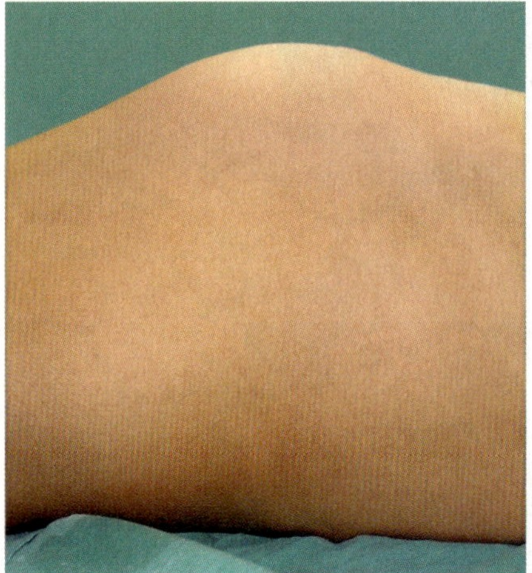

**Fig. 58.19:** Distension of the abdomen due to ascites—in such cases, there is uniform distension and shifting dullness is positive

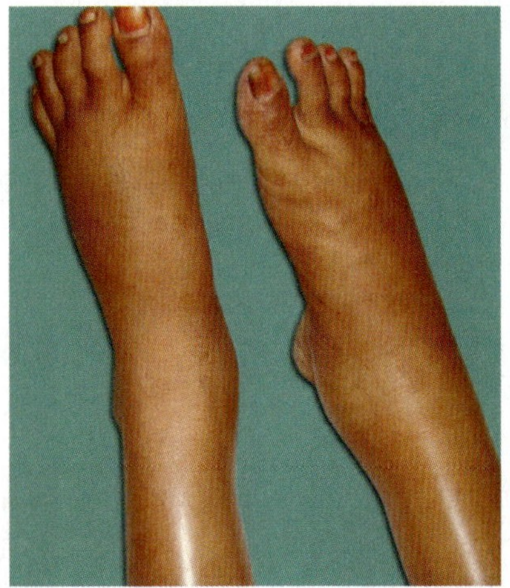

**Fig. 58.20:** Severe hypoproteinaemia—you can see bilateral pedal oedema. Such cases are mistaken for nephrotic syndrome and were treated also

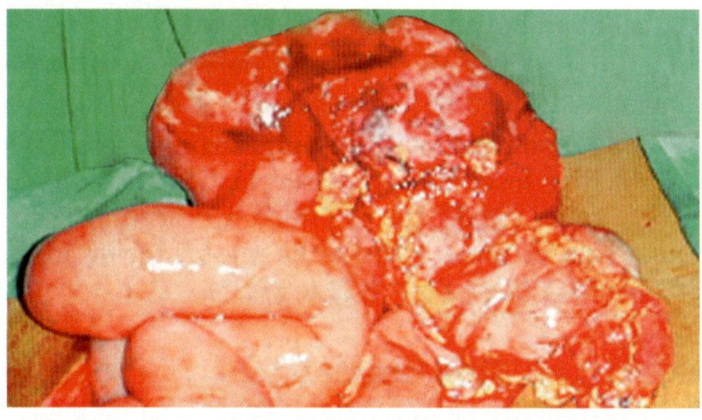

Fig. 58.21: Mass in the right iliac fossa—hyperplastic variety

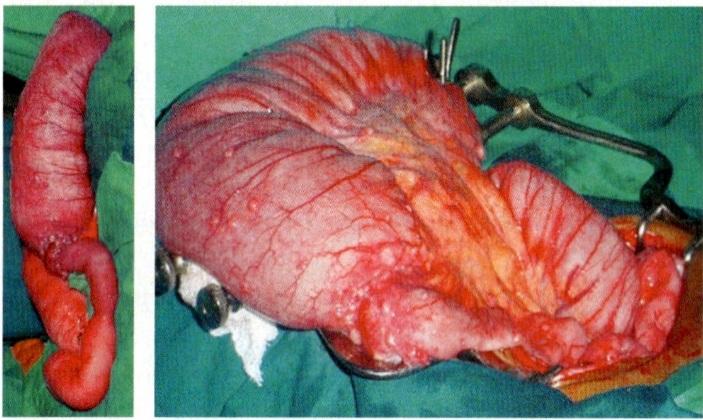

Figs 58.22 and 58.23: Tuberculous stricture with intestinal obstruction—observe the stricture, tubercles and massive proximal dilatation

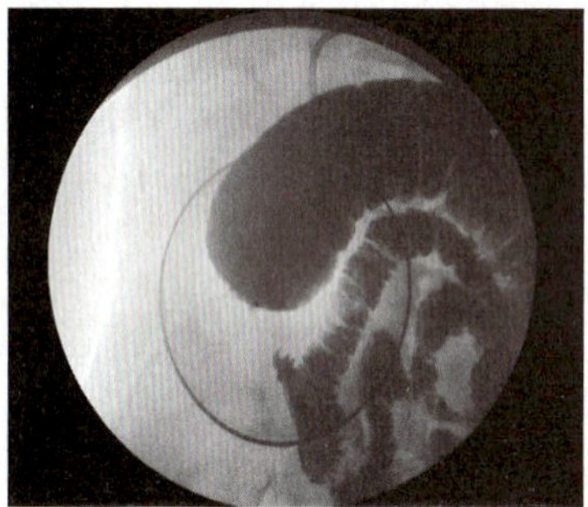

Fig. 58.24: Enteroclysis showing stricture of the jejunum with proximal dilatation

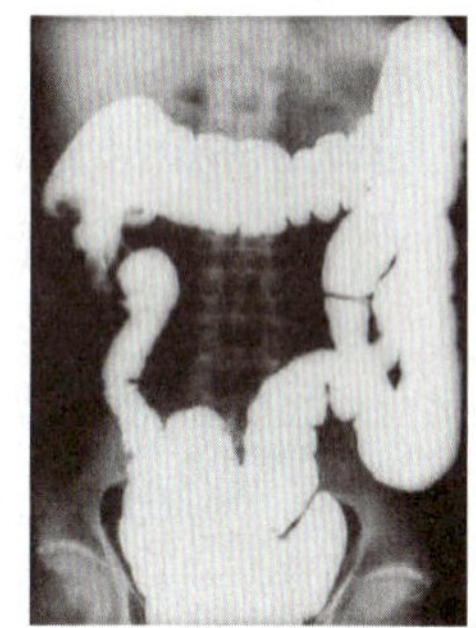

Fig. 58.25: Barium enema—'pulled up' caecum

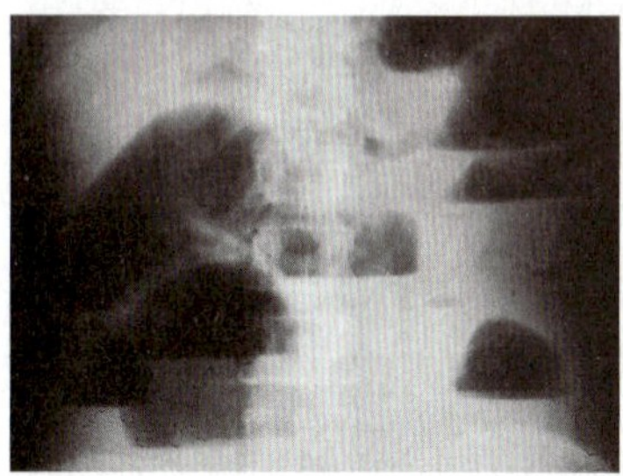

Fig. 58.26: Plain X-ray showing dilated air fluid levels

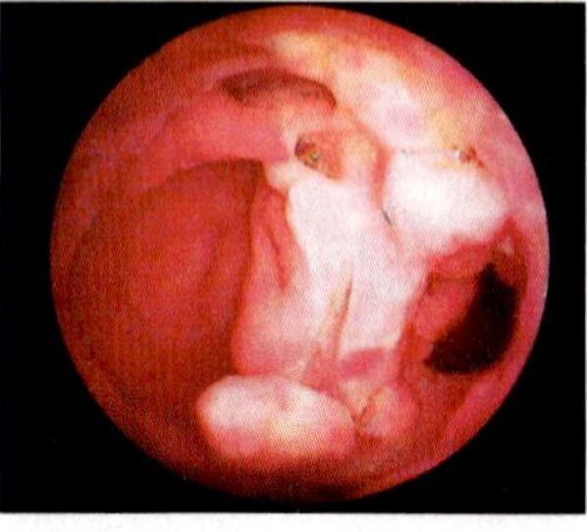

Fig. 58.27: Colonoscopy showing nodular leison in the ascending colon. Biopsy proved tuberculosis

## Management of Intestinal Tuberculosis

1. **No evidence of intestinal obstruction:** Antituberculous treatment.
2. **With obstruction (stricture): More details are given in the chapter of intestinal obstruction.**
   A. **Solitary stricture:** It is best treated by stricturoplasty by incising the stricture longitudinally and suturing it transversely (Fig. 58.28).
   B. **Multiple strictures** at long intervals: Stricturoplasty is the ideal treatment.
   C. **Multiple strictures within a short segment.** Resection is the ideal treatment (Fig. 58.29).
3. **Surgical treatment of hyperplastic tuberculosis:** Limited resection is the treatment of choice. It includes removal of terminal 8–10 cm of the diseased ileum, caecum with appendix, diseased portion of the ascending colon, followed by ileocolic anastomosis. All these cases have to be given antituberculous treatment for a period of 6 months. Some give it for 9 to 12 months. Decision of extending beyond 6

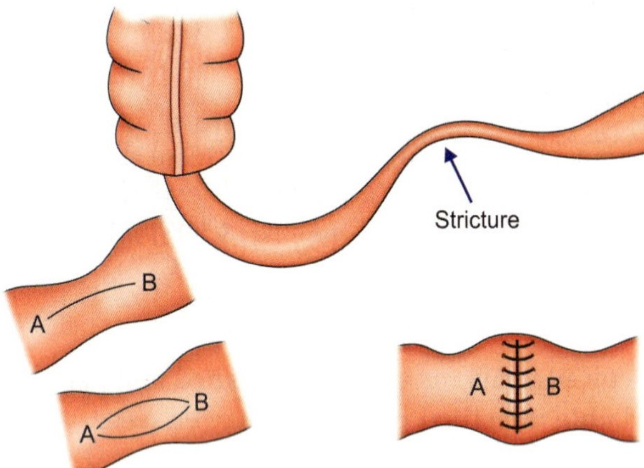


Fig. 58.28: Stricturoplasty

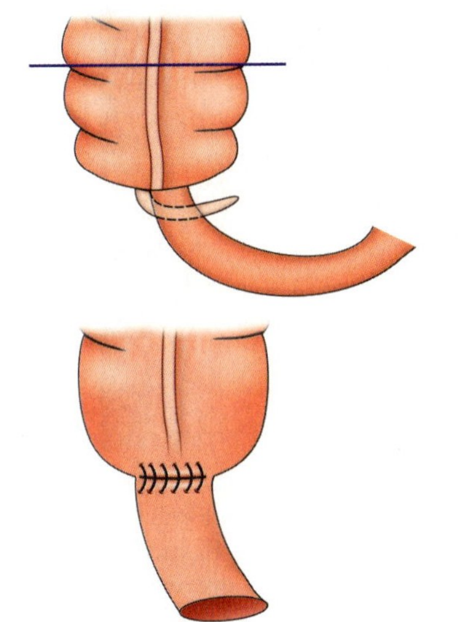

Fig. 58.29: Limited colectomy followed by ileocolic anastomosis

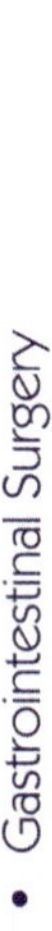

months also depends upon clinical improvement in the form of relief of symptoms and improvement in hemoglobin levels, nutrition (albumin) and ESR. Nutritional supplementation to improve albumin and haemoglobin levels and, if necessary, blood transfusion before and after surgery help in smooth recovery in the postoperative period.

*Pearls of Wisdom*

Stricture within 10 cm from the ileocaecal junction is best resected.

### Complications of Abdominal Tuberculosis

1. **Intestinal obstruction:** Usually it is ileal or jejunal obstruction—details have already been discussed.
2. **Perforation:** It is not uncommon. Carries 6–8% mortality rate specially in late cases with peritonitis.
3. **Malnutrition:** Diarrhoea, loose stools, and blind loop syndromes contribute to malnutrition.
4. **Faecal fistula** usually occurs following resection and anastomosis for intestinal tuberculosis. In such cases, anastomotic dehiscence may result in faecal fistula. The faecal fistula is not due to direct internal involvement of viscera unlike in Crohn's disease.
5. **Disseminated tuberculosis** *per se* from abdominal tuberculosis is not common. Most of such cases have fulminant pulmonary tuberculosis. This happens in untreated cases and immunocompromised cases.

## INFLAMMATORY BOWEL DISEASES

**SU28.13.5:** Understand the vascular anatomy of small and large intestines and apply the same pathologies like congenital, inflammatory, traumatic, benign and malignant, etc.

### Introduction

These are the diseases involving small and large bowel, of unknown aetiology, characterised by multiple ulcerations in the bowel, clinically manifesting as blood and mucus in stools. Ulcerative colitis and Crohn's disease (regional enteritis) are included under this heading. Both diseases can present as acute abdomen with intestinal obstruction and complications such as perforation toxaemia, etc. Also both are premalignant conditions for carcinoma colon. **Ulcerative colitis is a mucosal disease and Crohn's is a transmural disease.**

## ULCERATIVE COLITIS

### Aetiology

1. **Autoimmune factor:** Even though exact mechanism of ulcerative colitis is not clear, there are some factors which may point out to autoimmune reaction. They are:
   - Presence of **cytotoxic T lymphocytes** against colonic epithelial cells in the lamina propria of the bowel.
   - Presence of **anticolon antibodies**.
   - Whatever be the immune mechanisms, activation of inflammatory mediators such as cytokines, growth factors and arachidonic acids takes place and they are responsible for the disease.
2. **Dysfunctional immunoregulation** in the intestinal wall results in inappropriate production of **cytokines**. This creates an imbalance between various interleukins resulting in inflammatory changes.
3. **Psychosomatic and personality factors:** Ulcerative colitis is more common in western women. Emotional stress, family stress, and stress from divorce are the contributing factors. Periods of activity and remission is common.

*Pearls of Wisdom*

Western, white, worrying women's disease is ulcerative colitis.

4. **Dietary factors**
   - Westernisation of the diet which is rich in red meat has been blamed. Vegetarian diet is supposed to protect the colonic mucosa.
   - **Allergy to milk protein** is responsible for ulcerative colitis in a few patients.
5. **Defective mucin production** and a defective mucosal immunological reaction is considered as a chief factor responsible for ulcerative colitis.

*Pearls of Wisdom*

Appendicectomy and smoking have been protective factors for development of ulcerative colitis.

6. **Genetic:** 15% of patients have first degree relatives with ulcerative colitis.

### Pathology (Key Box 58.8)

- The disease always starts in the rectum and spreads in a backward manner, thus involving the entire colon in majority of cases. In 5% of cases, terminal ileum can also be involved—**back wash ileitis**.
- **Anus is not involved in ulcerative colitis.**
- The disease manifests as multiple, small superficial ulcers—**pinpoint ulcers**.
- As the disease progresses, inflammation spreads into the submucosa of the colon.
- Destruction of muscle is described as myocytolysis. Attempt at healing may produce **pseudopolyp**. There are areas of epithelial hypertrophy in between the

ulcers, resembling polyp. Healing with fibrosis results in a narrow, contracted colon, called **pipe stem colon**.

- Microscopy: **Pus** (abscess) in the crypts and pus cells (inflammatory cells) in the lamina propria are typical of ulcerative colitis.
- Long-standing cases will change into dysplasia of the epithelium—dysplasia associated lesion (DAL).

Key Box 58.8

**Pathology of Ulcerative Colitis**

**P**inpoint ulcers
**P**seudopolyposis
**P**ipe stem colon
**P**us cells

*Observe* **4 Ps**

## Clinical Features

- More common in females. Female:male ratio is 2:1.
- Age: Common age of presentation is 3rd decade followed by 4th and 2nd decades.
- The disease is characterised by passage of 15–20 stools per day and contains blood and mucus. Sometimes, it may be watery diarrhoea (Key Box 58.9). As the rectum loses elasticity and lumen collapses, tenesmus occurs.
- Relapses and remissions are common and are related to emotional disturbances. Tenesmus, urgency with severe inflammation result in incontinence.
- Severe dehydration, malnutrition, anaemia, hypoproteinaemia are late features.
- Acute fulminating attack is associated with high grade fever, bloody dysentery, distension and tenderness all over the abdomen with profound weakness. Hypokalaemia, acidosis, anaemia and shock are the other features.

**Clinical findings in severe disease**
Temperature
Tachycardia
Tender colon—abdomen
Tenesmus—anaemia, hypoproteinaemia
Terrific disease—dehydration, hypokalaemia, acidosis, shock

Key Box 58.9

**Types—Depending Upon Severity**

- **Mild colitis:** Refers to <4 stools/day without systemic signs and symptoms.
- **Moderate colitis:** Refers to <6 stools/day without systemic toxicity.
- **Severe colitis:** Refers to >6 stools/day with systemic toxicity—fever over 37.5°C, tachycardia more than 90/min, hypoalbuminaemia less than 3 g/dl, weight loss more than 3 kg.

## Types of Ulcerative Colitis
(depending upon the extent of the colon involved)

1. **Proctitis:** In about 20–25% of the patients, the disease involves only rectum. In such patients, stools are semisolid because of absorption of water by normal colon. Also, the intensity of the disease is not severe and risk of cancer is 2–5%.
2. **Left-sided colitis:** It is found in 15% of patients. It presents as severe recurrent attacks of diarrhea with blood in stools, without systemic toxicity (Fig. 58.30).
3. **Total proctocolitis:** It is seen in about 25% of the patients. Severe bloody diarrhoea and hypoproteinaemia are its features. Chances of cancer and complications are high in this group (Fig. 58.31).

## Complications

1. **Toxic megacolon:** It is an abdominal emergency encountered with fulminating colitis. Severe abdominal pain and tenderness, toxaemia, high fever, tachycardia and leucocytosis are the features. Plain X-ray abdomen which shows colon with a diameter more than 6 cm gives the diagnosis. It requires emergency treatment by laparotomy and colectomy. Local inflammatory mediators such as interleukins and nitric oxide are released from smooth muscles. Activities of macrophages are also increased. This results in colonic dysmotility and toxic dilatation. As a result, mucosal sloughing, bacterial translocation,

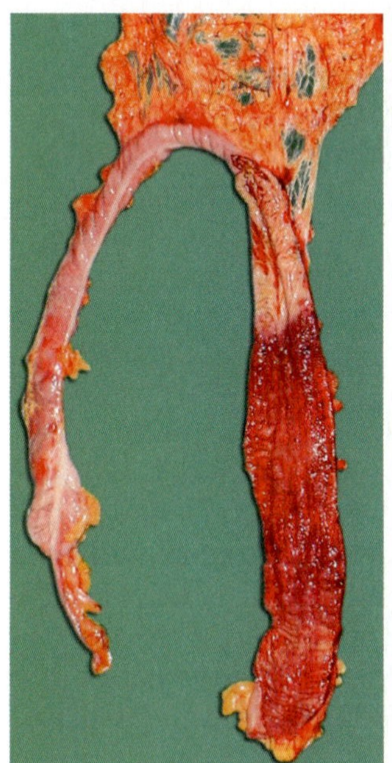

**Fig. 58.30:** Sharp demarcation at the splenic flexure may be due to an incomplete marginal artery ending at point of demarcation. Case of left-sided colitis

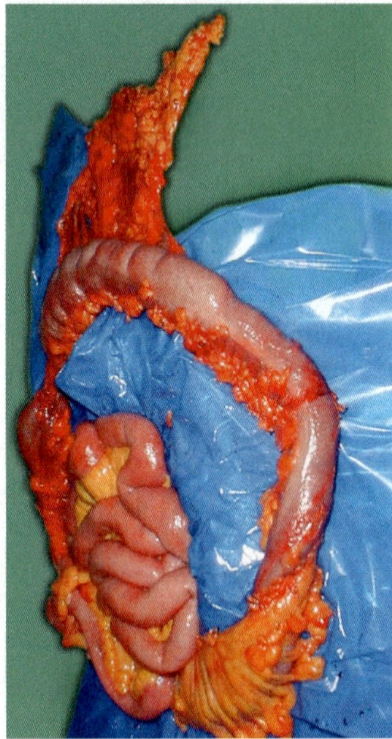

**Fig. 58.31:** Fully mobilised colon. Observe loss of haustrations. Total proctocolectomy with ileal pouch to anal anastomosis was done. A case of total proctocolitis

perforation/septicaemia and death can occur in untreated cases. Antidiarrhoeals, anticholinergics, narcotics, and hypokalaemia exaggerate this condition. Supportive treatment and intravenous corticosteroids are necessary (Key Box 58.10 and Figs 58.32 and 58.33).

2. **Massive haemorrhage** per rectum is uncommon. It is treated by blood transfusion.
3. **Perforation** is treated as peritonitis with resection of colon. Mortality rate is around 25–50%. Steroids may mask the symptoms. In an emergency situation, saving life is more important. Hence, resection followed by ileostomy should be done.

Key Box 58.10

**Factors Precipitating Toxic Megacolon**

- Barium enema
- Opiates, antidiarrhoeal drugs, anticholinergic agents
- Not known
- Ulcerative colitis, salmonella colitis
- Pseudomembranous colitis, amoebic colitis

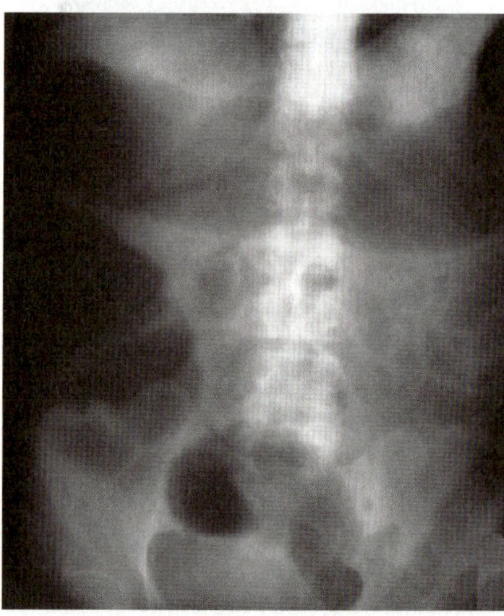

**Fig. 58.32:** Plain X-ray abdomen showing dilated transverse colon more than 6 cm is suggestive of toxic megacolon

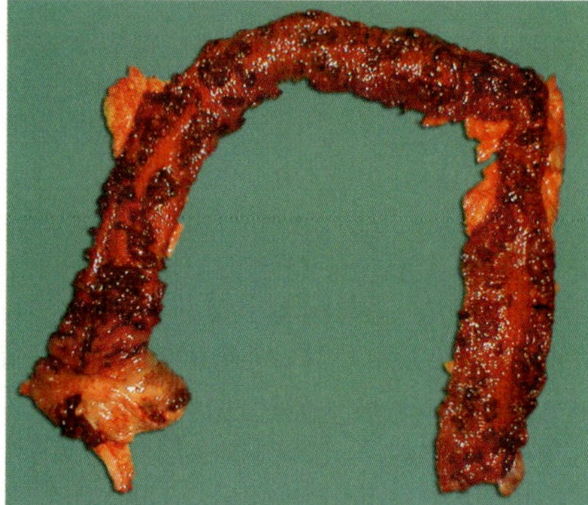

**Fig. 58.33:** Total colectomy for toxic megacolon specimen showing pseudopolyposis

4. **Carcinoma of the colon** (Key Box 58.11)
   - Overall incidence is 3% when the disease has been present for 15 years.
   - At the end of 25 years, the incidence may be around 20%.
   - Hence, routine sigmoidoscopy and biopsy have to be done when the disease is present for more than 10 years and if it shows epithelial dysplasia, it should be considered as premalignant.
   - Incidence is more in total proctocolitis and when the disease has started in the early age group.

Key Box 58.11

**Ulcerative Colitis (UC) and Colorectal Cancer (CRC)**

- CRC is more aggressive
- Multicentric and synchronous cancers
- UC patients with primary sclerosing cholangitis (PSC) have increased risk of CRC
- More advanced stage at the time of presentation
- Risk increases with duration of the disease
- Malignancy develops on a background of dysplasia [dysplasia associated lesion or mass **(DAL-M)**]

5. **Recurrent perianal abscess** resulting in perianal fistula, occurs in about 15–20% of patients.
6. **General complications (extraintestinal)**
   - **Protein malnutrition** resulting in cirrhosis. Primary sclerosing cholangitis is also found in many cases. Fatty acid infiltration is seen in 40% of cases. It is reversible after control of disease.
   - **Skin ulcerations**, pyoderma, erythema nodosum, etc. reflect protein malnutrition.
   - Conjunctivitis, iritis, arthritis involving large joints are also other features.
   - Incidence of **bile duct cancer** is high in these patients.

*Pearls of Wisdom*

Peripheral arthritis and ankylosing spondylitis are the two most common extraintestinal manifestations.

## Differential Diagnosis

- **Crohn's disease** should be ruled out first. The differences between the two inflammatory bowel diseases have been discussed at the end of the chapter. In general, diarrhoea and bleeding are more common with ulcerative colitis than Crohn's disease.
- **Dysenteries:** Bacillary dysenteries, shigellosis, salmonellosis, amoebiasis and other dysenteries have to be kept in mind specially in developing countries including tuberculosis which has been already discussed.
- **Diverticular disease of the colon:** However, when complications including bleeding occur, diverticular

disease of the colon and in cases of perforations, malignant perforation must be considered as a differential diagnosis.

## Investigations

1. **Stool:** It is done mainly to rule out various causes of infective diarrhoea—amoebiasis, *Shigella, Clostridium difficile.* Most common cause of infective colitis in UK is *Campylobacterium.*
2. **Sigmoidoscopy** (Key Box 58.12): Can demonstrate inflammatory changes in the mucosa. Mucus, pus and blood are visible. Multiple ulcers are visible with bleeding.

Key Box 58.12

**Sigmoidoscopy—Findings**

| Amoebic ulcer | Ulcerative colitis |
|---|---|
| Large | Small, pinpoint |
| Deep, flask shaped | Superficial |
| Mucosa in between ulcer is healthy | Mucosa in between ulcers unhealthy |

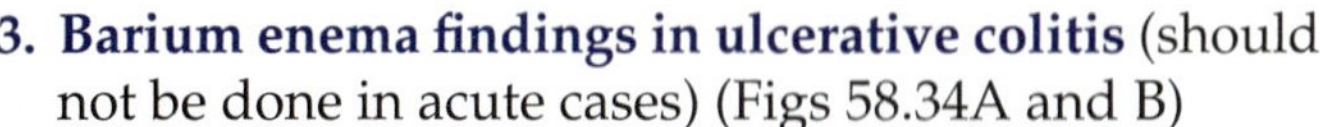

3. **Barium enema findings in ulcerative colitis** (should not be done in acute cases) (Figs 58.34A and B)
   - Contracted colon/pipe stem colon
   - Absence of haustrations and mucosal irregularity
   - Pseudopolyposis appears as stippled appearance
   - Retrorectal space is increased.
4. **Colonoscopy** (Figs 58.35 and 58.36)
   - To confirm the diagnosis by biopsy
   - To find out the extent of involvement of colon
   - To follow up patients who are on treatment
   - To rule out carcinomatous changes
5. **Plain X-ray abdomen:** To rule out megacolon and perforation.
6. **C-reactive protein:** Its levels are very high in case of acute fulminating attack or toxic megacolon.
7. Electrolytes, albumin levels are low. They have to be corrected especially in severe cases.

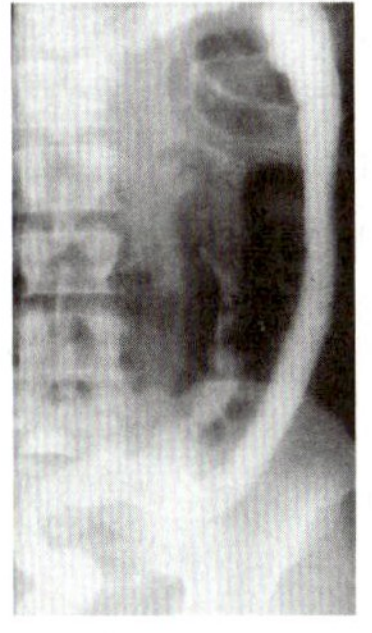

**Fig. 58.34A:** Barium enema showing pipe stem colon

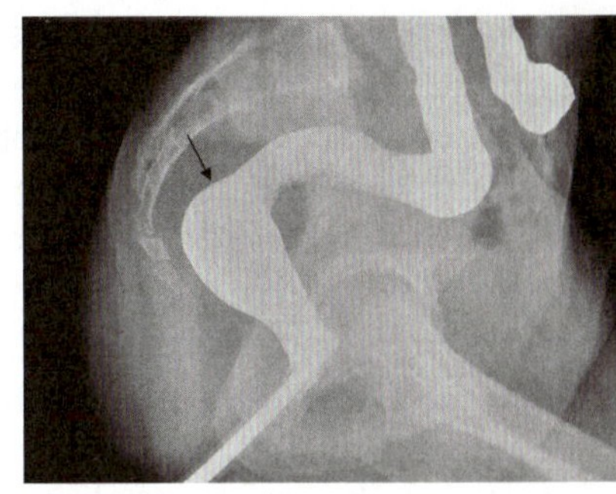

**Fig. 58.34B:** Barium enema demonstrating increased space between the rectum and sacrum

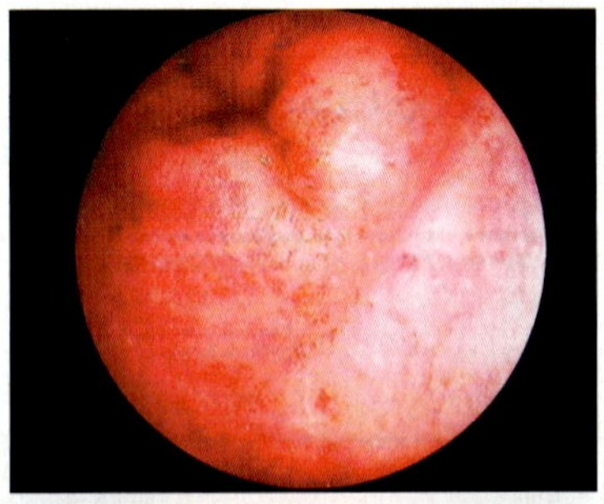

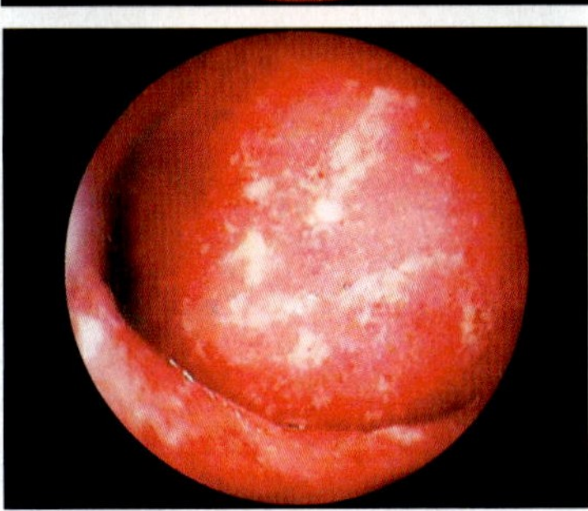

**Figs 58.35 and 58.36:** Colonoscopy—pinpoint ulcers with bleeding (*Courtesy*: Dr Filipe Alvares, Former Medical Gastroenterologist, KMC, Manipal)

## Treatment of Ulcerative Colitis

### *I. Conservative Line of Management* (Table 58.3)

- Hospitalisation and bed rest
- Correction of fluid and electrolyte imbalance
- Blood transfusions to correct anaemia and TPN for hypoproteinaemia (Fig. 58.37).
- **Salazopyrines** are given in the dose of 2 g/day. Mode of action: When given orally, it gets split into 5-aminosalicylic acid and sulphapyridine in the colon. This suppresses activity of prostaglandins $E_1$ and $E_2$ and thus reduces inflammation. They are used mainly to induce remission. They act as inhibitors of the cyclooxygenase enzyme system.
- **Corticosteroids:** Less severe cases not responding to salazopyrin are given a trial of oral prednisolone 60 mg/day. They decrease the frequency of stools. The dose is tapered off over 3–4 weeks.
- In acute attacks, IV hydrocortisone 100 mg is given.
- Prednisolone retention enema: 20 mg in 200 ml saline in intractable diarrhoea. It avoids systemic toxicity. Prednisolone 20–40 mg/day can also be given orally for 3–4 weeks.
- **Role of cyclosporine:** Those patients who do not respond to corticosteroids, can be given IV cyclosporine 4 mg/kg/day. It can induce remission.
- **Role of monoclonal antibodies:** These drugs act against antitumour necrosis factor alpha. They regulate inflammatory cascades. Infliximab or adalimumab are drugs. Vedolizumab is a rescue agent which blocks integrins.

| TABLE 58.3: Pharmacotherapy in ulcerative colitis | | |
|---|---|---|
| **Drug** | **Dose** | **Mode of action** |
| 1. Salazopyrin—**first choice** | • 2–4 g/day<br>• Anti-inflammatory<br>• Immunosuppressive | Suppresses $PGE_1$ and $E_2$ |
| 2. Steroids—refractory cases | • IV hydrocortisone 100 mg 8th hourly<br>• Prednisolone enema<br>• After acute illness, prednisolone 40–60 mg/day | Anti-inflammatory |
| 3. Immunomodulators<br>• Cyclosporine used in refractory cases | Azathioprine 6-mercaptopurines | Act at DNA level and inhibit T lymphocyte functions |
| 4. Monoclonal antibody–Antitumour necrosis factor-alpha (TNF-α) Infliximab | | Antitumour necrosis |
| 5. Anti-inflammatory (salicylic acid) | • Olsalazine (Dipentum)<br>• 500 mg 1–2 times/day | Directly targeted/released into the colon |

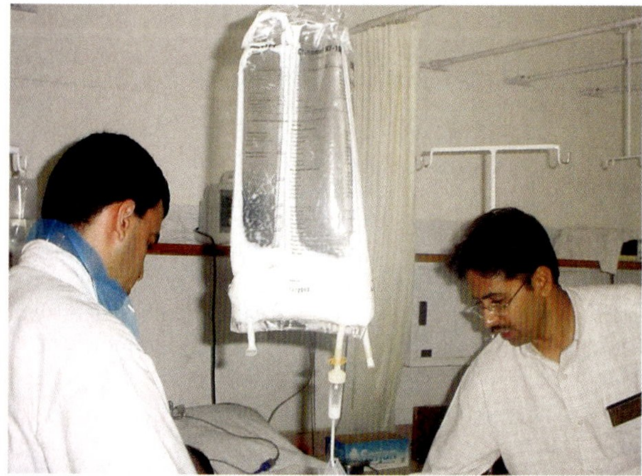

**Fig. 58.37:** Total parenteral nutrition (TPN) before and after surgery for ulcerative colitis plays an important role in the recovery of the patient, as these patients are grossly emaciated and hypoproteinaemic

### *II. Surgery*

*Indications for Surgery*

- Complications—toxic megacolon, perforation.
- Active disease in spite of medical line of management
- Severe disease not responding to medical treatment
- Dysplasia on biopsy
- Steroid dependence
- Haemorrhage

*Pearls of Wisdom*

Failure to improve within 7 days of maximum medical treatment with steroids and cyclosporine is an indication for surgery.

1. **Restorative proctocolectomy** with ileal pouch:
   - This can be done as one- or two-stage procedure.
   - Total proctocolectomy is done first.
   - A mucosectomy of the upper anal canal is done.
   - A pouch is created by anastomosing the loops of ileum. A J-shaped pouch is the most popular followed by W pouch (Figs 58.38 to 58.41).
   - The pouch is anastomosed to the dentate line (junction of upper and lower anal canal) by using stapler or by hand sutures.
   - Protective ileostomy is done and it can be closed after two months.
2. **Total proctocolectomy** followed by permanent ileostomy (ileoanal anastomosis should not be done because of incontinence). Ileostomy is connected to ileostomy bag. Adhesive obstruction and chronic perineal sinus are late complications. This is the procedure with least complications (Figs 58.42 and 58.43).

**Advantages of a pouch**

- Avoids ileostomy.
- Continence is preserved and patient is able to pass the stools *via* naturalis.
- At the same time, all the diseased **mucosa** has been removed. Thus, the risk of cancer is negligible.
  - Pouchitis is a complication.
  - *See* Table 58.4 also.

**Complications of pouch**

- Inflammation of the pelvis due to leak.
- Adhesion causing postoperative intestinal obstruction.
- Pouch—vaginal fistula.
- Frequency of the stools around 4 to 10 times/day.
- Pouchitis: It is inflammation of the pouch. Seen in about 30% of patients. Features represent original disease such as tenesmus, frequency of stools, toxicity, etc. Metronidazole can be used to treat.

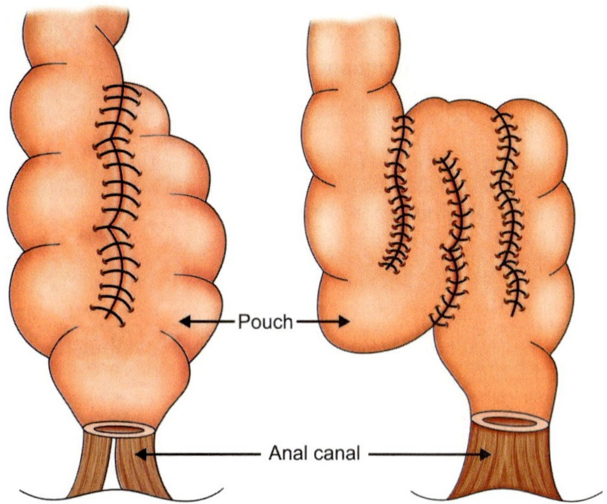


**Fig. 58.38:** J pouch

**Fig. 58.39:** W pouch

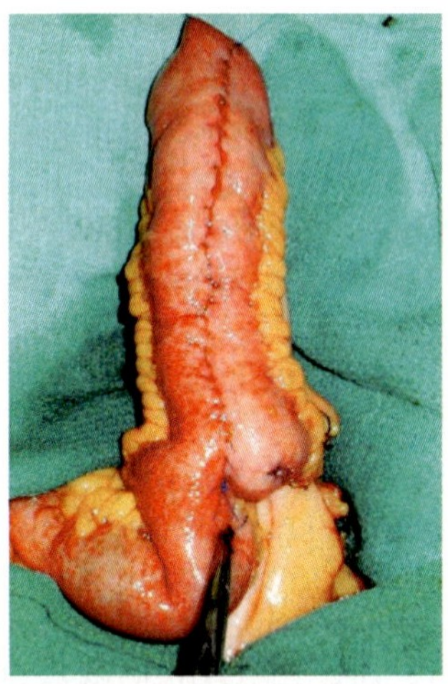

The length of the pouch is generally 15 cm and capacity around 300 ml when distended. Note that it is a two-layered anastomosis to create the pouch. The same can be achieved by linear stapling device.

**Fig. 58.40:** J pouch (*Courtesy*: Dr TLVD Prasad Babu, Ramcharan Thyagarajan, Srikanth Gadiyaram, Prof Sadiq S Sikora, Department of Surgical Gastroenterology, Manipal Hospital, Bengaluru)

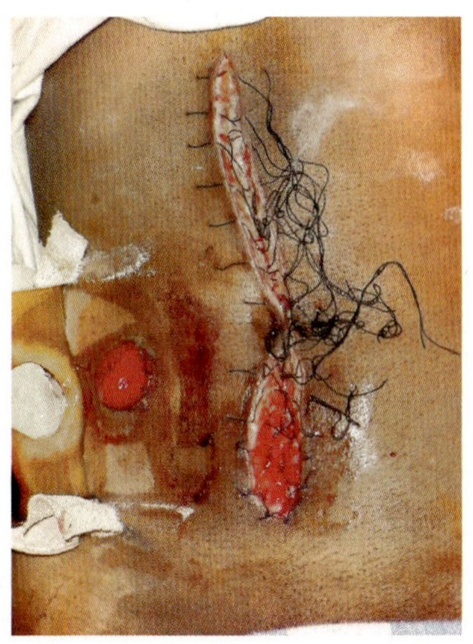

Wound was sutured after 48 hours because wound infection is a common complication after this surgery

**Fig. 58.41:** Total proctocolectomy with a pouch and protective ileostomy was done here

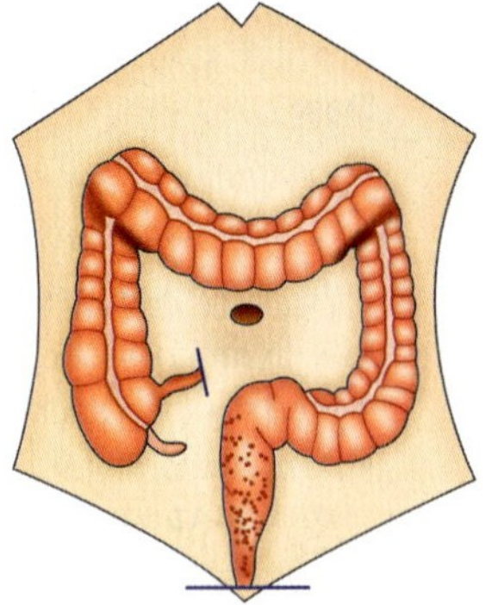

**Fig. 58.42:** Total colectomy

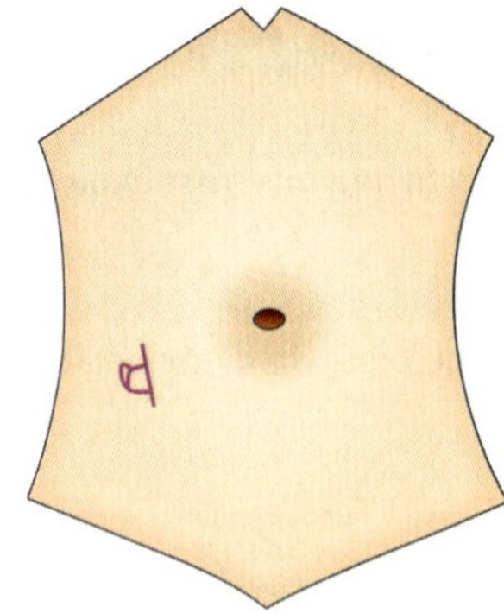

**Fig. 58.43:** Ileostomy

**TABLE 58.4:** Treatment of ulcerative colitis

| | **Mild** | **Moderate** | **Severe** |
|---|---|---|---|
| Admission | Not required | Not required | Required |
| Rectal steroid | Yes | Yes | No |
| Oral Prednisolone | 20–40 mg | Yes | IV hydrocortisone 100–200 mg/ 4 times/day |
| 5-ASA | Can be given | Can be given | Not given |
| **Nutrition** | **Oral** | **Oral** | TPN/**oral/high calorie diet** |
| Fluid/ electrolyte balance | Normal | Normal | Imbalance is very common |
| Blood transfusion | No | Yes | Yes |
| Surgery | Not done | Not done | No response for 3–5 days—**surgery** |

5-ASA: Amino salicylic acid; TPN: Total parenteral nutrition

## Prognosis

In general, emergency colitis is required in about 25% patients with severe attacks. Perforation has a mortality rate of up to 40% because of faecal contents and toxicity. Incidence of carcinoma colon is about 10–15%. Longer the duration of the disease, higher is the incidence.

## Dietary Advice

- High protein, carbohydrates, whole grains, and good fats. Meat, fish, poultry, and dairy products, breads and cereals; fruits and vegetables may be consumed.
- For vegetarians: Dairy products and plant proteins—such as soya bean products may be consumed.
- To avoid: High fibre high residue diet—thus to control diarrhoea.
- To avoid: Caffeine—coffee, dried fruits and nuts, alcohol, meat, spicy food, oily food, soda, etc.

## ILEOSTOMY

- Ileostomy is a surgical procedure wherein a loop of the ileum or end of the ileum is brought to the exterior (surface of the body).
- Two types are usually done: End ileostomy and loop ileostomy.
- End ileostomy is done following total proctocolectomy. It is a permanent ileostomy. The ileum is brought out through the lateral edge of rectus abdominis. It should project at least 5 cm outside (Figs 58.44A and B).
- Loop ileostomy is done to divert gastrointestinal contents to protect ileo-pouch anastomosis. It is a temporary ileostomy which is closed after 6–8 weeks.
- Permanent ileostomy is also required following total colectomy for carcinoma colon. It is an end ileostomy (Figs 58.45 to 58.47).
- Ileostomy care includes maintenance of fluid and electrolyte balance, use of disposable ileostomy bag and skin protection.
- Complications of an ileostomy are similar to that of colostomy—retraction, prolapse, bleeding, stenosis.
- Precautions—living with an ileostomy.
  1. Ileostomy bag has to be fitted well to the body surface. It needs to be adjusted often.
  2. Ileostomy has to be emptied 4–6 times depending upon the requirement.
  3. Chewed and masticated food is better.
  4. Avoid gas forming diet. Patients will learn slowly what to take and what not to take.
  5. Long-term complications include—gallstones, kidney stones, adhesions and intestinal obstruction.

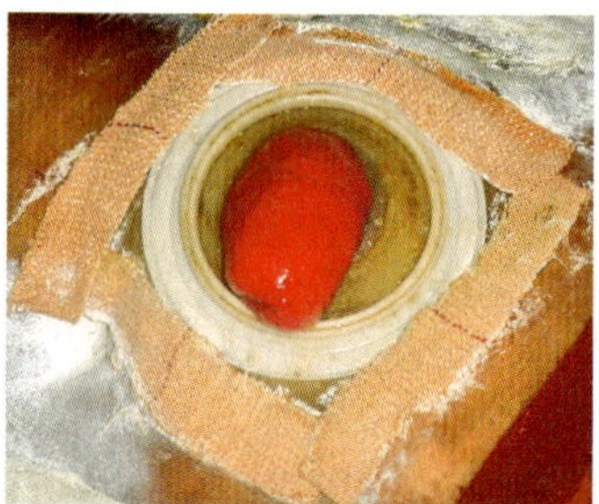

**Fig. 58.44A:** Ileostomy: It should project out for at least 5 cm

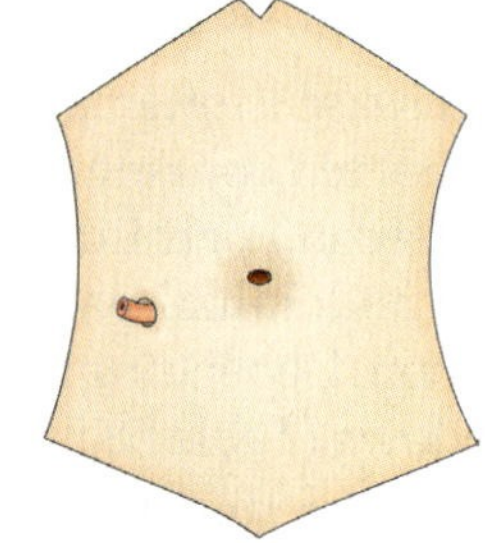

**Fig. 58.44B:** End ileostomy: Following total protocolectomy

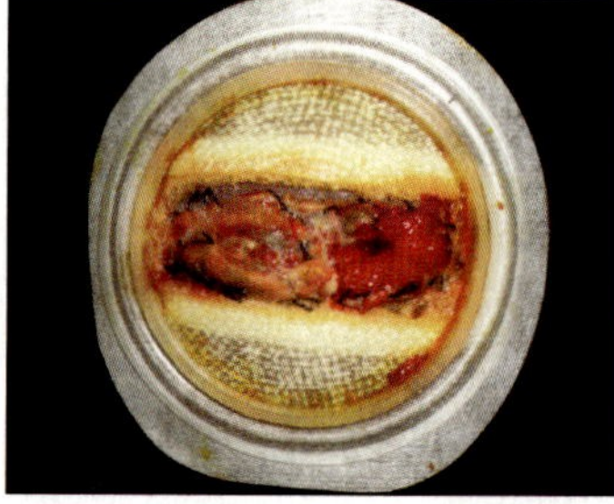

**Fig. 58.45:** Doubtful viability—complication of the ileostomy

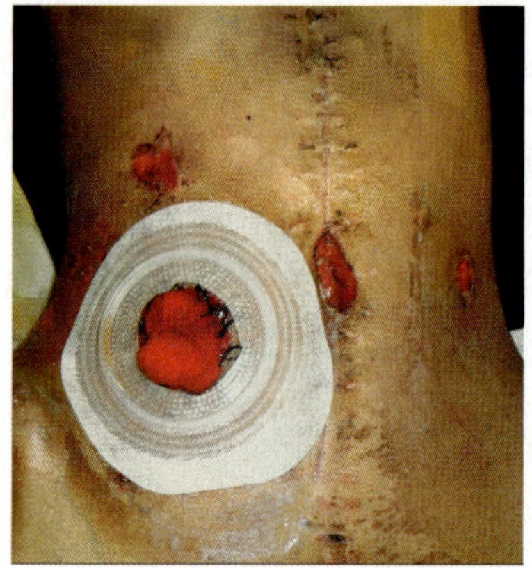

**Fig. 58.46:** An 18-year-old girl was diagnosed with acute appendicitis. At exploration, tuberculosis of ileum was diagnosed. Limited colectomy was done following which ileum was brought outside as temporary ileostomy

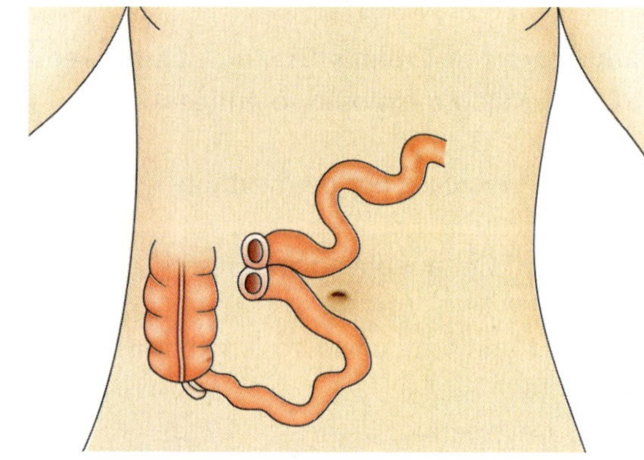

**Fig. 58.47:** Loop ileostomy is done following resection of perforated enteric ulcer. Distal ileum was friable and oedematous. Hence, it was brought out. This is a safer option

## CROHN'S DISEASE

It was called regional ileitis because the disease was first reported in the terminal ileum. However, today it is called **regional enteritis** because the disease can occur in jejunum, ileum, colon, oesophagus, etc. Involvement of ileum is more common, followed by colon. More common in North America and Northern Europe. Incidence is 8/100000 population and in UK incidence is 145/100000 population.

### Definition

Crohn's disease is a chronic transmural inflammatory disease of the gastrointestinal tract of unknown aetiology. It is neither neoplastic nor tuberculous.

### Aetiology

1. **Infectious agents:** *Mycobacterium paratuberculosis* and measles virus have been proposed as potential causes of Crohn's disease. However, it should be noted that antimicrobial therapy has not been effective in eradicating Crohn's disease (unlike ATT in TB). Also, no immunological reaction has been found.
2. **Immunologic factors:** Similar to UC. Focal ischaemia due to autoimmune reaction has also been considered.

3. **Genetic factors:** Single strongest risk factor for development of Crohn's is a relative with Crohn's disease.
   - Relatively high incidence is found in Ashkenazi jaws.
4. **Smoking:** It increases the risk of Crohn's disease threefold unlike its protective effect against ulcerative colitis.
5. **Diet and Crohn's disease:** Increased intake of carbohydrates and diet rich in refined food have been blamed for. Increased intake of animal protein, milk protein and increased ratio of omega-6 to omega-3 polyunsaturated fatty acids have also been blamed.

## Pathogenesis of Crohn's Disease

**Pathogenesis of Crohn's Disease—Early Events**

Mucosa exposed to antigens
↓
Increase gut permeability
↓
Cell-mediated response
↓
Interleukin-2 and tumour necrosis factor are released
+
Defective suppressor T cells
(Normally, it prevents escalation of this response)
–
Inflammation

## Pathology (Key Box 58.13)

- Disease **starts in terminal ileum** as ulcerations of intestine in about 60% of cases.
- There is extensive inflammatory oedema and mucosal ulcers are present. Fibrotic thickening of the intestine results in **hose pipe rigidity** of the intestine.
- There are **skip areas** which are characteristic of Crohn's disease (segments of intestine are normal in between).
- **Mesenteric nodes are enlarged.** They can be calcified but do not show any caseation.
- **Intense infiltration of mononuclear cells** and lymphoid hyperplasia is common.
- As the disease progresses, there is cicatrizing granuloma of the bowel wall. This results in narrowing of lumen causing intestinal obstruction. **Caseation is characteristically absent.**
- Once inflammation spreads to the serosa, adhesions develop between bowel loops or other structures. Abscesses occur in the mesentery which rupture resulting in internal fistula (Fig. 58.48).

*Pearls of Wisdom*

Transmural inflammation is characteristic of Crohn's disease.

Key Box 58.13

**Pathology of Crohn's Disease**

**T**ransmural inflammation
**R**eticulation cobblestone
**A**phthoid ulcers
**N**oncaseating cicatrising granuloma
**S**kip lesions
**M**esenteric lymph nodes enlarged
**U**lcers are in ileum, jejunum, colon, etc.
**R**igidity—Hose pipe
**A**dhesions occur soon
**L**inear ulcers

*Remember as* **TRANSMURAL**

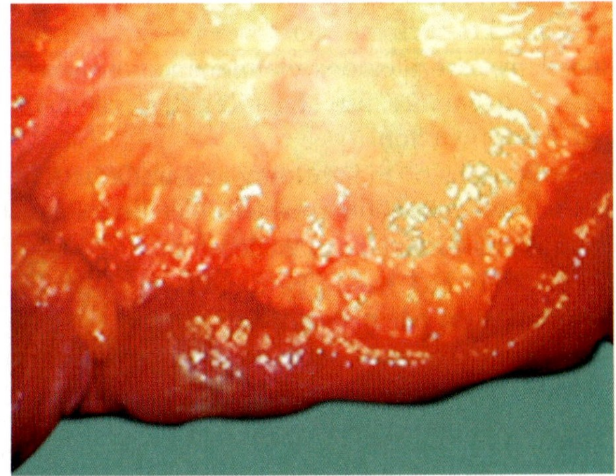

**Fig. 58.48:** Crohn's disease—creeping fat (*Courtesy*: Dr Ramesh Rajan, Gastrointestinal Surgeon, Trivandrum Medical College, Kerala)

## Clinical Features

(Key Box 58.14 and Figs 58.49 to 58.51)

The disease is often **insidious**, slowly progressive with a protracted course and commonly affects young adults in the second or third decade of life. Intermittent colicky lower abdominal pain, diarrhoea and weight loss are common. Depending upon symptoms, it can be classified as follows (Table 58.5):

1. **Stage of ileocolitis:** Clinically, it presents as pain abdomen and mucus in stools. It is seen in younger patients. It may be associated with fever. Presence of

Key Box 58.14

**Various Stages/Complications of Crohn's Disease**

**C**olitis—ileocolitis
**R**ectal—anorectal disease
**O**bstruction due to stricture
**H**ollow viscus fistulae
**N**utritional deficiencies

*Remember as* **CROHN**

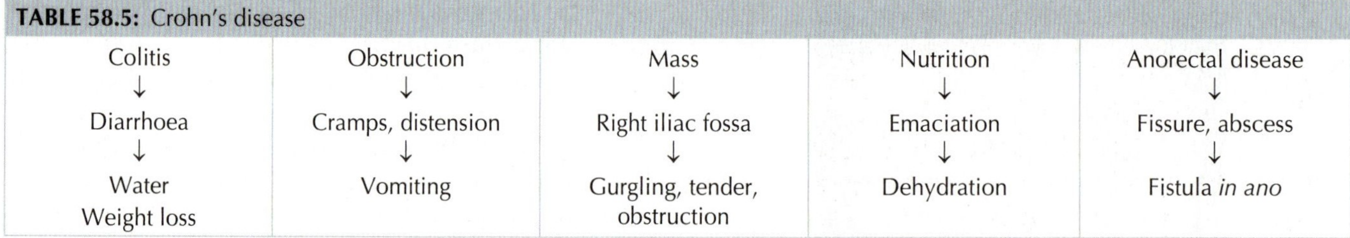

**TABLE 58.5:** Crohn's disease

| Colitis | Obstruction | Mass | Nutrition | Anorectal disease |
|---|---|---|---|---|
| ↓ | ↓ | ↓ | ↓ | ↓ |
| Diarrhoea | Cramps, distension | Right iliac fossa | Emaciation | Fissure, abscess |
| ↓ | ↓ | ↓ | ↓ | ↓ |
| Water<br>Weight loss | Vomiting | Gurgling, tender, obstruction | Dehydration | Fistula *in ano* |

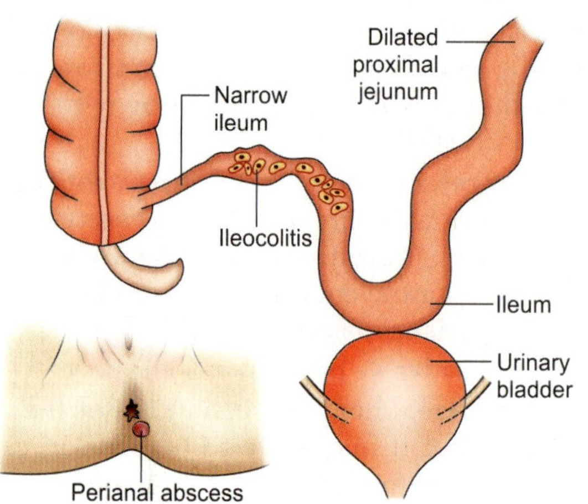


**Fig. 58.49:** Clinical features of Crohn's disease (*Courtesy*: Ms Vidushi, MBBS student, KMC, Manipal)

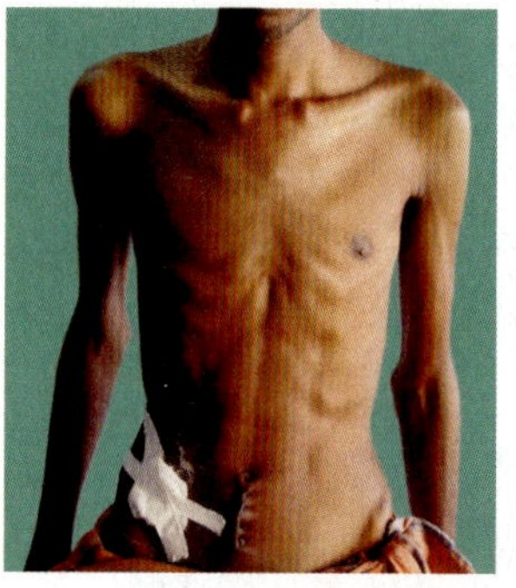

**Fig. 58.50:** An emaciated patient who underwent appendicectomy, only to present later with features of Crohn's disease

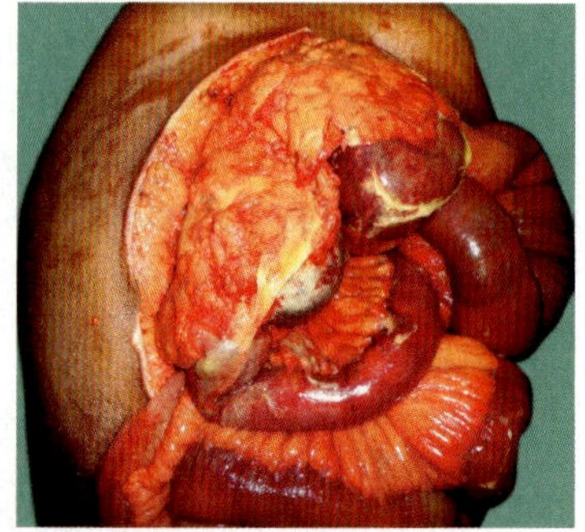

**Fig. 58.51:** Congested bowel loops, area of perforation, dilated loops of bowel are seen in this picture

pain and tenderness in the right iliac fossa mimics appendicitis. If there is a mass, it may be confused for an appendicular mass.

2. **Stage of subacute intestinal obstruction** occurs due to stricture of the terminal ileum. Strictures can be multiple. They are not reversible.
3. **Stage of fistula formation:** It can be enteroenteric or enterocutaneous. Following are the examples of fistulae encountered in Crohn's disease—ileovesical, ileocolic, ileoileal, ileovaginal, etc.
4. **Perianal disease** in the form of multiple ulcers in the anorectal region, perianal abscesses, multiple fistulae in ano are much more common than in ulcerative colitis. Repeated infection of anal crypt due to diarrhoea is common.

## Extraintestinal Complications

- Skin: Pyoderma gangrenosum, erythema nodosum
- Joints: Arthritis, ankylosing spondylitis
- Bile duct: Sclerosing cholangitis
- Eyes: Iritis, uveitis
- Nephrotic syndrome
- Pancreatitis
- Amyloidosis
- Crohn's disease that affects the ileum—increased risk of **gallstones**. This is due to a decrease in bile acid resorption in the ileum.

*Pearls of Wisdom*

Anal fissure is the most common anal problem in Crohn's disease. Noncaseating granuloma is most common in anorectal disease.

## Differential Diagnosis

1. **Ulcerative colitis:** However, colonic symptoms are more with ulcerative colitis.
2. **Tuberculosis:** In India, tuberculosis should be considered first and ruled out.
3. **Appendicitis:** Acute pain in the right iliac fossa can be confused for acute appendicitis. For benefit of the doubt, the patient can undergo laparotomy. Laparoscopy and appendicectomy will be better.
4. **Intestinal obstruction:** Other causes of obstruction have to be kept in mind.

## Investigations

1. **Small bowel enema:** Enteroclysis.
   - **Cobblestone** reticulation because of multiple ulcers with islands of normal mucosa in between.
   - Absence of peristalsis in terminal ileum.
   - **String sign of Kantor** is demonstrated in terminal ileum due to narrowing of the lumen.
   - Multiple strictures and dilated segments in between can be demonstrated.
2. **Sigmoidoscopy and colonoscopy** may demonstrate inflamed mucosa, which is granular with **aphthoid ulcers**, which are **discrete** (Fig. 58.52).

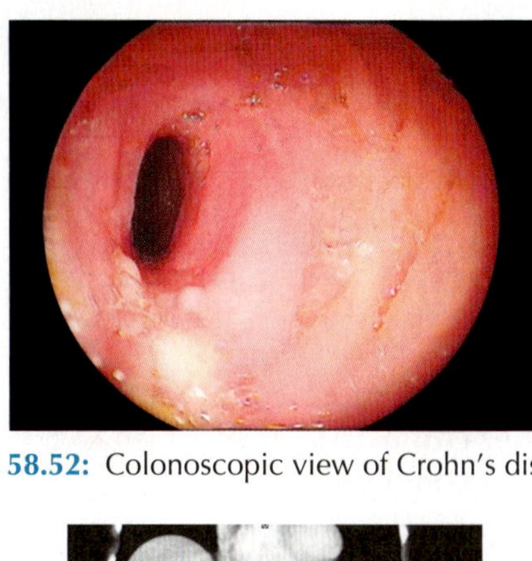

Fig. 58.52: Colonoscopic view of Crohn's disease

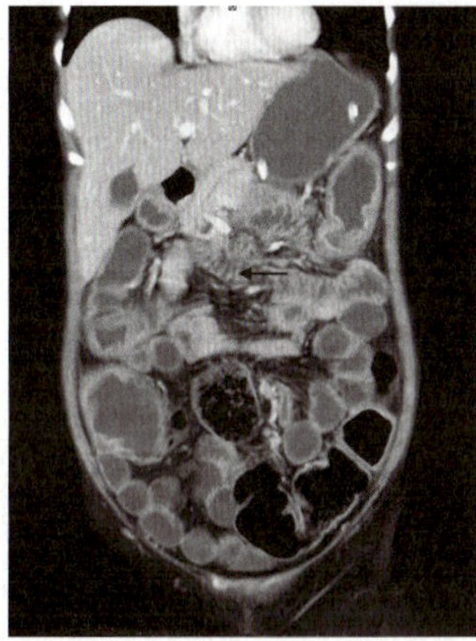

Fig. 58.53: CECT scan: Crohn's disease showing thickening of intestinal loops

3. **Fistulography** to localise the internal fistula.
4. **CT scan:** It is done to detect thickening of bowel and extraintestinal disease (Fig. 58.53).
5. Remember to investigate upper GI tract with gastroduodenoscopy and capsule endoscopy (*see* page 1006).

## Treatment

**I. General principles**

- Complete rest, avoid stress and emotions.
- A low residue, high caloric diet such as high protein diet.
- Some patients may require total parenteral nutrition—some at home called home parenteral nutrition.

**II. Conservative (medical) treatment** is similar to ulcerative colitis.

- Steroids are the mainstay of treatment. They are effective in inducing remission in 70 to 80% of cases.
- Steroids are most effective in treating small intestinal disease. They are anti-inflammatory. They do control diarrhoea, induce remissions. Prednisolone is used for short-term treatment. Long-term use can give rise to toxicity such as immunosuppression, bone loss, delayed wound healing, etc.
- Salazopyrines can be used especially in maintenance cases also.
- Even though salazopyrines and corticosteroids have been beneficial in Crohn's disease, salazopyrines do not induce remissions. They are used in acute ileocolitis. Steroids can be used for anorectal disease.
- Immunosuppressive therapy using azathioprine and 6-mercaptopurine are also effective.
- They are effective in treatment of colonic disease. The main concern is bone marrow toxicity. 6-mercaptopurines are known to produce pancreatitis.
- Most recent and promising drug is **infliximab**—a monoclonal antibody to tumour necrosis factor $\alpha$ (TNF-$\alpha$). It mainly helps in **closure of fistula**. It is given intravenously and is used for intestinal and perianal disease.
- Metronidazole has shown some benefit.

**III. Surgical treatment:** Resection is not the aim of surgery but it may have to be done in cases of obstruction, perforation, intra-abdominal abscesses, internal fistulae, bleeding and malignancies. Depending upon the involvement of the bowel, various resections are possible. Examples:

1. Stricture—stricturoplasty or resection
2. Ileocaecal resection (Figs 58.54A and B)
3. Colectomy and ileorectal anastomosis
4. If the fistulae are present, they are disconnected from the bowel and excised.

Comparison of intestinal tuberculosis, ulcerative colitis and Crohn's disease is given in Table 58.6.

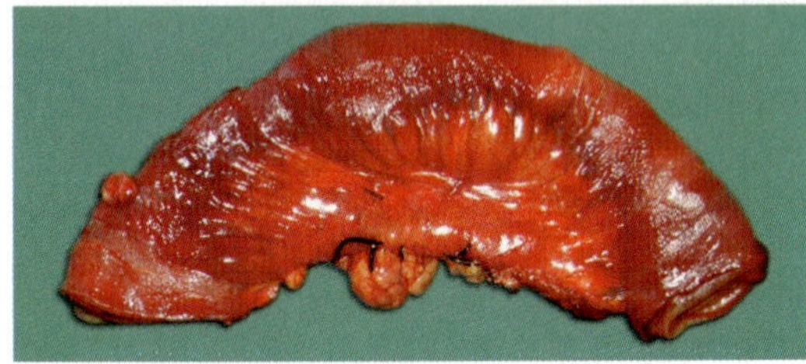

Fig. 58.54A: Resected specimen of small intestine. The patient had intestinal obstruction

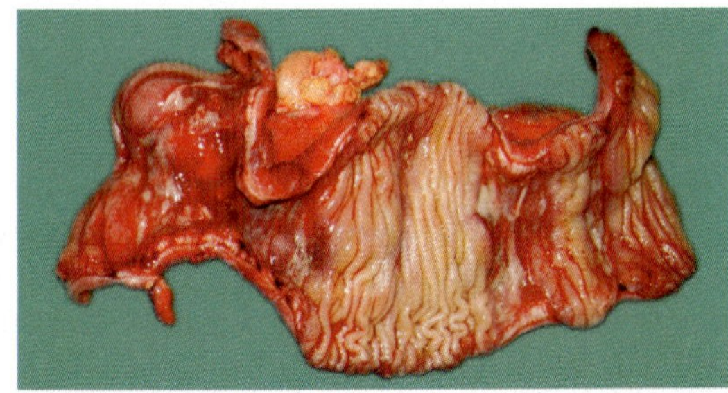

Fig. 58.54B: Opened specimen showing stricture. Biopsy proved Crohn's disease

**TABLE 58.6:** Summary of tubercular ileocolitis, ulcerative colitis and Crohn's colitis

| | Tuberculosis | Crohn's | Ulcerative colitis |
|---|---|---|---|
| 1. Bacteria | Mycobacterium | No | No |
| 2. Pathology | Continuous spread. Caseating granuloma, lymph node caseation. Transmural inflammation present | Skip areas. Cobblestone granuloma present. No caseation. Deep longitudinal ulcers. Transmural inflammation | Continuous, pseudopolyposis. Pinpoint ulcers. Crypt abscesses. Superficial ulcers. Mucosa and submucosa involved |
| 3. Site | Ileocaecal | Terminal ileum and colon | Rectum and colon |
| 4. Bowel wall | Thick and fibrotic | Thick fibrotic | Thin |
| 5. **Clinical** | | | |
| Bleeding | Uncommon | Uncommon | Very common |
| Diarrhoea | Uncommon | Very common | Very common |
| Fever | Common | Common | Rare |
| Mass | Very common | Common | Rare |
| Anal disease | Rare | Very common | Rare |
| Toxic megacolon | Never | Rare | More common |
| Fistulae | Uncommon | Very common | Uncommon |
| Stricture | Common | Common | Rare |
| 6. Malignancy | No | Can predispose (low) | High incidence |

### Prognosis

- In spite of various treatment, there is no cure for the disease. About 10–20% patients come with relapses and recurrent symptoms.
- Despite for repeated treatment including surgical procedures, survival is still good as compared to general population without the disease.

### A few observations in Crohn's disease

- Ileum is the most common site.
- Small bowel alone is affected in 20–30% of the patients.
- Both small bowel and large bowel in 50–60% patients.
- Duodenum, stomach, oesophagus can also be involved.
- Inflammatory cells and mediators of the inflammation such as cytokines, interleukins, tumour necrosis factors produce the inflammatory changes resulting in granuloma.
- Sometimes, it is very difficult to differentiate clinically and pathologically between tuberculosis and Crohn's disease.
- Anus is involved in Crohn's colitis, not in ulcerative colitis.

## SURGICAL COMPLICATIONS OF ENTERIC FEVER

During the third week of enteric fever, *Salmonella typhi, paratyphi* (enteric bacilli) multiply in Peyer's patches and can give rise to the following problems:

1. **Haemorrhage** is seen in about 5–10% of cases due to ulceration of Peyer's patches. It can be occult, obvious or rarely massive bleeding. It is managed conservatively in majority of cases.
2. **Perforation of terminal ileum:** An oval, vertical perforation results in peritonitis. Enteric perforation need not give rise to all signs of peritonitis. Guarding and rigidity can be minimal because of poor, immunocompromised nature of the disease and due to **Zenker's degeneration** of abdominal wall muscles. It is a single perforation in about 85% of the cases. It is situated in the antimesenteric border of the terminal ileum. Typically, it occurs in the third week of enteric fever. Bradycardia, dehydration, toxicity are the other features.
   - **Hyperplasia of reticuloendothelial system** including lymph nodes, liver and spleen is characteristic of typhoid fever (Key Box 58.15).
   - **Diagnosis of perforation** is based clinically on the acute abdominal pain, bleeding per rectum with/without guarding and rigidity. High grade fever, toxicity and bradycardia are other features that help in the diagnosis.
   - **Plain X-ray abdomen** may not reveal gas because of small sealed off performation.
   - **The most useful investigation is CT scan** which can reveal not only pneumoperitoneum but also pericolic collection, which can be missed by ultrasound (*see* the clinical notes).

*Pearls of Wisdom*

- When you suspect peritonitis, there is no guarding or rigidity.
- When you suspect perforation, there is no gas under diaphragm.
- When you suspect toxicity, there is no tachycardia but bradycardia, **suspect enteric ulcer.**

Key Box 58.15

**Typhoid Fever—Salient Features**

- **T**oxic—dehydrated delirious patient with diarrhoea—green pea soup stools
- **Y**oung patient
- **P**oor tone of the abdominal muscles due to Zenker's degeneration
- **H**igh grade fever
- **O**ther—hepatosplenomegaly, rose spots
- **I**mmunocompromised status
- **D**ecreased pulse rate—Faget sign

*You can remember as* **TYPHOID**

**Treatment:**

- Third generation cephalosporins are used.
- **Emergency laparotomy, resection of bowel** and end-to-end anastomosis or closure of the perforation by using non-absorbable sutures. Abdomen is closed with a tube drain kept in the right iliac fossa. Wound infection is common in such cases. Multiple fistulae are also common (Figs 58.55 to 58.58).
- **Small bowel exteriorisation:** This can be considered in cases after resection when both ends of the intestine are friable. This is a very safe option. After 1–4 weeks, relaparotomy and anastomosis of resected ends is done.

3. **Paralytic ileus** due to toxic dilatation of intestine results in distension of abdomen. It is managed by drip and suction.
4. **Typhoid cholecystitis** is not uncommon. It starts within 2 to 4 days fever. Chances of gallbladder perforation are present.
5. **Typhoid pyelonephritis,** cystitis, epididymo-orchitis.
6. **Typhoid osteomyelitis**
7. **Typhoid conjunctivitis**
8. **Thrombosis** of the common iliac vein occurs probably due to sluggish blood flow.
9. **Perforation** of large intestine can occur in paratyphoid 'B' infections.

Most of these complications occur due to bacteraemia produced in the early septicaemic phase of enteric fever. Liver, spleen, bone and bowel are commonly affected. Metastatic abscesses are common.

## INTESTINAL AMOEBIASIS

- This disease is caused by *Entamoeba histolytica* and transmitted mainly by contaminated drinking water.
- After the cysts are swallowed, they are broken down in the intestine by trypsin into trophozoites which produce inflammation of the colon. **Trophozoites swallow red blood cells and multiply by mitosis. They enter into crypts of Lieberkuhn.** They produce multiple submucous loculi which later result in multiple ulcers. These ulcers are **flask-shaped (bottle neck) ulcers** with healthy intervening mucosa.

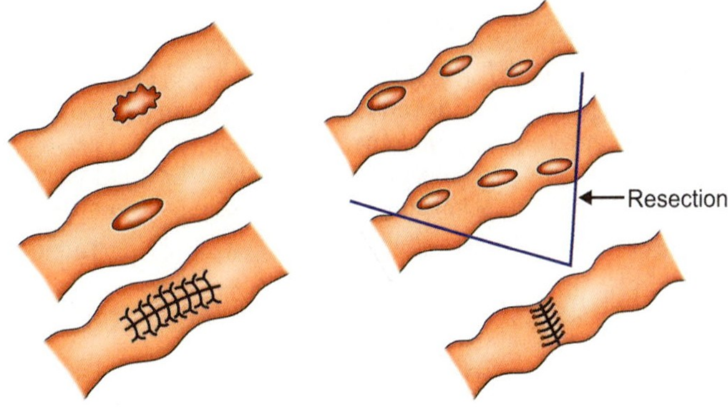


**Fig. 58.55:** Single ulcer, simple suturing

**Fig. 58.56:** Multiple ulcer—resection and anastomosis

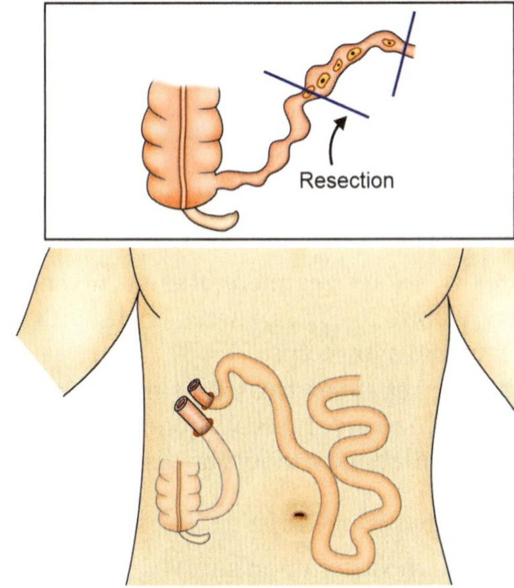


**Fig. 58.57:** Both ends brought outside—small bowel exteriorisation (*Courtesy*: Dr Vidushi, MBBS student, KMC, Manipal)

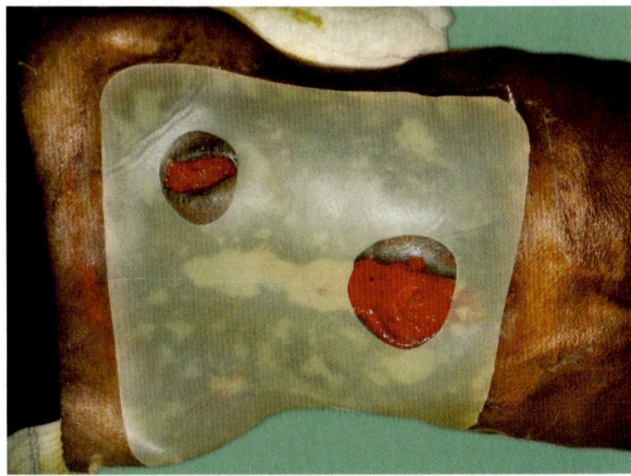

**Fig. 58.58:** Multiple bud fistulae developed following resection and anastomosis of typhoid ulcers treated with ostomy bags

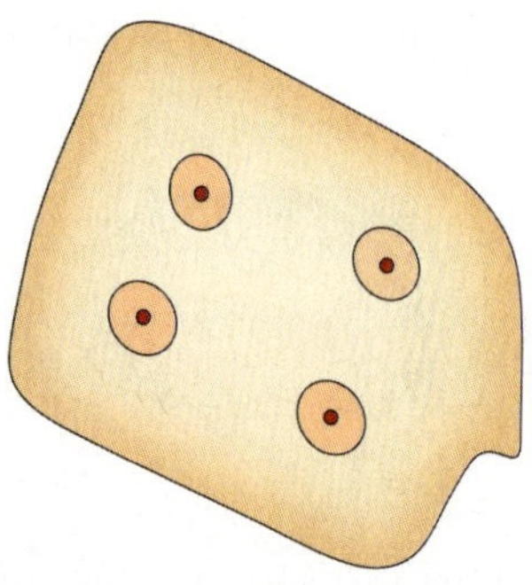

Fig. 58.59: Quadrinucleate cyst of entamoeba

- Some trophozoites are transformed into cysts and excreted outside (Fig. 58.59).
- Lower sigmoid and upper rectum are involved in 75% of cases.

## Clinical Features

1. **Amoebic typhlitis:** Inflammation of the caecum by amoeba is described as amoebic typhlitis. It produces pain in the right iliac fossa and it can be confused for appendicitis. However, in this condition, there is also tenderness in the left iliac fossa. A point on the left side corresponding to McBurney point on the right side is called **Sir Philip Manson-Bahr's amoebic point of tenderness** (Fig. 58.60) and is suggestive of involvement of rectosigmoid.
2. **Amoebic dysentery:** It can be acute or chronic. An acute attack is associated with gripping pain abdomen with blood and mucus in stool, an urgency to pass stools. High grade fever and tenesmus are the other features. Chronic dysentery is more common with 2–4 foul-smelling stools per day and mild to moderate colicky abdominal pain.
3. **Amoeboma:** Chronic, low grade, persistent inflammation of the caecum produces granulomatous hyperplasia of the caecum, with thickening of the pericaecal tissue (producing mass in the right iliac fossa) (Fig. 58.61). Amoeboma can also occur in rectosigmoid junction. This is, however, uncommon nowadays because of effective treatment with metronidazole.
   - Clinically, this manifests as mass in the right iliac fossa causing dull aching pain, vague ill health, tender palpable caecum with guarding. It can be confused for ileocaecal tuberculosis or carcinoma caecum.
   - It responds very well to metronidazole.
4. **Amoebic perforation of caecum** or sigmoid can occur resulting in pericolic abscess. Peritonitis needs emergency surgery.
5. **Massive bleeding per rectum** is rare. It occurs due to separation of the slough.

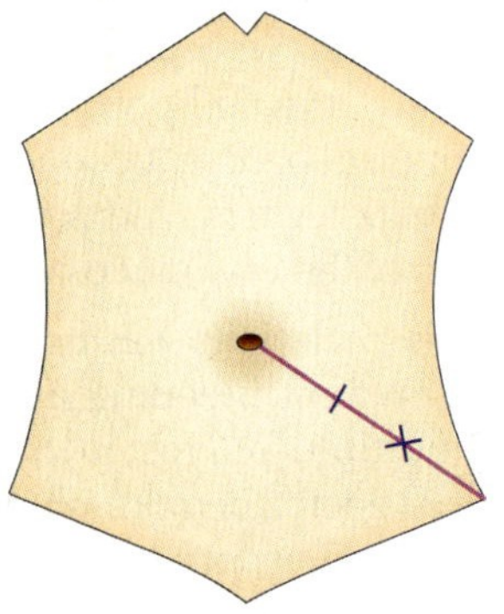

Fig. 58.60: Sir Philip Manson-Bahr's amoebic point

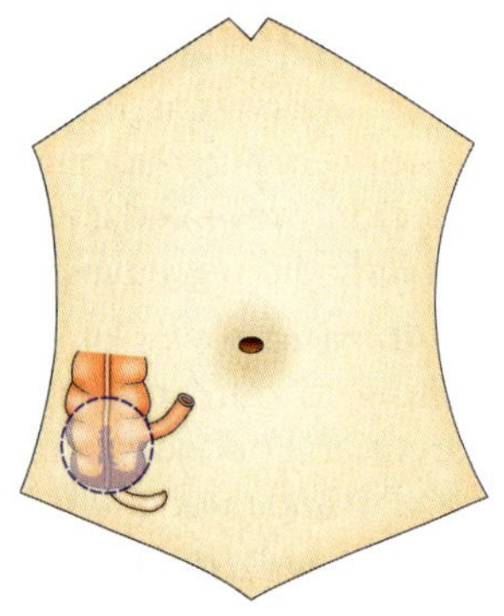

Fig. 58.61: Amoeboma is a tender thickened gurgling mass

## Treatment

1. **Metronidazole** 400–600 mg, 3 times a day for 10 days. It acts on amoebae present in the lumen and tissue.
2. Di-iodohydroxyquin 650 mg, 3 times a day for 20 days is another alternative.
3. Diloxanide furoate is ideal for chronic cases in the dose of 500 mg, 3 times a day for 10 days. It acts on luminal amoebae. It is the drug of choice in chronic cyst passers. Supportive treatment in the form of hospitalisation, correction of dehydration, antispasmodics and bedrest is also advised. Stool culture must be done before and after treatment with antiamoebic drugs.

# RADIATION ENTEROPATHY

Radiation damages rapidly growing cells of intestine also when they are exposed to it. It typically happens when radiation is given to the pelvis after rectal resections or radiation given to treat carcinoma cervix. Incidence is 5% after 4500 cGy units to 30% after 6000 cGy units. The chief factor is radiation-induced damage to the blood vessel supplying the bowel wall.

## Risk Factors

- Radiation dose more than 5000 cGy
- Previous laparotomy (if bowel loops are fixed due to adhesions)
- Pre-existing vascular disease
- Diabetes
- Hypertension

## Clinical Types

- **Acute:** It manifests as colicky abdominal pain, bloating, loss of appetite, diarrhoea, etc. It happens during 2nd week of treatment, because inflammatory changes are maximum during that period.
- **Chronic:** This occurs after 18 months and 6 years after radiotherapy.
- **Chronic intestinal ischaemia** occurs resulting in **stricture** and intestinal obstruction. Some cases are due to fibrosis, dense pelvic adhesions, bowel entrapment into the fibrosis, fistula formation and pelvic abscess.

- When there is no obstruction, conservative line of treatment is followed.
- If there is obstruction, laparotomy with resection, bypass or any other treatment depending upon the findings.
- Surgery can be difficult because of dense adhesions.

### Prevention

- Modern imaging and radiotherapy units.
- Radio-opaque markers such as titanium clips at the time of initial surgery.
- Decreasing the size of the radiation field.
- Reperitonisation of the bowel, using absorbable mesh cover over intestines, omental transposition also have been used.

### Treatment

- Sucralfate, mucosal protective agent, can be used in case of bleeding due to radiation proctitis.
- Antioxidants, probiotics, statins and angiotensin converting enzyme inhibitors are used when radiotherapy treatment is on.

## SMALL BOWEL TUMOURS

- Benign tumours such as lipoma, hamartoma, polyps can occur.
- Malignant tumours such as adenocarcinoma, gastrointestinal stromal tumours **(GIST)**, carcinoid and lymphoma can occur in the small intestine.

## PEUTZ-JEGHERS SYNDROME (FAMILIAL HAMARTOMATOUS POLYPOSIS)

This syndrome is characterised by:

1. **Familial** tendency
2. **Melanosis** of mucosa of lip, cheek, interdigital space and even perianal skin (Fig. 58.62 and Table 58.7).
3. **Multiple polyps** in the small bowel and large bowel mainly in the jejunum. They are hamartomatous polyps.
   - It is an autosomal dominant disease.

**TABLE 58.7:** Comparison of two hamartomatous polyposis syndromes

| Peutz-Jeghers syndrome | Cronkhite-Canada syndrome |
|---|---|
| Hamartomatous polyps | Hamartomatous polyps |
| Polyposis of small intestine (mainly) | Gastrointestinal polyposis |
| Melanin spots on the buccal mucosa and lips | Cutaneous pigmentation, finger nails atrophy, alopecia |
| Bleeding and intussusception are common complaints | Intestinal obstruction can occur |
| Rarely malignancy can occur | Severe malabsorption—protein-losing enteropathy |

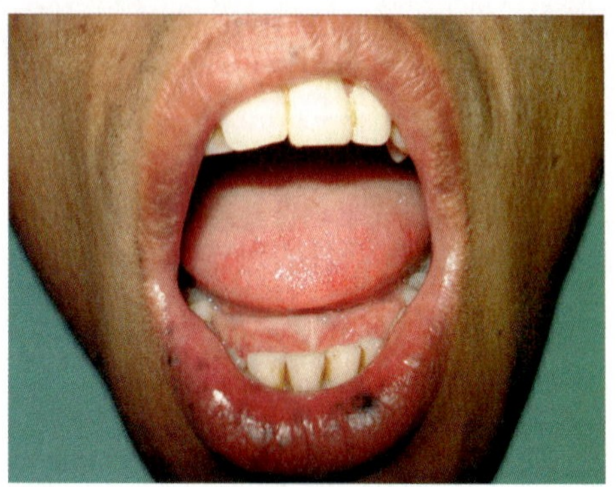

**Fig. 58.62:** This patient presented to hospital with abdominal pain. The registrar who examined the case reported that there was a mass abdomen. However, when he presented the case next day, there was no mass. The patient had undergone laparotomy 10 years back for similar complaints. A segment of bowel had been resected earlier. This photograph gives the clue to the diagnosis—pigmentation of lips and oral mucosa. The mass (appearing and disappearing) was due to intussusception (*Courtesy*: Prof Sreevatsa, Head, Prof Bharathi, Prof Bagli, Dr Srikar Pai, Department of Surgery, MS Ramaiah Medical College, Bengaluru, CME 2008)

### Clinical Presentation

- Runs in families.
- As a cause of bleeding per rectum, results in chronic anaemia.
- Can cause adult intussusception.
- Rarely, it can turn into malignancy.
- Female patients have increased chances of breast and cervical cancer (*see* clinical notes).

### Treatment

- Blood transfusion to correct anaemia
- Resection of that portion of bowel containing polyp, in cases of bleeding or intussusception.

#### Clinical Notes

A We had 3 interesting cases of Peutz-Jeghers syndrome.

**The first case** was of a boy of 14 years, who presented with acute intestinal obstruction. At laparotomy, there were 3 intussusceptions in the jejunum due to polyps. About 15 large polyps were removed after doing an enterotomy.

**The second case** was a 50-year-old lady, who presented with duodenal carcinoma. Endoscopy revealed polyps in the stomach and duodenum. Specimen of pancreaticoduodenectomy revealed it as a case of Peutz-Jeghers syndrome. This lady did not have pigmentation of the oral mucosa.

**The third case** was of a 35-year-old male who has been coming to our hospital with intermittent bleeding and anaemia. Endoscopy revealed multiple polyps in the stomach and duodenum. Small bowel enema demonstrated multiple polyps in the small bowel. Even proctoscopy showed multiple polyps in the rectum. He is being managed conservatively.

## ADENOCARCINOMA

- Incidence is 40% of small bowel tumours. Overall, small bowel tumours are rare. Reasons have been given in Key Box 58.16.
- Duodenum is the commonest site of adenocarcinoma. If it arises from first part and second part, it may require Whipple's pancreaticoduodenectomy. From the third part, early cases of adenocarcinoma can be resected without removal of pancreas.
- Some familial diseases predispose to adenocarcinoma. They are familial polyposis coli, adenomas, Crohn's disease, etc.
- Clinical features include vague features such as nausea, poor appetite, crampy abdominal pain, bleeding and intestinal obstruction.
- Diagnosis is by CT scan (Fig. 58.63).
- **Push enteroscopy** has the advantage of visualization of the growth and to take biopsy (Figs 58.64A and B).
- Other option is capsule endoscopy. It is time consuming and biopsy is not possible.
- Resection with at least 7 cm margin with lymphadenectomy is the treatment of choice (Figs 58.65 and 58.66).
- There is no role for radiotherapy and chemotherapy.

Key Box 58.16

**Malignancy in Small Intestine is Rare—Why?**

- No stasis, rapid transit of food
- Secretion of immunoglobulins—IgA
- Various carcinogens are diluted by secretions
- Comparatively low and inactive bacteria in the small bowel

## GASTROINTESTINAL STROMAL TUMOUR (GIST)

- Earlier called leiomyoma and leiomyosarcoma, they occur in jejunum or ileum. These are uncommon mesenchymal tumours (Figs 58.67 amd 58.68).
- **Stomach is the commonest site.** GISTs are rare in the oesophagus, whereas leiomyoma is more common.
- They constitute 20% of malignant neoplasms of the small bowel.
- More common in the 5th and 6th decades of life.
- They arise from **interstitial cells of Cajal** which are pacemaker cells that regulate motility and peristalsis.
- GISTs arise from muscularis propria. They tend to grow extramurally.

### Clinical Features

- They present as bleeding/mass/perforation.
- Very often massive bleeding may be the only presentation.

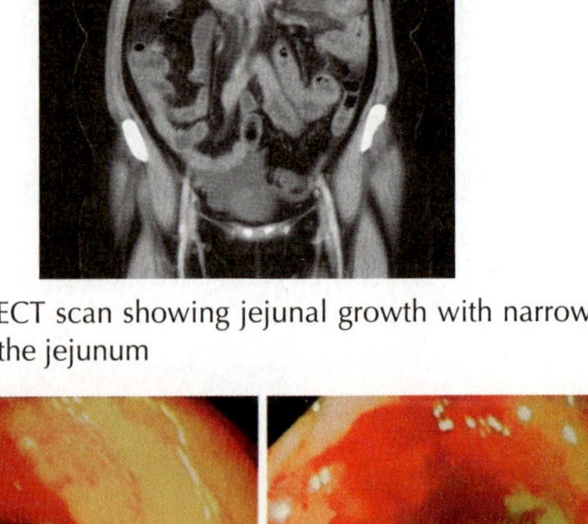

**Fig. 58.63:** CECT scan showing jejunal growth with narrowing of the lumen of the jejunum

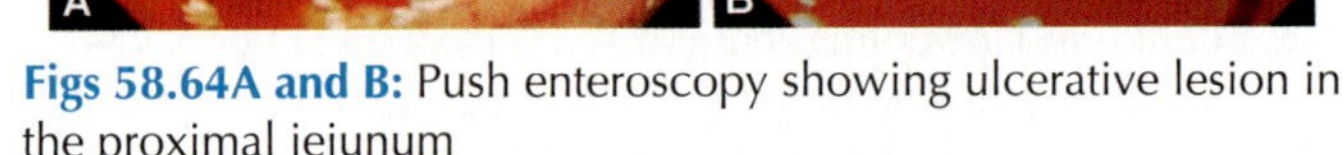


**Figs 58.64A and B:** Push enteroscopy showing ulcerative lesion in the proximal jejunum

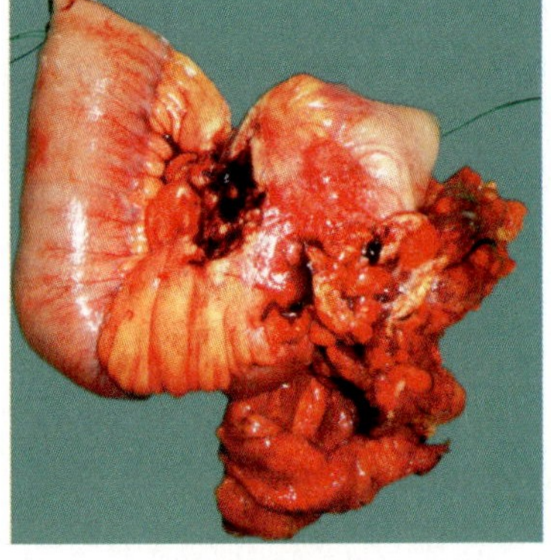

**Fig. 58.65:** Resection of the growth done with 6 cm margin with lymph nodes

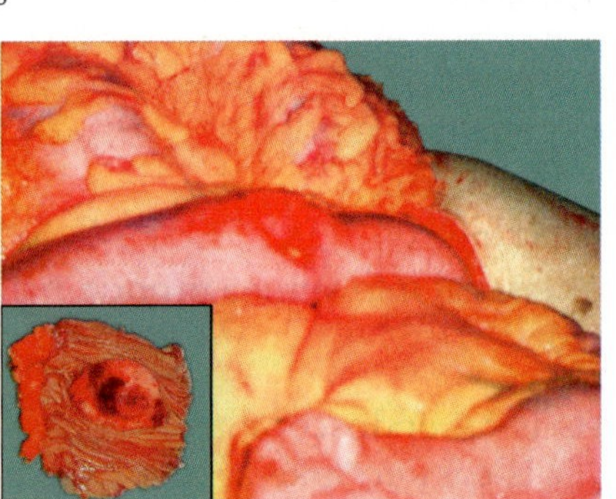

**Fig. 58.66:** This patient presented with abdominal pain, melaena and loss of weight. CT scan of the abdomen revealed mass in the jejunum. It was resected (inset). Mucosal surface showed ulceration. Histopathology report was adenocarcinoma

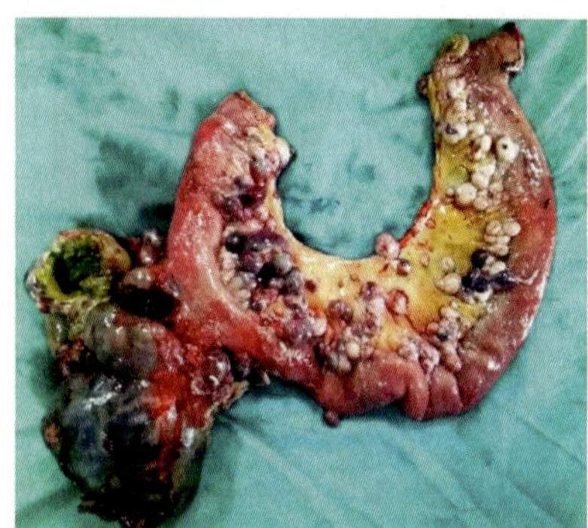

Fig. 58.67: Resected specimen of ruptured GIST of the jejunum. (*Courtesy*: Dr Jyothi, Head, Department of Surgery, GIMS, GADAG, Karnataka)

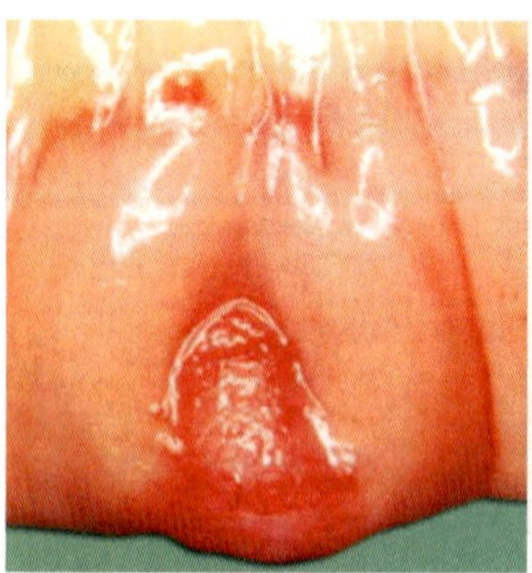

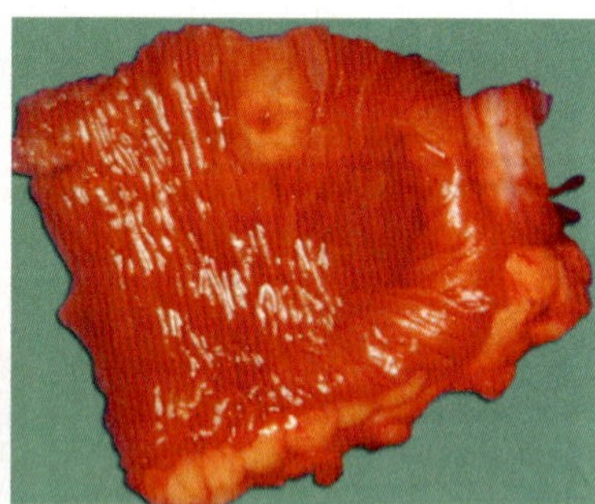

Fig. 58.68: GIST involving jejunum—resected specimen showing mucosal ulceration (*Courtesy*: Dr Padmanabha Bhat, Dept. of Surgery, KMC, Manipal, and Prof HD Shenoy, Father Muller's Medical College and Hospital, Mangaluru)

- **Carney's triad:** It consists of three components:
  1. GIST
  2. Pulmonary chondromas
  3. Extra-adrenal paragangliomas
- A palpable, mobile large nodular mass suggests GIST.

## Spread

- Spread is mainly locoregional. In malignant GIST of stomach, infiltration into the diaphragm is not uncommon. Haematogenous spread can occur into lungs and bone.
- Rarely lymphatic spread can occur.

## Prognosis

It depends upon three factors:

- Size more than 5 cm
- High mitotic index
- Tumour invasion into lamina propria.

## Diagnosis

- Diagnosis is by endoscopy and biopsy. If ulcer is present, it is easy to take a biopsy. If ulcer is not present, a biopsy on a biopsy should be taken. It is difficult in cases of GIST of small intestines.
- CECT scan can define the growth and infiltration with or without lymph nodes.

## Tumour Markers

They express CD117/CD34 antigen. **CD117 is known as C-kit receptor**.

## Treatment

- Treatment is in the form of resection. Diagnosis of malignancy is by mitotic figures: <10 mitoses/high power field (HPF) suggests a low grade malignancy. >10 mitoses/HPF suggests high grade malignancy.
- Increased incidence of C-kit has also been found in patients with neurofibroma.
- The drug of choice for GIST is Imatinib mesylate.

**Imatinib mesylate**

- It is a tyrosine kinase inhibitor.
- It is the first drug of choice in high-risk patients.
- Given as 400 mg/day for 3 years as adjuvant treatment.
- Not given for low-risk patients of R-O resection.
- It should be given, if tumour ruptures on table.
- It is the drug of choice for unresectable and metastatic tumours. Long-term side effects include abdominal cramp, bleeding wounds, gums, swelling of face and feet, etc.
- Imatinib with doxorubicin has shown some benefit in high grade tumours.

# NEUROENDOCRINE TUMOURS (NET)

- Its original name is **karzinoide**—means features resembling carcinoma.
- Today these carcinoid tumours are called **N**euro-**E**ndocrine **T**umours (NET).
- It arises from argentaffin/chromaffin cells which are present in the crypts of the villi of intestine. These cells are called **Kulchitsky cells**. These cells stain with ammonical silver salt solution to black colour. Hence, they are called argentaffinoma or chromaffinoma. They secrete 5-HT (serotonin or 5-hydroxytryptamine). They can be single or multiple and can be associated with adenocarcinoma.
- Median age of presentation is 63 years.
- NET are classified as:
  - Low grade: Grade 1, G1
  - Intermediate: Grade 2, G2
  - High grade: Grade 3, G3
- Symptoms occurring due to hormone secretion from these tumours together constitute carcinoid syndrome (Table 58.8).
- Midgut NET occurs within last 2 feet of ileum and secretes important hormones such as serotonin (5-HT) and substance-P.
- Location, pattern of growth, depth of invasion decide malignancy.

**TABLE 58.8:** Comparison of NET at various sites

| | **Foregut** | **Midgut** | **Hindgut** |
|---|---|---|---|
| **Site** | Duodenum, stomach, bronchus, pancreas, etc. | Jejunum, ileum, right colon | Rectum |
| **Incidence** | Rare | Common | Uncommon |
| **Hormones** | Low serotonin (5-HT), 5-Hydroxytryptophan + | 5-HT, prostaglandins, insulin, ACTH | Do not secrete 5-HT but somatostatin + |

*Bronchial carcinoid produces bronchial obstruction and produces carcinoid syndrome without secondaries in liver.*

- The tumour appears as a small firm submucosal nodule with large mesenteric lymph nodal mass. Tumour produces desmoplastic reaction resulting in fibrosis, intestinal kinking and intestinal obstruction.
- Intermittent recurrent colicky abdominal pain, diarrhoea and weight loss are the features.

## Sites

- *Appendix:* 65%. **It is the most common site.** It occurs more commonly in females. When the tumour occurs in the **appendix, it is usually benign,** hard and occurs in distal one-third of appendix (Key Box 58.17).
- **Terminal ileum:** 30%. Most of them are **malignant**. When the tumour occurs in the **ileum, it is usually malignant** and produces multiple bulky secondaries in the liver, even when primary is very small. Fibrosis of the mesentery results in kinking of bowel causing periodic abdominal pain.
- The hormones produced by the tumour **5-HT** (serotonin) are not metabolised because of the secondaries. So, they are absorbed into the circulation and produce various symptoms. This is called carcinoid syndrome.

Key Box 58.17

**'Most Common' for NET Appendix**

- Most common neoplasm of the appendix
- Mostly found in distal one-third of the appendix
- Mostly tumour is yellow staining at immunohistochemistry
- Mostly benign—very rarely metastasise
- Mostly appendicectomy is sufficient. Rarely, right hemicolectomy may be required

## Carcinoid Syndrome

- Usually malignant NET from ileum produces classical symptoms of vasomotor, cardiac and gastrointestinal involvement.
- Invariably it is associated with massive hepatomegaly due to metastasis.
- Hormones responsible for symptoms are serotonin, 5-HTP, histamine, dopamine, prostaglandins, etc.

## Signs and Symptoms

- **Vasomotor:** These are the most common findings seen in about 80% of cases. These can be erythromatous red flushing attacks, either involving entire body or limited to areas such as face, neck and upper chest.
- **Gastrointestinal:** Episodic watery diarrhoea is seen in about 70–75% of patients. It is caused by hormone serotonin. It responds to methysergide which is a serotonin antagonist.
- **Cardiac: Pulmonary stenosis is the most common cardiac lesion** followed by tricuspid insufficiency and tricuspid stenosis.

## Diagnosis

1. 5-hydroxyindole acetic acid (5-HIAA), a serotonin metabolite is elevated. It is measured in 24-hour urine sample.
2. Chromogranin-A (CgA) has a specificity around 95%. Thus a combination of 5-HIAA with CgA measurements is recommended.
3. CT scan: It can identify as NET—it appears to be solid, with spiculated borders and radiating strands. CT scan helps to locate NET and to define lymph nodal mass.
4. MRI is not used for diagnosis but can detect liver metastasis.
5. Scintigraphy is useful in detecting extra-abdominal disease. It can detect somatostatin receptor sites. Octreotide is used for scintigraphy.
6. 18FDG-PET (18F-fluorodeoxyglucose positron emission tomography) is useful only in high grade NET which has high Ki-67 expression.

## Surgery

- **Excision/resection** of the NET with intestinal segment for small primary tumours less than 1 cm in size.
- **Larger tumours:** Resection of tumour, intestine and mesentery.
- **Terminal ileal NET:** Right hemicolectomy.
- **Disseminated disease:** Surgical debulking.

## Pharmacotherapy

- Octreotide (somatostatin analogues) is the drug of choice in treating patients with symptoms. Mainly used in carcinoid syndrome to treat flushing and diarrhoea.

- Metastatic tumours are treated by debulking (if possible) with combination chemotherapy using Inj streptozotocin, 5-fluorouracil (5-FU) and cyclophosphamide.
- **Bromocriptine** 2.5 mg twice a day can be given to reduce the symptoms. Other agents which can be used are methysergide and diphenoxylate hydrochloride.
- Secondaries in the liver are treated by intra-arterial (hepatic artery) **streptozocin**. Localised liver metastasis can be treated with resection.
- **Therapeutic embolisation** of hepatic artery by using gel foam, etc. will reduce the size of the liver, thereby decreasing discomfort to the patient.
- Injection octreotide 100 mg IV is the drug of choice in cases of carcinoid crisis (severe bronchospasm).

**Octreotide in Carcinoid Syndrome**

1. It is used to suppress the tumour growth.
2. Control symptoms—flushing, wheezing, diarrhoea.
3. It controls the release of GI hormones.
4. Dose is 100 µg subcutaneously three times a day in patients with mild/moderate, non-life-threatening carcinoid syndrome.

### Summary of the NET (Key Box 58.18)

Key Box 58.18

**Summary of NET**

- They are APUDOMAS.
- Arise from enterochromaffin cells.
- They may be associated with multiple endocrine neoplasia (MEN) type 1 and type 2.
- About 15% of NET patients may have carcinoma elsewhere, e.g. carcinoma stomach, carcinoma lung or carcinoma colon.
- Common age is 40–50 years.
- Majority arise from midgut—almost 85% cases. They secrete 5-HT.
- Appendix is the most common site. Often appendicectomy is sufficient for malignant carcinoid tumour.
- Foregut NET do not secrete serotonin.
- Flushing and diarrhoea can be controlled by octreotide.
- Secondaries can be multiple and big, but slow growing similar to primary. Arterial embolisation has been tried in many cases.
- Since they are slow growing and prognosis is good, aggressive treatment in the form of surgery, octreotide, liver resections and rarely liver transplantation have been done.

## MALIGNANT LYMPHOMA

*Primary:* Arising from lymphoid tissue.

*Secondary:* Part of systemic lymphoma. **Ileum is the most common site of lymphoma** (Key Box 58.19).

Key Box 58.19

**Malignant Lymphoma**

1. **Western type**
   - Non-Hodgkin's, B cell type
   - Annular ulcerating lesion
   - Bleeding, obstruction, perforation and weight loss
2. **Primary lymphoma with celiac disease**
   - Increased incidence of lymphoma
   - It is a T cell lympoma
   - Diarrhoea, pyrexia are other features
3. **Mediterranean**—associated with alpha chain disease.[1]

[1]Alpha chain disease is a disorder characterised by the secretion of a defective α-heavy chain. Patients present with steatorrhoea, often progressive and fatal.

### Precipitating Factors

1. Crohn's disease
2. Celiac disease
3. Immunosuppression—AIDS—usually it is a non-Hodgkin's lymphoma of 'B' cell origin.

## SHORT GUT SYNDROME

**SU28.14.4:** Describe the clinical features and principles of management of short gut syndrome.

### Causes of Short Gut Syndrome (Key Box 58.20)

- **Short gut syndrome** occurs due to **massive resection** of the bowel resulting in loss of length of the bowel, loss of absorptive area of the bowel and loss of valves. Superior mesenteric artery being an end artery, thrombosis at its origin is invariably fatal.
- **Midgut volvulus** of neonates is congenital due to arrested rotation resulting in floating caecum and mobile intestine.

**Clinical Notes**

We had an interesting case of midgut volvulus in an 18-year-old boy consequent to a laparotomy done for perforated duodenal ulcer. While replacing the coils of bowel within the abdomen, the mesentery was probably twisted resulting in massive gangrene. This boy now has about 100 cm of the small bowel.

- **Necrotising enteritis** (enteritis necroticans) is a complication of infection of small bowel by *Clostridium perfringens*. It usually occurs after a heavy feast where pork is consumed. There is extensive suppuration of mucosal and submucosal layer of jejunum (also ileum). Serosa may show multiple dark bluish patches.

Key Box 58.20

**Short Gut—Causes**

- Mesenteric infarction
- Midgut volvulus
- Necrotising enteritis
- Crohn's disease[1]
- Radiation enteritis

[1]It is common cause in western countries

Massive resection is done for a necrotic, perforated, unhealthy bowel which results in short gut syndrome.

- **Radiation enteritis** or radiation enteropathy results in patients who receive radiotherapy to the abdominal and pelvic regions, e.g. carcinoma cervix. Arrest of cell division resulting in mucosal thinning, ulceration followed by oedema and later, fibrosis are characteristics of this condition. Endarteritis and vasculitis also add to these changes resulting in stricture, perforations, abscess, malabsorption and multiple resection, etc.

### Pathophysiological Effects

(Fig. 58.69 and Key Box 58.21)

It depends upon:

- Extent of resection
- Site of resection
- Presence/absence of ileocaecal valve
- Age of the patients

Key Box 58.21

**Effects of Short Gut**

- Severe malabsorption
- Gallstones
- Fatty infiltration of liver
- Urinary stones
- Gastric hyperacidity

- Infants tolerate extensive resections better than adults. Patients with less than 100 cm of the small bowel will develop severe nutritional deficiencies and may require parenteral nutrition.
  1. **Malabsorption of fat and fat-soluble vitamins:** Can occur after ileal resections due to interruption of enterohepatic circulation of bile salts. These bile salts enter the colon and are converted into secondary bile salts. These bile salts block absorption of water and electrolytes.
  2. **Gastric hypersecretion:** Due to delayed clearance of gastrin, as in proximal jejunal resections, there is increased gastric secretion of acid resulting in hyperacidity.
  3. **Liver disease:** Fatty infiltration of the liver and mild hyperbilirubinaemia are seen massive resections and jejunoileal bypass. Acute fulminant hepatic failure can also occur.
  4. **Gallstone formation:** There is increased incidence of cholesterol stones as a result of reduced bile salt pool, after ileal resection and jejunoileal bypass.

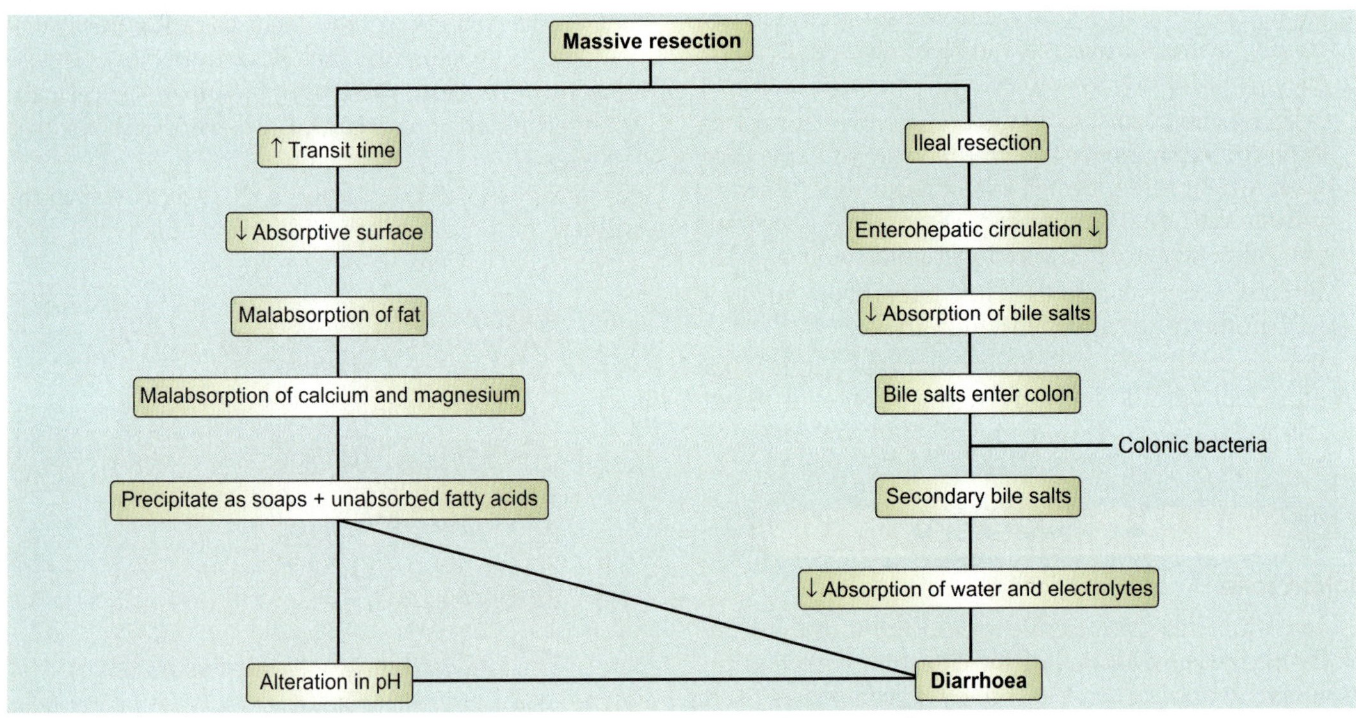


**Fig. 58.69:** Nutritional deficiency in short gut syndrome

**5. Urinary stones**

- All types of urinary stones are common due to low levels of calcium excretion in the urine and high levels of oxalate.
- Water and salt depletion, and loss of $K^+$ causes hyponatraemia and hypokalaemia.

### Adaptation (Key Box 58.22)

As a result of loss of significant bowel, dilatation of the remaining intestine and villous enlargement takes place. This is brought about by a humoral agent, entero-glucagon. In children, length of the bowel is increased. Also, the number of cells in the villi is increased (work hypertrophy). There is also evidence to suggest gradual slowing of the transit time.

Key Box 58.22

**Adaptation to Short Gut Syndrome**

- Villus—size
- Length of bowel
- Transit time
- Absorption from colon

### Treatment

- Treatment of short gut patients is difficult. It needs a special set up of dieticians who plan 'proper food' for these patients in consultation with treating surgeons. It is a gradual process of feeding the patient beginning with parenteral nutrition and progressing to normal, low fat diet after a few months.
- In the initial 2–3 months following massive resection, total parenteral nutrition including supplementation of fluid and electrolytes is the ideal treatment. Sips of plain water or oral hypotonic solutions can be allowed.
- After 2–3 months, when adaptation of bowel takes place, enteral feeding is started gradually with baby food, fat-free, fibre-free, protein-rich, liquid diet. Essential fatty acids should be supplied. Diarrhoea is a common problem and is treated with loperamide tablets.
- Enteral feeding can contain low fatty diet in addition to the other nutrients mentioned above.
- Small bowel transplantation is also being done when all measures fail specially when the bowel length is less than 50 cm. It is given in digital contents.

## INTESTINAL FISTULAE

### Introduction

- Intestinal fistulae are **abnormal communications** between two portions of the intestine, between the intestine and some other hollow viscus, or between the intestine and the skin of the abdominal wall.
- When it involves **skin and intestines, it is called enterocutaneous fistula.**
- Despite significant advances in their management, intestinal fistulae remain a major clinical problem, with an overall mortality rate of 15 to 25%.

### Classification

#### *Anatomical*

- Internal: Colovesical fistula
- External: Duodenal, jejunal fistula
- Mixed: Crohn's disease.

#### *Depending on the Contents*

- Low output <200 ml
- Moderate output 200–500 ml
- High output >500 ml.

### Aetiology

- **Iatrogenic (70%)—postoperative:** Injury to intestines unnoticed at the time of surgery or injury recognized at the time of surgery, sutured but has given way are prime causes of enterocutaneous fistula. **Anastomotic leak, partial or complete, is another important cause of enterocutaneous fistula. Meticulous surgical techniques, gentle handling of the bowel, usage of the proper suture material (Vicryl and silk), ensuring adequate blood** supply to the intestines which have to be anastomosed will largely prevent anastomotic leak (Fig. 58.70).
- **Stump blow out: Duodenal blow out: Typically happens 4–5 days following surgery** (*see* page 751).
- Inadequate resection of the **diseased segment:** In such situations, anastomosis may be in unhealthy bowel.
- **Instrumentation:** Oesophageal perforations are dangerous ones and can occur even with flexible scopies.
- **Spontaneous (30%):** Crohn's disease, diverticular disease of the colon, appendicitis are also known to give rise to fistulae.

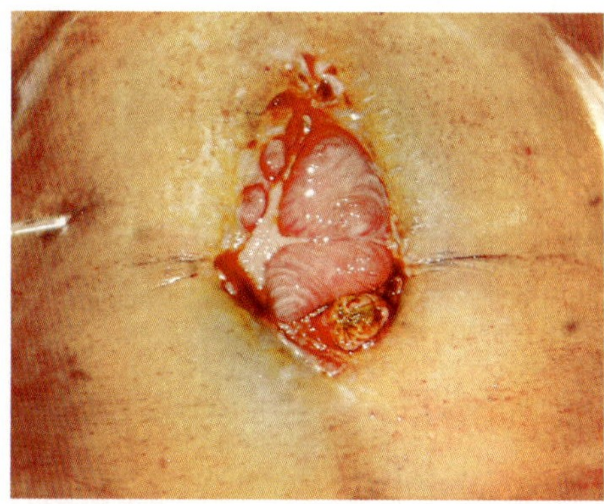

Fig. 58.70: Small intestinal fistulae due to anastomotic disruption and wound dehiscence

### Local Factors Precluding Spontaneous Closure

- Bleeding
- End fistula: Bowel discontinuity
- Foreign body: Swabs, tips of the suction tubes (detached), retained sponges or instruments
- Radiation
- Inflammation/infection/inflammatory bowel disease
- Epithelialisation of the tract is another important cause of the persistent fistula.
- Neoplasms
- Distal obstruction
- **Multiple fistulae** that do not heal as in Crohn's or typhoid perforations.
- **Lateral duodenal fistula** does not heal because large volume of contents are poured into the second part of duodenum and there is no rest to the part.
- When the **defect is more than 1 cm**, and the **track is more than 2 cm**, fistula does not close (*see* clinical notes).

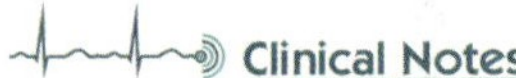
Clinical Notes

A 60-year-old man was operated for appendicitis. On the fifth postoperative day, he developed faecal discharge from the wound. Conservative management was done for 7 days with total parenteral nutrition and other measures. Fistula persisted. CT scan was done on the 14th day. It revealed a growth in the hepatic flexure almost encircling the lumen. Colonoscopy and biopsy proved adenocarcinoma colon. He underwent re-exploration and right hemicolectomy was done. The fistula stopped and he was discharged from the hospital after 10 days. This case highlights the fact that in the presence of a distal obstruction, fistula will not close. More importantly, what the patient had was not appendicitis but subacute intestinal obstruction! The pain was due to colic.

### Management: Principles

It can be discussed under the following headings.

1. Recognition and aetiology
2. Phase of stabilization
3. Nutrition—more details on page 38
4. Investigative phase
5. Phase of definitive management
   a. Surgery
   b. Skin care
   c. Abdominal wall defect

#### 1. Recognition and Aetiology

- Delay in recovery from paralytic ileus or a common phrase used—when the ***patient is not doing well*** are early indications of a leak or a breakdown of anastomosis. Once the fistula establishes, diagnosis is easy because the drain will start draining intestinal contents including food particles (if oral intake is started). Intra-abdominal collections, abscess, fever, sepsis are other features of leak.
- Recognising the cause is important because it can dictate treatment. To give an example: **If any foreign body is left in the abdomen, exploration and removal may be urgently required.**
- If a specific disease is suspected such as tuberculosis, antituberculous treatment may cure a fistula.

#### 2. Phase of Stabilisation

- Nil by mouth, total bowel rest, introduction of a nasogastric tube (Ryle's tube) with continuous drainage decreases fistula output.
- Proton pump inhibitors decrease gastric secretions.
- Protection of skin is by liberal zinc oxide application.
- Common fluid and electrolyte problems seen in patients with GI fistula include dehydration, hyponatraemia, hypokalaemia and metabolic acidosis. They have to be corrected.
- Drainage of collections by CT or ultrasound-guided aspiration or pig tail catheter insertions.
- Broad-spectrum antibiotics, with anaerobic coverage.

#### 3. Nutrition (more details on page 38)

- Nutrition has been discussed in detail in the Chapter 11 on Fluid-Electrolyte Balance and Nutrition. A few points worth mentioning are that more distal the fistula, less is the requirement of **total parenteral nutrition** (TPN). TPN is safe today. One may have to wait for 4–6 weeks with TPN for the final repair of complicated fistula such as lateral duodenal fistula or ileal fistula.
- Placement of **nasogastric, nasojejunal tubes, percutaneous gastrostomy or jejunostomy** for nutrition is an important step which can be done with the help of radiology and imaging department.

#### 4. Investigative Phase

**a. Routine biochemical and haematological investigations**

- Blood urea, serum creatinine, blood sugar
- Serum electrolytes
- Serum albumin, transferrin
- Blood culture helps in giving appropriate antibiotics
- Chest X-ray to rule out static pneumonia or ARDS, pleural effusions (source of sepsis also).

**b. Imaging studies**

- **USG:** Drainage of collections by catheters. If drainage persists, suspect fistulous communication.
- **Fistulograms** to define the exact site of fistula—proximal or distal—gastric or intestinal (Key Box 58.23).

Key Box 58.23

**Fistulogram/CT/Contrast GI Series**

- What is the cause of the fistula?
- Is the bowel completely disrupted or is it a lateral fistula with the bowel in continuity?
- What is the length of the fistula tract?
- Is there an abscess cavity?
- What is the size of the bowel wall defect?
- Is there a distal obstruction?

- **Contrast CT abdomen:** To detect collections, discontinuity, diseased segments, distal obstruction and foreign body. Extremely useful investigation in intestinal fistula.
- **Colonoscopy and barium enema** are other investigations used in specific situations such as colonic fistulae.

### 5. Phase of Definitive Management

**a. Surgical intervention**

- **Drainage or aspiration of pus** urgently when there is sepsis before doing an elective repair.
- **Feeding jejunostomy** as in high fistulae, e.g. duodenal or oesophageal fistula.
- **Diversion/exclusion/colostomy/bypass** are various other treatments depending upon the location of fistula (Fig. 58.71).
- **Definitive treatment:** It includes restoration of continuity—resection and anastomosis, internal diversion or exteriorisation of bowel as in suspicious viability (mesenteric ischaemia or enteric perforations—friable bowel, known for leak and releak).

**b. Methods of skin care** (Figs 58.72 and 58.73)

- Pouches, stoma bags of different sizes are available.
- Creams and ointments—zinc or petroleum-based

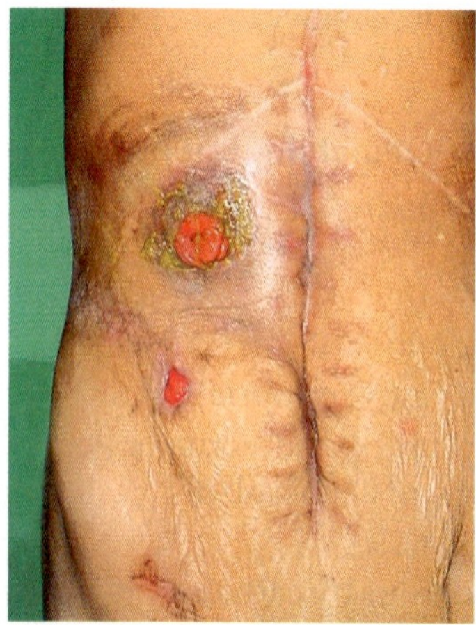

Fig. 58.71: Small bowel exteriorisation was done for enteric perforation after resection—safe option when there is gross contamination

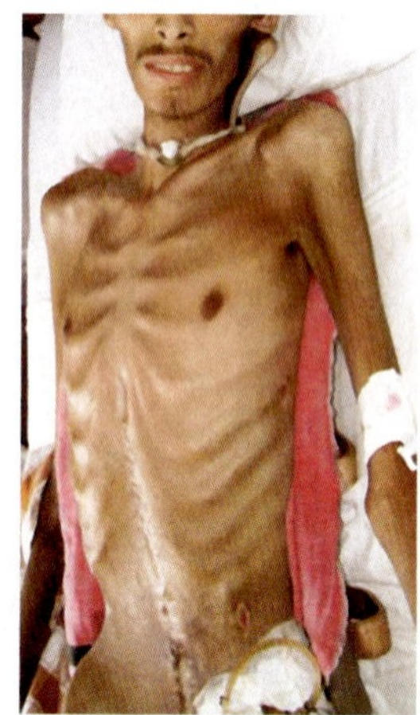

Fig. 58.72: Severe nutritional deficiency following duodenal fistula—autocannibalism

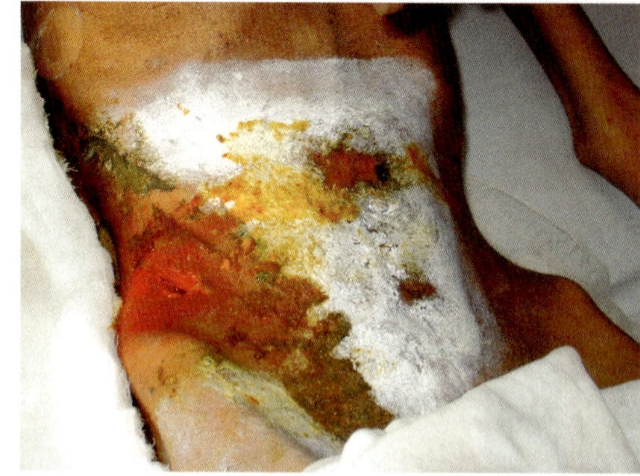

Fig. 58.73: Extensive excoriation of the skin in a faecal fistula. Zinc oxide has been applied to the abdominal wall

- Suction catheter placed *in situ*: Low pressure suction 60–80 mmHg.

**Generally, dressings need to be changed every 4 hours. Pouch/reservoir system should be employed.**

**c. Abdominal wall defects:** Depending upon the size of the defect, immediate or delayed closure can be achieved with tension-releasing incisions on the external oblique or laparostomy and secondary suturing, skin grafting or by using prosthetic mesh such as Marlex or Prolene.

## SMALL INTESTINAL DIVERTICULA

### Introduction

Small intestinal diverticula are far less common than colonic diverticula. Multiple sac-like mucosal herniations occur through weak points in the intestinal wall where blood vessels penetrate.

### Incidence

Diverticula are more common in duodenum than jejunum or ileum (Fig. 58.74).

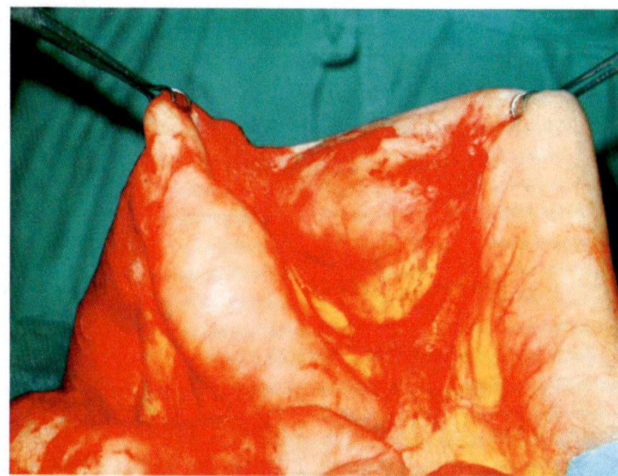

Fig. 58.74: Diverticula form mesenteric border of jejunum. It was the cause of anaemia due to occult blood loss

### Pathophysiology

- It is believed to develop as a result of abnormalities in peristalsis, intestinal dyskinesis and high segmental intraluminal pressures.
- **They occur in the mesenteric border unlike Meckel's which occurs in the antimesenteric border.**
- Diet low in fibre and rich in fat and some visceral myopathy have been blamed for development of diverticula.

### Clinical Features

- Asymptomatic
- Occult blood in the stools—positive
- Anaemia and symptoms such as fatigue, weakness, pedal oedema
- Malabsorption—diarrhoea, flatulence, weight loss
- Pain abdomen, signs of peritonitis such as tenderness, guarding or localised abscess.

### Investigations

- Specific investigations are enteroclysis and enteroscopy.
- CT with contrast is the ideal investigation.
- Often diverticula are not suspected but a CT scan obtained for some pathology in the abdomen may reveal a localised abscess. Later, at laparotomy, it can turn out to be diverticula (Figs 58.75 and 58.76).

### Treatment

Resection and anastomosis of the bowel containing diverticula.

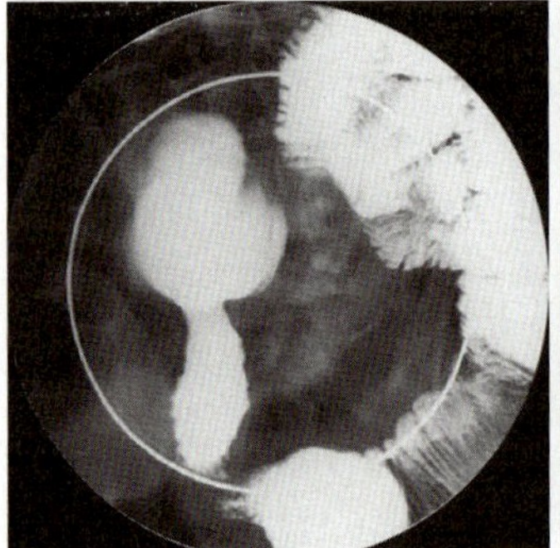
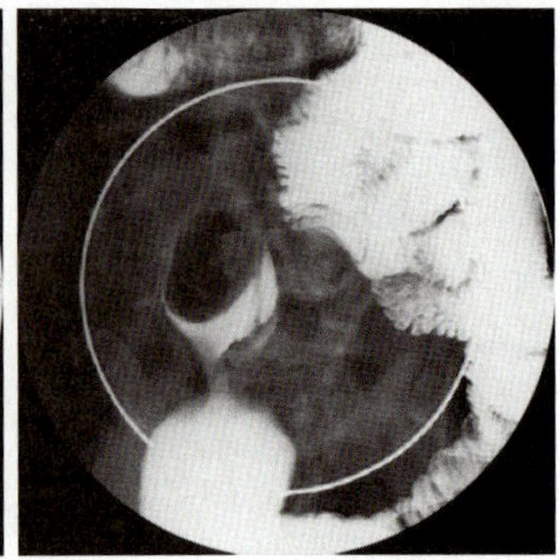

**Figs 58.75 and 58.76:** Enteroclysis. First picture showing filling defect and a clear view of diverticula in the second picture

**INTERESTING 'MOST COMMON' FOR INTESTINES**

- Most common site of gastrointestinal tuberculosis is ileocaecal region.
- Most common site of ulcerative colitis is rectum.
- Most common extraintestinal manifestations of ulcerative colitis are peripheral arthritis and ankylosing spondylitis.
- Most common site of gastrointestinal perforation in enteric fever is terminal ileum.
- Most common neoplastic lesion of small intestine is lymphoma.
- Most common anal problem in Crohn's disease is fissure in ano.
- Most common site of adenocarcinoma in intestines is duodenum.
- Most common site of malignant carcinoids is terminal ileum.
- Most common site of carcinoid in intestines is appendix.

## CLINICAL CASE CAPSULE 7: Management Oriented Discussion in Surgery (MODS)

A 50 years old lady presented with lower abdominal distension, fever and weight loss since 3 months. On further questioning she also said vague ill health, occasional cough and easy fatigue since 3 months. She was pale. No significant lymphadenopathy. Abdominal examination findings: Lower abdominal distension as visible in the picture. Vague firm mass was palpable with gurgling in mid and lower abdomen. Shifting dullness was present. Rest of the examination was normal. Adventitious sounds were heard in the respiratory system.

**Discussion:** Initial history and clinical examination a chronic debilitating illness. Tuberculosis, malignancy of ovary or even a lymphoma were considered. After abdominal examination: Shifting dullness suggests fluid and a vague mass with lower border was easily palpable so ovarian pathology was largely ruled out. Imaging findings prompted the diagnosis of tuberculosis. Aspirated fluid was exudate (rich in proteins). Chest X-ray findings also suggested fluid. Thinking of 2 cavities with fluid–first diagnosis comes to mind is tuberculosis or intra-abdominal malignancy with pleural effusion-may be metastasis including/pleura. It

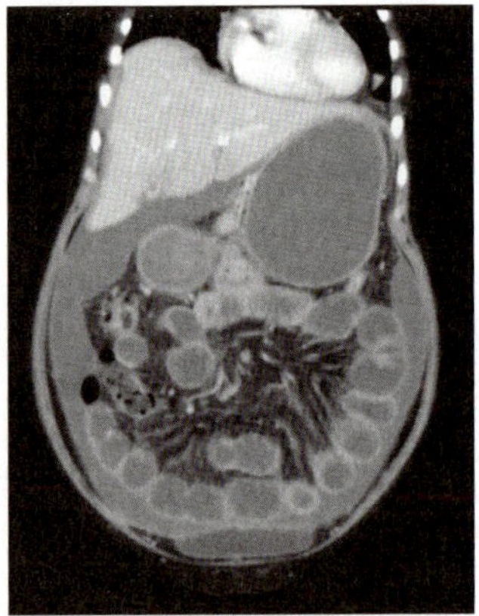

**Fig. 58.77:** CECT scan findings: Fluid in the peritoneal cavity, shortened mesentery, few dilated intestinal loops *(Contd.)*

(*Contd.*)

was left sided pleural effusion. If patient had ascites, right sided pleural effusion and ovarian mass, rare Meigs's syndrome (Ovarian fibroma) was considered. Right side pleural effusion is more common than left side because the transdiaphragmatic lymphatic channels are larger in diameter on the right than left side. Diagnostic laparoscopy gave the classical findings with caseating nodules which proved to be due to tuberculosis. Cartridge Based Nucleic Acid Amplification (CBNAAT): Test results were positive. It is to check rifampicin resistance. She was given ATT and she is asymptomatic after 6 months of treatment. At the end of 1 year she has no complaints.

Contrast-enhanced computed tomography (CECT) scan revealed large loculated high attenuation ascites associated with prominent vasa recta and linear striations along the mesentery and omental thickening and nodularity features–possibly peritoneal tuberculosis (wet type) (Fig. 58.77).

**Chest X-ray:** Left mild pleural effusion and subsegmental collapse of underlying lung segments (Fig. 58.78).

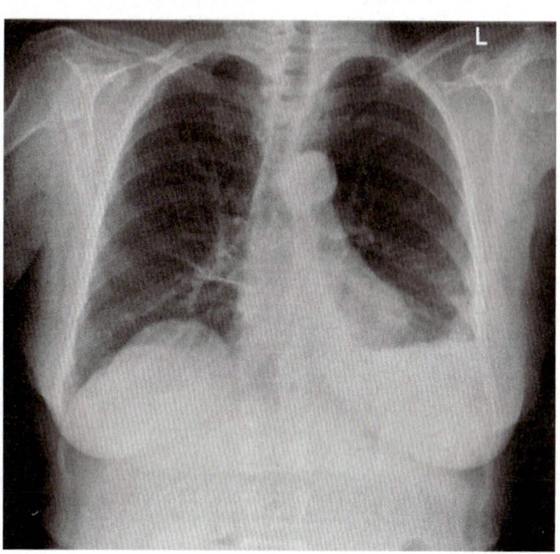


**Fig. 58.78:** Chest X-ray showing pleural effusion

Fluid was aspirated from peritoneal cavity with ultrasound guidance. It was exudate with proteins 7 g/dl and high LDH: 298U/L.

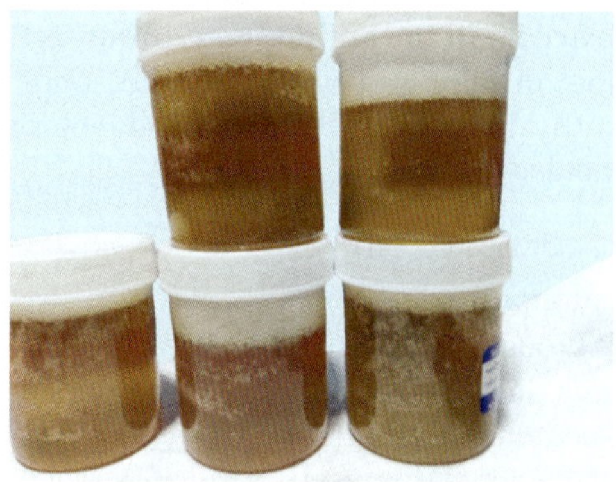

**Fig. 58.79:** Fluid drawn from ascites

**Diagnostic laparoscopy:** Extensive adhesions between abdominal wall and intestines were found and they were released. Multiple caseating tubercles were identified and biopsy taken (Figs 58.79 and 58.80).

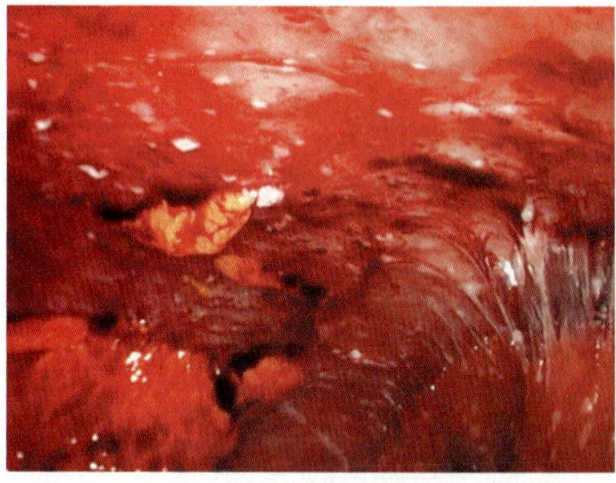

**Fig. 58.80:** TB abdomen

Histopathology reported as tuberculosis. With ATT standard care of 6 months, she made a very good recovery.

## MULTIPLE CHOICE QUESTIONS

**1. Pathology of ulcerative colitis includes all of the following, *except*:**
A. Punched out ulcers
B. Pseudopolyposis
C. Pipe stem colon
D. Pus cells

**2. Toxic megacolon is seen in the following, *except*:**
A. Intestinal tuberculosis
B. Ulcerative colitis
C. Amoebic colitis
D. Salmonella colitis

**3. String sign of Kantor is seen in:**
A. Crohn's disease
B. Tubercular enteritis
C. Typhoid enteritis
D. Amoebic colitis

**4. Guarding and rigidity can be minimal in enteric perforation of terminal ileum because:**
A. The perforation is usually small
B. It is self-sealing and self-limiting
C. Zenker's degeneration of abdominal muscles
D. Occurs in the antimesenteric border of the terminal ileum

**5. Flask-shaped (bottle neck) ulcers are a feature of:**
A. Intestinal tuberculosis
B. Crohn's disease
C. Intestinal amoebiasis
D. Typhoid enteritis

**6. Malignancy in small intestine is rare because:**
A. Bacteria in the intestine are protective
B. Blood supply is very good
C. No stasis, rapid transit of food
D. Low levels of immunoglubulins

**7. Most common site of gastrointestinal perforation in enteric fever is:**
A. Duodenum B. Jejunum
C. Colon D. Terminal ileum

**8. Adaptation to short gut syndrome includes all of the following, *except*:**
A. Decreased transit time
B. Increased villus size
C. Absorption from colon
D. Increased length of bowel

**9. The symptoms of carcinoid syndrome is due to:**
A. Histamine B. Serotonin
C. Prostaglandins D. Epinephrine

**10. Tenderness in the Sir Philip Manson-Bahr's point is a feature of:**
A. Rectosigmoid involvement in amoebic colitis
B. Acute appendicitis
C. Acute cholecystitis
D. Crohn's disease

**11. The commonest site for gastrointestinal stromal tumour is:**
A. Oesophagus B. Stomach
C. Duodenum D. Jejunum

**12. Carney's triad includes all of the following, *except*:**
A. Gastrointestinal stromal tumours
B. Pulmonary chondromas
C. Extra-adrenal chondromas
D. Familial hamartomatous polyposis

**13. One of the drugs used in the treatment of carcinoid syndrome is:**
A. Metronidazole B. Bromocriptine
C. Streptomycin D. Serotonin

**14. The most common site for a carcinoid tumour is:**
A. Stomach B. Duodenum
C. Appendix D. Rectum

**15. Causes of short gut syndrome include all of the following, *except*:**
A. Mesenteric ischaemia
B. Necrotising enterocolitis
C. Crohn's disease
D. Radiation enteritis

**16. C-kit receptor is expressed in:**
A. Gastrointestinal stromal tumour
B. Peutz-Jegher syndrome
C. Carcinoid syndrome
D. Crohn's syndrome

**17. The most recent and promising drug used in the treatment of Crohn's disease is:**
A. Trastuzumab B. Infliximab
C. Monteleukast D. Fab antibodies

**18. Most common anal problem in Crohn's disease is:**
A. Anal fistula
B. Haemorrhoids
C. Anal fissure
D. Perianal abscess

**19. Transmural inflammation is characteristic of:**
A. Crohn's disease
B. Tuberculous enteritis
C. Typhoid enteritis
D. Ulcerative colitis

**20. 'Hose pipe rigidity' is a feature of:**
A. Crohn's disease
B. Tuberculous enteritis
C. Typhoid enteritis
D. Ulcerative colitis

**21. The most common symptomatic presentations of Meckel's diverticulum in children of 2 years of age is:**
A. Haemorrhage
B. Perforation
C. Diverticulitis
D. Intestinal obstruction

**22. The drug used to control diarrhoea in neuro-endocrine tumour is:**
A. Streptozotocin
B. Sunitinib
C. Methysergide
D. Octreotide

**23. Investigation of choice for gastrointestinal NET is:**
A. Ultrasound
B. CT scan
C. MRI scan
D. FDG–PET scan



## Answers

| | | | | | | | | | |
|---|---|---|---|---|---|---|---|---|---|
| **1.** A | **2.** A | **3.** A | **4.** C | **5.** C | **6.** C | **7.** D | **8.** A | **9.** B | **10.** A |
| **11.** B | **12.** D | **13.** B | **14.** C | **15.** D | **16.** A | **17.** B | **18.** C | **19.** A | **20.** A |
| **21.** A | **22.** C | **23.** B | | | | | | | |

Chapter 59

# Large Intestine (Colon)

- Surgical anatomy
- Colonic function
- Tumours of the large intestine
  - Polyps
  - Familial polyposis coli
  - Hereditary nonpolyposis colorectal cancer
- Carcinoma colon
  - ERAS
- Colon screening
- Diverticular disease of colon
- Faecal fistula
- Colonic stricture

## SURGICAL ANATOMY

**SU28.13.1:** Appreciate anatomy and physiology of the large intestine.

Colonic blood supply is given here but resections and correlation with blood supply is given on page 940 operative surgery section.

- Large intestine extends from ileocaecal valve to anus. It has five segments: Right colon, left colon, transverse colon, sigmoid colon, rectum and anal canal (Fig. 59.1).
- Average length is about 135–150 cm.
- Interestingly, alternating portions of the colon are mobile and fixed. Ascending colon and descending colon are fixed but caecum, transverse colon and sigmoid colon are mobile. Mobile structures can undergo twisting (volvulus).
- Layers of colon: Mucosa, submucosa, muscularis propria and serosa. Inner circular and outer longitudinal muscle layers constitute muscularis propria. In spite of 4 layers, wall of the colon is thin. Hence, it distends much more in obstruction.

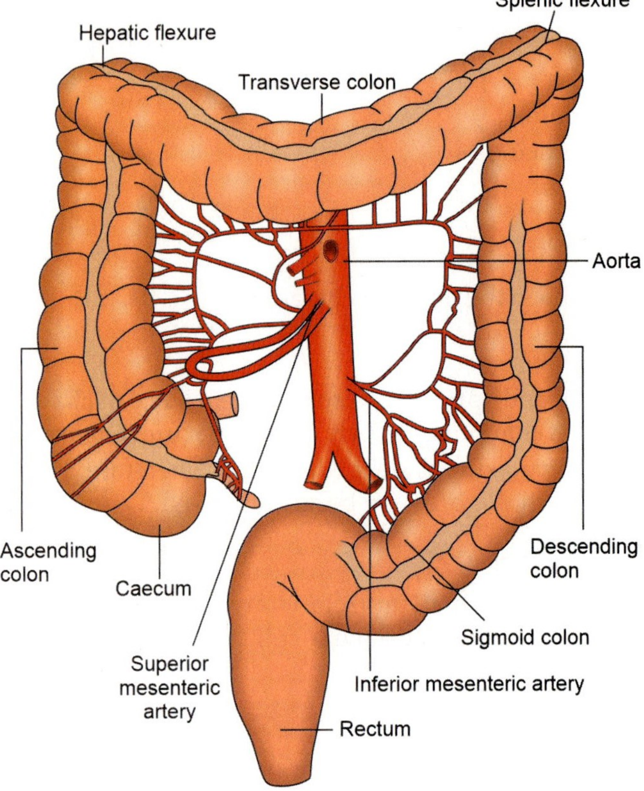


**Fig. 59.1:** Anatomy of the colon and parts

### Caecum

- 7.5 cm in both length and breadth
- Blind pouch
- Completely covered by peritoneum except posterior surface
- Mobile

*Diseases*

- Carcinoma
- Tuberculosis
- Amoebic typhlitis
- Intussusception
- Volvulus—rare.

### Ascending Colon (15 cm Long)

- Caecum continues as ascending colon.
- Covered by peritoneum in front and on both sides.
- In 25% of patients, it has a mesentery.

- Right paracolic gutter is deep on the lateral aspect of ascending colon—space for paracolic abscess in cases of perforation peritonitis.

### Transverse Colon (50 cm Long)

- Most mobile part of large intestine.
- It is suspended by transverse mesocolon, loops down and is adherent to the posterior wall of omental bursa.

*Diseases*

- Cancer
- Ulcerative colitis.

### Descending Colon (25 cm Long)

- Continues as sigmoid colon
- Retroperitoneal (like ascending colon)
- Also has paracolic gutter.

### Sigmoid (40 cm Long)

- S-shaped
- Ends as rectosigmoid junction where taenia coli ends.

*Diseases*

- Volvulus
- Diverticulosis
- Cancer

### Right Colon (Table 59.1)

Big and hepatic flexure is broad.

### Left Colon

- Small and splenic flexure is acute. Hence, **ischaemic colitis commonly affects splenic flexure** (Table 59.1).
- Splenic flexure is deeply situated. Therefore, malignancy in this area can be easily missed.

### *Muscle Coat*

Outer longitudinal muscle is arranged in the form of **three strips** called **taenia coli**. All three join at the rectosigmoid junction and form a complete longitudinal layer of the rectum. **These three taenia coli converge at the base of the appendix**. This is an important method to localise appendix. Inner circular muscle coalesces distally to form internal anal sphincter. **No taenia over the rectum**.

**Recognise large intestine by:**

1. Taenia coli
2. Omental appendices—appendicular epiploicae
3. Haustrations
4. Large diameter (calibre).

**Names of three taenia coli**

1. Mesocolic: Transverse colon and sigmoid colon are attached by this.
2. Omental: To which omental appendices attach.
3. Libera (free): Nothing is attached.

*Pearls of Wisdom*

Since taenia are shorter than intestine, the colon becomes sacculated between taenia forming haustra.

### Arterial Supply (Fig. 59.2)

1. **Superior mesenteric artery,** a branch of abdominal aorta, arises at the level of first lumbar vertebra (L1). It supplies the entire small bowel and the right colon up to proximal 2/3rds of transverse colon. **Branches** of superior mesenteric artery (SMA) supplying colon are:
   A. **Middle colic artery** supplies ascending colon, hepatic flexure and the transverse colon mainly. It divides into right and left branches.
   B. **Right colic artery** supplies right colon.
   C. **Ileocolic artery** supplies the terminal ileum and ascending colon. It divides into anterior and posterior caecal branches and supplies caecum and appendix through appendicular artery.

**TABLE 59.1:** Comparison between right colon and left colon

| Right colon | Left colon |
|---|---|
| 1. Big | 1. Small |
| 2. Hepatic flexure is broad | 2. Splenic flexure is acute and narrow—mobilisation is difficult |
| 3. Hepatic flexure is not deep | 3. Splenic flexure is deep |
| 4. Paracolic space is broad | 4. Left paracolic space is narrow |
| 5. Luminal diameter is big | 5. Luminal diameter is narrow |
| 6. Contents are liquid | 6. Contents are solid |
| 7. Growth pattern is usually ulceroproliferative | 7. Growth is annular stricture |
| 8. Obstruction is not common | 8. Hence, obstruction is common |
| 9. Growth is more common in women | 9. Growth is more common in men |

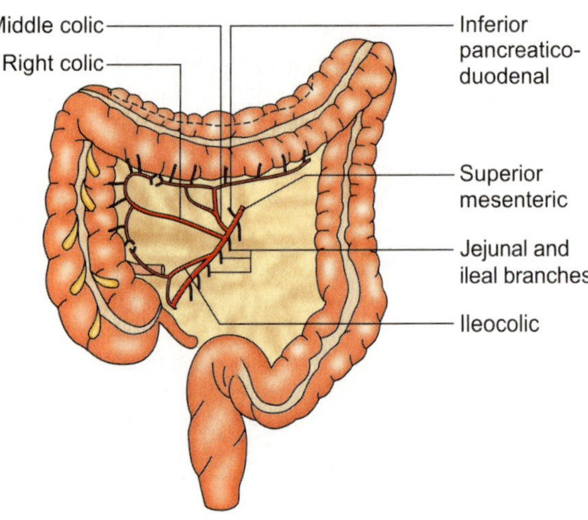


Fig. 59.2: Blood supply of the right colon

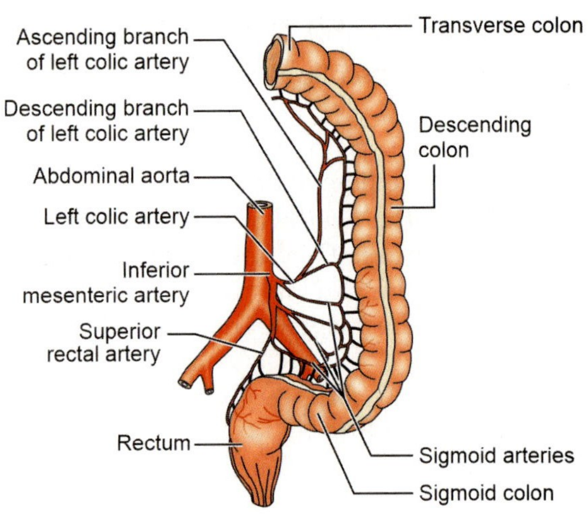


Fig. 59.3: Arterial supply of left colon

2. **Inferior mesenteric artery (IMA),** a branch of abdominal aorta arising at the level of L3, supplies the left colon up to mucocutaneous junction at the lower end of anal canal (Hilton's line). Its branches are (Fig. 59.3):
   A. **Left colic artery** which anastomoses with branches of middle colic artery. It divides into upper and lower branches supplying the descending colon.
   B. **Three sigmoidal branches** supply sigmoid colon. Narrow point of blood supply between the first sigmoidal artery and left coelic artery is called **Sudeck's point**.
   C. **Superior haemorrhoidal artery** (rectal).
      - The anastomotic branches form **marginal artery of Drummond,** which is relatively narrow in the region of splenic flexure (another reason for development of ischaemia). That narrow point is called **Griffith's point**.
      - **Arc of Riolan** is the anastomotic arcade formed between branches of IMA and SMA.

### Venous Supply

- Follows the corresponding artery and empty into superior and inferior mesenteric veins, ultimately draining into the portal vein (Fig. 59.4).
- Thus, if the colorectal area gets infected secondary to inflammatory conditions or after surgical procedure, the infection can easily spread to the portal vein and result in portal pyaemia.

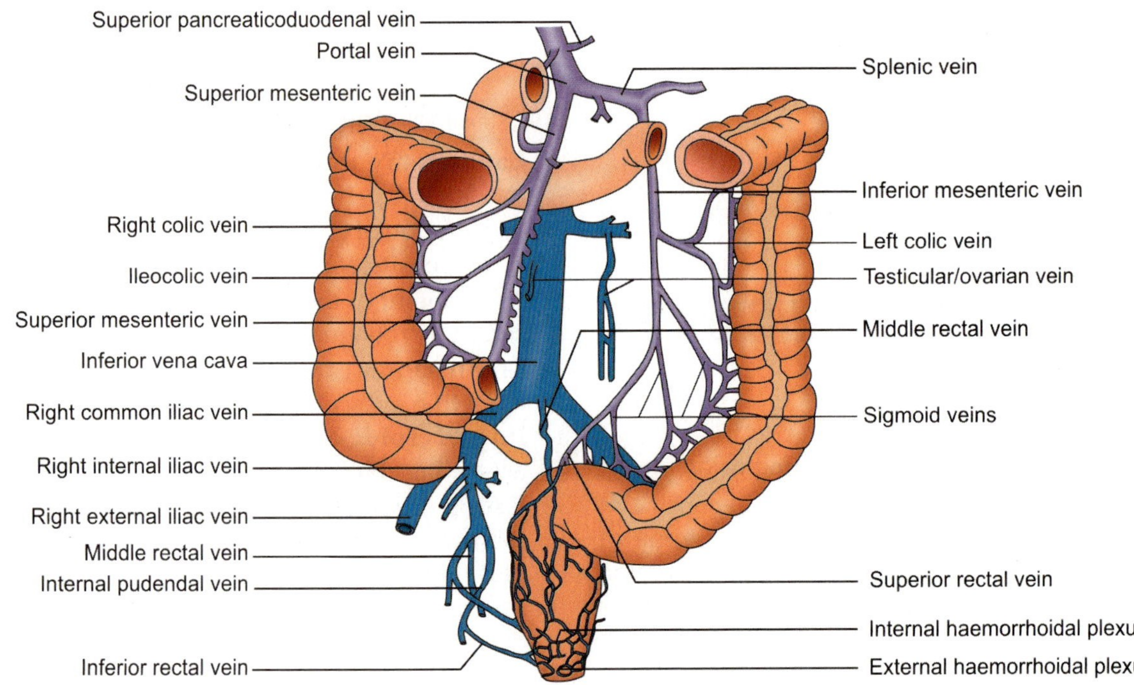


Fig. 59.4: Venous drainage

### Lymphatic Drainage (Fig. 59.5)

- **N1:** Epicolic, paracolic nodes are the first to get involved.
- **N2:** Nodes at the origin of ileocolic and middle colic arteries—intermediate nodes.
- **N3:** Nodes at the origin of superior and inferior mesenteric arteries. They are involved in approximately 50% of the patients with carcinoma colon at presentation to the hospital. These are called principal nodes.

### Colorectal Nerve Supply

- Sympathetic (inhibitory) arise from T10–T12 and L1–L3.
- Parasympathetic (stimulation).
  A. Vagus nerve supplies right and transverse colon.
  B. Sacral nerves (S2–S4 which form nervi erigentes) supply distal colon, i.e. splenic flexure onwards.

**Significance**

Colonic pseudo-obstruction starts from splenic flexure. Transition zone of vagal supply to sacral nerve supply.

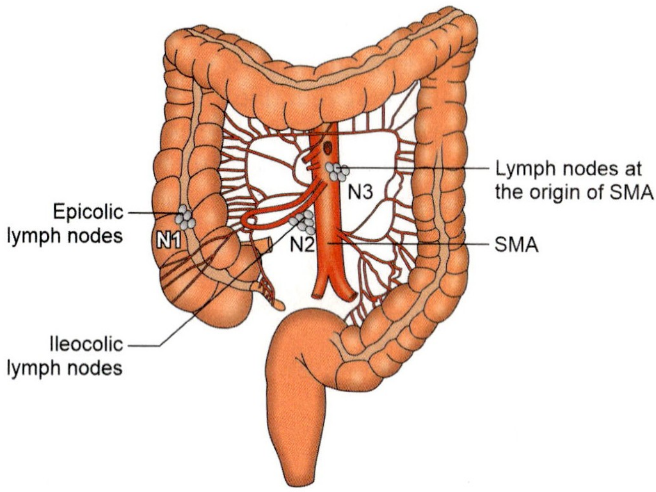


**Fig. 59.5:** Lymphatic drainage (*see* text for description of N1, N2 and N3)

## COLECTOMY

### RIGHT HEMICOLECTOMY

### Indications

1. Carcinoma of the caecum or ascending colon
2. Tumours of appendix
3. Extended right hemicolectomy for carcinoma of hepatic flexure and proximal 1/3rd transverse colon and for closed loop obstruction in carcinoma of the transverse colon.
4. Modified right hemicolectomy for tuberculosis, Crohn's disease involving terminal ileum (Fig. 59.6).

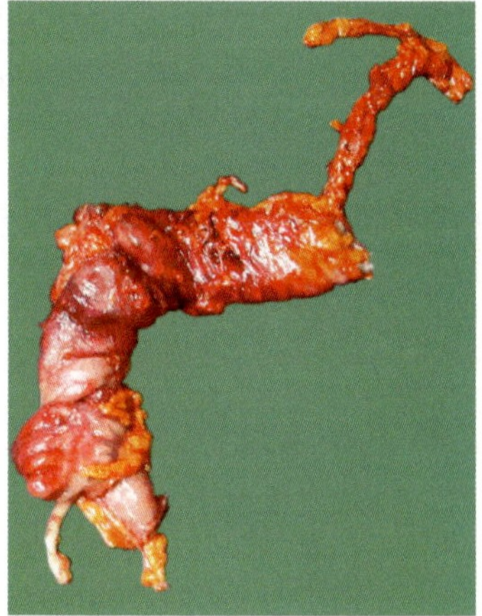

**Fig. 59.6:** Right hemicolectomy

### Structures Removed

1. Terminal 5–10 cm of ileum
2. Caecum
3. Ascending colon
4. Proximal 1/3rd of transverse colon with hepatic flexure.
5. Extended right hemicolectomy—all the above structures with the proximal two-thirds of the transverse colon.
6. **Modified right hemicolectomy**—all the above structures with variable length of hepatic flexure or proximal transverse colon preserved.

### Vessels Ligated

1. Ileocolic vessels
2. Right colic vessels
3. Right branch of middle colic vessels
4. Ileal vessels are ligated last.

### Surgical Techniques

1. **Laparotomy** through midline/right paramedian incision.
2. **Exploration** of the abdomen for liver deposits, peritoneal deposits, ascites and other synchronous lesions.
3. **Assessment** of the tumour for site, extent, mobility, serosal involvement and local extension.
4. **Mobilisation of the right colon** done by incising along the avascular lateral peritoneal fold or **white line of Toldt** and rotating the caecum and the ascending colon anteriorly and medially.
5. **Retroperitoneum is entered** through the incision and dissection carried up towards the third and fourth part of duodenum.
6. Retroperitoneal structures encountered during dissection are the right kidney with **ureter, right gonadal vessels and duodenum**. Care must be taken to avoid injury to these structures.

7. **Turnbull's technique or no touch isolation technique**—early ligation of the vessels before manipulation of the tumour should be followed to prevent dissemination of the tumour cells during handling.
8. Ileocolic, right colic, right branch of middle colic and lastly ileal **vessels are isolated, ligated and divided**. Ileocolic and right colic vessels are ligated at the origin to include all the associated lymph nodes.
9. Ileum is transected at 5–10 cm from the ileocaecal junction and transverse colon at the junction of the proximal 1/3rd and distal 2/3rds. This is followed by an **ileotransverse colon anastomosis**.
10. Abdominal wall is closed in layers.

## LEFT HEMICOLECTOMY

### Indications

1. Carcinoma of the descending colon
2. Carcinoma of the splenic flexure
3. High-risk polyps.

### Structures Removed

#### *Carcinoma of the Descending Colon*

1. Distal 1/3rd of transverse colon
2. Splenic flexure
3. Descending colon
4. Sigmoid colon.

#### *Carcinoma of the Splenic Flexure*

1. Distal 2/3rds of transverse colon
2. Splenic flexure and descending colon.

### Vessels Ligated

1. Left branch of middle colic vessels
2. Left colic vessels
3. Inferior mesenteric and sigmoidal vessels in case of carcinoma of descending colon.

### Surgical Techniques

1. Laparotomy through midline/left paramedian incision.
2. Exploration of the abdomen for liver deposits, peritoneal deposits, ascites and other synchronous lesions.
3. Assessment of the tumour for site, extent, mobility, serosal involvement and local extension.
4. Mobilisation of the left colon done by incising along the avascular lateral peritoneal fold or white line of Toldt and rotating the descending colon and the sigmoid colon anteriorly and medially. Splenic flexure is mobilised by dividing the gastrocolic ligaments and phrenicocolic ligaments.
5. **Retroperitoneum is entered** through the incision and dissection carried medially towards the ligament of Treitz.
6. Retroperitoneal structures encountered during dissection are the **left kidney with ureter and left gonadal vessels.** Care must be taken to avoid injury to these structures.
7. **Turnbull's technique** or no touch isolation technique—early ligation of the vessels before manipulation of the tumour should be followed to prevent dissemination of the tumour cells during handling.
8. **Left colic and left branch of middle colic vessels** are isolated, ligated and divided in case of carcinoma of splenic flexure. Inferior mesenteric and sigmoidal vessels are also ligated in case of carcinoma of descending colon.
9. **Level of colonic transection and anastomosis:**
   - Carcinoma of the splenic flexure: Proximally at the junction of right 1/3rd and left 2/3rds of transverse colon and distally at the junction descending and sigmoid colon. Colocolic anastomosis is done.
   - Carcinoma of the descending colon: Proximally at the junction of right 2/3rds and left 1/3rd of transverse colon and distally at the rectosigmoid junction.
   - Colorectal anastomosis is done.
10. **Abdominal wall is closed in layers.**

## TRANSVERSE COLECTOMY

### Indication

Carcinoma of transverse colon.

### Structures Removed

Whole of the transverse colon including the hepatic and splenic flexures.

### Vessels Ligated

1. Middle colic vessels
2. Left branch of right colic vessels
3. Right branch of left colic vessels.

### Surgical Techniques

1. Laparotomy through midline incision
2. Exploration of the abdomen for liver deposits, peritoneal deposits, ascites and other synchronous lesions.
3. Assessment of the tumour for site, extent, mobility, serosal involvement and local extension.
4. Mobilisation of the hepatic flexure is done by incising along the right avascular lateral peritoneal fold or white line of Toldt and rotating the hepatic flexure anteriorly and downwards. Splenic flexure is mobilised by dividing the gastrocolic ligaments and phrenicocolic ligaments.

5. **Turnbull's technique or no touch isolation technique**—early ligation of the vessels before manipulation of the tumour should be followed to prevent dissemination of the tumour cells during handling.
6. Isolation of middle colic, left branch of right colic and right branch of left colic vessels done and ligated.
7. Proximal transection is done just proximal to the hepatic flexure and the distal transection is done just distal to the splenic flexure.
   - Colocolic anastomosis is done
8. Abdominal wall is closed in layers.

## SIGMOID COLECTOMY

### Indications

1. Carcinoma sigmoid colon
2. Diverticular disease
3. Sigmoid volvulus.

### Structures Removed

1. Sigmoid colon
2. Associated mesosigmoid
3. Lymph nodes in malignancy.

### Vessels Ligated

1. Inferior mesenteric vessels distal to the origin of left colic vessels.
2. Sigmoidal vessels.
3. Left branch of left colic vessels.

### Surgical Techniques

1. **Laparotomy through midline**/left paramedian incision.
2. Exploration of the abdomen for **liver deposits**, peritoneal deposits, ascites and other synchronous lesions.
3. **Assessment of the tumour** for site, extent, mobility, serosal involvement and local extension.
4. **Mobilisation of the left colon** is done by incising along the avascular lateral peritoneal fold or white line of Toldt and rotating the descending colon and the sigmoid colon anteriorly and medially.
5. **Retroperitoneum is entered** through the incision and dissection carried medially towards the origin of inferior mesenteric artery.
6. Retroperitoneal structures encountered during dissection are the **left ureter and left gonadal vessels**. Care must be taken to avoid injury to these structures.
7. **Turnbull's technique or no touch isolation technique**—early ligation of the vessels before manipulation of the tumour should be followed to prevent dissemination of the tumour cells during handling.
8. **Inferior mesenteric vessels** distal to the origin of left colic vessels, sigmoidal vessels and left branch of left colic vessels done are isolated, ligated and divided.
9. **Colonic transection** done proximally at the junction of descending colon and sigmoid colon and distally at the rectosigmoid junction. Colorectal anastomosis is done.
10. Abdominal wall is **closed in layers**.

## COLONIC FUNCTION

### Absorption

Water content of faecal matter is reduced to 1000–1500 ml per day. Thus stools become solid. Similarly, sodium, potassium and bile salts are also absorbed. Significance of this is in cases of diarrhoea, there is loss of water, sodium, potassium and other electrolytes (choleretic diarrhoea). Amino acids and fatty acids are also absorbed slowly in the colon. After ileal resection, bile salts enter the colon irritate the colon resulting in diarrhoea.

### Secretion

Colon also secretes $K^+$ and $Cl^-$. It is increased in colitis. Chloride secretion is increased in cystic fibrosis.

### Motility

Colon has four types of motility: Propulsive, retropulsive, mass peristalsis and gastrocolic reflux. Thus, contents travel aborally. Retropulsive activity is more in the right colon, these allowing the contents to 'churn' more and more. Mass contractions are found more in left colon—especially after meals.

*Factors which stimulate the colonic motility*

- Dietary fat, rich fibre diet, less water intake
- Physical activity—walking, change in posture, exercises
- Emotional activity

*Constipation* (Key Box 59.1)

- It depends upon several factors such as food habits, genetic, social customs.
- Generally a patient is said to have constipation, if he passes less than 2 stools per week.
- In addition to the low fibre diet, emotional feelings and many rectal diseases also cause constipation. Example—prolapsed rectum, solitary rectal ulcer syndrome. Colonic disease such as megacolon—Hirschsprung disease is an important cause of constipation in children.
- Increasing constipation in elderly patient suggest carcinoma in left colon. Needs to be evaluated by colonoscopy.

Key Box 59.1

**Constipation**

- Defective digestion and absorption
- In a child—Hirschsprung's disease
- Adult women—idiopathic/following child birth
- Middle-aged women—following hysterectomy
- Elderly man—carcinoma left colon
- Constipation with severe pain—anal fissure
- Depression patient—psychotropic drugs—used to treat schizophrenia, antidepressants and antiepileptic drugs

### Recycling

- Recycling of various nutrients takes place in the colon. Examples: Fermentation of carbohydrates, short-chain fatty acids and urea cycling.
- Butyrate is the main product of bacterial fermentation. It is required mainly as a fuel for colonic epithelium.
- To accomplish this, the colon depends highly on its bacterial flora, especially for degeneration and fermentation ability.
- So broad-spectrum antibiotics inhibit production of butyrates and produce diarrhoea.

*Pearls of Wisdom*

More distal the colon—more is the protein metabolism and putrefaction resulting in carcinogens and greater exposure to colonic mucosa. Hence, two-thirds of colonic cancer occur in the left colon.

### Colonic Bacteria

- **Anaerobic bacteria:** They constitute more than 99%. The most common pathogen is *Bacteroides fragilis* ($10^{10}$/g of faeces). Other organisms are clostridia, cocci, etc.
- **Aerobic bacteria:** *Escherichia coli* is the most common organism about $10^7$/g of faeces. Other organisms are *Klebsiella, Proteus* and *Enterobacter.*
- **Normal function:** Bacteria degrade bile pigments, thus resulting in brown-coloured stools. They also help in colonic motility and absorption. Fatty acids produced by bacteria supply nutrition to colonic epithelium. Bacteria also supply vitamin K to the host.

### Prebiotics and Probiotics

- **Prebiotics** are non-digestible food ingredients that stimulate the growth and/or activity of bacteria in the digestive system in ways claimed to be beneficial to health. Traditional dietary sources of prebiotics include soybeans, inulin sources (such as Jerusalem artichoke, jicama, soya and chicory root), raw oats, unrefined wheat, unrefined barley, and yacon.
- **Probiotic** is defined as a "live microbial feed supplement which beneficially affects the host animal by improving its **intestinal microbial balance**". They are non-degradable oligosaccharides. They stimulate the growth of beneficial intestinal bacteria.
- Probiotics are dietary supplements which contain live cultures of bacteria and yeast that are beneficial to colonic and host function. The common species used as probiotics are *Lactobacillus* and *Bifidobacterium.* Probiotics stimulate immune function, exhibit anti-inflammatory property and suppress pathogenic organism.
- **Clinical application:** When a person takes antibiotics, both the harmful bacteria and the beneficial bacteria are killed. Bacterial change in flora alters carbohydrate metabolism with decreased short-chain fatty acid absorption and results in osmotic diarrhoea. In a similar fashion, antibiotic therapy causes increase in the growth of *Clostridium difficile.* Thus, probiotics have been recommended in antibiotic-induced diarrhoea. Also, they have been used to treat diarrhoeas in ulcerative colitis, in pouchitis (inflammation of the pouch after total proctocolectomy for ulcerative colitis) and in necrotising colitis in children.

## EXAMINATION OF COLON

**Anoproctoscopy:** One can examine up to 10–12 cm of anal canal and rectum. Rubber band ligation (for piles) and polypectomy can be done with this instrument.

**Flexible sigmoidoscopy:** The scope measures about 60 cm in length. One can easily reach up to splenic flexure. Bowel wash or an enema is given before the procedure. No sedation is required (Figs 59.7 and 59.8).

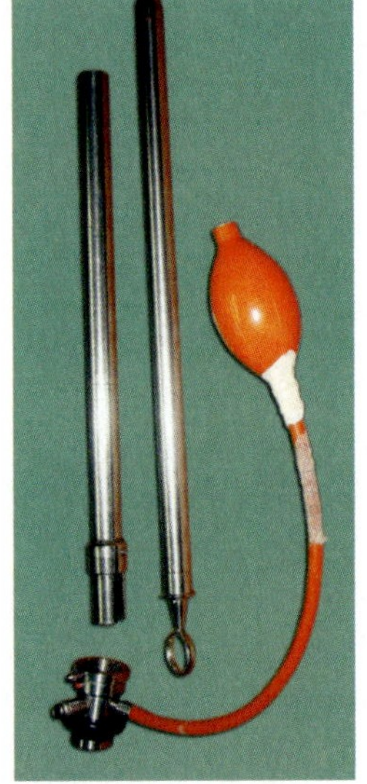

**Fig. 59.7:** Rigid sigmoidoscope

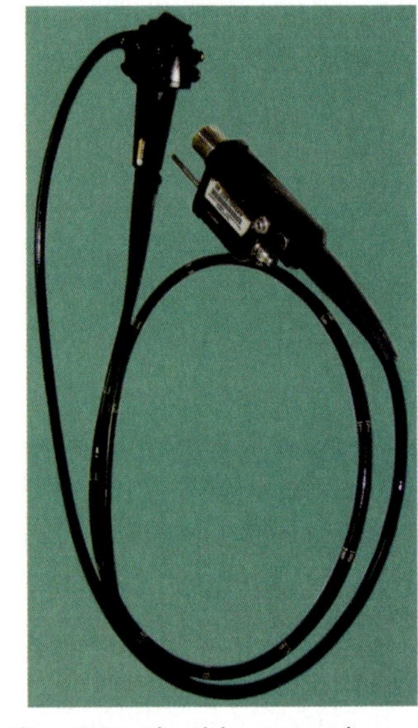

**Fig. 59.8:** Flexible sigmoidoscope

**Fibreoptic colonoscopy** can assess the entire colon. It is 100–160 cm in length. Usually, there will be multiple polyps varying from a few millimetres to centimetres. Biopsy has to be taken. Polyps are visible after 15 years and certainly by the age of 30 years.

- It is the investigation of choice in most of the large intestinal lesions.
- It permits examination of entire colon and terminal ileum.
- Colon is prepared by polyethylene glycol given orally.
- Risk of perforation of colon is less than 0.1%.

## Indications

### *Diagnostic*

- Lower gastrointestinal bleeding
- Inflammatory bowel diseases
- Abnormal finding in barium enema
- Family history of colorectal cancers
- Biopsy of caecum/ileum in suspected cases of cancer
- Ileocaecal tuberculosis—to take biopsy.

### *Therapeutic*

- Control of bleeding—coagulation or injection sclerotherapy
- Snaring of polyps
- Removal of foreign body
- Detorsion of volvulus
- Decompression of pseudo-obstruction.

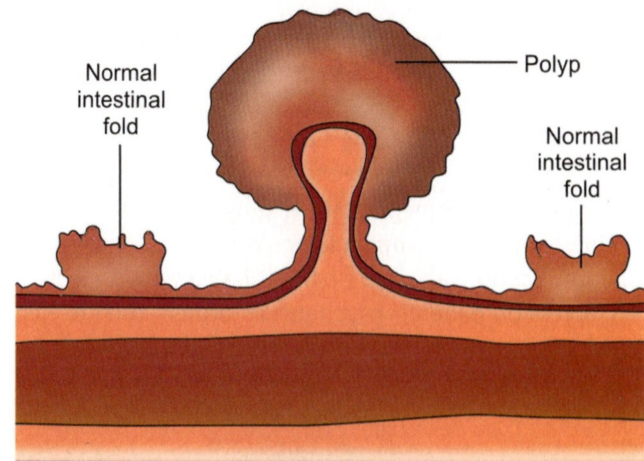


**Fig. 59.9A:** Polyp

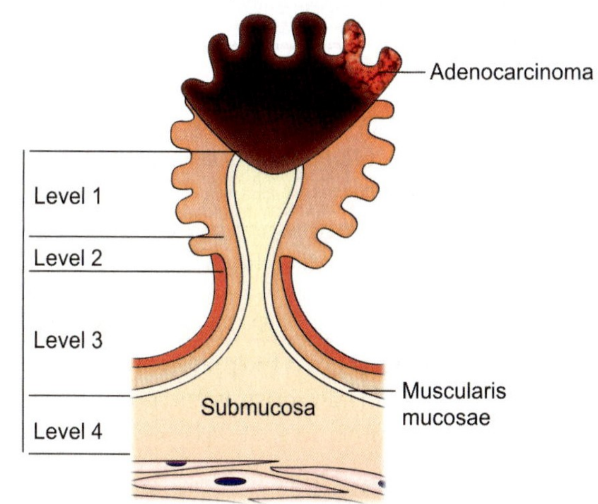


**Fig. 59.9B:** Pedunculated adenoma

## TUMOURS OF THE LARGE INTESTINE

> **SU28.13.5:** Understand the vascular anatomy of small and large intestines and apply the same pathologies like congenital, inflammatory, traumatic, benign and malignant, etc.
>
> Ulcerative colitis is discussed under inflammatory bowel diseases. Polyps, colonic cancer, diverticular diseases and colonic stricture are discussed here.

## Classification of Colonic Diseases

1. Congenital: Hereditary polyposis coli
2. Inflammatory: Ulcerative colitis
3. Infective: Tuberculosis, amoebic dysentery, bacillary dysentery, etc.
4. Neoplastic: Benign—Polyps-Juvenile, hamartomatous (Rarely can be malignant), hyperplastic polyps.
   Malignant: Carcinoma, lymphoma, stromal tumours
5. Motility: Adult Hirschsprung, diverticular disease
6. Miscellaneous: Ischemic colitis, angiodysplasias, AV malformations.

Benign tumours (Figs 59.9A and B) are usually referred to as polyp, which means **elevated from the surface**. Adenomatous polyps have got malignant potential. A few criteria have been incorporated into a system when malignancy develops in the polyp.

- It takes into consideration the level of invasion.
- **Haggitt classification of polyps:** Haggitt's level 0 is absence of invasive carcinoma.
- Level 1: In this, carcinoma is limited to the top of the polyp. From the mucosa, it is invading through muscularis mucosa into the submucosa.
- Level 2: Carcinoma at the junction of head and stalk.
- Level 3: Carcinoma confined to anywhere in the stalk.
- Level 4: Infiltration into submucosa.

## ADENOMATOUS POLYP (Key Box 59.2)

- It may be a villous adenoma which is a flat lesion or a tubular adenoma having a pedicle. Tubular is more common.
- They give rise to bleeding, mucus diarrhoea and hypokalaemia.

Key Box 59.2

**Adenomatous Polyps**

- Most of the neoplastic polyps occur in elderly patients (>50 years).
- Most of them are pedunculated.
- Most pedunculated polyps are removed by colonoscopic snaring.
- Most common polyps have malignant potential.
- Adenomas larger than 5 mm in diameter carry risk of malignant potential.
- More the polyps, more chances of synchronous carcinoma.
- Flat sessile adenomas also carry malignant potential.

- They can be single or multiple.
- They are dysplastic.
- They are premalignant and the risk of malignancy is greater with increase in the size of the adenoma. Large colonic adenomas more than 3 cm in size have a focus of invasive malignancy in almost 30 to 35 % patients.
- They can be removed with the colonoscope—polypectomy.
- Malignant potential of ***villous adenoma*** is more than tubular adenoma (Fig. 59.10).
- Adenoma less than 1 cm—risk of malignancy is 1%; 1–2 cm is 10%; >2 cm is 30%.
- Symptoms and signs of polyps: Bleeding per rectum is the most common symptom. Fresh bleeding is seen in rectal polyps. Typically, it is painless. It is intermittent. If it is associated with change of bowel habits means probably a malignant change. These changes include mucus discharge, tenesmus, sometimes constipation. In children, polyp may project outside the anus. In such cases, it has to be distinguished from prolapsed rectum.

### Treatment

- Colonoscopy and polypectomy is the standard treatment.
- If specimen shows invasive carcinoma, radical surgery needs to be done.

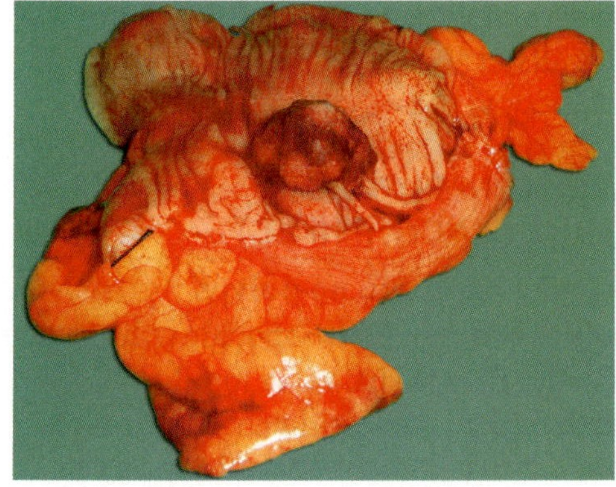

**Fig. 59.10:** Carcinoma in polyp

*Pearls of Wisdom*

Although most neoplastic polyps do not evolve to cancer, most colorectal cancers originate as a polyp.

## HAMARTOMATOUS POLYP (JUVENILE POLYP)

- This can occur in the colon as in Peutz-Jeghers syndrome. Risk of malignancy is very limited. Symptomatic polyps need to be treated.
- **Juvenile polyps** are usually single and occur in children. They give rise to bleeding and are easily resected. They do not have malignant potential.

## FAMILIAL POLYPOSIS COLI (FPC) OR FAMILIAL ADENOMATOUS POLYPOSIS (FAP)

- FAP is a genetic disorder inherited as a Mendelian dominant. The gene APC (adenomatous polyposis coli) is located on the short arm of chromosome 5. **Prevalence:** 1 in 10,000. It is clinically defined by the presence of more than 100 colorectal adenomas (Figs 59.11 and 59.12).
- It is transmitted from both sexes. The incidence is same in either sex.
- When it is associated with desmoid tumour, craniofacial osteoma, epidermoid cysts, congenital hypertrophy of retinal pigment epithelium, it is described as **Gardner's syndrome** (Key Box 59.3).
- When familial polyposis coli is associated with central nervous system tumour and glioblastoma, it is called **Turcot's syndrome**.
- 50% of them have benign gastric polyps and 90% of them have duodenal polyps.

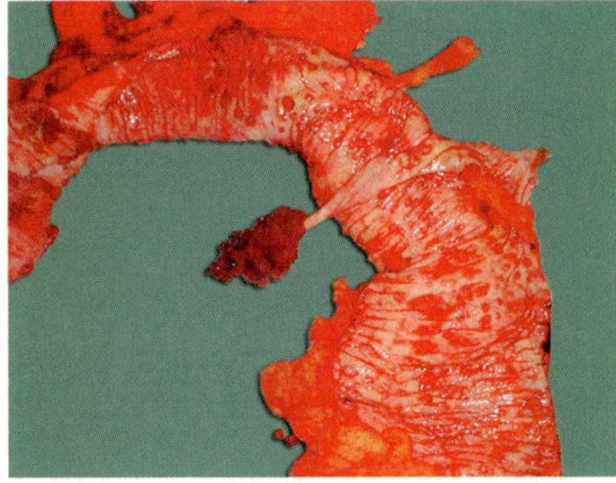

**Fig. 59.11:** Thousands of polyps. One of them is 2 cm and is pedunculated

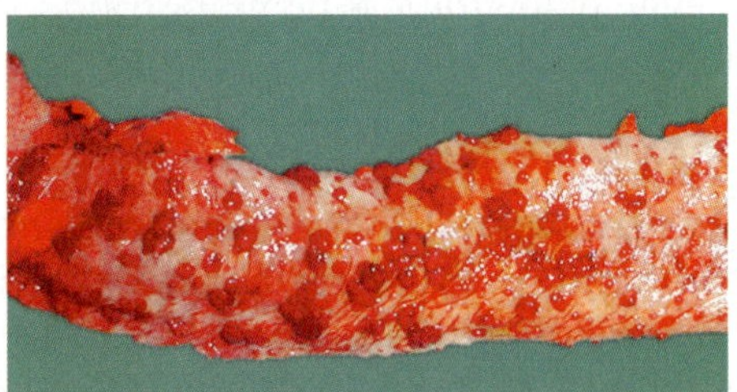

**Fig. 59.12:** Close-up view of the polyps

Key Box 59.3

**Familial Polyposis Coli—Summary**

- **P**olyps are more than 100 (colorectal adenomas).
- **O**ther mesodermal tumours—desmoid tumours, osteoma, epidermoid cysts can be present (Gardner's syndrome).
- **L**arge bowel is predominantly involved.
- **Y**ear of development of carcinoma—mean age 39 years.
- **P**olyposis gene—autosomal dominant APC gene.
- **O**ther syndrome—Turcot
- **S**igmoidoscopy from age of 15 at intervals is the investigation of choice.
- **I**leoanal anastomosis with pouch—restorative proctocolectomy—recommended above the age of 30.
- **S**urgery is the only means of preventing colonic cancer.

*Remember as* **POLYPOSIS**

### Clinical Features

- Runs in families; other members of the family are affected.
- Manifests at the age of 20 in the form of blood and mucus in the stool, loose stools, etc. It produces crampy lower abdominal pain.
- Anaemia, weight loss and protein malnutrition occur slowly.
- Mean age of development of carcinoma is 29 years.

### Complications of FAP

Malignancy (100% risk).

### Investigations

Colonoscopy—to confirm the diagnosis, involvement of colon, detection of polyps. Suspicious polyps need to be biopsied. If malignancy is detected it is an urgent indication for surgery. Biopsy is not always indicated because these patients require elective surgery after age of 30.

### Treatment

- **NSAIDs: Sulindac** 300 mg, twice a day and **aspirin** 325 mg once a day have been found to decrease the size of polyps.
- Patients with FAP who are above the age of 30 have high chances of having a carcinoma in the colon. Hence, even when there is no malignancy, surgery is advisable.

### Types of Surgery (Figs 59.13 and 59.14)

- Many patients do not like ileostomy. Hence, a subtotal colectomy with ileorectal anastomosis can be done. This is done provided that rectum is examined frequently and endoscopic snaring of the polyps is done regularly, especially in a young patient.

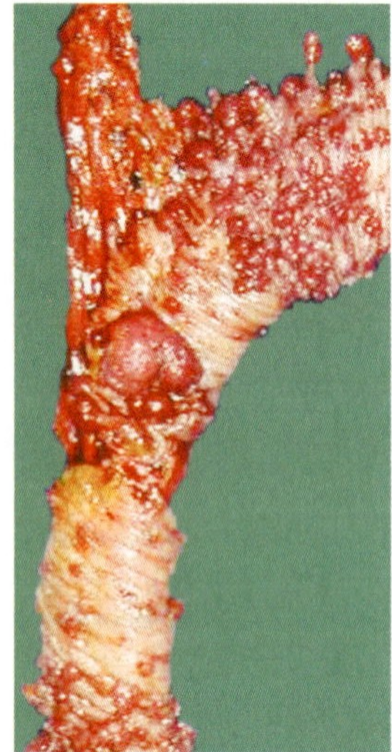

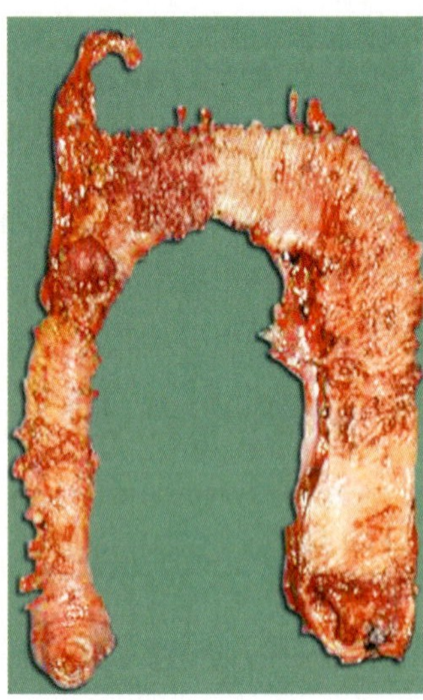

**Figs 59.13 and 59.14:** Familial adenomatous polyposis with two malignancies—lower rectum and hepatic flexure. This patient was being treated for chronic diarrhoea for 7–8 years with various medications. 'He underwent colonoscopy for the first time in our hospital.' Total proctocolectomy specimen (*Courtesy*: Dr Challa Srinivas Rao, Professor, Department of Surgery, and Dr Ravi, Konaseema Institute of Medical Sciences (KIMS), Amalapuram, Andhra Pradesh)

- **Restorative proctocolectomy** with ileoanal anastomosis by using a pouch is another alternative. However, it is a major surgical procedure and should be undertaken only by an experienced surgeon.

### Screening

Starts from the age of 10–12 years, repeat every 1–2 years until the age 35.

*Pearls of Wisdom*

If there are no adenomas by the age of 30 years, FAP is unlikely.

## METAPLASTIC POLYP

They are also called as hyperplastic polyps. Generally, they are considered as benign with no malignant potential. However, few subtypes can have malignant potential especially with KRAS/BRAF mutations. Such polyps are also called as serrated polyps. Such polyps should be removed.

## HEREDITARY NONPOLYPOSIS COLORECTAL CANCER (HNPCC)

- Autosomal dominant, **no polyps**
- **Lynch's syndrome I:** Site-specific colorectal cancer.
- **Lynch's syndrome II:** Cancer family syndrome—they have extracolonic cancers such as endometrial cancer, ovarian cancer, transitional cell cancer, etc.
- Lifetime risk of developing colorectal cancer is 80%.

- **Synchronous carcinoma means more than one cancer at the time of diagnosis. Metachronous carcinoma which means appearance of second carcinoma after 6 months.**

### Diagnostic Criteria (Amsterdam Criteria II)

1. At least 3 members in a family should have colorectal cancer—two of whom are first degree relatives.
2. At least two consecutive generations.
3. At least one relative should have had colorectal cancer by less than 50 years of age.
4. Exclusion of FAP.

### Screening

Increased incidence of **proximal colonic cancer**.

## CARCINOMA COLON

### Introduction

It is the second most common cancer and cancer-related death cases in the Western world next only to lung cancer. The incidence increases with age. Multiple synchronous lesions (more than 1 malignancy at the time of diagnosis) are found in about 5% of the patients. Colon is also one of the sites of metachronous cancer (new malignancy appearing after 6 months of curative surgery). More than 95% are adenocarcinoma and surgery remains the most effective treatment. Survival has improved because of early diagnosis and multi-modality of the treatment.

Over a period of years, the understanding of development of carcinoma has changed and more and more molecular biology of colonic cancer is being discussed. The **Fearon-Vogelstein adenoma–carcinoma multistep model** of colorectal neoplasia represents one of the best known models of carcinogenesis (Fig. 59.15).

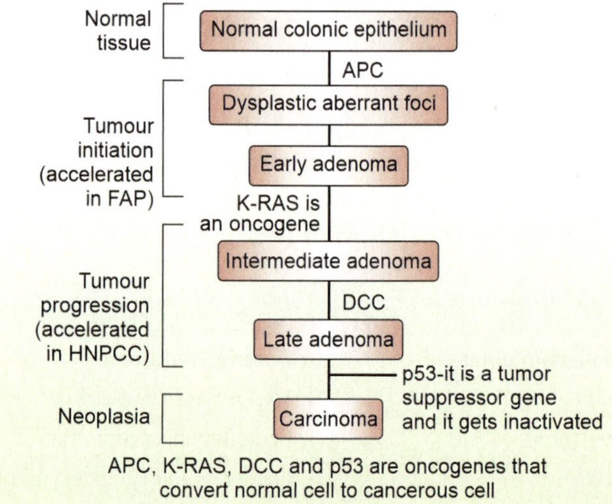


**Fig. 59.15:** Fearon-Vogelstein Model

- **Terminology:** Before we start the discussion on carcinoma colon, we shall study a few terminologies used in carcinoma colon. They are synchronous carcinoma, metachronous carcinoma, familial colorectal carcinoma.

## SYNCHRONOUS CARCINOMA

- **Moertel's definition:** Synchronous cancers as those occurring within 6 months of the first primary cancer, or two or more histologically distinct simultaneously detected malignancies or more than one malignancy at the time of initial diagnosis. This will happen especially in cases of colon and upper aerodigestive tract wherein the stimulus or aetiological factor for malignancy affects different parts of the organ.
- Colon, head and neck, oesophagus are the sites of synchronous carcinomas.
- In cases of carcinoma colon with specific aetiological factors such as familial polyposis coli, ulcerative colitis, hereditary non-polyposis cancer, often carcinoma is synchronous.
- Thus, it is important to do a complete colonoscopy when a patient comes with colonic carcinoma because he/she may be having another synchronous carcinoma elsewhere. *See* the clinical notes.

**Clinical Notes**

A 68-year-old lady was admitted with large bowel obstruction. Plain X-ray abdomen showed intestinal obstruction. Exploratory laparotomy was done. A 3 cm constricting growth was identified at rectosigmoid junction and high anterior resection and anastomosis was done. On the 4th postoperative day, the patient was allowed liquid diet. Distension increased. For another 3 days, distension went on increasing. Plain X-ray abdomen revealed obstruction with more gas than before. The patient was having colicky abdominal pain. Exploratory laparotomy was done. Findings at 2nd laparotomy—anastomosis was intact. Transverse colon was hugely dilated. Careful palpation of splenic flexure revealed one more growth. A resection and anastomosis was done again. Patient was discharged after 10 days. The first surgeon agreed that after finding the rectosigmoid growth, he did not look for any other lesions (mistake). This was obviously a case of synchronous carcinoma.

## METACHRONOUS COLONIC CANCER

- Metachronous cancer was defined as those cancer occurring more than 6 months following resection of one malignancy.
- A few examples of metachronous site are: Colorectum, breast, kidney.

- Family history of hereditary, nonpolyposis colorectal cancer (HNPCC or Lynch syndrome), an autosomal dominant disease, also can present with both synchronous or metachronous colorectal cancers.
- It is more common in females.
- Common usually at young age.
- The associated genetic defect lies at the mismatch repair genes, responsible for the correction of DNA bases mismatch.
- The coexistence of adenomatous polyps is also considered a risk factor for the development of metachronous lesions. Thus, after treating one carcinoma, example—carcinoma sigmoid, annual colonoscopy is recommended. If polyps are detected, patients have to be informed about the polyps and their potential of malignancy.
- Survival is better.

## FAMILIAL COLORECTAL CANCER

- All these have a carrier gene and thus, run in families. Malignancies occur in young age group. Often they are synchronous. Metachronous lesions are not uncommon.
- Certain criteria have been laid upon for the diagnosis of these conditions which have been discussed already.
- Genetic instability is the chief factor responsible. The instability can be at chromosomal level called chromosomal instability or **at DNA level called microsatellite instability—MSI.** As a result of this after the cell division by duplication, mismatched genes develop. These genes cannot be repaired. This predisposes to mutation, results in a cancer gene.
- **Familial polyposis coli** accounts for about 1% of colorectal cancers. However, incidence of malignancy is 100%. Gardner's and Turcot's syndromes are the variants of FPC.
- **HNPCC** accounts for about 5 to 10% of colorectal cancers. They also have extracolonic cancers such as endometrial, ovarian and urinary bladder cancers.
- Other familial syndromes are **Cronkhite-Canada syndrome.** It is more common in females. Multiple polyps develop in stomach, duodenum and in the colon. Diarrhoea is the clinical presentation. Other features include pigmentation, alopecia, loss of weight and cachexia. Chances of developing malignancy is about 15%.

## PRECANCEROUS CONDITIONS (Key Box 59.4)

1. **Polyps:** Environmental and genetic factors favour the development of colonic polyps and their transformation into malignancy. The incidence of malignancy is increased when the polyp is more than 1 cm, polyps are multiple or flat (Table 59.2).

Key Box 59.4

**Risk Factors Associated with Colon Cancer**

| Risk factor | Incidence of cancer |
|---|---|
| Familial polyposis coli | 100% chances of colorectal cancer |
| HNPCC | 80% chances |
| Ulcerative colitis | 10–20% after 20 years |
| Crohn's colitis | 5% after 10–20 years |
| Adenomatous polyps | 1–20% depending upon the size |

*Pearls of Wisdom*

Familial polyposis coli has 100% chance of carcinoma.

2. **Inflammatory bowel disease:**
   - A. **Ulcerative colitis** is a definite precancerous condition. Presence of dysplasia diagnosed by colonoscopic biopsy is an indication for colectomy. At the end of 20 years of ulcerative colitis, 10 to 15% increased risk of developing ulcerative colitis is present.
   - B. **Crohn's** involving colon also has a mildly increased risk of developing carcinoma when compared to ulcerative colitis.
   - C. **Schistosomal colitis:** The risk of colorectal cancer is increased in patients with long-standing schistosomal colitis. Long-standing cases are associated with mild to severe grades of colonic epithelial dysplasia. Thus ulcers or pseudopolyps can occur. These dysplastic changes are considered as premalignant.
   - D. **Radiation exposure:** Usually, it is mucin-secreting adenocarcinoma with poor prognosis.
   - E. **Ureterosigmoidostomy** increases risk of colonic cancer over 100–500 times.

**TABLE 59.2:** Summary of colonic polyps and malignant potential

| Type | Cause | Malignant potential | Features/syndrome |
|---|---|---|---|
| 1. Adenomatous polyp | Benign tumour | 1–10% | Hypokalaemia, diarrhoea |
| 2. Hamartomatous polyp | "Misfire" | Negligible | Peutz-Jeghers syndrome |
| 3. Familial polyposis coli | Genetic disorder | 100% | Gardner's and Turcot's syndrome |
| 4. Metaplastic polyps | Hyperplasia | Nil | Asymptomatic |

## AETIOLOGICAL FACTORS

**SAD factors:** It is sad to know that **SAD** factors are responsible for carcinoma colon. They are **S**—Smoking, **A**—Alcohol, **D**—Dietary factors. Diet rich in red meat has high animal fat. This alters intestinal bacteria, which convert primary bile acids into secondary bile acids. ***This is the beginning of formation of carcinogenic polycyclic aromatic compounds.*** After cholecystectomy, there is increase in free bile acid concentration, thus increasing the risk of colonic cancer. Thus increased roughage is associated with increased transit time which in turn reduces exposure of mucosa to carcinogens.

- Increase incidence is found in western countries wherein diet rich in animal fat is consumed in large quantity. Incidence is more after the age of 50 years. Obesity, poor exercise and smoking are the contributing factors.
- Some interesting observations are also found in females with colonic cancer which have been depicted in Key Box 59.5.

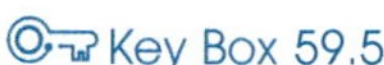

Key Box 59.5

**Women and Colonic Cancer**

- **Caecum** is more commonly involved than other parts.
- Women with **breast cancer** have increased incidence of colonic cancer.
- Women **smokers** have increased chances of colonic cancer.
- Women who have undergone **cholecystectomy** have increased chances of colonic cancer.
- Metastasis to ovary is mostly haematogenous (1 to 10%).

*Pearls of Wisdom*

Calcium salts are protective. They form insoluble bile salt complexes, thus reducing the concentration of bile acids in the colon. After cholecystectomy, the proximal colon has a greater absorption of secondary bile acid and more exposure to carcinogenic metabolites. So, the incidence of proximal colon cancer is higher.

## PATHOLOGICAL TYPES (Figs 59.16A to D)

- It is an adenocarcinoma—columnar epithelium. Rectum (40%) and sigmoid (20%) take a major share in colorectal carcinoma followed by caecum (12 to 15%). Multiple synchronous cancers are also common in the colon.

  A. **Annular stricture:** Common in left colon (splenic flexure, pelvic colon). So, obstruction is common.

  B. **Tubular stricture:** Common in left colon and at the rectosigmoid junction.

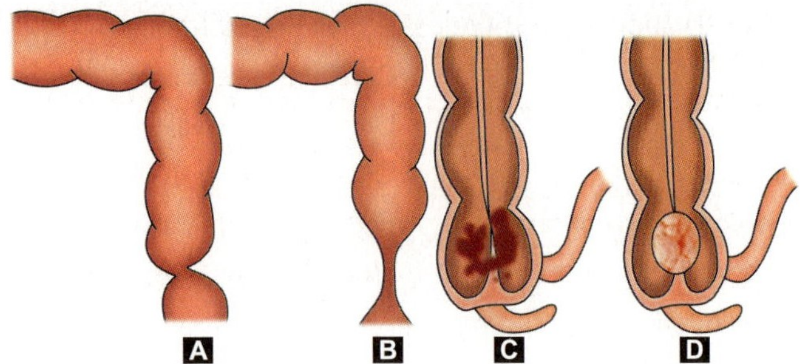


**Figs 59.16A to D:** Types of carcinoma colon

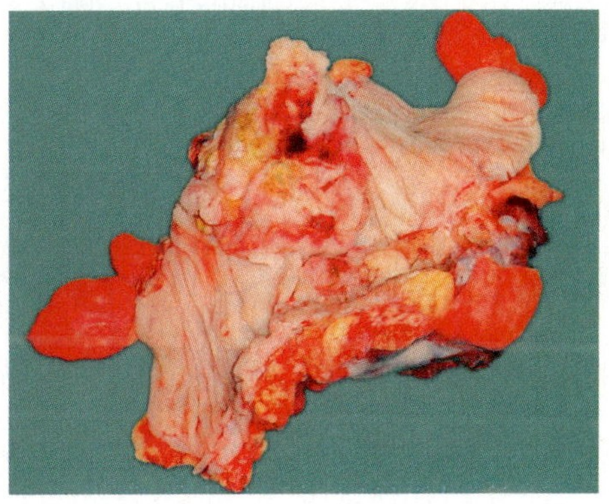

**Fig. 59.17:** Ulceroproliferative growth in the descending colon

  C. **Ulcerative lesion:** Ascending colon or caecum, they present with anaemia.

  D. **Proliferative growth:** More in right colon, the least malignant, fleshy and bulky polypoid lesion (Fig. 59.17).

- It is a columnar cell adenocarcinoma. In about 5% of cases, it undergoes mucoid degeneration. Such tumours carry poor prognosis. They spread to the liver very fast and secondaries produce mucoid material.

## CLINICAL FEATURES OF CARCINOMA COLON

(Figs 59.18A to C and Table 59.3) (*Mnemonic:* **TMA Pai**)[1]

1. **Tumour:** The mass produced by carcinoma caecum, ascending colon and even hepatic flexure is palpable. It is firm to hard, irregular and with or without fixity.
   - Cancer of sigmoid colon may be palpable on the left side with some mobility.
   - However, on left-sided constrictive lesions, growth is not often felt. It is the hard faecal matter and lymph nodes which are felt as a mass.
2. **Metastasis:** 5–10% of the patients present with metastasis to liver (mucoid adenocarcinoma), lungs, ascites, etc. Distant metastasis is not common (Fig. 59.19).
3. **Anaemia** is an important feature of carcinoma caecum. It may be due to blood loss or a proliferative

[1]Late Padmashree Dr TMA Pai, was the founder of Kasturba Medical College which he started in 1953. He was also a banker and educationist. He is called 'Modern Architect of Manipal', where Manipal Academy of Higher Education (MAHE)—deemed to be the university is situated.

**TABLE 59.3:** Comparison of right colon versus left colon

| | Carcinoma right colon | Carcinoma left colon |
|---|---|---|
| Presentation | Unexplained weakness, anaemia | Change in bowel habits |
| Bleeding | Occult blood in stools | Gross blood in stools |
| Abdominal discomfort | Right side and dyspeptic symptoms also | Constipation and obstruction |
| Incidence | More common in women | More common in men |
| Frequency | About 10–20% | About 60–70% (including rectum) |
| Pathology | Ulcerative/proliferative lesion | Strictures (rectosigmoid) |
| Investigation | Colonoscopy | Flexible sigmoidoscopy |
| Complication | Obstruction—less common | Obstruction, perforation, pericolic abscess—common |

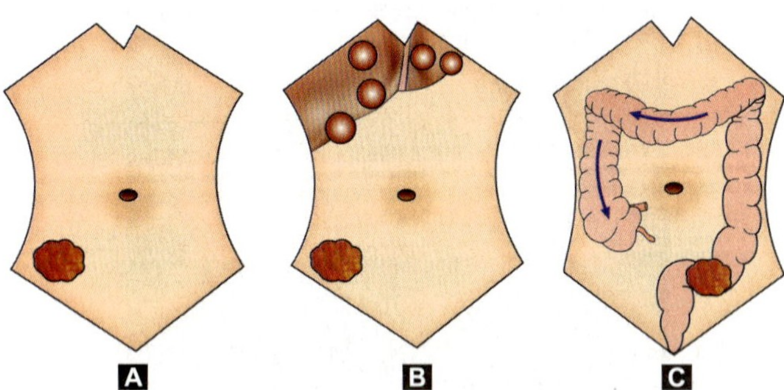


**Figs 59.18A to C:** (A) Carcinoma caecum; (B) Carcinoma caecum with secondaries in the liver; (C) Carcinoma left colon with intestinal obstruction

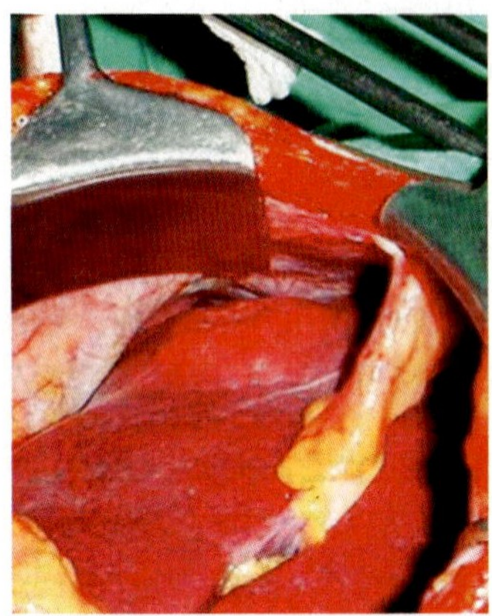

**Fig. 59.19:** Large secondary in the liver. Look at the umbilication resulting due to central necrosis of the secondary

growth secreting toxins causing suppression of bone marrow. Other explanations for anaemia are: 'Chronic anaemia resulting from an anti-erythropoietin factor, reduction in mean RBC life, and poor iron availability'. Asthaenia and anorexia are the other features.

4. **Pain abdomen:** Dull aching pain may be present. Colicky pain is due to chronic obstruction as in left-sided growths (napkin ring stricture).
5. **Alteration in the bowel habits:** A recent constipation, increase in the dose of laxatives followed by attacks of diarrhoea can be due to carcinoma colon. Diarrhoea is due to hard faecal balls, irritating the colonic mucosa resulting in increased secretion of mucus produced by proximal colon.
6. **Intestinal obstruction** is caused by constricted left-sided lesions (Fig. 59.20). On the left side, diameter of the colon is narrow, contents are solid and growth is constrictive. Lower abdominal distension, right to left peristalsis are the late features. Carcinoma sigmoid colon can cause colovesical fistula.

### *To Summarise*

- **Early cases:** It can be easily missed—such as change in bowel habits such as diarrhoea, vague ill health, weakness (due to anaemia), intermittent bleeding per rectum, often attributed to piles or some other cause. Mass is usually not palpable.
- **Late cases:** It can present with obstruction (recto-sigmoid junction growth), perforation, intussusception (right-sided tumours), mass abdomen, secondaries in the liver, left supraclavicular nodes (Troisier's sign), etc.

*See* Key Boxes 59.6 to 59.8.

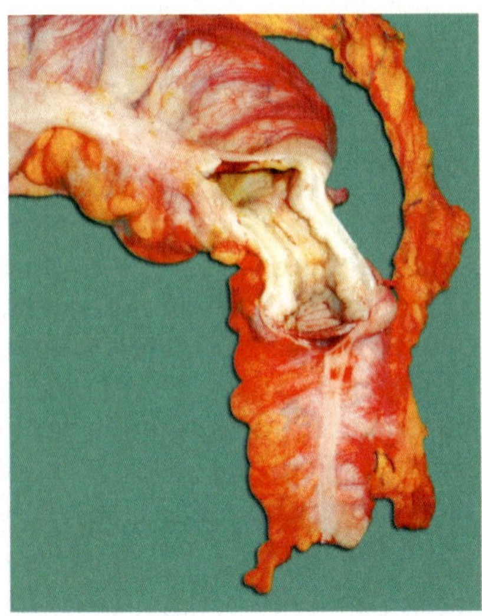

**Fig. 59.20:** Tubular stricture at rectosigmoid junction—cut opened specimen after resection

Key Box 59.6

**Peculiarities of Carcinoma of Caecum**
(Figs 59.21 to 59.27)

- Incidence is more in females.
- Presents with anaemia and a mass.
- Can present as acute appendicitis when the lumen of appendix is obstructed—called secondary appendicitis (in elderly patients).
- It is a cause of intussusception (secondary).
- Can present with flexion of hip due to infiltration of iliopsoas.

Key Box 59.7

**Peculiarities of Carcinoma Splenic Flexure**

- Presents as obstruction.
- It is easily missed unless carefully looked for.
- Carries poor prognosis as many cases present with obstruction.
- Often, it is inoperable. Reasons may be Perforation, extensive local; spread, peritoneal spread etc.

Key Box 59.8

**Peculiarities of Carcinoma Sigmoid**
(Figs 59.28 and 59.29)

- Commonly presents as **obstructive lesion**—constipation and intestinal obstruction.
- **Colovesical fistula:** Carcinoma sigmoid is the 2nd commonest cause. 1st cause is diverticulosis.
- It can cause **colovaginal fistula**.
- It can also **infiltrate ureter, uterus and ovary**.
- It can present as **abscess in the lateral abdominal wall**.

*Pearls of Wisdom*

Obstructed and perforated carcinoma colon have poor prognosis.

## Spread

1. **Local:** For a long time, the lesion is confined to mucosa and submucosa. They grow in annular fashion and later longitudinally. Once serosa is involved, spread occurs rapidly into neighbouring structures such as ureter, bladder, uterus, etc. The involvement of these structures is **not a contraindication** for surgery (TNM staging).
   - Local perforation may result in pericolic abscess.
   - Hollow viscus perforation results in internal fistula.
2. **Lymphatic spread** (*see* next page TNM staging).
3. **Blood spread:** It occurs late, resulting in secondaries in the liver, lungs, etc. Cannonball in lung, nodule in the liver.

A few clinical photographs, staging pictures and operative pictures have been given in the next page.

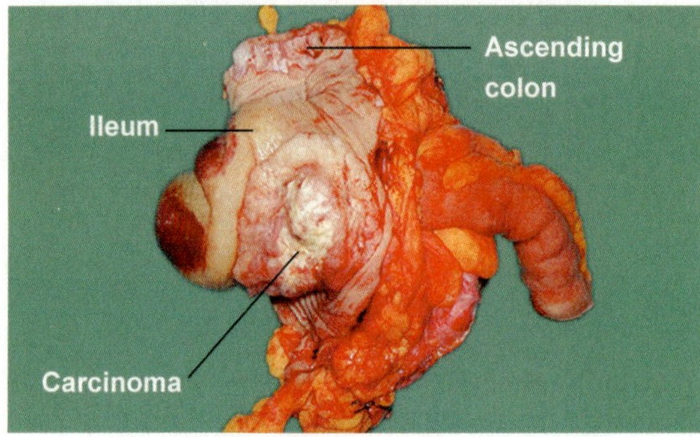


**Fig. 59.21:** Intussusception due to carcinoma caecum

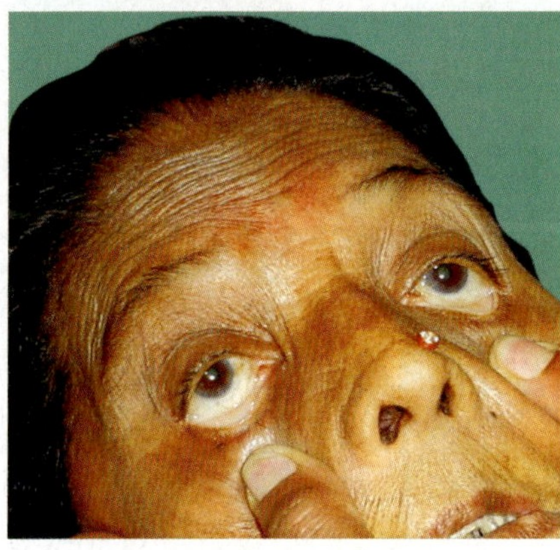

**Fig. 59.22:** Pallor disproportionate to the blood loss—typical of carcinoma caecum

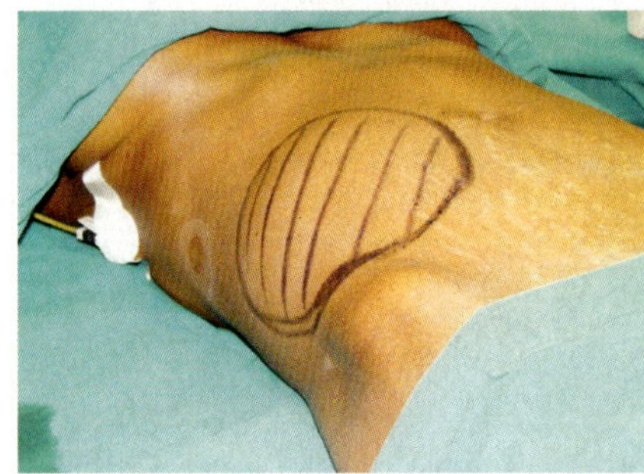

**Fig. 59.23:** A 34-year-old lady presented to the hospital with mass in the right iliac fossa with slight flexion of the right hip. Mass was hard and irregular. She also had anaemia

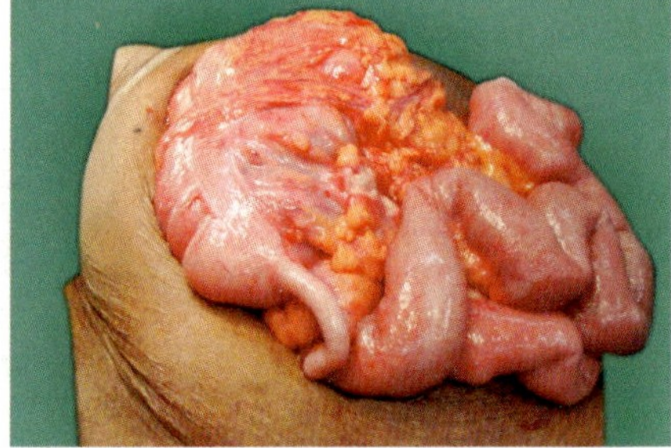

**Fig. 59.24:** Exploration of the mass (caecum). It was mobile. Entire right colon is mobilised by incising right paracolic gutter and dividing colophrenic ligament

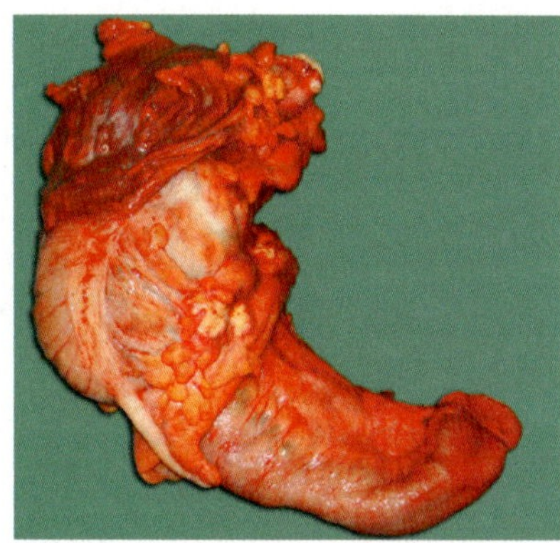

Fig. 59.25: Right hemicolectomy specimen—a case of carcinoma caecum

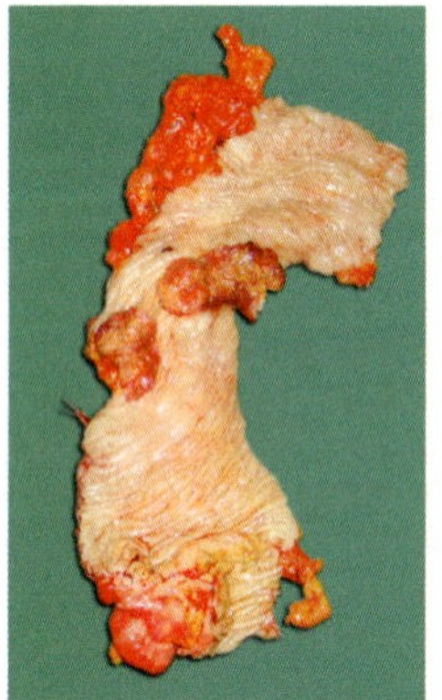

Fig. 59.26: Carcinoma hepatic flexure with partial obstruction

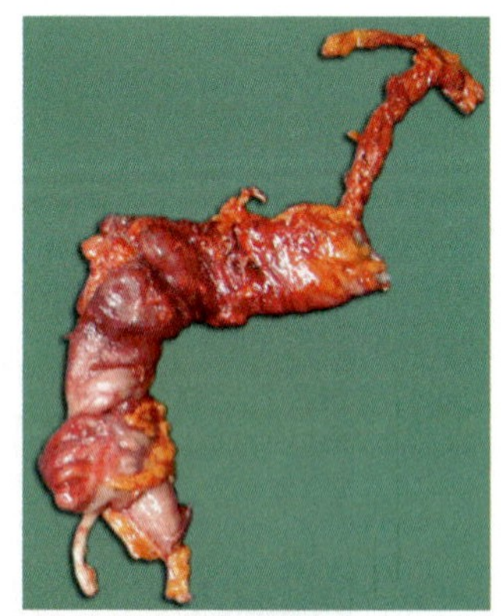

Fig. 59.27: Extended right hemicolectomy specimen

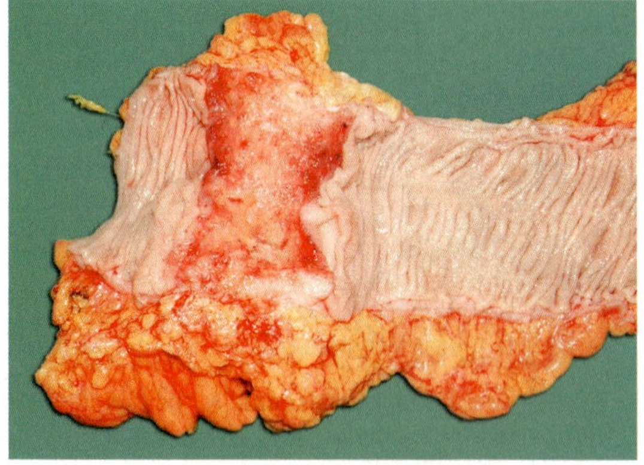

Fig. 59.28: Rectosigmoid stricture. Patient underwent high anterior resection. 5 cm proximal margin is enough for radical cure

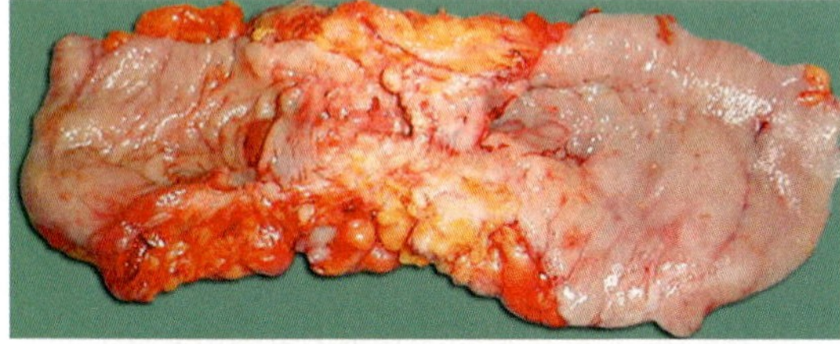

Fig. 59.29: Intestinal obstruction due to rectosigmoid stricture—a common complication. **Tumour rarely goes beyond 2 cm from the edge of the tumour** unless there is concomitant spread to lymph nodes

*Pearls of Wisdom*

Because of the drainage into the portal system, colonic cancers spread to the liver first. On the other hand, rectal cancers spread to the lungs because of drainage into inferior vena cava.

## Staging/Classifications

There are many classifications and staging for carcinoma colon/rectum. They are not important. A few important ones have been given here.

### *Dukes' Staging for Colorectal Cancer*

- **Stage A:** Invasion of but not breaching the muscularis propria.
- **Stage B:** Breaching the muscularis propria but not involving the lymph nodes.
- **Stage C:** Lymph nodes are involved.

A few authors describe a stage D for metastatic disease. Since it has not been described by Duke, it is called modified Dukes' staging.

### *TNM Staging*

**TNM Classification of Colonic Cancer–UICC (Union for International Cancer Control, 8th edition)**

**Tumour—T**

Tx—Primary tumour cannot be assessed

T0—No evidence of tumour

Tis—Carcioma *in situ*—intraepithelial/invasion into lamina propria

T1—Invasion into submucosa

T2—Invasion into muscularis propria

T3—Invasion into pericolorectal tissues/fat

T4a—Invasion into surface of the visceral peritoneum

T4b—Direct invasion or adherent to adjacent structures/organs

**Regional nodes—N**

Nx—Nodes cannot be assessed

N0—No nodal spread

N1—Regional nodes 1–3 involved

- N1a—1 regional node
- N1b—2 to 3 regional nodes
- N1c—Tumour deposits in serosa/mesentery/non-peritonealised pericolic or perirectal tissue without regional nodes

N2a—Regional nodes 4 or more involved

- N2a—4–6 regional nodes
- N2b—7 or more regional nodes

*(Contd.)*

(*Contd.*)

**Distant metastases M**

M0 No distant spread
M1 Distant spread present
M1a Spread confined to one organ or site—liver/lung/ovary/nonregional nodes
M1b Spread to more than one organ or site/peritoneum
M1c Peritoneal spread

**Histological grade G**

Gx—Grade cannot be assessed
G1—Well-differentiated
G2—Moderately differentiated
G3—Poorly differentiated
G4—Undifferentiated

**Residual tumour R**

R0—No residual tumour after resection
R1—Microscopic residual tumour after resection
R2—Macroscopic residual tumour after resection

**Stage Group**

0—Tis N0 M0
1—T1 N0 M0; T2 N0 M0
IIA—T3 N0 M0
IIB—T4a N0 M0
IIC—T4b N0 M0
IIIA—T1-2 N1-1c M0; T1 N2a M0
IIIB—T3-4a N1-1c M0; T2-3 N2a M0; T1-2 N2b M0
IIIC—T4a N2a M0;T3-4a N2b M0;T4b N1-2 M0
IVA—Any T any N M1a
IVB—Any T any N M1b
V0—No venous invasion; V1—presence of venous invasion
L0—No lymphatic vessel invasion; L1—presence of lymphatic vessel invasion

## Complications (Fig. 59.30)

1. **Intestinal obstruction**
2. **Pericolic abscess:** Advanced cases and untreated patients develop perforation of the caecum resulting in pericolic abscess. Tenderness is a feature and pyrexia may be present. Small perforation may get unnoticed. However, free perforation into the peritoneal cavity results in peritonitis which demands urgent laparotomy and resection anastomosis and drainage of peritoneal cavity. Pain is present in the tumour site and may radiate to back, leg or hip as in caecal perforations. It is due to irritation of the psoas muscles or due to irritation of femoral nerve.
   - Diagnosis is confirmed by ultrasound/CT scan.
   - Percutaneous aspiration, followed by elective resection is the best treatment.

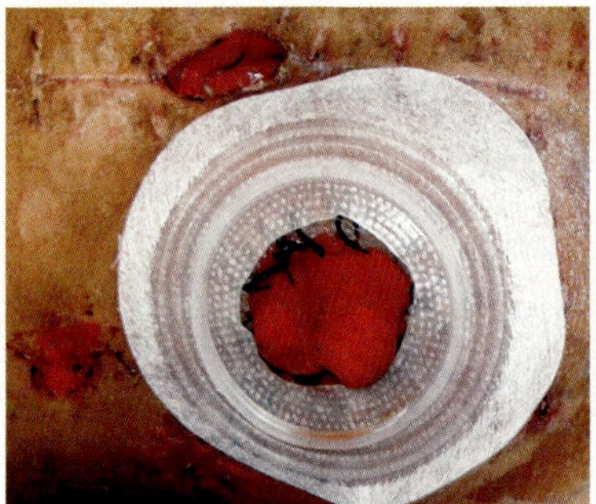

**Fig. 59.30:** Limited colectomy leak—managed by refashioning of the stoma followed by ileostomy

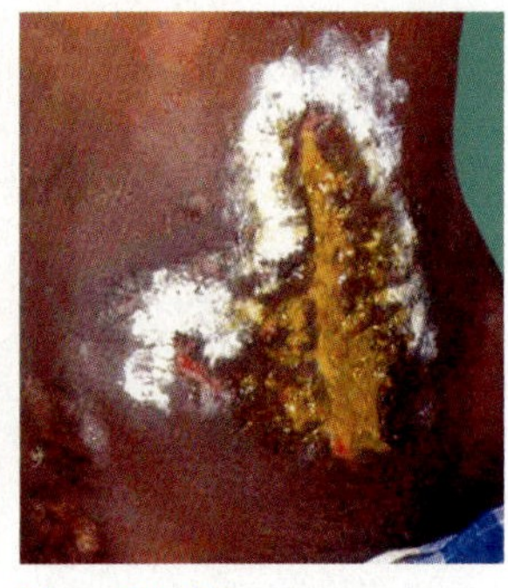

**Fig. 59.31:** Carcinoma colon perforated—pericolic abscess which on draining resulted in faecal fistula

3. **Faecal fistula** (Fig. 59.31)
   - Pericolic abscess when it is incised or drained to the exterior may result in faecal fistula, if there is malignancy.
   - Carcinoma caecum may result in appendicitis and appendicectomy may invariably result in faecal fistula.
4. **Internal fistula:** Colovesical (commonest), colocolic, coloenteric are not uncommon complications of malignancies. They are managed by resection. However, preoperative assessment of fistulae by investigations should be done.

*Pearls of Wisdom*

Involvement of local structures is not a contraindication for radical resection.

## Investigations (Fig. 59.32)

1. **Complete blood picture**—demonstrates low Hb%
2. **Occult blood** in stools.

*Pearls of Wisdom*

Occult blood in the stools may be the finding which gives a 'clue' in many cases of 'anaemia for evaluation'.

3. **Ultrasound:** It is the first baseline investigation to be obtained.
   - It can detect colonic mass.
   - It can detect hydronephrosis, liver metastasis, ascites, para-aortic nodes.
   - Ultrasound-guided biopsy is possible in advanced cases.
   - Definitely it cannot pick up early mucosal lesions or lesions which have not penetrated up to muscularis mucosa or serosa.
4. **Flexible sigmoidoscopy:** 60 cm of colon can be visualised. It is an outpatient procedure. It is indicated in rectal bleeding. An enema is given before the procedure.

**Carcinoma colon—investigations**

**Routine tests/general fitness**
1. **Complete blood count**
   - Hb%: Low indicating anaemia
   - TC, DC: If it is high, it indicates perforation, pericolic abscess
   - ESR: May be increased
2. **Stool:** Occult blood positive
3. Liver function tests, renal function tests and blood sugar estimation
4. Cardiac ECHO/ECG for fitness before surgery

ECOG performance score—page 740

**Diagnostic tests**
1. **Ultrasound:** Simple, baseline noninvasive investigation
   - Can pick up 'colonic mass'
   - Can detect liver metastasis
   - Can demonstrate ascites, para-aortic nodes
2. **CT scan**
   - Objective, more precise about mass, infiltration to vascular pedicles, lymph nodes, ureters
3. **Colonoscopy**
   - Invasive but diagnostic and **Gold standard investigation**
   - Biopsy should be taken for final confirmation

**Metastatic workup—investigations to know spread**
1. Chest X-ray to look for cannonball secondaries
2. CEA: Gross elevation may suggest advanced stage
3. CT is also done to know local and distant spread
4. PET scan: If CEA levels start increasing during follow-up of cases of carcinoma colon

**Fig. 59.32:** Carcinoma colon—investigations

5. **Colonoscopy** is done to take a biopsy from growth and also to rule out synchronous malignancy as seen in 5% of the cases (more than one malignancy at the time of diagnosis). Six biopsy pieces have to be taken for histopathological examination. If biopsy cannot be taken, as in obstruction, brush cytology can be taken (Figs 59.33A and B).
   - Small risk of perforation is present and it is invasive procedure.
   - **Virtual colonoscopy** can pick up polyp of 6 mm size also but biopsy cannot be taken.
6. **CT scan in carcinoma colon**
   - Other than a biopsy, it has all the advantages and it is the investigation of choice after colonoscopy.
   - Anatomical location of the tumour, involvement of serosa.
   - Infiltration of local adjacent structures like ureter (right side)—preoperative stenting is required in such cases.
   - Metastasis in the liver, ascites, para-aortic nodes.

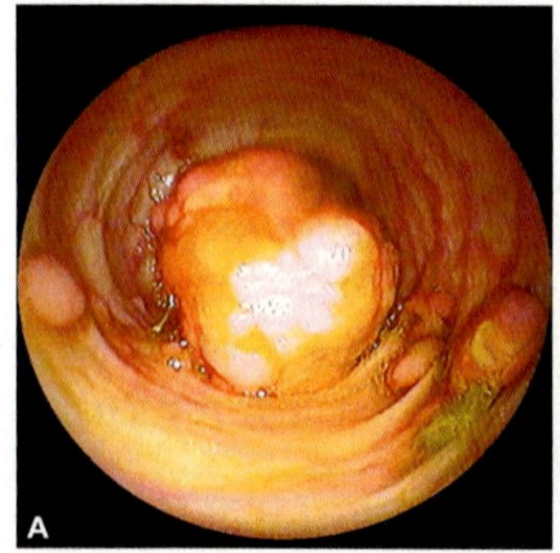


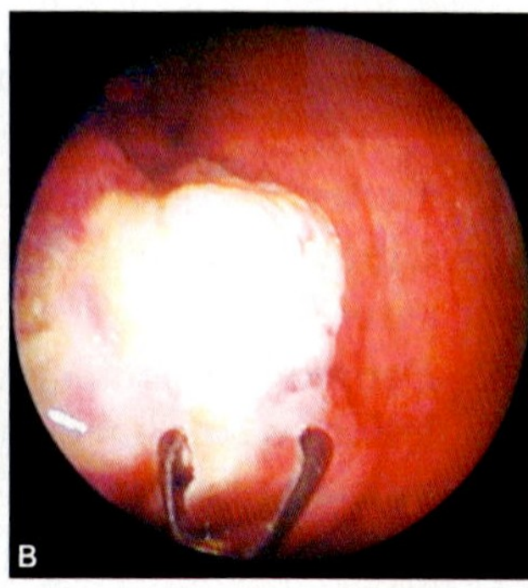


**Figs 59.33A and B:** Colonoscopy shows growth and biopsy is being taken (*Courtesy*: Dr Filipe Alvares, Consultant, Medical Gastroenterologist, KMC, Manipal)

   - Other associated diseases especially in elderly such as aortic aneurysm, gallstone, hiatus hernia, etc.
   - 90% and 95% sensitivity and specificity in detecting liver lesions greater than 1 cm.
7. **Carcinoembryonic antigen (CEA)** (Key Box 59.9).
   - It is a foetal glycoprotein, not present in normal human beings (minute quantities). It is present in the cell membranes of many tissues including colorectal cancer.
   - It is present in the last trimester in the foetus.
   - It has a prognostic rather than a diagnostic value. After treatment of the primary, CEA level should come back to normal. If it does not come back to normal, it indicates residual disease. If it is increased, it suggests either recurrent tumour or secondaries in the liver.

Key Box 59.9

**Carcinoembryonic Antigen—CEA**

- Discovered by Gold and Freedman.
- It is a surface glycoprotein.
- Produced by colorectal epithelium but cleared by Kupffer cells of liver. Its half-life is prolonged (normal—10 days) in cholestasis and hepatocellular dysfunction.
- Normal levels: 0–4 mg/ml.
- Significant increase in the levels is also found in pancreatic carcinoma, gastric carcinoma, lung carcinoma, breast carcinoma.
- Increased CEA in the follow-up period of colorectal cancer suggests metastasis. PET scan may help in these patients when CT/US are normal.
- It has very low sensitivity.
- If preoperative CEA is increased in node-negative colonic cancer, chemotherapy is recommended.

8. **Role of PET scan**
   - Routine use of PET—positron emission tomographic scanning in the primary management of colorectal cancer is not recommended.
   - It is useful in the follow-up cases wherein CEA levels are increasing and the actual cause for the rise is being evaluated.
   - **Chest X-ray:** Colonic carcinoma spreads more often to lungs than carcinoma of stomach giving rise to cannonball secondaries.
9. **Double contrast barium enema** may show irregular filling defect—intrinsic, persistent. It may also show an apple core deformity (Figs 59.34 and 59.35; Key Box 59.10) not routinely done.

Key Box 59.10

**Barium Enema**

- Gives good anatomic and topographic information.
- Can detect associated diverticular disease.
- Small ulcerative lesions can also be diagnosed.

### Prognostic Factors of Carcinoma Colon

- **Spread:** If it is limited to mucosa and there are no nodes, 5-year survival is 90–100%.
- **Age:** Younger patients have poor prognosis.
- **Grade:** Poorly differentiated tumours have worse prognosis.
- **Obstruction and perforation:** Poor prognosis is due to dissemination of malignant cells.
- **Blood transfusion:** Perioperative blood transfusion has poor prognosis.

*Pearls of Wisdom*

Blood transfusion increases number of suppressor T lymphocytes, thus causing immunosuppression. Hence, follow bloodless surgery or autologous blood transfusion.

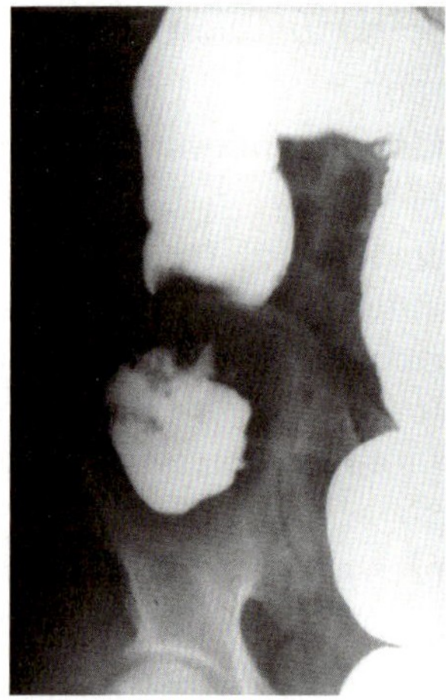

**Fig. 59.34:** Barium enema showing apple core deformity

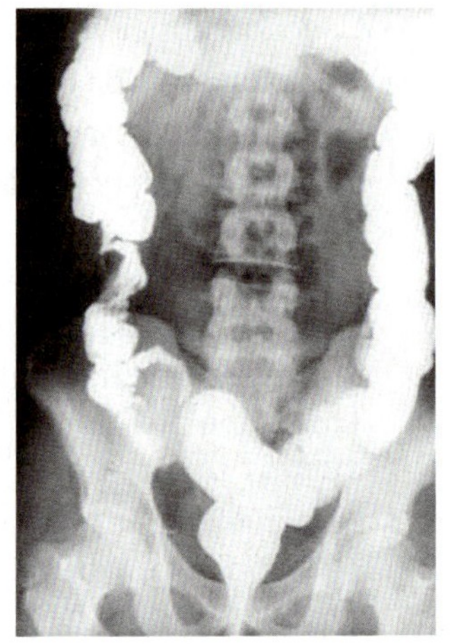

**Fig. 59.35:** Intrinsic, irregular, persistent filling defect

## PREOPERATIVE PREPARATION IN COLONIC SURGERY

1. **Mechanical bowel preparation (MBP):** It was believed that mechanical bowel preparation had the following benefits: It decreases intraoperative contamination, prevents disruption of anastomosis, improves the handling of the bowel, prevents postoperative infectious complications such as wound infection, intra-abdominal abscess and anastomotic leak, and reduces the bacterial count within the colon. However, studies have proved that often liquid faecal matter is present at the site of anastomosis. Liquid faeces are more difficult to handle than solid faeces and spillage of liquid faeces results in increased chance of contamination. MBP damages colocytes, causes oedema and inflammation of colon and facilitates bacterial translocation and anastomotic leak. MBP does not reduce colonic bacterial count/surgical site infection (SSI). The patient needs prior hospitalization and it delays fast-track colonic surgery. In addition to this, MBP prolongs postoperative ileus. In spite of this, many surgeons still use mechanical bowel preparation by using polyethylene glycol (PEG). It is the agent used for cleansing of the gut. PEG is an osmotic laxative and is a balanced solution that is not absorbed. Hence, it is safe for patients with electrolyte imbalances (i.e. renal failure patients) or patients who may not be able to tolerate fluid shifts (i.e. congestive heart failure patients, patients with ascites from liver disease). In addition, **PEG solution is the method of choice for bowel cleansing of infants and children.**
2. **Oral antibiotics:** Colorectal resections have a higher SSI rate than other elective abdominal operations because of the high bacterial load present within the colon lumen, estimated to be $10^{12}$ colony-forming units per gram of stool. Metronidazole 500 mg given may be substituted for erythromycin for better tolerability. Metronidazole has excellent anaerobic activity, enterohepatic circulation, and has been shown to be clinically effective.

   Preoperative intravenous antibiotics + oral antibiotics, with or without mechanical bowel preparation, should represent the standard of care for patients undergoing elective colorectal surgery.
3. **Parenteral antibiotics:** There is a little doubt among surgeons that administration of preoperative parenteral antibiotics prevents SSI. Second generation cephalosporins with metronidazole are given 0 to 2 hours before incision. The dose needs to be repeated in 2 to 6 hours depending upon the antibiotic used and the duration of surgery. **Do not continue these drugs after their use for surgical prophylaxis.**
4. **Diet:** Patients are routinely fasted before an anaesthetic but the required duration of fasting varies with

substances ingested. Fasting for 2 hours is advised for clear fluids. The patients must abstain from taking solid food and milk for 6 hours before surgery. Fried/ fatty food or meal needs a longer time for gastric emptying. Hence, they should fast for 8 hours after fatty food meal. Prolonged fasting is not advisable and hence, **ingestion of carbohydrate-rich clear fluids is recommended until 2 hours prior to surgery**. Advantages of carbohydrate-rich drink are that it reduces postoperative thirst, reduces postoperative hunger and decreases anxiety. It also reduces postoperative insulin resistance and postoperative weight loss. In anabolic state, postoperative nitrogen and protein losses are reduced and hence, lean body mass and muscle strength are better maintained.

5. **Thromboprophylaxis:** Patients undergoing colorectal resections are considered moderate to high-risk group for deep vein thrombosis (DVT)/pulmonary embolism (PE) and, therefore, should receive thromboprophylaxis as a rule. Chemical thromboprophylaxis is given using low molecular weight heparin—enoxaparin/ dalteparin. Unfractionated heparin is equally effective but APTT needs to be monitored. Mechanical thromboprophylaxis can also be done in the operation theatres by using DVT stockings. **The drug used for thromoprophylaxis must be continued for minimum 4–6 weeks in the postoperative period**.
6. **Nasogastric tube:** It is not recommended routinely. Presence of a nasogastric tube will keep the oesophagogastric junction sphincter open and may cause increased chances of aspiration pneumonia. It may delay recovery from paralytic ileus. However, it is definitely indicated in cases of obstructed colon.

**Preoperative Preparation of the Colon**

| | |
|---|---|
| 1. Mechanical bowel preparation | Yes/No |
| 2. Oral antibiotics | May be/yes |
| 3. Fasting for 6 hours | Yes |
| 4. Thromboprophylaxis | Yes |
| 5. Intravenous antibiotics prophylaxis | Yes |
| 6. Nasogastric tube | No |

## Surgery

Over a period of years, radical resections for carcinoma of colon have become less radical pertaining to the extent of bowel resection. For example: One need not remove terminal 30 cm of ileum for carcinoma caecum today. Only 6–8 cm of ileum removal is sufficient in a right hemicolectomy.

**TEN COMMANDMENTS OF SURGERY FOR CARCINOMA COLON—OPEN SURGERY**

1. Should mark the ostomy site preoperatively—Example: after resection anastomosis of left colonic obstructed tumours as diversion stoma (Ileostomy).
2. Should do diagnostic laparoscopy to look for peritoneal nodules. If present, may abandon the procedure, chemotherapy is given and resection attempted later.
3. Should assess the resectability of the growth-fixity to adjacent structures-to do colectomy with or without organ involved, e.g. ureter in right sided lesions.
4. Should remove the growth with at least 7 cm margin, with all groups of regional nodes, chief lymph nodes (origin of superior mesenteric artery and veins), intermediate lymph nodes (branches of the above said vessels-right colic, left colic, etc. and pericolic (vicinity of growth) lymph nodes. Fat fascia and lymphatics called *en block* resection—R-0 resection.
5. Should do the resection without touching or handling the tumour—follow no touch technique of Turnbull.
6. Complete mesocolic excision with central vascular ligation (CME–CVL) is the standard operative principle.
7. Should ensure the cut ends bleed well before anastomosis.
8. Should ensure there is no tension at the suture line.
9. Should do one stage procedure in all elective cases—resection and anastomosis.
10. Should consider, thromboprohylaxis.

## Different Types of Surgery

1. **Carcinoma right colon including caecum:** If it is operable, the treatment is right radical hemicolectomy. Structures removed in this operation are (Fig. 59.36):
   - **Terminal 6–8 cm of ileum**[1]
   - Caecum, appendix and ascending colon
   - One-third of transverse colon
   - All 3 levels of lymph nodes and minimum of 12 lymph nodes should be removed.
   - If the growth is fixed to posterior abdominal wall and common iliac vessels, ileostomy is done first followed by neoadjuvant chemotherapy is given to downstage the tumour followed by resection. This is the only indication for neoadjuvant chemotherapy in carcinoma colon.
   - However, in advanced cases and elderly patients with poor performance status, palliative ileotransverse colostomy can be done.

[1]Removal of a foot of ileum is not necessary unless it has a doubtful vascularity after ligation of pedicles.

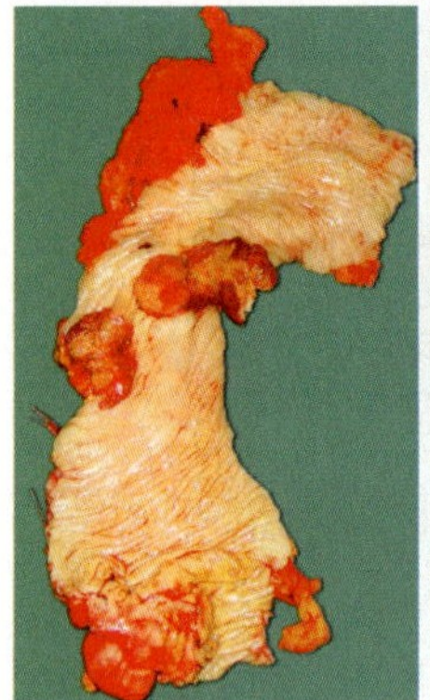

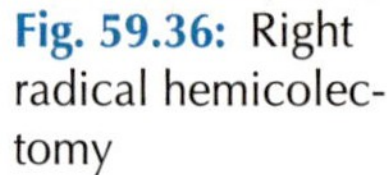

**Fig. 59.36:** Right radical hemicolectomy

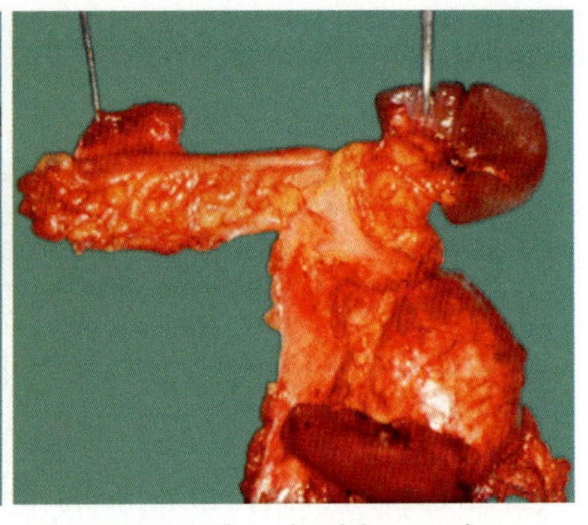

**Fig. 59.37:** Left radical hemicolectomy including removal of the spleen as the growth was infiltrating the spleen—routine removal of spleen should not be done

2. **Carcinoma transverse colon**—'V' resection. The area supplied by middle colic artery is removed followed by end-to-end anastomosis. The patient may need removal of entire transverse colon depending upon lesion.

   When lesion is at hepatic flexure or in the transverse colon, extended right hemicolectomy should be done.
3. **Carcinoma left colon**—left radical hemicolectomy.

   Left half of the transverse colon and descending colon are removed followed by anastomosis of transverse colon to sigmoid colon—this is the area supplied by left colic artery (Fig. 59.37).
4. **Carcinoma sigmoid colon**—radical sigmoid colectomy followed by anastomosis of descending colon to the rectum (colorectal anastomosis). In a few cases, left hemicolectomy may have to be done.
5. **Left-sided colonic tumours with intestinal obstruction**—an emergency temporary transverse colostomy is done to divert the faecal matter and to relieve intestinal obstruction (for more details on colostomy, *see* page 1025). Resection is not done because many patients are elderly with comorbid illness such as diabetes, hypertension, and cardiac illness.
   - General condition of the patient is poor with gross abdominal distension and dehydration.
   - Left colon is loaded with faecal matter. Hence, high chances of anastomotic leakage and faecal peritonitis are present.
   - After 2 weeks, laparotomy is done once again. The primary tumour is resected and end-to-end anastomosis done.
   - This is followed by closure of the colostomy 8 weeks later—**three-stage operation**.
   - Single-stage resection can also be done provided, thorough colonic irrigation through appendicular stump (after appendicectomy), is given and it should be successful in cleaning the entire colon. This is the concept of on-table irrigation and lavage. Indicated in left sided resections more in obstructed colons, after resection.

---

**Note:** *A few diagrammatic representations of the colectomies are shown in the next page* (Figs 59.38 to 59.43).

## ENHANCED RECOVERY PROGRAMME

Enhanced **Re**covery After **S**urgery **(ERAS)**

- It is also described as ERP (enhanced recovery programme), also called **fast track surgery**.
- Traditionally hospital stay following colorectal surgery is about 10–14 days. Now, with a few important steps taken in the pre-, peri- and postoperative periods, it is possible to decrease hospital stay to 2–5 days.

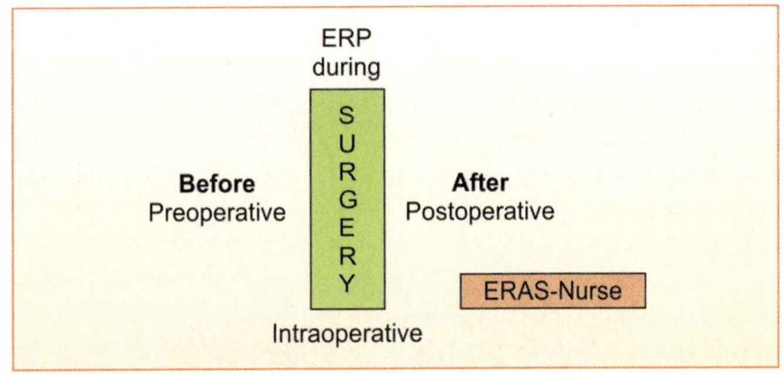


### Preoperative Steps

- Metabolic response to injury/surgery produces increasing metabolic demands and nitrogen consumption. A few days in the postoperative period, there will be catabolic phase resulting in loss of muscle mass. Carbohydrate loading done a few hours before surgery decreases postoperative complication by decreasing postoperative insulin resistance and negative nitrogen balance.
- Only patients with anterior resection need to have bowel preparation. For all other colonic surgery, a single enema is more than enough.

### Perioperative Steps

- Laparoscopic surgery gives the best results in the form of less pain, less wounds, less manipulation, less handling of bowel, no exposure to environment. (Thus recovery is fast.) Anaesthetic requirements are less including analgesia.
- Avoid long-acting narcotic analgesics.
- Avoid pre-medication.
- Mid-thoracic epidural block can be offered.
- Avoid tubes and catheters such as nasogastric tube (Ryle's tube) unless there is distension, postoperative drains (unless suspicious of doubtful anastomosis).

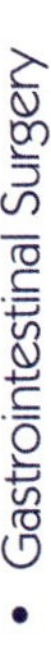

## SURGERIES IN A CASE OF CARCINOMA COLON (Figs 59.38 to 59.43 and Table 59.4)

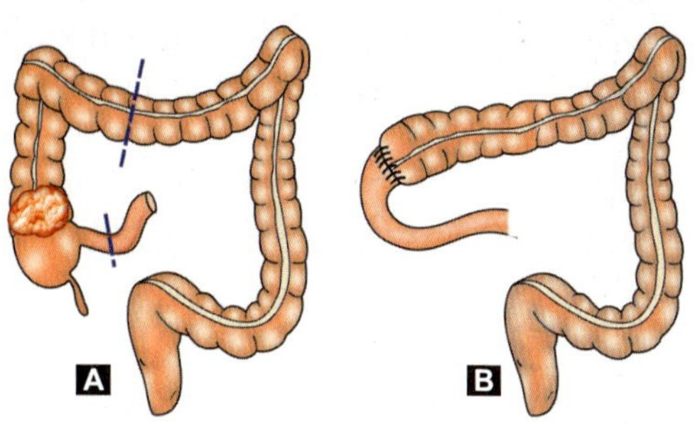


**Figs 59.38A and B:** Right hemicolectomy followed by end-to-end anastomosis—ileocolic

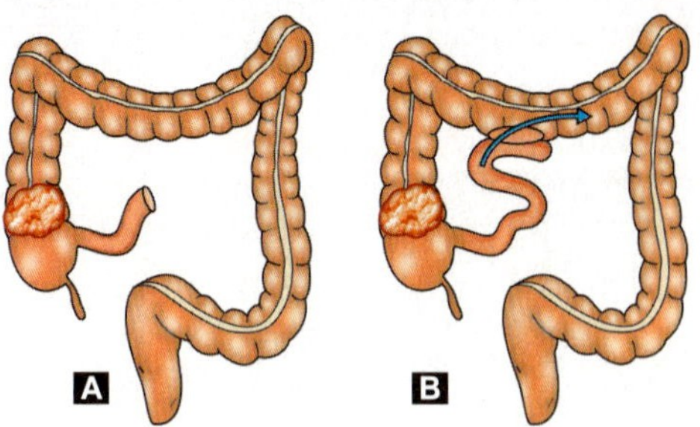


**Figs 59.39A and B:** Palliative ileotransverse anastomosis inoperable case

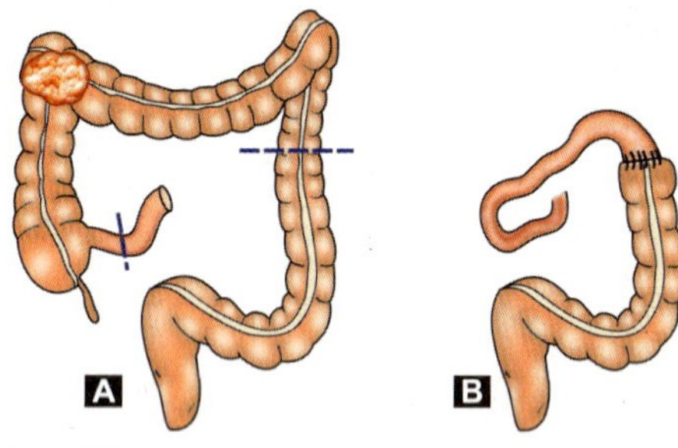


**Figs 59.40A and B:** Extended right hemicolectomy—growth in the hepatic flexure

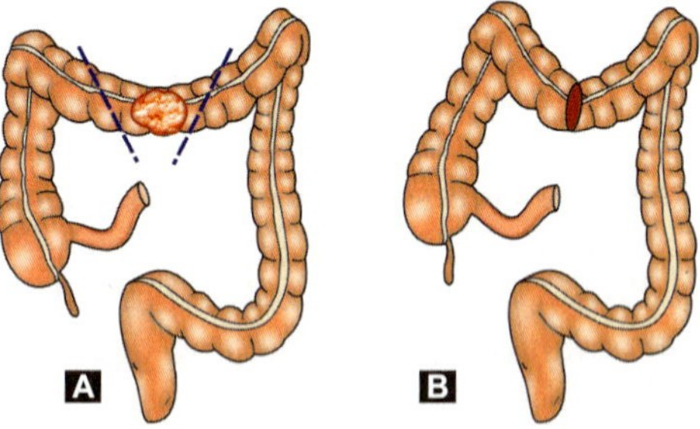


**Figs 59.41A and B:** Transverse colectomy followed by colocolic anastomosis

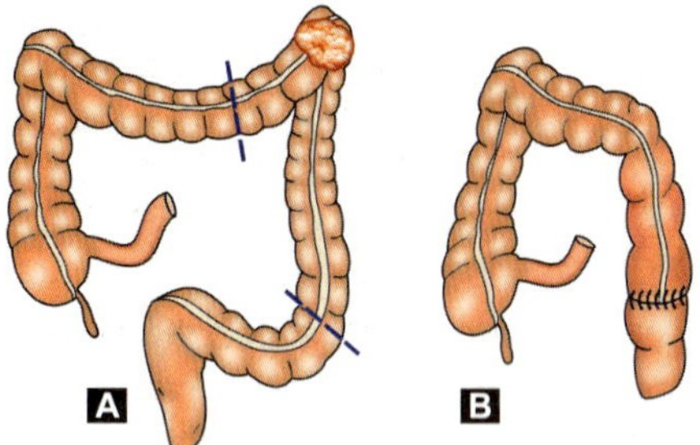


**Figs 59.42A and B:** Left hemicolectomy for growth in the splenic flexure

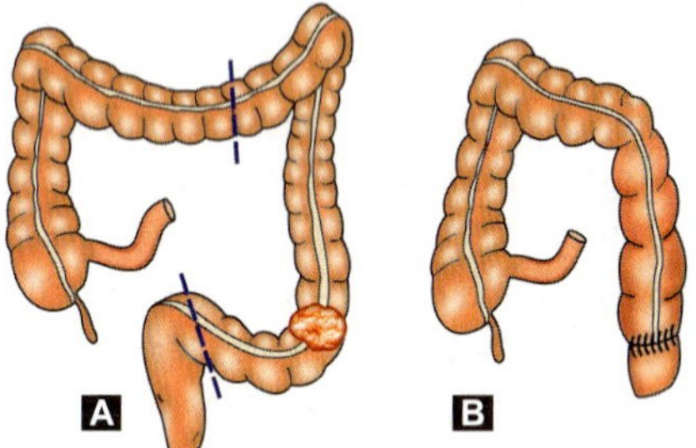


**Figs 59.43A and B:** Resection of rectosigmoid growth followed by colorectal anastomosis

(Figures 59.38 to 59.43 are contributed by Ms Vidushi, MBBS student, KMC, Manipal)

**TABLE 59.4:** Summary of the resections for carcinoma colon

| Site of the tumour | Name of surgery | Part of the bowel resected | Artery supplying | Safe margin |
|---|---|---|---|---|
| Caecum | Right hemicolectomy | Terminal ileum to midtransverse colon | Ileocolic, right colic<br>Right branch of middle colic | 5 cm |
| Ascending colon | Right hemicolectomy | Terminal ileum to midtransverse colon | Ileocolic, right colic<br>Right branch of middle colic | 5 cm |
| Hepatic flexure | Extended right hemicolectomy | Terminal ileum to descending colon | Ileocolic, right colic<br>Middle colic | 5 cm |
| Transverse colon | Extended right hemicolectomy | Terminal ileum to descending colon | Ileocolic<br>Right colic<br>Middle colic | 5 cm |
| Splenic flexure | Extended left hemicolectomy | Right flexure to rectosigmoid | Middle colic<br>Left colic<br>IMA | 5 cm |
| Descending colon | Left hemicolectomy | Left flexure to sigmoid | IMA<br>Left branch of middle colic | 5 cm |

- Avoid central line and arterial lines.
- Preoperative-fluid restrictions—do not overload with water and sodium. Fluids should be less than 2 litres.
- Meticulous technique decreases the time taken for surgery, decrease in number of ports and small incisions for retrieval of specimen—all matters in ERAS.

### Postoperative Steps

- Analgesics should be planned well—epidural blocks.
- Early mobilisation.
- Look for ileus/complications. If present, one should ready to manage.
- Early feeding—carbohydrate liquids.

## POSTOPERATIVE CHEMOTHERAPY

1. pT1-2N0M0 do not require any adjuvant treatment, such patients can be kept on follow-up with routine 3 monthly CEA and annual CECT thorax/abdomen/ pelvis.
2. pT3N0M0 or node positive disease requires adjuvant treatment in the form of concurrent chemoradiotherapy and chemotherapy. 2 cycles of FOLFOX (5-FU + Leucovorin + Oxaliplatin) → Concurrent 5-FU/ Leucovorin and radiation → 2 more cycles of FOLFOX. Oral Capecitabine can be used in place of IV 5-FU.
3. It is preferable to add Oxaliplatin in the chemotherapy regimen, if nodes are positive for metastatic disease. In older population (>65–70 years), it might be of less benefit.
4. Oxaloplatins have been shown to downsize liver metastasis. Chief complication of Oxaliplatins is peripheral neuropathy.

Following are various treatment modalities for colorectal cancer.

**Surgery:** Radical colectomy: All stations of lymph node and complete mesorectal excision is done. Majority are managed without a stoma in elective cases.

Indications for chemotherapy have been given in Key Box 59.11.

Key Box 59.11

**Indications for Chemotherapy**

- All node positive patients. If less than 12 nodes are harvested, it is inadequate lymph node clearance
- In node negative patients, if:
  - T4 lesions are involving free mesothelial surface
  - Major microscopic vein involvement
  - **Signet cell carcinoma**
  - High preoperative CEA
  - Aneuploidy on flow cytometry
  - Microsatellite instability

## POSTOPERATIVE RADIOTHERAPY

Adenocarcinoma colon does not respond well to radiation. Routinely, it is not given. Small bowel is adjacent to the large bowel and so it cannot tolerate high dose of radiation without developing radiation enteritis. Surgery remains the gold standard for carcinoma colon. Soft tissue infiltration into psoas muscle or abdominal wall or inoperable recurrent tumours are indications for radiotherapy.

## METASTATIC DISEASE WITHOUT OBSTRUCTION

Patients with isolated liver/lung secondaries should also undergo treatment with a radical approach as even in these cases with resection of the primary and adequate liver/lung resection, a good disease control can be achieved.

1. A typical course of neoadjuvant therapy comprises concurrent 5-FU/Capecitabine and radiation in cases of large lesions abutting the abdominal wall or down into the pelvis. A dose of 45–50 Gy is used to treat the pelvis including the growth and the draining lymphatic regions followed by 5 Gy boost to the tumour itself.
2. Following neoadjuvant therapy, patient should be re-evaluated using CT/MRI for possibility of resection.
3. Surgery is usually considered after 6–8 weeks following neoadjuvant therapy as the maximal response to the treatment may take up to 2 months.
4. Further adjuvant treatment is to be given following surgery depending upon the histopathological report.

## MANAGEMENT OF LIVER SECONDARY

- CT scan and PET scan are done to evaluate local/ systemic disease. Provided there is no systemic spread, liver secondaries have to be treated aggressively. Pattern of recurrence in colonic carcinomas is more commonly distant, i.e. they tend to recur more commonly at distant sites such as liver, and lungs. As a result, systemic treatment is essential.
- Liver-directed therapies such as hepatic arterial chemotherapy infusion/embolisation, radiofrequency-ablation, radiotherapy should be used in treatment of isolated liver metastasis.
- Isolated liver metastasis is not a contraindication for definitive resection of the primary.
- Indications for liver resection are given in Key Box 59.12.

Key Box 59.12

**Indication for Resection of Liver Metastasis**

- Solitary metastasis or metastasis confined to one lobe
- <3 metastasis in both lobes
- Absence of extrahepatic disease

### Novel Agents in Colorectal Cancers

1. Bevacizumab—anti-VEGF (vascular endothelial growth factor) monoclonal antibody. It has anti-angiogenesis property, thereby controlling the tumour growth.
2. Cetuximab and panitumumab—anti-EGFR (epidermal growth factor) monoclonal antibody is given, only if K-RAS is negative.

### Follow-up (Key Box 59.13)

Most of the colonic cases are curable, if diagnosed and treated early. Also metachronous lesion can occur in the rest of the colon. Hence, certain tests are necessary during follow-up.

Key Box 59.13

**Follow-up of Colorectal Cancer**

| Tests | Duration | In years |
|---|---|---|
| 1. Haemo-occult | Once in 3–6 months | 3 |
| 2. Colonoscopy | 6 months after surgery, later once in a year | 3 |
| 3. Alkaline phosphatase | Once in 3–6 months for 3 years | 3 |
| 4. CEA | Once in 6 months | 3 |
| 5. CECT chest and abdomen | Yearly | 3 |

## TREATMENT OF RECURRENT OR METASTATIC CANCER

- Recurrence or metastasis is suspected during follow-up by abnormal values of investigation.
- Recurrent tumour should be resected *en bloc*—it may amount to a more radical procedure including resection of duodenum, liver, kidney.
- Metastasis in the liver (*see* Key Box 59.12).

## CHEMOPREVENTION OF COLONIC CANCER

1. **Folic acid:** It is an important vitamin with many functions. In the absence of folic acid, hypomethylation can occur. As a result of this overexpression of proto-oncogenes such as K-RAS and c-Myc can occur. Deficiency of folic acid causes imbalances in the nucleotide pool leading to DNA break and mutation. Thus folic acid supplementation should be given in adenoma specially when baseline levels of folic acid is low.
2. **Dietary fibres:** Fibres decrease the transit time, they dilute the carcinogens and are used to present development of cancer. Cellulose, hemicelluloses and pectin are a few examples. Fibres also produce short chain in fatty acids causing fermentation by faecal flora. Thus colonic pH becomes more acidic which in turn inhibits carcinogenesis.
3. **Aspirin, calcium, and sulindac** also have been used to prevent cancer developing in an adenoma.

## COLON SCREENING

- Large bowel is the 4th most common site for cancer after lung, stomach and breast.
- More common in North America, North Europe and Australia. Lowest rates in Africa, India.
- 75% of CRC develop in people with no known risk factors apart from older age.

### Screening Options

1. **Faecal occult blood test (FOBT)**
   - It is guaiac test which will detect elevated level of blood in stool. It requires two samples from each of three consecutive stools which are smeared onto cards.
   - **False positive:** Vegetables, fruits, red meat, aspirin or any other bleeding lesion proximal to colon screening, FOBT has shown to decrease mortality by 20 to 30%.
2. **Flexible sigmoidoscopy (FS)**
   - Reduces incidence and mortality of distal CRC by around 60%.
   - Single FS at the age of 60 is recommended in UK.
   - In US, 5-yearly screening is being done.
3. **Colonoscope screening**
   - Should be done if there is distal adenoma (chances of proximal adenoma are high).
   - 70% of all advanced colorectal neoplasia will be detected with this strategy.
   - Procedure is painful, requires sedation and analgesics.
   - Chances of perforation are 1 in 500 to 2000 cases.
   - It requires skills of an experienced endoscopist.
4. **Virtual colonoscopy**
   - It is an alternative but not yet become popular because of time, cost and preparation.
   - It is done with the help of CT scan.
   - Biopsy cannot be taken.

## DIVERTICULAR DISEASE OF COLON

It is an acquired condition, in which colonic mucosa herniates through the circular muscle fibres at weak points, where blood vessels penetrate the colonic wall. Since, it is acquired, it lacks the muscle coat. They are thin, more prone for infections and perforation. Hence, they are termed pseudodiverticuli.

### Aetiopathogenesis

- The disease is common in western population wherein diet is very **poor in fibres** because of refining of sugar and flour. **Nonstarch polysaccharides (NSP)** or low dietary fibres are the chief factor for **diverticulosis of colon** (Key Box 59.14).

Key Box 59.14

**NSP and Diseases**

- Diverticular disease
- Obesity and diabetes mellitus
- Constipation, and piles
- Breast cancer and colonic cancer

- It requires very high pressure for propulsion of faecal matter and this is believed to cause characteristic thickening of muscles and herniation of mucosa (Figs 59.44A and B). Hence, it is called pulsion diverticulum.
- In Africans and Indians, the disease is rare because of high fibre content of the diet.
- The disease starts after the age of 40. Any stress or emotional disorders may add to the constipation already caused by dietary factors and result in diverticular formation.
- **90% of them affect sigmoid colon.** Rectum is spared in majority. Rarely, it affects right colon.
- Diverticulae project between antimesenteric and mesenteric borders with taenia but they never penetrate taenia (Fig. 59.45).
- There is **muscle hypertrophy,** which project into the lumen as obstructive folds. The mucosa is essentially normal. Slowly, luminal diameter is narrowed.
- **Inflammation** occurs in the pericolonic tissue with or without abscess formation.

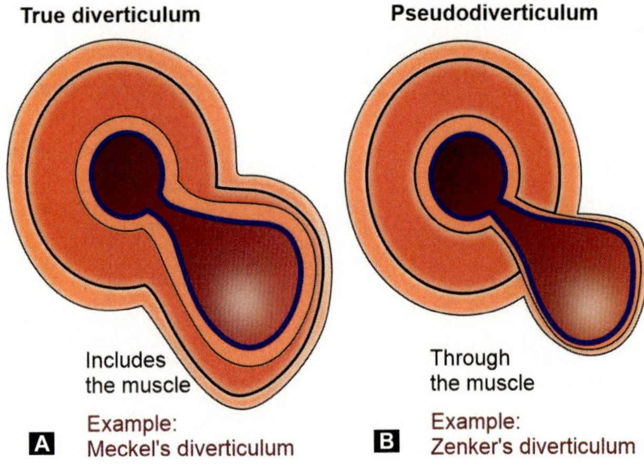


**Figs 59.44A and B:** Diverticulum

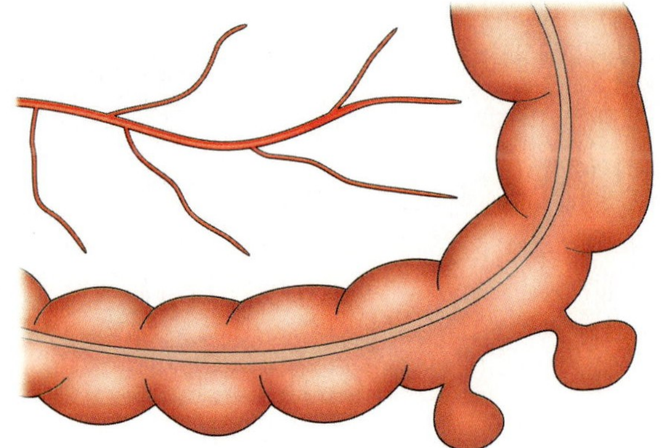

**Fig. 59.45:** Sigmoid diverticulae

## Structural Changes in Colonic Wall of Patients with Diverticulosis

- Mycosis
- Thickening (neither hypertrophy nor hyperplasia) of the circular muscle layer.
- Shortening of the taenia coli
- Luminal narrowing
- ↑ elastin deposition in taenia coli
- ↑ type III collagen synthesis
- ↑ collagen cross-linking

## Segmentation

- Law of Laplace: Pressure = K × Tension/Radius
- Sigmoid colon has small diameter resulting in highest pressure zone.
- Segmentation = motility process in which the segmental muscular contractions separate the lumen into chambers.
- Segmentation → increased intraluminal pressure → mucosal herniation → diverticulosis.
- May explain why high fibre prevents diverticuli by creating a larger diameter colon and less vigorous segmentation.
- Collagen connective tissue diseases such as Ehlers-Danlos syndrome, Marfan's syndrome, and autosomal-dominant polycystic kidney disease result in structural changes in the bowel wall, leading to decreased resistance of the wall to intraluminal pressures and thus allowing protrusion of diverticula.

## Clinical Features (Fig. 59.46)

1. **Diverticulosis:** It refers to presence of diverticulosis without much symptoms. But on careful questioning, patients do have lower abdominal distention, heaviness, flatulence, etc. Vague abdominal pain is also felt in the left iliac fossa.
2. **Diverticulitis:** Left-sided lower abdominal pain, moderate to severe, is associated with passage of loose stools. The pain is partially relieved on passing flatus.
   - Bleeding per rectum can be the presenting feature, sometimes it can be massive.
   - Low-grade fever, tenderness, rigidity and even mass may be present in the left iliac fossa (like left-sided appendicitis). The mass is thickened, inflamed, tender and sigmoid. Such attacks result in abscess which rupture into hollow organs and give rise to fistulae (Fig. 59.47).

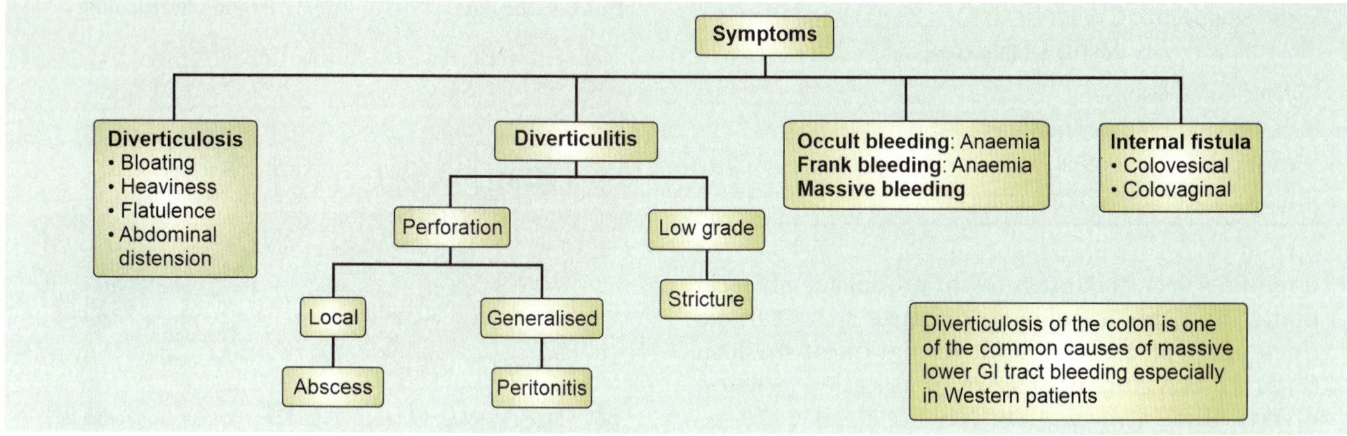


**Fig. 59.46:** Summary of diverticular disease

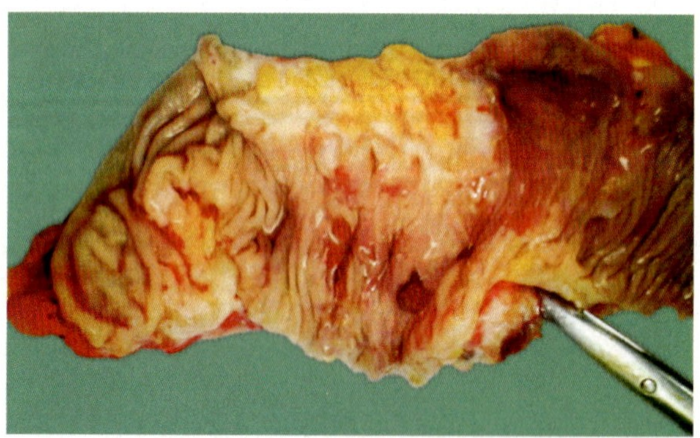

**Fig. 59.47:** Perforated diverticula at surgery—resected specimen (*Courtesy*: Dr Ramesh Rajan, Surgical Gastroenterologist, Trivandrum Medical College, Kerala)

3. **Internal fistulae:** Colovesical fistulae (commonest) give rise to pneumaturia (flatus in the urine) and rarely faeces in the urine (Key Box 59.15). Other fistulae are colovaginal, coloenteric, and colocutaneous.

Key Box 59.15

**Causes of Internal Fistulae**

- Diverticular disease of colon (commonest)
- Carcinoma of colon
- Crohn's disease
- Radiation
- Tuberculosis

For summary of diverticular disease *see* Fig. 59.46.

## Classification/Staging System

### *Hinchey Classification* (Fig. 59.48)

I. Pericolic abscess
II. Walled off pelvic abscess
III. Generalised purulent peritonitis
IV. Generalised faecal peritonitis

Hinchey stages I and II may be treated by sigmoid colectomy and primary anastomosis (a one-stage operation).

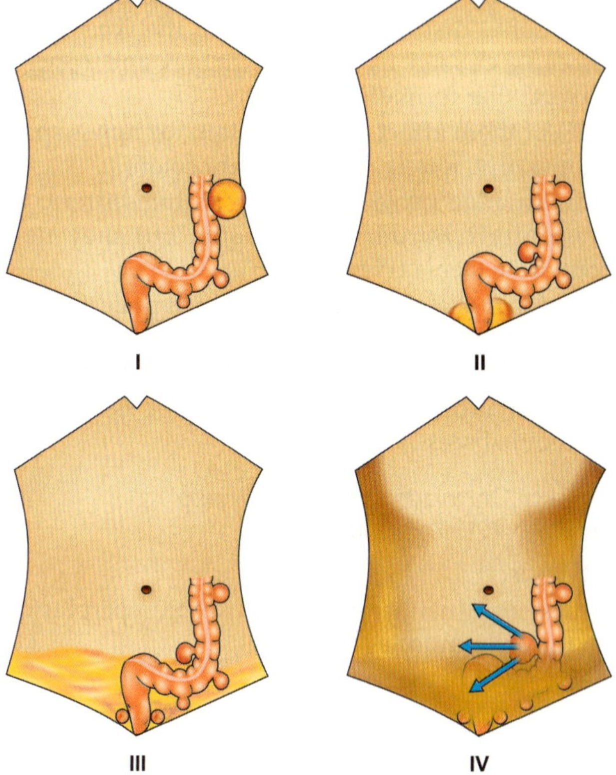


**Fig. 59.48:** Hinchey classification

Hinchey stages III and IV are treated by sigmoid colectomy followed by end-colostomy and Hartmann pouch.

*Pearls of Wisdom*

The most common fistula in acute diverticulitis is colovesical followed by colovaginal fistula.

## Investigations in Elective Cases

1. **Sigmoidoscopy:** Mucosa may be normal or may show erythematous and oedematous changes. Ulcers are absent. Opening of diverticulae can be seen.

2. **Barium enema: Contraindicated in acute cases.**
   - It may show **saw-tooth** appearance due to muscle hypertrophy.
   - It may show a long stricture.
   - **Champagne glass sign:** Partial filling of diverticula by barium with stercolith inside the diverticula.
3. **Colonoscopy** to confirm the findings and to rule out **carcinoma colon** (Figs 59.49 and 59.50). It is the investigation of choice in diverticulosis.

*Pearls of Wisdom*

Sigmoidoscopy, colonoscopy and barium enema are contraindicated in acute diverticulitis.

4. **Ultrasound and CT scan** (Key Box 59.16) are the investigations of choice in acute diverticulitis (Fig. 59.51).

Key Box 59.16

**CT Scan Acute Diverticulitis**

- Can detect thick muscular folds—confirms the diagnosis.
- Detects an abscess and can confirm complication.
- Detects extraluminal air or contrast—confirms perforation.
- Can rule out other causes—acute pancreatitis with pericolic collection, etc.
- **It is the investigation of choice in acute diverticulitis.**
- Thickened colonic wall >4 mm.
- Pelvic abscess can be diagnosed.

## Complications

1. **Massive haemorrhage** per rectum: Haemorrhage is due to vessels in the base of diverticulae, more so in atherosclerotic or hypertensive patients.
2. **Stricture** of sigmoid colon can develop due to recurrent attacks resulting in intestinal obstruction.
3. **Perforation** may result in peritonitis, pericolic abscess or pelvic abscess (Fig. 59.52 and Key Box 59.17).
4. **Fistula formation:** Internal fistulae occur due to inflammatory adhesions and abscess formation which ruptures resulting in fistulae. Thus, colovesical, colovaginal, colointestinal fistulae can occur.

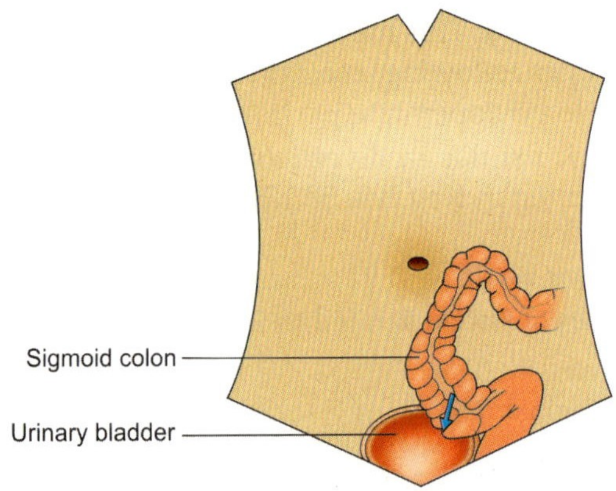


**Fig. 59.49:** Colovesical fistula (arrow)

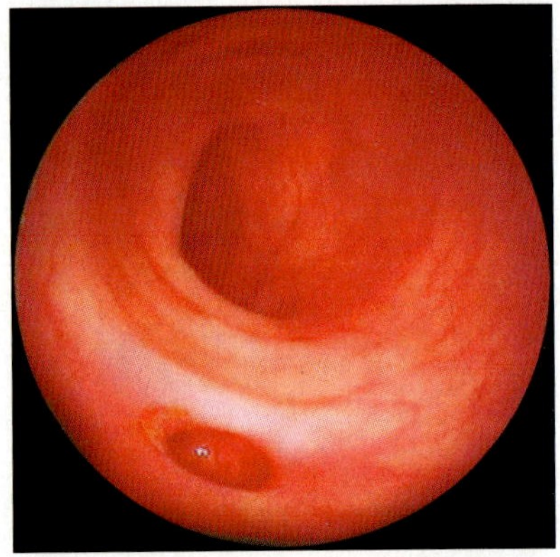

**Fig. 59.50:** Colonoscopy showing opening of diverticula

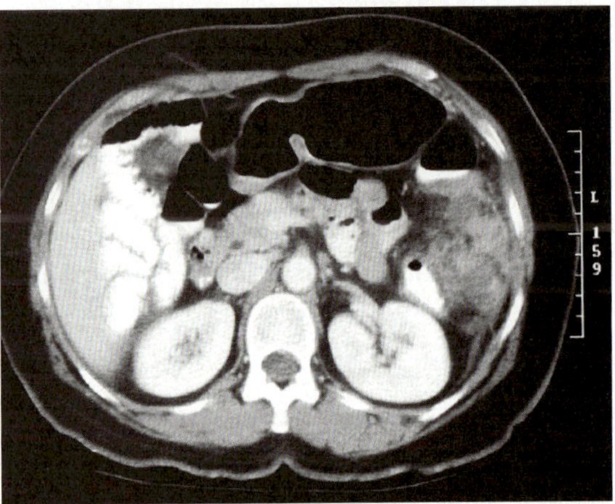

**Fig. 59.51:** CT scan showing pericolic abscess on the left paracolic space

Key Box 59.17

**Pericolic Abscess**

- Abscess depends on the ability of the pericolic tissues to localise the spread of the inflammatory process.
- Intra-abdominal abscesses are formed by—anastomotic leakage: 35%—diverticular disease: 23%.
- Limited spread of the perforation forms an inflammatory phlegmon, while further (but still localised) progression creates an abscess.
- Signs and symptoms: High grade fever with or without leukocytosis despite adequate antibiotics, tender mass.
- Treatment:
  - A. **Small pericolic abscess:** 90% will respond to antibiotics and conservative management alone. Often it is retrocolic. May present as swelling in the loin.
  - B. **Percutaneous abscess drainage** (PAD) is the treatment of choice for small, simple (>4 cm), well-defined collections. 100% success in simple unilocular abscesses.
  - C. **Open drainage:** In cases of multilocular collection, abscesses associated with enteric fistulas, and abscesses containing solid material, drainage of pus, resection and Hartmann's operation is the ideal choice. Closure of colostomy is done after 6–8 weeks.

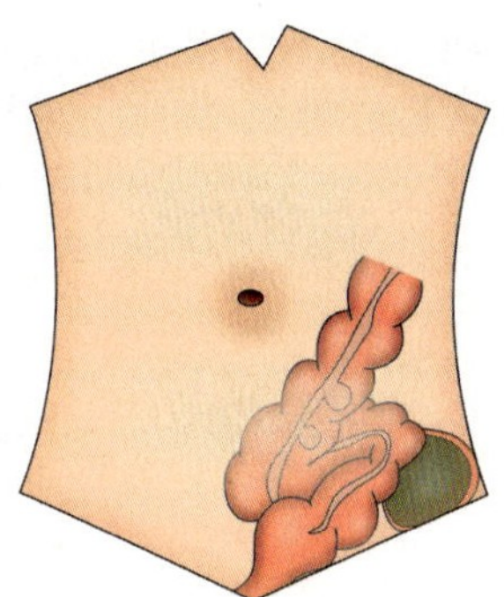

Fig. 59.52: Pericolic abscess

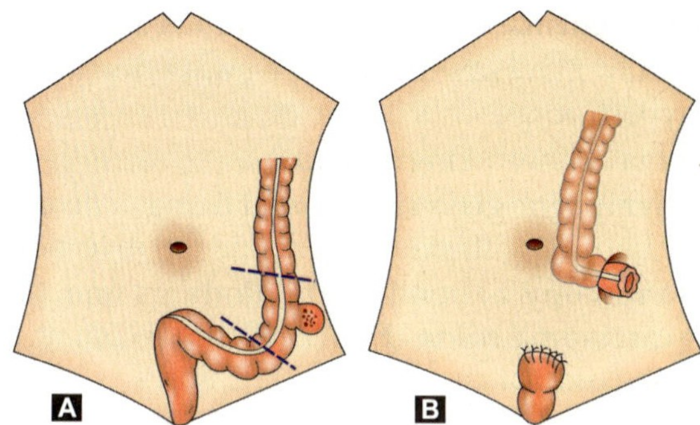


Figs 59.53A and B: Hartmann's procedure

## Differential Diagnosis

- Carcinoma of the colon
- Inflammatory bowel disease
- Ischaemic colitis
- Irritable bowel syndrome
- Pelvic inflammatory disease.

## Indications for Surgery

1. Failure to respond to conservative/dietary advice
2. Two attacks of diverticulitis
3. Complications.

## Treatment

1. **Stage of diverticulosis** or in those patients who have recovered from one attack of diverticulitis.
   - High residue diet
   - Fruits and vegetables
   - Whole meal bread and flour
   - Bulk purgative
   - To avoid constipation

   *Diet*
   - High fibre diet, optimal amount of daily fibre is unknown.
   - 20 to 30 g per day is widely recommended.
   - Recommendation to avoid seeds, nuts and popcorn.
2. **Acute diverticulitis with pericolic abscess**
   - Rest, hospitalisation, correct hydration
   - IV antibiotics: Bactericidal against gram –ve and anaerobes.
   - Abscess is aspirated under ultrasound guidance.
   - After 4–6 weeks, elective sigmoid colectomy and anastomosis is done.
3. **Diverticulitis with peritonitis**

   A. **Hartmann's procedure** is the choice: Sigmoid colon is resected, end-colostomy is done by using descending colon followed by closure of rectal stump (Figs 59.53A and B).
   - After 4–6 weeks, colorectal anastomosis is done.

   B. However, if a **perforation is small** and the general condition is good after the resection, the colon is irrigated with 8–10 litres of saline till the contents are clear. This is followed by colorectal anastomosis in the same sitting.
4. **Treatment of fistulae:** As an elective procedure, with good preparation, after confirming the site of fistula, resection of the sigmoid colon with closure of fistula can be done.

## MISCELLANEOUS

## FAECAL FISTULA

### Classification

#### *Depending upon the Nature of the Disease or a Surgical Procedure*

I. **Primary or type I fistula:** It develops as a result of an underlying disease affecting gut. Example: Carcinoma colon infiltrating urinary bladder resulting in colovesical fistula or rupture through the skin resulting in pericolic abscess, fistula.

II. **Secondary or type II fistula:** It occurs after injury to otherwise normal gut. Examples: Left colonic/right colonic injury in percutaneous nephrolithotomy (PCNL) for renal stones or following anastomotic leak.

#### *Depending upon the Site of the Fistula*

A. **Lateral fistula:** It occurs after a colocolic or ileocolic anastomosis wherein a few sutures would have given way in the immediate postoperative period.

B. **End fistula:** This means both ends of the intestines are open following resection and anastomosis giving rise to postoperative peritonitis.

- A few fistulae in diverticular disease of the colon are given in Key Box 59.18.

Key Box 59.18

**Types of Fistula Related to Diverticular Disease**

- Colovesical: 65%
- Colovaginal: 25%
- Colocutaneous
- Coloenteral

### Bacterial Flora

- More than 99% of faecal bacterial flora are **anaerobic**.
- Most common anaerobe is ***Bacteroides fragilis,*** with a count of $10^{10}$/g of wet faeces. Clostridia, Lactobacillus are other organisms.
- ***E. coli*** is the predominant **aerobic organism**. Count is $10^7$/g of faeces. Klebsiella, Proteus, and Enterobacter are other **aerobes**. ***Streptococcus faecalis*** is the principal enterococcus.

### Clinical Manifestations

- Postoperative patient 'not doing well'—prolonged paralytic ileus, faeculent discharge from wound or drainage site, etc. is an indication of faecal fistula.
- Features of septic shock: Often patient may not complain of abdominal pain but manifestations can be of renal failure, tachycardia, tachypnoea and hypotension.

### Diagnosis

- Total counts are elevated—it indicates infection.
- Creatinine and urea values are high indicating renal failure.
- Ultrasound to detect any collection.
- CECT can detect intraperitoneal collection, pneumoperitoneum, anastomotic leak. However, creatinine should be normal before doing CT scan. Often patients are in sepsis with renal failure.

### Treatment (Figs 59.54 to 59.56)

- Control of infection
- Drainage of sepsis—laparotomy, resection and anastomosis, ileostomy or colostomy may be necessary.
- Lateral fistula may heal with total parenteral nutrition provided there is no distal obstruction (TPN).
- End fistula may require resuturing with or without proximal diversion colostomy/ileostomy.

## COLONIC STRICTURE

### Causes

1. Malignant: Adenocarcinoma colon is the commonest cause of stricture colon (rarely lymphomas, carcinoid).
2. Tuberculosis: Uncommon cause of stricture in the ascending colon.
3. Ischaemic: Uncommon/rare cause—left colon may be affected.
4. Inflammatory bowel disease: Any ulcers, including amoebic, may heal with fibrosis resulting in stricture.
5. Diverticular stricture
6. Radiation stricture
7. Endometriomas: Ectopic endometriosis tissue responds to cyclic hormonal stimulation causing inflammation and fibrosis.

### Clinical Features

- Progressive constipation
- Change in bowel habits
- Bleeding per rectum
- Features of large bowel obstruction
- Mass may/may not be felt.

### Investigation

Colonoscopy and biopsy.

### Treatment

- Single-stage resection and end-to-end anastomosis.
- Treatment of the cause.

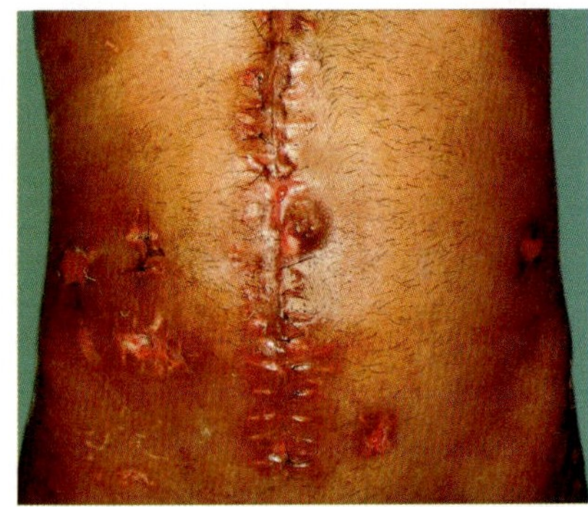

**Fig. 59.54:** This patient underwent three surgical procedures for treatment of fistula. Initial surgery was right hemicolectomy for ileocaecal tuberculosis. Second surgery was resection and a proximal diversion ileostomy because of the leak and finally after two months, closure of ileostomy was done followed by ileotransverse anastomosis

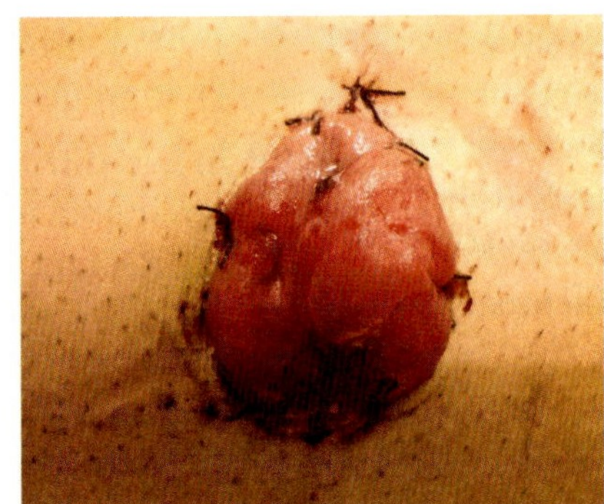

**Fig. 59.55:** Ileostomy was done to divert the proximal intestinal contents. To have the maximum benefit it should be an end ileostomy and the distal end can be brought out as mucus fistula. However, often during exploration of this type of cases, it is not possible

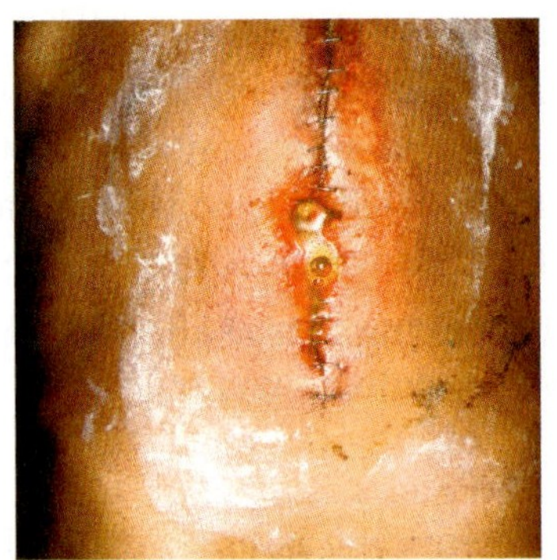

**Fig. 59.56:** A case of faecal fistula following ileal resection for obstruction caused by a band. Following resection anastomosis on the fifth postoperative day, air-mixed faecal matter started coming out from the wound. CT scan revealed small lateral fistula. The patient responded to conservative treatment with TPN given for 14 days. Fistula subsided

## MULTIPLE CHOICE QUESTIONS

1. **The following feature is true of adenomatous polyps of the large intestine:**
   A. Most are sessile
   B. Most can be removed by colonoscopic snaring
   C. Adenoma smaller than 15 mm in diameter do not carry the risk of malignant potential
   D. Young people are more likely to have these polyps
2. **Common premalignant conditions for colonic cancer include the following, *except*:**
   A. Familial polyposis coli
   B. Ulcerative colitis
   C. Adenomatous polyp
   D. Peutz-Jeghers syndrome
3. **Flexion of the hip can be caused by:**
   A. Carcinoma splenic flexure
   B. Carcinoma caecum
   C. Carcinoma sigmoid colon
   D. Carcinoma hepatic flexure
4. **Abscess in the lateral abdominal wall can be a feature of:**
   A. Acute pancreatitis
   B. Perforated carcinoma caecum
   C. Diverticular perforation
   D. Meckel's diverticular perforation
5. **Mechanical bowel preparation is best given using:**
   A. Plenty of saline
   B. Oral mannitol
   C. Glycerine enema
   D. Whole gut irrigation using oral polyethylene glycol
6. **Which one of this is true in surgery for malignancy of colon?**
   A. No touch technique of Turnbull
   B. Right-sided lesions are treated by colostomy
   C. Left-sided lesions are treated by resection
   D. Removal of 30 cm of ileum along with colon
7. **Following is true about prognostic factors of carcinoma colon, *except*:**
   A. Elderly patients have poorer prognosis
   B. Perioperative blood transfusion has poor prognosis
   C. Survival is good if it is limited to mucosa and there are no nodes
   D. Obstruction and perforation is associated with poor prognosis
8. **In familial polyposis coli, colonoscopy is done to look for**
   A. Stricture of colon
   B. Look for ileal disease
   C. Look for perforation
   D. Look for polyps and malignancy
9. **Proliferative growth is more common in the _______ colon:**
   A. Right B. Left
   C. Rectosigmoid D. Splenic flexure
10. **The 'Gold standard' investigation for detection of colonic cancer is:**
    A. Ultrasound abdomen
    B. CT scan
    C. Barium enema
    D. Colonoscopy and biopsy
11. **Following are the features of intestinal tuberculosis, *except*:**
    A. It can be secondary to pulmonary tuberculosis
    B. Terminal ileum and caecum are commonly involved
    C. Ulcers are transverse
    D. Ulcers do not result in stricture
12. **In which of the following malignancies anaemia is an important method of presentation?**
    A. Malignant melanoma
    B. Carcinoma breast
    C. Carcinoma caecum
    D. Carcinoma pancreas
13. **The most common fistula in diverticulitis is:**
    A. Colovesical B. Colovaginal
    C. Colorectal D. Colocolic
14. **Which of the following is a true diverticulum?**
    A. Sigmoid diverticulum
    B. Meckel's diverticulum
    C. Parabronchial diverticulum
    D. Laryngeal diverticulam
15. **In hereditary nonpolyposis colorectal cancer, which carcinoma is more often seen?**
    A. Rectum
    B. Rectosigmoid
    C. Transverse colon
    D. Caecum and ascending colon
16. **Incidence of malignancy in familial polyposis coli is:**
    A. 10% B. 30%
    C. 50% D. 100%
17. **Following are true for carcinoembryonic antigen, *except*:**
    A. It is a glycoprotein
    B. It is tumour marker for carcinoma colon

C. It should be done in all cases of carcinoma colon before surgery
D. Produced by colorectal epithelium and cleared by kidney

**18. Following are true for right hemicolectomy for carcinoma caecum, *except*:**

A. Right one-third of transverse colon is also removed
B. Greater omentum should be removed
C. Terminal 30 cm of the ileum should be removed
D. Duodenum can get injured during surgery

**19. Indications for postoperative chemotherapy following colectomy for carcinoma include following, *except*:**

A. Signet ring carcinoma
B. Lymph nodes are positive
C. Lymphovenous involvement
D. Involvement of muscularis propria

**20. The most common aerobic organism present in a sigmoid colonic faecal fistula is:**

A. Clostridia
B. Lactobacillus
C. Bacteroides fragilis
D. *E. coli*

**21. What is the chief complication of Oxaliplatins**

A. Agranulocytosis
B. Peripheral neuropathy
C. Hepatitis
D. Cardiomyopathy

**22. What is Hartmann's procedure?**

A. Low anterior resection
B. Resection of sigmoid followed by colostomy and closure of rectal stump
C. Sigmoid resection followed by colostomy and open the rectum to exterior
D. No resection but the sigmoid which is gangrenous is brought out

**23. Which one of the following is true for adenomatous polyps?**

A. Tubular adenomas have high risk of malignancy
B. Pedunculated lesions have more malignant potential
C. Failure of elevation after injection of solution into polyp suggest malignancy.
D. They are uncommon causes of polyps in the colon

**24. Which one of following is true for CECT scan for colonic cancer?**

A. In every patient who had rectal bleeding it is done
B. It is ideal investigation to detect peritoneal disease
C. It is a good investigation to know the layers of colon involvement
D. It is a diagnostic investigation in patients with palpable mass

**Answers**

| | | | | | | | | | |
|---|---|---|---|---|---|---|---|---|---|
| **1.** B | **2.** D | **3.** B | **4.** D | **5.** D | **6.** A | **7.** A | **8.** D | **9.** A | **10.** D |
| **11.** D | **12.** D | **13.** A | **14.** B | **15.** D | **16.** D | **17.** D | **18.** C | **19.** D | **20.** D |
| **21.** B | **22.** B | **23.** C | **24.** D | | | | | | |

Chapter 60

# Intestinal Obstruction

- Pathophysiology, basic principles in management
- Sigmoid volvulus
- Meckel's diverticulum
- Adhesions and bands
- Gallstone ileus
- Intussusception
- Mesenteric vascular occlusion
- Hirschsprung's disease
- Atresia and stenosis
- Arrested rotation with bands
- Volvulus neonatorum
- Meconium ileus
- Anorectal anomalies
- Imperforate anus
- Paralytic ileus
- Pseudointestinal obstruction
- Intestinal obstruction in pregnancy
- Ileosigmoid knotting
- Iliac graft site hernia
- Internal hernia
- Food bolus obstruction
- Capsule obstruction
- Malrotation and midgut volvulus

## INTRODUCTION

- Intestinal obstruction is a challenging surgical emergency encountered by general surgeons. This can affect any age group starting from neonate to an old man. It can affect a school going boy, working woman or a man during their peak of life. Sometimes it can be fatal either due to delay in the diagnosis, delay in the treatment or complications related to surgery. Abdomen is a Pandora's box. Sometimes, it is difficult to pinpoint the cause of obstruction.
- Adhesions and hernia are the two most common causes of intestinal obstruction. Adhesions are more common than hernias nowadays. Laparoscopic surgery has definitely decreased incidence of adhesions. In Western countries more than 50% cases of intestinal obstruction are due to adhesions and only 10–15% are due to obstructed hernia (Fig. 60.1). However, students should be able to diagnose intestinal obstruction, resuscitate the patients and refer the patient for further surgical treatment. With the availability of sophisticated investigations such as CT scan, diagnosis can be established in majority of cases before surgery. However, in other cases, **'exploratory laparotomy'** will give the diagnosis.

*Pearls of Wisdom*

Fatty female with fatty fold of abdomen concealing a small femoral hernia. In all cases of intestinal obstruction, examine hernia orifices.

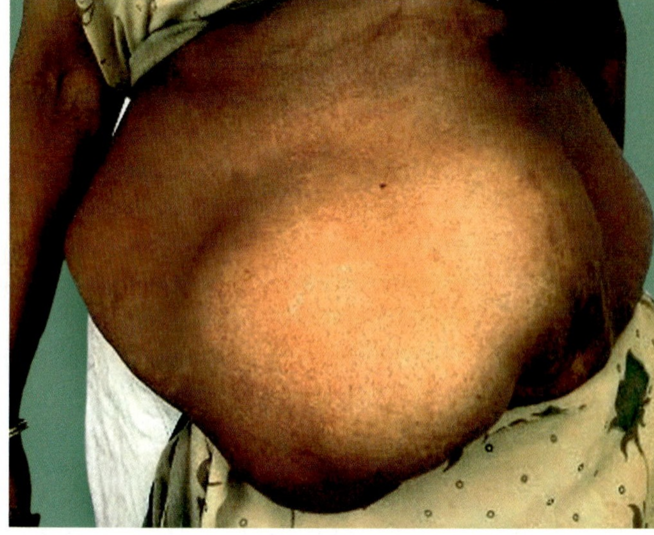

**Fig. 60.1:** Obstructed incisional hernia (*Courtesy:* Prof. (Late) Manjunath Shenoy, JSS Medical College and Hospital, Mysuru)

## DEFINITION

When the intestinal contents fail to move distally, it is called intestinal obstruction. It is the most common surgical disorder (emergency) of the intestines.

*A few important facts about intestinal obstruction:*

- 80% occur in small bowel
- 20% occur in large bowel
- Majority (more than 80%) of small bowel obstructions are benign in nature.

- In the large bowel, more than 70% of colonic obstruction is due to malignancy—others being inflammatory bowel diseases, ileocaecal tuberculosis, volvulus, etc.

## Classification

### I. Depending upon the Nature of Obstruction

(Key Box 60.1)

A. Dynamic obstruction/mechanical obstruction.
B. Adynamic obstruction—paralytic ileus or neurogenic ileus.

Key Box 60.1

**Commonly used Terminology**

- **Mechanical obstruction:** There is a physical barrier which prevents the normal progress of intestinal contents.
- **Paralytic ileus:** There is no physical barrier but failure of peristalsis to propel intestinal contents due to neurogenic causes.
- **Simple obstruction:** It refers to obstruction to lumen only (early cases).
- **Strangulated obstruction:** It refers to obstruction with impairment of blood supply to the gut.
- **Closed loop obstruction:** In this condition, the intestine is occluded in two places. More chances of gangrene and perforation are present, e.g. volvulus.
- **Pseudo-obstruction:** No mechanical cause.

### II. Depending on the Blood Supply

A. **Simple obstruction:** Blood supply is not seriously impaired.
B. **Strangulated obstruction:** Blood supply is seriously impaired, resulting in gangrene of the bowel and gram-negative shock.
C. **Closed loop obstruction:** It means both proximal and distal ends are blocked. This occurs in carcinoma of hepatic flexure—the right colon with constrictive lesions. If the ileocaecal valve is competent and the obstruction is total, the intraluminal pressure within the colon increases. As a result of this, the caecum may perforate. Thus, closed loop obstruction can be dangerous (Fig. 60.2). Another example is sigmoid volvulus.

**SU28.14.6:** List the causes of small bowel and large bowel obstruction. Refer Fig. 60.4.

### III. Depending upon Severity of Obstruction

A. **Acute obstruction:** Signs and symptoms appear very early. Usually, it affects small bowel, obstructed hernia, bands.
B. **Chronic obstruction** (e.g. carcinoma colon) affects large bowel (colic comes first, distension later). Diverticular disease also produces chronic obstructions.
C. **Acute on chronic obstruction** develops in carcinoma colon, wherein an acute obstruction suddenly results due to the accumulation of faecal matter in the proximal bowel.

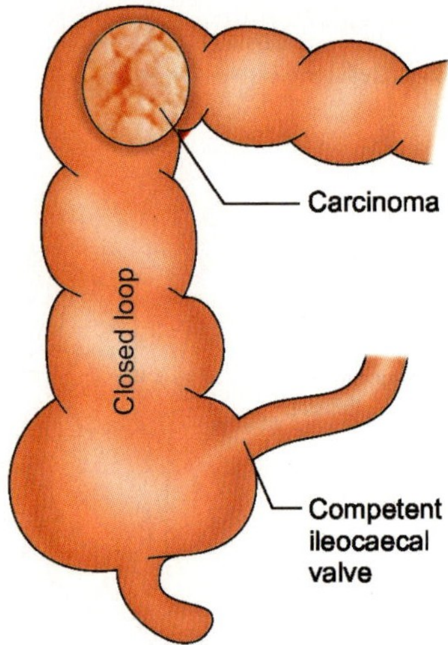


**Fig. 60.2:** Closed loop obstruction: In 40% of patients, ileocaecal valve is competent

## Pathophysiology

**SU28.14.5:** Differentiate pathophysiology of dynamic and adynamic intestinal obstruction.

### A. Pathophysiology of Dynamic Obstruction

- As a result of obstruction, the proximal bowel undergoes hyperperistalsis which is responsible for colicky pain abdomen. The peristalsis may continue for a few days and later the intestine may be paralysed and flaccid. After 3–4 hours, distal to the obstruction, all physiological activities of the bowel are stopped. Intestine becomes contracted, pale and does not exhibit peristalsis. After a few hours, the proximal bowel gets dilated secondary to obstruction (Fig. 60.3).

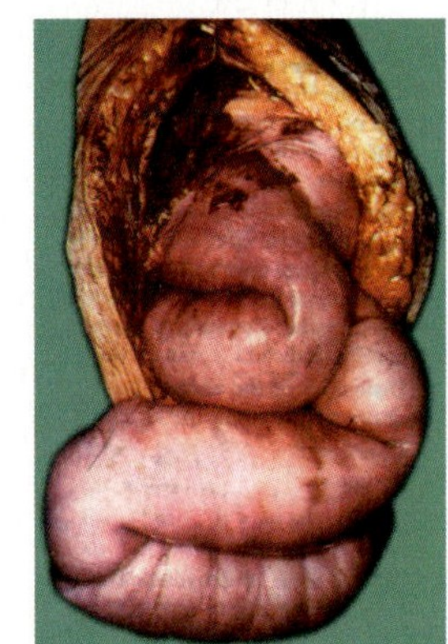

**Fig. 60.3:** Dilated small intestinal loops in a case of ileal obstruction

- The causes of distension of intestinal loop are:

**A. Gaseous distension**

- Swallowed air (70%). Because of colic and anxiety, the swallowed air is increased. Oxygen is absorbed and nitrogen remains as it cannot be absorbed. This results in distension.

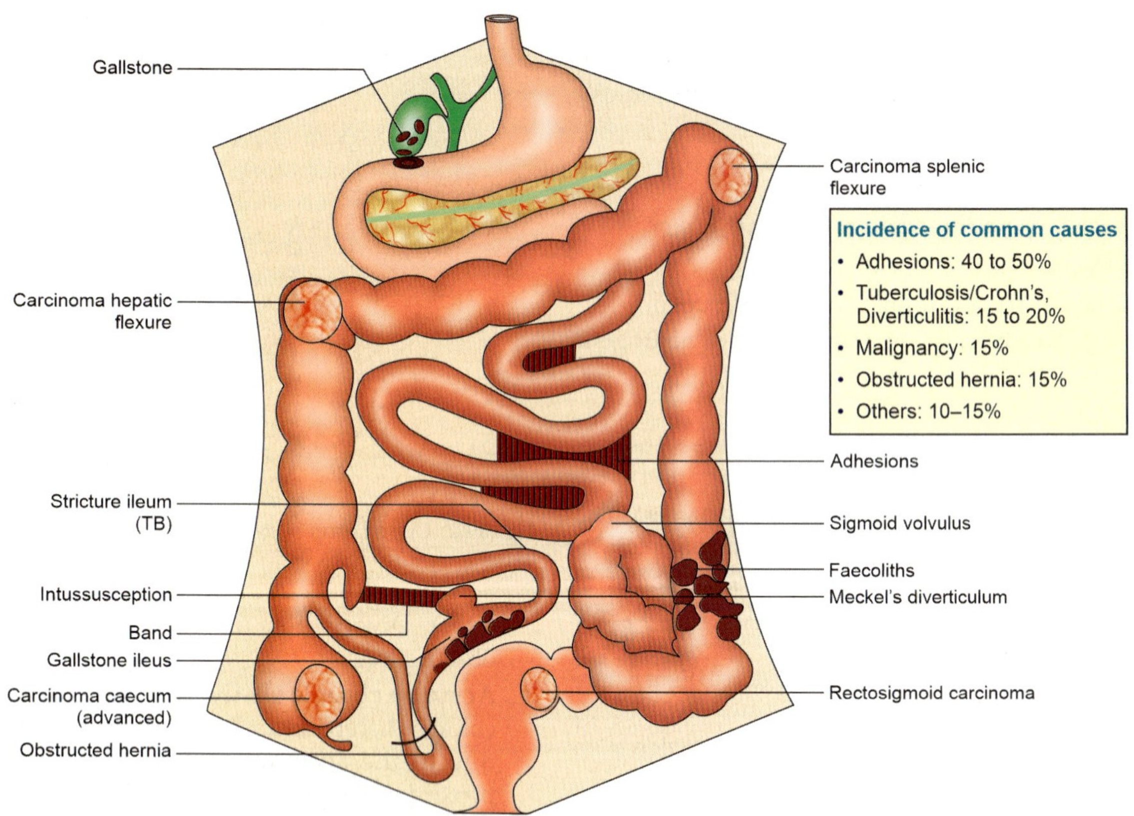


**COMMON CAUSES OF SMALL INTESTINAL OBSTRUCTION**
- Adhesions
- Obstructed hernia
- Stricture
- Intussusception
- Ileocaecal tuberculosis
- Gallstone ileus
- Bands
- Worm ball—in children
- Ileal atresia—in children

**COMMON CAUSES OF COLONIC OBSTRUCTION**
- Carcinoma colon
- Sigmoid volvulus
- Faecal impaction
- Mesenteric ischaemia
- Hirschsprung's disease in children
- Anorectal malformations in children
- Stricture colon—rare

**COMMON CAUSES OF GANGRENE**
- Volvulus
- Intussusception
- Obstructed hernia
- Mesenteric vascular occlusion
- Twisting around a band
- Necrotising enterocolitis in children

**In the lumen of the gut**
- Gallstone ileus
- Food bolus obstruction
- Roundworm mass
- Foreign body (rare)
- Meconium ileus

**In the wall of the gut**
- Stricture, e.g. tuberculosis
- Crohn's disease
- Carcinoma
- Atresia
- Adhesions

**Outside the wall of the gut**
- Volvulus, intussusception
- Congenital bands
- Meckel's diverticulum with band
- Obstructed hernia

**Fig. 60.4:** Differential diagnosis of intestinal obstruction—diagrammatic representation



- Diffusion of air from the blood into bowel lumen increases carbon dioxide which diffuses very rapidly.
- Gas due to bacterial activity releases $H_2S$, $NH_3$, etc.

**B. Distension due to fluids**
- 1500 ml of saliva
- 2 litres of gastric juice
- 3 litres of intestinal secretions
- 1 litre of bile and pancreatic juice

Normally, all this fluid is absorbed in the bowel. In cases of intestinal obstruction, this fluid absorption is delayed. It accumulates in the intestinal loop. Excretion of water and electrolytes into the lumen is also increased.

**C. Role of nitric oxide:** Activated neutrophils and macrophages accumulate within the muscular layer of the bowel wall due to dilatation and inflammation of the bowel wall z. This damages the secretory and motor processes by release of reactive proteolytic enzymes and cytokines. Net result is increase in **the local release of nitric oxide**, itself a potent inhibitor of smooth muscle tone. It further aggravates the intestinal dilatation.

**D. Role of bacteria**
- Bacterial colony count increases following obstruction resulting in stasis. From less than 106 in jejunum and from 108 in ileum, counts increase.

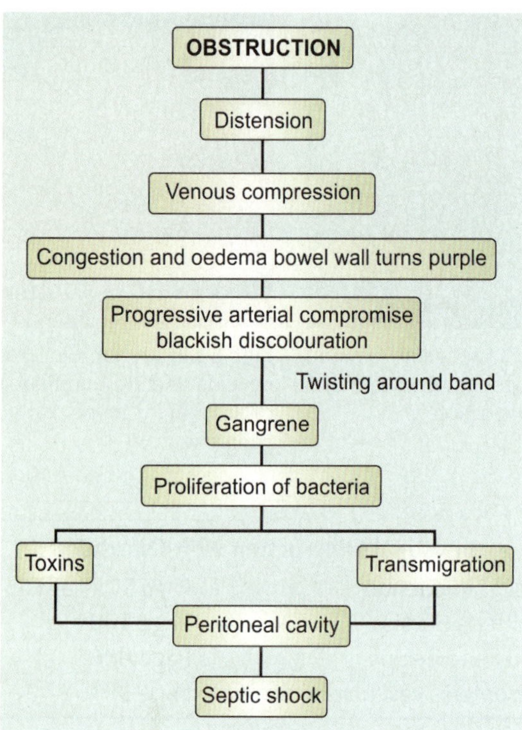


**Fig. 60.5:** Pathophysiology of intestinal obstruction

- **Bacterial translocation** can occur even in simple obstruction without strangulation. Thus, bacteria can enter into lymph nodes and into systemic circulation. Abdominal distension, hypovolaemia, renal failure and sepsis set in. In addition to these changes, diaphragm gets elevated, respiration is impaired which result in respiratory complications such as atelectasis and basal pneumonia. Summary of pathophysiology is given in Fig. 60.5.

**E. Strangulation** (Fig. 60.6 and Key Box 60.2)

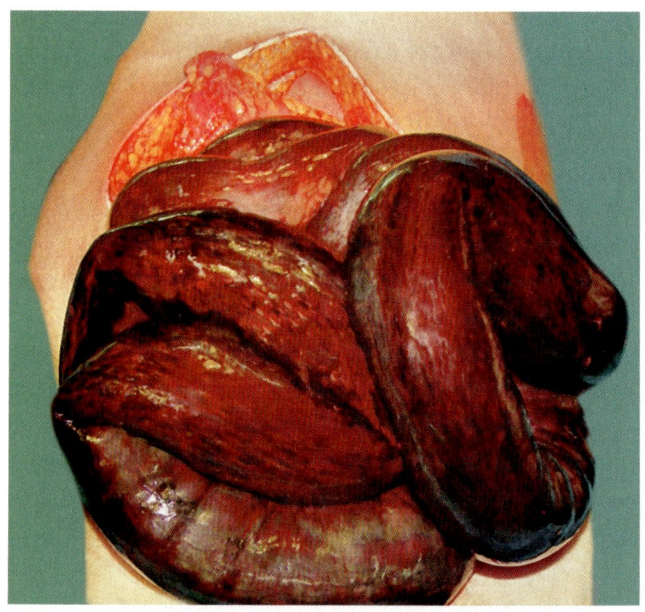

**Fig. 60.6:** Gangrene of the intestine due to bands

Key Box 60.2

**Factors Predisposing to Ischaemia**

- Volvulus
- Mesenteric ischaemia
- Necrotising enterocolitis
- Intussusception
- Progressive distension—long standing
- Extrinsic compression by adhesions, bands, etc.

- Interference with blood supply: As the tension within the loops becomes more and more, venous congestion takes place resulting in oedema of the bowel wall. In doubtful cases of viability, if facilities are available, a test called **fluorescein** test can be done. 1000 mg of fluorescein is injected into peripheral vein and bowel is inspected under wood light. If loops are nonviable, resection and anastomosis is done.
- If the obstruction is not relieved, capillary rupture and haemorrhage into bowel may ensue. **In cases of volvulus and intussusception,** the **arterial supply gets compromised rapidly causing gangrene of bowel wall** very early. Bacterial proliferation takes place and endotoxins are released.
- **Transmigration** (translocation) of gram-negative organisms, anaerobes and gram-positive organisms through the gangrenous bowel into the peritoneal cavity (without perforation) results in peritonitis.
- The organisms release **powerful endotoxins** which are absorbed from the peritoneal surface. It results in septic shock, multiorgan failure and death, if left untreated.
- Early gangrene without obstruction is a feature of mesenteric thrombosis or embolism.
- Loss of blood volume is an important feature of massive gangrene.

### *B. Pathophysiology of Adynamic Ileus-Paralytic Ileus*

- As a result of adynamic obstruction (no peristaltic activity), contents within the lumen do not get absorbed. Saliva, gastric and intestinal contents secreted in the lumen further add to the volume resulting in volume of fluid loss, distension and difficulty in breathing. Hypovolemia worsens and also hypokalemia resulting in further distension.
- If not treated, distension results in stretching of intestinal wall, ischaemia, even perforation and septic shock.
- Difficulty in breathing results in basal atelectasis/pneumonia.
- Fluid and electrolyte imbalance.
- Nutritional deficiencies.

**SU28.14:** Describe the clinical features, investigations and principles of management of small bowel and large bowel obstruction.

## Clinical Features (Key Box 60.3)

1. **Pain abdomen:** Central abdominal pain is a feature of small intestinal obstruction and peripheral pain is a feature of large intestinal obstruction. The pain is colicky in nature, lasts for 5–10 minutes and is intermittent. On pressure, it decreases.
   **Sudden symptoms**—spasmodic pain (due to peristalsis) and continuous pain suggest strangulation.
2. **Vomiting** is due to reverse peristalsis. Vomitus consists of stomach contents initially, then bile, followed by faeculent matter. **Faeculent is not faecal matter** but **terminal ileal contents which undergo bacterial degradation** and **fermentation** resulting in the smell of faecal matter. Vomiting of altered blood indicates haemorrhage and gangrene. Frequent vomiting reflects jejunal obstruction (Fig. 60.7 and Table 60.1).

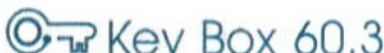

### Key Box 60.3

**Cardinal Features of Intestinal Obstruction**

- Colicky abdominal pain
- Vomiting
- Abdominal distension
- Absolute constipation

*Pearls of Wisdom*

Vomiting of faeculent contents indicates terminal ileal obstruction.

3. **Distension of the abdomen:** It may be central abdominal distension as seen in ileal obstruction, peripheral abdominal as in large bowel obstruction, or localised to one or two quadrants as in sigmoid volvulus.
4. **Constipation** occurs because the distal bowel does not move. Constipation to faeces and flatus is called obstipation. Exceptions are given in Key Box 60.4.
5. **Late (advanced cases):** Oliguria indicates renal failure, tachypnoea indicates acidosis due to sepsis, altered sensorium indicates sepsis, hypoxia, electrolyte imbalances suggest impending gangrene (Fig. 60.8).

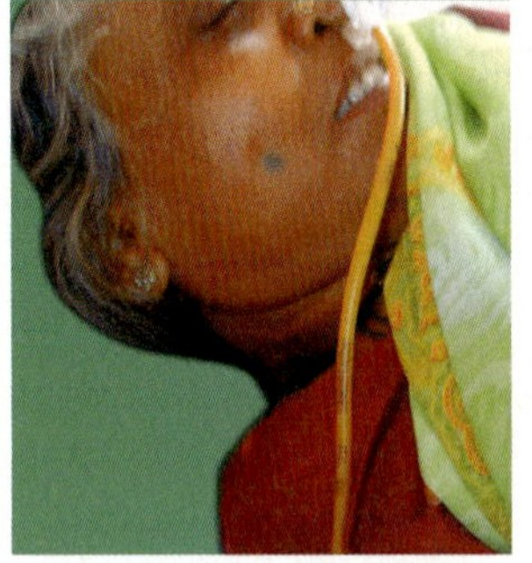

**Fig. 60.7:** Faeculent vomiting is pathognomonic of terminal ileal obstruction

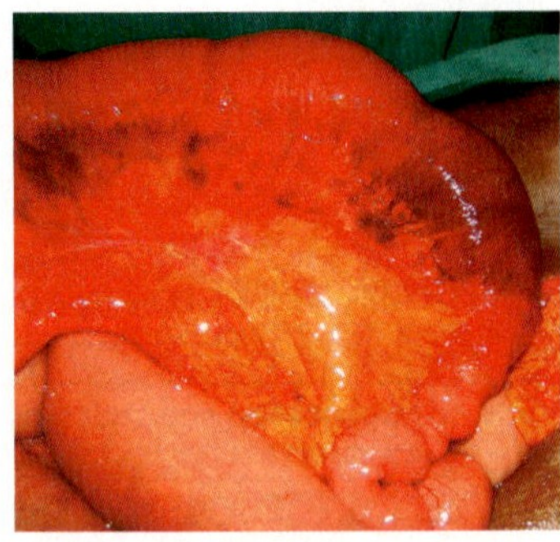

**Fig. 60.8:** Ischaemic area may develop stricture (intestinal stenosis of Garré) or may progress to gangrene

### Key Box 60.4

**Intestinal Obstruction with Diarrhoea**

- Faecal impaction : Page 970 (*see* Fig. 60.4)
- Richter's hernia : Page 1099
- Gallstone ileus : Page 986
- Mesenteric vascular occlusion : Page 991

## Signs

1. **General signs of dehydration** such as dry skin, dry tongue, sunken eyes, feeble pulse, low urinary output are seen. Dehydration occurs due to persistent vomiting and sequestration of fluid and electrolytes. Hypokalaemia is an important finding.
2. **Abdominal findings**
   - Distension, tympanitic note on percussion
   - Step ladder peristalsis (Figs 60.9 and 60.10) is seen in terminal ileal obstruction. Right to left colonic peristalsis is seen in left-sided colonic obstruction, large bowel obstruction.
   - On auscultation—loud, noisy intestinal sounds are heard. They are called **borborygmi**.
   - All hernial orifices have to be examined, especially for a femoral hernia in females.

## Signs of Strangulation

- It should be suspected when features of obstruction are present along with features of shock.
- Features of **septic shock**—fever, hypothermia, renal failure, respiratory failure (Key Box 60.5).

**TABLE 60.1:** Comparison of clinical features at different levels of intestinal obstruction

| | High (jejunum) | Distal (ileum) | Low (colon) |
|---|---|---|---|
| Vomiting | Frequent, bilious | Moderate bilious, faeculent | Late vomiting, faeculent |
| Distension | No | Moderate distension | Marked distension |
| Pain | Intermittent, not crescendo type | Intermittent, crescendo type, colicky | Variable pain, not classical crescendo |
| Constipation | Not initially | Not initially | Initially present |
| Peristalsis | Not seen | Step ladder peristalsis | Right to left peristalsis may be seen |

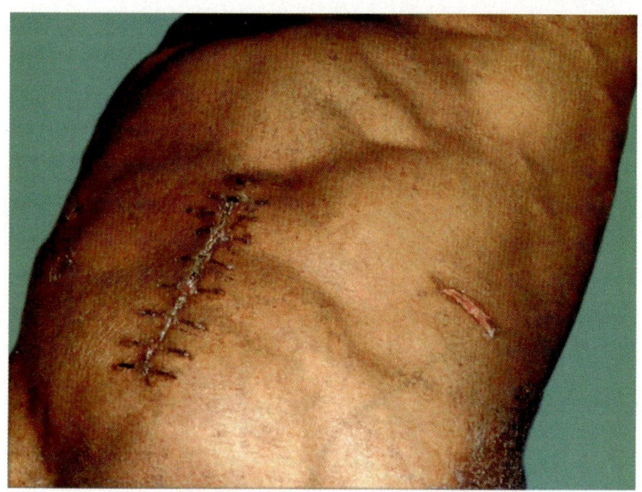

Fig. 60.9: Step ladder peristalsis

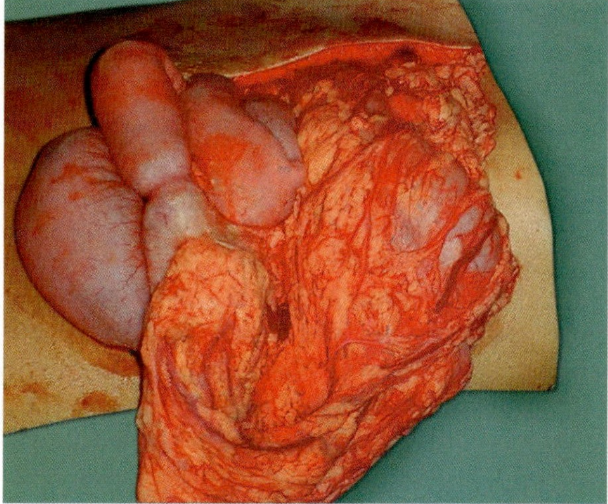

Fig. 60.11: Perforation due to obstruction

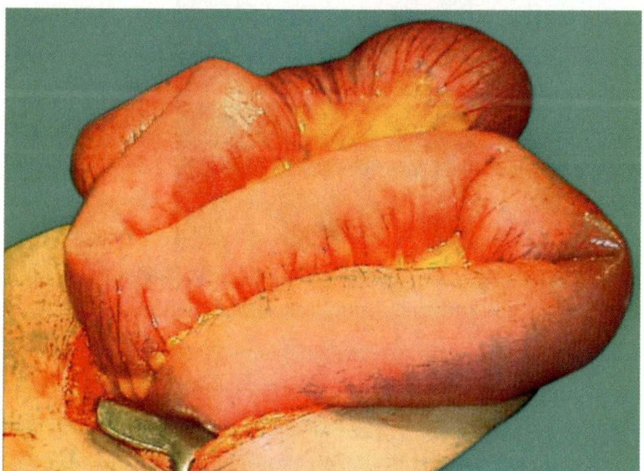

Fig. 60.10: Dilated intestinal loops

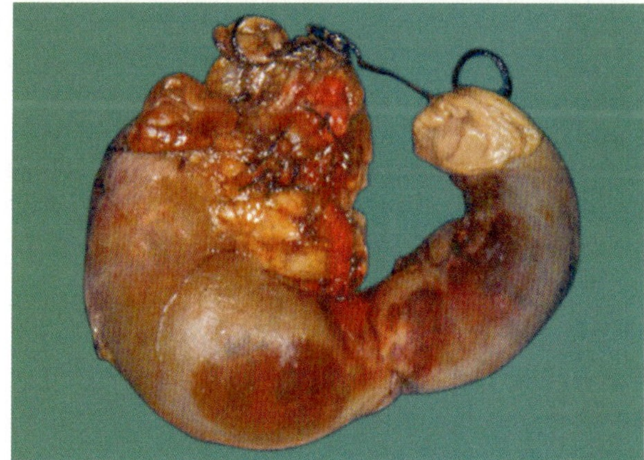

Fig. 60.12: Gangrene due to intussusception

Key Box 60.5

**Features of Strangulation**

- Tachycardia
- Tenderness
- Temperature—fever
  - Delayed cases result in septic shock and multiorgan failure
- Acidosis
- Drowsiness
- Altered sensorium
- Tense abdomen
- Rebound tenderness

- **Rebound tenderness:** It is called **Blumberg's sign**. It is a classical sign of peritonitis.
- Guarding and rigidity of the abdominal wall.
- **Absent bowel sounds** because rest of the bowel loops undergo paralytic ileus.
- Features of strangulation and perforation occur quickly in cases of closed loop obstruction (Figs 60.11, 60.12 and Key Box 60.6).

Key Box 60.6

**Closed Loop Obstruction**

- This occurs when the bowel is obstructed at both proximal and distal points.
- Proximal bowel is not distended as much in this condition.
- Gangrene and perforation can occur fast.
- Retrograde thrombosis of mesenteric vein, can result in distension of the bowel.
- A few examples of closed loop obstruction include sigmoid volvulus, strangulated hernia, carcinoma right colon.

## Rectal Examination

- In small bowel obstruction, **rectum is empty** and is often ballooned out.
- Carcinomatous growth with or without stools can be felt.
- The finger may be stained with blood.
- Altered foul blood indicates gangrene of the bowel.
- Located colon/hard masses indicate pseudo-obstruction.

## INVESTIGATIONS

- **Complete blood picture:** Low Hb% indicates underlying malignancy. Increased total WBC count indicates infection and sepsis (perforation and gangrene).
- Electrolytes: Most of the electrolytes are low in cases of intestinal obstruction and require correction preoperatively. Strangulation may be associated with deranged potassium, amylase or lactic dehydrogenase.
- **Plain X-ray abdomen in the erect position may show multiple gas fluid levels.** Gas levels appear earlier than fluid level. Normally, two insignificant fluid levels can be present, one in the terminal ileum and another in the first part of the duodenum (Key Box 60.7). Supine films indicate the distal limit of obstruction (Figs 60.13 and 60.14).

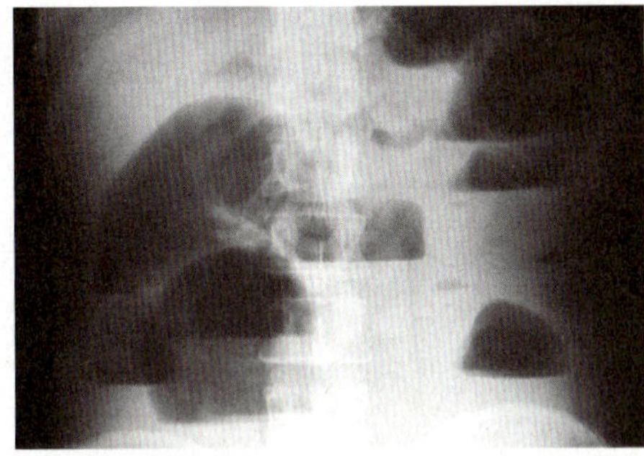

Fig. 60.13: Multiple gas fluid levels—plain X-ray erect abdomen

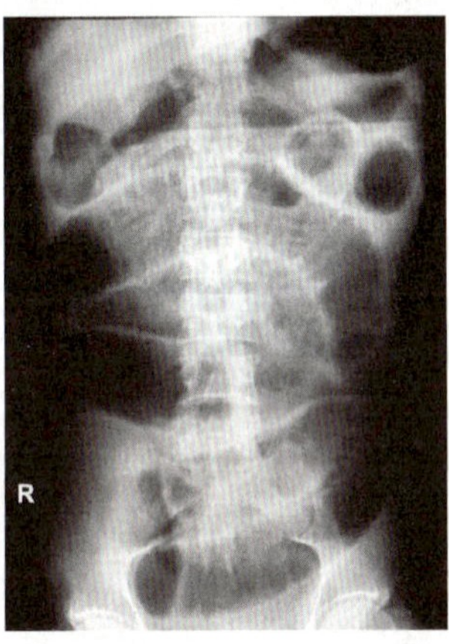


Fig. 60.14: Plain X-ray abdomen supine—distended intestines. Supine X-ray will indicate distal limit of obstruction

Key Box 60.7

### Plain X-ray Findings Upright and Supine

- First get supine films. They indicate distal limit of obstruction. Erect films are asked if any doubt exists about obstruction.
- Jejunum is characterised by regularly placed mucosal folds called **valvulae conniventes** (Fig. 60.15) placed opposite to each other **(Herringbone pattern)**. They are produced by **valves of Kerckring**.
- Large bowel is characterised by **haustrations** (Fig. 60.16): Incomplete, large mucosal folds, not placed opposite to each other.
- **Caecum has no haustrations.** It appears as a round gas shadow in the right iliac fossa.
- Ileum has no characters—**characterless loop of Wangensteen.**
- Plain X-ray may demonstrate gallstone ileus or foreign body.
- Gas is absent in the small bowel as in mesenteric vascular ischaemia.
- Sigmoid volvulus appears as a large dilated loop—inverted 'U' shape.

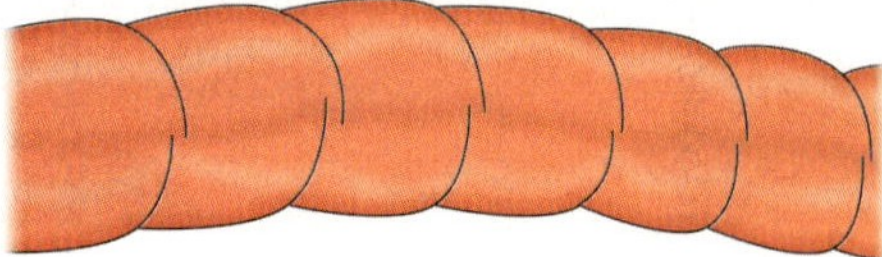

Fig. 60.15: Valvulae conniventes—typical of jejunum

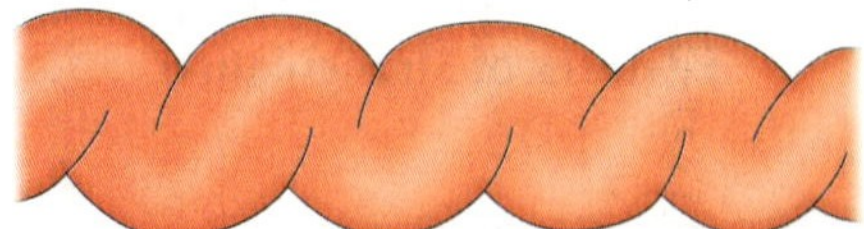

Fig. 60.16: Haustrations—typical of colon

- The small intestine is considered dilated if loops of bowel measure more than 3 cm in diameter. Measurements for the large bowel vary among different anatomic segments, with a relative threshold of 9 cm in diameter for the proximal colon and 5 cm for the sigmoid colon.
- Barium studies should not be done in acute intestinal obstruction. It may result in perforation and fatal barium peritonitis. Thin barium can be used in cases sub-acute obstruction wherein diagnosis could not be achieved by other tests. Figure 60.17 indicates pulled up caecum—a case of ileo-cecal tuberculosis.
- Ultrasound can diagnose few conditions (Key Box 60.8). Enteroclysis can diagnose strictures ( Fig. 60.18).
- CECT scan scan diagnose not only mass lesions but early ischaemia, pneumotosis and stricture also (Fig. 60.19, Box 60.9).

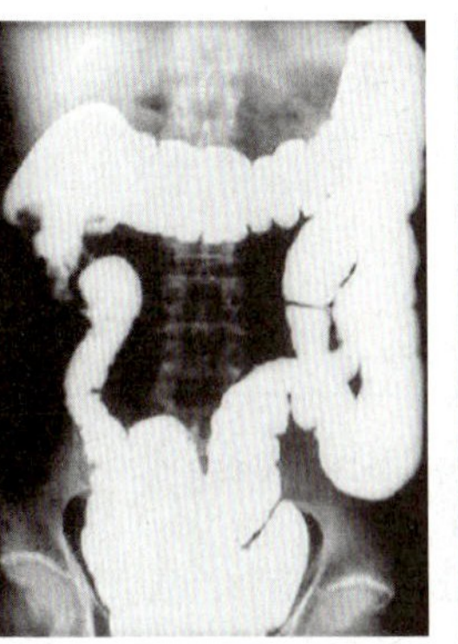

Fig. 60.17: Barium enema showing pulled up caecum—an increase in the ileocaecal angle from acute to obtuse

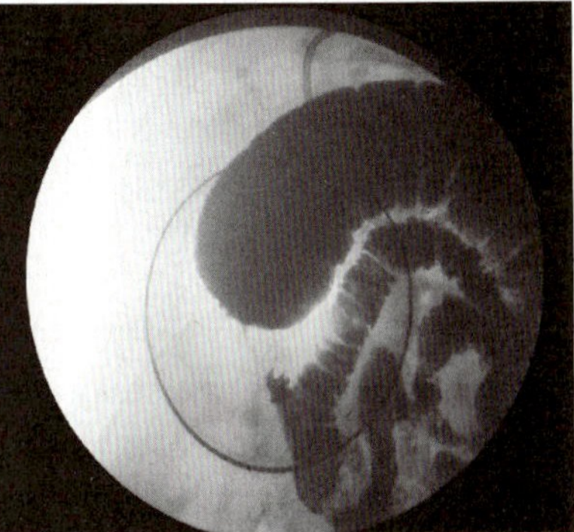

Fig. 60.18: Jejunal stricture due to tuberculosis—enteroclysis picture. You can see grossly dilated jejunal loops proximally.

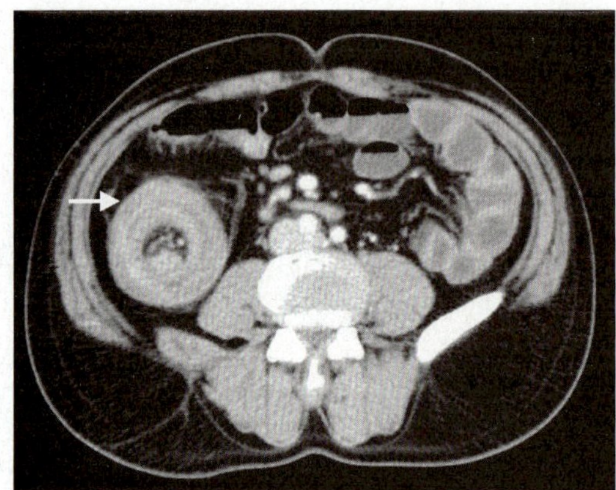

Fig. 60.19: Ileocolic intussusception—observe 'target sign' on the right side

Key Box 60.8

**Ultrasound**

- It is not the investigation of choice or it may not be required

**However, a good sonologist can diagnose:**

a. Dilated loops of intestine
b. Presence of fluid in the abdomen
c. Gallstone ileus
d. Infarcted/ischaemic bowel/gas in the portal vein or intrahepatic gas.
e. Intussusception and can assess vascularity with the help of duplex scan.
f. It can also rule out other causes.

**Being a noninvasive investigation, it has more benefits.**

Key Box 60.9

**CT Scan in Intestinal Obstruction**

- Can detect dilated intestines proximally and collapsed bowel distally.
- If bowel wall is thick and air is present **(pneumatosis)**, strangulation is likely mesenteric ischaemia
- It can detect portal venous gas (suggesting gangrene)
- CT can detect **mass lesions**—carcinoma sigmoid, caecum or ileocaecal mass (TB).
- CT has low sensitivity in detecting low grade or partial small bowel obstruction. Sensitivity increases in total obstruction.

## MANAGEMENT PRINCIPLES

Preoperative preparation includes correction of aggressive fluid resuscitation with Ringer lactate–may range from 125 to 150 ml/hour. Check pulse volume, urine output and diameter of inferior vena cava by bedside ultrasound, electrolytes and broad spectrum antibiotics. Principles in the management of intestinal obstruction are as follows: **Mnemonic: A, B, C, D, E, F.**

**A. Aspiration with Ryle's tube:** This is the most important step in the management of intestinal obstruction. It helps in decreasing the distension and also prevents vomiting. This will help in preventing respiratory complications due to aspiration following general anaesthesia.

**B. Bowel care:** No purgatives because purgation can cause perforation. Do not stimulate bowel by drugs or food. Arrange blood in appropriate patients.

**C. Charts:** Temperature, pulse, respiration and intake output chart. In cases of conservative management such as obstruction due to adhesions, change in temperature and increasing pulse rate suggest perforation or gangrene. These cases have to be explored immediately. Oliguria can also be a feature of early sepsis due to gangrene. Monitor carefully.

**D. Drugs** (antibiotics) to cover gram-positive, gram-negative and anaerobic organisms.

**E. Exploratory laparotomy** is done and depending upon the findings, obstruction is treated (Box 60.10 and Fig. 60.20). You will get to know more details in subsequent pages.

**F. Electrolytes** should be given before, during and after surgery. It forms the most important treatment of intestinal obstruction.

Key Box 60.10

**Principles of Exploratory Laparotomy**

- Ideally done within 6–8 hours
- Long midline incision
- Resection of gangrene and anastomosis
- Adhesions—release
- Bands—divide
- Gallstone ileus—remove the stone/stones
- Volvulus—untwist or resection
- Obstructed hernia—reduce/resect if gangrene
- Stricture—resection or stricturoplasty
- Advanced malignancy (inoperable)—bypass

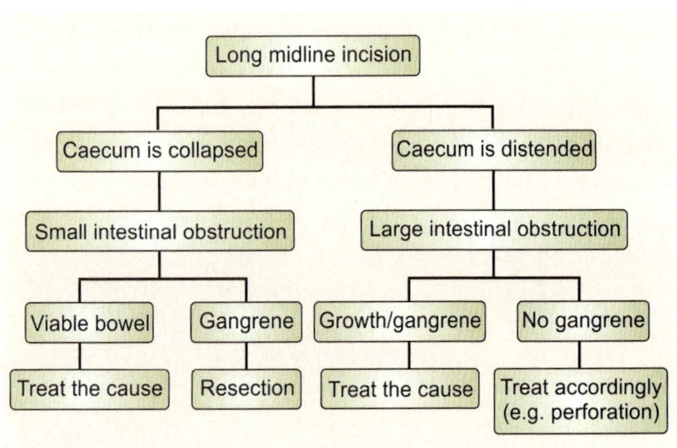


Fig. 60.20: Principles of management of intestinal obstruction

## APPROACH TO THE MANAGEMENT OF INTESTINAL OBSTRUCTION—MORE DETAILS

Ask the following questions to yourself and proceed.
1. What is the probable cause of obstruction?
2. Is it small bowel obstruction at laparotomy?
3. Is it large bowel obstruction at laparotomy?
4. Is it simple obstruction?
5. Is it strangulation?
6. Is it some kind of a surprise or a difficult case?
7. Can I manage conservatively?

### 1. Probable Cause of Obstruction

- A previous **laparotomy scar** may indicate that it could be an adhesive obstruction (most common).
- An obvious obstructed hernia (inguinal/umbilical/incisional or femoral) can be managed with inguinal approach (Figs 60.21 to 60.23). It is treated by reducing contents, repair: Suture/mesh and resect, if gangrene is present.
- An elderly man, hypertensive and atherosclerotic, with features of blood in the stools and acute abdominal pain may be having superior mesenteric ischaemia.
- A constipated, elderly man in poor health, with acute or chronic obstruction may be having carcinoma of the colon.

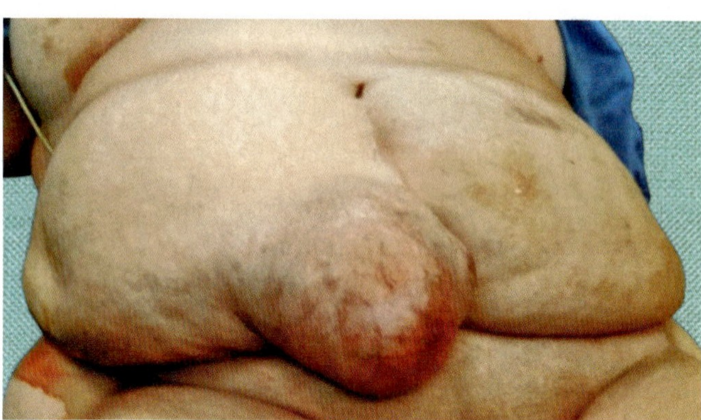

**Fig. 60.21:** Obstructed incisional hernia

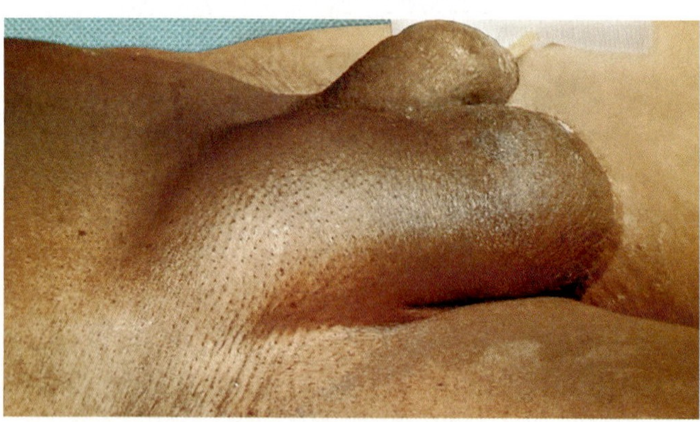

**Fig. 60.22:** Obstructed inguinal hernia

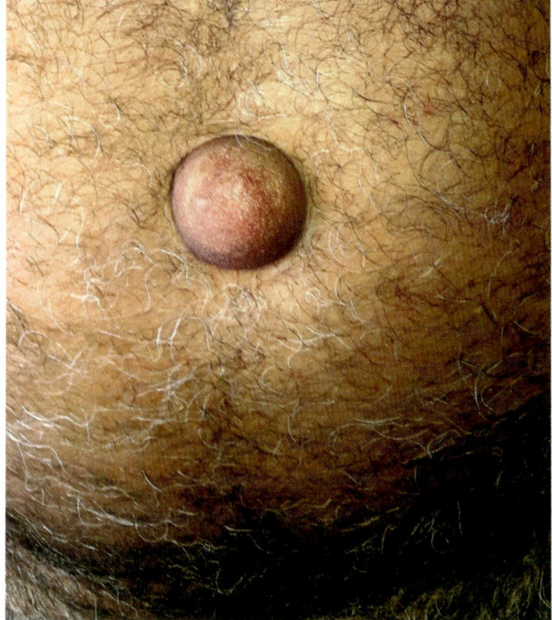

**Fig. 60.23:** Obstructed umbilical hernia

### 2. Diagnosis of Small Bowel Obstruction at Laparotomy

- Caecum is collapsed
- Dilated loops of small intestine are present.
- A stricture or a mass lesion may be obvious at laparotomy.

### 3. Diagnosis of Large Bowel Obstruction at Laparotomy

- Caecum is distended.
- A growth may be palpable and obvious in the transverse colon or in the hidden colon, i.e. splenic flexure.
- It is very important to examine the entire colon (synchronous carcinoma is more common).

### 4. Diagnosis of Simple Obstruction

- Here, the bowel is not gangrenous.
- In doubtful cases, because of long-standing ischaemia, wrapping the bowel with warm and moist pack and administration of 100% oxygen may help the bowel to recover from ischaemia.
- Pink bowel, peristalsis is seen, peritoneal sheen and pulsations indicate healthy bowel.

### 5. Diagnosis of Strangulation

(Fig. 60.24 and Key Box 60.11)

- Black, dark, foul-smelling bowel is seen as soon as laparotomy is done.
- Peritoneal fluid contains blood-stained fluid.
- Precautions must be taken not to contaminate peritoneal cavity when gangrenous segment is removed.

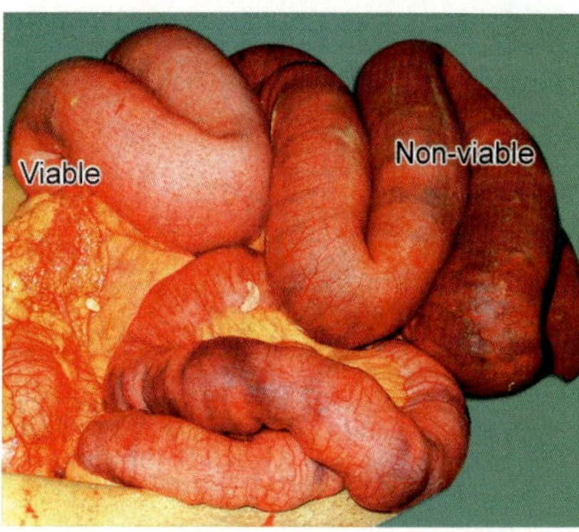


**Fig. 60.24:** Viable and non-viable bowel

Key Box 60.11

**Viable Bowel—Features**

- Normal peristalsis
- Normal peritoneal sheen is present
- Normal pulsations are visible or felt at the mesentery
- Normal pink colour is present

**Do not hesitate to take the help** of senior experienced surgeons in treating an uncommon situation such as massive ischaemia and gangrene of small bowel and colon (due to mesenteric vascular occlusion), synchronous carcinoma and ileosigmoid knotting, etc.

### 6. It is a Surprise (Look for clues-Key Box 60.12)

Surprises are well known in intestinal obstruction. Congenital bands, foreign bodies, internal herniation, strictures are a few examples.

Key Box 60.12

**Intestinal Obstruction**
**'Clues' to the Causes of Obstruction**

| Clue | Cause |
|---|---|
| Operative scar | Adhesions |
| Groin swelling | Obstructed hernia |
| Gross distended intestinal loop | Sigmoid volvulus |
| Stepladder peristalsis | Small intestinal obstruction |
| Red currant jelly stools | Intussusception |
| Deformed umbilicus in child | Meckel's diverticulum with band |
| Melanosis of lips, mucosa | Intussusception in adults (PJ syndrome) |
| H/o constipation/bleeding per rectum | Colonic obstruction (cancer) |
| Emaciated, young patient with loose stools/weight loss/fever | Ileocaecal tuberculosis (TB) stricture |
| Elderly, hypertensive, severe abdominal pain, tachycardia, tachypnoea, acidotic | Mesenteric vascular occlusion |

### 7. Can I Manage Conservatively?

In these cases, a long intestinal tube called Miller-Abbott tube can be passed to decompress intestines (Key Box 60.13) conservatively.

Key Box 60.13

**Intestinal Obstruction Conservative Treatment**

1. **Partial small bowel obstruction** mostly due to adhesion: Wait for 48 to 72 hours. They may show improvement. If not, surgery is required.
2. **Early postoperative obstruction:** Let us study in more detail about a few common conditions presenting as acute abdomen with diagnosis of intestinal obstruction. It rarely progresses to strangulation. Hence, nonoperative management can be extended to many days (3–7), provided there is no evidence of peritonitis.
3. **Intestinal obstruction in Crohn's disease:** Aim in Crohn's disease is to 'preserve' bowel as it may respond to medications.
4. **Carcinomatosis:** Disseminated malignancy with obstruction. The aim is nonoperative treatment as nothing much can be achieved with laparotomy.

### 8. Acute Large Bowel Obstruction

Details about the causes of large bowel obstruction, pathophysiology and the treatment are given in Chapter 59. However, a few important points have been given in ten commandments.

**TEN COMMANDMENTS WHILE TREATING INTESTINAL OBSTRUCTION**

1. Should rule out pseudo-obstruction before exploring the abdomen.
2. Should do limited contrast study or CECT scan
3. Should resuscitate the patient before surgery
4. Should take into account, the general condition of the patient before resection anastomosis.
5. Should consider right hemicolectomy or extended hemicolectomy for right-sided growth which is operable.
6. Should consider single stage resection anastomosis also for left-sided growth provided general condition of the patient is good and on table lavage is given before the anastomosis.
7. Should consider exteriorisation of gangrenous bowel in a very sick patient.
8. Should consider a simple diversion colostomy in moribund patients with rectosigmoid obstruction (it is a common problem).
9. Should not do anastomosis in cases with faecal contamination, peritonitis, haemodynamic instability or possible ischaemia of the remaining colonic segments.
10. Should mark the probable stoma site.

## CAUSES OF INTESTINAL OBSTRUCTION AS PER AGE

### NEONATES: 0 TO 7 DAYS AND IN YOUNGER CHILDREN

1. Atresia and stenosis
2. Hirschsprung's disease
3. Arrested rotation with bands
4. Volvulus neonatorum
5. Meconium ileus
6. Imperforate anus
7. Malrotation
8. Intussusception
9. Worm ball (Fig. 60.25)

Refer page 996 for more details

### Young Patients: Up to 40 Years

1. Obstructed hernia
2. Adhesions
3. Tuberculous stricture and fibrous adhesions
4. Crohn's disease of ileum
5. Meckel's diverticulum with band
6. Adult intussusception

### Middle-aged Patients: 40 Years Onwards

1. Adhesions
2. Obstructed hernia
3. Carcinoma left colon
4. Diverticulosis with stricture left colon
5. Gallstone ileus
6. Sigmoid volvulus
7. Mesenteric vascular occlusion

## DIFFERENTIAL DIAGNOSIS OF INTESTINAL OBSTRUCTION

### STRICTURES

- Common causes are tubercular stricture of the ileum or jejunum in India (Fig. 60.26) and Crohn's disease in the Western world.
- Malignant strictures. Carcinoma rectosigmoid junction (Fig. 60.27).
- Radiation stricture, ischaemic strictures and non-specific strictures (Fig. 60.28) are the other causes.
- Recurrent, intermittent abdominal pain, frequent vomiting ball rolling sensation helps in the diagnosis.
- Investigations have been discussed earlier such as X-rays and CT scans. In selected patients, (Fig. 60.29 to 60.33) enterocylsis, diagnostic laparoscopy and balloon enteroscopy can be used. Primary aim is to relieve obstruction. Resection in tubercular, radiation

Fig. 60.25: Worm ball obstruction

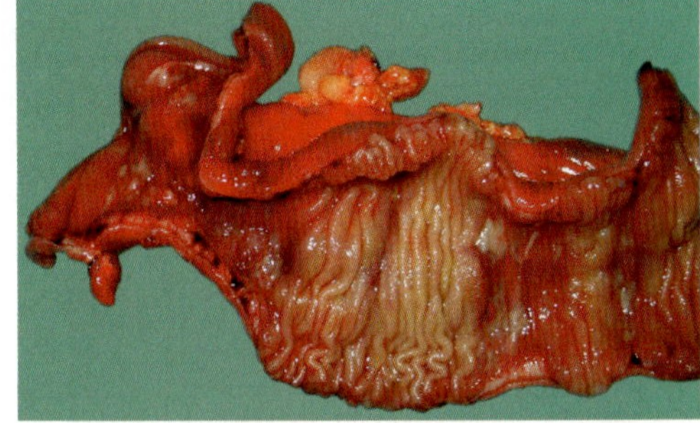

Fig. 60.26: Tubercular stricture—annular stricture

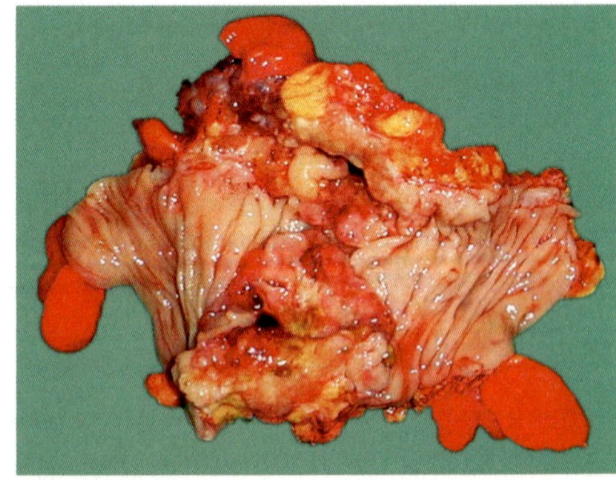

Fig. 60.27: Sigmoid stricture due to carcinoma

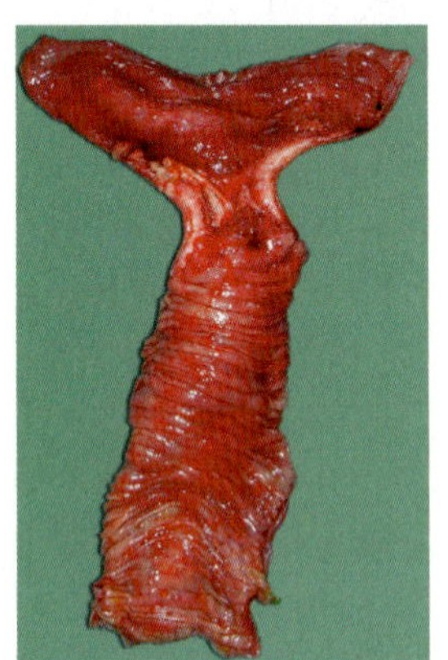

Fig. 60.28: Non-specific stricture

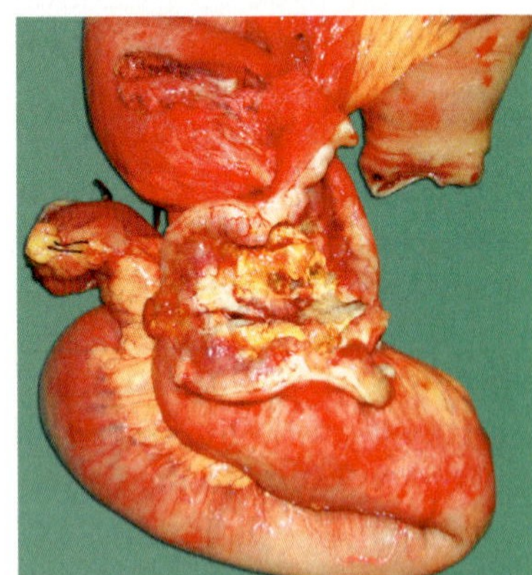

Fig. 60.29: Peritoneal metastasis causing narrowing of lumen resulting in obstruction

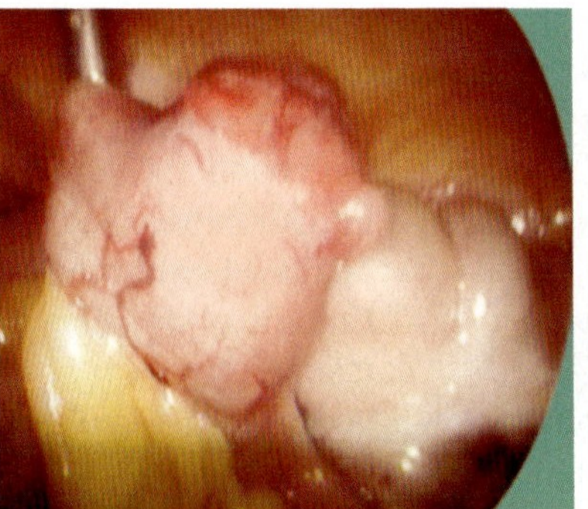

Fig. 60.30: Laparoscopy detected a lesion in the small intestine. On opening the abdomen turned out to be a jejunal GIST with obstruction

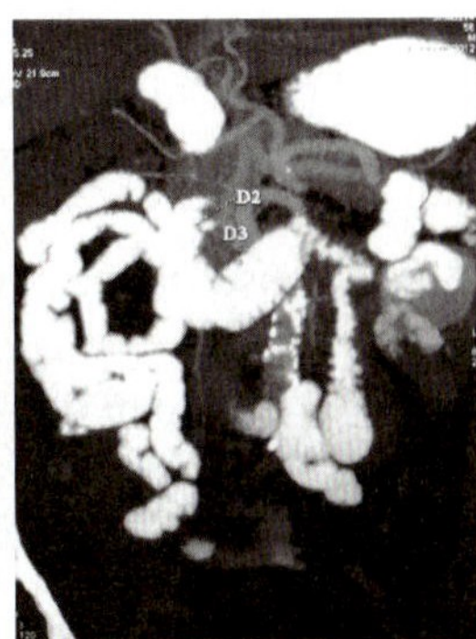


Fig. 60.31: Enteroclysis showing jejunal narrowing and aortic calcification

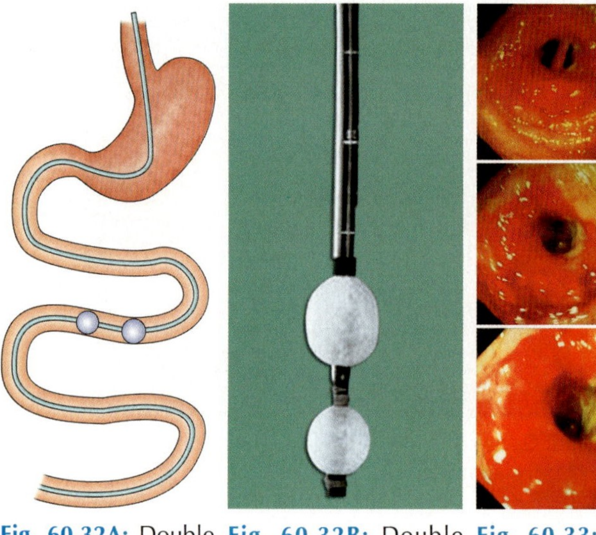

Fig. 60.32A: Double enteroscopy representation

Fig. 60.32B: Double balloon enteroscopy

Fig. 60.33: Balloon enteroscopy showing jejunal ulcers

and malignant strictures. In Crohn's disease, aim is to preserve the bowel as much as possible. Few may respond to medications, non-responders can be treated with stricturoplasty or resection.

## VOLVULUS OF THE SIGMOID COLON

- Common in North India (Punjab), Eastern Europe, Uganda.
- In certain parts of India as mentioned above, it is one of the common surgical emergencies in elderly population (Key Box 60.14).

Key Box 60.14

**Certain Facts about Sigmoid Volvulus**

- More common in males.
- 2/3rd of the cases are sigmoid volvulus and 1/3rd are caecal volvulus.
- Common in middle age and >60 years.
- It accounts for about 10 to 15% of cases of intestinal obstruction in India.
- More common in rural population.
- It is not an uncommon event during pregnancy.

### Precipitating Factors (Fig. 60.34)

Sigmoid volvulus is a definite occurrence in mentally disturbed patients, hypothyroidism, Parkinson's disease, multiple sclerosis, etc. probably due to severe constipation due to medications.

*Pearls of Wisdom*

Ogilvie's syndrome precipitates volvulus.

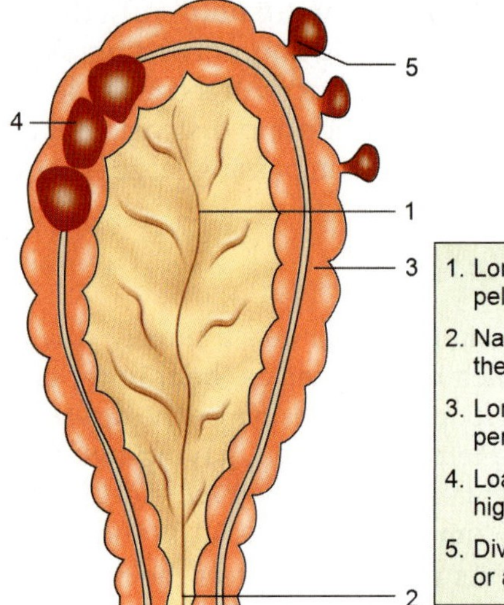


Fig. 60.34: Causes of sigmoid volvulus

### Clinical Features

1. **Acute sigmoid volvulus (fulminant)** presents as intestinal obstruction. It starts usually after straining at stools. Volvulus is usually in anticlockwise direction and after one and a half turns, the entire loop becomes gangrenous.

   **Enormous distension of the abdomen takes place,** which gives a tympanitic note all over the abdomen. It is due to **diffusion of $CO_2$** (Fig. 60.35). Due to gross distension, severe hypovolaemic shock develops within 6–8 hours of volvulus. Gangrene sets in, which gives rise to features of strangulation. A dilated loop can be seen and felt. Features of peritonitis are seen within 1–2 days. Per rectal examination shows rectum to be empty.

*Pearls of Wisdom*

Distended tympanitic drum-like abdomen—sigmoid volvulus.

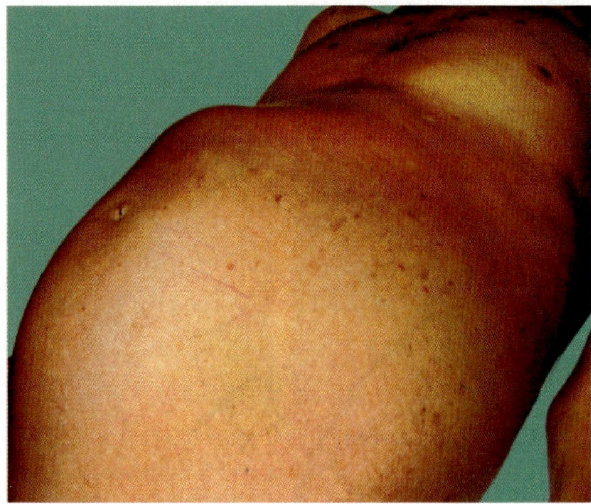

Fig. 60.35: Uneven distension due to sigmoid volvulus

2. **Chronic (indolent) recurrent sigmoid volvulus:** It occurs due to partial twisting and untwisting of the bowel. Elderly patients present with recurrent lower abdominal pain on the left side and distension of the abdomen which is relieved on passing large amount of flatus.

### Diagnosis

- **Plain X-ray abdomen erect** shows a hugely dilated sigmoid loop which is described as **'bent inner tube sign'**. The dilated loop may be visible on the right side, centre and to the left of abdomen, having two fluid levels, one on right side and one on left side. This is also described as **'omega sign'** (Figs 60.36 and 60.37).
- **Contrast enema:** As the barium enters the rectum, it tapers into the sigmoid colon—**Bird's beak sign** (not to be done in acute cases).

## TREATMENT

### I. Nonoperative

A successful passage of flatus tube or sigmoidoscope up to 25–30 cm results in release of a large amount of flatus and fluid, and obstruction is relieved. If obstruction is completely relieved or if there is no gangrene and the general condition of the patient improves, an elective resection is done after 7 days. If resistance is found while passing flatus tube, instill barium for guidance.

### II. Operative Treatment

1. **Single-stage resection:** This can be done, provided general condition of the patient is good. If the loop is gangrenous, resection followed by end to end anastomosis is done, after giving 'on table' lavage using saline washes till the contents of the colon are clear. Sigmoid colon is hugely dilated (Fig. 60.38).

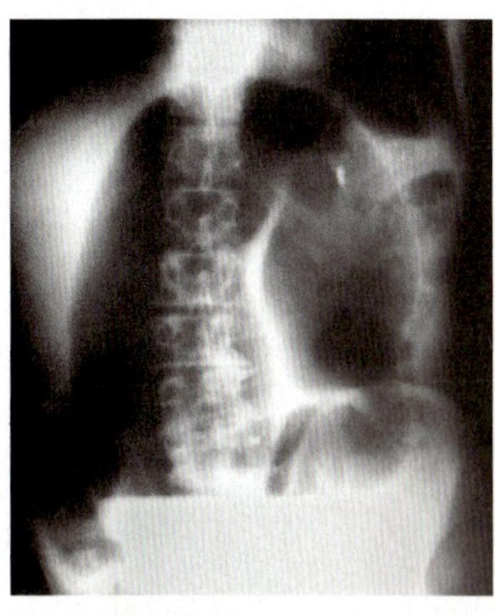

**Fig. 60.36:** Plain X-ray abdomen showing distended sigmoid loop

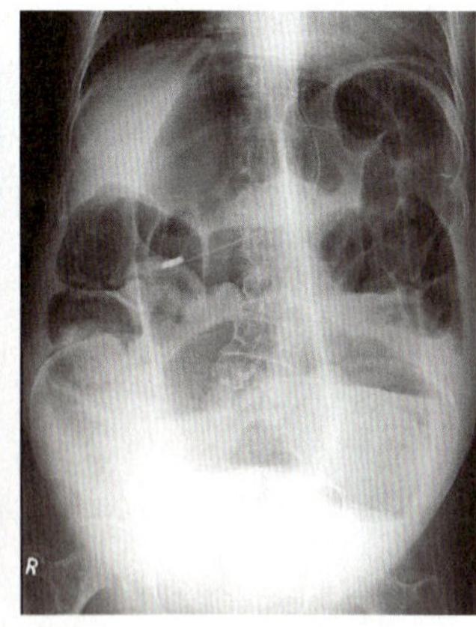


**Fig. 60.37:** An 84-year-old patient with sigmoid volvulus, managed by sigmoidoscopic decompression

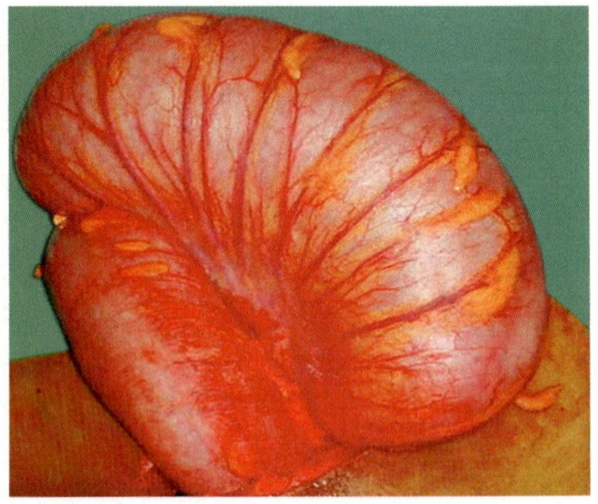

**Fig. 60.38:** Sigmoid colon at surgery—huge distension results in severe hypovolaemic shock

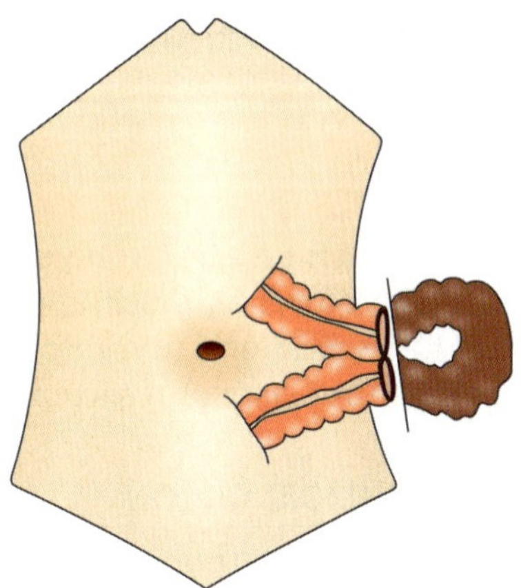

**Fig. 60.39:** Paul-Mickulicz procedure

2. **Hartmann's procedure:** If the loop is gangrenous and proximal bowel is loaded with faecal matter, resection of the sigmoid colon is done. Proximal descending colon is brought out as an end colostomy and rectum is closed (Hartmann's procedure). After 6 weeks, colorectal anastomosis is done.
3. **Sigmoidopexy:** If the loop is not gangrenous, untwist the sigmoid loop and fix the sigmoid to the posterior abdominal wall (sigmoidopexy). If the mesentery is long, it can be made short by plication.
4. **Exteriorisation:** Paul-Mickulicz procedure is done when general condition of the patient is poor as in elderly patients or in a severely dehydrated patient with impending septicaemia. In such cases, the gangrenous loop is brought outside and resected, with a proximal colostomy and a distal mucous fistula (Fig. 60.39).

## CAECAL VOLVULUS AND BASCULE

- It is a rare cause of intestinal obstruction (Figs 60.40 to 60.43 and Key Boxes 60.15 and 60.16).
- Presumably, it is more likely to occur following any surgical procedure which might require some degree of medial visceral rotation or disruption of the fusion

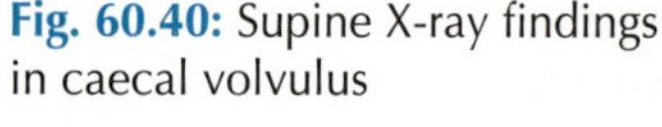

Fig. 60.40: Supine X-ray findings in caecal volvulus

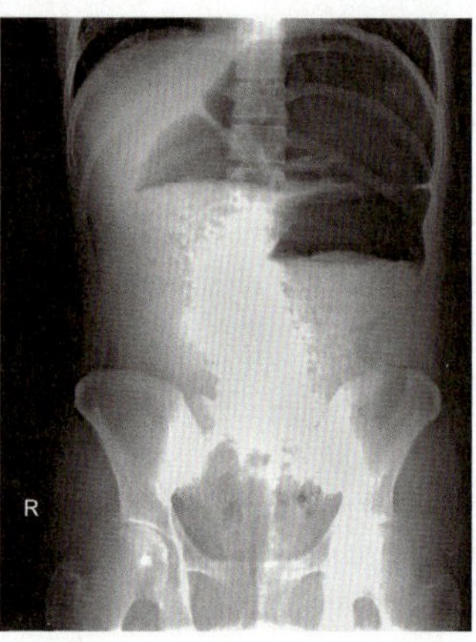


Fig. 60.41: Erect X-ray showing distended loop. Caecum was palpable in the left hypochondrium

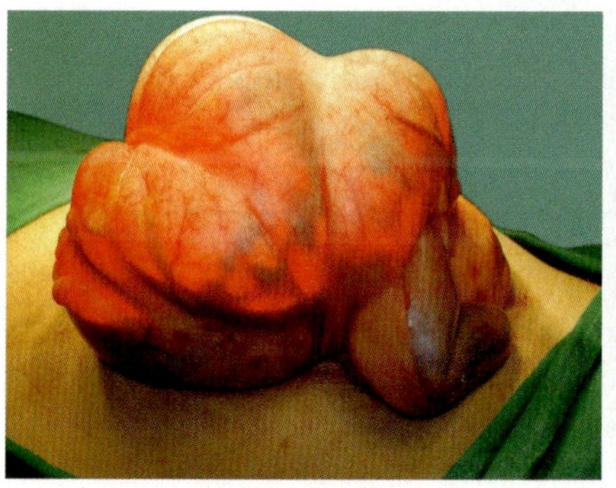

Fig. 60.42: Distended caecum at surgery. (*Courtesy:* Dr Basavaraj Patil, Dr Hartimath, Dr Rasheed, Dr Nikil, Department of Surgery, KMC, Manipal)

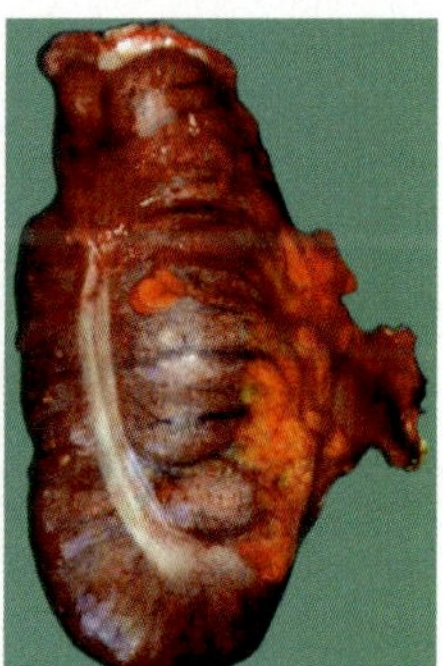

Fig. 60.43: Caecal volvulus with gangrene

Key Box 60.15

**Caecal Bascule**

- Caecum folds anteromedial to the ascending colon, with production of a flap-valve occlusion at the site of flexion.
- Caecum will be markedly distended and will be found in the centre of the abdomen.
- Occasionally, it is associated with malrotation of the gut.
- There will be a constricting band across the ascending colon.
- It is also argued that caecal bascule can also be due to lack of fixation of large bowel. Resection is ideal even though fixation (caecopexy) is also another alternative.
- Bascule is a French term for seesaw and balance

plane between the caecum or ascending colon with the lateral peritoneum, providing sufficient mobility allowing caecal volvulisation to occur.

- A constant feature of **caecal bascule** is the presence of a constricting band across the ascending colon. This may be found at laparotomy.
- In a plain X-ray abdomen, caecum produces round shadow in the centre of the abdomen.
- Resection is the ideal treatment.

Key Box 60.16

**Comparison of Caecal Volvulus and Sigmoid Volvulus**

| Caecal volvulus | Sigmoid volvulus |
|---|---|
| Rare | Common |
| Clockwise twist | Anticlockwise |
| Mobile caecum | Long mesentery is the cause |
| Middle-aged | Elderly, debilitated |
| Kidney-shaped gas shadow with single fluid level on the leftside | Omega sign or coffee shaped. Two fluid levels can be found. |
| Treated only by surgery | Nonoperative treatment should be attempted in all cases, provided there is no ischaemia. |

*Pearls of Wisdom*

If loop is gangrenous, do not derotate—clamp the mesentery first, then detorsion can be done to avoid reperfusion injury.

## MECKEL'S DIVERTICULUM WITH A BAND

It is a congenital diverticulum which occurs due to persistent intestinal end of vitellointestinal duct. **Being congenital, it has all the layers of the bowel**. Hence, it is a true diverticulum.

### Anomalies of Vitellointestinal Duct (Figs 60.44A to F)

A. **Fibrous band** results when entire duct is obliterated and bowel can twist around the band, resulting in volvulus.

B. **Persistent intestinal end:** Meckel's diverticulum.

C. **Meckel's diverticulum with the band** attached to the umbilicus can give rise to intestinal obstruction.

D. **Umbilical fistula** results when entire duct is patent. Even though it is connected to the terminal ileum, the opening is very small. The discharge is rarely faecal. Often, it is the mucus secreted from the lining of the duct **(omphaloenteric fistula)**.

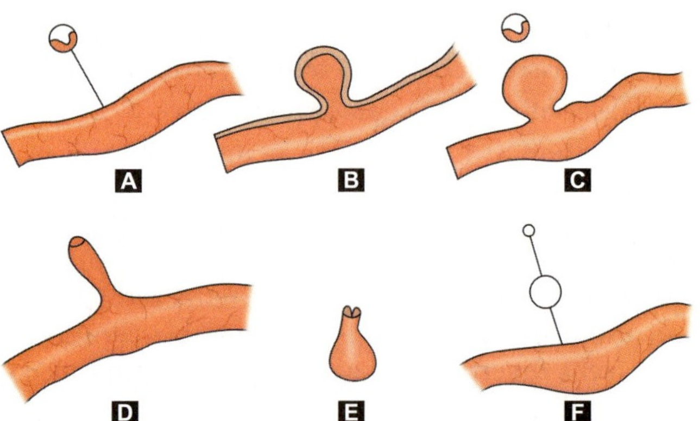


Figs 60.44A to F: Anomalies of vitellointestinal duct (A to F *see* text for details)

**E. Umbilical sinus** results due to persistent umbilical end discharging mucus. Slowly umbilical adenoma occurs and epithelial lining of the sinus gets everted.

**F. Intra-abdominal cyst** results when both ends are obliterated. The central portion of the duct persists and secretes mucus. This is very, very rare.

## MECKEL'S DIVERTICULUM

- It is present in 2% of the cases, 2 inches long, 2 feet away from ileocaecal region in the antimesenteric border (ileal duplication can occur in the mesenteric border). It is two times more common in females.
- Symptomatic cases are below 2 years of age.
- In 12% of the patients, heterotopic gastric tissue is found which can produce peptic ulceration. In a few other patients, it can contain pancreatic and colonic tissue. Other anomalies (Key Box 60.17).

Key Box 60.17

**Meckel's[1] Diverticulum and other Associated Anomalies**

- Angiodysplasia of the caecum
- Anorectal atresia, atresia of the oesophagus

[1]The most common congenital anomaly of small intestine

### Clinical Presentation

- **Massive bleeding per rectum:** In the form of melaena, it is not uncommon. In many other patients, mild chronic bleeding can result in anaemia. Blood is maroon coloured.
- **Acute Meckel's diverticulitis:** Factors which precipitate diverticulitis are:
  - Peptic ulceration due to ectopic gastric mucosa of the diverticulum
  - Ingested foreign material, e.g. stalk of vegetable, seeds, fish or chicken bones
  - Faecolith (not common in ileum), tumours, worms causing stasis and bacterial infection
  - Inflammation and ischaemia caused by torsion due to an associated band—mesodiverticular band
  - Association with acute appendicitis
- **Perforation:** It is impossible to differentiate it from ruptured appendix. This is treated by laparotomy and resection of diverticulum along with adjacent intestine. In majority of appendicular perforations, local abscess will occur because of retrocaecal position of the appendix (70%). However, perforation of Meckel's diverticulum, even though a rare cause of peritonitis, has a high mortality rate. This is because infection spreads very fast as **diverticulum is intraperitoneal and contents are faeculent**.

**RULE OF 2 FOR MECKEL'S DIVERTICULUM**

- Incidence: 2%
- Location: 2 feet proximal to ileocaecal junction
- Length: 2 inches long
- Ectopic tissue: 2 types—gastric and pancreatic
- Presentation: 2 years or below 2 years is the most common age
- Male: female ratio—1:2

- As a cause of **intestinal obstruction**, when it is associated with a band or due to volvulus. It is the most common presentation in adults (Key Box 60.18).

Key Box 60.18

**Meckel's Diverticulum and Intestinal Obstruction**

- Intussusception
- Volvulus due to band
- Internal herniation beneath mesodiverticular band
- Diverticulitis with band
- Littre's hernia

*Pearls of Wisdom*

Older child, deformed umbilicus, scarless abdomen with intestinal obstruction—cause may be Meckel's diverticulum. Hernia of Littre is a hernial sac containing Meckel's diverticulum (Key Box 60.18).

- **As a cause of intussusception:** Here also, inflamed heterotopic tissue can be found in the diverticulum (2% cases).
- **Pain** can occur due to chronic peptic ulceration.
- **Neoplasm:** Carcinoids and GIST are more common in Meckel's diverticulum than elsewhere in the small intestine although presence of Meckel's diverticulum itself is rare.

### Investigations

1. CECT abdomen is the investigation in cases of acute abdomen. In Meckel's diverticulitis, round or tubular air-fluid structures communicating with small bowel can be seen. Mural wall thickening and enhancement also can be made out.
2. **$^{99m}$Tc-labelled pertechnetate** when given IV, may localise the heterotopic gastric mucosa in the Meckel's diverticulum, in about 90% of patients.
   - This radionuclide is taken up by **mucin-secreting cells** and **parietal cells** and it is secreted immediately. Thus, if $^{99m}$Tc appears in the stomach as well as in other part of bowel, it indicates functioning heterotopic tissue.
   - Even acute bleeding: This is the investigation of choice even when bleeding is at a rate of 0.1 ml/minute, it can detect Meckel's diverticulum. Hence, it is superior to angiography.

*Pearls of Wisdom*

The pertechnetate anion $^{99m}$Tc is selectively taken up by gastric mucosal cells, thyroid, salivary glands and choroid plexus.

### Treatment (Fig. 60.45)

1. Incidentally found Meckel's during laparotomy for some other causes can be left alone, provided it has a wide mouth. However, a note of it must be made in the operation register (Key Box 60.19).
2. Meckel's diverticulum with bleeding, band, perforation and narrow mouth is treated by removal of diverticulum with adjacent intestine because the gastric tissue may often line the adjacent intestine also (Figs 60.46 and 60.47).

Key Box 60.19

**Indications for Removal of Incidentally found Meckel's Diverticulum**

- Children under 2 years of age
- Meckel's with a band
- Meckel's with adhesions
- Meckel's with narrow base
- Long Meckel's diverticulum

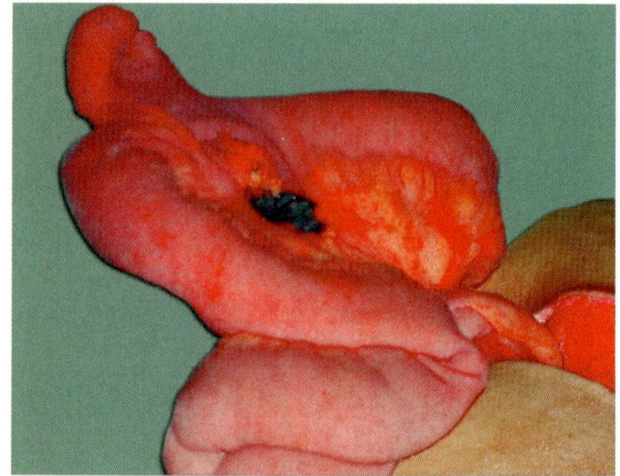

**Fig. 60.45:** Inflamed Meckel's diverticulum of surgery

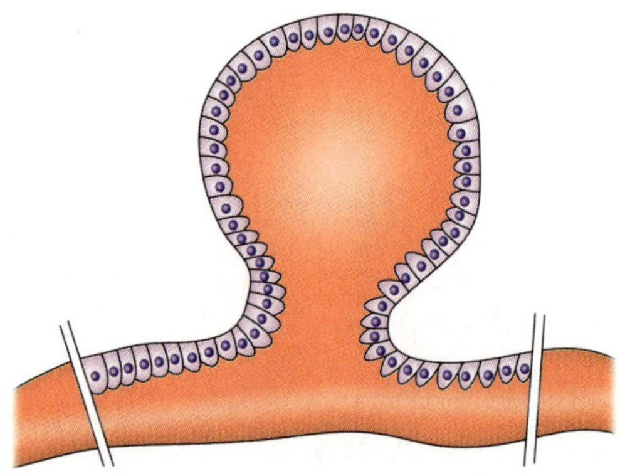

**Fig. 60.46:** Meckel's diverticulectomy should include normal intestine also

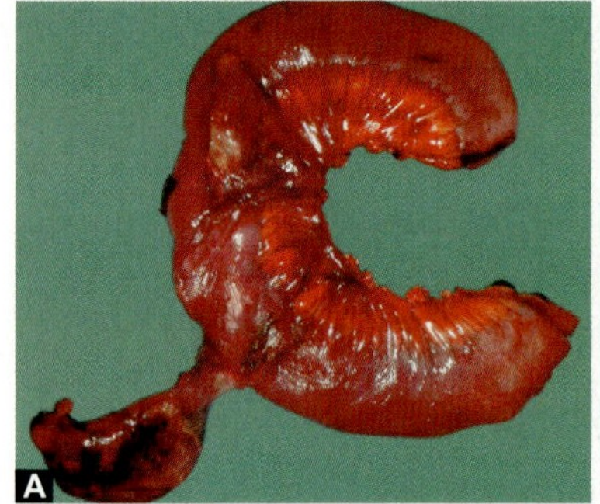


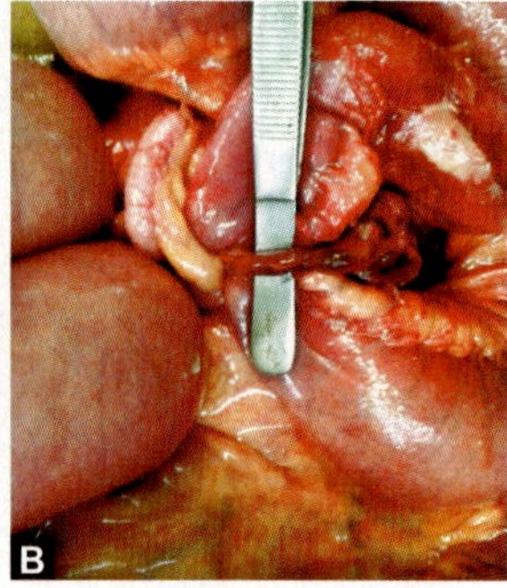


**Figs 60.47:** (A) Resected Meckel's diverticulum with normal intestine; (B) Meckel's diverticulum with band and obstruction (*Courtesy:* Dr Pramod K, Dr Deviprasad Shetty, Kasturba Hospital, Manipal)

## ADHESIONS AND BANDS

### Adhesions

**Introduction:** Intra-abdominal adhesions develop after abdominal and pelvic surgery as part of the normal healing processes that occur after damage to the peritoneum. Open adnexial surgery, ileal pouch surgery and open abdominal hysterectomy are the most common surgeries causing intestinal obstruction. The early balance between fibrin deposition and degradation seems to be the critical factor in adhesion formation. They also cause significant morbidity, including adhesive small bowel obstruction, infertility and increased difficulty with reoperative surgery. Thus, high chances of causing intestinal fistula after reexploration.

**Definition:** Peritoneal adhesions can be defined as abnormal fibrous bands between organs or tissues or both in the abdominal cavity that are normally separated. They are common causes of intestinal obstruction in the western world.

*Pearls of Wisdom*

It is important to realise that secondary infertility in women and ectopic gestation can occur due to adhesions.

### Causes: Remember the Important 5 I s

1. **Infection:** Laparotomy done for acute appendicitis with or without perforation, perforation peritonitis, intra-abdominal abscess have higher incidence of adhesions. Surgery is the commonest cause of peritoneal adhesions.
2. **Ischaemia:** Lack of blood supply, particularly venous occlusion can cause adhesions, e.g. mesenteric vascular occlusion.
3. **Iatrogenic:** It refers to talc, silk thread, foreign body (mop), etc. used for surgery which can induce extensive adhesions due to foreign body reaction (spilled gallstone also).
4. **Injury** to the bowel can result in adhesions.

5. **Irradiation** enteritis is becoming common due to irradiation for carcinoma of the cervix.

## Pathogenesis

Ischaemia and irritation of the intestines are the chief factors responsible for adhesions (Key Box 60.20).

Key Box 60.20

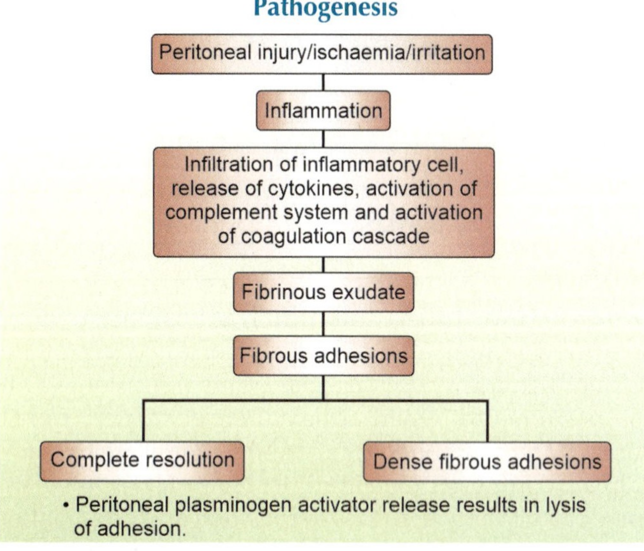


## Types (Fig. 60.48)

1. **Fibrinous adhesions** (bread and butter adhesions): They are the causes of early postoperative obstruction, which settles down within 3–5 days. Majority of them disappear in due course of time.
2. **Fibrous adhesions:** If the infection is continuing or if foreign body is present, the fibrinous material is converted to fibrous band. They also occur at the site of ischaemia. They will cause late intestinal obstruction (Fig. 60.49).
3. **Tuberculous adhesions** are dense adhesions that result in matting of intestinal coils. Separating them at laparotomy is extremely difficult (Fig. 60.50).
   Congenital band is the 4th type of band (not due to adhesion).

*Pearls of Wisdom*

A congenital band, omental band, a string band of bacterial peritonitis or a fibrous band of tuberculosis is responsible for obstruction (Fig. 60.51, and Key Box 60.21).

Key Box 60.21

**Types of Band**

- Congenital : Transduodenal band of Ladd
  : Vitellointestinal duct associated band
- Acquired : Following peritonitis
  : Diverticulum
  : Greater omentum as a band

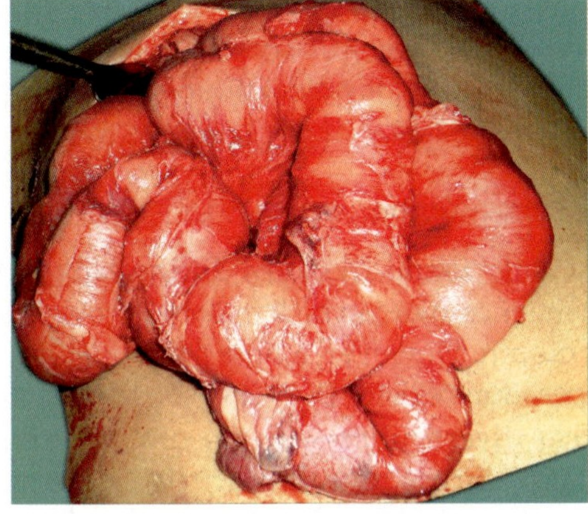

**Fig. 60.48:** Bread and butter adhesions—case of perforation peritonitis

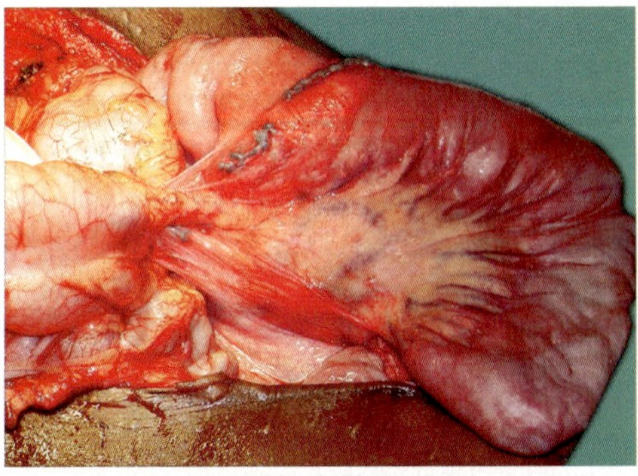

**Fig. 60.49:** Postappendicectomy band causing obstruction

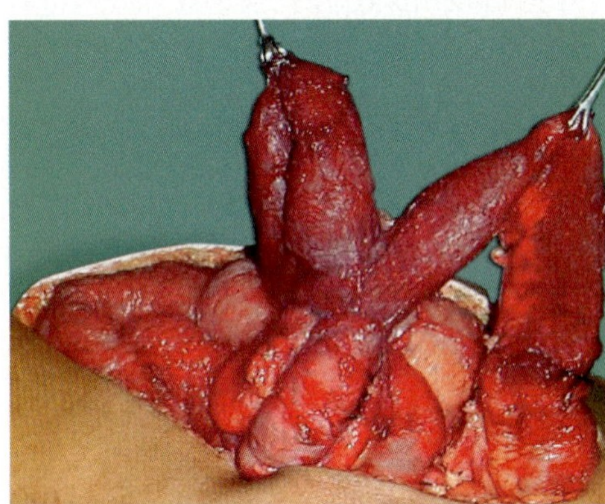

**Fig. 60.50:** Tuberculous adhesions and bands causing intestinal obstruction

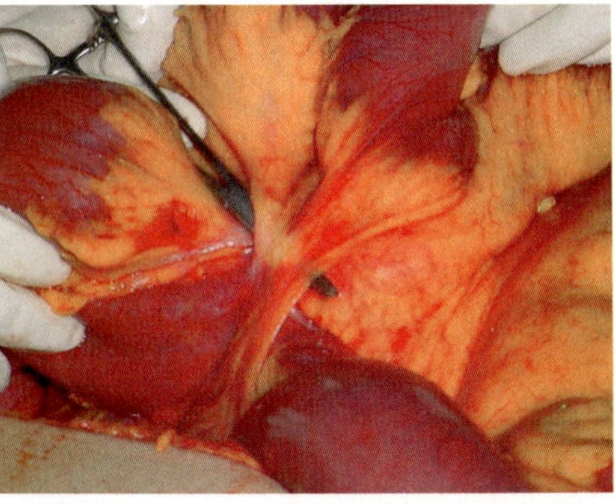

**Fig. 60.51:** Congenital band causing obstruction

### Clinical Features

- Recurrent abdominal pain, vomiting and distension are the typical features. Often the attacks are mild and self-limiting. However, persistent symptoms require monitoring and treatment.
- There may be peristalsis as in cases of terminal ileum.
- Gangrene is not common in cases of adhesive obstruction (Fig. 60.51). However, these cases have to be closely monitored for any changes in the type of pain or new abdominal signs. Severe pain, tachycardia, temperature, tachypnoea and tenderness in the abdomen indicate gangrene or perforation (Figs 60.52 and 60.53).

Gilroy Benan triad of adhesive pain:
- Pain gets aggravated or relieved on change of posture.
- Pain in the region of old abdominal scar.
- Tenderness elicited by pressure over the scar.

### Investigations

Plain X-ray abdomen.

### Treatment

#### *I. Conservative Treatment*

- In the form of nasogastric aspiration, IV replacement of fluids and electrolytes to correct dehydration may be successful in early postoperative obstruction. If it is not successful, reoperation is required. Generally 48–72 hours is the waiting period in patients who present to the hospital as late adhesive obstruction.

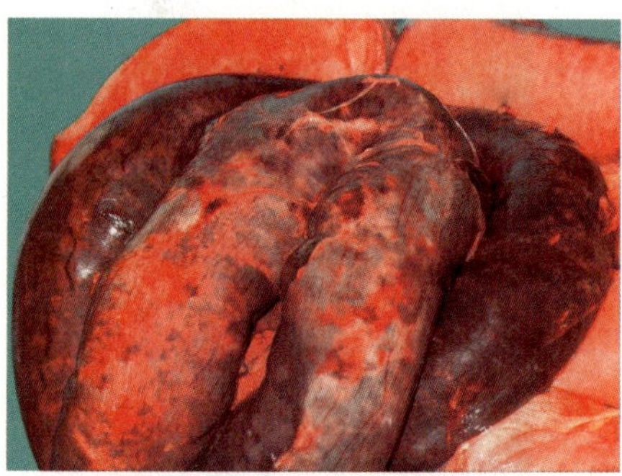

**Fig. 60.52:** Close up view of gangrene

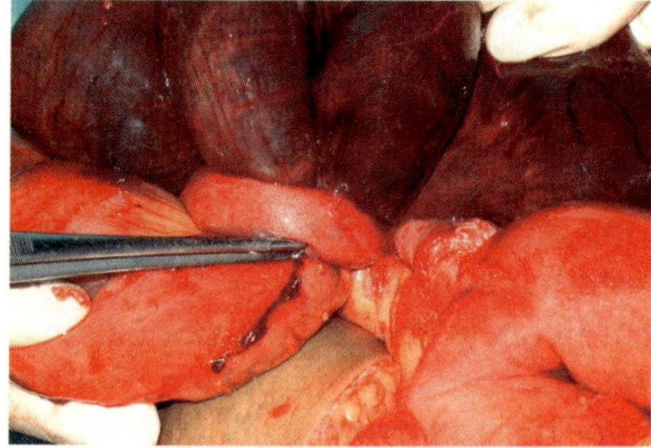

**Fig. 60.53:** Band secondary to peritonitis causing gangrene

Further delay may result in perforation or gangrene of the bowel.
- Record pulse rate, blood pressure, abdominal girth and intake output. Increasing pulse rate, hypotension, increasing abdominal girth and oliguria in spite of adequate IV fluids will suggest gangrene. Such cases need to be explored immediately.

#### *II. Surgical Methods* (Key Box 60.22)

- Where fibrous bands are the cause, they need to be divided to relieve obstruction.
- Laparoscopic adhesiolysis is more often being used and it is indicated in pelvic adhesion, selected cases of abdominal adhesion, single band adhesion and obstruction with mild distension.

Key Box 60.22

**How to Decrease Adhesions?**

- Handle the bowel carefully. Good suturing without tension. Avoid anastomotic leak.
- Raw peritoneal areas should not be sutured.
- Thorough peritoneal toilet in cases of peritonitis with saline or dextran to drain pus, bile, blood clots.
- Avoid spillage of contents—bile, faecal matter.
- Prefer a Pfannenstiel incision to midline incision.
- Noble's plication (Fig. 60.54)
- Laparoscopic method produces decreased adhesions than laparotomy.
- Membrane barriers.

#### *III. Prevention of Adhesion* (Key Box 60.23)

A. Recently **absorbable and nonabsorbable membrane barriers** such as expanded polytetrafluoroethylene **(PTFE)** and membrane composed of hyaluronic acid and carboxy-methyl cellulose have been used.

B. **Noble's plication:** By suturing loops together so that they are fixed in a suitable relation to one another (not very successful) (Fig. 60.54).

Key Box 60.23

**Membrane Barriers**

- The bioresorbable membrane called seprafilm is currently the most effective membrane barrier.
- It consists of hyaluronic acid and carboxymethylcellulose.
- At the completion of surgery, these films are placed at the potential sites of adhesion formation—such as pelvis, between the intestinal loops.
- Mechanism of action: Within the next 24 to 48 hours, the seprafilm membrane hydrates to form a gel-like barrier. It slowly resorbs within 7 days.
- These barriers should not be used to cover the anastomosis—chances of leak rates are high.

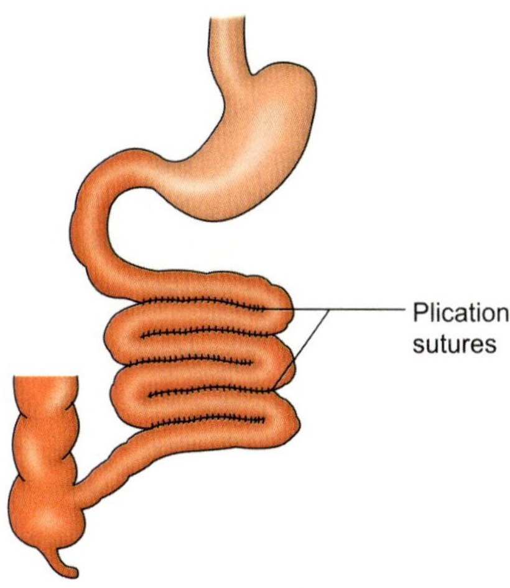


Fig. 60.54: Surgery for adhesions

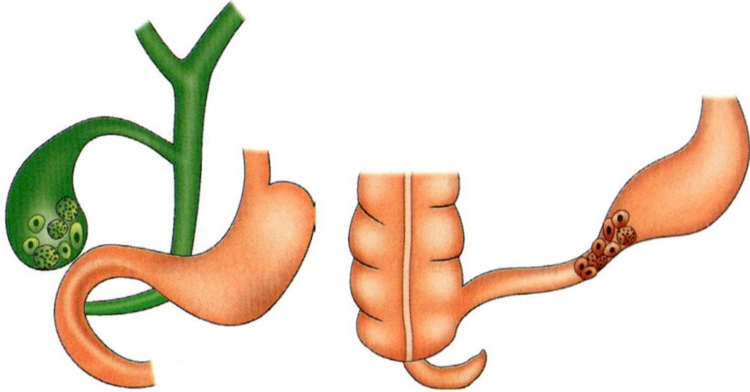

Fig. 60.55: Cholecystoduodenal fistula caused by gallstones

Fig. 60.56: Gallstones ileus (*Courtesy:* Both these figures are contributed by Ms Vidhushi, Kasturba Medical College, Manipal)

Key Box 60.24 describes summary of adhesive obstruction.

Key Box 60.24

**Adhesive Intestinal Obstruction**

- It is the most common cause of intestinal obstruction (in the West).
- The most common cause of adhesion is inflammatory peritonitis.
- It is the cause of recurrent intestinal obstruction—often partial.
- Conservative treatment is successful in majority of cases.
- One can wait for 3–4 days with careful monitoring before a decision of laparotomy is undertaken (worsening situation).
- Repeated X-ray abdomen and CT scan will show changes and progression of the obstruction.
- Most valuable clinical signs of ischaemia/gangrene are tachycardia and tenderness.
- Adhesiolysis/resection is the treatment.

## GALLSTONE ILEUS—GALLSTONE OBTURATION

**Introduction:** Gallstone ileus is more common in women and accounts for 1–4% of all presentations to hospital with small bowel obstruction. The term gallstone ileus is a misnomer, as the condition is a mechanical obstruction of the gut and not a true ileus.

- It should be suspected in a patient who has gallstones and present with intestinal obstruction.
- Elderly females above the age of 60 are usually affected.
- Gallstone reaches the terminal ileum by forming 'cholecystoduodenal fistula' due to recurrent attacks of cholecystitis (Figs 60.55 to 60.58).
- Due to recurrent inflammation, adhesions develop between gallbladder and duodenum (common) or gallbladder and colon or stomach (rare). Large stones cause pressure necrosis, resulting in formation of a cholecystoduodenal fistula.
- Terminal ileum is the narrowest portion of the gut wherein gallstone gets impacted. Sometimes, the stone may ulcerate from gallbladder into jejunum, colon, etc.

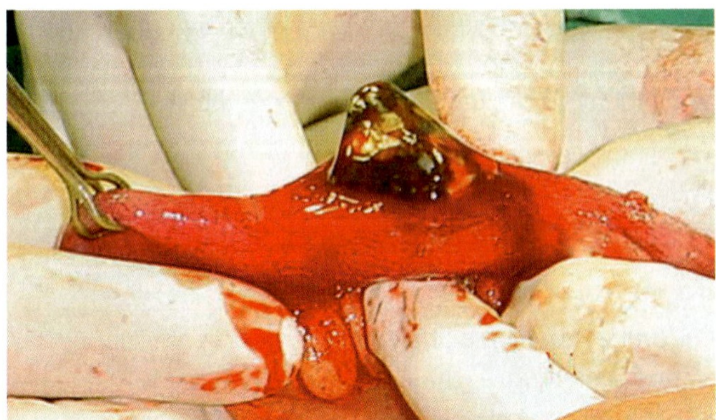

Fig. 60.57: Gallstone ileus (*Courtesy:* Prof MG Shenoy and Dr GN Prasad, KMC, Manipal)

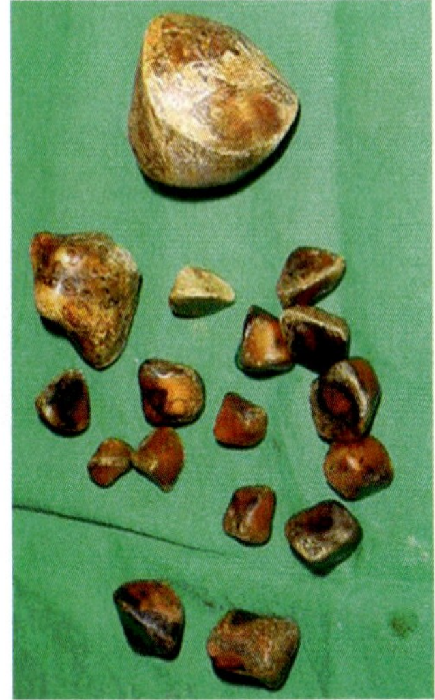

Fig. 60.58: 17 Gallstones were removed in this case

- *Clinical features:* They are suggestive of small intestinal obstruction—abdominal pain is severe, vomiting and distension. Step ladder peristalsis may be seen. History suggestive of recurrent cholecystitis may be present.

***Rigler's triad:*** **Pneumobilia**, the **presence of an aberrant gallstone** and **enteric obstruction** (Fig. 60.59). *Bouveret syndrome: It is a gastric outlet syndrome secondary to stone lodged in proximal duodenum due to cholecystoduodenal fistula. Proximal migration of the stone will precipitate obstruction.

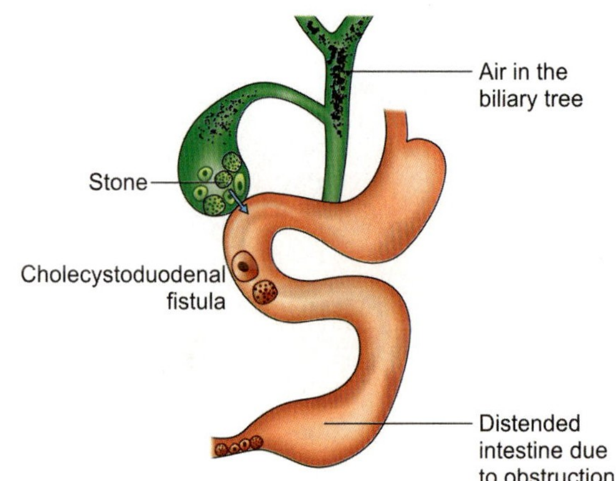


**Fig. 60.59:** Rigler's triad

## Investigations

1. **Plain X-ray abdomen** (erect position) may demonstrate multiple gas and fluid levels and stone in the gallbladder and also in the lower abdomen suggesting gallstone ileus.
   - **Air may be found** in the biliary system.
2. **Small bowel enema** may demonstrate partial obstruction.
3. **Computed tomography (CT)** scanning is the investigation of choice. It has preoperative diagnosis of gallstone ileus with a sensitivity of 93%. It will also indicate any inflammation of the gallbladder, fistula—air pockets in the gallbladder, distal stone and proximal dilatation.

## Treatment

There is difference of opinion regarding what is the ideal surgery to be done in case of gallstone obstruction. It is because many patients are elderly, with co-morbidity and they have intestinal obstruction (dehydration, bowel oedema, bacterial proliferation, etc). Whatever it is, the first step is always to do enterolithotomy by incising the ileum and deliver the stone/stones. It may be possible to crush the stone and pass it onto caecum, avoiding enterolithotomy. Search the proximal intestine for any other stones. What must be done next? Two types are described.

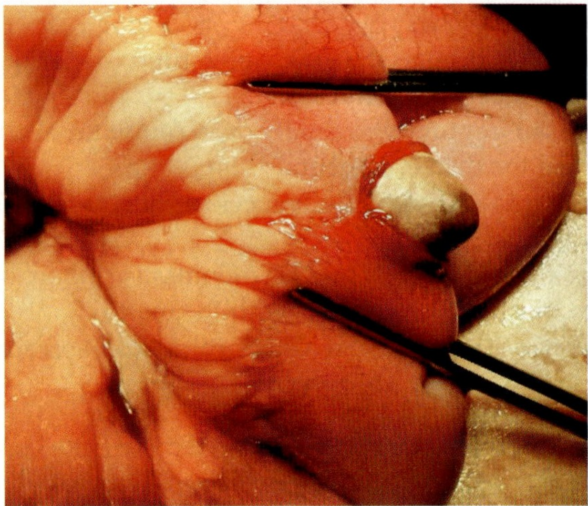

**Fig. 60.60:** Enterolithotomy and removal of stone

1. **Single stage procedure:** If general condition of the patient is good, and gallbladder is gangrenous or inflamed (more chances of perforation), enterolithotomy, cholecystectomy followed by closure of the duodenal fistula is done.
2. **Two-stage procedure:** If general condition is not good or with no active inflammation of the gallbladder, enterolithotomy is the procedure of choice, followed 6 weeks later by cholecystectomy with closure of the duodenal fistula (Fig. 60.60).

## INTUSSUSCEPTION

### Definition

Invagination of one segment of intestine into another (usually the proximal into distal) is called intussusception.

*Pearls of Wisdom*

It is the most common cause of intestinal obstruction in infants aged 6 to 18 months.

**Incidence:** 2–4/1000 live births.

### Types

1. **Simple ileocolic** is the most common type, followed by ileoileal or colocolic.
2. **Compound**—ileo-ileocolic
3. **Retrograde jejunogastric intussusception**, a complication of gastrojejunostomy (GJ) is a rare but interesting type of intussusception (*see* page 748).

*Cholecystoduodenal fistula, choledochoduodenostomy, sphincteroplasty, emphysematous cholecystitis are a few other conditions wherein air is found within biliary tree.

## Parts (Fig. 60.61)

1. **Intussuscipiens:** It is the outer tube (distal bowel which receives the intestine).
2. **Intussusceptum:** Proximal bowel (inner tube) which enters the distal segment.
3. **Apex** is the part which advances further into the distal bowel.
4. **Neck**, the narrowest portion of intussusception, is the junction of entering layer with the mass.

   The whole mass that develops is called intussusception.

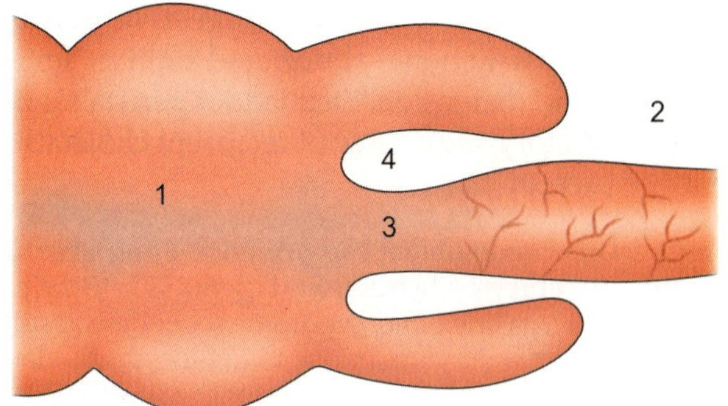


**Fig. 60.61:** Parts of intussusception: 1. Intussuscipiens, 2. Intussusceptum, 3. Apex, 4. Neck

## Aetiopathogenesis

1. **Idiopathic intussusception:** Actual cause is not known. It is seen in infants. Possible factors (Key Box 60.25).
   - **Dietary factor:** Around the age of 6–9 months, weaning of breast milk is done. Weaning causes alteration in the bacterial flora in the GIT, causing enlargement of the Peyer's patches. These protrude into the terminal ileum and may precipitate intussusception.
   - **Infective factor:** It usually follows upper respiratory tract infection with virus (Adeno rotaviruses) which produce inflammation of Peyer's patches.

Key Box 60.25

**Predisposing Factors**

- Recent viral infection (upper respiratory)
- Recent operation
- Henoch-Schönlein purpura
- Cystic fibrosis
- Coeliac disease
- Haemophilia

2. **Adult intussusception (secondary):** In adults, there is always a cause for intussusception (Key Box 60.26 and Figs 60.62 and 60.63).

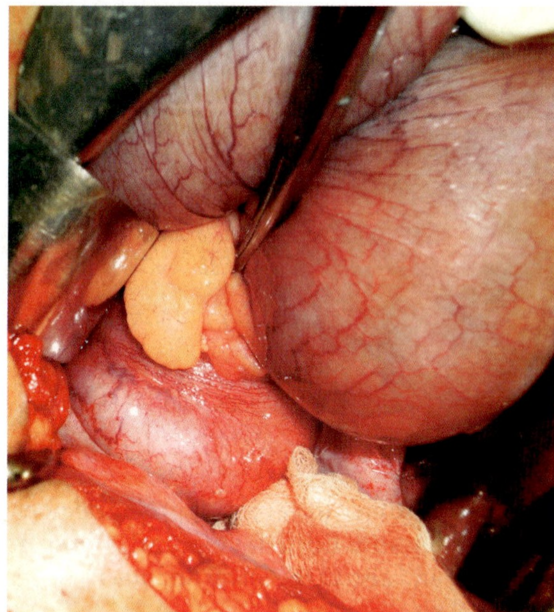

**Fig. 60.62:** Carcinoid of the ileum with intussusception

Key Box 60.26

**Adult Intussusception**

- Meckel's diverticulum
- Polyps, tumours, submucous lipoma
- Carcinoma colon (caecum, transverse colon)

## Pathophysiology

- As the apex advances, it drags the mesentery containing blood vessels which get obstructed at the neck resulting in mucosal ulcers and haemorrhages. Marked lymphadenopathy and hypertrophy of Peyer's patch is found at operation.
- If the neck is too tight, gangrene sets in very early, as in ileocolic intussusception.
- All other features of strangulation, dehydration, distension and septicaemic shock develop later.

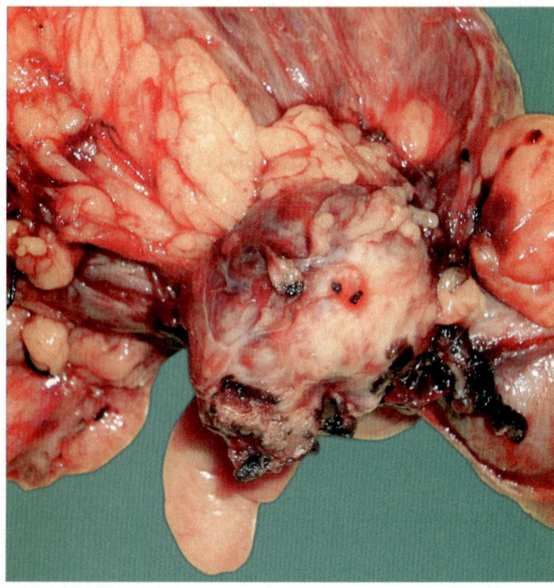

**Fig. 60.63:** Carcinoid of the ileum causing intussusception—resected specimen

### Clinical Features

A. In children, B. In adults

**In children:** First born male infants between 6 and 9 months are commonly affected. Boys : Girls—3 : 2.

- **Child screams** with abdominal pain[1] (intestinal colic) which is associated with facial pallor.
- One attack of **red currant jelly stools** is characteristic. Bleeding is due to mucosal ulcer (venous infarction). Mucus secretion is due to irritation of intestines. This is followed by absolute constipation. **Red currant jelly stools are not found in adult intussusception.**
- Vomiting 3–4 times, initially due to pylorospasm. Later, due to obstruction.
- In between the spasms, the child sleeps but gets up suddenly with pain.

### Signs

- The mother is asked to feed the baby in sitting position and examination of the baby's abdomen is done with the left hand, standing in front of the mother.
- A contracting, hardening mass in and around the umbilical region can be felt (**sausage-shaped,** Fig. 60.64).

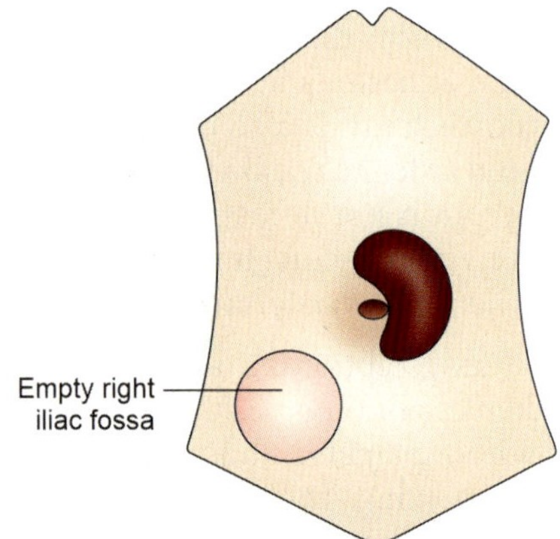


**Fig. 60.64:** Sausage-shaped mass—resonant, mobile

- **Emptiness in the right iliac fossa** (Dance's sign—*signe de dance*).
- There may be a **visible step ladder peristalsis.**
- Rarely, intussusception can be seen **outside the anus** due to long mesentery.
- Rectal examination reveals **blood-stained mucus** on the examining finger.
- Features of peritonitis occur in untreated cases.

### Investigations

- **Ultrasound** (Fig. 60.65) is the investigation of choice. It can detect target sign and detect mass **(Doughnut sign)**. With Doppler, it can be used to assess vascularity of the bowel also. Thus, barium enema has become obsolete.
- **CT scan:** It is the most sensitive imaging modality in the diagnosis of intussusception. Sausage-shaped mass, with blood vessels within bowel lumen are typical findings (*see* Fig. 60.66 to 60.68). Gangrene can be detected.
- More useful in adults.
- **Barium enema:** 'Claw (pincer) ending' (Fig. 60.69) is diagnostic of intussusception. This is also called '**meniscus sign**'. If there is any suspicion of gangrene, this test should not be done. This test is not done nowadays.

### Treatment

**A. *In children***

***I. Conservative Treatment*** (Key Box 60.27)

- Hydrostatic reduction can be attempted when the gangrene is ruled out as in early intussusception. A lubricated catheter is introduced into the rectum and 1–2 litres of saline from a height of 1–2 metres is allowed to run. Catheter is removed and buttocks are pressed together. 50–70% of cases are reduced by this method, 1:3 barium sulphate in warm isotonic saline can also be used.

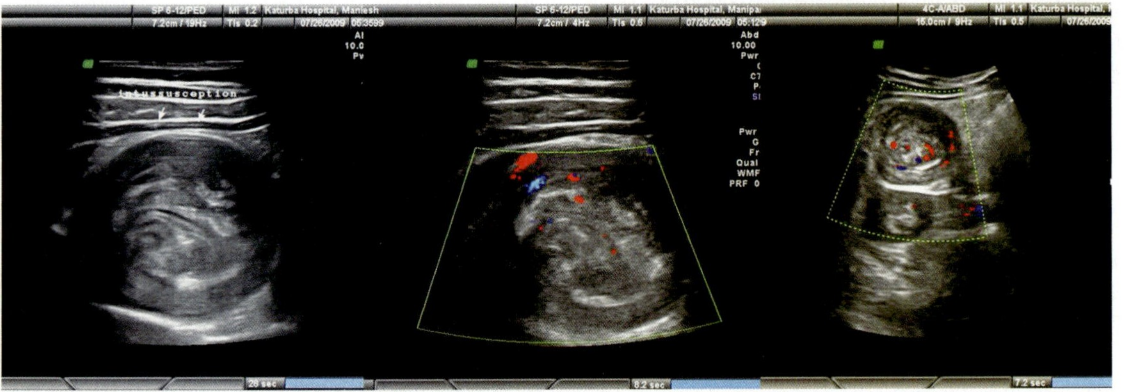

**Figs 60.65:** Ultrasound—pseudokidney sign, target sign, Duplex—assesses vascularity also

[1]Hindi speaking mother says; *'Baccha sota hai aur rota hai.'*

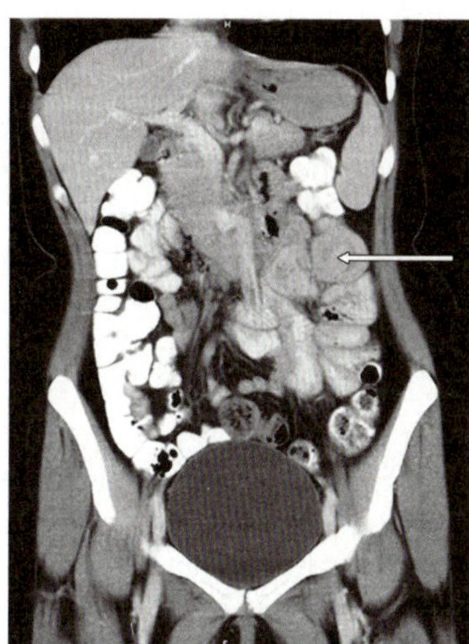

Fig. 60.66: Intussusception due to polyp (arrow)

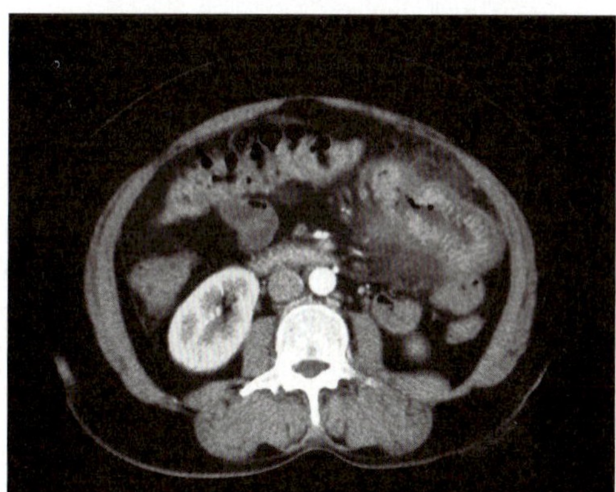

Fig. 60.67: Jejunal carcinoma—CT coronal section

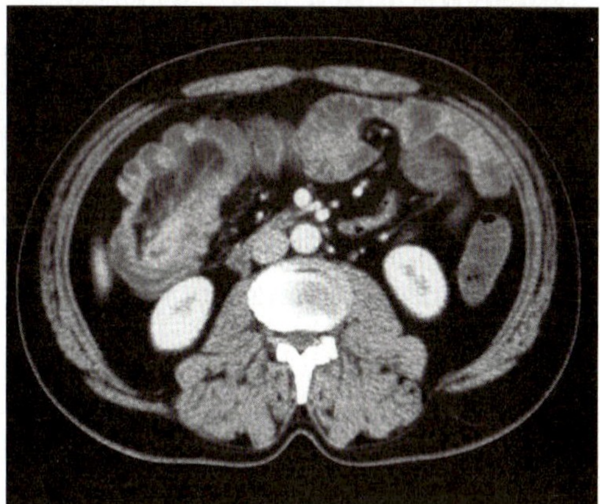

Fig. 60.68: Ileocolic intussusception CT

Key Box 60.27

**Hydrostatic Reduction is Successful when**

1. Flatus and faeces are passed with barium
2. Child is symptom-free and comfortable
3. Small bowel loops are filled with contrast

**Advantage**

- Easy, nonoperative method

**Complication**

- Rarely, colonic perforation

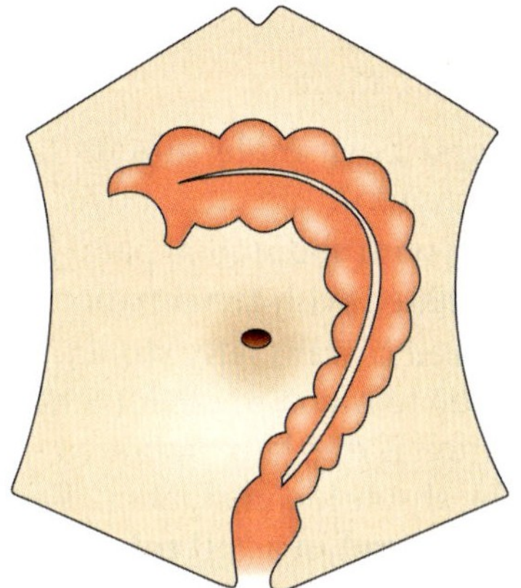

Fig. 60.69: Claw ending

- Air contrast enema will not reduce gangrenous bowel. Air is pumped into the colon at a pressure of 60–80 mmHg.

  **Contraindications**
  - Peritonitis with shock
  - Total intestinal obstruction.

***II. Surgical Treatment*** (Figs 60.73 to 60.75)

**Laparotomy and reduction of intussusception**

Intussusception is reduced by milking (squeezing) the colon in opposite direction, which is facilitated by breaking the adhesions at the neck using the little finger. Appendicectomy is also done, as it avoids any future confusion as to the reason for the abdominal scar. Fixing the caecum is not necessary because idiopathic intussusception rarely recurs. If the loop is gangrenous, resection and ileocolic anastomosis is done.

**B. *In adults:*** Intussusception is due to a pathology such as a polyp or other lesions (Figs 60.70 to 60.75). Presentation in adults is with a palpable abdominal mass, resonant and may be contracting. They are always resected after examining rest of the bowel especially when you suspect polyps. This is because there may be many more such

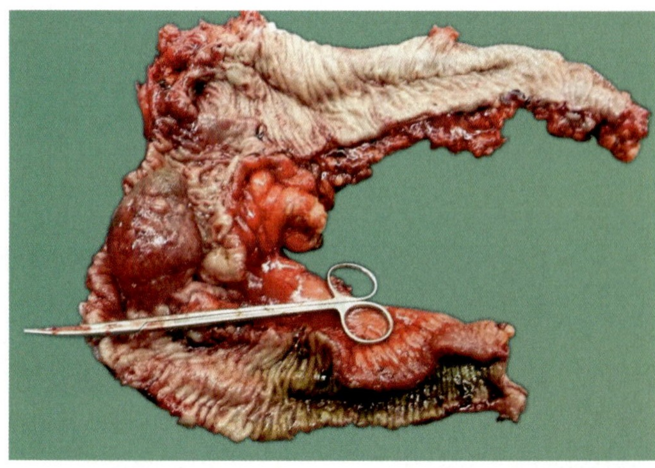

Fig. 60.70: Opened specimen showing polyp

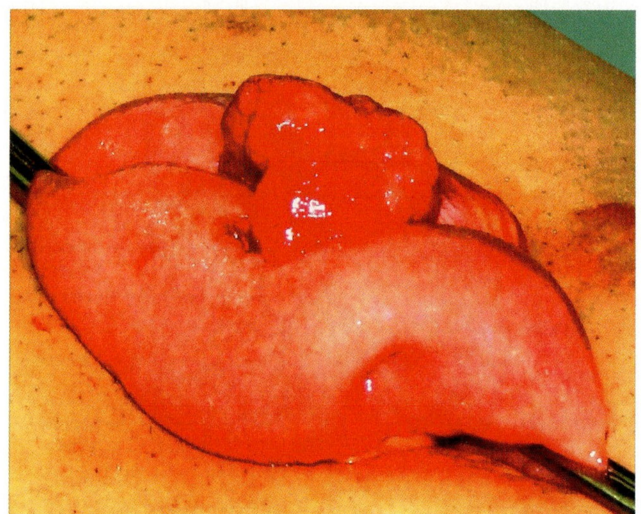

**Fig. 60.71:** Intussusception due to polyp. Enterotomy is done, pedunculated polyp delivered, ligated and enterotomy is closed. (*Courtesy:* Dr Kshama Hegde, Dr Sunilkrishna, Department of Surgery, KMC, Manipal)

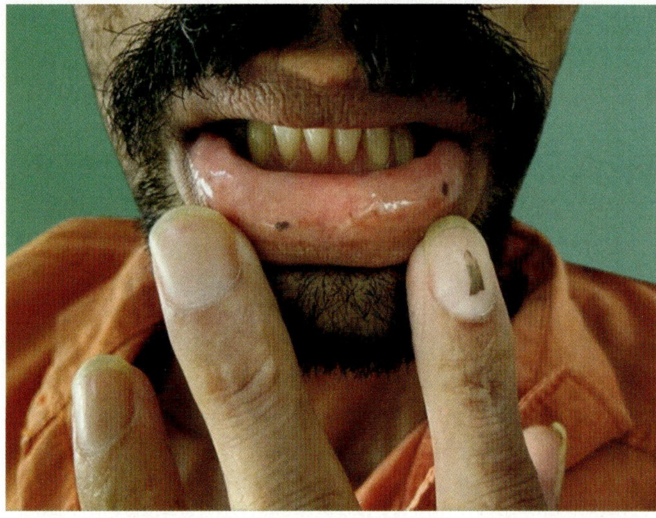

**Fig. 60.72:** Patient with jejunal intussusception and pigmentation of lips-case of Peutz Jeghers syndrome (*Courtesy:* Dr Bharath SV, Dr Sanketh Bhat, Dr Nanda Yashaswi, Dept of surgery, KMC Manipal)

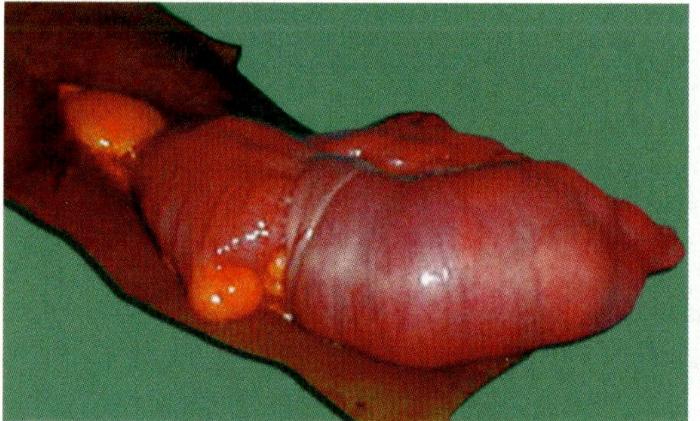

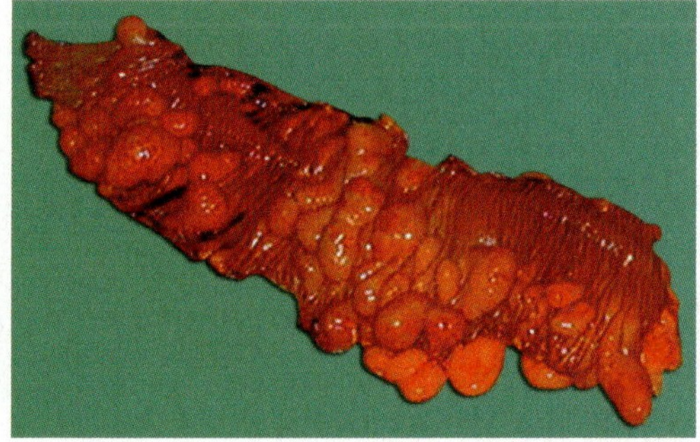

**Figs 60.73 and 60.74:** Adult intussusception due to jejunal lipomatosis. This patient was 24-year-old male who presented with intestinal obstruction. A mass was palpable in the umbilical region at laparotomy. This mass was resected. Opened specimen showed extensive segmental lipomatosis (*Courtesy:* Dr Gabriel Rodrigues, Dr Mahesh Gopa Setty, Dr Lavanya K, KMC, Manipal)

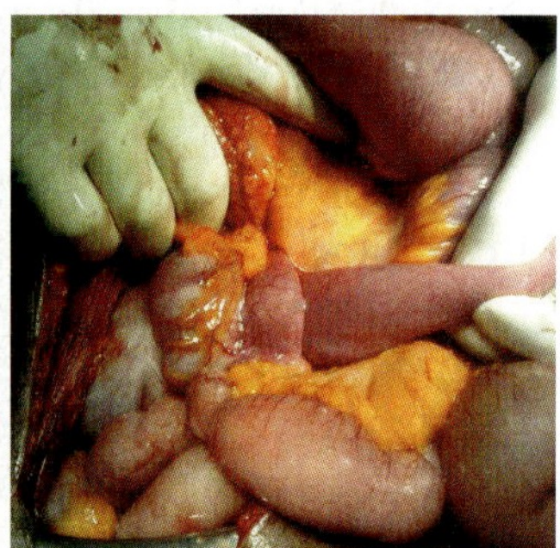

**Fig. 60.75:** Intussusception is reduced at surgery

polyps. In such cases, treatment is more complicated—multiple enterotomies, snaring of pedunculated polyps, on table entroscopy, and snaring, etc.

**Recurrent intussusception is rare:** If it occurs, terminal ileum is sutured to the side of the ascending colon.

Key Box 60.28 for some interesting "more common" about intussusception.

Key Box 60.28

**Acute Intussusception—Most Common**

- Most common in children between 5 and 10 months of age
- Most common cause of intestinal obstruction in children
- Most common cause is idiopathic (90%)
- Most common variety is ileocolic variety
- Most commonly hypertrophied Peyer's patches are reported
- Most common type of nonoperative reduction is by using air and barium enema

## MESENTERIC VASCULAR OCCLUSION

### DEFINITION

Acute mesenteric ischaemia is an abrupt reduction in blood flow to the intestinal circulation of sufficient magnitude to compromise the metabolic requirements and potentially threaten the viability of the affected organs (Key Box 60.29).

Key Box 60.29

**Types**

1. Acute mesenteric ischaemia (AMI): It is a sudden occlusion of artery or vein resulting in gangrene. It has a mortality rate of 60 to 90%.
2. Chronic mesenteric ischaemia (CMI): It is associated with stenosis of coeliac artery, superior mesenteric artery or inferior mesenteric artery.

**SU28.13.2:** Understand and differentiate different parts of small and large intestines depending on length, size, vascular anatomy, mesentery and their attachment.

## Anatomy of Mesenteric Vasculature

The mesenteric arterial and venous circulation of the abdominal viscera form an extensive vascular network. There are a large number of collateral pathways that protect against ischaemic changes. The three major branches of aorta responsible for the arterial supply of the intestine are: Coeliac artery supplies **foregut**, superior mesenteric artery (SMA) supplies **midgut** and inferior mesenteric artery supplies **hindgut**. The venous drainage includes the superior and inferior mesenteric vein.

## Normal Anatomy and Variations

- **Coeliac axis:** Normal coeliac axis anatomy is seen in only 55% of patients. An anomalous right or left hepatic artery has been reported in about 50% of patients.
- **Superior mesenteric artery:** It supplies the entire small intestines and right one-third of transverse colon (Fig. 60.76).
- **Inferior mesenteric artery (IMA):** It supplies left colon including rectum and surgical anal canal. The IMA arises at the level of the third lumbar vertebra supplies the large bowel from mid-transverse colon to upper rectum. Several collateral networks exist in the branches of IMA. These collaterals are important when rectosigmoid or splenic flexure resection is performed (Fig. 60.77).
- **Collaterals:** Like collaterals in the leg, many collaterals exist between 3 major branches—coeliac artery, SMA and IMA. Because of this extensive collaterals, patients remain asymptomatic with normal bowel function may have chronic occlusion of one or two mesenteric vessels.

***Griffiths' point:*** Between branches of left colic and SMA.
***Sudeck point:*** Sigmoidal arteries and superior rectal vessels.

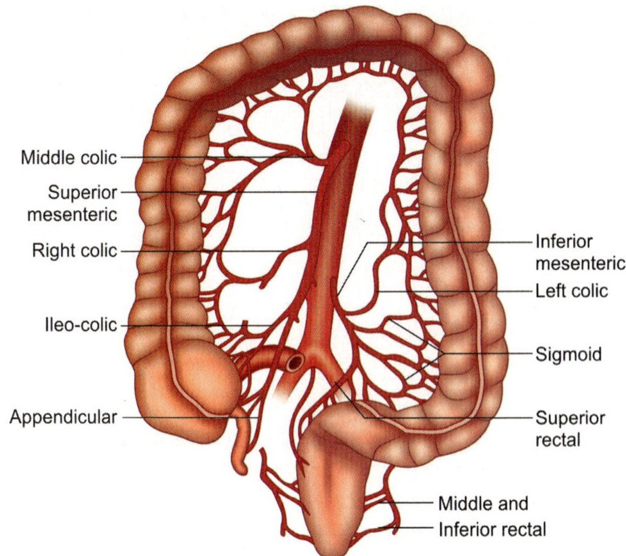


**Fig. 60.76:** Superior mesenteric artery and its branches

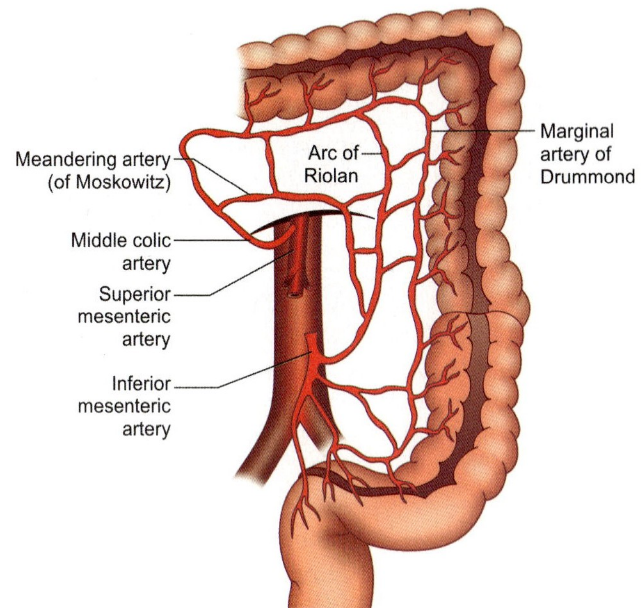


**Fig. 60.77:** Inferior mesenteric artery and its branches

## Types (Fig. 60.78)

1. **Acute mesenteric ischaemia (AMI):** It is a sudden occlusion of artery or vein resulting in gangrene. It has a mortality rate of 60 to 90%.
2. **Chronic mesenteric ischaemia (CMI):** It is associated with stenosis of coeliac artery, superior mesenteric artery or inferior mesenteric artery.
3. **NOMI:** Non-occlusive mesenteric ischaemia.

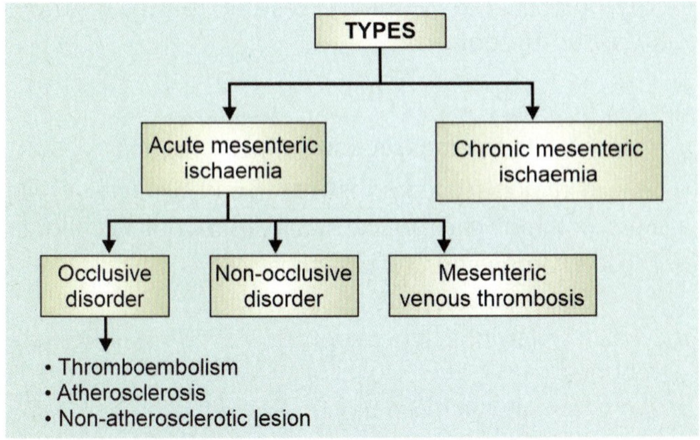


**Fig. 60.78:** Types of mesenteric ischaemia

## Pathogenesis

Ischaemic damage to the intestine occurs with decreased blood supply to a level at which delivery of oxygen and various nutrients cannot maintain oxidative metabolism.

Cell integrity is lost resulting in cell death. In low-flow states, blood is shunted from arterioles to venules near the base of the villus resulting in necrosis of the intestinal villi.

## ACUTE SMA THROMBOEMBOLIC MESENTERIC ISCHAEMIA

SMA takes off at less obtuse angle than the celiac axis. Hence thromboembolism most commonly involves the SMA. Ischaemia affects the mucosa first—most sensitive to hypoxia. Subepithelial oedema occurs within 30 min, loss of epithelial cells along the villus in 1 hour and total loss of villi with sloughing of mucosa in 2 hours. Within 4 hours gangrenous changes start. Thus the condition is rapidly fatal (Key Box 60.30).

Key Box 60.30

**Ischaemic Injury**

Vascular occlusion

↓

Inflammatory cell infiltrate

↓

Loss of capillary integrity

↓

Bowel wall oedema

↓

Breakdown of mucosal barrier

↓

Bacterial translocation

↓

Endotoxaemia

↓

Sequestration of fluid within bowel lumen

### Aetiopathogenesis

- It is common in elderly patients who are hypertensive and usually obese.
- It is due to atherosclerosis causing thrombosis of the superior mesenteric artery or due to emboli which originate from atheromatous plaques or from the infarcted heart.
- Smokers are more often affected by this condition.
- **Superior mesenteric vein** can also get thrombosed due to injury during pancreatectomy or thrombosis as a result of oral contraceptive pills.

### Effects

The pathological effects of arterial occlusion and venous occlusion are the same. Superior mesenteric artery supplies the entire midgut starting from the duodenojejunal flexure to right one-third of the transverse colon. It is an end-artery. As a result of thrombosis, the entire small bowel and portion of the large bowel becomes gangrenous (if there is a thrombus at the origin of superior mesenteric artery).

### Splanchnic Circulation

- It is better to have some idea about the splanchnic circulation to understand the effects of ischaemia to the gut.
- The splanchnic circulation receives approximately 25% of the resting and 35% of the postprandial cardiac output.
- 70% of the mesenteric blood flow is directed to the mucosal and submucosal layers of the bowel. Hence early cases present with bleeding due to mucosal ulcerations.
- 30% supplies the muscularis and serosal layers.
- Blood flow is regulated by intrinsic (metabolic and myogenic) and the extrinsic (neural and humoral) factors.
- Reactive hyperaemia and hypoxic vasodilation are considered intrinsic controls and are responsible for instantaneous fluctuations in splanchnic blood flow.
- An imbalance between tissue oxygen supply and demand will raise the concentration of local metabolites (e.g. hydrogen, potassium, carbon dioxide, and adenosine), resulting in vasodilation and hyperaemia.

### Causes of Acute Mesenteric Ischaemia

1. **Arterial emboli** are the most frequent cause of AMI and are responsible for approximately 40 to 50% of cases. Most mesenteric emboli originate from a cardiac source. They lodge in the superior mesenteric artery (SMA) because it emerges from the aorta at an oblique angle. A few emboli lodge in the origin of middle colic artery.

**Embolic:** Majority of emboli originate in the heart
- Valvular heart disease
- Dilated left atrium
- Recent myocardial infarction
- Atrial arrhythmias
- Ventricular dilatation with mural thrombus
- Atheroemboli
- Aneurysm

2. **Acute mesenteric thrombosis** accounts for 25 to 30% of all ischaemic cases. Atherosclerotic disease is the cause of thrombosis. It typically occurs at the origin of the superior mesenteric artery. Gangrene is more extensive in cases of thrombosis than embolism.

3. **Nonocclusive mesenteric ischaemia (NOMI):** Typically happens in cases of hypotensive patients. Low cardiac output, ICU patients on vasoconstrictors and inotropes precipitate the problem. Splanchnic vasoconstriction occurs in response to hypovolemia. Vasoactive drugs, particularly digoxin, have been implicated in the pathogenesis of NOMI.
4. **Mesenteric venous thrombosis (MVT)** is the least common cause of mesenteric ischaemia, representing up to 10% of all patients with mesenteric ischaemia related to primary clotting disorders. Thrombi usually originate in the venous arcades and propagate (Key Box 60.31).

Key Box 60.31

**Aetiology of Mesenteric Venous Thrombosis**

- Hypercoagulable states (e.g. polycythaemia vera, protein C and S deficiencies)
- Visceral infection
- Portal hypertension
- Blunt abdominal trauma
- Pancreatic malignancy
- Pancreatitis
- Women taking oral contraceptives
- Post-splenectomy
- Smokers

## Clinical Features

### *Symptoms*

1. **Abdominal pain:** Severe, poorly localised, unresponsive to narcotics, out of proportion to the physical findings (Fig. 60.79).
2. Onset may be abrupt (embolism) or insidious (thrombosis).
3. **Gastrointestinal emptying:** Vomiting, diarrhoea, with occult or frank bleeding once infarction sets in.

Condition presents as severe abdominal pain which is sudden onset, constant and more in the periumbilical region. It is often preceded by palpitations, arrhythmia, catheterization or myocardial infarction. There is urge to defecate. Loose stools develop within 2–3 hours of onset of symptoms. Attack of melaena indicates gangrene. Patients often present in an agitated or anxious state.

### *Signs*

- Abdomen is flat or scaphoid with a little to no pain on palpation. Abdomen is often soft and "Pain out of proportion to the signs" is often typical of AMI. Peripheral pulses may be feeble as it is common to have multiple emboli.
- Peritoneal signs with guarding and rigidity is a late sign and implies bowel gangrene and perforation.
- Very soon septic shock develops with dehydration, cold clammy extremities, hypotension, desaturation, acidosis, oliguria.

*Pearls of Wisdom*

Sudden event, sudden bleeding, sudden collapse, severe pain, silent abdomen, shock progressing to sepsis is mesenteric ischaemia.

## Investigations

1. **Total counts** are raised, in about 75% of cases >15,000 cells/mm$^3$.
2. **Plain X-ray abdomen** (erect) reveals absence of gas within the bowel loops and intramural gas. Blunt plicae are seen. This is called **thumb printing** (Figs 60.80 and 60.81).
3. **Metabolic acidosis** in > 50% of cases.
4. **Serum phosphate** levels are raised within 3–4 hours following ischaemia as smooth muscle layer of small bowel is rich in phosphates.
5. **D-dimer** is elevated in all cases.

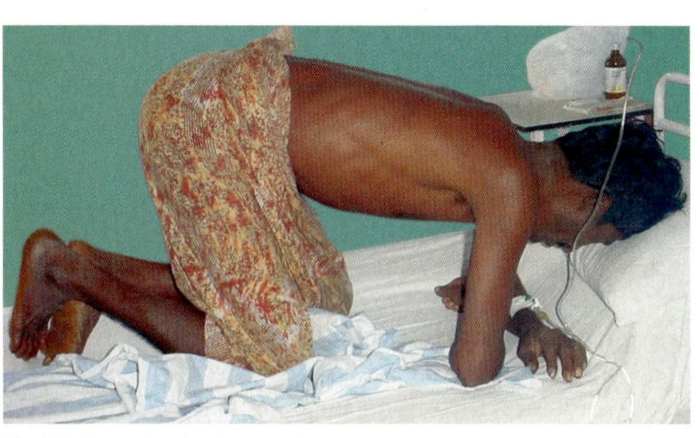

**Fig. 60.79:** Attitude of a patient with severe ischaemia due to superior mesenteric vascular occlusion. In these cases, the pain is disproportionate to the abdominal signs

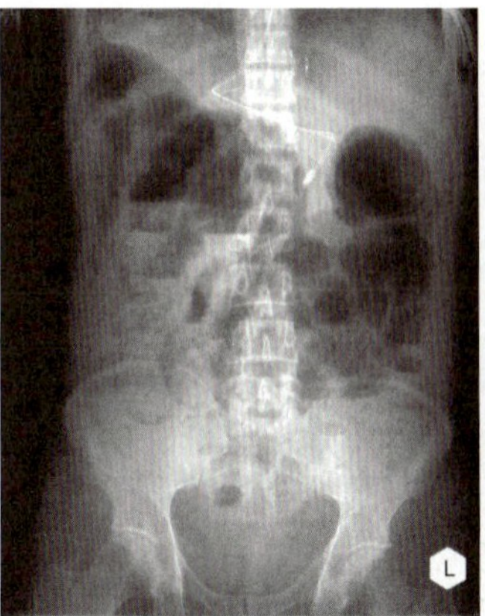


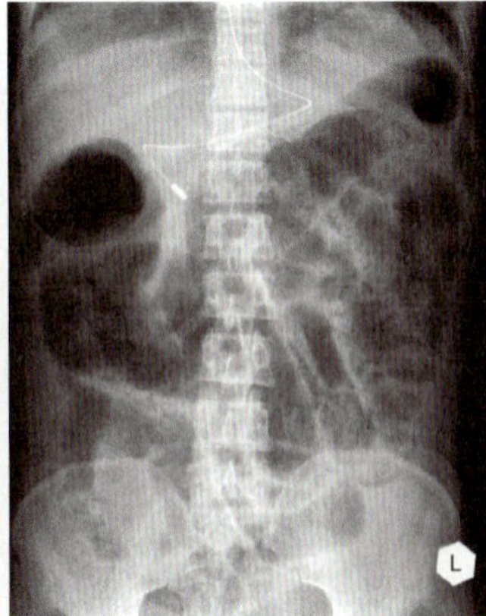


**Figs 60.80 and 60.81:** Plain X-ray showing presence of air in the bowel wall

6. **CT angiogram** is the investigation of choice. It can detect **intramural air pockets** in the bowel wall, air within biliary radicle, perforation, etc. It can also detect thrombus or narrowing of superior mesenteric artery or superior mesenteric vein (Figs 60.82 and 60.83).
7. **Hypercoagulability disorders**—protein C and protein S, antithrombin III, factor V, anticardiolipin antibody (MVT).

## Treatment

- Patient is admitted in intensive care unit.
- Resuscitation is done. Nasogastric tube is inserted. Antibiotics started, heparinisation heparin given.
- Once CT confirms the diagnosis, exploratory laparotomy is done.
  1. Majority of the patients present late with massive gangrene. Massive resection of the gangrenous bowel followed by end to end anastomosis is done. These patients suffer from short bowel syndrome *(vide infra)*, if they survive.
  2. If patients come within 4–6 hours of ischaemia, emergency angiography followed by papaverine infusion (30 to 60 mg/h) into the superior mesenteric artery can be tried. Otherwise, emergency laparotomy is done and the superior mesenteric artery is explored. A Fogarty catheter is introduced and embolectomy is done. These patients may require a **second look operation within 24–48 hours** to rule out gangrene developing later due to rethrombosis of the artery (Fig. 60.84). Before resection check for bowel viability.

     *Assessing bowel viability*
     - Doppler (84%)
     - Absent arterial flow on antimesenteric border of bowel.
     - Absent mesenteric arterial flow
     - Fluorescein test (100%)
       - Sodium fluorescein 1 g administered IV over 30 to 60 seconds and the bowel examined using a hand-held long wave UV Wood's lamp (yellow).
  3. Other vasodilator agents used are: Tolazoline, glucagon, nitroglycerine, nitroprusside, prostaglandin E, phenoxybenzamine, isoproterenol.
  4. Sympathetic epidural block

**Recent advances** in cases of mesenteric ischaemia
- Catheter directed thrombolysis
- Percutaneous transluminal angioplasty

## Prognosis

Majority of the cases present with massive gangrene. Even after massive resection, they succumb to the sepsis and multiorgan failure (Fig. 60.84).

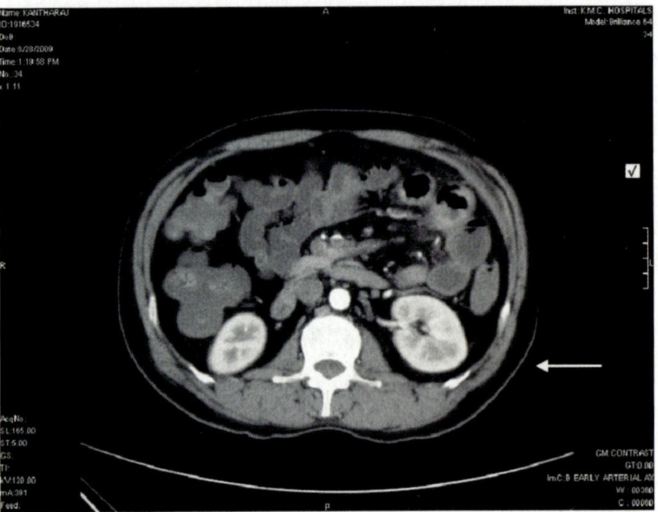

**Fig. 60.82:** CT showing SMA thrombosis

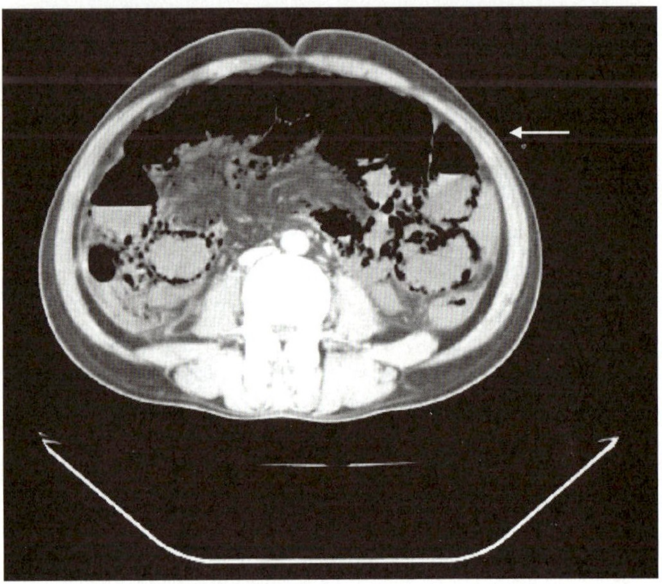

**Fig. 60.83:** CT confirming the same. A case of superior mesenteric arterial thrombosis with massive gangrene (*see* Fig. 60.84) with pneumotosis intestinalis

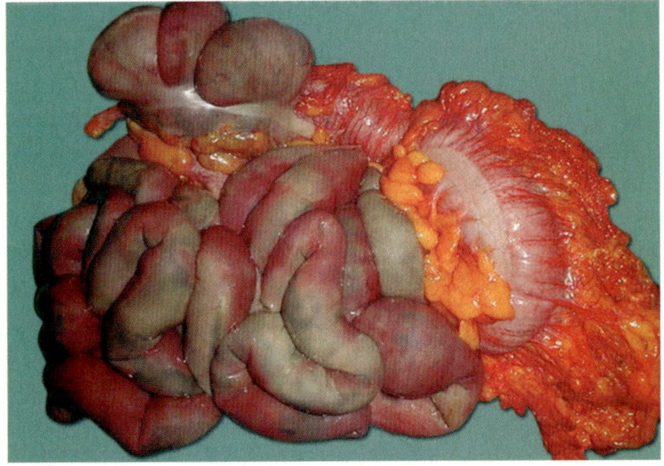

**Fig. 60.84:** Massive gangrene of small intestines and right side of the colon due to thrombosis at the origin of superior mesenteric artery

## NON-OCCLUSIVE MESENTERIC ISCHAEMIA (NOMI)

It is a discrete clinical entity where mesenteric flow is impeded due to arterial spasm.

- Causes of NOMI are given below in Key Box 60.32.
- Typically these patients are critically ill in intensive care units (ICU), intubated. The pathology resides in the mesenteric arcades where severe spasm has limited flow. Like AMI, they can have loose and bloody stools, abdominal pain out of proportion to signs. Tenderness is present.

  Diagnostic arteriography is the only way to demonstrate the small vessel mesenteric arterial spasm that leads to NOMI.
- **Treatment:** Direct catheter delivery of papaverine (30–60 mg/hour) may have to be given for a few days. Systemic anticoagulants are given. Vessel spasm can be overcome by maximizing cardiac output. Peritonitis or clinical evidence of bowel perforation mandates exploration and resection of ischaemic segment. Also, primary cause of acute illness is treated.

Key Box 60.32

**Etiology**

- **Pharmacotherapy**
  - Digoxin
  - Digitalis
  - Cocaine
  - Alpha agonists
  - Vasopressin
- **Sympathetically mediated stress response**
  - Hypovolaemia or haemorrhagic shock
  - Haemodialysis
  - Cardiopulmonary bypass
  - CCF
  - Arrhythmias
  - Pancreatitis
  - Septic shock
  - End-stage renal disease

## CHRONIC MESENTERIC ISCHAEMIA (CMI)

It is a form of severe atherosclerotic disease affecting multiple mesenteric arteries. Most of patients are asymptomatic due to rich collateral network. Most common cause—atherosclerosis. Other causes are vasculitides—Takayasu disease, coarctation of aorta. Women are more commonly affected than men. When patient is not eating, the circulatory demands of the resting bowel are easily met and there is no pain.

- After eating, in times of high demand, pain occurs. Hence called **postprandial pain**. Pain typically begins 15 to 45 minutes after eating and is described as crampy, affecting the upper and periumbilical abdomen. It is due to a phenomenon called **"Gastric steal"** phenomenon. Metabolically active stomach "steals" from the splanchnic circulation. Fixed proximal arterial obstruction does not allow for blood volume to compensate. Small bowel ischaemia and pain follow.
- Patients develop an aversion to eating or "food fear" as the disease progresses.
- Over a period of time, significant weight loss occurs.
- **Triad of CMI: Postprandial pain, food fear and weight loss.**
- CT angiography is the investigation of choice.
- Endovascular therapy and stenting and bypass grafts can be used. Endarterectomy can also be done if significant thrombus is present in the SMA.

## NEONATAL INTESTINAL OBSTRUCTION
(Figs 60.85 to 60.92)

**SU28.14.3:** Describe the clinical features, investigations and principles of management of neonatal obstruction.

### Causes

1. **Hirschsprung's disease**—congenital megacolon
2. Atresia and stenosis
3. Arrested rotation with bands
4. Volvulus neonatorum
5. Meconium ileus
6. Imperforate anus

## HIRSCHSPRUNG'S DISEASE: CONGENITAL MEGACOLON

Hirschsprung's disease is also called congenital megacolon, aganglionic megacolon or primary megacolon. It is one of the common causes of neonatal intestinal obstruction.

### Pathophysiology (Fig. 60.93)

- The disease always involves the anus and rectum wherein parasympathetic ganglion cells are absent in the neural plexus of the intestinal wall. The defect involves internal sphincter.
- As a result of this, there is a terminally constricted, non-relaxing segment, in the rectum and sigmoid (lower part), above which the pelvic colon (sigmoid) is enormously dilated. Rectosigmoid area is involved in 80% of cases.
- Circular muscle hypertrophy, mucosal hyperaemia and ulcers are present in the dilated segments.
- In between, there may be a transition zone (cone), which contains a few parasympathetic ganglion cells.
- Rarely, Hirschsprung's can also involve the entire sigmoid colon or even the entire colon.
- Hirschsprung's rarely occurs in adults also.

### Types of Hirschsprung's Disease (Fig. 60.94)

1. **Ultrashort segment:** Anal canal and terminal rectum are aganglionic.

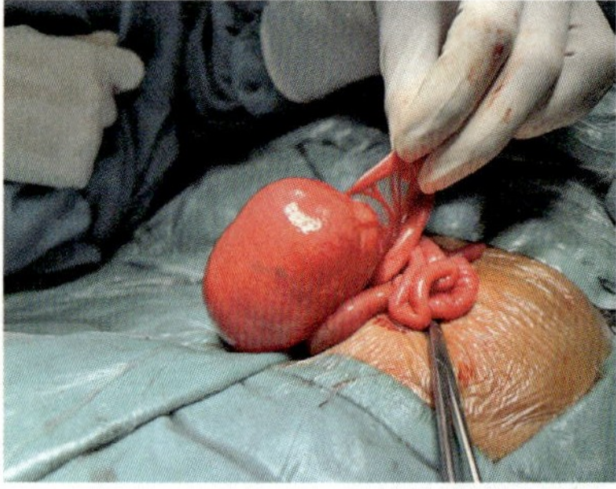
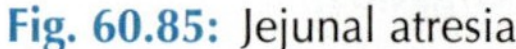

Fig. 60.85: Jejunal atresia

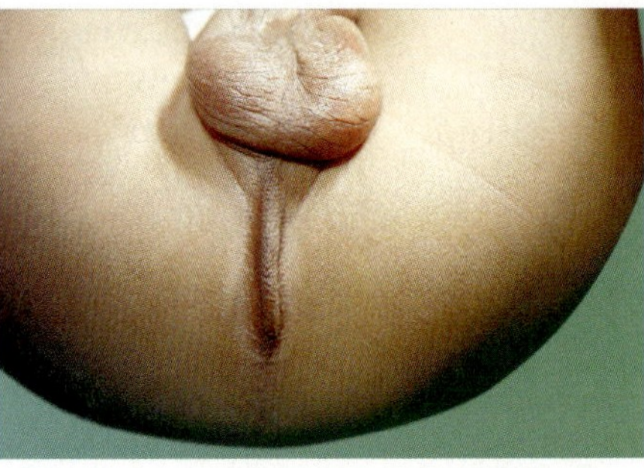

Fig. 60.86A: Anorectal malformation

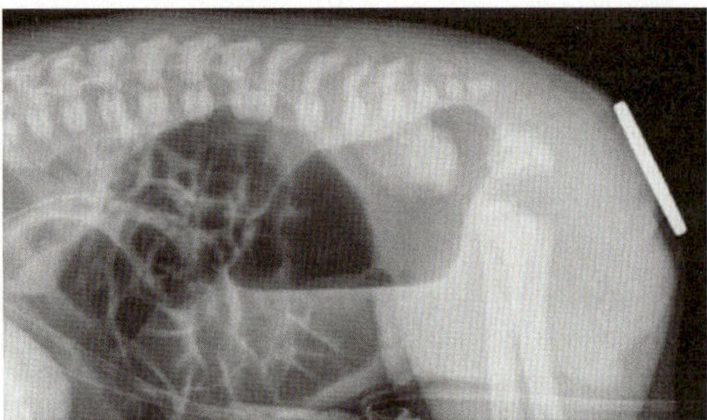

Fig. 60.86B: Prone position showing high anomaly

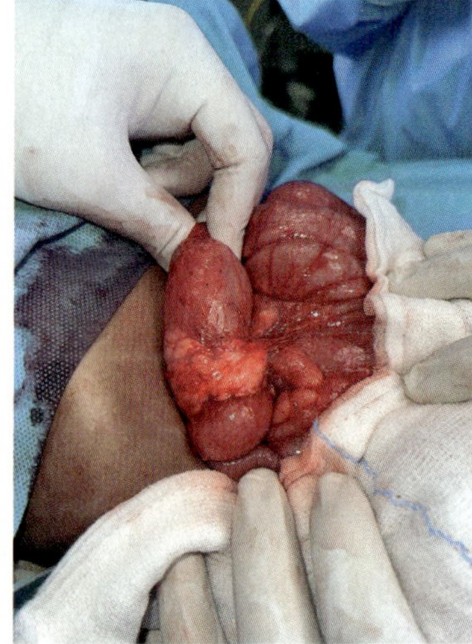

Fig. 60.87: Annular pancreas

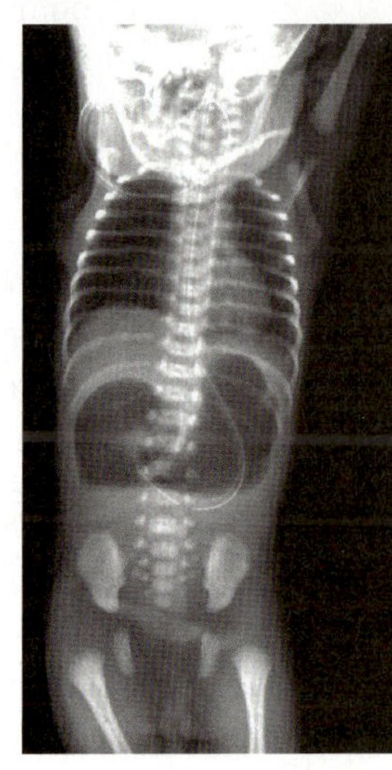

Fig. 60.88: Double-bubble appearance

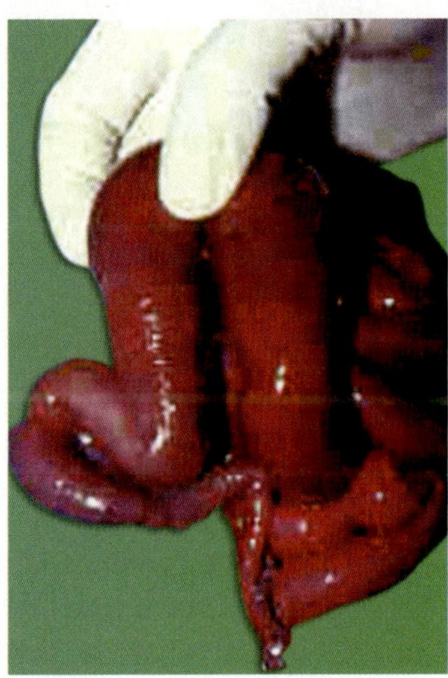

Fig. 60.89: Hirschsprung's disease

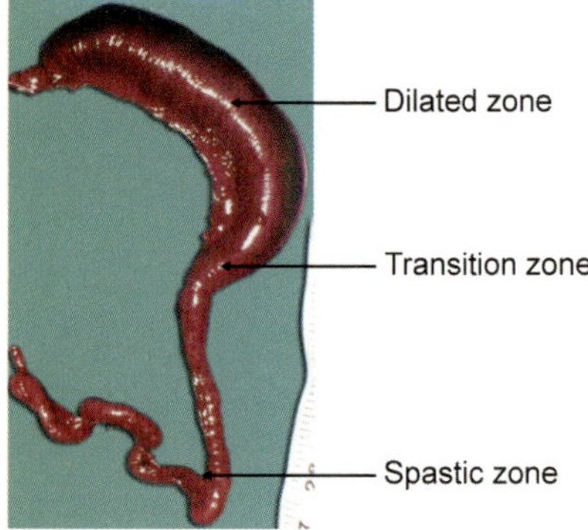


Fig. 60.90: Various segments of the large intestine in Hirschsprung's disease

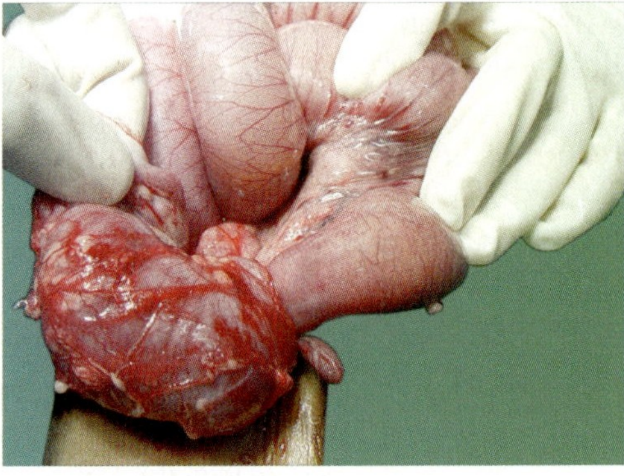

Fig. 60.91: Ileocaecal intussusception

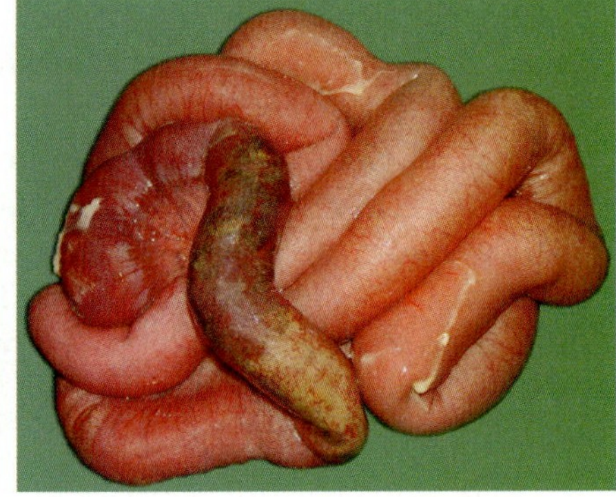

Fig. 60.92: Necrotising enterocolitis with patchy gangrene

(*Courtesy:* Vijaykumar, Professor and Head, Department of Paediatric Surgery, KMC, Manipal)

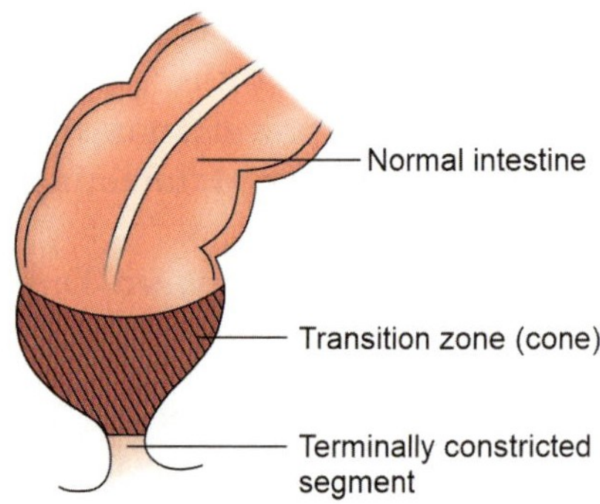


Fig. 60.93: Pathophysiology

2. **Short segment:** Anal canal and entire rectum is completely involved.
3. **Long segment:** Anal canal, rectum and part of colon involved.
4. **Total colonic:** Anal canal, rectum and whole length of colon is involved.

## Clinical Features

- Male children are commonly affected, when compared to females.
- **Incidence:** 1 in 4000 to 5000 live births.

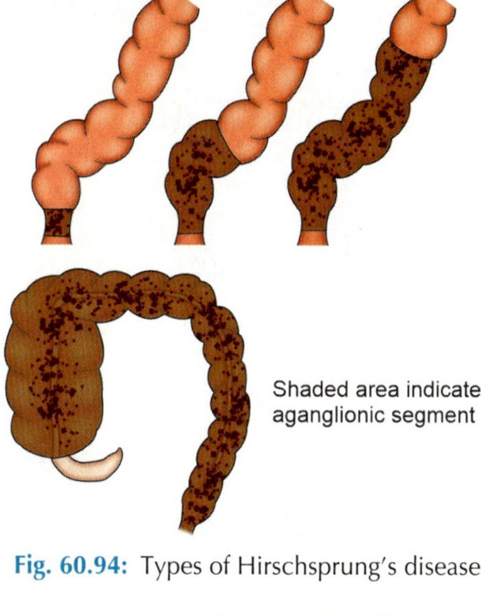


Fig. 60.94: Types of Hirschsprung's disease

*Pearls of Wisdom*

The most common associated anomaly with Hirschsprung's disease is Down's syndrome (5 to 10%).

- The child presents with acute neonatal intestinal obstruction as manifested by failure to pass meconium or delay in passing meconium with abdominal distension.
- Within 12–24 hours, all features of intestinal obstruction can be found. If it is complicated by enterocolitis, it may result in perforation and septicaemia. A severe diarrhoea with blood and mucus, abdominal distension and vomiting can occur within a few hours, followed by hypovolaemic shock.
- Rectal examination reveals that the rectum is empty, finger is gripped by anal sphincter and there is no perianal soiling (Fig. 60.95). On the other hand, in acquired megacolon, rectum is loaded with faecal matter, perianal soiling is present and there is no sphincter activity (Fig. 60.96).

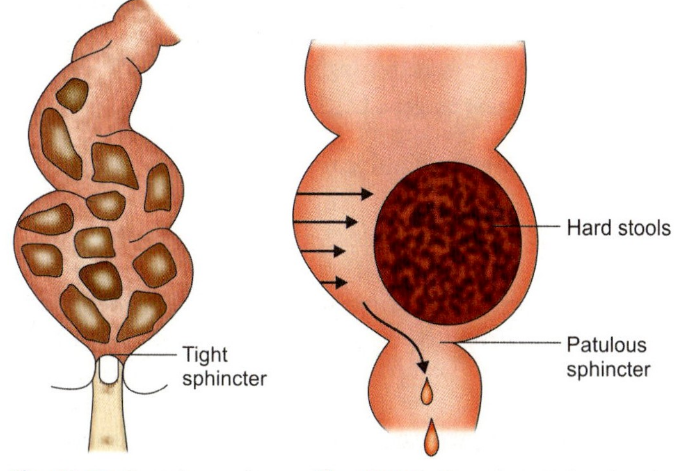


Fig. 60.95: Rectal examination in congenital megacolon

Fig. 60.96: Rectal examination in acquired megacolon

- **Chronic variety:** Chronic constipation manifesting in the first few weeks of life. The child may be brought with abdominal distension. Stools are goat pellet-like.

## Differential Diagnosis (Key Box 60.33)

**Acquired megacolon:** Usually manifests by one to two years of age. Rectum is loaded with faecal matter.

Key Box 60.33

**Differential Diagnosis**

- Hypothyroidism
- Meconium plug syndrome
- Intestinal pseudo-obstruction
- Colonic neuronal dysplasia

## Complications

- Intestinal obstruction, perforation, peritonitis
- Enterocolitis
- Growth retardation

## Investigations

1. **Full thickness rectal wall biopsy** under GA demonstrates absence of parasympathetic ganglion cells and hypertrophic nerve fibres in the nerve plexus. It should be taken above the anorectal junction. Today submucosal suction biopsy is more popular than biopsy since it avoids haemorrhage, infection and scarring.
2. **Barium enema:** 3.6% solution of barium is used, the intermediate zone appears as a cone with proximal dilatation and a distal narrow zone which is characteristic of Hirschsprung's disease.

## Treatment

### *I. Emergency Cases*

- Right transverse loop colostomy: In most of the cases, aganglionic segment is limited to rectosigmoid region.
- A full thickness biopsy of the colostomy is sent for histopathological examination.

### *II. Definitive Surgery*

- Can be done usually between the age of 3 and 6 months (8 to 10 kg of weight).
- Resection of aganglionic bowel (anorectum) followed by a pull-through procedure. **Maintaining continence is the main aim.**
- A few points of comparison between 'Duhamel's and Swenson's pull-through' are mentioned below.

| Duhamel's | Swenson's |
|---|---|
| • Retrorectal pull-through | • Endorectal pull-through |
| • Technically easy | • Difficult |

### Steps of Duhamel's Pull-through Surgery

1. The rectum is transected above the peritoneal fold and is closed.
2. The proximal ganglionic segment is pulled down behind the rectum (retrorectal space created by using blunt dissector).
3. An incision is made in the posterior wall of the anorectum above the dentate line and is deepened through the entire bowel wall.
4. The end of the proximal colon is sutured to the opening in the posterior anal canal all around.
5. The adjacent walls of rectum (posterior wall) and colon (anterior wall) are crushed by using a Kocher's forceps which falls off by itself by the 14th day.
6. The open end of the rectum (above) is closed end to side to the colon.

   **Other types of surgery:** Soave's mucosectomy and pull-through operation.

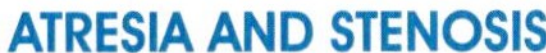

## ATRESIA AND STENOSIS

- Commonly, it affects the duodenum, followed by ileum and jejunum (Fig. 60.97).
- There may be single/multiple atresia.
- Incidence: 1 in 10,000 live births.

*Pearls of Wisdom*

Duodenal atresia is the most common cause of intestinal obstruction in neonates.

## DUODENAL ATRESIA (Key Box 60.34)

### Types

**Type I: Complete atresia**—it is the commonest atresia. The proximal dilated segment and distal collapsed segment are completely separated.

**Type 2:** There is no separation of the two parts. However, a **fibrous band** is in between.

**Type 3:** It is incomplete obstruction: There may be a web or stenosis.

Key Box 60.34

**Duodenal Atresia—Associated Lesions**

- Annular pancreas, incomplete rotation of the gut
- Down's syndrome (trisomy 21)
- Maternal hydramnios
- Congenital heart disease
- Anorectal malformations

**Windsock deformity:** An incomplete diaphragm, with central aperture (hole) with proximal dilatation

- *Anastomosis:* A special anastomosis named after Kimura is being described. It is a diamond-shaped

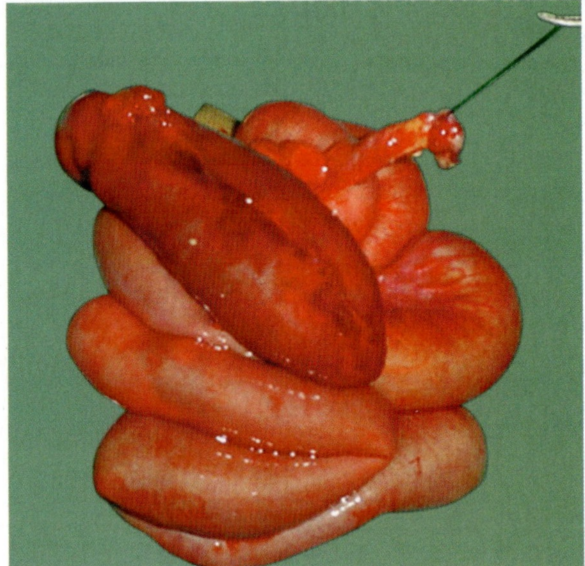

**Fig. 60.97:** Ileal atresia at surgery

anastomosis between upper pouch (duodenum) which is opened transversely and lower pouch (distal duodenum) which is opened longitudinally.
- The general condition of the patient has to be taken care of with supportive therapy including fluid and electrolytes, total parenteral nutrition, nasogastric decompression and adequate urinary output.
- Clinical features of obstruction manifest within 48–72 hours in the form of obstruction.
- Atresia means imperforation; stenosis means narrowing.
- Duodenal atresia presents as vomiting with or without bile, minimal distension and visible gastric peristalsis.
- Jaundice
- **X-ray abdomen erect: Double-bubble** in duodenal atresia.

### Treatment

**Duodenal atresia:** Duodenojejunostomy by anastomosing dilated duodenum above the atresia to the jejunal loop.

## SMALL INTESTINAL ATRESIA

### Salient Features

- It can affect jejunum (common) or ileum.
- Like duodenal atresia, it can be associated with maternal hydramnios or malrotation of the gut.
- Exact reasons for atresia are not known. However, vascular variations in the mesentery such as V-shaped mesentery or due to occlusion of vessels in the intrauterine life are the possible factors.
- Like any obstruction, proximal bowel is dilated and distal bowel is collapsed. The colon is very small—microcolon.

## GRIES FIELD MODIFICATION OF MARTIN'S CLASSIFICATION

- **Type I:** Simple stenosis. Mesentery is normal. It is mucosal atresia (Fig. 60.98).
- **Type II:** Proximal and distal bowels are connected by a fibrous band which has no lumen—atretic segment. Here again, mesentery is normal (Fig. 60.99).
- **Type III:** Further divided into 2 types. IIIa refers to atresia with V-shaped loss of mesentery in between, IIIb refers to complete jejunal atresia with coiled ileum. It has been called Christmas tree deformity (Figs 60.100A and B).
- **Type IV:** Multiple atretic segments including mesentery (Fig. 60.101).

***Please note:*** Apple-peel or Christmas tree deformity. Here, obstruction is usually in the proximal jejunum, which is supplied by the entire superior mesenteric artery (SMA). This results in a gap in the mesentery. So, rest of the small intestine is coiled around the ileocolic branch of the SMA.

### Treatment

Resection, anastomosis—aim is to conserve as much as possible.

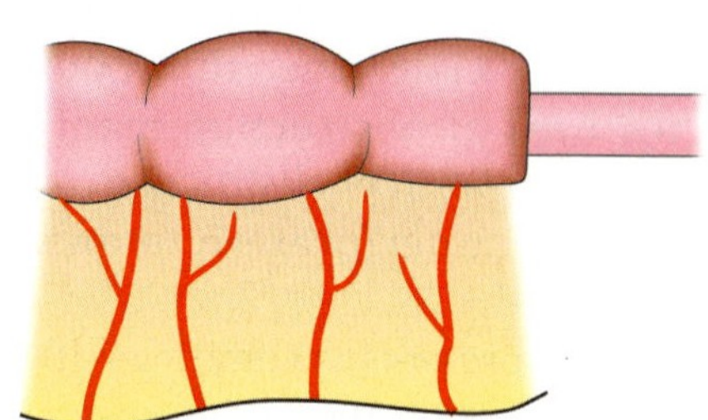

Fig. 60.98: Type I

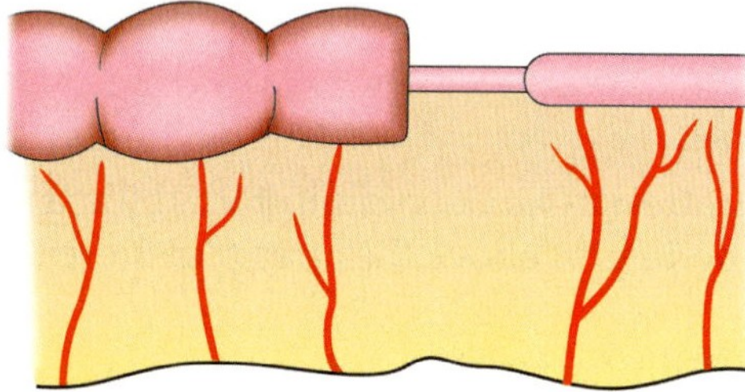

Fig. 60.99: Type II

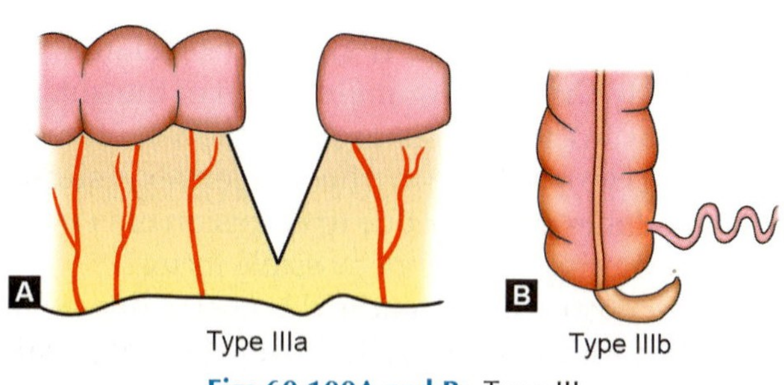


Figs 60.100A and B: Type III

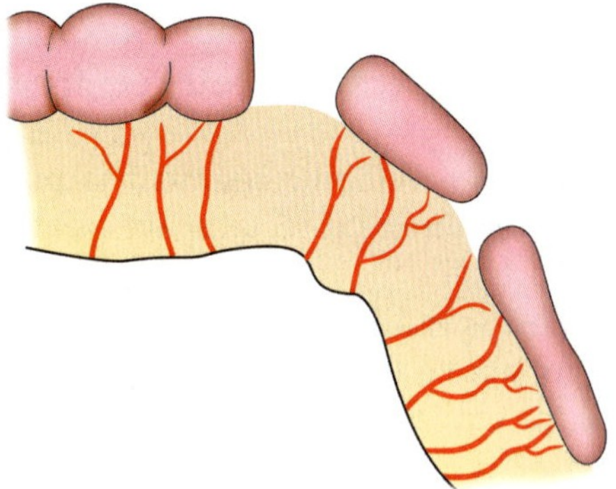

Fig. 60.101: Type IV

## ARRESTED ROTATION WITH BANDS

- It is a congenital anomaly wherein the caecum and right colon are found on the left side (Fig. 60.102).
- As a result of this, there are peritoneal bands which run across from left to right and cause intestinal obstruction (duodenal obstruction).
- One such band is called **transduodenal band of Ladd** which compresses the second part of duodenum and gives rise to obstruction (features similar to duodenal atresia).
- Differential diagnosis is duodenal atresia.

### Treatment

Laparotomy, division of band and fixation of the caecum in the right iliac fossa.

## VOLVULUS NEONATORUM

Volvulus neonatorum—it is a complication of arrested rotation with bands which pre-disposes to midgut volvulus (small bowel). These unfortunate infants undergo massive resection of the bowel if it is gangrenous (Fig. 60.103). Such massive resections give rise to short gut syndrome. Thus, the patient becomes a digestive cripple. If the loop is not gangrenous, it is treated by laparotomy, untwisting of bowel and division of bands.

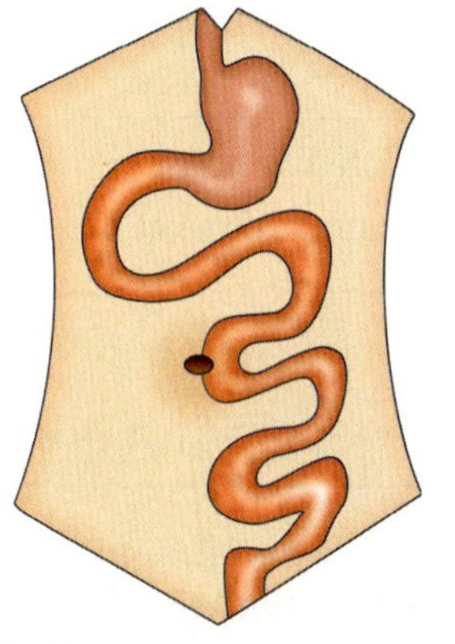

Fig. 60.102: Arrested rotation—malrotation

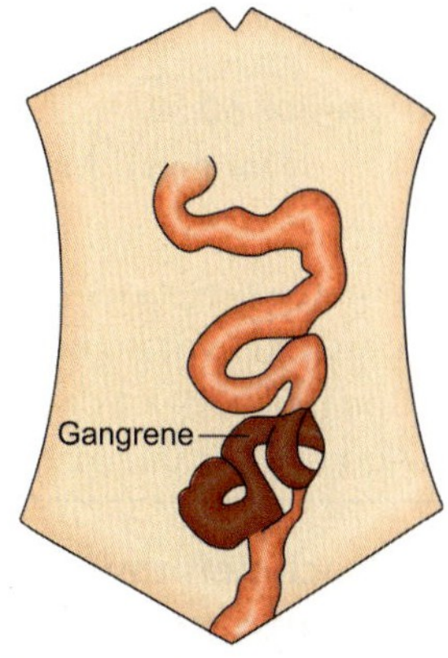


Fig. 60.103: Volvulus neonatorum

## MECONIUM ILEUS

- Meconium ileus—it is a neonatal manifestation of **mucoviscidosis** of the pancreas wherein the mucus is thick and viscid. This, along with meconium, produces obstruction. **There may be ileal atresia**, which might have precipitated meconium ileus (Fig. 60.104). Majority of meconium ileus is coupled by complications such as **gangrene, perforation** and **peritonitis**. As a sequel to peritonitis, calcification and adhesive meconium obstruction develop.
- Infants present with abdominal distension, bilious vomiting and failure to pass meconium.
- Plain X-ray shows distended bowel and **mottling** due to calcification.
- **Soap bubble sign** or **Neuhauser's sign:** Ground glass appearance in the right lower quadrant due to viscid meconium mixed with air.
- **Ultrasonography:** Dilated loops of bowel filled with echogenic material are highly suggestive of meconium ileus rather than ileal atresia.
- If perforation is ruled out, barium enema can be done which shows microcolon.

### Treatment

#### I. Conservative Treatment

It is indicated if there is no peritonitis, general condition of the child is reasonably good or if there is partial obstruction. Dilute gastrograffin is introduced into the colon as enema. It fills up terminal ileum. It absorbs fluid from the interstitial space into the lumen because it is hyperosmolar. Consequently, the meconium becomes soft and it is rejected naturally. Hypervolaemia is to be corrected during this.

#### II. Nonresectional Procedures

**A. Bishop-Koop operation** (Fig. 60.105)

- Ileum is divided in the proximal healthy part. This proximal ileum is anastomosed to the ascending colon to relieve obstruction—end-to-side anastomosis.
- Distal ileum containing thick meconium pellets is brought outside as a fistula and regular saline washes are given to dilute the meconium. Mucous fistula needs to be closed after a few weeks.

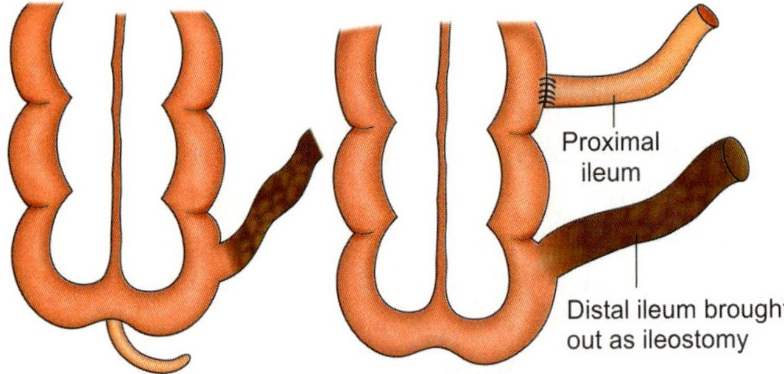


**Fig. 60.104:** Meconium ileus **Fig. 60.105:** Bishop-Koop operation

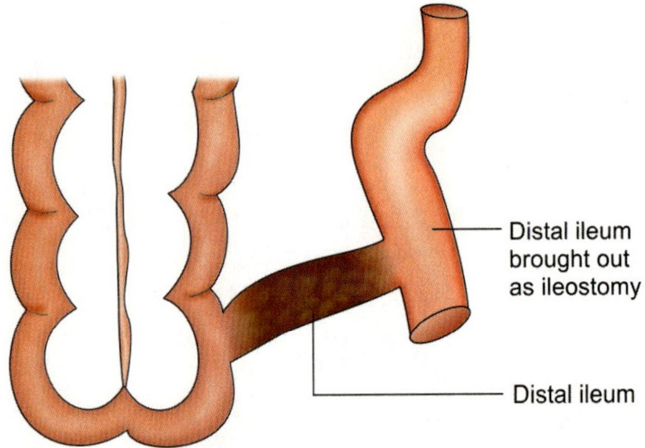


**Fig. 60.106:** Santulli operation

**B. Santulli operation** (Fig. 60.106)**:** In this operation, proximal ileum is brought out as ileostomy. Distal ileum is anastomosed to proximal ileum as end-to-side anastomosis.

#### III. Resection

**Resection is the surgery of choice today** as more cases present with short segment obstruction. Long-term results and complications are much less than nonresectional procedures.

## ANORECTAL ANOMALIES

**SU28.16.2:** Describe clinical presentation, diagnosis and management of imperforate anus and other congenital anorectal malformations.

### Developmental Anatomy

- To start with, there is a common chamber called cloaca, which is later divided into 2 chambers, anteriorly allantois gives rise to urinary bladder and posteriorly, postallantoic gut gives rise to rectum and upper 2 cm of anal canal.
- Postallantoic gut fuses with proctodeum, thus giving rise to anal canal. If there is a defective fusion of this, it results in imperforate anus.

## IMPERFORATE ANUS

### Incidence

1:4500 live births. Common in female children.

### Types of Imperforate Anus

**I. Low anomalies:** It refers to termination of the bowel below the anorectal bundle.

1. **Covered anus** (Fig. 60.107A): The anal orifice is covered by a tag of skin.
2. **Membranous anus** (Fig. 60.107B): Covered with a thin membrane.

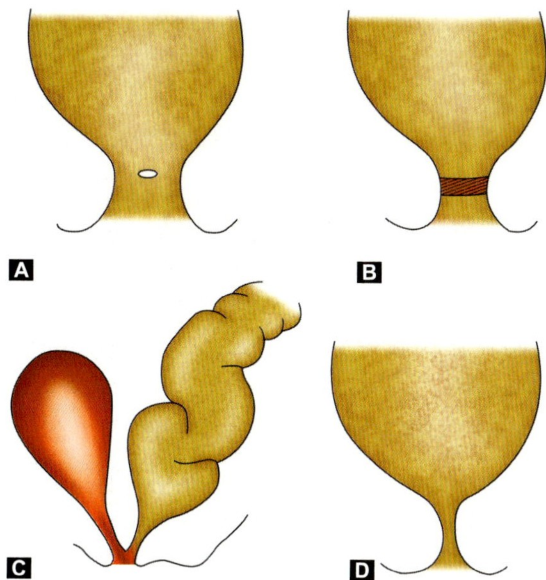

Figs 60.107A to D: Low anorectal anomalies

3. **Anterior ectopic anus** (Fig. 60.107C): Anus is situated anteriorly.
4. **Stenosed anus** (Fig. 60.107D): Anal orifice is microscopic.

II. **High anomalies:** They are supralevator—the bowel terminates above the anorectal bundle.

Anorectal and agenesis, with fistula: Rectovesical, rectovaginal, rectourethral fistulae (Figs 60.108A and B).

### Diagnosis

12 hours after birth, the child is put in the prone position (*see* Fig. 60.86B) (12 hours is the time for the gas shadow to reach the distal portion of the gut). A metal coin is strapped to the site of anus and X-ray is taken. If the gas shadow is above the pubococcygeal line, it is a high anomaly. If the distance between the coin and gas shadow is more than 2.5 cm, it is a high anomaly. If the gas shadow is below the pubococcygeal line, it is a low anomaly. Pubococcygeal line is called Stephen's line.

### Treatment

I. **Low anomaly:** Easy to treat, division of membrane or skin followed by dilatation is all that is required with some amount of plastic reconstruction (anoplasty is necessary).

II. **High anomaly:** Repaired by 3-stage procedure:
- 1st stage: Preliminary transverse colostomy to relieve intestinal obstruction.
- 2nd stage: When the child is 8–10 kg of weight, a "pull-through" operation is done with division of fistula.
- 3rd stage: After 2 months, colostomy is closed.

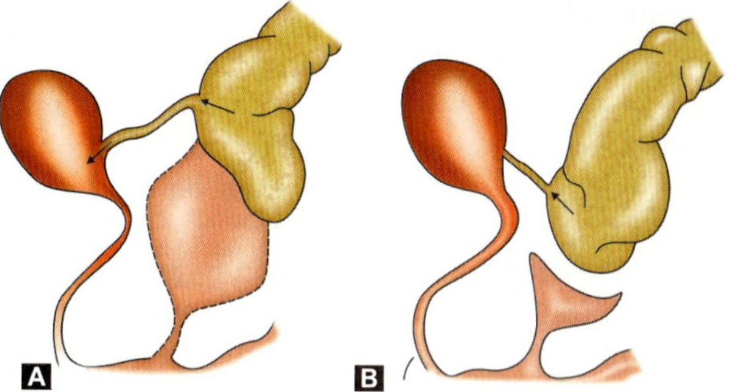

Figs 60.108A and B: High anorectal anomalies

## PARALYTIC ILEUS (NEUROGENIC ILEUS)

In this condition, there is a failure of transmission of parasympathetic impulses from one segment to the other. That means, there is a failure of parasympathetic mechanism, which results in paralysis of bowel. It gives rise to a large collection of fluid and gas within the bowel resulting in distension.

### Causes/Etiology

- During surgery, stimulation of sympathetic nerves that inhibits gastrointestinal movement results in autonomic nervous system dysfunction(s) causing ileus.
- In sepsis, a few inflammatory mediators like *nitric oxide, prostaglandins, vasoactive intestinal peptide-VIP* are released. They cause some motility problems to the gut. Inflammation also results in leukocyte infiltration and this factor also adds to paralytic ileus.
- Hypokalaemia: Potassium is responsible for depolarization in nerve cells that innervate muscle of the small intestines, hence hypokalemia causes paralytic ileus.
- Hypocalcaemia: Calcium is associated with smooth muscle contraction, hence hypocalcaemia can give rise to paralytic ileus (it is uncommon).
- Metabolic: Uraemia, diabetes (gastropathy).
- Drugs: Central-acting drugs—loperamide, phenothiazine, tricyclic antidepressants, and anti-Parkinson's drugs. Peripherally acting drugs—anticholinergic group, calcium-channel blocker group (e.g. verapamil), alpha-2 adrenergic agonist group (e.g. clonidine), etc.

### Clinical Features

1. **Abdominal distension** is gross. Tympanitic note all over is a feature. Respiratory and cardiac functions are impaired.
2. **No colicky pain abdomen** (in dynamic obstruction, colicky pain is a feature). Dull pain occurs due to distension of the abdomen.
3. **Failure to pass flatus,** effortless vomiting is also characteristic of paralytic ileus.

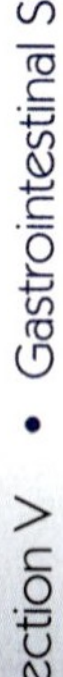

4. On auscultation, **tinkling sounds** are heard due to shift of fluid from one coil of bowel to the other (Key Box 60.35).
5. Severe fluid, electrolyte and protein depletion occur.

Key Box 60.35

**Three Types of Bowel Sounds**

- Normal: Once in 20 seconds, low pitch.
- Borborygmi: Loud, noisy, which occurs once in 5–10 seconds.
- Tinkling sounds: Mild metallic sounds as in paralytic ileus.

### Investigations

1. Plain X-ray abdomen erect demonstrates distended loops of bowel (Fig. 60.109).
2. Electrolyte study and correction of any abnormality.

### Treatment

- Basic principle of treating paralytic ileus is **drip and suction.**
- The cause of paralytic ileus has to be treated first, e.g. if there is **hypokalaemia, supplement potassium**. If there is pus in the peritoneal cavity, **drain** it.
- **Ryle's tube aspiration,** to give rest to the gut.
- Intravenous fluids, supplementation of ions, correction of dehydration, oliguria, etc. Such treatment is continued for 3–4 days.
- Ryle's tube is removed when abdomen is soft, bowel sounds are heard and patient has passed flatus. Clear oral fluids are started for 2–3 days followed by soft diet. Small bowel activity returns within 12–18 hours, followed by colon which starts functioning within 36–48 hours. However, gastric functions may return ranging from 18 hours to 4 days.

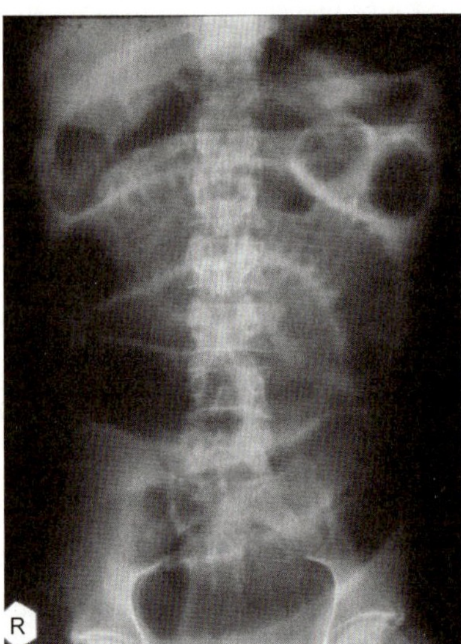


**Fig. 60.109:** Plain X-ray abdomen showing dilated bowel loops

## PSEUDOINTESTINAL OBSTRUCTION

Acute colonic pseudo-obstruction (ACPO) is also called **Ogilvie's syndrome**. It is massive colonic distension in the absence of a mechanically obstructing lesion.

### Pathogenesis

It occurs mainly due to **malfunctioning of sacral parasympathetic nerves (S2–S4)**. It results in atony of the descending colon resulting in functional obstruction. It is interesting to note that the **junction of the dilated and collapsed bowel is near the splenic flexure. This is the place wherein parasympathetic supply by vagus ends and sacral autonomic nervous system starts**. An increased sympathetic tone results in colonic dilatation due to inhibition of contraction (Key Box 60.36).

Key Box 60.36

**Causes of Colonic Pseudo-obstruction**

1. Retroperitoneal irritation
   - Blood
   - Urine
   - Fracture spine and pelvis
2. Drugs
   - Levodopa
   - Tricyclic antidepressants
3. Metabolic
   - Uraemia
   - Diabetes
   - Myxoedema
   - Hypokalaemia
4. Viral infections

### Clinical Features

- Elderly bedridden patient with cardiac/lower respiratory illness are the victims. Aerophagia and drugs which decrease colonic mobility are precipitating factors.
- Failure to pass faeces and flatus for several days.
- Tachypnoea due to elevation of the diaphragm due to distended colon is common.
- Rectal examination reveals some faeces (in cases of mechanical obstruction, rectum is empty).
- Plain X-ray abdomen erect may or may not show one or two air fluid levels. Distension is mainly colonic.
- Carcinoma colon is to be differentiated by barium enema.
- Caecal perforation is a dangerous complication. Hence, look for right iliac fossa tenderness.

### Treatment

- It is conservative, provided acute abdomen is ruled out.

- Colonoscopic decompression is the method of choice.
- Prokinetic drugs such as cisapride or mosapride have been tried in selected cases.
- Rarely, even after colonoscopic decompression, caecal tenderness continues. If distension persists, laparotomy followed by tube caecostomy may have to be done.

## INTESTINAL OBSTRUCTION—UNCOMMON CAUSES

### INTESTINAL OBSTRUCTION IN PREGNANCY

- The commonest cause of intestinal obstruction in pregnancy and puerperium is **adhesive bands**.
- **Volvulus** is the second commonest cause of intestinal obstruction—intestine volvulates around an adhesive band and that is why the primary cause is adhesive bands (Fig. 60.110).
- **Inguinal hernia** and **intussusception** are the other causes.
- The consequences of intestinal obstruction in pregnancy **do not differ** from those found in nonpregnant women except that in the pregnant patient, a second entity, the foetus, is also threatened.
- Most of the intestinal obstructions tend to occur in the **third trimester**.
- Maternal **mortality** for intestinal obstruction in pregnancy (10–33%) is **higher** than in nonpregnant patients.
- In the first half of the pregnancy, nausea, vomiting and episodes of constipation are quite common. Hence, they are confused for hyperemesis gravidarum, acute duodenal ulcer and gastritis.
- **In the second half of the pregnancy,** symptoms can be confused for toxaemia, constipation, Braxton Hicks contractions, etc.

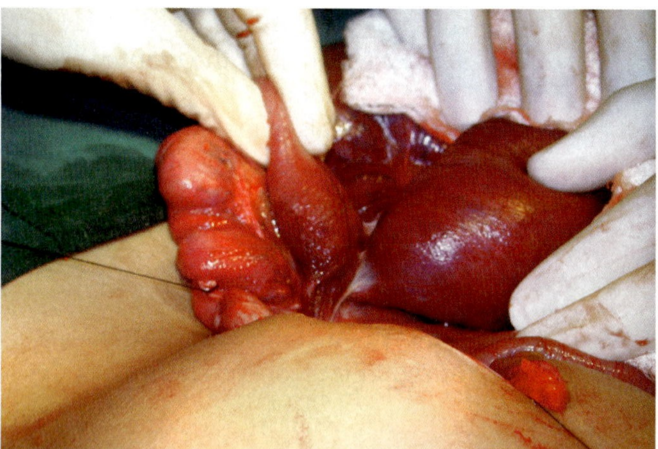

**Fig. 60.110:** Pregnant lady with adhesions causing intestinal obstruction

- **Ultrasound** can help in the diagnosis by detecting dilated intestinal loops, fluid in the peritoneal cavity and intussusception. It also helps to rule out ovarian torsion, gallstone disease, etc.
- **Premature labour can be prevented with tocolysis (abolition of uterine contraction).**
- **Abdominal surgery in the third trimester does not induce labour.**
- Negative laparotomy carries a small risk of disturbing the pregnancy.
- **Volvulus and intussusception** are the two major causes of small intestinal obstruction in pregnancy. Both can give rise to gangrene. Hence an intervention is required before gangrene sets in.
- ***The diagnosis and treatment of a pregnant patient suspected of having a bowel obstruction should be no different from those given to a nonpregnant one.***

### ILEOSIGMOID KNOTTING

It is rare type of knotting between sigmoid and ileum carrying significant mortality if not treated timely (Key Box 60.37).

Key Box 60.37

**Ileosigmoid Knotting**

- It is also called compound volvulus.
- Predisposing factor is long pelvic mesocolon.
- The ileum twists around the sigmoid colon resulting in gangrene of ileum or sigmoid colon or both.
- Even though sigmoid is also twisted, features are similar to small intestinal obstruction—not massive distension as seen in sigmoid volvulus.
- Resection anastomosis of gangrenous segment followed by anastomosis of the bowel (ileoileal/colic and colocolic).

### ILIAC CREST GRAFT HERNIA WITH OBSTRUCTION

- This is also a rare hernia following bone graft removal from the iliac crest for treatment of fractures.
- Iliac crest is the common donor site of bone graft. If the bone graft removed is large, the intestines can herniate resulting in intestinal obstruction.
- Tenderness in the surgical site scar can cause diagnostic difficulty.
- It is confused for haematoma.
- CT scan gives the diagnosis.

Following is the case report of a patient who had undergone iliac crest bone graft and developed hernia (Figs 60.111 and 60.112).

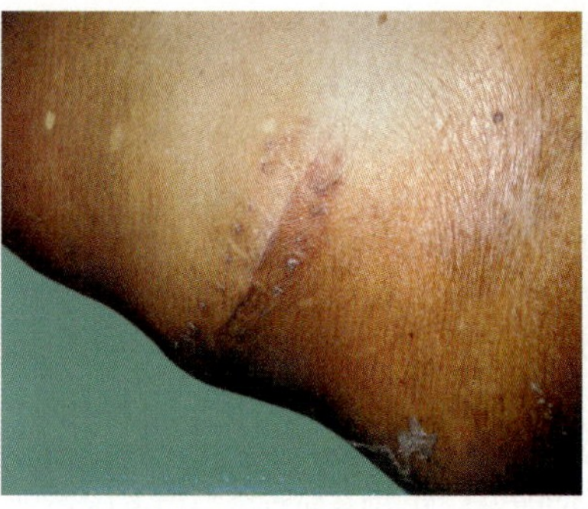

**Fig. 60.111:** Iliac bone graft site hernia

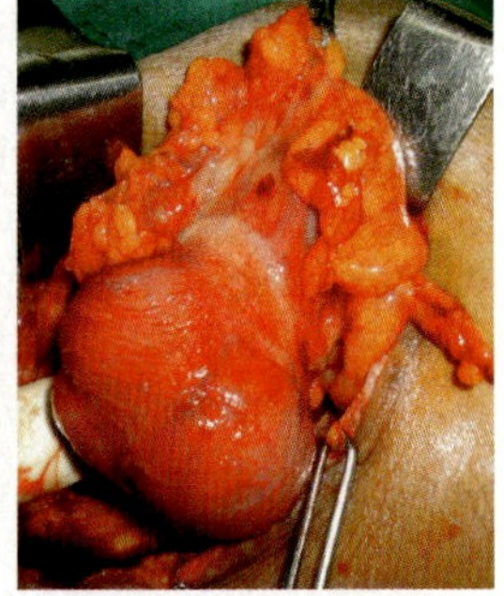

**Fig. 60.112:** Caecal herniation

**Clinical Notes**

A 50-year-old man presented to the casualty with abdominal pain, vomiting and distension. Features were suggestive of intestinal obstruction. On examination, there was a bulge in the region of right iliac fossa—more lateral. There was a scar of bone graft incision. On questioning the patient, he says that he had fracture humerus. Two months back, nailing and bone grafting had been done. Ultrasound revealed bowel loops. CT scan showed a large bone graft defect with herniation of intestines resulting in intestinal obstruction. Emergency surgery, reduction of hernia contents and mesh repair was done. Recovery was uneventful.

## FOOD BOLUS OBSTRUCTION

This complication can occur, particularly when a GJ or partial gastrectomy is done.

### Factors Precipitating this Condition

- Unmasticated, undigested particles
- Coconut pieces, jackfruit seeds and gulped coins, etc.
- They get impacted in the terminal ileum which is the narrowest portion of the gut.

### Treatment

Squeeze the bolus into the caecum. Otherwise, enterotomy and removal may be necessary.

## OBSTRUCTION DUE TO INTERNAL HERNIA

### *Syn: Stammer's Hernia*

1. These are rare causes of intestinal obstruction. Due to some congenital defect in the mesentery, the floating, mobile intestines can herniate (Key Box 60.38). The defect may be in:
   - Mesentery
   - Transverse mesocolon or
   - Broad ligament
   - Foramen of Winslow

   Hence, whenever a surgical procedure is done for resection of the bowel or GJ, etc. Once the anastomosis is completed, the rent in the mesocolon as in GJ or rent in the small bowel mesentery should be closed.
2. Herniation can also occur through one of the potential spaces (fossae) in and around a viscus.

**Key Box 60.38**

**Internal Hernia**

- Wherever a defect is present which is an anatomically present recesses or congenital or following surgery, loop of small intestine can herniate resulting in hernias.
- They are difficult to diagnose. The diagnosis is by exclusion.
- Triggering factors: Inflammation in the vicinity with or without an adhesion and band trigger herniation and complications.
- Most of these cases present as acute abdomen with features of intestinal obstruction.
- CT scan is the best investigation in such cases.
- It should be remembered that an important vessel runs in the close vicinity of these sites in most of the cases.
- Treatment is reduction, suturing the defect or resection anastomosis if the intestine is gangrenous taking care not to damage the vessel. Decompression without dividing the constricting ring may be required.

### Duodenal Fossa

- Left paraduodenal fossa: Inferior mesenteric vein lies very close to the free border here.
- Right duodenojejunal fossa: Superior mesenteric artery runs in its free border.

### Colonic Fossa

- Superior ileocaecal fossa
- Inferior ileocaecal fossa
- Sigmoid fossa

*Pearls of Wisdom*

These are the rare causes of intestinal obstruction to be kept in mind.

## ABDOMINAL COCOON SYNDROME

- It is characterized by small bowel encapsulation by a fibro-collagenous membrane or "cocoon". It is a rare cause of intestinal obstruction secondary to kinking and/or compression of the intestines within the constricting cocoon.
- **Three types have been recognized.**

A. **Primary form** is probably caused by a subclinical peritonitis leading to the formation of a chemical peritonitis was caused by retrograde menstruation, leading to the formation of a cocoon. This was first reported by Foo[1] KT, *et al.* and he coined the term "abdominal cocoon" in 1978.

[1]Foo KT, Ng KC, Rauff A, Foong WC, Sinniah R. Unusual small intestinal obstruction in girls: The abdominal cocoon. Br J Surg 1978;65:427–30.

B. **Secondary** causes include the placement of Le Veen shunts for refractory ascites, continuous ambulatory peritoneal dialysis, systemic lupus erythematosus, use of povidone iodine for abdominal wash-out, an adrenergic blocker practolol, etc.

C. **Tuberculosis** also has been found to be a factor in a few cases.

- Diagnosis is established by CECT scan and treatment is separation of bowel loops and removal of the membrane in toto or in pieces.

## CAPSULE OBSTRUCTION

Capsule endoscopy is done for evaluation of small intestines, major indication being occult bleeding or diarrhoea—causes can be tumours or tuberculosis or Crohn's disease, etc. Capsule can get stuck at the site of ulcer or stricture or a bent intestinal loop due to adhesions (Fig. 60.113). In such patients, it needs to be removed along with intestine.

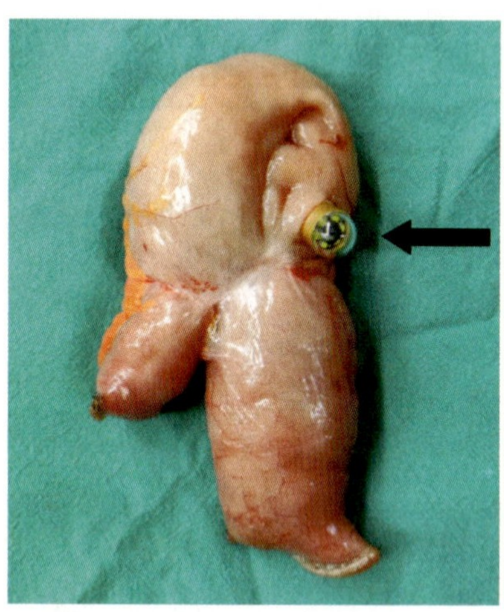

**Fig. 60.113:** Capsule obstruction (*Courtesy:* Dr Bharath Bhat, Dr Jegan, Dr Sridevi, Department of Surgery, KMC, Manipal)

## MALROTATION AND MIDGUT VOLVULUS

### Introduction

- The incidence of malrotation is 1 in 500 infants.
- The male to female ratio is 2 : 1.
- Malrotation with midgut volvulus may become rapidly life-threatening. The previously healthy infant with bilious vomiting is a characteristic presentation of malrotation. Usually, it presents with bilious vomiting, failure to thrive and features of intestinal obstruction (Fig. 60.113).
- In approximately 60% of patients, malrotation presents by one month of age. Another 20–30% of patients present at age 1–12 months. Thereafter, it can present at any age, and is seen in adults and even the elderly.

### Basic Pathophysiology

- A volvulus is a complete **twisting of a loop of intestine around its mesenteric attachment site.** This can occur at various locations of the GI tract, including stomach, small intestine, caecum, transverse colon, and sigmoid colon. Midgut malrotation refers to twisting of the entire midgut about the axis of the superior mesenteric artery (SMA).
- **Malrotation is any deviation from the normal 270° counterclockwise rotation** of the bowel that occurs during embryogenesis (Figs 60.114 and 60.115).
- At the fourth week of gestation, the gastrointestinal system is a straight tube centrally located in the abdomen. During the ensuing 8 weeks, the midgut rotates and becomes fixed to the posterior abdominal wall. **Arrest of development at any stage narrows the**

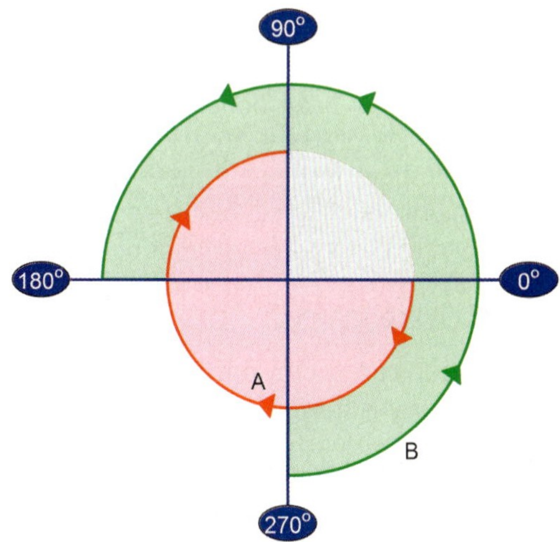


**Fig. 60.114:** Midgut volvulus: A. Clockwise rotation resulting in superior mesenteric ischaemia shown in red line, B. Anticlockwise untwisting to be done at surgery is shown as green line

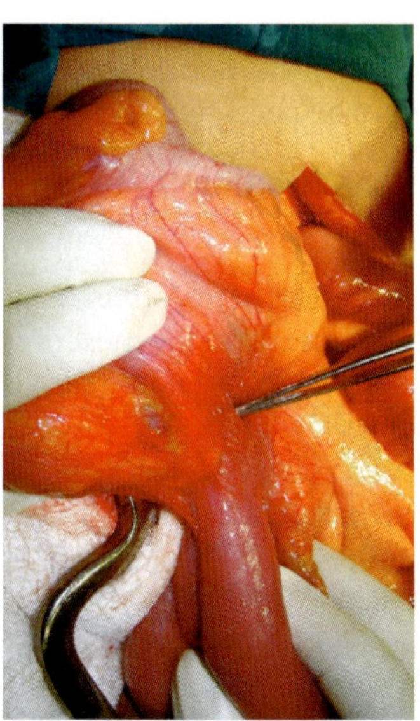

**Fig. 60.115:** Malrotation with band

**mesenteric base and impairs fixation, leaving the bowel at high risk for volvulus.**

- The resultant shortened mesenteric pedicle predisposes to midgut volvulus, a clockwise rotation around the superior mesenteric artery axis that can lead to bowel ischaemia.

## Investigations

- Conventional radiographs are neither sensitive nor specific for malrotation.
- On the upper GI series, it is crucial to locate the position of the duodenojejunal junction (DJJ). The DJJ must be at least over (but more reassuringly lateral to) the left vertebral pedicle and at the same height as the duodenal bulb on a well-centred view. If the DJJ does not meet these two criteria, malrotation is diagnosed.
- **Signs of midgut volvulus include an abrupt termination, or break of the contrast column and the corkscrew (apple peel, or barber pole) sign.**
- On ultrasound (US) and computed tomography (CT), the superior mesenteric artery (SMA) and superior mesenteric vein (SMV) relationship may be reversed.
- Normally, the SMV is to the right of the SMA; with malrotation, the SMV may occupy a position directly anterior or to the left of the SMA.

## Treatment

- **The Ladd procedure** remains the cornerstone of surgical treatment for malrotation today.
- ***A classic Ladd procedure*** is described as reduction of volvulus (if present), division of mesenteric bands, **placement of small bowel on the right and large bowel on the left of the abdomen, and appendicectomy.**
- A laparoscopic variation of the Ladd procedure has been used in some centres, with the general advantage of decreased adhesions and scarring, but good visualisation of the entire bowel is necessary.

## CLINICAL CASE CAPSULE 8: Management Oriented Discussion in Surgery (MODS)

We had a 30-year-old man with nil previous history of abdominal pain or any illness, presented to the hospital with colicky abdominal pain, 2 times bilious vomiting and distension. On examination tympanitic vague mass was palpable in the right iliac fossa. X-ray was suggestive of intestinal obstruction. Abdominal ultrasonography revealed clustering of the small bowel loops in the right iliac fossa. CECT was reported as intestinal obstruction secondary to internal herniation. Emergency exploratory laparotomy was done. A cocoon with matted loops were found in the right iliac fossa (Fig. 60.116). An attempt to separate the cocoon resulted in multiple tears, it was not possible, hence resection and anastomosis of about 20 cm of the ileum followed by ileocolic anastomosis was done. Patient recovered completely from obstruction and was discharged.

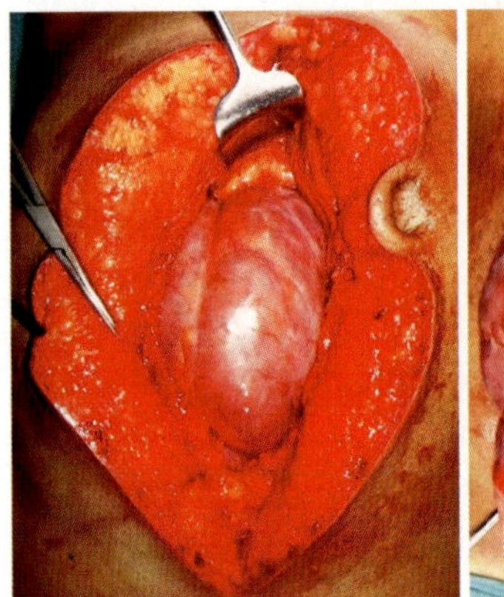
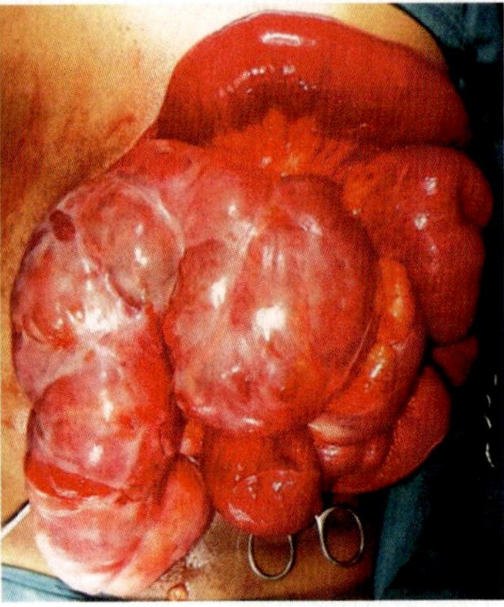

**Fig. 60.116:** Abdominal cocoon (*Courtesy:* Dr Sunil Krishna, Dr Keertan Upadhya, Dr Ameena, Department of Surgery, KMC, Manipal)

Section V • Gastrointestinal Surgery

## MULTIPLE CHOICE QUESTIONS

1. **Which of the following is true for closed loop obstruction?**
   A. Can occur with constrictive growth in the hepatic flexure
   B. Ileocaecal valve is incompetent
   C. Perforation of the sigmoid colon is common
   D. Occurs with partial obstruction
2. **Which of the following is not the cause of gangrene in intestinal obstruction?**
   A. Ileocaecal tuberculosis
   B. Mesenteric vascular occlusion
   C. Necrotising enterocolitis
   D. Volvulus
3. **Faeculent vomiting is pathognomonic of:**
   A. Jejunal obstruction
   B. Terminal ileal obstruction
   C. Duodenal obstruction
   D. Colonic obstruction
4. **Cardinal features of intestinal obstruction include all of the following, *except*:**
   A. Colicky abdominal pain
   B. Vomiting
   C. Diarrhoea
   D. Abdominal distension
5. **The following is true in a plain X-ray of abdomen in intestinal obstruction:**
   A. Caecum can appear as round shadow
   B. Ileum has valvulae conniventes
   C. Jejunum is characterless
   D. Sigmoid appears shapeless
6. **Features of strangulation includes all of the following, *except*:**
   A. Tachycardia
   B. Disappearance of pain abdomen
   C. Fever
   D. Acidosis
7. **The features of viable bowel includes all of the following, *except*:**
   A. Normal peristalsis
   B. Normal pulsations are visible
   C. Normal pink colour is present
   D. Peritoneal sheen is absent
8. **Conservative treatment is advocated in intestinal obstruction when there is:**
   A. Disseminated malignancy with obstruction
   B. Complete obstruction with adhesions
   C. Postoperative obstruction with peritonitis
   D. Crohn's disease unresponsive to medications
9. **'Bent inner tube design', 'Omega sign', 'Bird's beak design' are all seen in:**
   A. Sigmoid volvulus
   B. Caecal volvulus
   C. Meckel's diverticulum
   D. Bascule
10. **The most common cause of intestinal obstruction in infants aged 6–18 months is:**
    A. Worms B. Bands
    C. Intussusception D. Adhesions
11. **Red currant jelly stools are characteristic of:**
    A. Worms B. Bands
    C. Intussusception D. Adhesions
12. **Dance's sign (signe de dance) is a feature of:**
    A. Worms B. Bands
    C. Intussusception D. Adhesions
13. **The investigation of choice in mesenteric vascular occlusion is:**
    A. Ultrasound abdomen
    B. Plain X-ray abdomen
    C. CT with or without angiogram
    D. MRI
14. **The most common cause of intestinal obstruction in neonates is:**
    A. Bands B. Duodenal atresia
    C. Imperforate anus D. Meconium ileus
15. **The most common congenital anomaly of small intestine is:**
    A. Bands B. Duodenal atresia
    C. Stenosis D. Meckel's diverticulum
16. **Features of paralytic ileus include the following, *except*:**
    A. Gross abdominal distension
    B. Pain abdomen
    C. Failure to pass flatus
    D. Tinkling sounds
17. **Melanosis of lips and mucosa with intestinal obstruction should arouse the suspicion of:**
    A. Gardner's syndrome
    B. Turcot's syndrome
    C. Peutz-Jeghers syndrome
    D. Down's syndrome
18. **Which is the factor precipitate sigmoid volvulus?**
    A. Short colon
    B. Broad attachment at the base
    C. Empty colon
    D. Long mesentery of the colon

**19. Common factor precipitating sigmoid volvulus in patients with parkinsonism, multiple sclerosis, hypothyroidism is:**
A. Diarrhoea
B. Constipation
C. Drugs
D. Long mesentery of the colon

**20. Investigation of choice for detecting bleeding Meckel's diverticulum is:**
A. CT scan B. PET scan
C. MRI scan D. Technetium scan

**21. Presence of intramural air is diagnostic of:**
A. Gallstone ileus B. Sigmoid perforation
C. Duodenal atresia D. Intestinal gangrene

**22. Following complications can occur after gastro-jejunostomy, *except*:**
A. Dumping syndrome
B. Intussusception
C. Volvulus
D. Stomal ulcer

**23. Following are the causes of adult intussusception, *except*:**
A. Meckel's diverticulum
B. Submucous lipoma
C. Carcinoma caecum
D. Hypertrophy of Peyer's patches

**24. The most common anomaly associated with Hirschsprung's disease is:**
A. Down's syndrome
B. Hypothyroidism
C. Meckel's diverticulum
D. Anorectal atresia

**25. Following are causes of paralytic ileus, *except*:**
A. Anastomotic leak B. Retroperitoneal irritation
C. Hyperkalaemia D. Fracture spine

**26. Investigation of choice for Meckel's diverticulitis is:**
A. CECT scan B. PET scan
C. MRI scan D. Technetium scan

**Answers**

| | | | | | | | | | |
|---|---|---|---|---|---|---|---|---|---|
| 1. A | 2. A | 3. B | 4. C | 5. A | 6. B | 7. D | 8. A | 9. A | 10. C |
| 11. C | 12. C | 13. C | 14. B | 15. D | 16. B | 17. C | 18. A | 19. B | 20. D |
| 21. D | 22. B | 23. D | 24. A | 25. C | 26. A | | | | |

Chapter

61

# Rectum and Anal Canal

- Surgical anatomy
- Surgical anatomy of anal canal
- Carcinoma rectum
- Anorectal physiology
- Anal incontinence
- Prolapse rectum
- Haemorrhoids
- Anorectal abscess
- Fistula *in ano*
- VAAFT
- Fissure *in ano*
- Pilonidal sinus
- Sacrococcygeal teratoma
- Malignant tumours of anal canal
- Stricture of anal canal and rectum

**SU28.16.1:** Describe applied anatomy including congenital anomalies of the rectum and anal canal.

## SURGICAL ANATOMY OF THE RECTUM

The rectum starts at the rectosigmoid junction, opposite the third piece of sacrum. It descends in the sacral hollow, passes through the pelvic floor, and ends in the anorectal junction, which is about 4 cm away from the anal verge. Anorectal junction is encircled by puborectalis muscle posteriorly and in the lateral aspects. **The rectum is 12–15 cm in length** (Key Box 61.1).

### Peritoneal Covering

- Upper one-third is **completely covered** by peritoneum (>11 cm from anal verge) (Figs 61.1 and 61.2).

Key Box 61.1

**Some Interesting Features of Rectum**

1. Rectum means straight, but it is not
2. Coverings of the peritoneum are different at different levels.
3. Even though it is a part of the large intestine, taenia, appendices epiploicae and sacculations are absent.
4. Middle curve marks the anterior peritoneal reflection. It is about 12–15 cm above anus.
5. Rectal carcinoma has high recurrence rates because of lack of serosal layer and close relation to other pelvic viscera.
6. Principal route of lymphatic drainage is upwards towards para-aortic nodes.

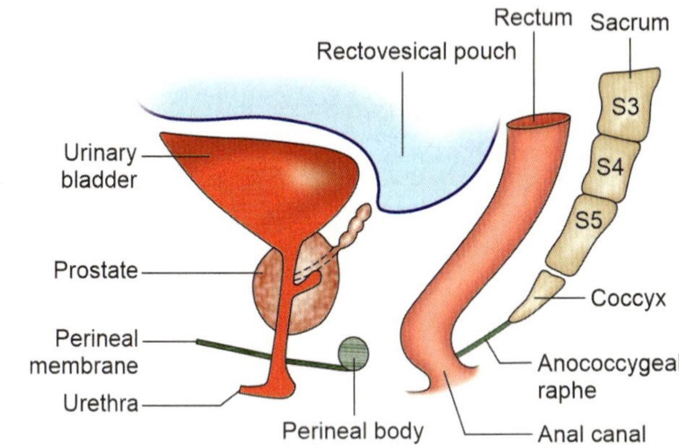


**Fig. 61.1:** Sagittal section through the male pelvis showing the location of the rectum and some of its anterior and posterior relations

- Middle one-third is **covered in front and lateral aspects** (6–11 cm).
- Lower one-third (0–6 cm) has **no extraperitoneal covering** but has two fascial condensation layers. Posteriorly, the strong **Waldeyer's** layer separates the rectum from lower sacral pieces and coccyx. At surgery, **stripping of this fascia results in uncontrollable bleeding from sacral plexus of veins,** which is underneath the Waldeyer's fascia.
- Anteriorly, the weak **Denonvilliers'** fascia separates the rectum from prostate and bladder. **Stripping of this fascia results in troublesome bleeding from prostatic venous plexus.**
- Rectum is attached to side wall of pelvis by **lateral ligaments,** which contain middle haemorrhoidal vessels. These need ligation or coagulation during mobilisation of lower rectum.

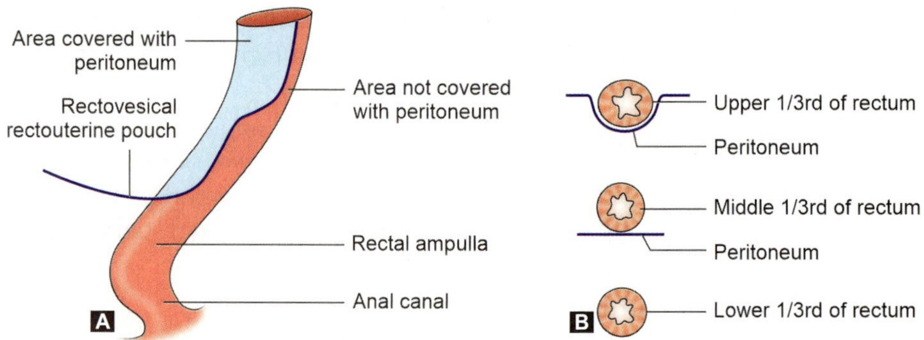


**Figs 61.2A and B:** Peritoneal relations of the rectum

- **Valves of Houston:** Despite the name rectum means straight, it is **never straight in adults**. It has 2 convexity on the left side and 1 convexity on the right side. There are **3 valves of Houston** (prominent mucosal folds), two on the left and one on the right.
- That portion of the rectum resting on the pelvic floor is called **ampulla**—dilated portion of the mid-rectum.

**Rectovesical pouch** (Key Box 61.2)

Key Box 61.2

**Rectovesical Pouch—Rectouterine Pouch**

- After investing the upper rectum, pelvic peritoneum is reflected anteriorly in males onto the urinary bladder, thus forming into rectovesical pouch. In females, it reflects onto uterus to form rectouterine pouch.
- It is one of the sites of transcoelomic spread of malignant cells.
- Malignant cells settle down in this most dependent part of the abdominal cavity and grow.
- They are palpable by rectal examination, a shelf-like finding—popularly called Blumer's shelf.
- Thus, if per rectal or per vaginal examination findings suggest presence of Blumer's shelf—it means hard deposits are felt and the case is inoperable.
- Rectovesical pouch is also the site of pelvic abscess.
- Pelvic abscess is diagnosed by per rectal or per vaginal examination.
- Pus can be drained through the rectum or posterior fornix.
- Aspiration of blood from rectovesical pouch through posterior fornix indicates intraperitoneal bleeding—may be ruptured ectopic.

## Arterial Supply

1. **Superior haemorrhoidal artery** is a branch of the superior rectal artery which is the continuation of the inferior mesenteric artery. It divides into right and left branches. The right branch divides into anterior and posterior branches which supply the rectum (Fig. 61.3).
2. **Middle haemorrhoidal artery**, a branch of internal iliac artery, runs in the lateral ligament of the rectum.

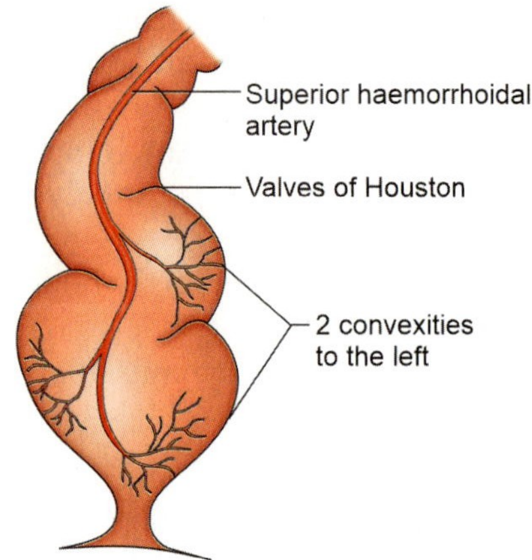


**Fig. 61.3:** Arterial supply of rectum

3. **Inferior haemorrhoidal artery,** a branch of internal pudendal artery, supplies the lower rectum.

## Venous Return (Fig. 61.4)

The rich submucous plexus of veins surrounding the ampulla forms external rectal plexus. The venous drainage from here flows in two directions.

1. **Upwards** to drain into **superior rectal veins**. These join inferior mesenteric veins, which in turn drain into the portal system.

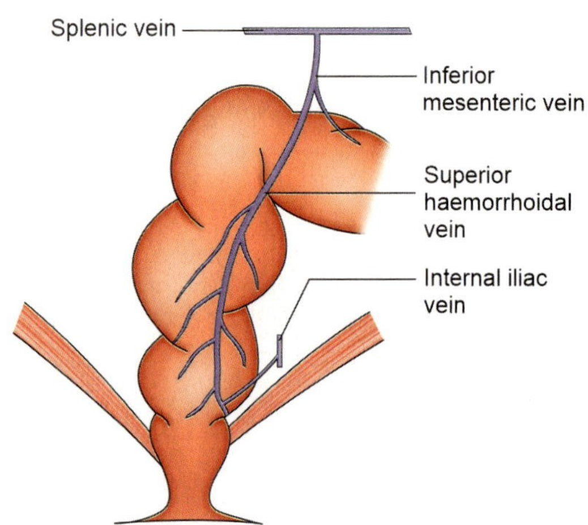


**Fig. 61.4:** Venous return

2. **Across** to drain into middle rectal veins, which run in the lateral ligament of the rectum along with middle rectal artery. Hence, the lateral ligaments have to be ligated and divided during resection of rectum. These veins drain into internal iliac veins (systemic circulation). Hence, rectum is a site of portosystemic anastomosis.

### Lymphatic Drainage of Rectum (Fig. 61.5)

- **Upper one-third of rectum** is completely enclosed by peritoneum and the **middle one-third of rectum** is covered in front and on the sides by peritoneum. From these areas, lymphatic drainage always occurs in the **upward direction,** first to **(A)** pararectal nodes of Gerota followed by superior haemorrhoidal nodes, middle haemorrhoidal nodes and nodes at the origin of inferior mesenteric artery.
- From **lower one-third of rectum**, lymphatics spread in the **lateral direction** and can involve **(B)** internal iliac nodes.
- Lymph nodes are also present in the hollow of sacrum along median sacral artery **(C)**.

  Lymphatics are present in the muscularis mucosa.

### Nerve Supply

- **Sympathetic:** The fibres come from hypogastric plexus, which is located at the aortic bifurcation at the level of L5. Injury to this can cause absence of erection or dry orgasm. Fibres also come along with inferior mesenteric artery and superior rectal artery.
- **Parasympathetic:** (S2, S3, S4) by means of nervi erigentes from the hypogastric plexus and supply motor fibres to detrusor. Pain and ability to distinguish flatus and faeces is because of these fibres. Loss of the rectal mucosa results in the loss of these sensations. During division of lateral ligaments or during anterior dissection of the bladder base, injury to nervi erigentes can occur.
- External anal sphincter and puborectalis are innervated by inferior rectal branches of internal pudendal nerve (somatic).

## SURGICAL ANATOMY OF ANAL CANAL

Anal canal is 3 cm long, starts as the continuation of rectum, passes through pelvic diaphragm and ends at the anal verge (skin).

### Internal Anal Sphincter (IAS) (Fig. 61.6)

- It is the continuation of circular muscle fibres of rectum and ends 0.5 cm below the pectinate line.
- It is involuntary and 2.5 cm long.
- The IAS is a muscular ring that surrounds about 2.5–4.0 cm of the anal canal. Its inferior border is in contact with, but quite separate from, sphincter ani externus muscle.
- Internal sphincter with fibres of external sphincter and puborectalis which maintains the anorectal angle, form the **anorectal bundle, and maintains continence.**
- Its fibres are transversely placed. Motor fibres come from presacral plexus.

### External Sphincter

- It is formed by **striated muscle fibres** intermingled with longitudinal muscle fibres of the rectum which are attached to the skin of perianal region.
- It has superficial, deep and subcutaneous portions.
- The funnel-shaped configuration of the paired levator ani muscles form the major part of the pelvic floor, and their fibers decussate medially with the contralateral side to fuse with the perineal body around the prostate or vagina.

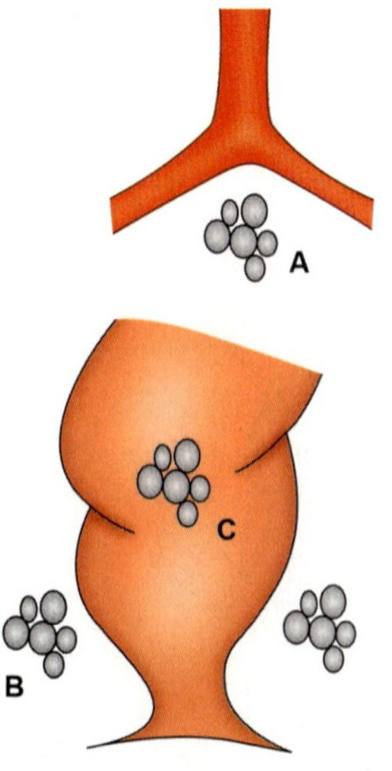


**Fig. 61.5:** Lymphatic drainage

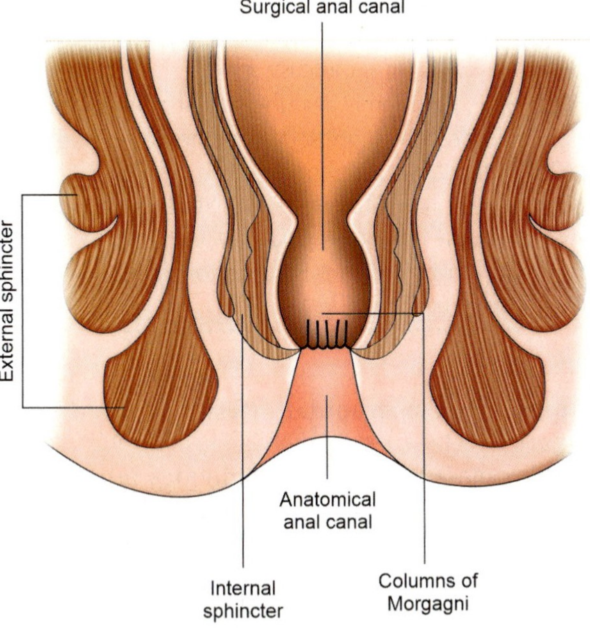


**Fig. 61.6:** Anatomy of the anal canal

- Nerve supply (motor) comes from inferior haemorrhoidal branch of internal pudendal nerve and perianal branch of the 4th sacral nerve (motor to levator ani also).
- It is voluntary and gives temporary continence.

## Development

- Anal canal is developed from fusion of **post-allantoic gut** with **proctodeum**.
- The junction of these is the dentate line or pectinate line. **Anal valves of Ball** are remnants of proctodeal membrane.
- At the level of dentate line, the mucosa is folded in the form of longitudinal columns—***columns of Morgagni***.
- In between the columns of Morgagni, 4–8 anal glands open into small anal sinuses.

## Lining Epithelium

- The mucosa of the upper anal canal, like that of the rectum, is pinkish and is lined by columnar epithelium, whereas the mucosa distal to the dentate line is paler and lined by squamous epithelium devoid of hair and glands.
- The change between the two types of epithelium is called transitional zone. It lies immediately proximal to the dentate line and consists of layers of cuboidal cells with a few columnar cells.
- Thus diseases affecting the rectal mucosa, such as ulcerative colitis, can extend to the transitional zone but not distal to the dentate line. *Cancers proximal to the dentate are typically adenocarcinomas, and those distal are squamous cell carcinoma.*
- Thus even after total proctocolectomy and pouch procedures for ulcerative colitis, carcinoma can occur in the transitional zone.
- At the anal verge, characteristics of normal skin with its apocrine glands are present. This is where infectious complications of the apocrine glands—hidradenitis suppurativa can occur. This differentiation helps in sensory perception, which influences the surgical approaches to anorectal conditions. *To give an example, internal hemorrhoids can be treated with rubber band ligation without the need for local anaesthesia. On the other hand, excision of external hemorrhoids requires the application of local anaesthesia.*

## Blood Supply, Lymphatic Drainage and Nerve Supply

- The superior portion of the anal canal (i.e. superior to the dentate line) is supplied by the superior haemorrhoidal artery. Below the dentate line, the inferior haemorrhoidal arteries supply the inferior most part of the anal canal. Between the two, the middle haemorrhoidal arteries form anastomoses.
- Above the dentate line, internal haemorrhoidal venous plexus drains into the superior haemorrhoidal vein. Below, veins drain into the inferior haemorrhoidal vein. Also, middle haemorrhoidal veins drain the muscularis externa and anastomose with the superior and inferior haemorrhoidal veins.
- **The lymphatic drainage:** Above the dentate line, the lymphatics drain into the internal iliac lymph nodes and below the dentate line, lymphatics drain into the superficial inguinal lymph nodes.
- **Nerve supply:** The anal canal has differing nervous innervations above and below the dentate line. Above the dentate line, the nerve supply comes from the inferior hypogastric plexus (visceral). This part of the anal canal is sensitive to stretch. Below the dentate line, the nerve supply is somatic, receiving its supply from the inferior haemorrhoidal nerves (branches of the pudendal nerve). It is sensitive to pain, temperature, and touch (refer to Table 61.1).

***Please note:*** Congenital anomalies of rectum and anal canal are given on page 1010.

## Examination of Rectum and Anal Canal (Table 61.2)

These are the common anal/perianal conditions which can be diagnosed by inspection (only), or palpation or per rectal examination/proctoscopic examination (Fig. 61.10).

**TABLE 61.1:** Comparison of anal canal above and below the dentate line

| | Above the dentate line | Below the dentate line |
|---|---|---|
| Nomenclature | Surgical anal canal | Anatomical anal canal |
| Epithelium | Cuboidal epithelium | Skin—squamous epithelium, without hair and sweat glands |
| Nerve supply | Parasympathetic. Hence, painless | Spinal nerves, inferior haemorrhoidal nerve, very painful |
| Venous drainage | Portal system | Systemic veins (external iliac vein) |
| Colour | Pink | Skin colour |
| Development | Post-allantoic gut | Proctodeum |
| Lymphatic drainage | Para-aortic nodes | Superficial and deep inguinal nodes |

| **TABLE 61.2:** Examination of rectum and anal canal | | |
|---|---|---|
| **Digital rectal examination** (Fig. 61.7) | **Proctoscopy (Kelly's)** (Fig. 61.8) | **Flexible sigmoidoscopy** (Fig. 61.9) |
| • Lubricate the finger with lignocaine jelly<br>• **Sim's position: Left lateral** is ideal position<br>• Explain to the patient what you plan to do<br>• Gently apply pressure on the external sphincter (anal opening) and slowly introduce the finger<br>• Polyps, carcinomatous growths, strictures, thrombosed piles can be felt<br>• Sphincter tone is poor in prolapse rectum and lumbosacral myelopathy | • Do a per rectal examination and rule out painful condition (fissure *in ano*)<br>• Proctoscope with obturator is introduced to full length<br>• Piles are seen bulging into lumen as **obturator is withdrawn**<br>• Biopsy from growth can be taken<br>• Piles can be injected with sclerosants<br>• Pelvic abscess can also be drained | • Flexible sigmoidoscope is 60 cm long<br>• An enema is given before the procedure<br>• Growth, ulcers, bleeding diverticulae, polyps, colitis can be diagnosed and biopsy can be taken<br>• Do not force instrument—it may perforate colon<br>• It may deflate and derotate sigmoid volvulus—therapeutic use of sigmoidoscopy |

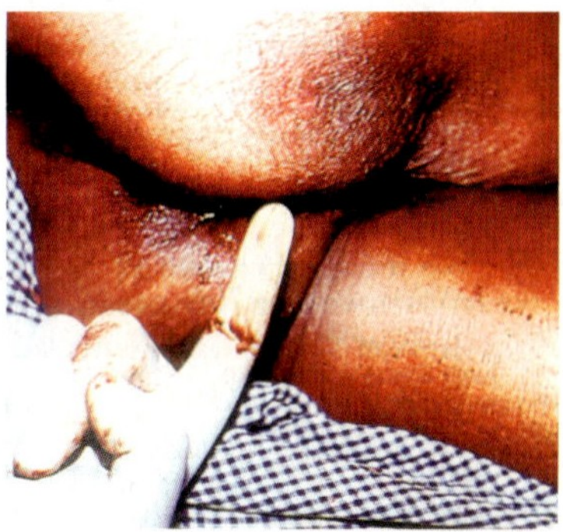

**Fig. 61.7:** Digital rectal examination

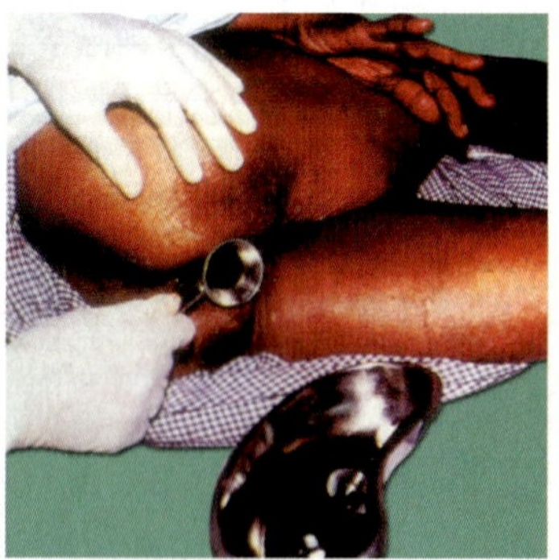

**Fig. 61.8A:** Proctoscopy

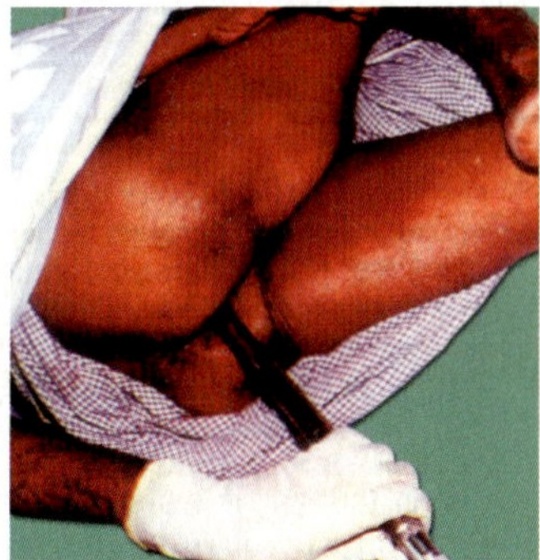

**Fig. 61.8B:** Rigid sigmoidoscopy

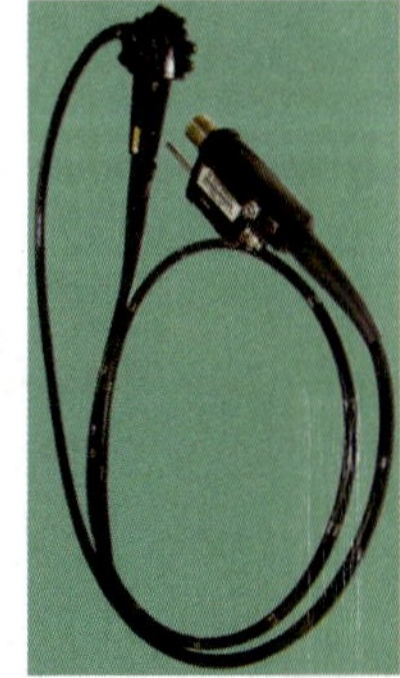

**Fig. 61.9:** Colonoscopy

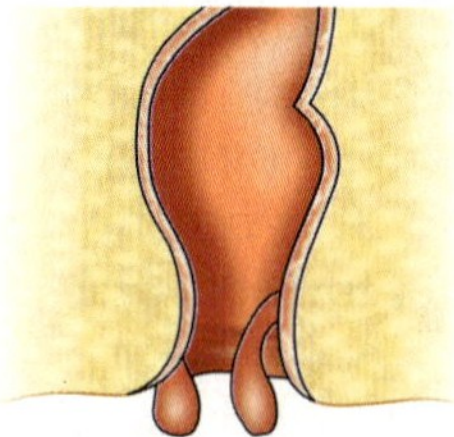

Haemorrhoids—painless

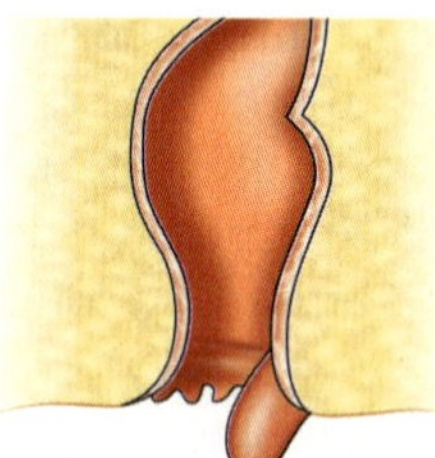

Thrombosed external haemorrhoids—painful

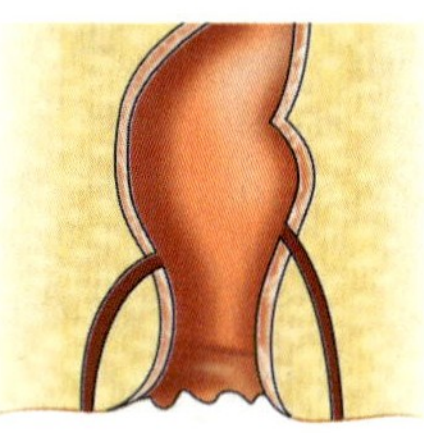

Fistula *in ano*—painless/painful

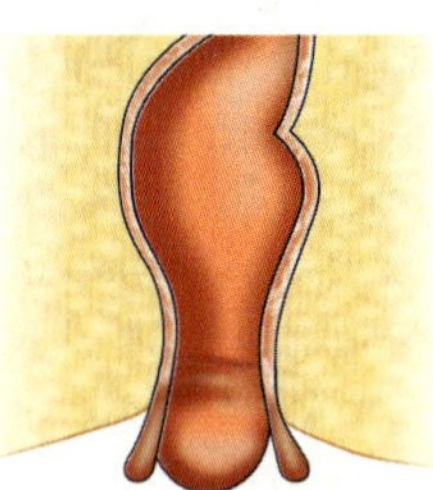

Rectal prolapse—painful/painless

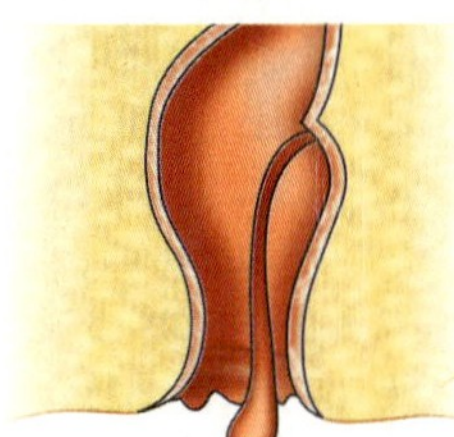

Pedunculated polyp—painless

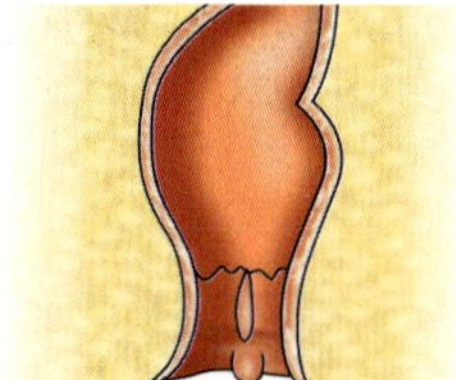

Anal fissure—painful

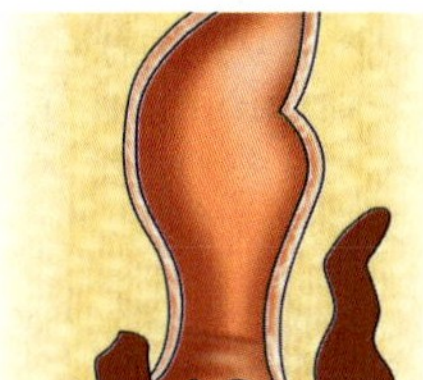

Perianal abscess—painful

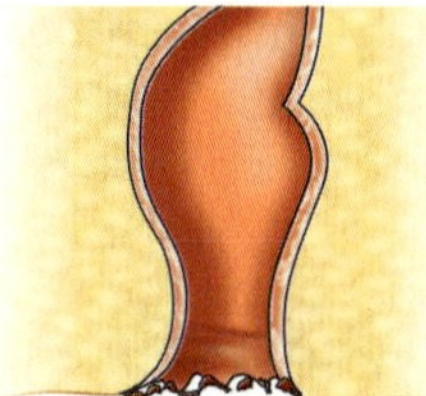

Perianal warts—painless

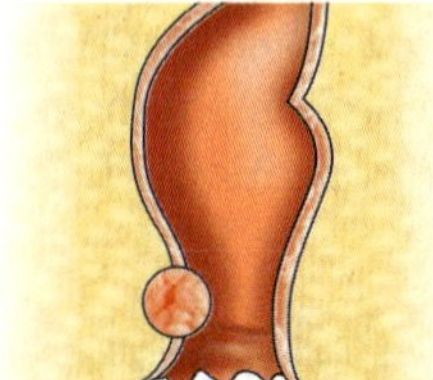

Carcinoma anal canal—painless

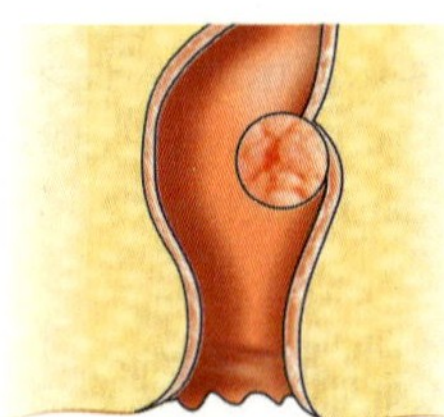

Carcinoma rectum—painless

**Fig. 61.10:** Common diseases of anorectum

## RECTAL POLYPS

Polyps are discussed in the chapter of large intestines. Adenomatous polyp of more than 1 cm in diameter has increased chances of invasive carcinoma. All adenomas should be removed. Villous adenomas are more common than tubular adenomas. Serrated adenomas are found in the right colon. Familial polyposis coli has 100% chances of malignant potential. Hence when the disease is present more than 10 years, treatment is warranted. Juvenile polyps are bright red pedunculated tumour in children. It has no malignant potential. Rectal polyps can be removed by endoscopic snaring or endoscopic submucosal resections.

## CARCINOMA RECTUM

**SU28.17.5:** Describe pathology, clinical features, diagnosis and principles of treatment of carcinoma rectum.

**Aetiopathogenesis:** Similar to carcinoma colon events such as adenoma—dysplasia and carcinoma. However, a few precancerous conditions and risk factors are given as follows.

### Pathogenesis

**Genetic:** Adenoma to invasive carcinoma is associated with genetic alterations—like in colonic cancers, mutation of *APC* gene (Adenomatous polyposis gene). APC mutations are also seen in sporadic colorectal cancers. Abnormal methylation of DNA causing silencing tumour suppressor genes thus may lead to malignant transformation. Other genes are KRAS oncogene, mutation of *MSH2* genes. Net result is in high frequency microsatellite instability-(H-MSI).

**Environmental and diet:** Increased incidence has been found in patients with diet rich in red meat, low fibres, low intake of fruits and vegetables. Alcohol, smoking and obesity are also few other factors.

**Inflammatory bowel disease:** Ulcerative colitis and Crohn's disease are associated with increasing incidence of colorectal cancers. Incidence increases with duration of disease.

### Risk Factors

- **Smoking:** Smokers have 30 to 40% more likely to die of colorectal cancer.
- **Obesity:** Obesity and lack of exercises are associated with rectal cancers.
- **Alcohol:** Definite increase has been found in breast and colon cancers. Alcohol damages the cells and prevents repair of cells, thereby increases the risk of malignancy.
- **Genetic:** Familial adenomatous polyposis gene: In hereditary forms of colorectal cancers such as Lynch syndrome (*see* page 946) **mutation** in one of the DNA mismatch repair genes is responsible.

### Pathological Types

1. **Annular** variety is common at the **rectosigmoid** junction. It presents with constipation and intestinal obstruction. It takes about a year for the growth to completely encircle the lumen of the gut (napkin ring deformity) (Fig. 61.11).
2. **Polypoidal** lesions are common in the **ampulla** of the rectum (Fig. 61.12).
3. **Ulcerative** lesions can occur anywhere in the rectum with **raised edges** and growth occurs in the transverse direction.
4. **Diffuse** variety is similar to linitis plastica. It develops from ulcerative colitis. It has a poor prognosis.
5. **Colloid** variety is rare. The tumour contents are **gelatinous** due to increased mucus production. This variety is seen in young patients. The cell is filled with mucus and nucleus is displaced. It is called **'signet ring' carcinoma**. It is associated with poor prognosis (Fig. 61.13).

### Clinical Features of Carcinoma Rectum

- **Constipation** requiring increasing doses of purgatives due to annular growth at rectosigmoid junction. Always a sense of incomplete evacuation and altered bowel habits.
- **Bleeding per rectum,** frank blood or mixed with stools is common. It is painless, never massive and is the

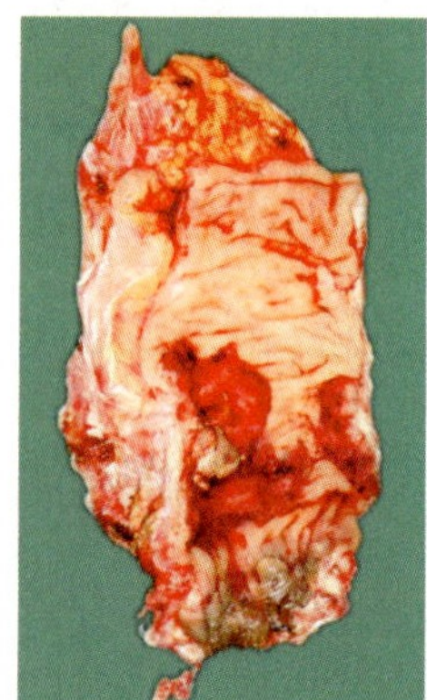

**Fig. 61.11:** Annular constricting lesion—patient presents with colonic obstruction

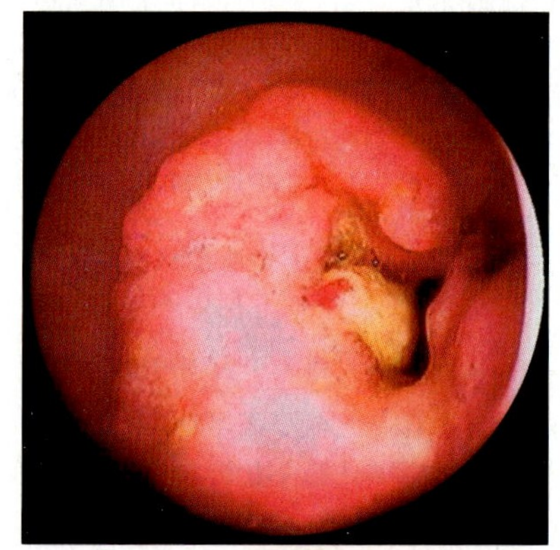

**Fig. 61.12:** Fibreoptic sigmoidoscopy showing growth in the upper rectum—biopsy proved signet ring carcinoma

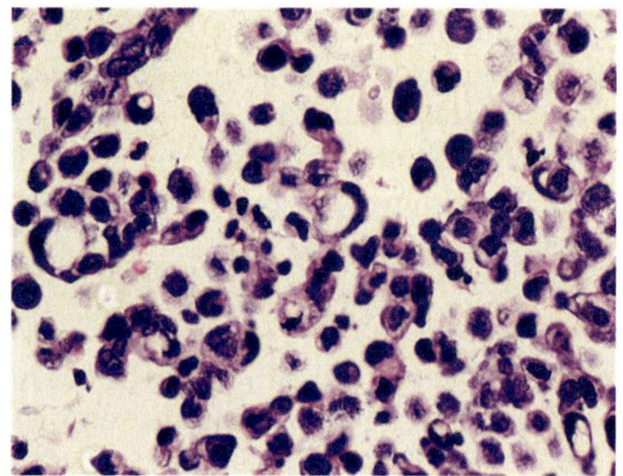

**Fig. 61.13:** Signet ring carcinoma colon—relatively poor prognosis (*Courtesy*: Dr Laxmi Rao, Head, Department of Pathology, KMC, Manipal)

earliest symptom of carcinoma rectum. Very often, it is confused for haemorrhoids.

- **Early morning spurious diarrhoea** is due to accumulation of mucus overnight in the ampulla of rectum (dilated middle portion of rectum), which causes an urgency to pass stools but results in passage of only mucus with minimal stools. It is associated with a sense of incomplete defaecation.
- **Tenesmus**
  - **Painful, incomplete defaecation** associated with **bleeding** is called tenesmus.
  - This symptom is common with stricturous growths.
- **Bloody slime** (Key Box 61.3): An attempt at defaecation results in mucus mixed with blood.
- **Loss of appetite,** loss of weight due to **liver secondaries** (cancer cachexia) and abdominal distension due to obstruction are late features.

Key Box 61.3

**Correlation of Symptoms to Carcinoma Rectum**

| Symptom | Probable site of lesion/explanation |
|---|---|
| Constipation | Rectosigmoid |
| Bleeding | Cauliflower-like growth |
| Tenesmus | Rectosigmoid stricture |
| Early morning spurious diarrhoea | Growth in the ampulla of rectum |
| Bloody slime | Blood and mucus |
| Sciatica-like pain | Sacral plexus infiltration |
| Abdominal distension | Large bowel obstruction |
| Loss of weight/ abdominal distension | Liver metastasis, ascites, etc. |
| Strangury | Infiltration of the bladder base anteriorly |

## ABCDEF of Rectal Carcinoma—Symptoms

1. **A**ltered bowel habits
2. **B**leeding per rectum and bloody slime—upper rectum.
3. **C**onstipation increasing—annular carcinoma at rectosigmoid junction.
4. Incomplete **d**efaecation
5. **E**arly morning spurious diarrhoea—midrectum
6. **F**atigue, weight loss

## Clinical Examination

- **Digital rectal examination:** In every patient with bleeding per rectum, rectal examination has to be done. More than 90% of cases of carcinoma rectum can be diagnosed by rectal examination. Always feel for the ulcer or growth, nodularity, induration, fixity to posterior sacrum, anterior bladder base and laterally to lateral ligaments. Look for the blood stains especially in ulcerative cases. It is also possible to feel the lymph nodes in the mesorectum in cases of lower third carcinomas.
- **Vaginal examination:** When the growth is situated in the anterior wall of the rectum, accurate assessment of the growth can be done with one finger in the rectum and the other in the vagina. Large Krukenberg tumours, if present, can also be felt by vaginal and rectal examinations.
- **Evidence of metastasis:** Palpable nodular liver, paraaortic lymph nodes, ascites and enlarged left supraclavicular nodes **(Troisier's sign).**

*Pearls of Wisdom*

Rectal cancer presenting as fistula *in ano* is the equivalent to a perforated colonic cancer. It is a bad prognostic sign.

**Histology:** They are adenocarcinomas—well differentiated, moderately differentiated and poorly differentiated. However, a few special types of adenocarcinomas are colloid carcinoma rectum and signet ring carcinoma. In colloid carcinoma, colloid-like substance is produced which can be detected macroscopically. Signet cell cancer is **a rare (less than 1%) type of cancer that starts in glandular cells.**

Signet ring carcinoma and colloid carcinoma carry poor prognosis.

## Differential Diagnosis (Key Box 61.4 and Fig. 61.14)

1. **Villous adenomas (benign)** present as bleeding per rectum with occasionally mass per rectum. They have a frond-like appearance. They are very friable, bulky and easily bleed on touch. Biopsy is a must. If it is benign, it can be removed through the rectum—submucosally.
2. **Proctitis due to inflammatory bowel diseases:** Both ulcerative colitis and Crohn's disease produce diarrhoea, blood in the stools and multiple non-indurated ulcers. Regardless biopsy is a must before doing a major surgical resection. Ulcers in ulcerative colitis are typically described as pinpoint ulcers. In Crohn's, they are fissure type or patchy with a cobblestone appearance.

Key Box 61.4

**Rectal Ulcers**

1. Carcinoma rectum
2. Amoebic ulcers
3. Ulcerative colitis
4. HIV infection
5. Solitary rectal ulcers
6. Radiation proctitis

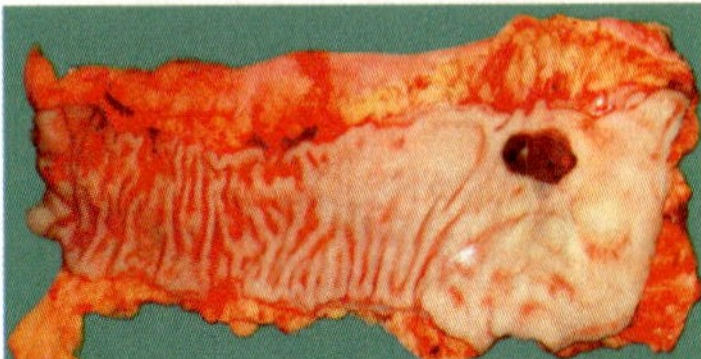

**Fig. 61.14:** Solitary rectal ulcers

**Clinical Notes**

A 22-year-old girl was treated with iron tablets for anaemia due to occasional bleeding per rectum. She was treated with metronidazole because she was passing mucus along with the stools. She developed intestinal obstruction after 6 months during which time a surgeon was consulted. Rectal examination revealed a large growth, fixed all around. She died 6 months later because of advanced disease. The case illustrates the importance of rectal examination and that carcinoma of the rectum often occurs in young patients also. Again to highlight the importance of rectal examination in a case of bleeding per rectum.

3. **Amoebic granuloma:** It is not common nowadays. It presents with a soft mass at rectosigmoid junction with or without obstruction. An ulcer over the surface will mimic carcinoma. Biopsy is mandatory because amoebomas are completely curable with antiamoebic treatment.
4. **Tuberculous proctitis:** Usually patients have pulmonary tuberculosis. Submucosal abscess ruptures and results in ulcers with undermined edges. Hypertrophic tuberculosis with stricture can also occur. Biopsy is mandatory before resection.
5. **Endometrioma:** It presents as constipation, bleeding per rectum especially during menstruation. Typically young females between the age of 20 and 40 years are affected. It produces a constricting lesion in the rectosigmoid junction. Mucosa is intact as seen by sigmoidoscopy. Treatment is biopsy followed by treatment of endometriosis.
6. **Solitary rectal ulcer syndrome (SRUS)** (*see* Box 61.4 and Fig. 61.14)
   - **Site:** Commonly occurs in the anterior wall of lower rectum, an area of mucosal change.
   - **Mucosa:** It is erythematous, heaped up and bleeds on touch.
   - It is a single, depressed ulcer.
   - The cause, even though not clear, is probably due to trauma by anal digitation. Today, it is believed that it is due to **internal intussusception** or **anterior wall prolapse**.
   - **Clinical features are** passage of blood and mucus in stools. Mucosal prolapse may also be a feature.
   - A biopsy must be done to rule out carcinoma rectum.
   - **Treatment is conservative:** Avoidance of constipation and straining may treat the prolapse.

## Spread of Carcinoma Rectum

1. **Local spread**
   - **It takes 18 months** for a growth to encircle the rectal lumen as in annular strictures at the rectosigmoid junction.
   - Then, it involves muscle coat and spreads into extrarectal tissues.
   - **Anteriorly,** it involves **prostate, seminal vesicles and bladder** base in males, vagina and uterus in females.
   - **Posteriorly, sacral plexus** gets involved in late cases and causes sciatica-like pain. Posterior sacral infiltration and anterior bladder base infiltration—surgery can be very difficult and dangerous (uncontrollable bleeding from sacral plexus of veins and prostatic plexus of veins in males. Hence, preoperative chemoradiotherapy followed by surgery is done.
   - Involvement of mesorectum carries poor prognosis. Hence, the **circumferential resected margin** is important.
2. **Lymphatic spread**—chief nodes are para-aortic nodes.
3. **Haematogenous spread:** It results in secondaries in the liver, lungs, etc. It is common in young patients with anaplastic variety and in colloid carcinoma.
4. **Peritoneal spread:** It results in ascites, carcinomatous nodules over the peritoneum, etc.

## STAGING

**SU28.17.2:** Describe investigations for diseases of the rectum including those used for staging of carcinoma rectum.

### I. Modified Dukes' Staging of Carcinoma of Rectum
(Fig. 61.15)

#### *Stages*

A. Growth confined to the rectal wall

B. Growth involving perirectal pad of fat and tissues. No nodes are involved.

B1: Invading muscularis mucosa

B2: Invading to or through serosa

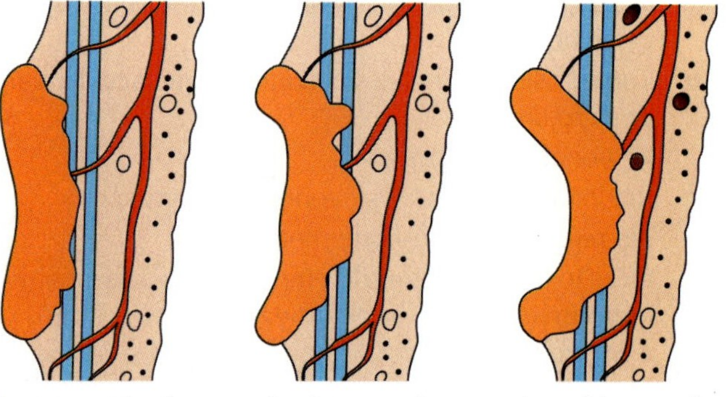

**Fig. 61.15:** The three cardinal stages of progression of the neoplasm

C. Nodes are involved

C1: Local lymph nodes—pararectal

C2: Distal lymph nodes—along the course of blood vessels

D. Distant spread—liver, lungs, etc.

## II. Astler-Coller Modification of Dukes' System

### Stages

| | |
|---|---|
| A | Limited to mucosa—no nodes |
| B1 | Extension into muscularis propria—no nodes |
| B2 | Extension into entire bowel wall—no nodes |
| B3 | Extension into adjacent organs—no nodes |
| C1 | Extension into muscularis propria—positive nodes |
| C2 | B2 + Lymph nodes |
| C3 | B3 + Lymph nodes |
| D | Distant metastasis |

### Prognosis as per Dukes' Staging

- Dukes' A: 5-year survival is 90 to 100%.
- Dukes' B: 5-year survival is 50 to 80%.
- Dukes' C: 5-year survival is less than 50%.

## III. TNM Staging

| TNM STAGING | |
|---|---|
| **T** | **Primary Tumour** |
| **TX** | Primary tumour cannot be assessed |
| **T0** | No evidence of primary tumour |
| **Tis** | Carcinoma *in situ*: Intramucosal carcinoma (involvement of lamina propria with no extension through muscularis mucosae) |
| **T1** | Tumour invades the submucosa (through the muscularis mucosa but not into the muscularis propria) |
| **T2** | Tumour invades the muscularis propria |
| **T3** | Tumour invades through the muscularis propria into pericolorectal tissues |
| **T4** | Tumour invades the visceral peritoneum or invades or adheres to adjacent organ or structure |
| **T4a** | Tumour invades through the visceral peritoneum (including gross perforation of the bowel through tumour and continuous invasion of tumour through areas of inflammation to the surface of the visceral peritoneum) |
| **T4b** | Tumour directly invades or adheres to adjacent organs or structures |
| **N** | Regional lymph nodes |
| **NX** | Regional lymph nodes cannot be assessed |
| **N0** | No regional lymph node metastasis |
| **N1** | One to three regional lymph nodes are positive (tumour in lymph nodes measuring ≥0.2 mm), or any number of tumour deposits are present and all identifiable lymph nodes are negative |
| **N1a** | One regional lymph node is positive |
| **N1b** | Two or three regional lymph nodes are positive |
| **N1c** | No regional lymph nodes are positive, but there are tumour deposits in the subserosa, mesentery or non-peritonealized pericolic, or perirectal/mesorectal tissues |
| **N2** | Four or more regional lymph nodes are positive |
| **N2a** | Four to six regional lymph nodes are positive |
| **N2b** | Seven or more regional lymph nodes are positive |
| **M** | **Distant metastasis** |
| **M0** | No distant metastasis by imaging, etc.; no evidence of tumour in distant sites or organs |
| **M1** | Metastasis to one or more distant sites or organs or peritoneal metastasis is identified |
| **M1a** | Metastasis to one site or organ is identified without peritoneal metastasis |
| **M1b** | Metastasis to two or more sites or organs is identified without peritoneal metastasis |
| **M1c** | Metastasis to the peritoneal surface is identified alone or with other site or organ metastases. |

- T1s: Does not penetrate muscularis mucosa.
- T1s: Intraepithelial carcinoma—but this term is not used.
- pT4a: It should not be used for non-peritonised portion of large bowel such as ascending and descending colon, lower rectum.
- Minimum of 12 nodes should be removed. If less number of lymph nodes are removed, even if they are negative, these patients should receive chemotherapy.
- M1a: Multiple metastasis in an organ, even paired organs (ovaries lungs) M1a disease.
- Stage grouping: **Stage I:** T1 or T2 N0 M0, **Stage IIA:** T3 N0 M0, **Stage IIB:** T4 N0 M0, **Stage IIIA:** T1 N2a M0, T3 or T4a N1/N1c M0, **Stage IIIB:** T2 or T3 N2a M0, T1 or T2 N2b M0, **Stage IIIC:** T3 or T4a N2b M0, T4b N1 or N2 M0, **Stage IV:** Any metastasis.

### Investigations

1. **Proctoscopy:** It should be done in all cases of bleeding per rectum. It is done as an outpatient procedure. The left lateral position with buttocks elevated on a small pillow is the ideal position for proctoscopy. However, knee-elbow position can also be used. The growth appears as an ulcer with everted edges. A biopsy is taken to confirm the diagnosis. The histological grading of the tumour is as follows:

   A. ***Well-differentiated carcinoma:*** Low-grade variety (10–15%).

   B. ***Moderately differentiated carcinoma:*** The most common variety (65%).

   C. ***Undifferentiated carcinoma:*** The most aggressive variety (20–25%).

2. **Sigmoidoscopy:** To take a biopsy from rectosigmoid growths, sigmoidoscopy is essential.

3. **Colonoscopy: To detect any** synchronous carcinoma. It can be present in about 8 to 10% of patients. It can also detect adenomas, polyps. Biopsy should be taken in all suspicious lesions.
4. **CEA:** Increased levels of carcinoembryonic antigen indicates metastasis.
5. **Ultrasound of the abdomen: It is done to know the** metastasis such as secondaries in the liver, ascites with para-aortic nodes, etc. Colloid carcinoma rectum is one of the types which can present as metastasis.
6. **Endorectal ultrasonography (EUS)** (Key Box 61.5) **Endoscopic ultrasound staging of rectal tumours**

| | |
|---|---|
| UT1 | Invasion confined to the mucosa and submucosa |
| UT2 | Penetration of the muscularis propria but not through the mesorectal fat |
| UT3 | Invasion into the perirectal fat |
| UT4 | Invasion into the adjacent organ |
| UN0 | No enlargement of lymph nodes |
| UN1 | Perirectal lymph nodes enlarged. |

Key Box 61.5

**EUS**

- It is also called **T**rans Rectal **U**ltra **S**onography **(TRUS)**
- To know the level of penetration
- Detect perirectal lymph node enlargement
- Invasion of adjacent structures—levator ani, bony pelvis, etc.
- It is superior in T-staging of rectal cancers.

7. **CECT scan: Contrast enhanced computed tomography**
   - It helps to detect the lesion, to know the extension of the tumour thus able to detect T staging.
   - To know the fixation to adjacent structures (ureter, uterus, bladder base, etc. hydronephrosis).
   - Importantly, to know nodal status
   - Detect metastasis in liver.
8. **MRI:** Both MRI and EUS are good for assessment of T-staging. MRI has the following advantages:
   - It is better for T3 and T4 stages.
   - High resolution MRI is better for assessment of circumferential resected margin (CRM).
   - It is also good for lymph nodal staging and phased array MRI can pick up small nodes.

## TREATMENT PRINCIPLES

1. Aim is to have a **curative resection.**
2. Radical surgery is described as **total mesorectal excision (TME)**—which improves quality of life (*see* Ten commandments and Key Box 61.6).

Key Box 61.6

**Total Mesorectal Excision—Advantages**

1. Mesorectum is the perirectal fat surrounding the rectum.
2. It preserves autonomic nerves.
3. Impotence, urinary incontinence and retrograde ejaculation are lesser after TME.

**TEN COMMANDMENTS OF TOTAL MESORECTAL EXCISION**

1. Should perform TME in all cases of mid and lower carcinoma rectum
2. Should excise the entire mesorectum (contains fat, lymph nodes and superior rectal blood vessels)
3. Should perform the dissection with electrocautery or scissors
4. Should open the posterior plane between visceral and parietal layers of endopelvic fascia—**holy plane of Heald or avascular plane** (refer to Figs 61.16A to D)
5. Should exert good traction and countertraction to develop the planes
6. Should excise the entire mesorectum circumferentially—minimum of 5 cm of the CRM
7. Should be inside the pelvic plexus laterally
8. Should excise Denonvilliers' fascia anteriorly
9. Should excise rectosacral ligament so as to reach the pelvic floor
10. Should perform proximal diversion ileostomy.

3. Even though surgical treatment is the main modality, **radiotherapy and chemotherapy** are beneficial.
4. **At surgery, ligation of vascular pedicle is done first to prevent tumour embolisation.**
5. **Ligation of bowel,** proximal and distal to the tumour helps to prevent transluminal dissemination.
6. **Distal surgical margin should be about 2 cm.** Proximal margin—minimum 5 cm.
7. A double-stapled anastomosis as described or a hand-sewn anastomosis is then performed. A diverting loop ileostomy is used routinely for these ultra low anastomoses.
8. **Palliative resection** is worth doing even in the presence of metastasis, when there is obstruction.
9. **Colonic pouch:** The splenic flexure is mobilised first. A 6 cm limb of sigmoid or descending colon is folded and a pouch is created. A colotomy is made at the apex of the pouch. Linear cutter is used to staple the pouch on itself to create a common lumen. A second fire of the stapler may be necessary. This pouch now acts like a neo-rectum.

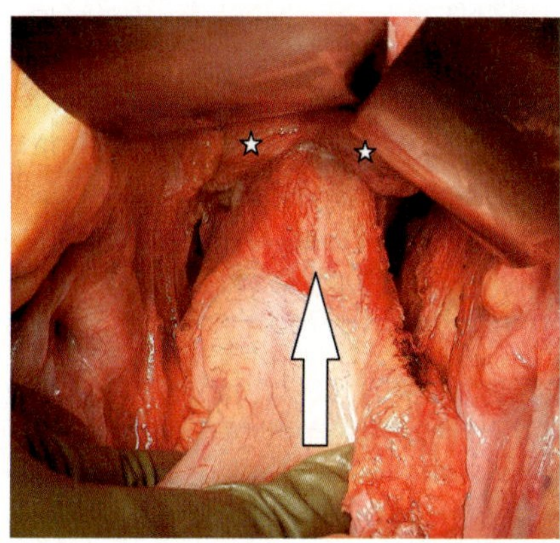

Fig. 61.16A: Anterior TME (holy plane) plane in male patient. Star (★) indicates right and left seminal vesicles. Arrow points mesorectum covered by Denonvilliers' fascia

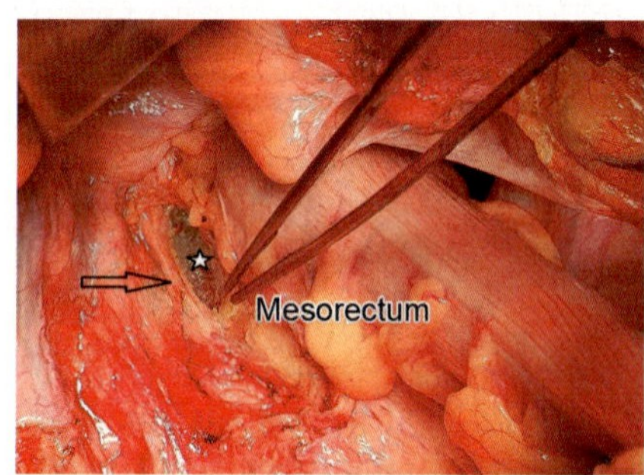


Fig. 61.16B: Left lateral dissection between lateral aspect of pelvic fascia and mesorectum. Arrow points to pelvic nerves. Forceps show plane of dissection. Star (★) indicates exact holy (TME) plane where dissection is to be done

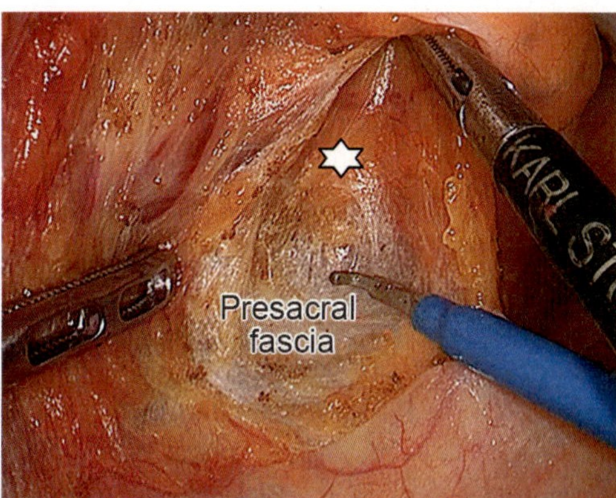


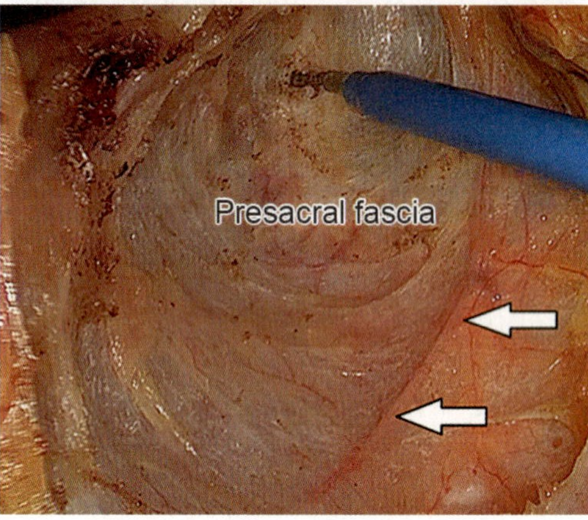


Fig. 61.16C: Posterior TME (holy) plane between presacral (Waldeyer's) fascia and mesorectum. Arrows point to pelvic nerves covered by pelvic fascia. Star (★) indicates mesorectum with all lymph nodes

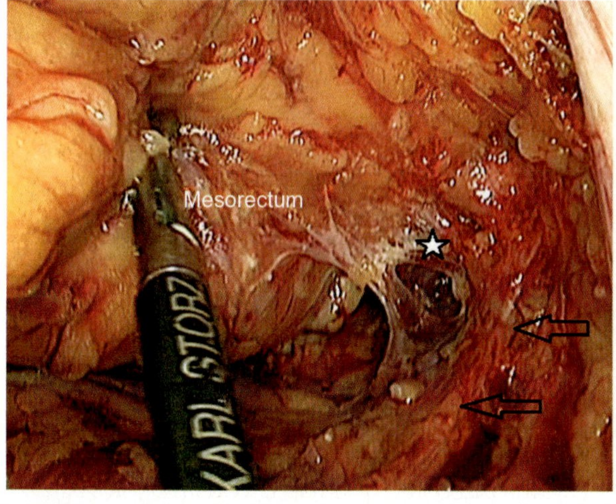


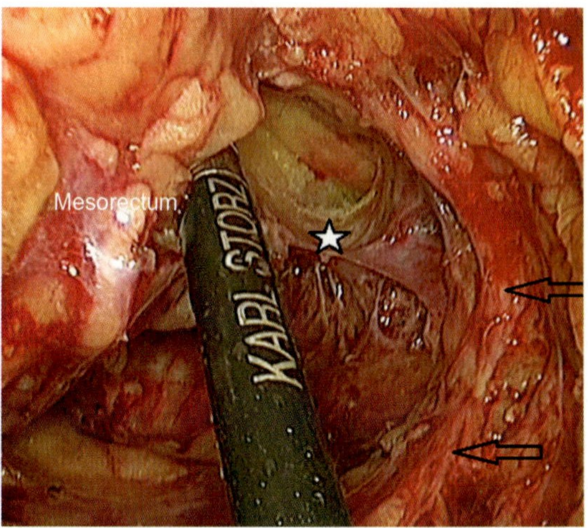


Fig. 61.16D: Right lateral dissection between mesorectum and pelvic fascia covering pelvic nerves. Arrow points to fascia covering pelvic nerves. Star (★) indicates exact plane of dissection (*Courtesy:* Figs 61.16A to D, Dr Vipin Goel, Basavatarakam Indo-American Cancer Hospital and Research Institute, Hyderabad)

## LAPAROSCOPIC MESORECTAL EXCISION

### Introduction

Laparoscopic anterior resection and total mesorectal excision are well-established procedures now. It is possible because of advances in the laparoscopic instruments, high definition cameras and improved technology.

### Advantages

- A 30° camera allows a beautiful magnified view of the entire dissecting field specially low down in the pelvis. Thus, no part of the laparoscopic procedure is blind.
- Laparoscopic surgery allows the surgeon to adopt the principle of no touch technique. At the same time with

better visualisation of the rectum and mesorectum all around, it permits a good dissection.

- It is not uncommon in the open method that the specimen gets torn due to traction. It has been proved that this tearing is much less in laparoscopy.
- Recovery is very fast after laparoscopy.
- Better preservation of the pelvic autonomic nerves, low anastomotic leak and low mortality rates.
- For laparoscopic low resections, one need not mobilise splenic flexure but sigmoid colon can be used for anastomosis.
- Wound infection, paralytic ileus are much less after laparoscopic surgery than open surgery.

### Disadvantages

- **Very low resection**—because of the limited space and the lack of proper curved instruments—open method has a slight advantage.
- **Port site recurrence:** Local tissue trauma due to trocars, tumour manipulation, tumour behaviour are the factors responsible for port site recurrence. Tumour spillage, tumour cell aerosolisation due to sudden loss of pneumoperitoneum, tumour spillage during extraction and immunosuppression during pneumoperitoneum are a few factors responsible for port site recurrence. This can be minimised by using bag for extraction, minimal handling of the tumour and avoiding tearing of the specimen.

## DIFFERENT TYPES OF SURGERIES FOR CARCINOMA RECTUM

### Carcinoma Upper One-third of Rectum (Fig. 61.17)

High anterior resection, which includes removal of growth along with the nodes, followed by colorectal anastomosis is the treatment of choice. This is the operation of choice when the growth is situated between **11 and 15 cm** from the anal verge. The lymphatic spread from upper one-third is always in the upward direction. Hence, the sphincter is saved. If the bowel is well prepared, protective colostomy is not necessary (sphincter-saving surgery). Stapler anastomosis is popular as there is a lesser incidence of leak.

### Carcinoma Lower One-third of Rectum (Figs 61.18 to 61.20)

This refers to growth within 4 cm from the anal verge. Two types of surgery can be done depending upon the degree of involvement of the growth with adjacent and surrounding tissues. When the sphincter is involved, **abdominoperineal resection** (APR) is done. In early cases, local excision can be done. In patients with low rectal cancers—T3 and T4 lesions, chemoradiation is

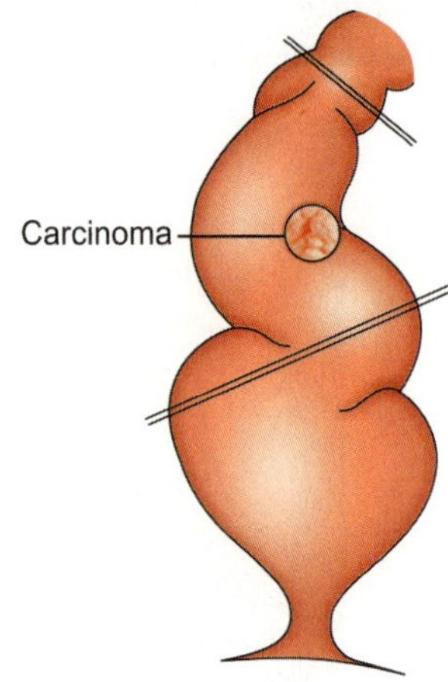


**Fig. 61.17:** Carcinoma upper rectum

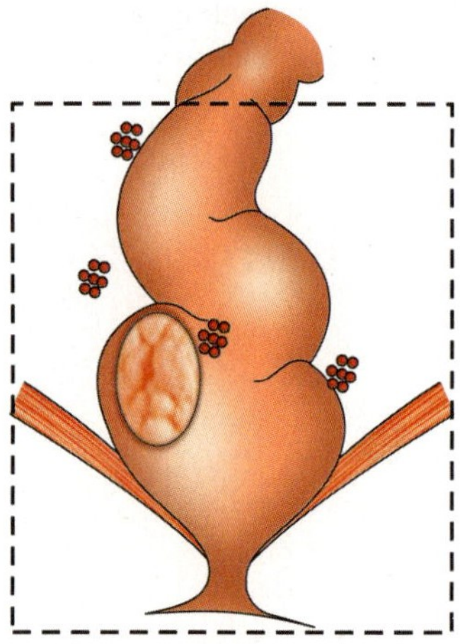

**Fig. 61.18:** The field of clearance in APR

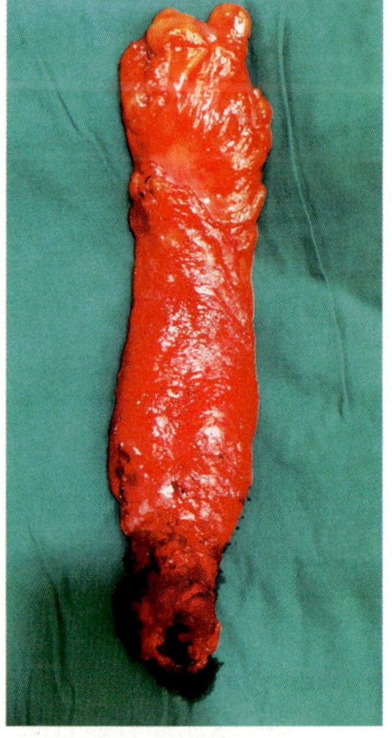

**Fig. 61.19A:** APR specimen showing appearance of baby bottom (*Courtesy*: Dr SS Prasad, Dr Rajendra, Dr Vijendra, Department of Surgery, KMC, Manipal)

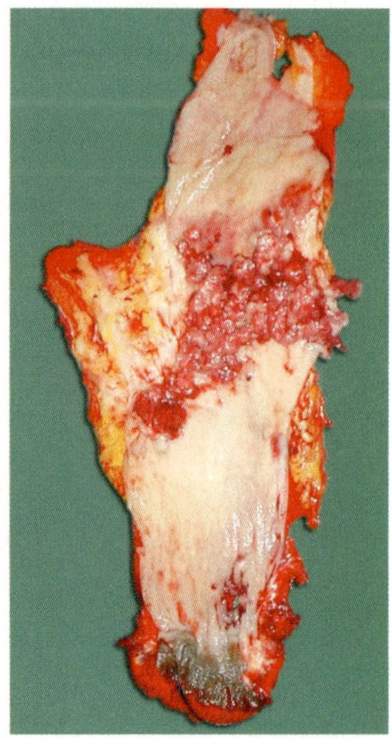

**Fig. 61.19B:** Nodular lesion 3 cm away from the anal verge buttock. (*Courtesy:* Dr Dinesh B, Dr Sunilkrishna, Department of Surgery, KMC, Manipal)

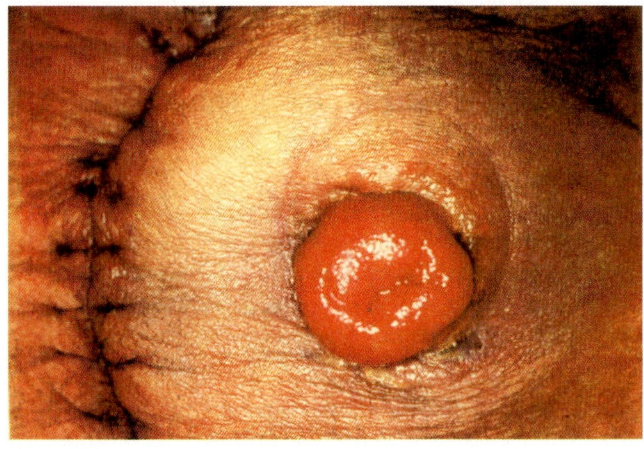

**Fig. 61.20:** Permanent end-colostomy following APR

## VARIOUS PHOTOGRAPHS OF CARCINOMA RECTUM AT SURGERY (Figs 61.21 to 61.25)

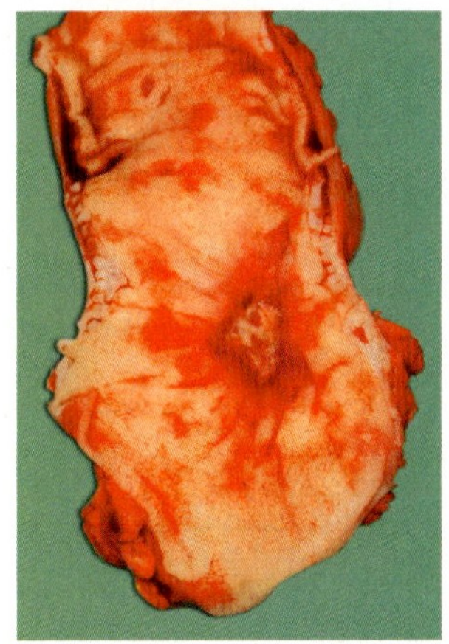

Fig. 61.21: This patient with carcinoma midrectum presented with bleeding per rectum. Low anterior resection was done. At least 3 cm margin could be achieved distally

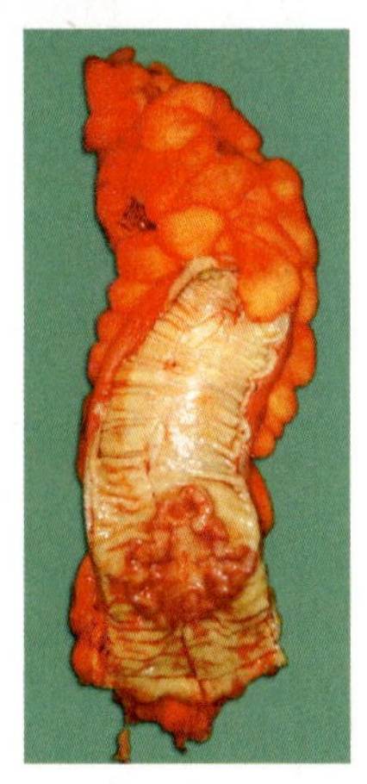

Fig. 61.22: Low anterior resection—see the lower margin

Fig. 61.23A: Low anterior resection is in progress. The rectum has been mobilised from urinary bladder anteriorly and sacrum posteriorly—carcinoma midrectum

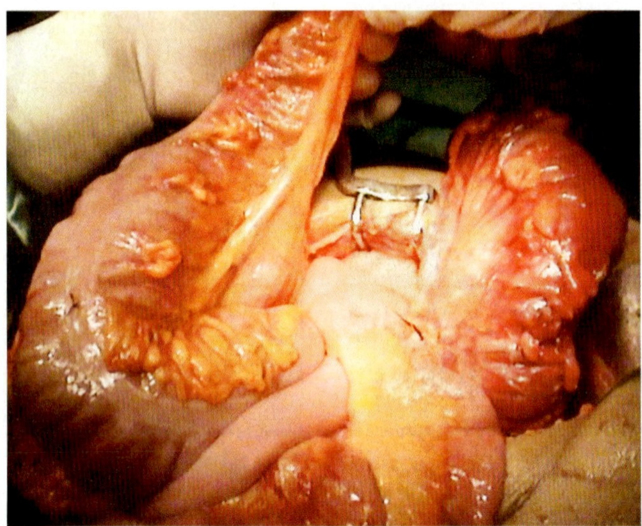

Fig. 61.23B: Proximal colon is mobilised up to the transverse colon so that it can be easily brought down without tension

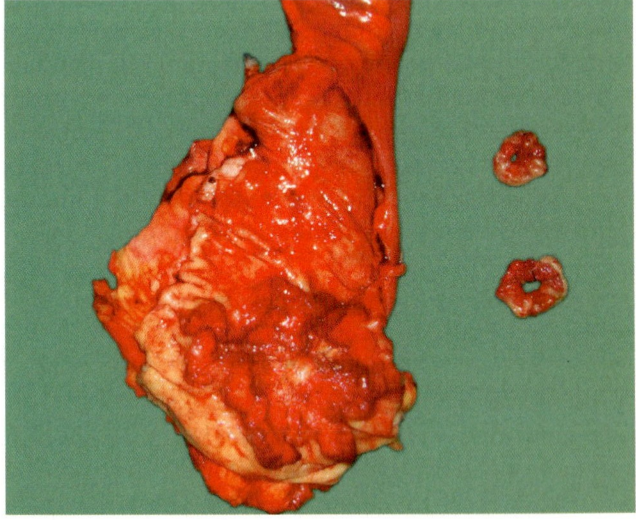

Fig. 61.24: Low anterior resection specimen—Stapler anastomosis has been done—you can see the complete doughnuts

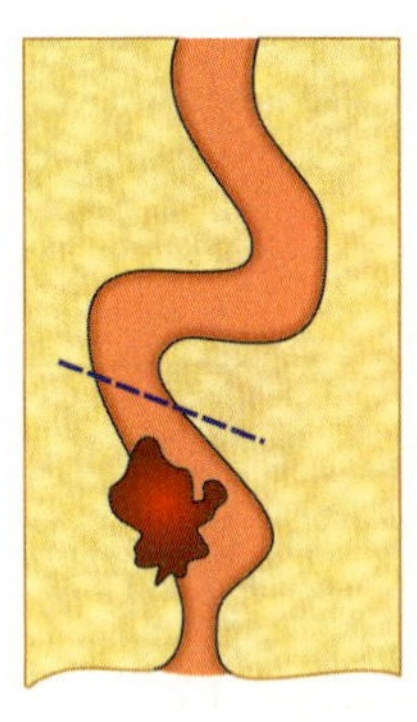

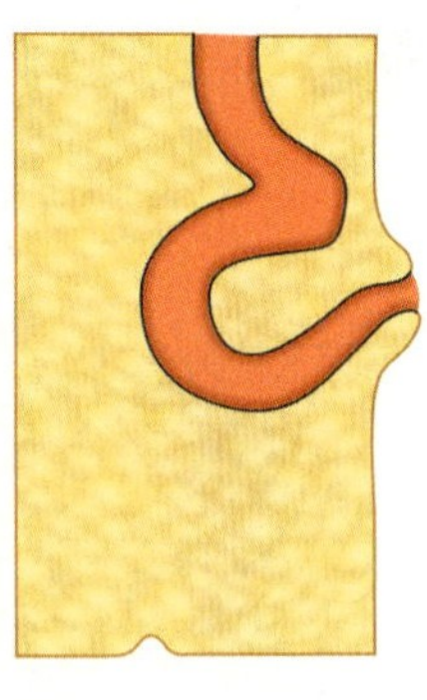

A

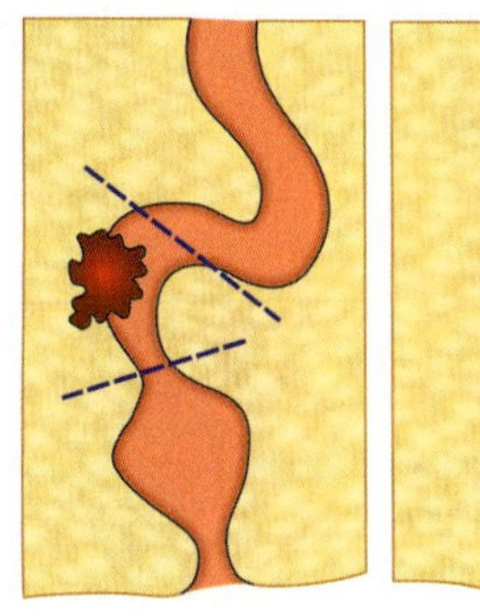

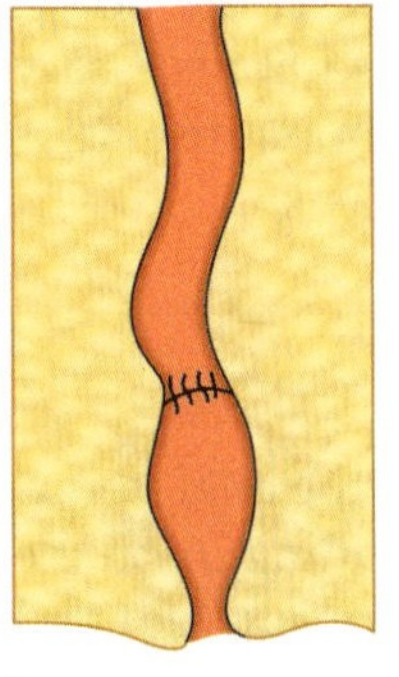

B

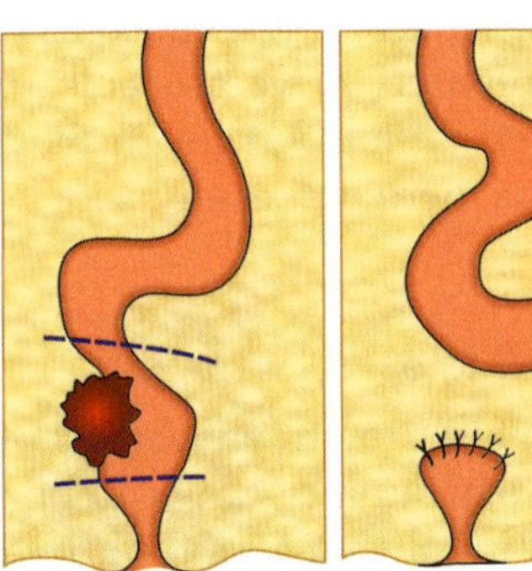

C

Figs 61.25A to C: Schematic representations of resection of the rectum: (A) AP resection followed by colostomy; (B) High anterior resection followed by anastomosis; (C) Low anterior resection with colostomy and closure of rectal stump—Hartmann's procedure—in large bowel obstruction. The colostomy is closed and colorectal anastomosis is done after 4 weeks

given before surgery. This method is also followed when sphincter is involved. This is called preoperative chemotherapy. Inoperable lesions may become operable, and, in a few patients, it is possible to save the sphincter. Details are given later.

A. **Radical surgery** is called **abdominoperineal resection** (APR) or Miles-Walker operation (Key Box 61.7). The patient is put in Lloyd-Davies position (supine with lithotomy). Two surgeons operate simultaneously, one from the abdomen and one from the perineum. Abdomen is opened first and the growth is mobilised from the sacrum and urinary bladder. At this stage, anus is closed by a perineal surgeon. Rectum and anal canal are mobilised. The entire specimen of rectum, anal canal and lymph nodes are removed followed by ***permanent endcolostomy*** by bringing the sigmoid colon out-side in the left iliac fossa (sphincter sacrificing surgery).

Key Box 61.7

**Structures Removed in APR**

- Growth with entire rectum and anal canal.
- Fascia propria with pararectal nodes.
- Two-thirds of the sigmoid colon and mesocolon with lymphatics and lymph nodes.
- Muscles and peritoneum of pelvic floor.
- Wide area of perianal skin, with part of ischiorectal fossa.

B. **Local excision:** In our country, 95% of low rectal cancers are offered and treated with abdominoperineal resection. Very small percentage of patients may be considered for local treatment—**local excision** (Key Box 61.8). This can be done only in selected group of patients.

C. **Ultra-low resection:** *Low anterior resection and ultra-low resection*
   - In female pelvis, broad pelvis, and even in thin males, a tumour measured at 5 cm by rigid proctoscopy, at surgery often may be moved to 8 cm from the dentate line, thus growth can be resected with a good margin and low resection can be done.

Key Box 61.8

**Local Excision of Carcinoma Rectum**

- Mobile tumours less than 4 cm in diameter
- Less than 40% of rectal wall involvement
- Located within 6 cm of anal verge
- Lesion should be T1 or T2 with node negative status
- No vascular or lymphatic invasion
- No nodal involvement—preoperative MRI or EUS.
- Well/moderately differentiated

- Now with availability of the staplers, if one can give a 2 cm distal margin, ultra-low resection can be done followed by stapler anastomosis.
- Stapler anastomosis is the choice for low and ultralow resections. A 30, 45, or 60 mm linear stapler is used. The bowel is clamped and transected just proximal to this point (Figs 61.26 to 61.28).

  A diverting loop ileostomy is done in any low anastomoses (<5 cm) from the dentate line, which are associated with anastomotic leak rates of up to 17%. Other risk factors for anastomotic leak include a history of radiation, malnutrition, elderly patients undergoing preoperative combined-modality therapy with planned postoperative chemotherapy.
- Coloanal anastomosis is done just above the anorectal ring. It usually causes increased frequency of stool, incontinence or soilage, and impaired quality of life owing to an insufficient reservoir. Diet restrictions and time after surgery usually will improve these symptoms. These complications can be minimised by creating a colonic pouch.

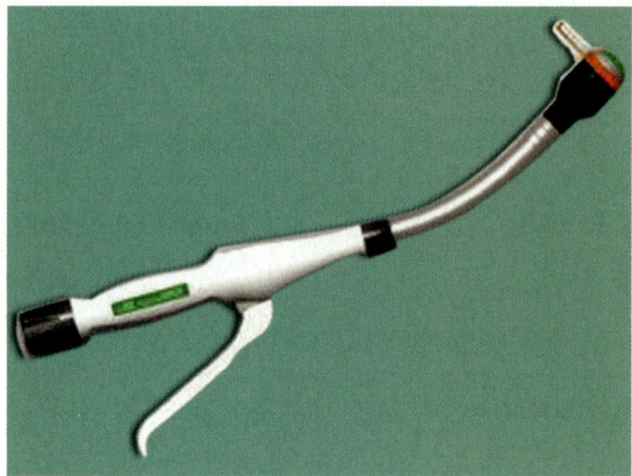

**Fig. 61.26:** Circular stapler used for anterior resection

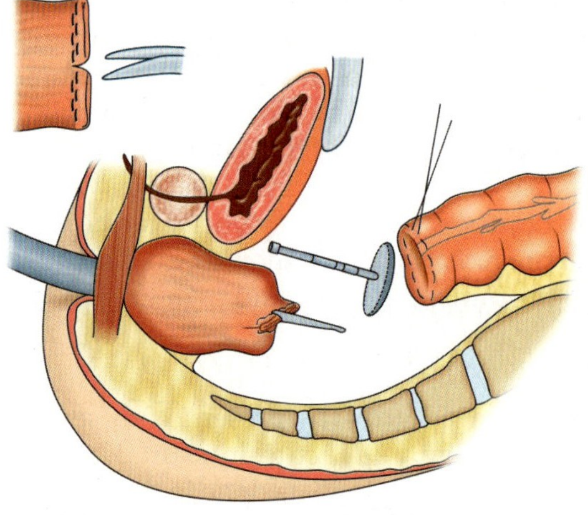

**Fig. 61.27:** Diagrammatic representation of anterior resection and use of staplers.

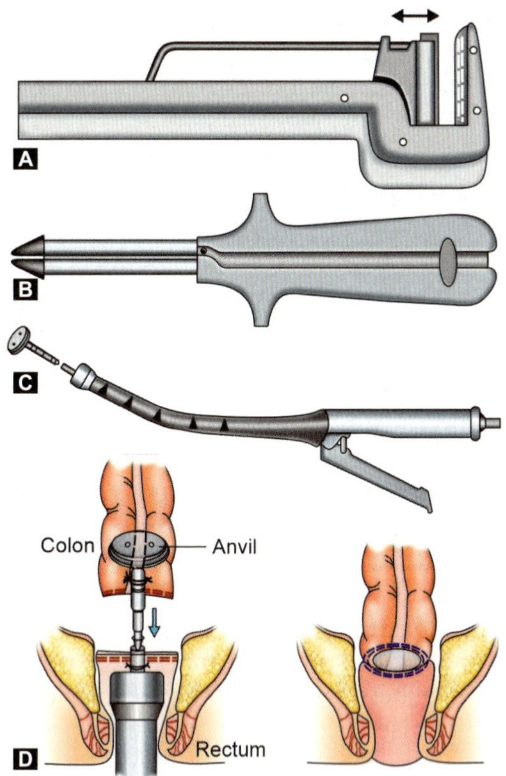


Figs 61.28A to D: (A to C) Parts of the stapler; (D) shows as the stapler is tightened, upper and lower rectum come together and the anvil fits in very well in the circular stapler

**Recent change in APR:** In the conventional APR, dissection is within the levator ani and levator ani is preserved. The change is APR with removal of levator ani—it is called Extra Levator Abdominoperineal Excision (ELAPE). The resected specimen has a waist—it is called cylindrical APR. Aim is to get adequate CRM.

### Carcinoma Middle One-third of Rectum

This refers to growth between **7 and 11 cm** from the anal verge. The decision to save the sphincter can be taken at laparotomy. In cases of well-differentiated carcinoma, 2 cm margin is adequate. **In anaplastic carcinoma, 5 cm clearance is necessary**. In female patients with broad pelvis after mobilisation of the rectum, the 7 cm growth may appear around 10 cm from the anal verge. Thus, sphincter can be saved. If the sphincter can be preserved, low anterior resection (LAR) should be done. (APR is also done, if the tumour is bulky and high-grade.)

### Inoperable Cases

Locally advanced growths present with severe pain, bleeding and with subacute intestinal obstruction. Temporary loop colostomy is done in the left iliac fossa by bringing the sigmoid colon outside. Postoperatively, radiation and chemotherapy are given.

### Hartmann's Operation (Fig. 61.29)

This is indicated in old and debilitated patients who may not withstand APR. The rectum is excised, the lower end of the rectum is closed and a colostomy is performed. When the growth is slow-growing, this operation gives good palliation.

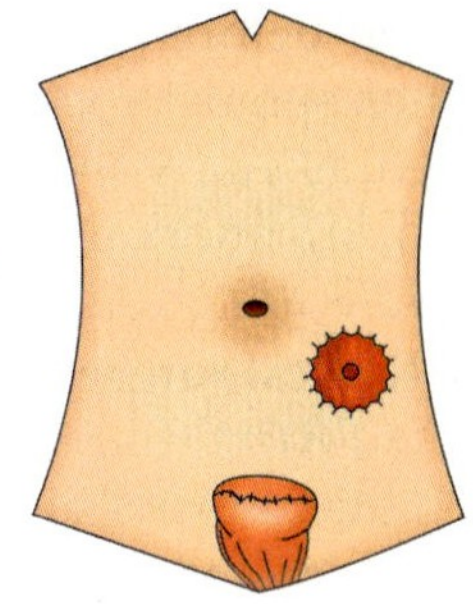

Fig. 61.29: Hartmann's operation

### Other Types of Surgeries

**TEM (transanal endoscopic microsurgery):** It involves wide anorectal retraction, followed by good visualisation of lesion using operating sigmoidoscope and distension of rectum by $CO_2$ followed by complete thickness excision and direct suturing. It can also be done by trans-sacral or trans-sphincteric approach.

## ENDOSCOPIC TREATMENT OF COLORECTAL LESIONS

- **Colonoscopic polypectomy:** All adenomas and potential adenomas should be removed. Pedunculated polyps are removed by snare. Small polyps can be removed by cold or hot forceps and hot or cold snare. Bleeding can be controlled by injection of epinephrine, electrocautery, clips or endoloops.
- **Endoscopic mucosal resection:** It is indicated for flat, sessile lesions, not more than 2.5 cm in diameter. First the lesion is elevated by injecting saline or hypertonic dextrose with epinephrine. The lesion is elevated, cut and removed or sucked and cut.
- **Endoscopic submucosal dissection:** Technically more difficult. Principle of the procedure is same. More chances of perforation.
- **Endoscopic stents for decompression for malignant obstruction:** Large bore colorectal decompression tubes are available. They can be passed with or without endoscope with a guidewire. They are used to relieve obstruction so that bowel preparation can be done and one stage treatment—resection and anastomosis can be done. Self-expandable metal stents—SEMS have been used as palliation in cases of large gut obstruction. Quality of life is slightly better but no increase in survival rate of patients. Stent migration, tumour ingrowth, overgrowth, perforation and bleeding are the other complications.
- **Bridge to surgery: In left colonic obstruction, this is used in operable and advanced lesions.** Self-expandable metal stents—SEMS is used to relieve obstruction or an emergency ostomy without resection. Advantages of this method is: Get time for correction of fluid/electrolyte imbalance, normalization of bowel caliber, mechanical bowel preparation, provides time for the multidisciplinary team to complete staging

workup. We can also screen for synchronous lesions, and initiate neoadjuvant therapy for the primary tumour, if needed. Advantage of diverting ostomy being, it offers a high success rate for relieving obstruction compared to stenting, no need for tumor manipulation, no potential risk of stent-related perforation or tumor spillage.

## ROLE OF RADIOTHERAPY AND CHEMOTHERAPY

### Postoperative Management

1. pT1-2N0M0 do not require any adjuvant treatment, such patients can be kept on follow-up with routine 3 monthly CEA and annual CECT thorax/abdomen/pelvis.
2. pT3N0M0 or node positive disease requires adjuvant treatment in the form of concurrent chemoradiotherapy and chemotherapy. Example: 2 cycles of FOLFOX (5-FU + Leucovorin + Oxaliplatin) → concurrent 5-FU/Leucovorin and radiation → 2 more cycles of FOLFOX. Oral Capecitabine can be used in place of IV 5-FU.
3. It is preferable to add Oxaliplatin in the chemotherapy regimen, if nodes were positive for metastatic disease. Although in older population (>65–70 years), it might be of less benefit.
4. Radiation portals should include the postoperative tumour bed, presacral nodes and internal iliac nodes. External iliac nodes should be included in T4 tumours. Radiation dose is usually 45–50 Gy given over 5 days a week for 5 consecutive weeks. Another 5–9 Gy boost to the tumour bed can be considered especially when there are adverse features such as lymphatic emboli, close margins, etc.

### Preoperative—Neoadjuvant Chemoradiation
(Key Box 61.9)

**Rationale:** In locally advanced cases where the surgeon feels that complete resection may not be feasible or sphincter saving will not be possible, neoadjuvant chemoradiation can be attempted thus saving the patient from having a permanent colostomy bag and also better curative outcomes.

Generally, clinically T3–T4 tumors which may or may not be node positive are eligible candidates for neoadjuvant (NACT) chemotherapy.

1. A typical course of NACT comprises concurrent 5-FU/Capecitabine and radiation. A dose of 45–50 Gy is used to treat the pelvis including the growth and the draining lymphatic regions followed by 5 Gy boost to the tumours itself.
2. Following NACT, patient should be re-evaluated using CT/MRI for possibility of resection.
3. Surgery is usually considered after 6–8 weeks of NACT as the maximal response to the treatment may take up to 2 months.
4. Further adjuvant treatment is to be given following surgery depending upon the histopathological report.

> **Key Box 61.9**
>
> **Advantages of Preoperative Radiotherapy**
>
> - Decreased tumour seeding at surgery
> - Increased radiosensitivity due to more oxygenated cells
> - Conversion of APR to LAR

> *Pearls of Wisdom*
>
> Rectal cancers are more radiosensitive and colonic cancers are more chemosensitive.

## LOCALLY RECURRENT RECTAL CANCER

- Major cause is a positive margin on the pelvic side wall. This is the reason why preoperative chemoradiotherapy should precede excision of T3 and T4 lesions with TME.
- Usually develops within 18 months.
- Presents as pelvic pain, mass and rectal bleeding.
- Pelvic CT, MRI, CEA levels are the required investigations.
- Chemoradiation, surgery, local palliative treatment, pelvic exenteration (resection of rectum and bladder—Brunschwig's operation) are alternative treatments available.

# COLOSTOMY

Opening of the colon to the exterior, either temporary or permanent, for the drainage of faecal matter is called colostomy.

## TYPES

### 1. Temporary Colostomy

A. In cases of acute left-sided colonic obstruction, proximal half of right transverse colon is brought out through the upper part of the right rectus abdominis muscle. Later, radical resection of the left colon is done followed by closure of the colostomy.

B. In cases of traumatic or congenital fistula affecting the left colon, temporary colostomy is indicated (*see* Fig. 61.37). The loop of the colon which is brought outside is held in place by a glass rod. This is passed through the transverse mesocolon and held by rubber tubing. This rod is removed after 10 days.

C. Colostomy/ileostomy is done, if a distal colorectal anastomosis gives way (Figs 61.30 and 61.31).

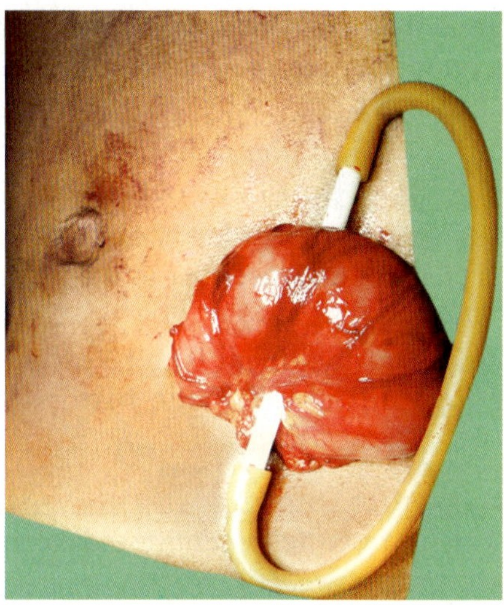

**Fig. 61.30:** Sigmoid colon is brought out and a glass rod connected to rubber tube is used to hold it out

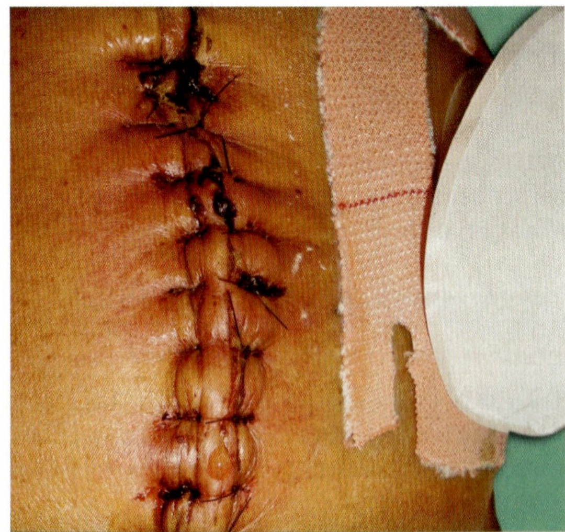

**Fig. 61.32:** End colostomy away from the main incision

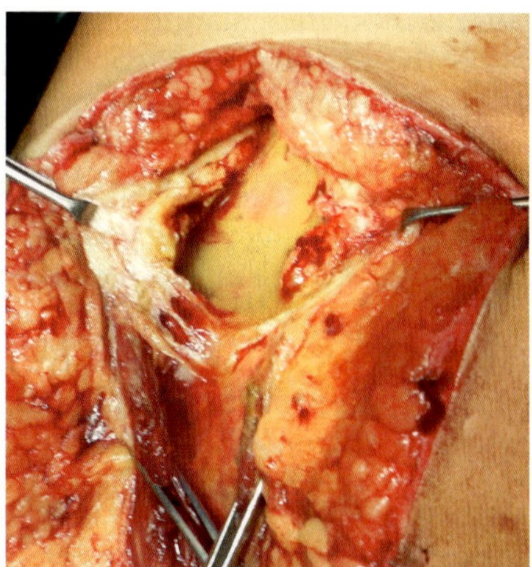

**Fig. 61.31:** Faeculent leak from failed anterior resection

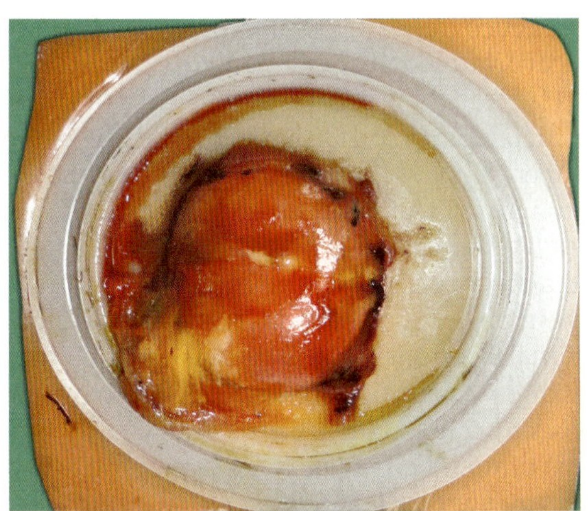

**Fig. 61.33:** Inspect for vascularity of colostomy following APR

**TEN COMMANDMENTS OF END COLOSTOMY**

1. Should mark the colostomy site in the standing and sitting positions.
2. Should be at least 3 cm away from the bony landmark (anterior superior iliac spine).
3. Should be at least 3 cm away from the midline incision. Otherwise, colostomy will contaminate the incision site (Fig. 61.32).
4. Should close the paracolostomy space within the abdomen to prevent herniation of the small intestines.
5. Colostomy should be opened after 2 or 3 days and midline incision should be protected from getting infected due to bowel contents
6. Should be in flush with skin surface in the left iliac fossa.
7. Should excise a disc of skin for permanent colostomy
8. The stoma should be brought out through the rectus muscle.
9. Should avoid bringing stoma outside through scar tissue.
10. Should examine the end of the colostomy for vascularity (Fig. 61.33).

*Pearls of Wisdom*

Transverse colostomy is bulky, contents are semiliquid and difficult to manage—try to avoid it.

## 2. Permanent Colostomy

It is indicated after abdominoperineal resection where the end of sigmoid colon is brought outside in the left iliac fossa as permanent colostomy (Figs 61.32 and 61.33, Key Box 61.10). The colostomy site should be 3 cm away from anterior superior iliac spine so that colostomy bag can be fitted properly (Figs 61.34 and 61.35).

Key Box 61.10

**Permanent Colostomy—Left Iliac Fossa**

- Avoid bony prominences
- Avoid belt lines
- Avoid marking in lying down position
- Avoid scars
- Avoid bringing out stoma lateral to rectus

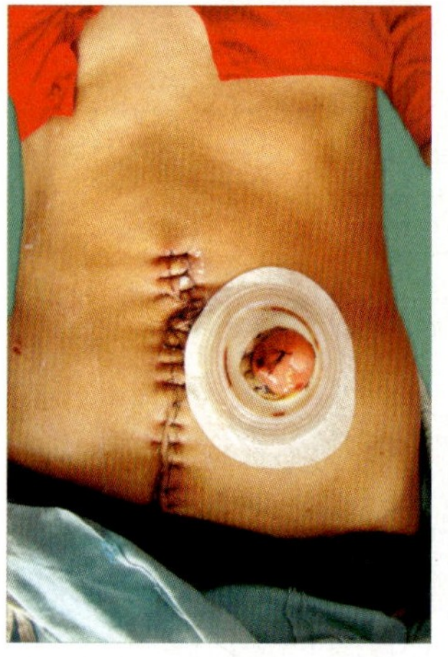

Fig. 61.34: Disposable colostomy bags are available with or without flange. Depending upon the size of the stoma, it can be cut open so as to fit into the colostomy

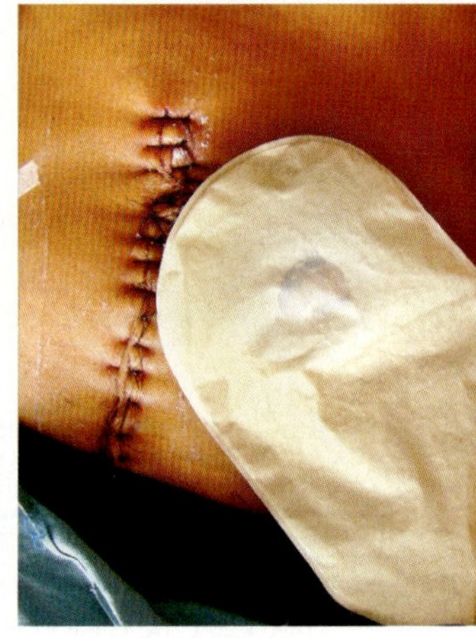

Fig. 61.35: A colostomy bag has been applied. It can be reused

### 3. Double-barreled Colostomy

In this, the adjoining walls of the intestine are crushed. Both ends of the loop are defunctioned. This type of colostomy is not frequently done now. It was done earlier for sigmoid volvulus, resection of colonic stricture, etc.

### Indications for Colostomy

- **Congenital:** In Hirschsprung's disease and anorectal anomalies, temporary colostomy is done first.
- **Carcinoma:** Following APR, permanent end-sigmoid colostomy is done.
- **Colonic fistulae:** Fistulae due to diverticulitis, Crohn's disease or tuberculosis.
- **Colonic injuries:** Trauma due to stab injuries or operative injuries following nephrectomy, pelvic operations, PCNL (percutaneous nephrolithotomy).

### Advantages of Colostomy

Distal bowel takes complete rest, regains normal size and bacterial colonisation is reduced. It becomes empty and sterile so that chances of leakage at a later operation is reduced.

### Complications of Colostomy (Figs 61.36 to 61.39)

- Bleeding, necrosis, retraction, prolapse, parastomal hernia and colostomy diarrhoea are some complications.
- Colostomy obstruction, gangrene.

*Pearls of Wisdom*

Colostomy should be done by an experienced surgeon as patient has to live with the colostomy life long.

Fig. 61.36: Paracolostomy hernia: Herniation of bowel from the side of colostomy. It can give rise to intestinal obstruction. This needs to be repaired by reduction of contents, closure of defect and sometimes mesh repair

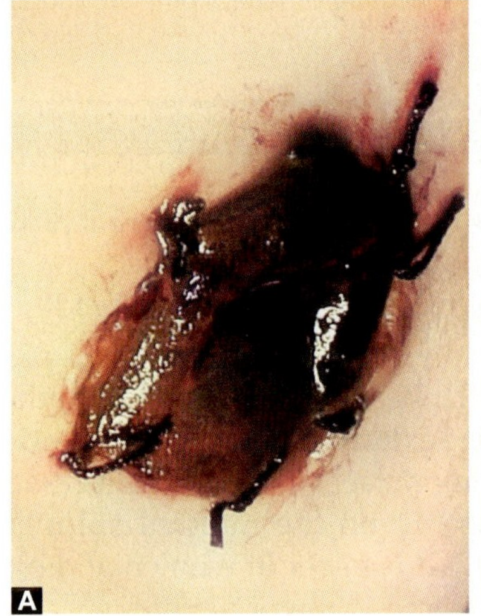

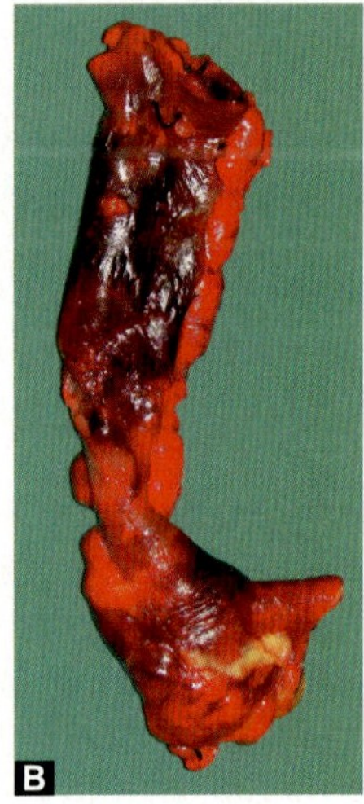

Figs 61.37A and B: Colostomy gangrene. It is mandatory to inspect the end of the colostomy everyday in the postoperative period to check for vascularity. If it is gangrenous and if it is retracted, it is better to open the abdomen again and refashion colostomy

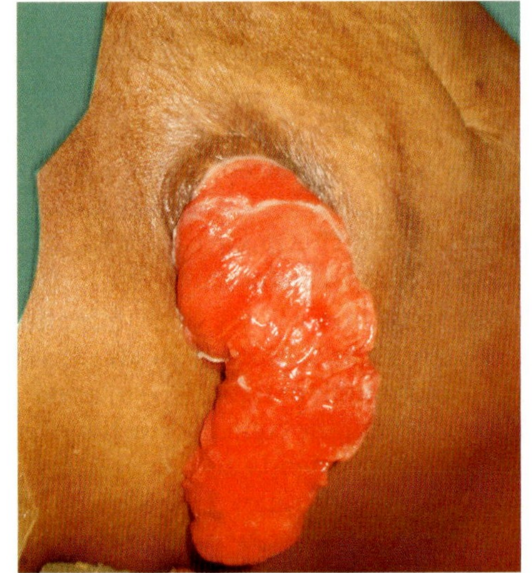

Fig. 61.38: Colostomy prolapse due to give way of sutures anchored to the aponeurotic layer. The patient also had violent cough in the postoperative period

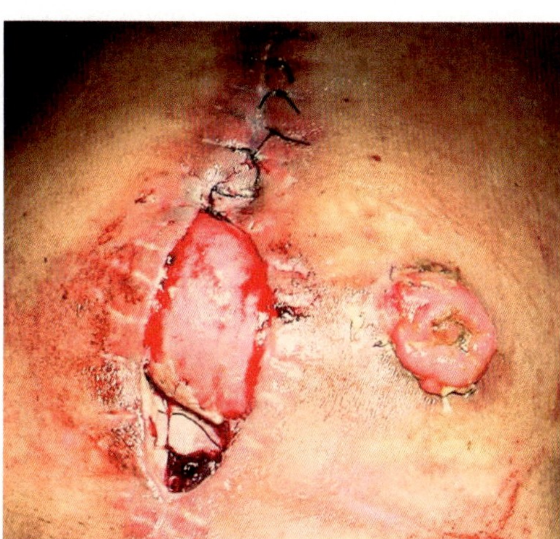

Fig. 61.39: Burst abdomen due to contamination of the wound from colostomy—proper care should be taken to isolate laparotomy site and colostomy till complete healing of laparotomy wound takes place

## ANORECTAL PHYSIOLOGY

**SU28.17.7:** Describe aetiology and management of anal incontinence.
(*Refer* Surgical Anatomy of Anal Canal, Page 1012)

- The anal canal which has length of 4 cm, lengthens with squeezing of the external sphincter and shortens with straining during defaecation. Resting pressure, which depends largely on the internal sphincter, averages 90 cm $H_2O$. It is lower in women and older patients than in men and younger patients.
- This high-pressure zone increases resistance to the passage of stool. The external anal sphincter and puborectalis muscle generate pressure, by contraction which is more than double the intra-anal canal resting pressure.
- The principal mechanism that provides continence is the pressure differential between the rectum (6 cm $H_2O$) and the anal canal (90 cm $H_2O$). The anorectal angle is produced by the anterior pull of the puborectalis muscle as it encircles the rectum at the anorectal ring. This angle may act as a flap valve or have a sphincter-like function.
- Anorectal sensation allows discrimination of the enteric contents (gas, liquids, or solids). It also detects the need to pass stools or flatus. The internal sphincter will relax when enteric contents reach the anal canal, while the rectum distends and contracts. It is called rectal anal inhibitory reflex. Transient relaxation of the internal anal sphincter brings the rectal content into contact with the sensory mucosa of the proximal canal so that it can be recognized.

### Act of Defaecation (Key Box 61.11)

Key Box 61.11

**Act of Defaecation**

Rectal distension
→ Faeces in the anal canal
→ Inhibition of external sphincter
→ Rectum and anal canal is straight | Pelvic floor is lowered | Peristaltic wave | Cerebral factor

## ANAL INCONTINENCE

### Mechanism of Anal Continence

- Distension of rectum causes **tonic contraction of external sphincter**. This is controlled by cerebrum and the centre is in the **lumbosacral region of the spinal cord**.
- Faeces in contact with anal canal stimulates the specialised nerve endings. Nerve endings are also present in the puborectalis.
- **High pressure** in the anal canal (25–120 mmHg) and angle between rectum and anal canal (80°) are the important factors which maintain anal continence.

### Anorectal Ring

- It marks the junction between the rectum and anal canal.
- It is formed by puborectalis, highest part of internal sphincter, longitudinal muscle and external part of sphincter.

### Causes of Anal Incontinence (Key Box 61.12)

1. **Traumatic:** Injury to the anorectum due to sharp penetrating objects occurs due to accidents.
2. **Surgical procedures**
   - Damage to the internal and external sphincter can occur due to Lord's dilatation[1], a procedure done for fissure *in ano*. However, most of it is temporary.
   - Division of high fistula *in ano* may result in incontinence.
   - Following pull-through procedures done for anorectal anomalies, Hirschsprung's disease.
   - Haemorrhoidectomy—very large pile masses.
   - Extensive small bowel resection
   - Rectal excision
3. **Mass in the anorectum:** Prolapse piles, prolapse rectum and carcinoma rectum may produce temporary incontinence which subsides after surgical procedures.

[1]Lord's dilatation or blunt sphincterotomy is no longer done.

Key Box 61.12

**Common Causes of Anal Incontinence**

- **T**rauma
- **R**epeated pregnancies
- **A**nal surgery
- **U**nnatural sex—anal intercourse
- **M**egacolon—congenital or acquired
- **A**geing or senility

*You can remember as* **TRAUMA**

4. **Neurological causes:** In females, **pudendal nerve neuropathy** which occurs due to chronic straining may result in incontinence. Spinal injuries, spina bifida, meningomyelocele are associated with anal incontinence.
5. **GI motility increase:** Inflammatory bowel diseases irritate bowel and produce temporary incontinence.
6. **Childhood/congenital causes:** Anorectal malformations, Hirschsprung's disease, spina bifida, abnormal behaviour.
7. **Miscellaneous:** Old age (senility), general debility and faecal impaction, Parkinson's disease, behavioural problem, etc.

### Treatment

I. **Temporary incontinence:** Reassurance. Perineal exercises to improve the tone of internal and external sphincter.

II. **Permanent incontinence:**

1. Divided sphincter can be reunited, followed by overlapping of the remaining muscles.
2. Intersphincteric repair of puborectalis sling and plication of the external sphincter.
3. Gracilis muscle can be used to create a new anal sphincter by transposing it followed by electrical stimulation using a pacemaker.
4. Using artificial sphincter.

## PROLAPSE RECTUM

**SU28.17.3:** Describe etiology, clinical features and management of rectal prolapse.

Protrusion of the mucous membrane or the entire rectum outside the anal verge. This condition is common in children and elderly patients.

### Types

Prolapse can be of two types: Partial prolapse and complete prolapse.

### Partial Prolapse

- In this variety, the protrusion is between 1.25 and 3.75 cm outside the anal verge (Fig. 61.40).
- It is usually a mucosal prolapse.

### Causes

1. In infants, it is due to **undeveloped sacral curve** and in children it can be secondary to **habitual constipation.**
2. It can follow an attack of **whooping cough or excessive straining** (Fig. 61.41).
3. It can follow an attack of diarrhoea resulting in **loss of fat** in the ischiorectal fossae, which supports the rectum.
4. In adults, it is common in females mostly due to **torn perineum** caused by obstetric trauma.

### Treatment

1. **Digital reposition:** In infants, partial prolapse is temporary. The mother is advised to push the prolapse inside after lubricating with lignocaine jelly.
2. **Injection of ethanolamine oleate** into the submucosa of the rectum. It causes aseptic fibrosis. Thus, mucosa gets tethered to the other layers.
3. Partial prolapse can be **excised**, after applying **Goodsall's ligature**.

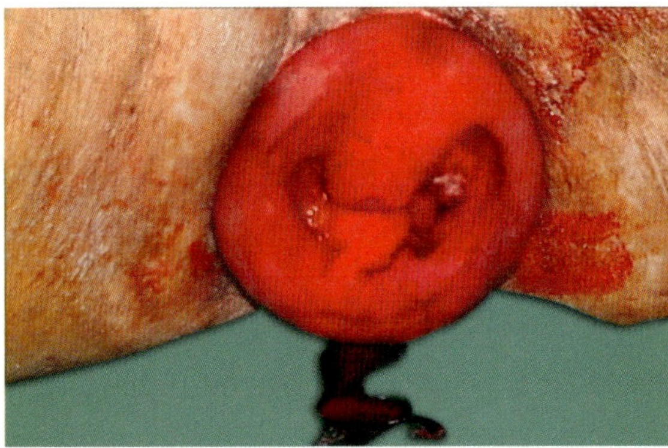

**Fig. 61.40:** Partial prolapse

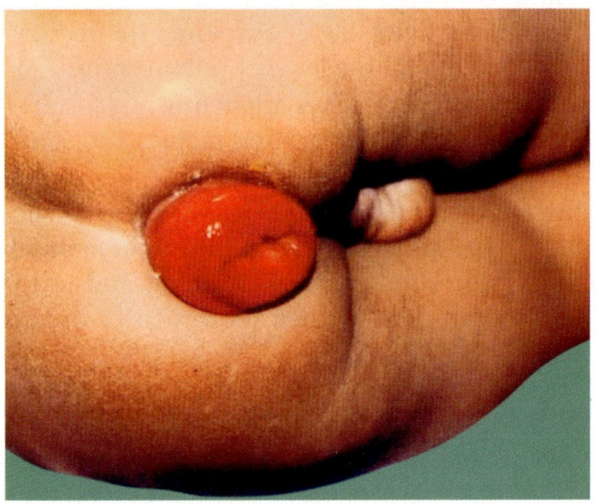

**Fig. 61.41:** Rectal prolapse in a child

## PHOTOGRAPHS OF PROLAPSE RECTUM

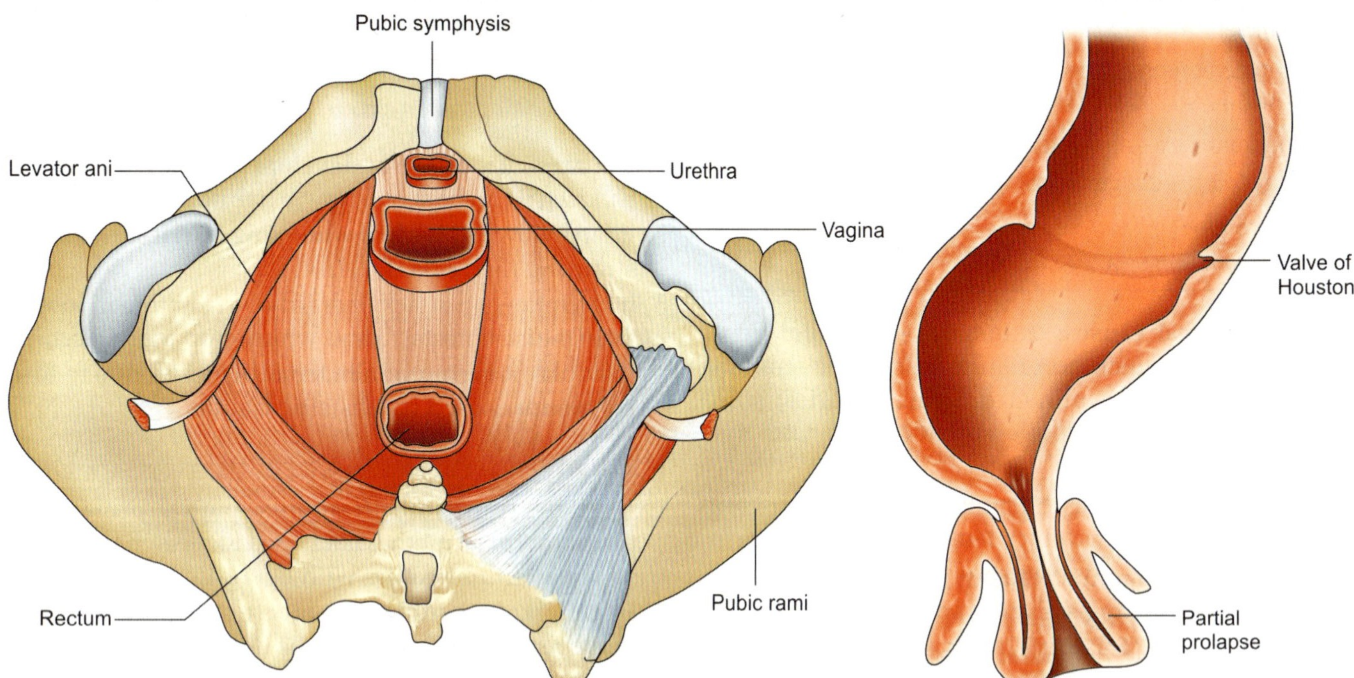


**Fig. 61.42:** Pelvic floor anatomy—weakness of the pelvic floor is an important cause of prolapse rectum

**Fig. 61.43:** Prolapsed rectum—diagrammatic representation, sometimes confused for prolapsed haemorrhoids

## COMPLETE/TOTAL PROLAPSE

- Full thickness prolapse is also called procidentia.
- It is defined as protrusion of the rectum for more than 3.75 cm outside the anal verge. Very often, it is the entire rectum which protrudes out on straining, sometimes along with the peritoneal sac.
- Often, it is associated with prolapse uterus.

### The Pelvic Floor—Surgical Anatomy (Fig. 61.42)

- It is composed of **two levator ani** and a **puborectalis** muscle.
- Levator ani originates from pelvic side walls and sacrospinous ligament. It **suspends** the rectum in a muscular sling till the level of puborectalis.
- Puborectalis muscle takes origin from posterior aspect of pubis, forms a sling around rectum and returns to posterior pubis.
- **Contracted puborectalis is responsible for normal acute anorectal angle and it is critical for maintaining continence.** Thus during coughing and sneezing, anorectal angle becomes more acute, increasing continence.

### Supports of the Rectum and Surgical Importance

Various supports keep the rectum in place. Failure of one or more of these factors may precipitate rectal prolapse (Fig. 61.43). They have been enumerated as follows.

1. **Pelvic floor:** Weakness of pelvic floor can be due to birth injuries or due to defective collagen maturation.
2. **Lateral ligaments:** These ligaments are either condensation of pelvic fascia on either side of the rectum. Excessive mobility of these ligaments may be the contributing factor for prolapse rectum.
3. **Fascia of Denonvilliers** (rectovesical fascia): **Deep rectovesical pouch** is often found in prolapse rectum. In all cases of complete prolapse rectum, please look for the deep rectovesical pouch and if present, it should be obliterated.
4. **Fat in the ischiorectal fossae** supports the rectum. Hence, any chronic illness and loss of fat may contribute to prolapse rectum.

### Anorectal Physiology and Investigation

These are useful in patients who have complaints of prolapse rectum, constipation, incontinence.

1. **Anorectal manometry**
   - Normal resting pressure in the anal canal—40–80 mmHg. (It is the function of internal anal sphincter.)
   - **Squeeze pressure:** It is maximum voluntary contraction pressure minus resting pressure. It is 40–80 mmHg above resting pressure. It reflects the function of external anal sphincter.
2. **Function of pudendal nerve and perineal nerve:** Injuries to the nerve are diagnosed by nerve conduction studies.

### Causes or Pathogenesis (Fig. 61.44)

1. **Common in elderly women who are multipara.** It is probably due to repeated **birth injuries** to the perineum causing damage to the nerve fibres. As age advances, muscles become weak (Key Box 61.13). This, together with fatty degeneration of the muscle, results in prolapse rectum.

Key Box 61.13

**Obstetric Trauma**

- Multiple vaginal deliveries—cause pudendal nerve stretch.
- Prolonged labour—disrupts sphincter and stretching of pudendal nerve.
- 3rd degree perineal tears—weaken the internal sphincter and pelvic floor.

2. **Excessive straining** causes weakness of the supports of the rectum.
3. **Defective collagen maturation** results in failure of rectal support by levators and pelvic fascia.
4. Presence of **deep rectovesical pouch** and excessive mobility of the rectum (mesorectum) predisposes to prolapse of the rectum.
5. Many people believe that prolapse of the rectum starts as an **intussusception** in the first stage, initiated by certain factors such as diarrhoea, constipation and disorder of the pelvic floor. The process starts with anterior wall of rectum, where supporting tissues are weakest (Broden–Snellman theory).

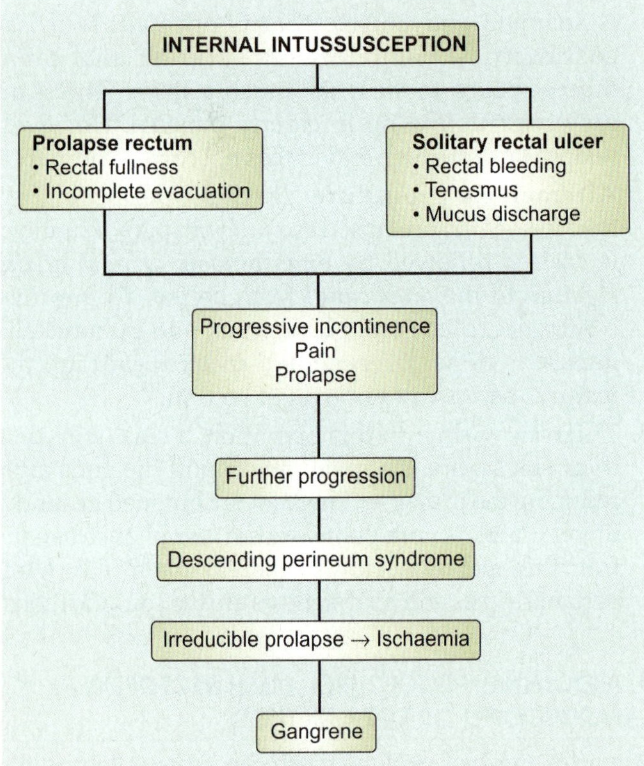


**Fig. 61.44:** Pathogenesis of prolapse rectum

### Beahrs Classification

A. Incomplete—mucosal prolapse
B. Complete—full thickness rectal prolapse
  1st degree—concealed
  2nd degree—externally visible on straining
  3rd degree—visible without straining.

### Clinical Features

- Female–male ratio is 6:1.
- Constipation is an important feature of rectal prolapse.
- Excessive mucus discharge causing irritation to the perianal skin. Tenesmus is also common.
- On asking the patient to strain at stool,[1] the rectum descends down, which clinches the diagnosis (Fig. 61.45).
- Some degree of incontinence of faeces and flatus is always present. It gives rise to urgency and perianal soiling.
- Rectal examination—lax anal sphincter and wide gaping on straining.
- Procidentia (Figs 61.46 and 61.47).
- Recurrent attacks of prolapse and negligence in seeking medical attention can give rise to gangrene. Such patients may require proctosigmoidectomy (Fig. 61.48).

*Pearls of Wisdom*

Palpation of prolapse between finger and thumb reveals double thickness of tissue, especially anteriorly because of deep pouch of Douglas.

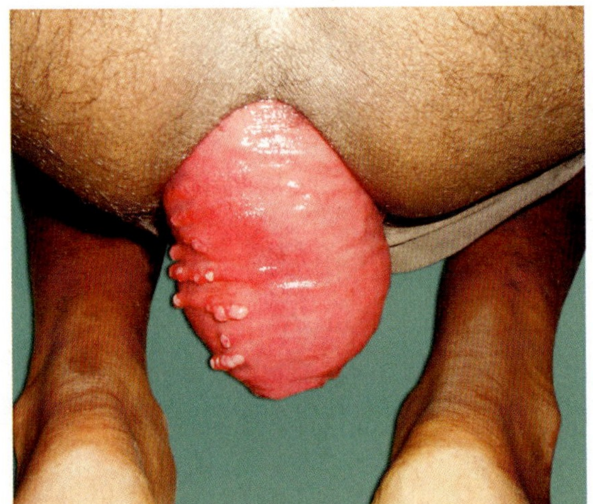

**Fig. 61.45:** Complete prolapse—should be tested by asking the patient to squat and strain

[1]In fact, the surgeon should see the prolapse of the rectum when patient strains to make a clinical diagnosis.

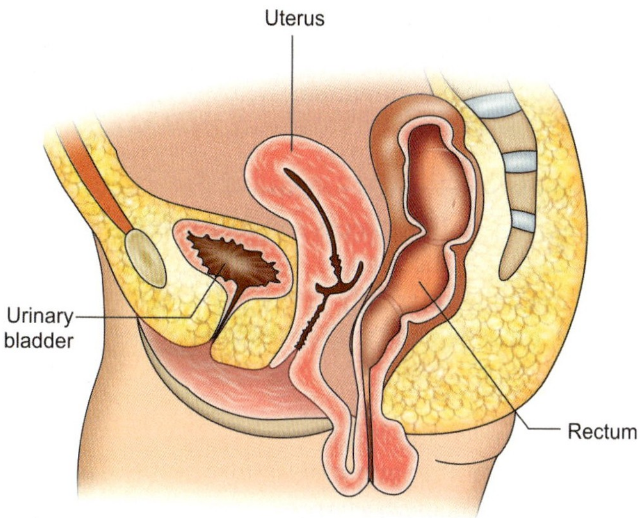


Fig. 61.46: Prolapse of the rectum with uterus: procidentia—not an uncommon presentation especially in multipara women

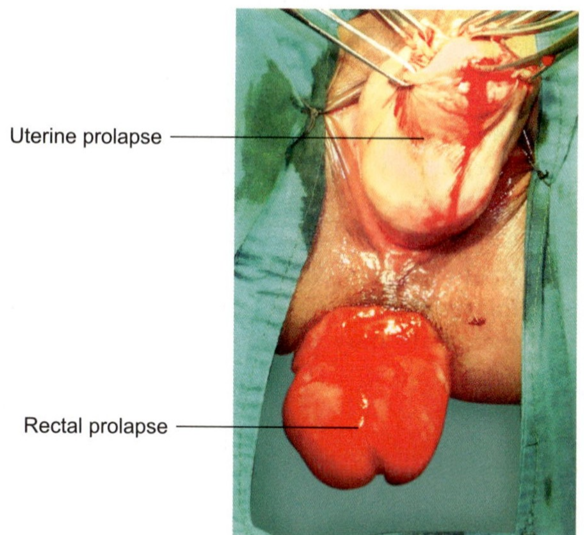


Fig. 61.47: Complete prolapse of the rectum with prolapse of uterus—procidentia

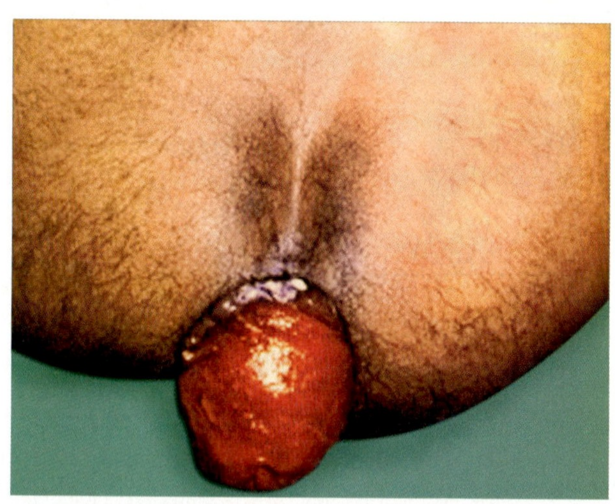

Fig. 61.48: Prolapsed rectum—slowly change in colour—would have become gangrene

### Differential Diagnosis

- Large third degree haemorrhoids—not circumferential and are blue in colour.
- Large polypoid tumour
- Prolapse of sigmoid colon

### Complications

- Proctitis, ulceration and rarely bleeding
- Gangrene of the rectum.

### Treatment

Medical management—prior to surgery, patients not fit for surgery or patients who refuse surgery

- Adequate fluid and fibre intake
- Enemas and suppositories for severe constipation.

### Surgical Procedures—Aim

1. Safe procedure to correct with minimal morbidity and without mortality. They are classified as **perineal procedures and abdominal procedures.**
2. To cure or to improve **incontinence.**

## I. PERINEAL PROCEDURES

(Preferred for High-Risk Patients)

1. **Delorme's procedure** (reefing the rectal mucosa): In this, the prolapse is completely everted, mucosa is stripped and muscle coat is plicated. Mucosal continuity is maintained by suturing anal canal mucosa below to the rectal mucosa above. This is an easy operation to do in elderly patients. However, relapse rates are high and it does not correct the defect.
2. **Altemeier's procedure:** In this operation, full thickness of the prolapsed rectum with part of sigmoid is *excised* followed by ***anastomosis of part of the sigmoid*** to the ***anal canal*** from below. To improve continence, plication of levator ani and puborectalis muscle is done. ***Urgency and incontinence*** are the features because of removal of rectum.
3. **Thiersch wiring:** In this operation, a steel wire or a thick silk suture is applied all around the anus after reducing the prolapse. The knot is tightened around a finger. Patients with poor surgical compliance benefit from this operation. However, breakdown of the wire, perianal sepsis and anal stenosis are the complications.

## II. ABDOMINAL PROCEDURE—MESH RECTOPEXY—LAPAROSCOPIC OR OPEN METHOD

A marlex mesh or prolene mesh can be kept behind the rectum. This is sutured behind, to the sacrum and then to the posterior and lateral surfaces of rectum. **Laparoscopic method of fixing the mesh has become popular. This**

**is the procedure of choice today.** Constipation is one of the complications of mesh rectopexy (Figs 61.49 and 61.50).

For summary refer Key Box 61.14.

Key Box 61.14

**Summary of Surgeries for Prolapse Rectum**

- Mesh rectopexy corrects/prevents prolapse but does not correct chronic constipation.
- Laparoscopic mesh rectopexy has become gold standard—fast recovery, less pain, short hospital stay.
- Mesh rectopexy with resection is ideal for patients with constipation or patients with a redundant sigmoid colon.
- High operative risk patients—Thiersch wiring—anal encirclement.
- Altemeier procedure done for perineum is an alternative in patients with incontinence. Here, perineal proctectomy and posterior sphincter enhancement is done.

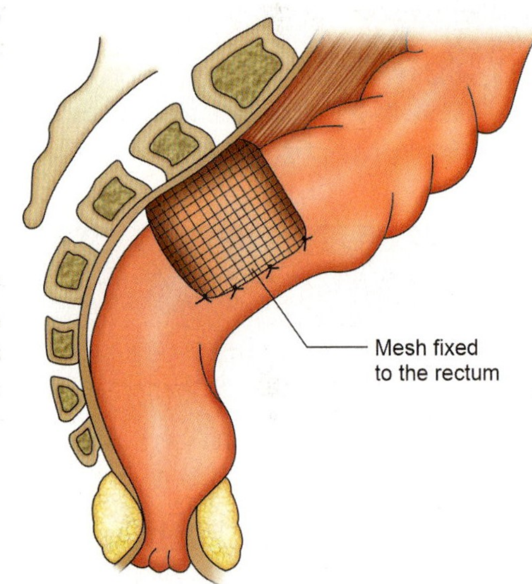


**Fig. 61.49:** Fixing the mesh to the rectum—mesh is sutured to the sacrum posteriorly and sutured to the sides of the rectum

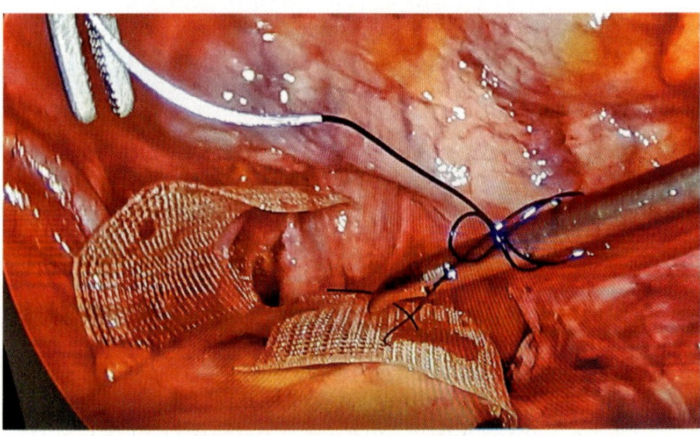

**Fig. 61.50:** Mesh rectopexy

## HAEMORRHOIDS (PILES)

**SU28.17.9:** Describe aetiology, clinical features, non-surgical management and surgeries for hemorrhoidal disease.

### Definition

Dilated plexus of superior haemorrhoidal veins, in relation to anal canal.

### Classification—Aetiological

#### *I. Primary/Idiopathic Haemorrhoids*

1. **Standing posture:** A famous saying goes-varicosity is the penalty for verticality against gravity. This holds true for haemorrhoids. It is true that animals do not develop haemorrhoids as well. Man's upright posture and absence of valves in the portal system with other factors precipitate development of haemorrhoids.
2. **Haemorrhoidal veins** and their branches are thin veins which pass through submucosa of the rectum. They get compressed due to contractions caused by rectal musculature (the sphincters) during the act of defaecation.
3. **Genetic/familial factors:** Absence of valves, or congenital weakness of the vessel wall are few other factors contributing for the haemorrhoids.
4. **Diet:** A diet deficient in fibres which prolongs the gut transit results in constipation and the hard pellet like stools. The hard stools compress veins and result in haemorrhoids.

#### *II. Secondary Haemorrhoids*

*Causes*

1. **Carcinoma of rectum**, by blocking the veins, can produce back pressure and can manifest as piles.
2. **Portal hypertension**—uncommon cause of rectal varices.
3. **Pregnancy**, due to compression of superior rectal veins or due to progesterone which relaxes smooth muscle in the wall of the veins, can cause haemorrhoids.

**Current view:** Normally, the anal cushions retract after defaecation. Latest theory is that haemorrhoids occur due to caudal displacement of anal cushions. It is due to recurrent trauma, shearing forces, loss of elasticity.

### Location

Classically situated in the 3, 7 and 11 o'clock positions (Fig. 61.51) (left lateral, right posterior and right anterior, respectively).

Superior haemorrhoidal artery gives 2 branches on right side and 1 branch on left side. Hence, piles are two on right side and one on left side.

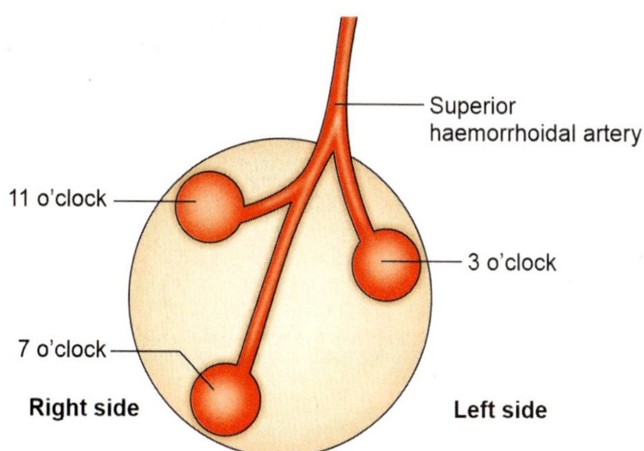


Fig. 61.51: Classic location of pile masses

## Clinical Features (Table 61.3)

- Painless bleeding—fresh bleeding occurs after defaecation—**splash in the pan**. This causes chronic anaemia. Haemorrhoids which bleed are called Grade I haemorrhoids.
- The capillaries of the lamina propria are protected by only a single layer of epithelial cells. Hence, minor trauma precipitates bleeding.
- As the straining increases, the haemorrhoids partly prolapse outside. After defaecation, it returns back (Grade II) or can be digitally replaced (Grade III haemorrhoids).
- Permanently prolapsed pile outside (Grade IV haemorrhoids). The patient complains of pain or discomfort.
- Most of the patients complain of constipation.
- Discharge of mucus and soiling of perianal skin—pruritus by prolapse of haemorrhoidal cushions and mucosa (Figs 61.52 to 61.54).

### *III. Depending upon the Location of Haemorrhoids*

1. **Internal haemorrhoids**—above the dentate line, covered with mucous membrane.
2. **External haemorrhoids**—at anal verge, covered with skin (Fig. 61.54).
3. **Interno-external**—both varieties together.

## Investigations

- Per rectal examination is done mainly to rule out carcinoma rectum or other causes of bleeding per rectum. Haemorrhoids cannot be felt by rectal examination unless they are thrombosed or fibrosed.
- **Proctoscopy:** As the obturator is removed, piles prolapse into the lumen of proctoscope as cherry red masses.
- **Sigmoidoscopy and proctoscopy are done to rule out proximal cancer.**

**TABLE 61.3:** Grades of haemorrhoids

| Grades features | Symptoms |
|---|---|
| I. Never prolapse | Bleeding per rectum |
| II. Prolapse on defaecation with spontaneous reduction | Mass per rectum descending down |
| III. Prolapse on defaecation requires manual reduction | Mass per rectum bleeding, mucus discharge, pruritus |
| IV. Permanent prolapse | Acute pain, throbbing discomfort |

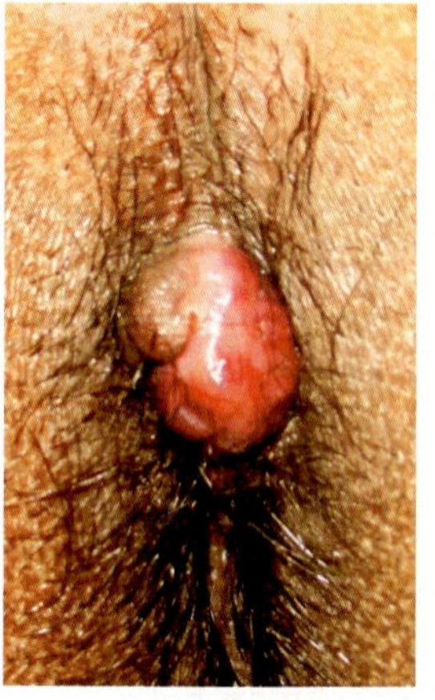

Fig. 61.52: Grade III haemorrhoids

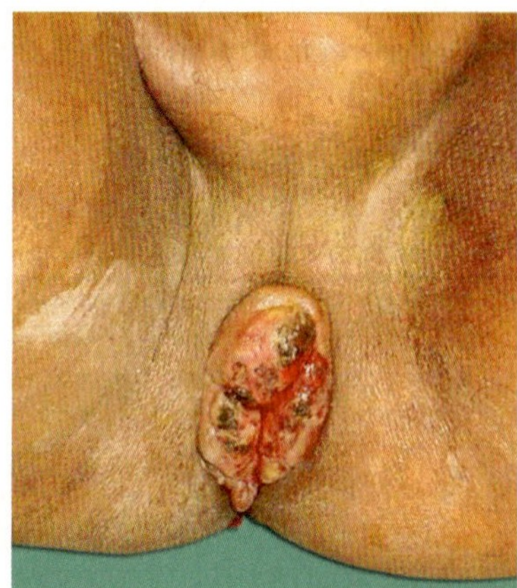

Fig. 61.53: Grade IV haemorrhoids

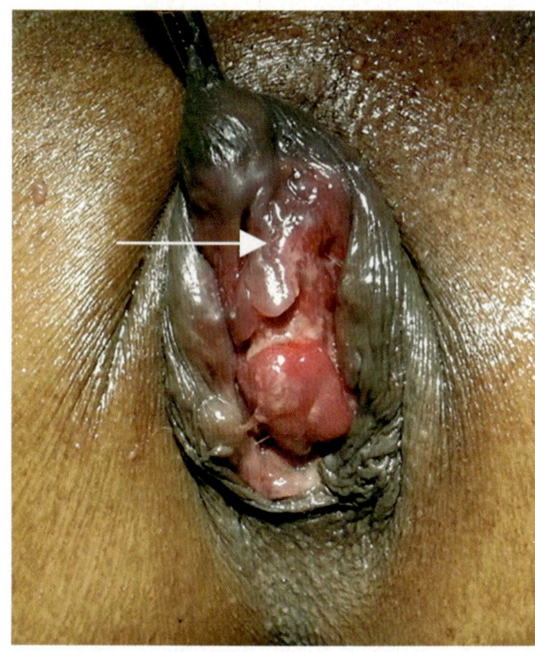

Fig. 61.54: External pile

## Complications of Haemorrhoids
(Figs 61.55 to 61.57)

1. It can cause **chronic anaemia**. Rarely, massive bleeding can occur because of portal hypertension.
2. A **prolapse** outside presents with severe pain in the perianal region—piles gripped by internal sphincter

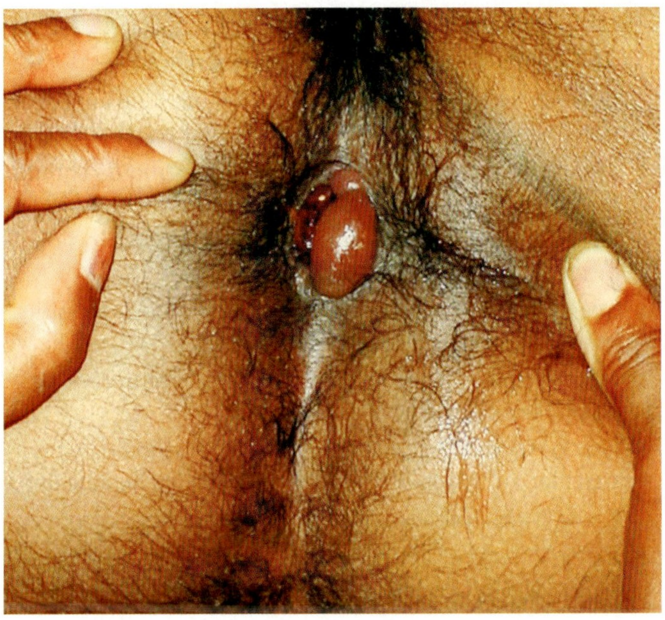

**Fig. 61.55:** Prolapsed piles—painful condition

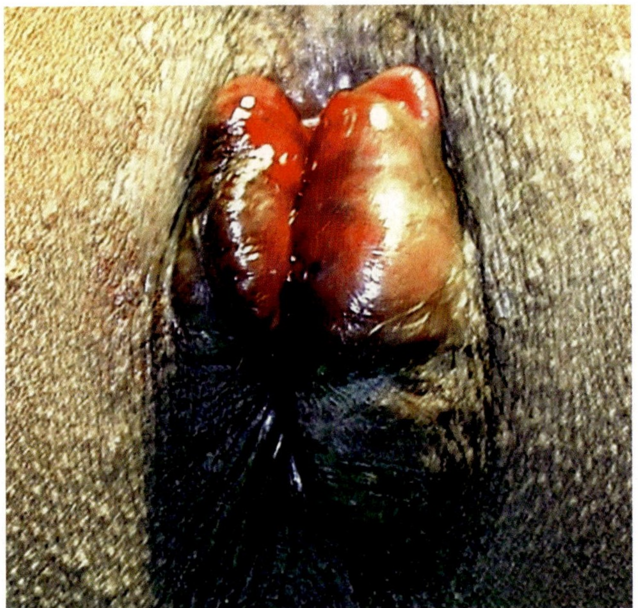

**Fig. 61.56:** Thrombosed pile mass

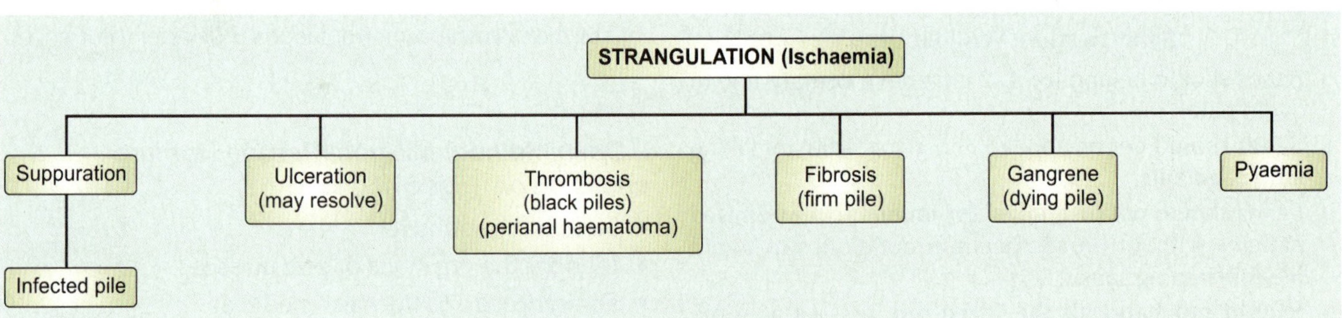


**Fig. 61.57:** Complications of piles

results in venous congestion and oedema followed by strangulation. Such patients are treated by:

- Elevation of foot end of bed
- Metronidazole 400 mg, 3 times a day for 5 days.
- Saline dressings to reduce oedema—glycerine $MgSO_4$
- Local lignocaine jelly application

3. **Ulceration** and secondary infection
4. **Thrombosis** and fibrosis.

## TREATMENT OF HAEMORRHOIDS

A. **Nonoperative treatment:** It is indicated in Grade I and Grade II piles which are not causing significant bleeding or discomfort (Key Box 61.15).

B. **Injection of sclerosant:** 5% phenol in almond oil is injected into **submucosa** above the dentate line. Hence, it is painless. It produces **aseptic thrombosis** of pile mass and is indicated in Grade I. The injection is **perivascular**.

Key Box 61.15

**Nonoperative Treatment**

- **F**ibre supplementation
- **I**ncreased fluid intake
- **B**ulk-purgative—laxatives—isabgol husk, etc.
- **R**eading in toilet to be discouraged (respond to call and do not strain)
- **E**ncourage to lose weight
- **S**itz-bath

*Remember as* **FIBRES**

C. **Barron's band application** (Figs 61.58 and 61.59)**:** It is indicated for Grade II and Grade III haemorrhoids, wherein bands are applied at the neck of the haemorrhoids. It causes necrosis and thus, piles get fibrosed. One or two can be banded at a time (Key Box 61.16).

D. **Operative treatment:** Haemorrhoidectomy. Open method, closed method, stapler haemorrhoidopexy.

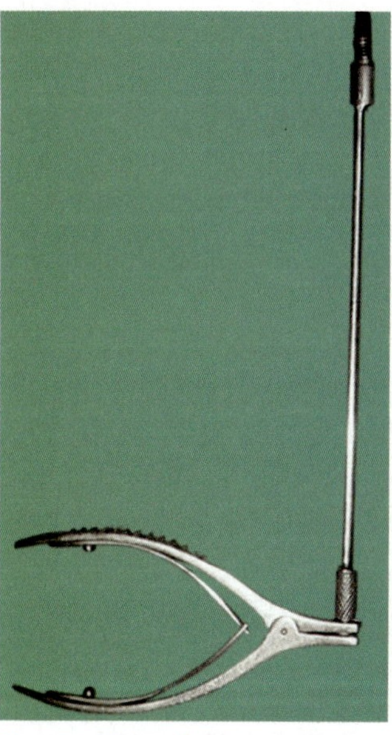

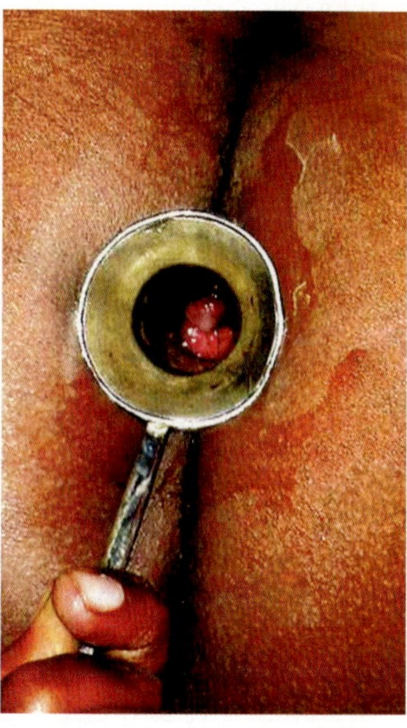

**Figs 61.58 and 61.59:** Barron's band ligator and band has been applied to one of the pile masses

Key Box 61.16

**Band Ligation: Wisdom Lines**

- Bands should be applied **1–2 cm above dentate** line to avoid pain.
- Bands should not be applied in patients who are taking **anticoagulants**.
- Bands **should not be applied for immunocompromised** patients without broad spectrum antibiotics to avoid life-threatening sepsis.
- **Should not band all the three pile** masses at same time. Quadrant by quadrant with a gap of 2 weeks is ideal.
- If severe pain, fever and urinary retention develop after band (sepsis), examine under general anaesthesia and remove band.

- Refer Key Box 61.17 for a few wisdom lines.

## HAEMORRHOIDECTOMY

Excision of the pile masses up to base is indicated in Grade II and Grade III haemorrhoids. It can be done by 3 methods: Open, closed and with stapler (*vide infra*).

Key Box 61.17

**Interesting Wisdom in Haemorrhoids**

- Haemorrhoids occur due to downward prolapse of vascular cushions into and beyond anal canal.
- Minimum ideal investigation for haemorrhoids should be flexible sigmoidoscopy.
- Preserve adequate mucocutaneous bridges in excisional procedures to prevent anal stenosis.
- Urgency and tenesmus following stapled haemorrhoidoscopy responds well to oral nifedipine.
- Metronidazole is the most important agent in reducing pain after haemorrhoid surgery.
- Grades I and II can be injected: Injections should be perivascular, submucosal and above the level of dentate line.
- Grade III requires haemorrhoidectomy or haemorrhoidopexy.
- Grade IV requires initial conservative treatment followed by surgical procedure.

*Pearls of Wisdom*

Excisional haemorrhoidectomy produces more discomfort (pain) than stapler haemorrhoidopexy but lesser recurrences.

### Types

#### *I. Open Method: Milligan-Morgan Ligature and Excision* (Figs 61.60 to 61.62)

- Stretch the sphincter
- Identify the positions of pile masses
- Dissection up to the base (pedicle)
- Transfixation ligature with **nonabsorbable silk**
- Excision of the piles with skin
- Trimming the wound
- Haemostasis obtained
- Wound packed with roller gauze
- A tube drainage is provided so that the blood (oozing) can escape outside.

*Pearls of Wisdom*

Always leave a bridge of skin in between the excised pile masses to prevent anal stenosis.

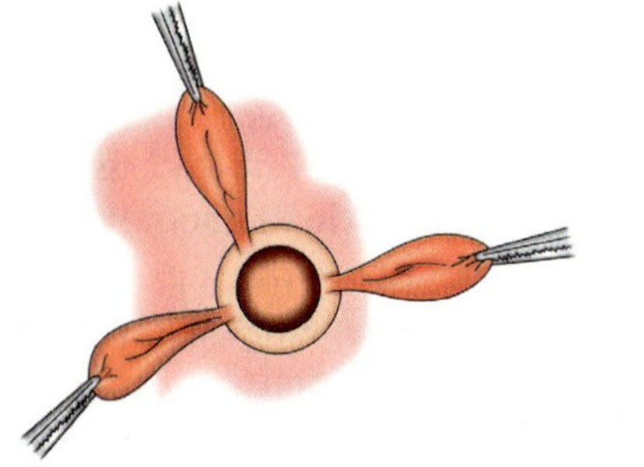

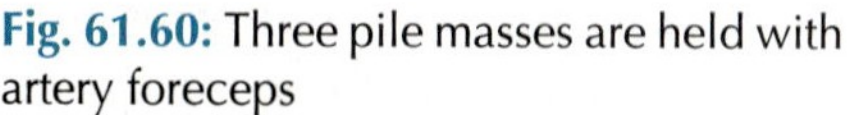

**Fig. 61.60:** Three pile masses are held with artery forceps

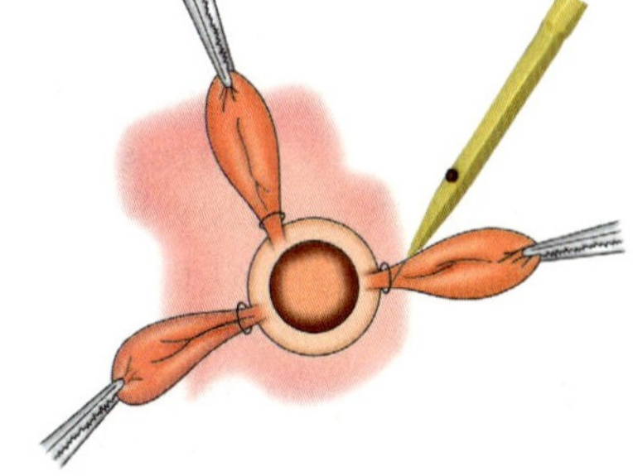

**Fig. 61.61:** Ligatures are applied at the base of the haemorrhoids and they are being cut with cautery

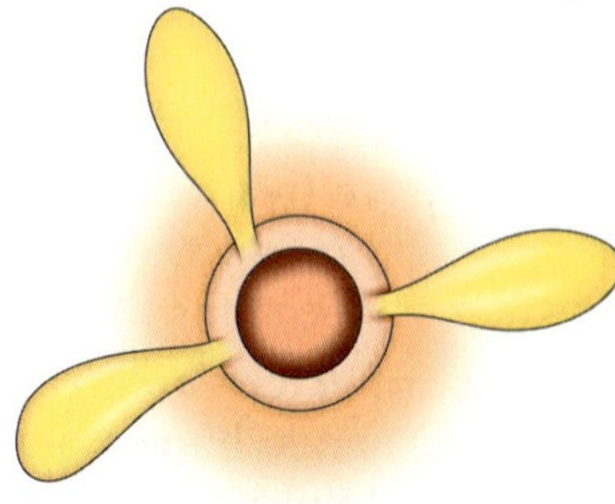

**Fig. 61.62:** After haemorrhoidectomy, the excised portion should look like a clover

#### *II. Closed Method (Hill-Ferguson)*

- Basic steps are the same as above.
- Cut mucosa and skin edges are sutured with absorbable catgut sutures.

### STAPLER HAEMORRHOIDOPEXY: NON-EXCISIONAL PROCEDURE (Figs 61.63 to 61.68)

- A novel method for 3rd and 4th degree haemorrhoids was introduced by Dr Antonio Longo in 1997.
- It is also called **P**rocedure for **P**rolapse and **H**aemorrhoids (**PPH**).
- After reduction of prolapsed piles, a prolene purse string suture is applied circumferentially, taking good mucosal bites 3 cm above dentate line.
- This is possible by using **C**ircular **A**nal **D**ilator (**CAD**).
- By maintaining traction in the tails of suture, the stapler is fully closed and fired.
- Slowly stapler is opened and withdrawn.
- **Look at 'doughnut'. If it is complete, nothing to worry.**
- Thus a circular ring of mucosal tissue above the level of dentate line is removed. Internal haemorrhoids are not removed, external haemorrhoids are also not removed (eventually they regress).
- Thus, **2 rows of staples** and **28 staples** are present.

#### Advantages

- Lesser operative time
- Less bleeding
- Lesser postoperative pain and need for analgesia
- Lesser postoperative stay at hospital, part of day care procedures
- Earlier return to normal activities
- No major postoperative short-term and long-term complications
- No long-term side effects such as anal stenosis or chronic pain as may happen with open haemorrhoidectomy.

#### Disadvantages

- High cost of instrumentation.
- Difficult technically and needs special training (learning curve).
- Rare complications such as intra- and postoperative bleeding. Occasional cases of postoperative fissures, mucosal discharge, persistent tenesmus, infection and long-term complications such as rectovaginal fistulae, polyps at stapler line and recurrence.

*Pearls of Wisdom*

In open haemorrhoidectomy: If wound is like clover, it is over. In stapler haemorrhoidectomy: If doughnut is complete, it is time to celebrate.

### DOPPLER-GUIDED HAEMORRHOIDAL ARTERY LIGATION

- Doppler principle is used to identify the feeding artery to the haemorrhoid mass and it is ligated.
- Doppler incorporated proctoscope is introduced and the artery is recognised by audible signal.
- After this, the needle is inserted into the lumen of the proctoscope.
- The artery is ligated by **figure of eight** suture. Thus, main artery supplying the haemorrhoid is blocked.
- The procedure is a simple outpatient procedure. There is no pain or blood loss. Anaesthesia is not required and recovery is early.
- Safe in all types of patients including patients with serious morbidity.

**External haemorrhoids**

- Described by Milligan as **5-day painful self-curing lesion.**
- Constipation and sudden straining at stools or lifting weights will result in a tender subcutaneous swelling at the anal margin.
- It is bluish in colour because it is a thrombosed vein or venule (external haemorrhoid).
- If tenderness is extreme, under local anaesthesia, incision can be given over the swelling and clot can be evacuated.
- In other cases, it will resolve within 5 days after fibrosis/suppuration.

#### Postoperative Management

1. Strong analgesics, in the form of injection pethidine or morphine, are given to reduce the pain.
2. Antibiotics along with metronidazole are given to prevent secondary infection.
3. Bulk purgatives are given to avoid constipation.
4. **Sitz bath** twice a day is given by using warm saline or $KMnO_4$ solution.

#### Postoperative Complications

They can be classified into early and late complications.

Acute retention of urine and haemorrhage are early complications. Anal stricture, anal stenosis, anal fissure and incontinence are the late complications. A few complications are described below.

1. **Retention of urine** is common in men due to severe pain. It can be managed by treating the pain and hot water fomentation in the suprapubic region. Catheterisation is done as a last resort.
2. **Reactionary haemorrhage** is more common. It is due to a loose ligature or some opened up bleedings. Generally stops by pressure packing. Otherwise, under anaesthesia, ligate or cauterise bleeding point.
3. **Secondary haemorrhage** can occur due to infection. It manifests 6 to 8 days later. If the bleeding is significant, exploration in the operation theatre may be necessary. It should be done under anaesthesia. With good

## STAPLER HAEMORRHOIDOPEXY

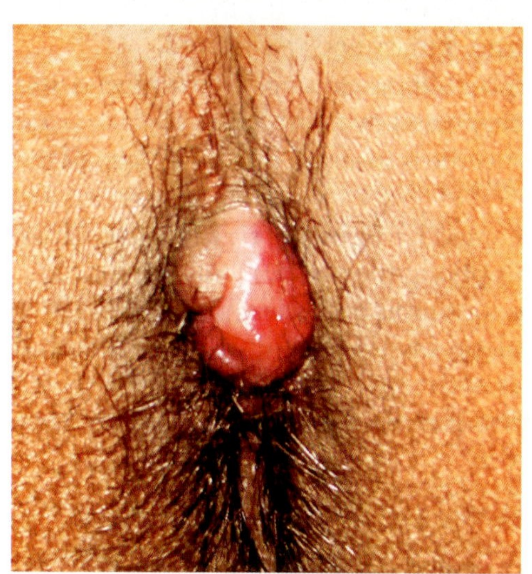
Fig. 61.63: Grade III haemorrhoids before surgery

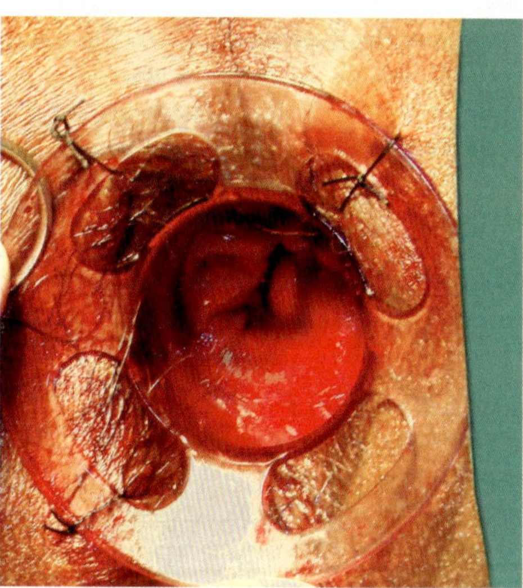
Fig. 61.64: Circular anal dilator is in place

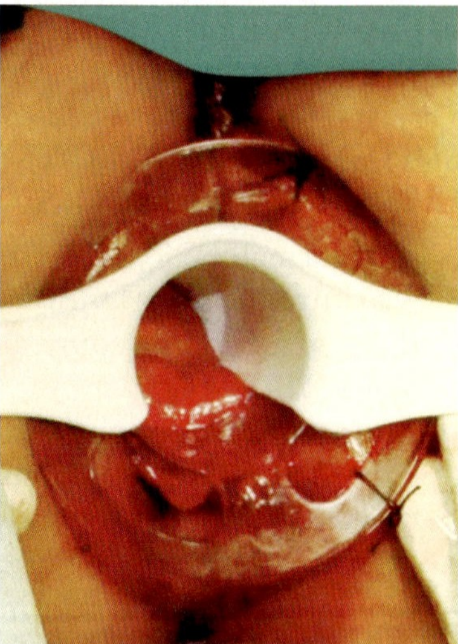
Fig. 61.65: Purse string suture is applied

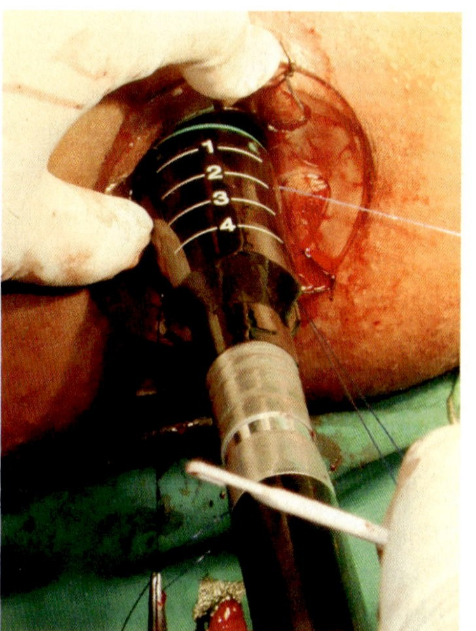


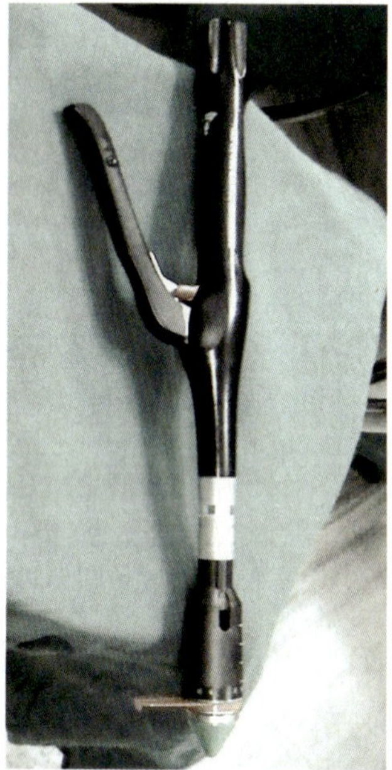

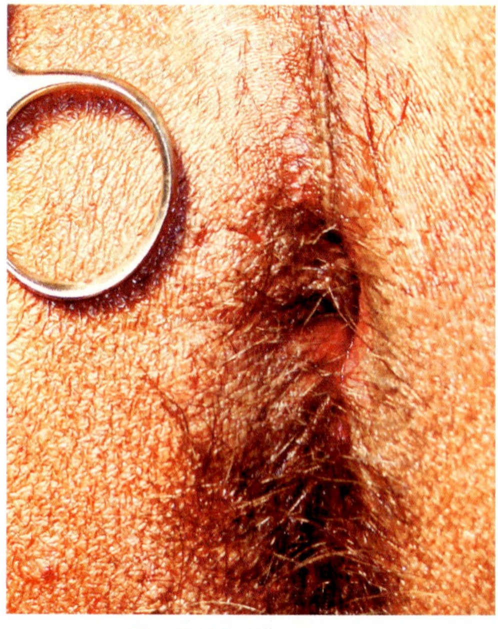

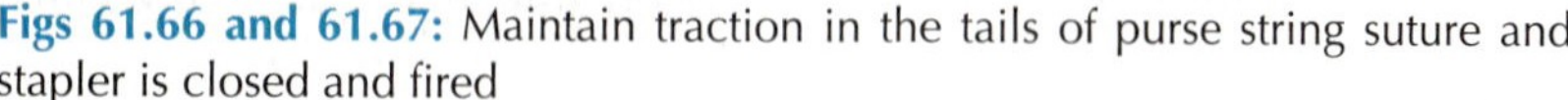
Figs 61.66 and 61.67: Maintain traction in the tails of purse string suture and stapler is closed and fired

Fig. 61.68: After surgery

*Courtesy:* Dr BH Anand Rao, Dr Vinayak Shenoy K, Dr Ramachandra L, Dr Hartimath B, Dr Prashanth Shetty, Dr Saritha Kanth (Consultants), and Dr Akshay Nadakarni (Registrar), Department of Surgery, KMC, Manipal.



illumination, it is possible to identify the bleeding points and ligate them.

4. **Anal stenosis** can occur, if too **much skin** is excised during haemorrhoidectomy. It needs regular dilatation.
5. **Anal fissure, submucous abscess, and incontinence** can occur after haemorrhoidectomy.
6. **Wound infection:** Minor degree of wound infection does occur and can be treated with sitz-bath, antibiotics and regular dressings.

## ANORECTAL ABSCESS

**SU28.17.10:** Describe aetiology, types, clinical features, complications of anorectal suppurative diseases.

### Acute Anorectal Suppuration—Anorectal Abscess

- More common in men especially diabetic. Bloodborne infection is common in diabetic patients.

- Mostly originate from the anal gland opening at the base of the anal crypts. This is **cryptoglandular theory of intersphincteric anal gland infection** described by Sir Allan Parks. From here, pus spreads along path of least resistance—thus form perianal abscess or ischiorectal abscess (Key Box 61.18).
- Other source of anorectal sepsis is foreign body, trauma, sexually transmitted diseases for lower level abscesses. Crohn's disease and carcinoma rectum with perforation may form pelvirectal abscess (supra-levator).

Key Box 61.18

**Causes of Anorectal Abscess**

- Infection
- Irritation (Crohn's disease, ulcerative colitis)
- Immunity low (diabetes, AIDS)

- Typically patients present with high grade fever with chills and rigors. On examination, a tender indurated swelling is found in the perianal region or in the ischiorectal fossa.
- Culture usually shows *E. coli* in about 70–80% of cases.
- *Staphylococcus aureus*, *Streptococcus*, *Bacteroides* are the other organisms.

## Types (Fig. 61.69)

### 1. Perianal Abscess

- It occurs due to infection of anal glands in the perianal region.
- It may be due to a boil, anal gland infection or thrombosed external pile.
- It produces severe pain, throbbing in nature and on examination a soft, tender, warm swelling is found.
- Rectal examination reveals a tender, boggy, swelling under the anal mucosa.

*Treatment*

Antibiotics, incision and drainage and excision of part of skin (roof).

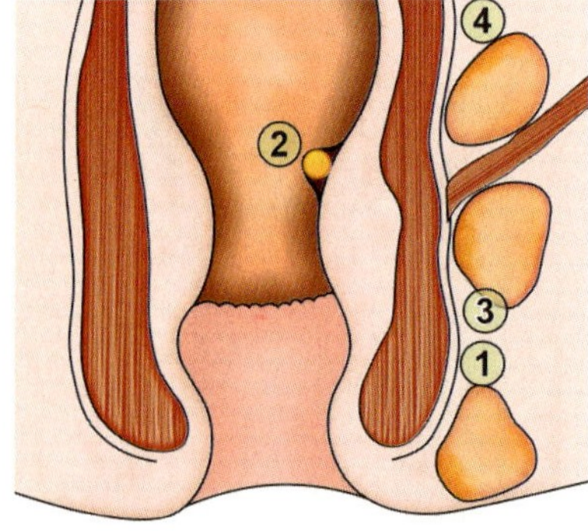


**Fig. 61.69:** Types of anorectal abscess (*see* text)

### 2. Submucous Abscess

- Collection of pus under the mucous membrane of rectum or anal canal.
- It can also be due to infection of injected haemorrhoids. It can be drained using proctoscope.

### 3. Ischiorectal Abscess

- Collection of pus in the ischiorectal fossa, which is lateral to rectum and medial to pelvic wall.
- Bounded above by levator ani and inferiorly by pad of fat in the ischiorectal fossa.
- Ischiorectal fat is poorly vascularised. Hence, it is more vulnerable to infection.
- Abscess occurs due to spread of perianal abscess or due to blood-borne infection.
- Diabetes is the precipitating factor.

*Clinical Features*

- Severe throbbing pain is characteristic of ischiorectal abscess.
- Induration in the ischiorectal fossa
- Common in diabetic men
- Frank evidence of abscess such as fluctuation need not be seen and is a late sign (Key Box 61.19).
- High grade fever with chills and rigors.
- Per rectal examination is painful and bogginess can be appreciated on the side of the lesion.

Key Box 61.19

**Deep Abscess without Fluctuation**

- Ischiorectal abscess
- Breast abscess
- Parotid abscess
- Prostatic abscess
- Midpalmar abscess

*Treatment*

Under anaesthesia, a cruciate incision (+) (Figs 61.70 and 61.71) is made and the 4 flaps are raised. All the pus is evacuated and the wound is packed with iodine roller gauze and left open. Edges of the skin are trimmed to leave an opening so that drainage of pus occurs freely. It heals with granulation tissue within 10–15 days. Appropriate antibiotics are given for a period of 5 to 10 days.

### 4. Pelvirectal Abscess

It is a pelvic abscess, which is drained through the rectum. The common causes are pelvic peritonitis, appendicitis, septic abortions, etc. The details of the causes, clinical features and the management are discussed on *see* page 882. *See* Key Box 61.20 for summary of anorectal abscess.

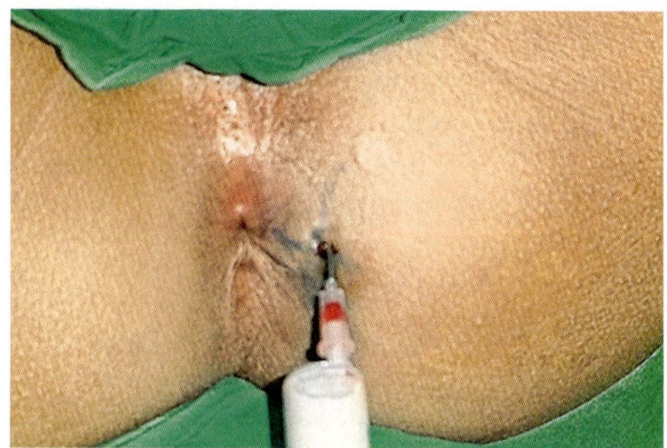

Fig. 61.70: Aspiration of ischiorectal abscess

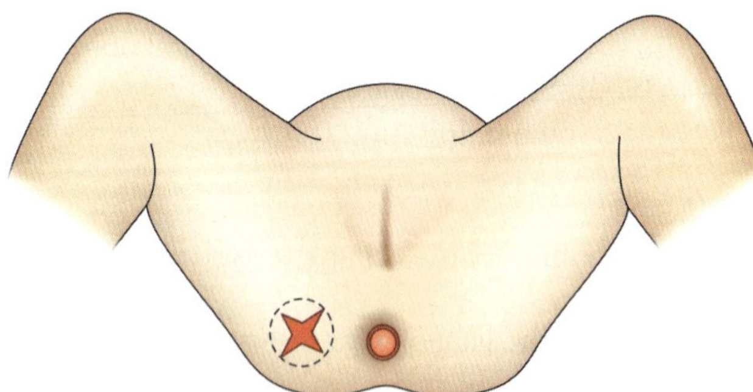

Fig. 61.71: Cruciate incision—drainage

Key Box 61.20

**Anorectal Abscess**

- Common causes such as boil or infected sebaceous cyst has to be ruled out first.
- Remember other causes such as infection following haemorrhoidal injection or band ligation.
- Uncommon causes such as foreign body or penetrating trauma also can give rise to anorectal abscess.
- Last but not the least, AIDS and diabetes have to be ruled out in all cases of anorectal abscess.

## FISTULA *IN ANO*

**SU28.17.11:** Describe aetiopathogenesis, clinical features and management of fistula *in ano*.

Abnormal communication between anal canal and rectum with exterior (perianal skin) is called fistula *in ano*. Even though multiple openings are seen in the perianal skin, **the internal opening is always single**.

### Aetiopathogenesis

1. They occur due to **persistent anal gland infection,** which results in anorectal abscesses, rupture inside as well as outside resulting in a fistula. Once a fistula occurs, it persists because of infection and absence of rest to the part. As there are many anal glands, often, problem persists in spite of initial treatment of one fistula.
2. In India, **tuberculosis** is common. Patients with pulmonary tuberculosis have 1–2% chances of developing multiple anal fistulae. Whenever a patient presents with multiple anal fistulae, it is but natural to think of tubercular aetiology. Such fistulae are **not indurated and there is watery discharge without pus.**
3. In Western countries, **ulcerative colitis and Crohn's disease** are responsible for multiple anal fistulae.
4. **Colloid carcinoma of rectum** can present as multiple fistulae *in ano*. This type of carcinoma has worst prognosis. Rectal examination should be done in every patient with anal fistula.

Other causes of anal fistula are given in Key Box 61.21.

Key Box 61.21

**Special Types of Fistula *In ano***

- **F**istula carcinoma
- **I**leitis—Crohn's
- **S**chistosomiasis
- **T**uberculosis
- **U**lcerative colitis
- **L**ymphogranuloma venereum
- **A**nal fissure abscess

*Students can remember as* **FISTULA**

### Classification

#### *I. Standard Classification* (Fig. 61.72)

1. Subcutaneous
2. Submucous
3. Low anal

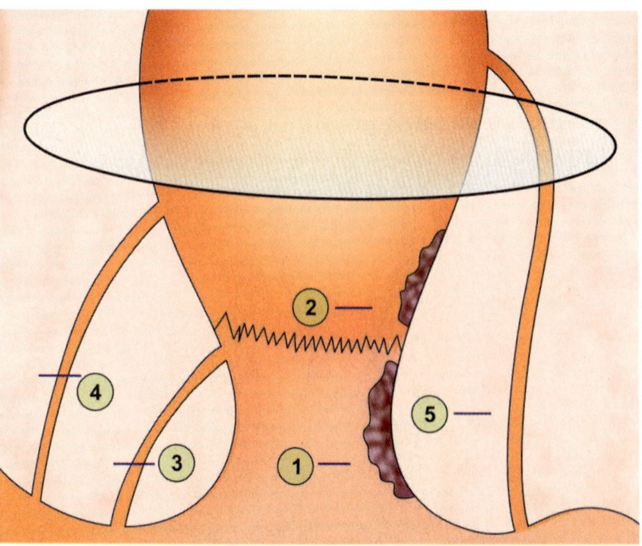


Fig. 61.72: Standard classification (*see* text)

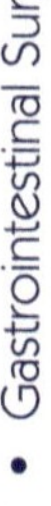

4. High anal
5. Pelvirectal

### *II. Park's Classification* (Fig. 61.73)

1. Intersphincteric
2. Trans-sphincteric
3. Supralevator (internal opening is situated above the anorectal bundle).

### Clinical Features

- Persistent seropurulent discharge, keeps the part always wet.
- Previous history of anal gland infection, with recurrent abscess.
- External opening can be single/multiple, with pouting granulation tissue, may discharge blood.
- Internal opening in carcinoma felt as a 'button hole' defect inside the rectum.
- **Goodsall's rule:** A fistula, with an external opening in the anterior half of anus within 3.75 cm tends to be direct type and in the posterior half, indirect type or curved and sometimes horseshoe type. It may communicate with the opposite side (Fig. 61.74).

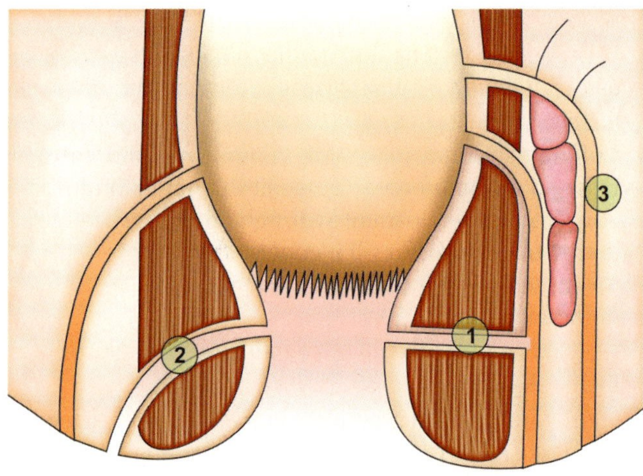


**Fig. 61.73:** Park's classification

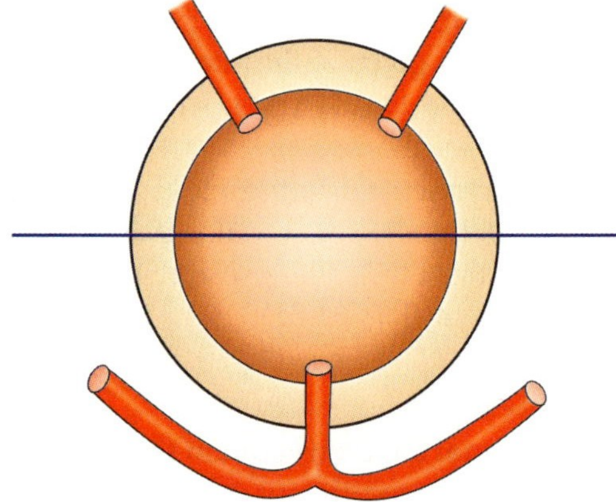

**Fig. 61.74:** Goodsall's rule

### Diagnosis

- External opening is found at the bottom of a depressed area or with granulation tissue or it is seen discharging pus.
- Internal opening may be felt on digital examination as **indurated** area or sometimes can be seen with proctoscopy or after sigmoidoscopy.
- The entire track may be palpable as indurated cord like structure.
- **Endorectal ultrasonography** and **MRI** seem to identify internal openings and fistula. However, they can be selectively used in deserving cases.
- Examination under general or regional anaesthesia.

## TREATMENT (Figs 61.75 to 61.80)

### I. Fistulotomy

It is indicated in low fistula (internal opening below the anorectal bundle). A probe is passed through the external opening into the rectum and along the length of this tract the fistula is laid open. It is done under anaesthesia. The wound is left open and allowed to

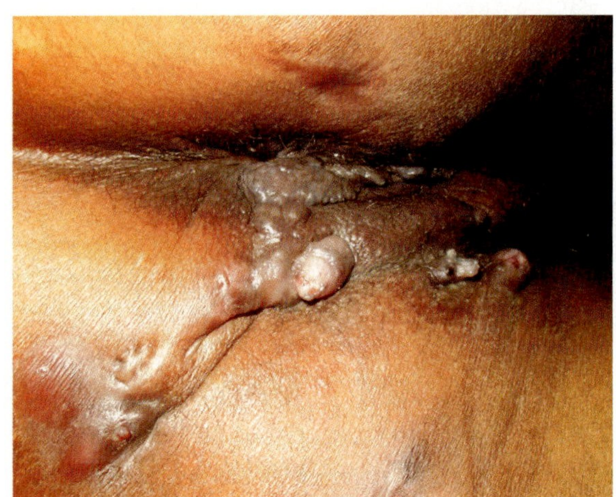

**Fig. 61.75:** Multiple recurrent fistula *in ano*—biopsy reported as tuberculosis

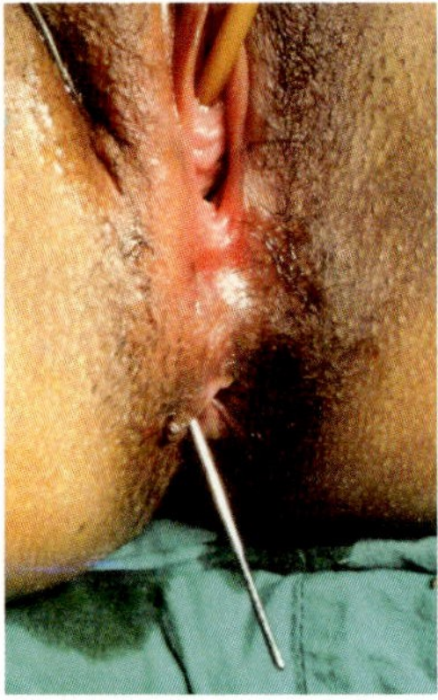

**Fig. 61.76:** Fistula—recto-vaginal fistula

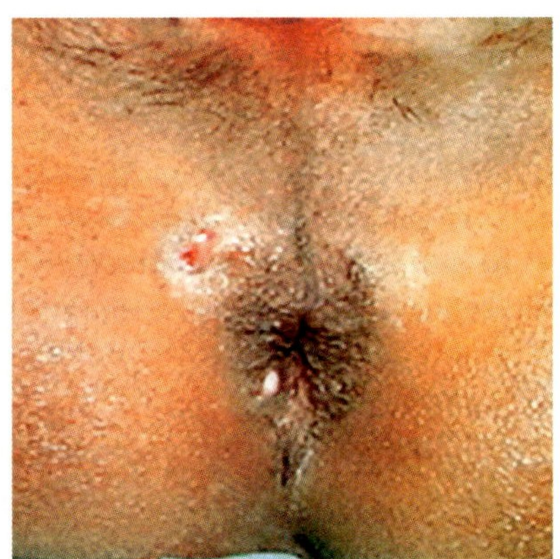

**Fig. 61.77:** Low fistula *in ano*

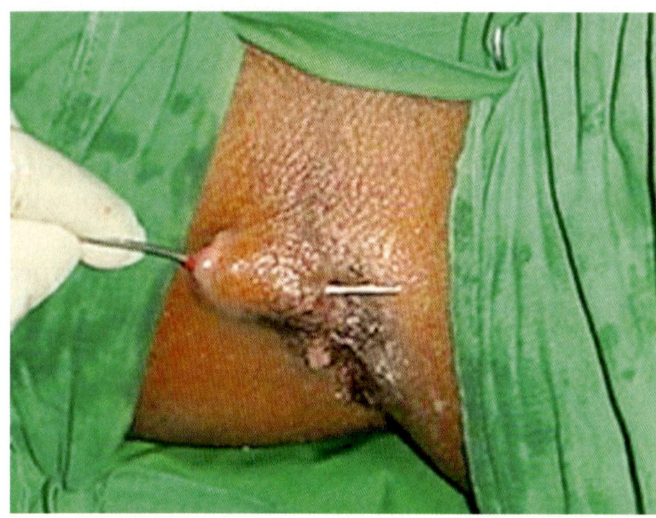

**Fig. 61.78:** Fistulotomy by passing a fistula probe

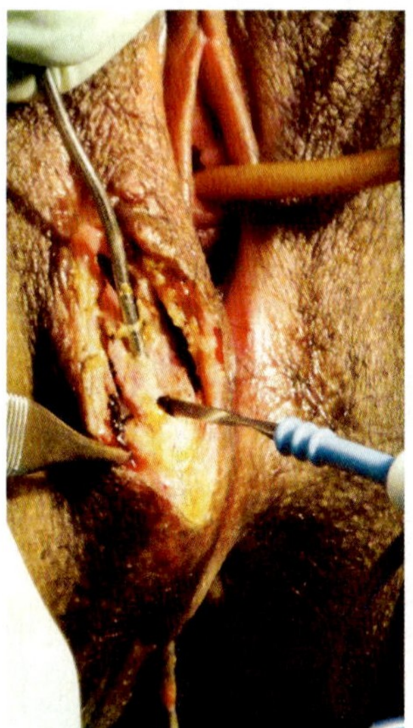

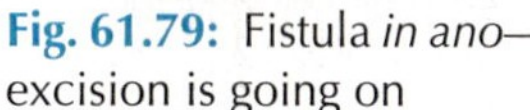

**Fig. 61.79:** Fistula *in ano*—excision is going on

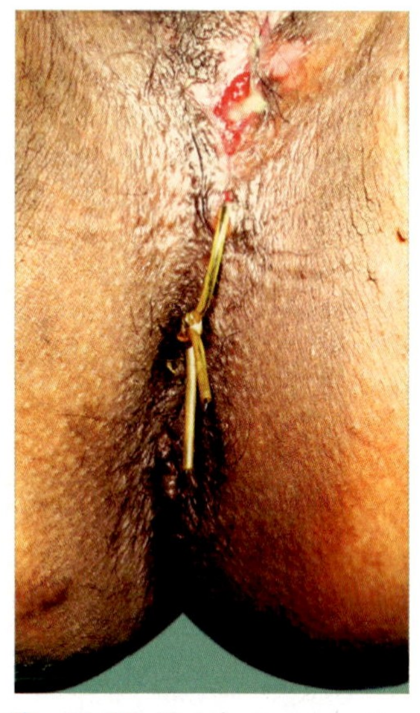

**Fig. 61.80:** Fistula *in ano*, seton in place

heal by granulation tissue developing from the floor of the fistula (marsupialisation). Intersphincteric and low trans-sphincteric fistulas of recent origin are treated by fistulotomy and marsupialisation.

### Advantages

- Least chances of recurrence
- Relatively easy procedure
- Minor degree of incontinence.

### II. Fistulectomy

All **chronic fistulae (low) are treated by fistulectomy** by excising the entire fibrous tissues and tract. Here also, the wound is kept open. This can also be done for **posterior semi-horseshoe and horseshoe** fistulae. Some incontinence can occur.

### III. Fistulectomy with or without Colostomy

It is indicated in high fistula *in ano*. The internal opening is situated above the anorectal bundle. Hence, during fistulectomy, there is a chance of injury to the anorectal bundle and may cause incontinence. Temporary or permanent colostomy may be necessary. If there is a cause, treat the cause. Surgery of intersphincteric fistula and trans-sphincteric fistula may result in incontinence.

### IV. Use of Seton or Medicated Thread (Ksharasutra)

Ksharasutra is an ayurvedic term. It is a medicated thread passed through the entire tract and both ends are tied and tightened once a week so that by 6 weeks it cuts through (Key Box 61.22).

Key Box 61.22

**Seton**

- It is a Latin word. Seton means bristle—material such as thread, wire, or gauze that is passed through subcutaneous tissues.
- Varieties of materials used as setons—plastic tubes, infant feeding tubes, prolene suture material, medicated thread used in Ayurvedic method—Ksharasutra. Ksharasutra is a Sanskrit phrase in which Kshar refers to anything that is corrosive or caustic; while sutra means a thread.
- Loose setons for long-term palliation. Examples: Fistulae associated with Crohn's disease, complicated recurrent fistulae.
- Cutting tight setons: Used in complicated high fistulae wherein a fistulotomy may result in anal incontinence. So, seton is tied, patient will tighten it everyday for a period of 8–12 weeks till it comes down. Once it comes down, seton is removed. This will decrease the chances of incontinence.
- Main advantage of seton is it eliminates sepsis by keeping the track open.
- Disadvantage is that patient will always feel a foreign body sensation in the rectum and anal canal.

### V. Ligation of Intersphincter Fistula Tact (LIFT)

It is a procedure done for high inter sphincteric fistula *in ano*. An incision is given in the intersphincteric groove and identifying the fistula tract. Internal opening is identified.

Entire fistula tract is ligated close to the internal opening. All the infected materials, granulation tissue is excised. Whatever defect present in the external sphincter is sutured (Fig. 61.81).

### VI. Video-assisted

**Video-assisted anal fistula treatment (VAAFT):** A novel sphincter-saving procedure for treating complex anal fistulae (more details on page 1241).

- **V**isualisation of the fistula tract using the fistuloscope.
- **A**im is correct localisation of the internal fistula opening under direct vision.
- **A** stapler or cutaneous-mucosal flap to close the internal opening after endoscopic treatment of the fistula.
- **F**istuloscopy is done under irrigation and followed by an operative phase of fulguration of the fistula tract.
- **T**otal closure of the internal opening and suture reinforcement with cyanoacrylate.

  *You can remember as* **VAAFT**
- Few new agents in treating fistula *in ano* (Key Box 61.23).

Key Box 61.23

**Recent Advances in Fistula Surgery**

**Biological agents:** The basic principle is to plug and seal the tract. It allows the ingrowth of healthy tissue. Thus initially fibrin glue was used but results are not good in long term. Porcine small intestinal mucosa or porcine dermal collagen also has been used. Results are not satisfactory.

### TEN COMMANDMENTS FOR FISTULA *IN ANO*

1. Should find out the internal and external openings.
2. Should try to define the type of the fistula in relation to sphincter.
3. Should define low or high fistula.
4. Should rule out special types of fistula.
5. Should conduct thorough examination again under anaesthesia before surgical procedure.
6. Should do MRI in difficult, recurrent and complicated fistula.
7. Should do fistulotomy in all intersphincteric fistulae and trans-sphincteric involving 30% of the voluntary musculature.
8. Should do fistulectomy in low fistula—it will open up the infected cavity better even though wound will be bigger than a simple fistulotomy wound.
9. Should use setons in high fistula or complicated fistula wherein a fistulotomy may result in recurrence or incontinence or when staged procedures are planned.
10. Should explain to the patient about possibility of some degree of incontinence and take consent for colostomy in high fistula.

## FISSURE *IN ANO*

**SU28.17.8:** Describe aetiopathogenesis, clinical features and management of anal fissure.

### Definition

Longitudinal tear in the lower end of anal canal results in fissure *in ano*. It is the **most painful condition** affecting the anal region. Commonly seen in young patients.

### Aetiopathogenesis (Fig. 61.81 and Key Box 61.24)

- 90% of anal fissures occur in the **posterior part of anal canal** and 10% anteriorly. It is initiated by hard stool causing a crack. As a result of this, defaecation results in pain. Anal fissure is more common posteriorly in the midline because of relative ischaemia.

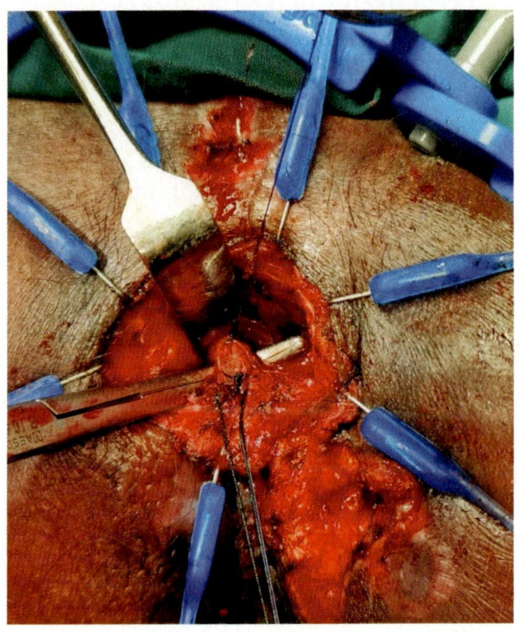

**Fig. 61.81:** Fistula LIFT

Key Box 61.24

**Various Factors which Precipitate Anal Fissure**

- **F**aeces—hard
- **I**schaemia
- **S**urgical procedures—haemorrhoidectomy
- **S**phincter hypertonia
- **U**nderlying diseases—Crohn's, sexually transmitted diseases, etc.
- **R**epeated childbirth
- **E**nthusiastic usage of ointments and abuse of laxatives

*Remember as* **FISSURE**

- **Due to pain, internal sphincter spasm** takes place which makes constipation worse resulting in a **chronic fissure**.
- **Anterior fissures** occur in elderly women secondary to repeated pregnancies. This is due to damaged pelvic floor and lack of support to anal mucous membrane. Acute fissure in females may occur after vaginal delivery.

*Pearls of Wisdom*

Fissure away from midline should raise the possibility of Crohn's disease, sexually transmitted diseases, etc.

## Clinical Features

- Severe pain during and after defaecation, burning in nature, lasting for about ½ to 1 hour because of which defaecation is postponed.
- Severe constipation is present.
- Stools are hard, pellet like and there is a drop of blood or streaks of fresh blood.

**Pearls of Wisdom**

Drop of blood is due to anal fissure. Splash of blood is due to haemorrhoids, bloody slime is due to carcinoma.

- Sentinel pile refers to tag of skin at the outer end of the fissure.
- In some cases, fissure may be associated with a small perianal abscess resulting in worsening of pain.

## Diagnosis (Table 61.4)

1. When the buttocks are spread apart, a longitudinal tear and a hypertrophied, thickened skin is seen near the lower end of fissure—**sentinel pile**.
2. Per rectal examination can be done (with lignocaine jelly application) and **sphincter spasm** can be appreciated.
3. Proctoscopy is contraindicated because the condition is very **painful**.

## Treatment (Table 61.5)

### *I. Conservative*

- Avoid constipation—encourage fibre diet, mild laxatives and not to postpone defaecation.
- Surface anaesthetic creams: Lignocaine jelly.
- Metronidazole and antibiotics.
- Sitz bath.

### *II. Agents which Decrease Sphincter Pressure*

- **Glyceryl trinitrate** (0.2%) topical application: Significant headache and 50% recurrence are drawbacks. It reduces spasm, increases vascular perfusion.
- **Purified botulinum toxin** injection into internal sphincter: It inhibits presynaptic release of acetylcholine from cholinergic nerve endings and cause temporary paresis of striated muscle. Cost, perianal thrombosis and sepsis are drawbacks. Injection produces **prolonged but reversible effects,** thus avoiding **permanent injury** (Key Box 61.25).
- **Calcium channel blockers:** Nifedipine, diltiazem oral and topical applications **(2%)** also have been used.

**TABLE 61.4:** Difference between acute fissure *in ano* and chronic fissure *in ano*

| Acute fissure | Chronic fissure |
|---|---|
| • Sudden onset—example after vaginal delivery or following hard stools<br>• Acute pain in the anal canal, severe burning after defaecation with bleeding<br>• No itching around anal opening<br>• Severe sphincter spasm, small crack in the lower anal canal<br>• No sentinel pile—tag of skin<br>• PR very painful<br>• Proctoscopes—better not try insertion<br>• Usually responds to conservative treatment—local application of glyceryl trinitrate (GTN) 0.2% 3–4 times a day or diltiazem 2% twice a day<br>• Emergency sphincterotomy may be required in a few patients | • A few months duration of symptoms<br>• Chronic pain in the anal canal, burning after defaecation with bleeding—a few exacerbations<br>• Itching is usually present due to ulcer or hypertrophied skin—sentinel pile<br>• Sphincter spasm, chronic canoe-shaped ulcer in the lower anal canal<br>• Sentinel pile—tag of skin<br>• PR painful<br>• Proctoscope—can be done with proper ligonocaine application to the anal canal<br>• Responds to conservative treatment but effect is temporary, surgery is the treatment of choice<br>• Lateral sphincterotomy or other procedures may be required |

**TABLE 61.5:** Treatment of chronic fissure *in ano*

| Pharmacological agents | Injection botulinum A toxin | Lateral sphincterotomy/flaps |
|---|---|---|
| • 0.2% **glyceryl trinitrate** ointment for local application<br>• Headache is a complication<br>• Still it is a popular treatment because it is simple<br>• Drug releases NO (nitric oxide) at a cellular level and mediates relaxation of internal sphincter<br>• **Oral nifedipine** 20 mg, twice daily. Topical nifedipine also helps | • Healing rate is 80% in chronic anal fissures<br>• 6% recurrence in 6 months<br>• Single injection, simple method, smooth recovery— chances of sepsis are present | • Gold standard<br>• Manometry of anal sphincter can be done before procedure especially in women because 30–40% of patients develop incontinence following lateral sphincterotomy<br>**Advancement flap**<br>Women—postpartum fissure—poor anal tone |

Key Box 61.25

**Role of Botulinum Toxin Injection**

- Achalasia cardia and other oesophageal motility disorders.
- Anal fissures
- Sphincter of Oddi dysfunction
- Frey syndrome

### *III. Surgical Treatment*

1. **Lateral anal sphincterotomy of Notaras** (or dorsal) is **the best alternative procedure.** Here internal sphincter is divided away from fissure either in right or left lateral positions. The procedure can be easily done by using a bivalved speculum in the anal canal. This is the procedure of choice. **Sphincterotomy should be limited to the length of fissure to avoid incontinence.**
2. **Fissurectomy and local advancement flap:** This is indicated in **persistent, chronic, nonhealing fissure.** After excision of the fissure, the resulting defect in the anal canal is closed by a small (**rhomboid**) advancement flap. This should be considered not as a first line of treatment. Recovery from this operation takes much more time than other treatments for anal fissures.
3. **Lord's dilatation:** It is also called **blunt sphincterotomy**—a few fibres of internal sphincter are divided. It relieves the spasm and the fissure heals. Rarely, in female patients, it may result in incontinence. **It is not a recommended treatment nowadays.**

*Pearls of Wisdom*

Lateral sphincterotomy is very popular and gives good results.

## PILONIDAL SINUS (JEEP-BOTTOM)

- Pilonidal sinus means **nest of hairs** in Greek. Also called **Jeep-bottom** because it was very common in jeep drivers.
- More common in dark people than fair people.
- It is an acquired condition, commonly found in hairy males.

  **It is acquired due to the following reasons:**
  - Appears between the age of 20 and 30 years.
  - Hairy men are more affected.
  - The **hair follicle is never demonstrated in the wall of the pilonidal sinus** but hair is the content of pilonidal sinus.
- Hair accumulates due to vibration and friction causing shedding of the hair. Thus, it accumulates in the gluteal cleft and enters the opening of the sweat glands.
- Pointed end of the dead hair is inside (blind end of the sinus).

### Clinical Features

- External opening of the sinus seen just above the anal verge in the midline over the coccyx (Key Box 61.26).
- History of discharge of pus
- History of recurrent abscesses which rupture, discharging pus.
- Can be asymptomatic.

Key Box 61.26

**Sites of Pilonidal Sinus**

- Midline over the coccyx
- Umbilicus
- Interdigital in barbers

### Diagnosis

Osteomyelitis of the coccyx is the only differential diagnosis for pilonidal sinus. Hence, X-ray of the coccyx should be taken.

### Treatment (Figs 61.82 to 61.85)

- Inject methylene blue to demonstrate branches of the sinus followed by **excision of the sinus**. The patient is positioned prone with buttocks elevated (**Jack knife position**).

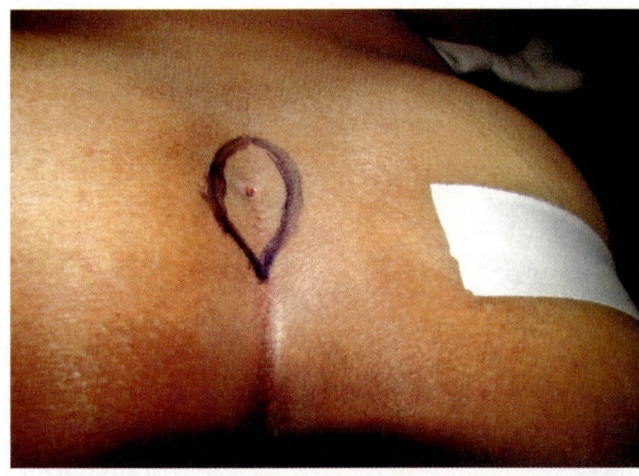

**Fig. 61.82:** A case of pilonidal sinus—methylene blue is first injected into the opening. The excision area is marked also with methylene blue

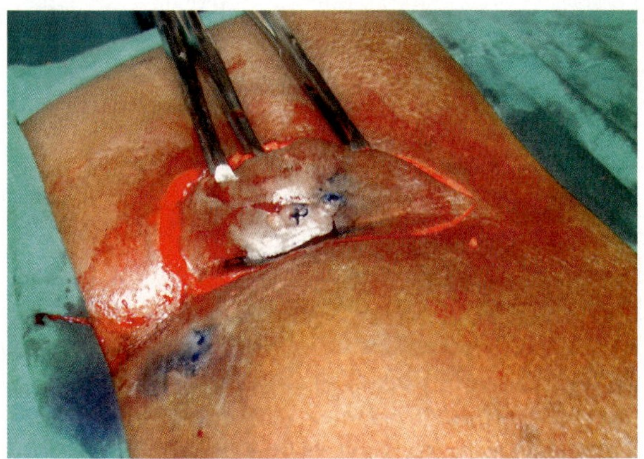

**Fig. 61.83:** Blue-stained tissues are dissected all around and removed

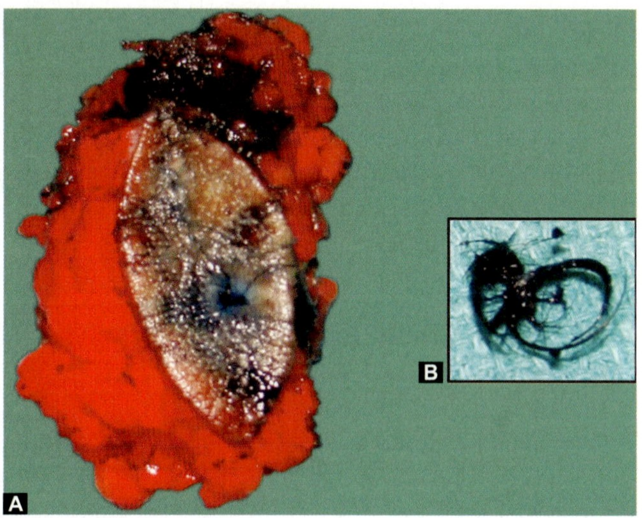

**Figs 61.84A and B:** (A) Specimen of excised tissue with sinus tract; (B) shows tuft of hair which was present within the sinus

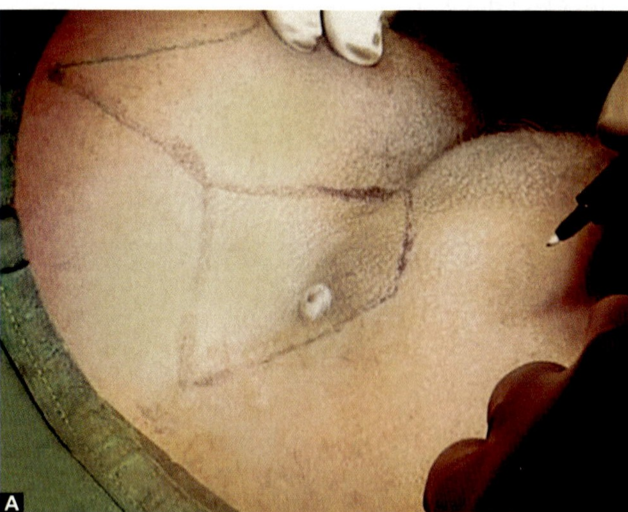

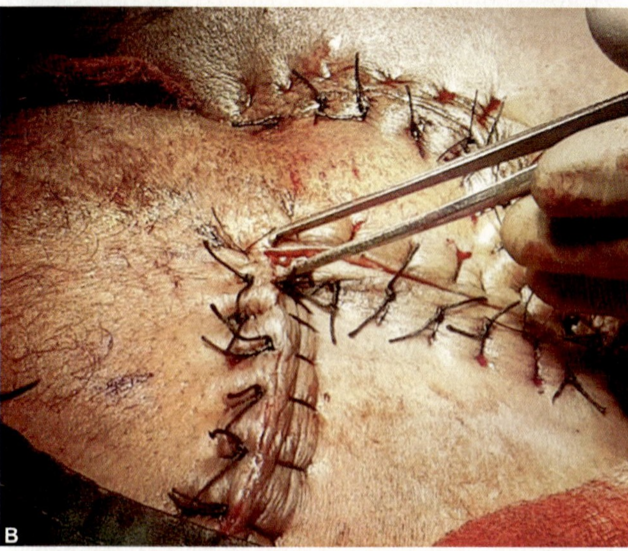

**Figs 61.85A and B:** (A) Pilonidal sinus excision. Limberg flap—marking done; (B) After excision, you can see the suture lines. (*Courtesy:* Dr Dayananda Nooli, Consultant Surgeon, Ex-Chairman ASI- Karnataka Chapter, Chikkodi, Karnataka)

- After excision, there are two methods to treat the wound—open and closed methods (Key Box 61.23).
- **Open method:** The wound is left open after excision followed by regular packing with iodine or eusol gauze pieces (Key Box 61.27).

Key Box 61.27

**Pilonidal Sinus**

- It is acquired condition—popularly called Jeep-bottom
- Common in hairy men
- Multiple sinuses communicating with each other
- They open to the exterior by multiple openings
- The direction of the sinuses is cephaloid
- Recurrent abscesses which rupture are common
- Excision with or without marsupialisation, flap closure or z plasty are the treatment options
- In spite of the adequate surgical procedures, recurrence is common.

- It may take 3–4 weeks for the healing of pilonidal sinus. Regular sitz bath is also given.
- This method carries the least recurrence.
- **Closed method:** The wound is closed by 'z' plasty. This method carries 10–20% chances of recurrence. Rhomboid flap (Limberg flap) can be raised to close the defect also.
- **Karydakis procedure:** Primary procedure is to remove all the sinus tracts and their branches till sacral bone. In this operation, semilateral incision is made around the sinuses and flaps mobilised to excise all the sinuses and their branches. Then tension free closure is done. Compared to elliptical incision, this incision and closure has decreased chances of skin necrosis.
- **Bascom's technique:** In this procedure, an incision is given laterally, not in the midline. After raising the flaps, wide excision of the infected sinuses and tracts is done followed by closure of the midline openings. Lateral wound is left open (in the conventional operation, midline wound is left open).

*Pearls of Wisdom*

Very, very rarely carcinoma can arise in a chronic pilonidal sinus.

## SACROCOCCYGEAL TERATOMA

- It is a congenital condition affecting the sacrococcygeal region.
- In this region, totipotential cells persist for a longer period compared to rest of the area. Hence, it is the site of teratomas.

### Clinical Features

- 20% of the cases are stillborn babies. It is common in a female child.
- Presents as a swelling in the sacrococcygeal region pushing the rectum anteriorly.
- The surface of the swelling ulcerates. Many cystic areas are present in the swelling.
- The swelling is fixed to the sacrum and coccyx from which it is impossible to separate/isolate.

### Complications

- Ulceration
- Secondary infection
- Haemorrhage
- Teratocarcinomatous change occurs by one year of age.

### Treatment

Excision of the teratoma with part of sacrum and coccyx.

## MALIGNANT TUMOURS OF ANAL CANAL

**SU28.17.12:** Describe aetiopathogenesis, clinical features, diagnosis and management of carcinoma of anal canal.

- They are not uncommon tumours which present with bleeding per rectum, burning and itching in the anal region.
- The diagnosis is obvious in many cases once buttocks are separated or by digital examination.
- Tissue diagnosis is a must before radical treatment.

### Types

1. **Squamous cell carcinoma:** Papillomas are the chief predisposing factors. Local excision or APR (abdominoperineal resection) is the treatment with external RT in appropriate cases (Fig. 61.86).

   For sphincter preservation—chemoradiation can be used. It is called Nigri's regime.

   Refer also to Key Box 61.28.

**Key Box 61.28**

**Anal Intraepithelial Neoplasia (AIN—Bowen's Disease)**

- It is squamous cell carcinoma *in situ* of the anus.
- It is precursor to an invasive squamous cell carcinoma.
- It is associated with human papillomavirus type 16 and 18 (HPV 16,18).
- Anoscopy, biopsy to be done.
- Dysplasia is an indication for resection/ablation.

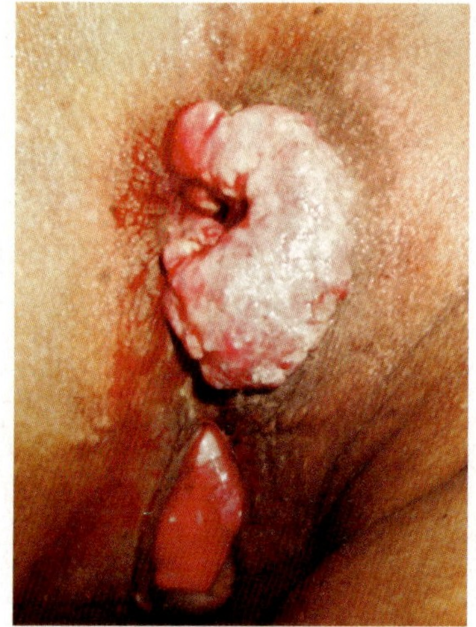

**Fig. 61.86:** Squamous cell carcinoma anal canal

2. **Basaloid carcinoma:** It is a highly malignant, non-keratinising, squamous cell carcinoma. Treatment is similar to squamous cell carcinoma.

*Pearls of Wisdom*

Basal cell carcinoma is very rare in the anal canal.

3. **Melanoma:** Beware of a patient who comes with bilateral groin nodes which are bulky. The patient may be having malignant melanoma of anal canal—bluish/blackish ulcer in the anal canal. APR is potentially curable in early cases of melanoma. If metastasis is present, the prognosis is poor. So, only local excision is done so as to provide palliation but colostomy is avoided (Figs 61.87 to 61.90).
4. **Adenocarcinoma** is rare. It can occur from the anal glands in pre-existing anal fistula. APR with 5-FU and radiation therapy is indicated.

*Pearls of Wisdom*

Please note that Bowen's disease, Paget's disease or verrucous carcinoma, squamous and basal cell carcinoma can also occur in the skin of anal margin.

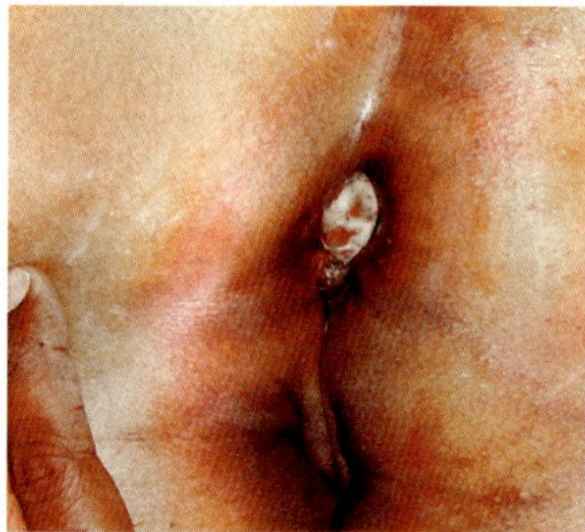

**Fig. 61.87:** Melanoma anal region

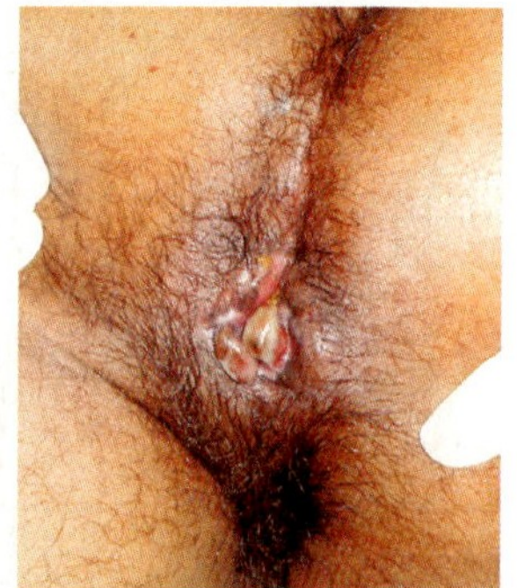

**Fig. 61.88:** Melanoma resembled prolapsed piles but pigmentation was evident on closer examination

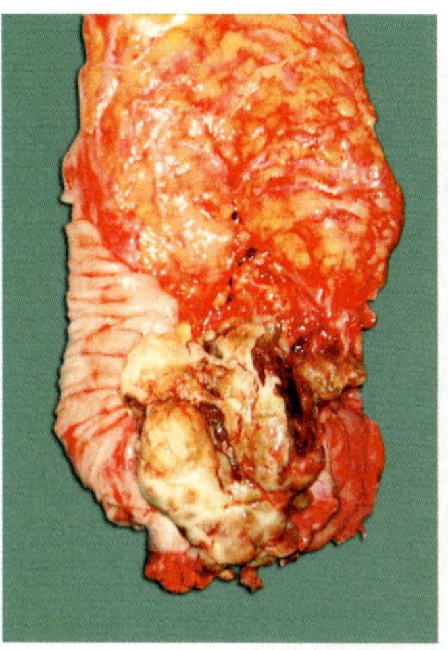
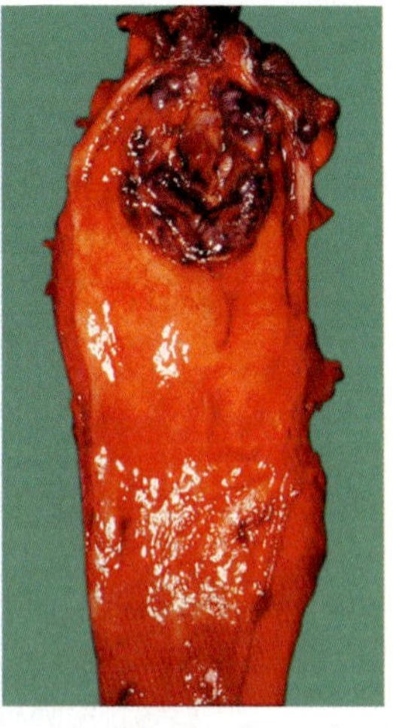

**Figs 61.89 and 61.90:** Malignant melanoma of the anal canal—APR specimens

## STRICTURE OF ANAL CANAL AND RECTUM

### Causes

1. **Postoperative:** Haemorrhoidectomy, pull-through operations, repeated diathermy fulguration of polyps.
2. **Irradiation:** It occurs one to two years after irradiation.
3. **Senile strictures**
4. **Lymphogranuloma inguinale:** A sexually transmitted disease affecting both male and female patients. Initially pararectal lymph nodes are enlarged followed by development of multiple rectal strictures.
5. **Inflammatory bowel diseases:** Both ulcerative colitis and Crohn's disease result in rectal strictures (5–10%).
6. **Rare:** Congenital, amoeboma, carcinoid, endometriosis, tuberculosis, CMV colitis (Figs 61.91 and 61.92).

### Clinical Features

Increasing constipation is the characteristic feature of stricture of the rectum. It may be associated with hard stools, bleeding and pain in some cases. Per abdominal examination may reveal loaded colon with scybalous masses. Rectal examination can detect a stricture.

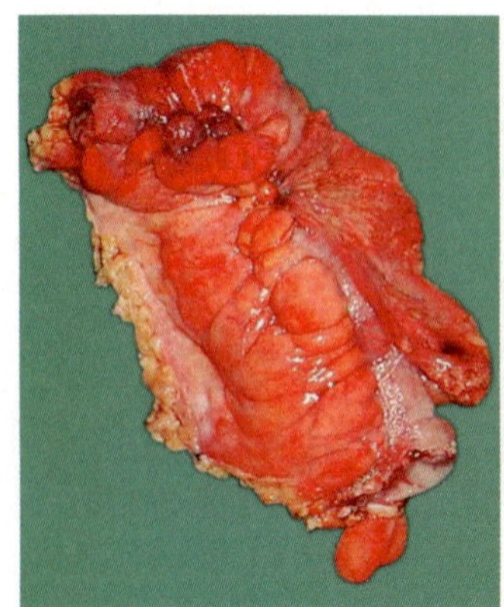
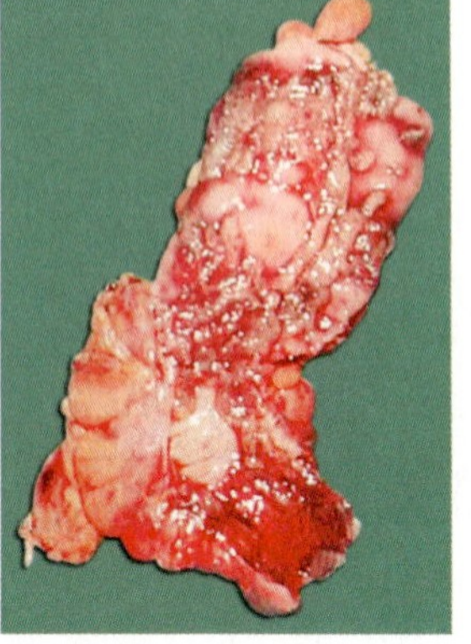

**Figs 61.91 and 61.92:** Rectal stricture due to CMV colitis (*Courtesy:* Dr Satyanarayana N, Dr Srinivas Pai, Dr Madhu, KMC, Manipal)

> *Pearls of Wisdom*
>
> It is mandatory to rule out carcinoma rectum which is the most common cause of stricture.

### Treatment

1. Conservative treatment includes bulk purgatives, a vegetable diet.
2. Regular dilatation may be necessary for the strictures situated low in the rectum and anal canal.
3. Intractable strictures need to be resected.
4. Treatment of the primary disease.

## PROCTALGIA FUGAX

- This condition is characterised by attacks of severe cramp-like pain arising in the rectum.
- Anxiety status, straining at stools or ejaculation are a few precipitating factors.
- The pain may be unbearable, may recur at irregular intervals. It is possibly due to segmental cramp in the pubococcygeus muscle. The pain usually lasts for a few minutes and subsides (fleeting perianal pain).
- Symptomatic treatment in the form of analgesics are given.

## PRURITUS ANI

### Definition

This is intractable itching around the anus.

### Causes

Perianal and anal discharge: Anal fissure, fistula *in ano*, prolapsed piles, polyps, genital warts are a few conditions which render the anus moist.

> *Pearls of Wisdom*
>
> Mucous discharge is an intense pruritic agent.

1. Poor hygiene, lack of cleanliness, excessive sweating and wearing tight and rough underclothing are common causes.
2. Parasitic causes—threadworms
3. Psychoneurosis
4. Allergy, diabetes are the other causes.

> *Pearls of Wisdom*
>
> Sexually transmitted diseases such as herpes, anal warts and HIV infection must be excluded.

**Treatment** (Key Box 61.29)

- Hygienic measures
- Prednisolone topical cream 1% with antifungal agent (miconazole nitrate 2%)
- Moisturising cream/lotion
- Antihistamine—promethazine hydrochloride 10–25 mg at night times.

*Pearls of Wisdom*

Pelvic floor dysfunction also referred to as nonrelaxing puborectalis syndrome is called ANISMUS. These patients present with constipation. It is a difficult problem to treat.

Key Box 61.29

**Pruritus Ani—Avoid**

- Toilet paper
- Soap
- Too tight underclothing
- Too many ointments
- Local anaesthetic cream

## HIDRADENITIS SUPPURATIVA

### Definition

It is a chronic recurrent suppuration of apocrine glands in the skin resulting in multiple abscesses which rupture causing multiple sinuses.

### Sites

Axilla, groin, back, buttocks and anal regions are common sites.

### Pathogenesis

- Occlusion of the gland ducts results in stasis, bacterial proliferation, abscess, rupture. Common organisms are *Staphylococcus aureus* and anaerobes (somewhat like breast abscess).
- Anogenital disease is more common in men. Hence, androgens may play a role in this condition.
- Obesity is another contributing factor.

### Clinical Features

- Common after puberty till the age of 40 years.
- Typically, it is a folliculitis presenting as multiple boils which are painful.
- Pus formation, rupture and persisting sinuses are common.
- Interestingly, it neither affects above the level of dentate line nor sphincters.

### Differential Diagnosis

All diseases resulting in multiple sinuses in and around perineum are the differential diagnosis such as Crohn's disease, tuberculosis, lymphogranuloma venereum, pilonidal sinuses, actinomycosis, etc.

### Treatment

- When in doubt, rule out other causes mentioned above and if necessary, a good biopsy from the sinus tract and from the edge of the sinus.
- General measures such as weight reduction, antibiotics, antiseptic medicated soaps, washing the part with warm saline or water.
- Surgery includes laying open all the openings or wide excision with or without skin (radical excision) and direct closure or skin grafting of flap reconstruction are the other choices.

## MULTIPLE CHOICE QUESTIONS

1. **Splash in the pan is classically described for bleeding from which condition?**
   A. Carcinoma rectum
   B. Fissure *in ano*
   C. Haemorrhoids
   D. Polyp
2. **Which of the following are causes of anorectal fistulae in males, *except*:**
   A. Crohn's disease
   B. Tuberculosis
   C. Ulcerative colitis
   D. Lymphogranuloma venereum
3. **Following are true about peritoneal coverings/fascia of the rectum, *except*:**
   A. Upper one-third is completely covered
   B. Middle one-third is covered anterolaterally
   C. Lower one-third is covered anteriorly
   D. Waldeyer's fascia separates the rectum from sacrum
4. **About signet ring carcinoma rectum, following are true, *except*:**
   A. It is seen in young patients
   B. Cells are filled with mucus and nucleus is displaced
   C. It carries bad prognosis
   D. Not an indication for chemotherapy
5. **Following are true for clinical features of carcinoma rectum, *except*:**
   A. Can give rise to tenesmus
   B. Can present as bloody slime
   C. Can present as liver secondaries
   D. Can cause closed loop obstruction
6. **The ideal surgical treatment for growth at 8 cm from the anal verge is:**
   A. Abdominoperineal resection
   B. Abdominosacral resection
   C. High anterior resection
   D. Total mesorectal excision
7. **On-table lavage of the intestines for resection and anastomosis can be done via:**
   A. Enterotomy
   B. Colotomy
   C. Enema from rectum
   D. Appendicular stump
8. **Local excision of malignant rectal tumour can be done, if:**
   A. The tumour is up to 6 cm size
   B. Up to 60% of the rectal wall involvement
   C. Lymphatic invasion is accepted
   D. Tumour is well differentiated
9. **Prolapse rectum is caused by several factors, *except*:**
   A. Birth injuries to the nerve fibres
   B. Defective collagen metabolism
   C. It does not start as intussusception
   D. Deep rectovesical pouch
10. **Below the dentate line, squamous epithelium has:**
    A. No basal cells
    B. Hair
    C. Sweat glands
    D. Pigment forming cells
11. **Above the dentate line, lymphatic drainage goes to:**
    A. Para-aortic nodes
    B. Superficial inguinal lymph nodes
    C. Deep inguinal lymph nodes
    D. Pudendal lymph nodes
12. **Following are true for prolapsed piles, *except*:**
    A. External sphincter grips the pile mass and cause gangrene
    B. Thrombosis can occur
    C. Portal pyaemia can be a complication
    D. Requires hemorrhoidectomy
13. **Which one of these precautions must be taken while applying band for haemorrhoids?**
    A. Bands are applied in grade 1 pile masses
    B. Bands are applied in grade 4 haemorrhoids
    C. Bands are applied below the dentate line
    D. Bands should not be applied in patients who are taking anticoagulants
14. **Anal stenosis is a complication of:**
    A. Stapler haemorrhoidopexy
    B. Open haemorrhoidectomy
    C. Too low application of the band
    D. Cryosurgery
15. **Following are true for injection line treatment of haemorrhoids, *except*:**
    A. It is given perivascular
    B. Given above the level of dentate line
    C. It is painful
    D. It is given in submucosal plane
16. **Following are true for stapler haemorrhoidopexy, *except*:**
    A. Recurrence rate is less
    B. Less discomfort than open haemorrhoidectomy
    C. Anal stenosis is not a complication
    D. Ideal for 3rd or 4th degree haemorrhoids

**17. In multiple fistula *in ano* and high fistula, which one of the following should not be done?**
   A. Biopsy of the track
   B. Colostomy
   C. Fistulogram
   D. Multiple fistulotomy

**18. Majority of the cases of fissure *in ano* are:**
   A. Anterior
   B. Posterior
   C. Anterolateral
   D. Posterolateral

**19. In lateral sphincterotomy:**
   A. Pecten fibres are ruptured
   B. It is blunt sphincterotomy
   C. External sphincter is divided
   D. Internal sphincter is divided

**20. In cases of pilonidal sinus:**
   A. Hair is demonstrated in the wall
   B. It is congenital
   C. It is known for recurrence
   D. It undergoes malignant change

**Answers**

| | | | | | | | | | |
|---|---|---|---|---|---|---|---|---|---|
| 1. C | 2. D | 3. C | 4. D | 5. D | 6. D | 7. D | 8. D | 9. C | 10. D |
| 11. A | 12. A | 13. D | 14. B | 15. C | 16. B | 17. B | 18. D | 19. D | 20. C |

Chapter 62

# Lower Gastrointestinal Bleeding



## Introduction

Lower gastrointestinal (LGI) bleeding refers to bleeding which occurs beyond the ligament of Treitz. Bleeding per rectum may be a manifestation of upper GI bleeding (UGIB), the causes of which have been discussed under haematemesis. In this chapter, bleeding per rectum due to lower GI causes will be discussed. LGI bleeding accounts for 1% of acute hospital admissions each year. Severe bleeding is that which continues for 24 hours after hospital admission or that which recurs 24 hours after resolution.

*Pearls of Wisdom*

In all, so-called the lower GI bleeding—rule out 3 important causes of upper GI bleeding, namely—oesophageal variceal bleeding due to portal hypertension, peptic ulcers—mainly duodenal ulcer bleeds and acute erosive gastritis or acute gastric mucosal lesions (AGML). Bleeding from these causes can be so massive, they result in fresh bleeding per rectum, thus adding confusion at the diagnosis. A **nasogastric tube lavage that yields blood or coffee-ground-like material confirms the diagnosis of upper GI bleeding**.

## Definition

**SU28.14:** Describe the clinical features, investigations and principles of management of disorders of small and large intestines. (*Please note:* This chapter deals with GI tract bleeding. You will come across important causes of bleeding).

- **Haematochezia:** Bloody stools (LGIB or rapid UGIB).
- **Melaena:** Black tarry stools from digested blood. The duration of bleeding is more than 8 hours.
- **Massive GI tract bleeding:** The bleeding which requires more than 3 units of blood transfusions in 24 hours or **25% of intravascular blood volume loss**.
- **Obscure:** Bleeding which persists or recurs after initial evaluation has failed (with EGD and colonoscopy). Two types:
  - A. *Obscure occult:* Iron deficiency anaemia, faecal occult blood positive, no visible bleeding. More than 80% resolve with **no treatment**.
  - B. *Obscure overt:* Recurrent and visible bleeding, e.g. angiodysplasia.

Investigating a case of lower GI bleeding is like investigating a 'crime' by CBI officer. One should not jump to conclusions as soon as one cause of bleeding is found. There are innumerable examples of 'piles' being treated for bleeding, totally missing a growth above in the rectum (Table 62.1 and Key Boxes 62.1 to 62.3).

## CAUSES

### Depending on Aetiology

#### I. Congenital

- Polyps: Congenital polyp, Peutz-Jeghers syndrome, familial polyposis coli (FPC).

**TABLE 62.1:** Differential diagnosis of lower GI bleeding: Incidence

| Colonic bleeding (90–95%) | Small bowel bleeding (5–10%) |
|---|---|
| Diverticular disease 30–40% | Angiodysplasia |
| Ischaemia 5–10% | Erosions or ulcers secondary to NSAIDs |
| Anorectal disease 5–15% | Crohn's disease |
| Neoplasia 5–10% | Radiation enteritis |
| Infectious colitis 3–8% | Meckel's diverticulum |
| Inflammatory bowel disease 3–4% | Neoplasia (adenocarcinoma, lymphoma) |
| Angiodysplasia 3% | |

Key Box 62.1

**Common Causes of Lower GI Bleeding**

- Most originate in the colon or rectum—haemorrhoids, polyps, carcinoma, and inflammatory bowel diseases are common causes.
- 10% from upper intestinal tract.
- Small intestinal haemorrhage is usually due to arteriovenous malformations (angiodysplasia), accounting for 70–80%.
- Jejunal diverticula, Meckel's diverticula, neoplasia, Crohn's disease, and aorto-enteric fistula following a previous aortic graft are other causes of bleeding from small intestines.

Key Box 62.2

**Lower GI Bleeding—Types**

**Depending upon the source:**

- Small bowel bleed—5%
- Colonic bleed—95%

**Depending upon the clinical manifestation:**

- *Melaena:* Passage of black tarry stools (altered blood) due to slow bleeding or more proximal source of bleed.
- *Haematochezia:* Passage of bright red stools with or without clots.

Key Box 62.3

**Bleeding Per Rectum with Acute Abdomen**

- Mesenteric ischaemia
- Intussusception
- Ischaemic colitis
- Necrotising enterocolitis

- Meckel's diverticulum
- Hereditary haemorrhagic telangiectasia (HHT)

*Pearls of Wisdom*

HHT is the most important inherited anomaly which produces bleeding.

### II. Inflammatory

- Tubercular ulcers
- Enteric ulcers
- Crohn's ileocolitis
- Ulcerative colitis
- Necrotising enterocolitis
- **Dysentery**—amoebic, bacillary, strongyloides infestation

### III. Neoplastic

- Papilloma of rectum
- Carcinoma colon, rectum
- GIST (*see* pages 746, 889)
- Lymphoma
- Carcinoma small bowel

### IV. Vascular

- Angiodysplasia
- Ischaemic colitis
- Vasculitis—polyarteritis nodosa
- Haemangioma

### V. Clotting Disorders

- Haemophilia
- Thrombocytopaenia
- Leukaemia
- Warfarin therapy
- Disseminated intravascular coagulopathy

### VI. Miscellaneous

- Piles, anal fissure
- Prolapse
- Injury to the rectum
- Diverticular disease

### Depending on Site of Bleeding

**I. Small intestine**

- Peutz-Jeghers polyps
- Meckel's diverticulum
- Tubercular ulcers
- Crohn's ulcers
- Leiomyoma
- Angiodysplasia

**II. Large bowel**

- Angiodysplasia right colon
- Carcinoma colon
- Ulcerative colitis
- Dysentery
- Diverticular disease

**III. Anorectal conditions**

- Haemorrhoids or piles
- Prolapse rectum
- Fissure *in ano*
- Polyps

Most of the causes have been discussed in the respective chapters.

## CLINICAL EXAMINATION

**1. Age of the patient**

- **Children and young boys:** Polyps, Meckel's diverticulum, necrotising enterocolitis.
- **Young age group:** Piles, tuberculosis, Crohn's colitis, dysentery.
- **Middle and old age:** Carcinoma, piles, prolapse, diverticular disease.

2. **Colour of blood**
- **Bright red:** Piles, fissure, polyp.
- **Altered blood:** Carcinoma, tubercular ulcer, Crohn's colitis, dysentery.
- **Maroon colour:** Meckel's diverticulum.

3. **Blood with mucus**
- Intussusception
- Dysentery
- Inflammatory bowel diseases
- Carcinoma

4. **Other special features**
- Severe pain with bleeding: Anal fissure
- Splash in the pan: Piles
- Red currant jelly stools: Intussusception
- Streaks of blood: Anal fissure
- Bloody slime: Carcinoma rectum
- Blood with cherry-red mass coming out: Piles, polyps.

5. **Palpable mass abdomen**
- Hard mass in the colon: Carcinoma colon.
- Firm to hard mass in the right iliac fossa: Ileocaecal tuberculosis.
- Contracting mass: Intussusception.

6. **Rectal examination** (Fig. 62.1)
- Very painful: Anal fissure
- Pedunculated mass: Rectal polyp (juvenile polyps)
- Ulcerations in the rectum: Solitary rectal ulcer
- Indurated ulcer or growth: Carcinoma rectum (Fig. 62.2).

7. **Evidence of bleeding tendencies**
- Purpuric spots
- Haematoma

## INVESTIGATIONS

1. **Proctoscopy** (Fig. 62.3)
   - Cherry red to pink mucosal bulges: Haemorrhoids
   - Bleeding ulcer or a growth: Cancer of rectum
   - Single anterior ulcer: Solitary ulcer rectum.

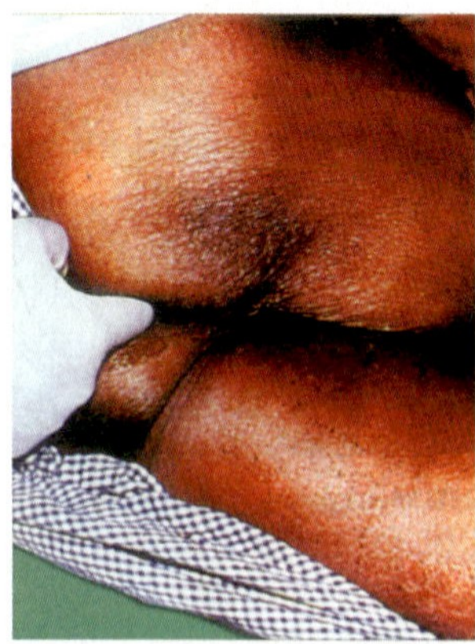

**Fig. 62.1:** Rectal examination

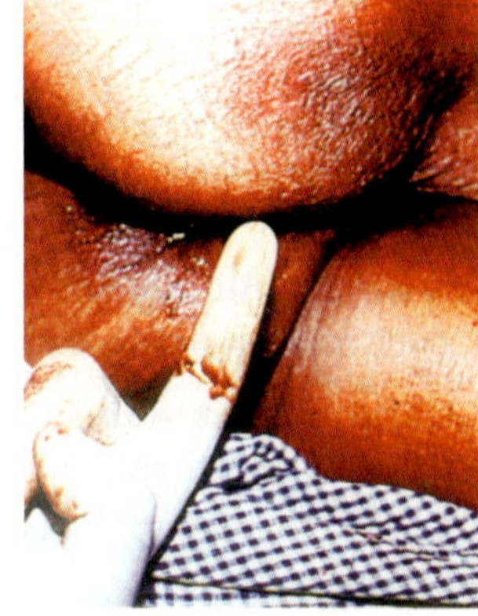

**Fig. 62.2:** Glove streaked blood–carcinoma rectum

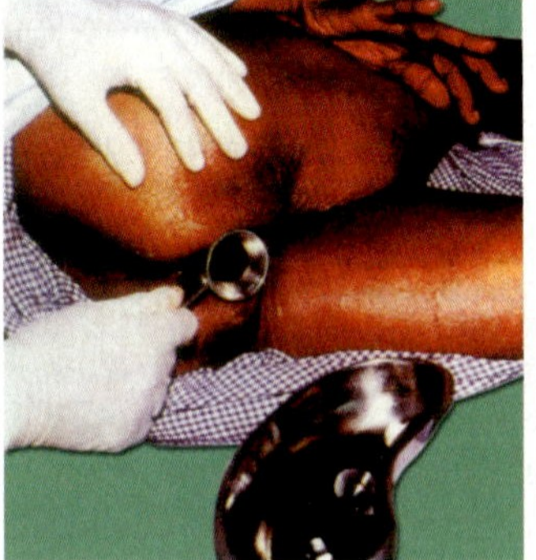

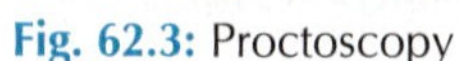

**Fig. 62.3:** Proctoscopy

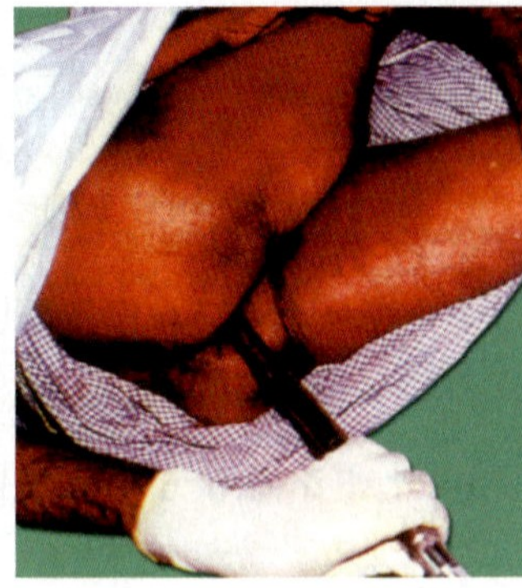

**Fig. 62.4:** Sigmoidoscopy

2. **Sigmoidoscopy** (Fig. 62.4): Rigid scopy has been replaced by flexible sigmoidoscopy. It is a simple outpatient procedure and can diagnose about 60% of cases of carcinoma colon. Few diseases and their characteristic findings are given below:
   - Multiple small pinpoint ulcers: Ulcerative colitis
   - Large deep flask-shaped ulcer: Amoebic ulcers
   - Multiple small polyps: Hereditary polyposis coli.

3. **Colonoscopy**
   - It is the gold standard investigation for lower GI bleeding. It can detect 3 important diseases: Carcinoma, inflammatory bowel diseases (IBDs) and diverticular diseases (Figs 62.5 to 62.18). It can also detect ischaemic colitis, polyps and angiodysplasia. It needs to be repeated. In massive bleeding, it can really tax an expert colonoscopist also.
   - Colonoscopic adrenaline injections, snaring and coagulation (argon plasma coagulation) are therapeutic advantages.

4. **Barium enema**
   - Irregular filling defect in the colon: Cancer colon.
   - Contracted pipe-stem colon: Ulcerative colitis.
   - Pincer ending: Intussusception.
   - Saw-tooth appearance: Diverticular disease.

5. **Stool examination**
   - Amoebiasis, bacillary dysentery
   - Hookworm infestations.

6. **Small bowel enema (enteroclysis)**
   - Diverticulum in the terminal ileum is Meckel's diverticulum. Multiple ulcers and stricture terminal ileum can be due to tuberculous ulcer.
   - Barium studies have a little value in the presence of acute haemorrhage. They can be used in intermittent or chronic bleeding wherein endoscopy has failed to detect the cause.

### Special Investigations

They are indicated when the diagnosis of lower GI bleeding cannot be made out. They are more useful where there is active bleeding or obscure bleeding.

## DIFFERENTIAL DIAGNOSIS OF LOWER GI BLEEDING (Figs 62.5 to 62.18)

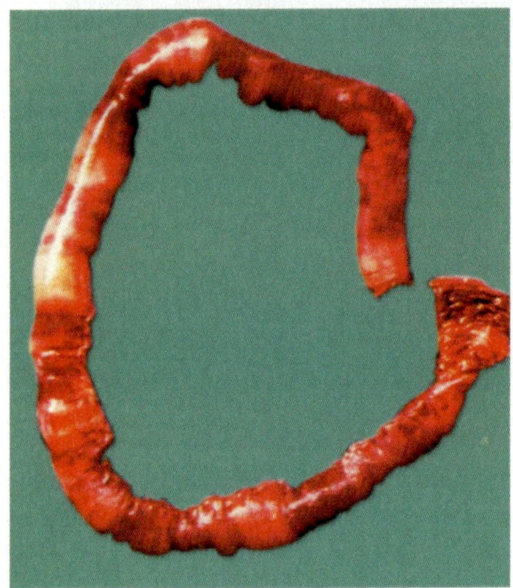

**Fig. 62.5:** Necrotising enterocolitis

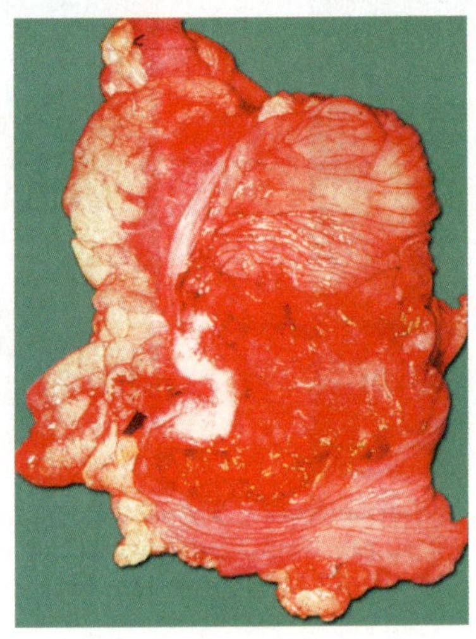

**Fig. 62.6:** Carcinoma colon

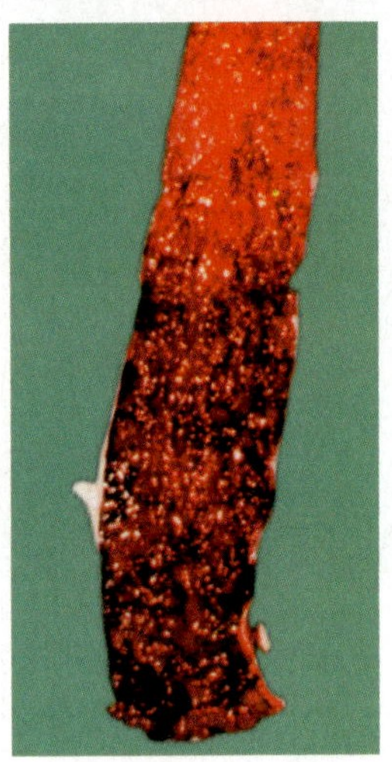

**Fig. 62.7:** Ulcerative colitis

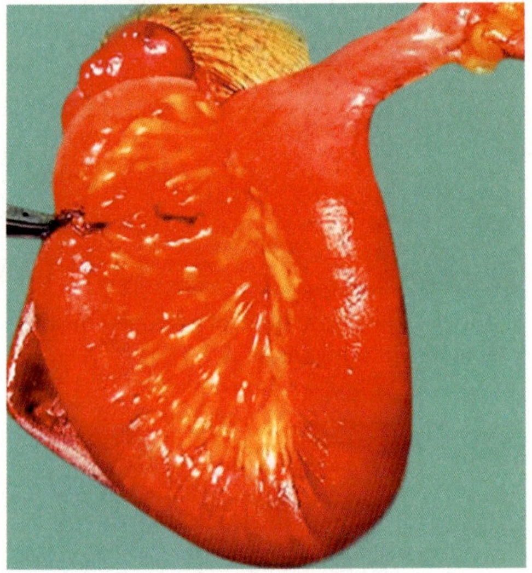

**Fig. 62.8:** Meckel's diverticulum (*Courtesy:* Dr Naaz Jahan Sheik, Senior Consultant Surgeon, Hospet, Karnataka)

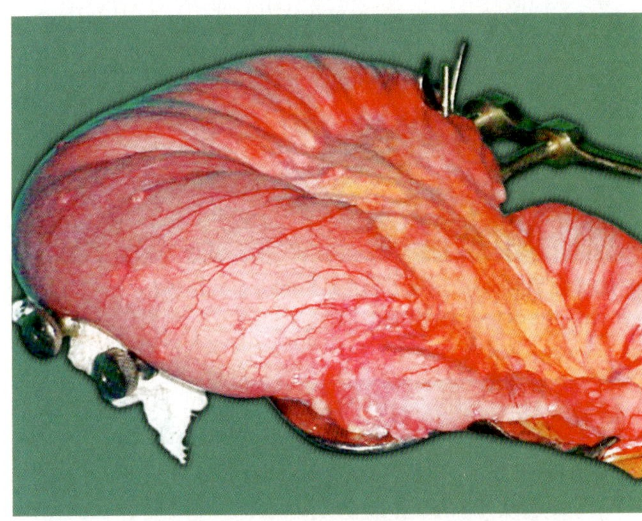

**Fig. 62.9:** Intestinal tuberculosis

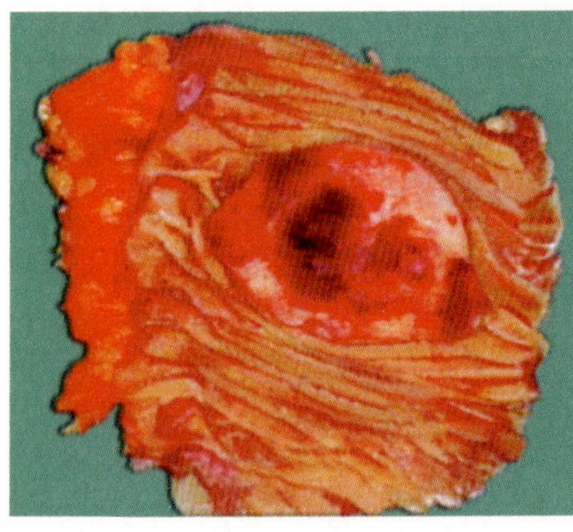

**Fig. 62.10:** Adenocarcinoma jejunum

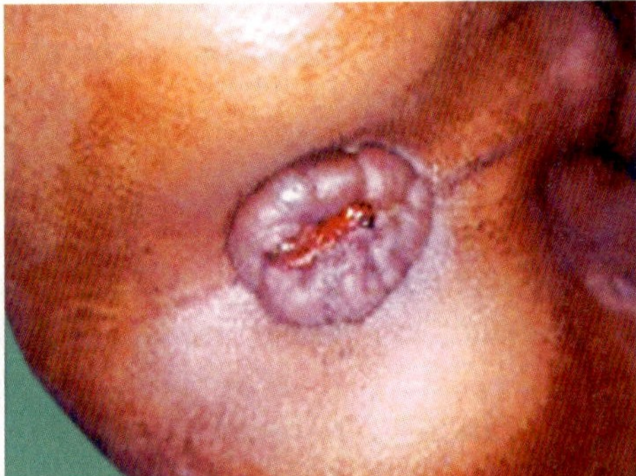

**Fig. 62.11:** Haemorrhoids

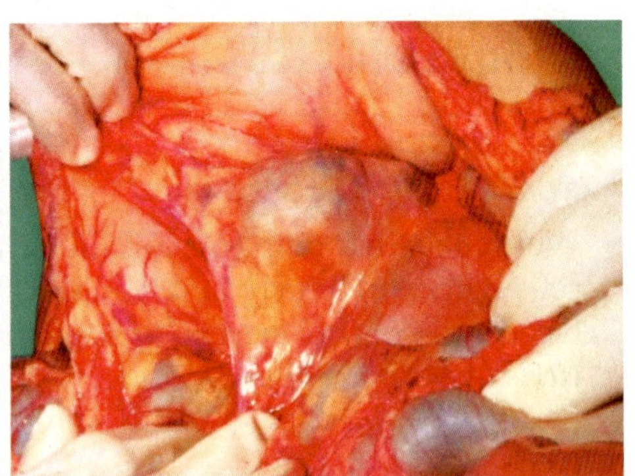

**Fig. 62.12:** Pancreatic pseudoaneurysm

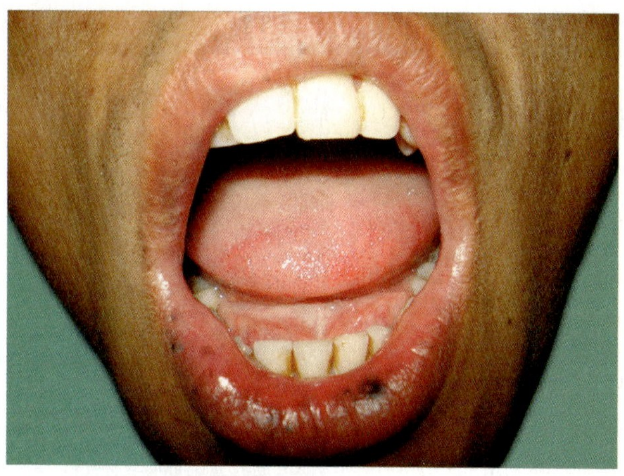

**Fig. 62.13:** Peutz-Jeghers syndrome (*Courtesy:* Dr Sreevatsa, Head, Department of Surgery, Dr Bharathi, Department of Surgery, MS Ramaiah Medical College, Bengaluru)

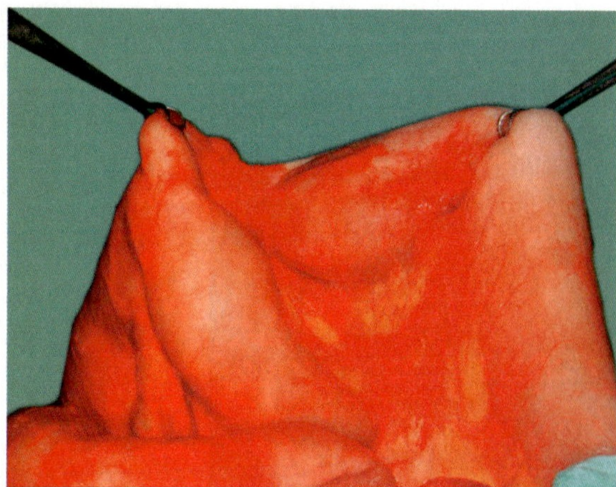

**Fig. 62.14:** Jejunal diverticulum from mesenteric border presented with occult blood in the stool—evaluation of anaemia, diagnosis was by enteroclysis

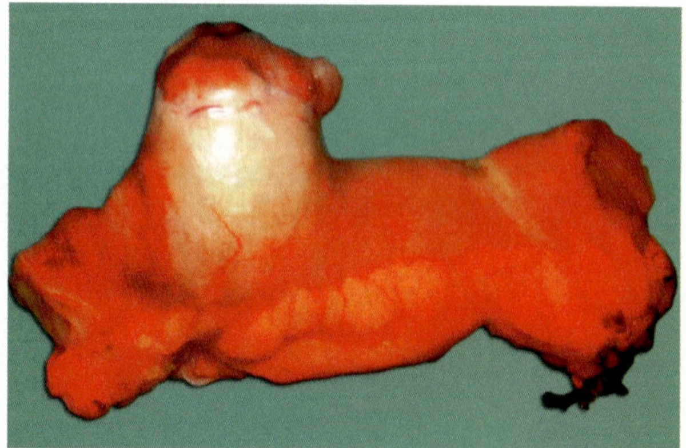

**Fig. 62.15:** Massive lower GI bleeding due to leiomyoma (GIST) of jejunum—resected specimen

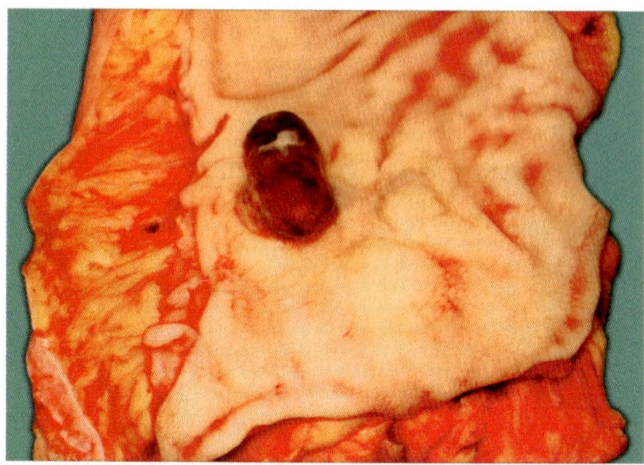

**Fig. 62.16:** Vascular malformation of rectum—misdiagnosed as solitary rectal ulcer with dysplasia

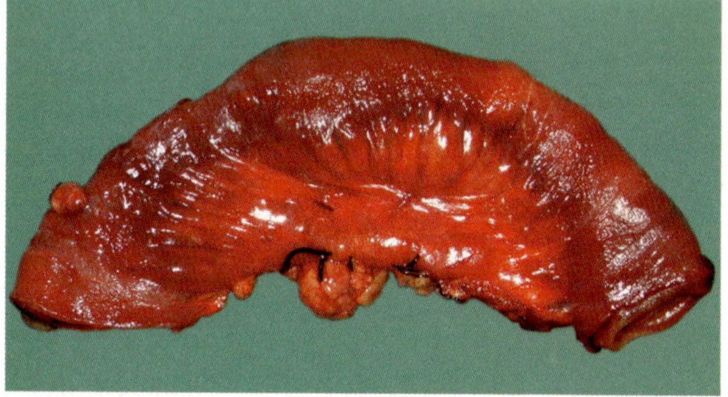

**Fig. 62.17:** Resected specimen of Crohn's disease

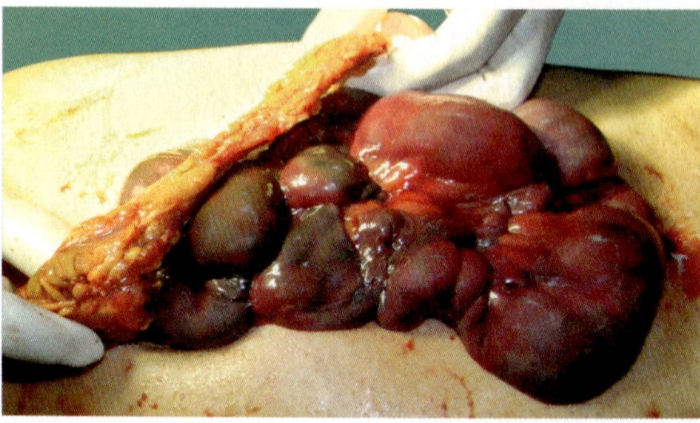

**Fig. 62.18:** Massive gangrene due to superior mesenteric arterial thrombosis



### A. Radionuclear Scanning

- 99mTc-labelled sulphur colloid or autologous red cells with 99mTc may be given which can detect the bleeding site. ***It is extremely sensitive, can detect as little as 0.1 ml/min of bleeding.***
- Less precise but less invasive with least complications. If 99mTc-tagged RBC scan is positive, then angiogram is used to localise the bleeding site.

### B. Visceral Angiography (Fig. 62.19)

- All three vessels—coeliac, superior mesenteric and inferior mesenteric arteries are used.
- Extravasation of contrast into the bowel lumen is suggestive of a 'lesion'.
- Bleeding rate should be at least 0.5 ml/minute.
- Thus, Meckel's diverticulum, angiodysplasia, small bowel tumours, vasculitis, etc. can be diagnosed.

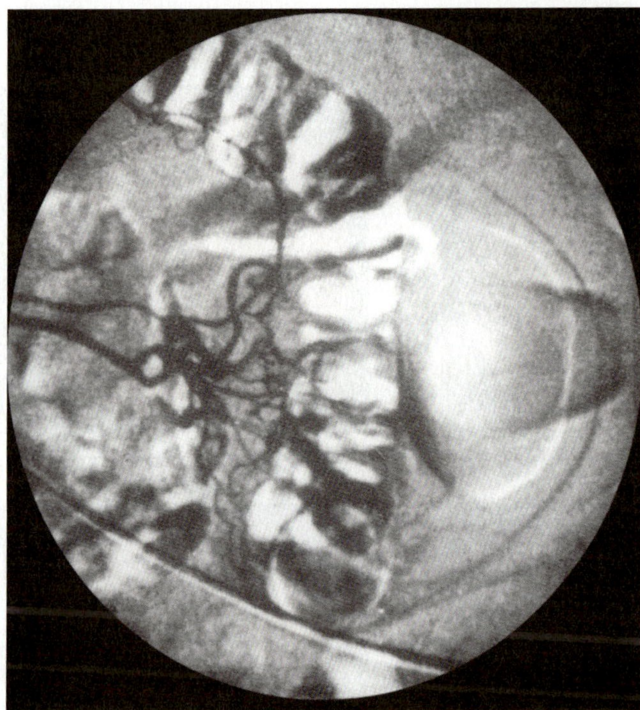

**Fig. 62.19:** Inferior mesenteric angiography showing leakage of dye into the lumen of sigmoid colon—sigmoid angiodysplasia

### C. Capsule Endoscopy

#### Definition

- It is an investigation wherein a small camera pill is swallowed to study the entire GI tract, in particular, small intestines.
- This **'camera pill'** that is swallowed is disposable.
- It weighs 4 grams and is 26 mm × 11 mm in size.
- Parts: Video camera, lens, colour camera chip, 6 light emitting diodes. As it passes through the entire gastrointestinal tract, images are taken.
- Capsule endoscopy is useful to detect (observe) small intestinal bleeds that are missed by routine upper GI scopy and colonoscopy. The procedure takes very long time for detection of the lesions.
- Such bleeds are called '**obscure**' bleeds. These are very difficult problems to treat because they tend to recur.

#### Procedure

- Patient should be fasting overnight.
- Patient swallows the pill.
- Capsule camera sends signals and pictures—2 pictures/second are taken.
- Capsule gets deactivated in 8 hours and is passed out in stools.
- The receiver tied over patient's waist receives signals and 'endo' pictures. This is connected to computer software and pictures are obtained.

#### Drawbacks

- Biopsy of the lesion cannot be taken.
- It cannot detect motility disorders which are very important in GIT.
- Expensive, not available in many centres.
- **Capsule** retention resulting obstruction can occur (*see* page 1006).

#### Conclusion

- Thus, it can detect polyps, inflammatory bowel disease (Crohn's disease), ulcers and tumours of the small intestine.
- Capsule endoscopy is an excellent tool in the patient who is haemodynamically stable but continues to bleed. Reported success rates as high as 90% in identifying small bowel pathology. It is usually well tolerated, although it is contraindicated in patients with obstruction or a motility disorder.

### D. Push Enteroscopy (see Figs 62.29 and 62.30)

- It employs 400 cm scope which is 'pushed' (hence push enteroscope) through duodenum, through DJ flexure into intestines. It needs lots of skill and expertise. It can detect leiomyoma of jejunum, small intestinal diverticular bleed causing chronic anaemia, etc.
- Extended enteroscopy is the same as enteroscopy but may take 6–8 hours till the scope travels distally with peristalsis. Up to 70% small intestine can be visualised.

> *Pearls of Wisdom*
>
> A tagged red blood cell scan can detect bleeds as low as 0.1 ml/minute but does not provide anatomical details. Angiogram can detect bleed at 0.5 ml/min. Embolisation with metal coils can be done to correct bleed. Methylene blue can be injected to stain target segment of intestine.

## MASSIVE LOWER GI BLEEDING

Massive lower GI bleeding is defined as haemorrhage distal to the ligament of Treitz that requires more than 3 units of blood in 24 hours (*see* Fig. 62.31).

### Common Causes

Diverticular disease, inflammatory bowel diseases, angiodysplasia, Meckel's diverticulum, haemobilia, etc.

**Signs of hypovolemia:**

- Mild to moderate hypovolemia: **Resting tachycardia.**
- Blood volume loss of at least 15%: **Orthostatic hypotension** (a decrease in the systolic blood pressure of more than 20 mmHg or decrease in diastolic pressure of more than 10 mmHg when moving from recumbency to standing).

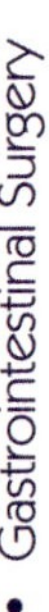

## ROLE OF COLONOSCOPY/ENTEROSCOPY (Figs 62.20 to 62.30)

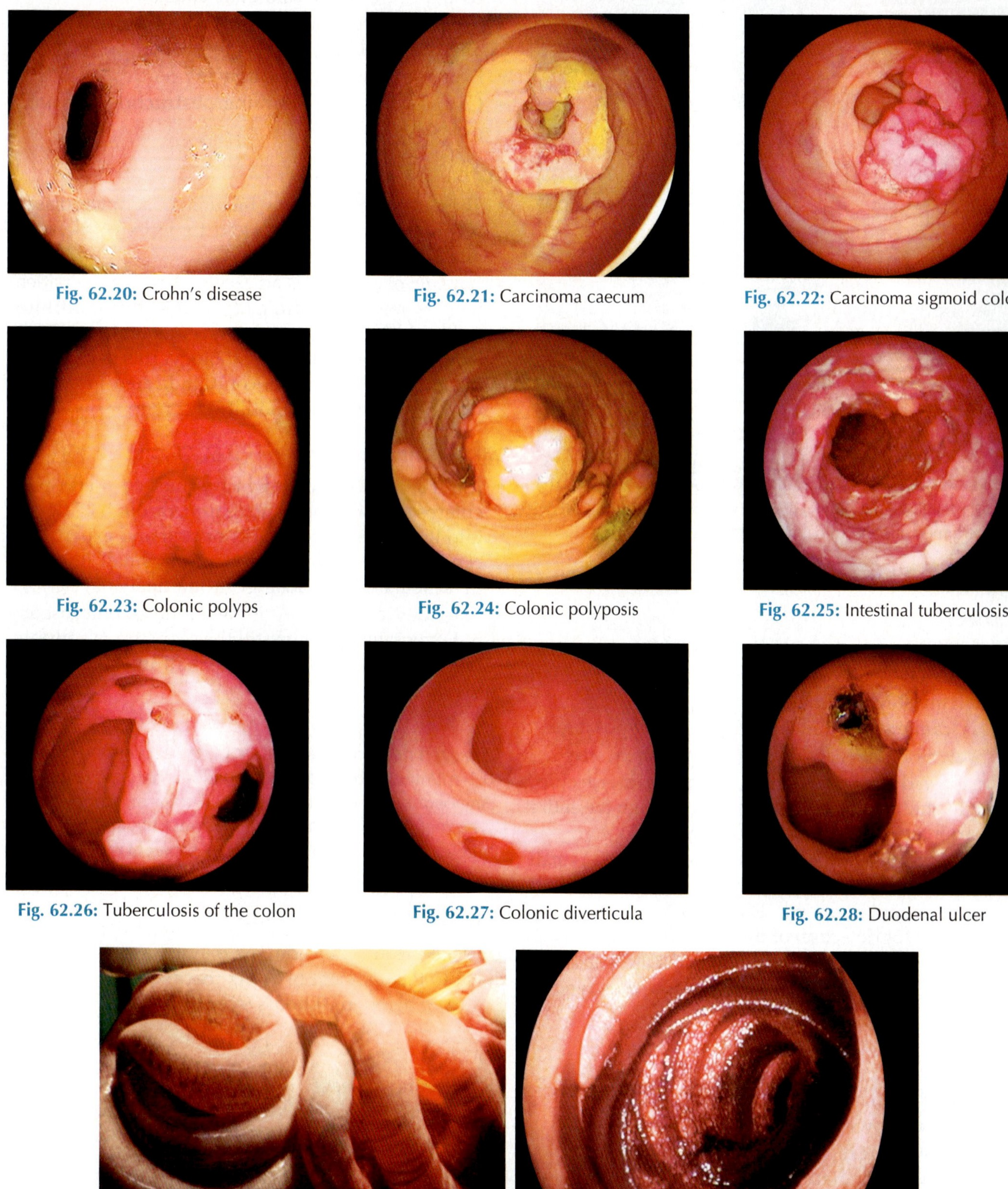

**Fig. 62.20:** Crohn's disease

**Fig. 62.21:** Carcinoma caecum

**Fig. 62.22:** Carcinoma sigmoid colon

**Fig. 62.23:** Colonic polyps

**Fig. 62.24:** Colonic polyposis

**Fig. 62.25:** Intestinal tuberculosis

**Fig. 62.26:** Tuberculosis of the colon

**Fig. 62.27:** Colonic diverticula

**Fig. 62.28:** Duodenal ulcer

**Figs 62.29 and 62.30:** Enteroscopy done at laparotomy for suspected case of angiodysplasia of the jejunum—resected successfully. (*Courtesy:* For all the endoscopic pictures: Dr Filipe Alvares, Gastroenterologist, ex-KMC, Manipal)

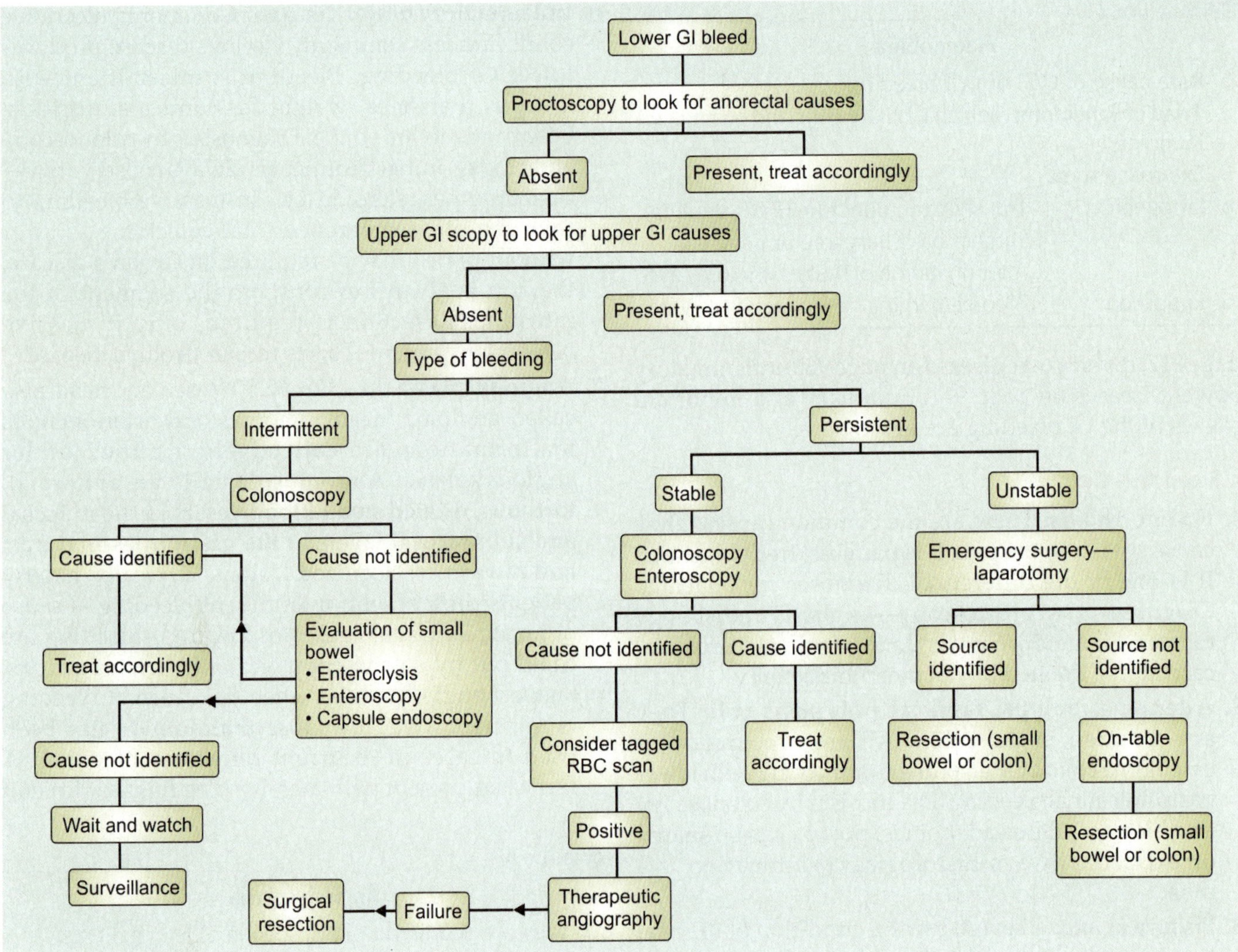


Fig. 62.31: Schematic representation of approach to lower GI bleeding (*Courtesy*: Dr Prasad S, Professor and Head, Department of Surgery, KMC, Manipal)

- Blood volume loss of at least 40%: **Supine hypotension.**
- **Refer to page 66 for more details about haemorrhagic shock and details about resuscitation.**

## Diagnosis

Diagnosis is established by colonoscopy, RBC tagged scan and angiography in most of the cases.

## Treatment

- Initial aggressive resuscitation by fluids, blood transfusion and treatment of shock.
- Emergency colonoscopy and vascular malformations, if detected, can be treated by argon plasma coagulation or by cauterisation.
- Therapeutic ***vasopressin*** infusion 0.2 units/minute via ***angiographic catheter*** with or without embolization will stop or arrest the lower GI bleeds in more than 85% of cases.
- Unstable patient should be subjected to urgent laparotomy.

## A Few Important Tips at Exploratory Laparotomy

- Laparoscopy is done first. If a lesion is identified, an example a stromal tumour, Meckel's diverticulum or polyps, the loop can be brought outside and can be dealt with accordingly. Otherwise, midline incision is **preferred**.
- Careful inspection and palpation of entire small and large bowel.
- Empty small bowel. Then palpate for hidden lesions.
- Intraoperative colonoscopy/enteroscopy, if no obvious lesion is found.
- Endoscopic evaluation of transilluminated gut wall.
- Rarely blind resection of suspected intestinal segment may be required.

## DIFFERENTIAL DIAGNOSIS

All the topics related to GI bleeding have been discussed in the respective chapters. Example: Haemobilia (Key Box 62.4) on page 1060, haemosuccus pancreatitis on

Key Box 62.4

**Haemobilia**

- Rare cause of UGI or LGI bleeding
- **Triad of Sandblom:** Melaena, biliary colic and obstructive jaundice
- External trauma
- Iatrogenic – Transhepatic puncture (PTC, stenting)
  - – Surgery on biliary tree or pancreas
  - – After dilatation of biliary strictures, etc.
- Endoscopy – Blood emerging from ampulla of Vater

page 817, diverticular disease on page 960, inflammatory bowel diseases on page 911. Summary and important causes of the GI bleeding are given here.

### I. From the Colon

1. **Haemorrhoids:** These are the common causes. They cause **splash in the pan**. It is painless, fresh bleeding. It is one of the differential diagnoses for anaemia. Diagnosis is by proctoscopy—as cherry red spongy masses. Sigmoidoscopy is done to rule out proximal carcinoma. Treated by haemorrhoidectomy.
2. **Adenoma, polyps, familial polyposis coli:** They are common in the colon. All are precursors for carcinoma colon. Often patients are young with lower gastrointestinal bleeding. Diagnosis is by colonoscopy and biopsy. Villous adenomas, polyps can be snared or excised. Always histological examination is a must.
3. **Fissure *in ano*:** A severe painful condition of the anal canal, results in constipation, hard pellet-like stools and drop of blood. Initial treatment is conservative in the form of local lignocaine-based ointments, sitz bath, stool softening agents, and good hydration. If conservative treatment fails, it is treated by lateral sphincterotomy.
4. **Carcinoma rectum/colon:** Fresh bleeding per rectum, bloody slime, loss of weight, anaemia, mass abdomen in an elderly patient suggests it could be carcinoma rectum/colon. Diagnosis is by colonoscopy and biopsy. Treated by colectomy or anterior resections or abdomino-perineal resections depending upon the location, involvement of sphincter and grade of the tumour.
5. **Diverticular disease of the sigmoid colon:** Common in Western patients, diet poor in fibre is mostly the cause. The diverticuli are acquired herniation of the mucosa, hence thin. Bleeding can be occult/intermittent or massive. Diagnosis is by colonoscopy. To visualise the bleeders, endotherapy can be done by injecting adrenaline into the bleeding vessel. In emergency situations, with massive lower GI bleeding, emergency colectomy is required.
6. **Inflammatory bowel diseases:** Commonly ulcerative colitis and less commonly Crohn's disease produces lower GI bleeding. Bleeding is intermittent with mucous diarrhoea, weight loss and malnutrition. Often patients are young. Diagnosis is by colonoscopy and biopsy. Initial treatment is always conservative—salazopyrines, steroids, etc. In massive bleeding to save the life—emergency total colectomy with or without pouch may be required. In Crohn's disease, the aim is always to conserve the segment of the intestine. Resection is required, only if massive bleeding is present. This is rare in Crohn's disease.
7. **Angiodysplasia** (Key Box 62.5): Vascular ectasia also called angioma, haemangiomas and arteriovenous malformations are collectively grouped under angiodysplasia. **Angiodysplasia is an abnormal, tortuous, dilated small blood vessel in the mucosal and submucosal layers of the gastrointestinal tract and always are acquired lesions.** Typically, elderly patients present with intermittent bleeding is cause of anaemia. Usual causes of lower GI bleeding are ruled out by colonoscopy and other investigations. Suspect angiodysplasia when the cause of bleeding is not identified, low dose thalidomide has been used in cases of recurrent refractory bleeding. A few cases present with massive bleeding—a difficult

Key Box 62.5

**Angiodysplasia**

- They are acquired lesions, seen in elderly patients.
- These lesions are seen in acute renal failure, von Willebrand's disease, HHT.
- Less rapid, but recurrent.
- Caecum and right colon are common sites—caecum is the most common site.
- Small bowel (proximal) is the second common site.
- Small red mucosal lesions between 2 and 10 mm, flat or raised lesions—dilated tortuous submucosal veins.
- Recurrent painless and self-limiting bleeding often **associated with aortic stenosis with angiodysplasia—Heyde's syndrome.**
- Colonoscopy is the investigation of choice.
- Enteroscopy, capsule endoscopy and intraoperative endoscopy are useful investigations.
- They can be treated endoscopically—Argon plasma coagulation ablation—is the most commonly used intervention, in which high-frequency energy is transmitted to tissues by ionized gas. Other modalities of treatment include: coagulation with heat probe, bipolar electrode or laser, etc. but recurrence or failure can occur.
- Surgery by resecting the segment is a definitive procedure.

problem to treat. Repeat colonoscopy, capsule endoscopy, angiography, on-table enteroscopy are the taxing investigations—all may provide no results: Endoscopic methods such as argon plasma coagulation is the first preferred method. In massive bleeding when all means fail: emergency colectomy or intestinal resection of the suspicious segment may be required.

8. **Ischaemic colitis:** Elderly, hypertensive patients present with diffuse abdominal pain, severe in nature, with blood in stools—it is often massive, sometimes moderate. On examination, tenderness may be present on the left side of the colon. Plain X-ray abdomen supine will show **thumb printing sign** due to mucosal oedema and submucosal haemorrhage. CT scan—colonic wall thickening with posterior fat shadowing. Colonoscopy may reveal ulcers or a few changes in the splenic flexure region. If conservative measures fail such as blood transfusion, segmental colectomy may be required.
   - Ischaemic colitis is a non-inflammatory condition affecting splenic flexure region resulting in ischaemia and lower GI tract bleeding.
   - Elderly hypertensive patients are commonly affected.
   - Often they are males.
   - The splenic flexure region can have relative less vascularity. The exact point is called **Griffith's point** (Fig. 62.32).
   - It is defined as the site of (a) communication of the ascending left colic artery with the marginal artery of Drummond, and (b) anastomotic bridging between the right and left terminal branches of the ascending left colic artery at the splenic flexure of the colon.
   - Anastomosis at Griffith's point is present in 48%, poor or tenuous in 9%, and absent in 43%.

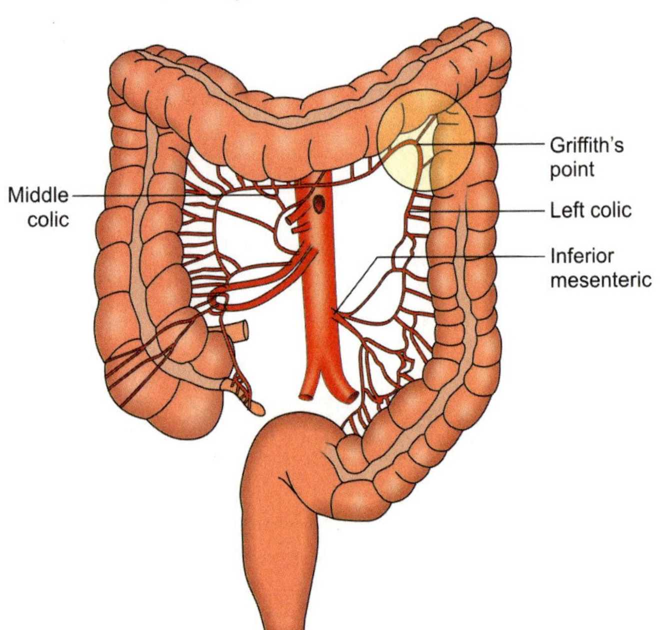


**Fig. 62.32:** Ischaemic colitis

9. **Dysentery:** Various dysenteries such as amoebic, bacillary, Shigella, HIV related—all produce ulcerations in the colon resulting in blood and mucus in the stools. Gripping pain, acute in nature with or without fever and tenderness over the colon—in the right iliac fossa and in the left iliac fossa are suggestive. Diagnosis is by stool examination and colonoscopy. Treated with antiamoebic drugs or antibiotics.
10. **Irradiation proctitis or telangiectasia:** Usually occurs with pelvic radiotherapy, example—radiation given to treat carcinoma cervix. Most common site is rectum. Tenesmus, mucus and blood in stool are common. Proctoscopy reveals ulceration. Treated with stool softening agents, 5-ASA (aminosalicylic acid) topical or steroid enema. Acute irradiation injury occurs within six weeks of therapy. Chronic radiation procto-sigmoiditis has a more delayed onset. The first signs often occur at approximately 9 to 14 months following radiation exposure, but may develop after more than two years in some patients.

## II. From the Small Intestines

1. **Tubercular ulcers:** They are never massive bleeders. Patients are between 20 and 40 years old with blood and mucus in the stools, loss of weight, crampy abdominal pain, evening rise of temperature with or without pulmonary tuberculosis. On examination, mass may be palpable, if caecum is also involved (ileocaecal tuberculosis). Visible step ladder peristalsis indicates obstruction from a tubercular stricture or obstruction due to mass. Colonoscopy with visualisation of the terminal ileum and biopsy is the key to the diagnosis. Obstructed cases can be treated with stricturoplasty in a single stricture or resection in appropriate cases. Cases without obstruction are treated with antitubercular treatment.
2. **Crohn's ulcers:** Ileum is the commonest site—rest of the bowel can also be affected. Transmural inflammation, multiple ulcers, skip lesions are other features. Diagnosis is by CT scan, push enteroscopy and biopsy. Treatment is as for ulcerative colitis (for more details *see* page 914).
3. **Enteric ulcers:** High grade fever—enteric fever patient who has bleeding after 15 days of fever may be having enteric ulceration of the Peyer's patches with bleeding. In majority of the cases, bleeding is occult and usually stops once the disease is treated, rarely exploration and resection of the segment may be required in cases of massive bleeding cases.

4. **Meckel's diverticulum:** Children or young patients, often bleeds are intermittent, maroon coloured with or without abdominal pain. Peptic ulceration in the ectopic mucosal site in the Meckel's diverticulum causes bleeding. Colonoscopy is normal. RBC-tagged technetium scan is the investigation of choice. It can pick up as little as 0.1 ml/min of bleeding. Exploration and excision of the Meckel's diverticulum is the treatment of choice.
5. **Angiodysplasias:** Small intestines are the most common sites of angiodysplasia. They are the differential diagnoses for obscure bleeds. Angiogram and small bowel push enteroscopy, capsule endoscopy are the investigations. Diagnosis is by exclusion.
6. **Small bowel tumours:** They are uncommon causes of lower GI bleeding. They have to be kept in mind when the common causes described above are ruled out one by one. Adenocarcinoma, lymphoma and stomal tumours (GIST—gastrointestinal stomal tumours) are a few examples. GIST can affect small intestine. The mucosal ulcerations cause GI blood loss. Bleeding is not massive—can be intermittent and result in anaemia. **Palpable mass sometimes massive which is bosselated, anaemia and bleeding are the triad of GIST.** CT scan is the investigation of choice. Resection almost cures the disease. Degree of malignancy is decided by the mitotic figures in pathology. Imatinib is the drug used in recurrent cases of GIST or GIST with metastasis. Patients with liver metastasis will live beyond 5–10 years with imatinib.

## MULTIPLE CHOICE QUESTIONS

**1. Lower GI tract bleeding refers to bleeding:**
A. Below ligament of Treitz
B. Below ampulla of Vater
C. Below Meckel's diverticulum
D. Distal to ileocaecal junction

**2. Most important inherited anomaly which produces bleeding is:**
A. Juvenile polyp
B. Meckel's diverticulum
C. Familial polyposis coli
D. Hereditary haemorrhagic telangiectasia

**3. The ideal investigation for bleeding Meckel's diverticulum is:**
A. CT scan
B. Colonoscopy
C. 99mTc-tagged RBC scan
D. Push enteroscopy

**4. Following facts are true for angiodysplasia, *except*:**
A. They are congenital lesions
B. Right colon is the common site
C. It is one of the causes of obscure bleeding
D. Small bowel is the second common site

**5. Following are true about capsule endoscopy, *except*:**
A. It is disposable pill
B. Ideal for small intestinal bleeds
C. Biopsy can be taken
D. Capsule retention can occur

**6. Following are true for jejunal bleeding lesions, *except*:**
A. Carcinoma
B. Meckel's diverticulum
C. Angiodysplasia
D. Hamartomatous polyp

**7. Following are true for haemobilia, *except*:**
A. It causes melaena
B. It causes biliary colic
C. Obstructive jaundice
D. Splenomegaly

**8. Which one of the following is the cause for massive lower GI bleeding?**
A. Carcinoma rectum
B. Crohn's colitis
C. Typhoid colitis
D. Diverticulitis of the colon

**9. Which one of these causes bleeding with septic shock?**
A. Carcinoma colon
B. Ulcerative colitis
C. Mesenteric ischaemia
D. Angiodysplasia

**10. Which one of these causes painless and massive bleeding per rectum?**
A. Angiodysplasia
B. Sigmoid volvulus
C. Necrotising enterocolitis
D. Mesenteric ischaemia

**Answers**

**1.** A **2.** D **3.** D **4.** A **5.** C **6.** B **7.** D **8.** D **9.** C **10.** A

Chapter 63

# Appendix



## Introduction

Acute appendicitis is the most common emergency encountered by the general surgeons. Men have slightly increased incidence of acute appendicitis compared to women. Incidence is 11 per 10,000 persons/year. The choice of surgery today is laparoscopic appendicectomy—one advantage being one can look into all quadrants of the abdomen—not to miss other causes such as perforated duodenal ulcer (*see* later **Valentino appendix**), etc. and very helpful to detect subhepatic appendicitis.

### Lessons Learnt from History

**Valentino appendix:** Rudolf Valentino was an Italian actor acting in Hollywood who was operated for right iliac fossa pain with features of peritonitis in the early 20th century. Following a few days of surgery, he died of sepsis. The actual disease was perforated duodenal ulcer. This is a typical case scenario that holds true even today. The contents from upper abdomen after perforation or pancreatitis, gravitate down along right paracolic gutter. The symptoms and signs mimic appendicitis. CT scan is the investigation needed to rule out other causes.

## Historical Events Related to Appendix

| | |
|---|---|
| Claudius Amyand (1736) | Removed inflamed appendix from hernia sac |
| Reginald Fitz (1886) | Coined term appendicitis |
| Charles McBurney (1889) | Described McBurney point |
| Kurt Semm | Did first laparoscopic appendicectomy |
| **Santiaggo Horgan and Mark A Talamini** | **Transvaginal removal of the appendix a procedure called NOTES—Natural Orifice Transluminal Endoscopic Surgery** |

## DEVELOPMENT AND ANOMALIES

Embryologically, the appendix and caecum develop as outpouchings of the caudal limb of the midgut loop in the sixth week of human development. By the fifth month, the appendix elongates into its vermiform shape, hence called vermiform appendix. At birth, the appendix is located at the tip of the caecum but due to unequal elongation of the lateral wall of the caecum, the adult appendix typically originates from the posteromedial wall of the caecum, caudal to the ileocaecal valve. A few anomalies are given below.

1. **Duplication of the appendix** is one anomaly which is further divided as follows:
   Type A: Single caecum—partial duplication
   Type B: Single caecum and 2 separate appendices
   Type C: Double caecum with each one having one appendix (Figs 63.1 and 63.2).
2. **Situs inversus:** In this condition, appendix is found on the left side. Adds confusion to the diagnosis of acute appendicitis.

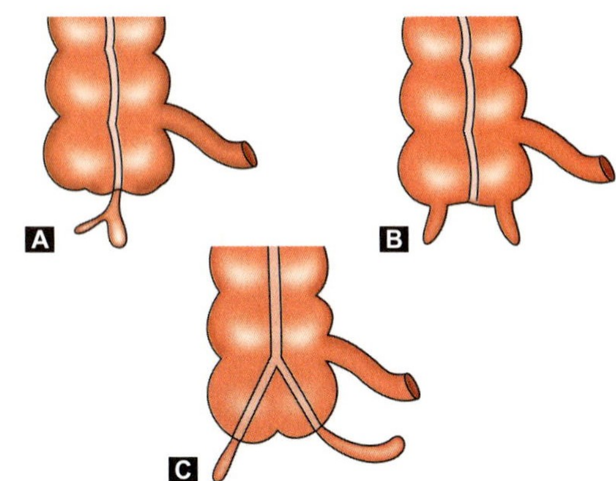


**Figs 63.1A to C:** Anomalies of the appendix (*see* text for details)

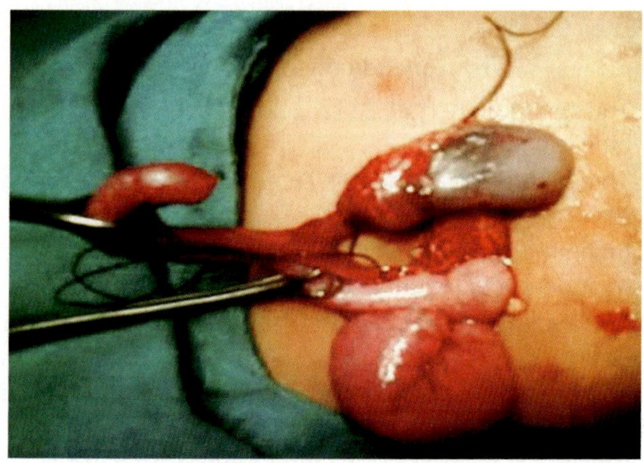

Fig. 63.2: Appendicular duplication and gangrene in one of the moieties

3. **Subhepatic appendix:** It happens in malrotation of the gut. Patients with subhepatic appendicitis may complain of pain in the right lower quadrant. A McBurney incision is usually given only to find no appendix in that location. Laparoscopy has the advantage of looking into all quadrants of the abdomen.
4. **Congenital absence of the appendix** is rare.

## SURGICAL ANATOMY OF THE APPENDIX[1]

**SU28.15.1:** Describe applied anatomy of vermiform appendix.

- It is 8–10 cm long, may vary from 3 to 30 cm in length.
- It is situated 2 cm posteromedial to ileocaecal junction, at the point of convergence of the three taeniae coli.
- It is the primary cause of lower abdominal pain on the right side.

### Positions of the Appendix (Fig. 63.3)

1. Retrocaecal in about 70% of patients (12 o'clock)
2. Pelvic in 20% of cases (4 o'clock)
3. Preileal and postileal (2 o'clock)
4. Subcaecal (6 o'clock)
5. Paracaecal
6. **Subhepatic appendix** is associated with subhepatic caecum. It occurs due to **malrotation of the gut.** (This position is not depicted in the figure.)

### Layers of the Appendix

- Mesoappendix is the continuation of mesentery of the ileum above. It comes down carrying blood vessels in the mesoappendix.
- Appendix has a serosa and a mucosa lined by columnar epithelium (similar to intestinal mucosa) between which are the circular and longitudinal muscle fibres. Crypts are present in the mucosa but less and argentaffin cells (Kulchitsky). They can give rise to neuroendocrine tumours.
- **Submucosa has rich lymphoid follicles** (lamina propria). The lymphatic tissue decreases as age advances. Hence, incidence of **appendicitis is less after the age of 30 years**.
- Appendicular orifice is occasionally guarded by an indistinct semilunar fold of mucous membrane, known as ***valve of Gerlach***.

### Blood Supply of the Appendix

- Appendicular artery is a branch of ileocolic artery. Accessory appendicular **artery of Seshachalam** (a branch of posterior caecal artery) is a branch of ileocolic artery, which runs in the mesoappendix (Fig. 63.4).
- Veins follow the artery and end in the superior mesenteric vein, thus draining into portal vein. This is the reason for development of pylephlebitis in cases of suppurative appendicitis.
- Pylephlebitis means thrombophlebitis of portal veins or its branches.

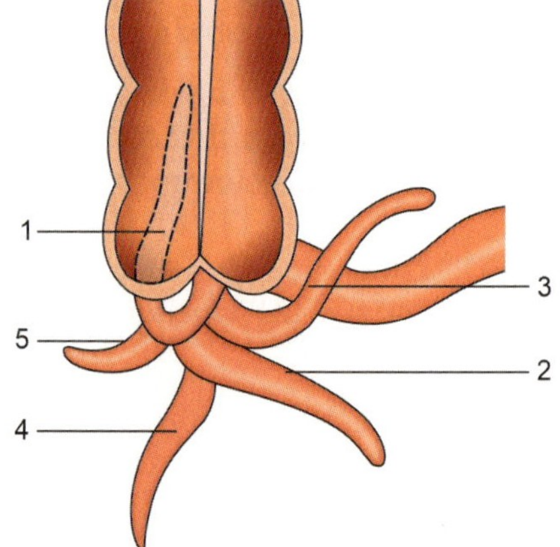


Fig. 63.3: Positions of the appendix (see text for numbers)

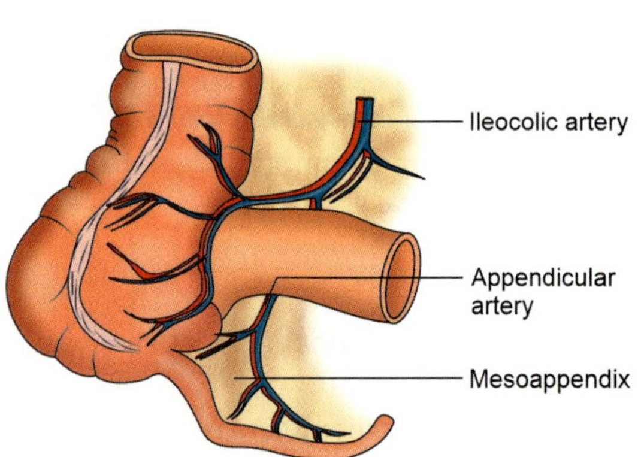


Fig. 63.4: Anatomy of the appendix

[1]Appendix secretes immunoglobulins particularly IgA. So, it is not considered as a vestigial organ anymore. However, appendicectomy is not associated with any immunological compromise.

### Locating the Appendix

Trace the taenia coli or trace ileal loops at laparotomy. Taenia coli point to the base of the appendix. However, surface marking of the appendix is done as follows: Draw a line from anterior superior iliac spine to the umbilicus. The junction of lateral 1/3rd and medial 2/3rds of this line indicates the location of appendix. This is the point of maximum tenderness in appendicitis. This is called **McBurney's point** (Fig. 63.5).

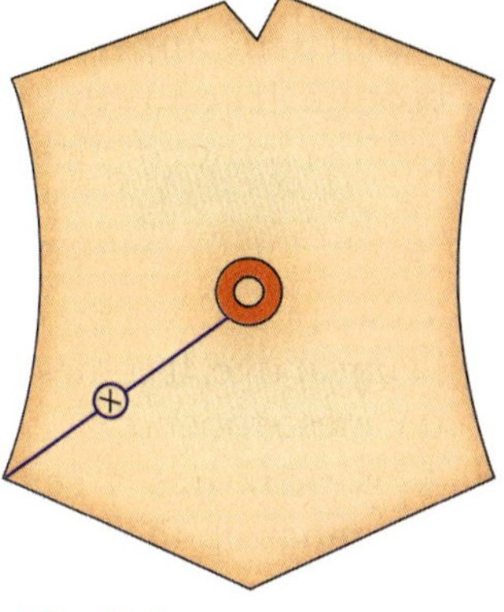

**Fig. 63.5:** McBurney's point

### Surgical Anatomy and Significance

1. **The area of the maximum tenderness** in acute appendicitis is called McBurney's point—corresponds to the site of appendix in vast majority of the cases. This is the site selected for incision in open method.
2. Appendicular artery must be ligated in open or laparoscopic method—**to free mesoappendix**.
3. Severe inflammation of the appendix can spread to portal vein via ileocolic vein and can result in **portal pyaemia,** a very dangerous condition.
4. **Malrotation of the gut**—appendix may be in subhepatic region—to be kept in mind in cases wherein appendix is not found in the right iliac fossa.
5. Appendix has thin muscle coat and lumen is very narrow, easily perforates (Key Box 63.1)

### Lymphatics

The lymphatic channels which are 4 to 6 in number drain into ileocolic nodes, ileocaecal nodes and appendicular nodes in mesoappendix.

## ACUTE APPENDICITIS

It is one of the most common surgical emergencies encountered by general surgeons.

### Definitions

- **Acute appendicitis:** Sudden appearance of signs and symptoms of appendicitis.
- **Recurrent appendicitis:** Recurrent attacks of acute appendicitis—incidence is 15 to 25%.
- **Grumbling appendicitis:** Low grade recurrent bouts of colics, vomiting with frequent admission, self-limiting cases.

Key Box 63.1

**Why Appendicitis is Dangerous?**

- The appendix is a cul-de-sac (closed at one end) and can be easily blocked.
- The appendicular artery is an end-artery (gangrene can occur fast).
- Inflammatory oedema causes easy and early thrombosis of appendicular artery.
- The appendix has thin muscular coat. Hence, perforates easily.
- The lumen of the appendix is very narrow—1–3 mm in diameter.
- Closed loop obstruction: Intraluminal pressure builds up as the appendicular mucosa secretes fluid resulting in mucosal ischaemia. Slowly bacterial overgrowth and translocation occurs.

- **Simple appendicitis:** If duration of symptoms is less than 48 hours or imaging does not show any abscess or phlegmon.
- **Complicated appendicitis:** Acute appendicitis with perforation or large abscess/phlegmon.
- **Pseudoappendicitis:** Acute ileitis mimics appendicitis following ***Yersinia* infection**. It can also be due to **Crohn's** disease.
- **Stump appendicitis:** It is the inflammation and infection of residual appendicular stump (postoperative cases). To avoid stump appendicitis, one should not leave appendicular stump **longer than 3 mm.**
  - Everybody should be aware of this condition.
  - Symptoms are similar to acute appendicitis.
  - More in laparoscopic appendicectomies because of lack of a three-dimensional perspective and absence of tactile feedback.
  - This can happen, if the exact junction of appendix with caecum is not clearly identified.
  - CECT is the best investigation.
  - It may require stump appendicectomy.

**Prevention:** It is important to ligate and divide at the base of the appendix to avoid this complication (more so in laparoscopic appendicectomy).

**SU28.15.2:** Describe etiology, pathogenesis, clinical symptoms and signs of acute appendicitis.

### Aetiology

**1. Racial and dietary factors**

- It is more common in white race than in coloured persons. Young males are affected more often.
- It may be related to **Westernization** of food—a diet rich in meat precipitates appendicitis and ***a diet rich in fibre (cellulose) protects the person from appendicitis.***

2. **Familial susceptibility:** It is related to having a ***long retrocaecal appendix*** in which case the blood supply is diminished to the distal portion and may precipitate appendicitis.
3. **Socioeconomic status:** Appendicitis is common in middle class and rich people. The exact reasons are not known.
4. **Obstructive theory:** Obstruction to the lumen of the appendix due to faecoliths, worms, ova and cysts. Obstruction *can also be due to lymphoid hyperplasia or neoplasm. Entamoeba* causes obstructive appendicitis. Faecolith is seen only in one-third of cases (Fig. 63.6).
5. **Non-obstructive theory:** It is due to bacteria such as *E. coli*, enterococci, Proteus, Pseudomonas, Klebsiella and anaerobes which produce diffuse inflammation of appendix and cause appendicitis. This seems to be more common cause than obstruction.

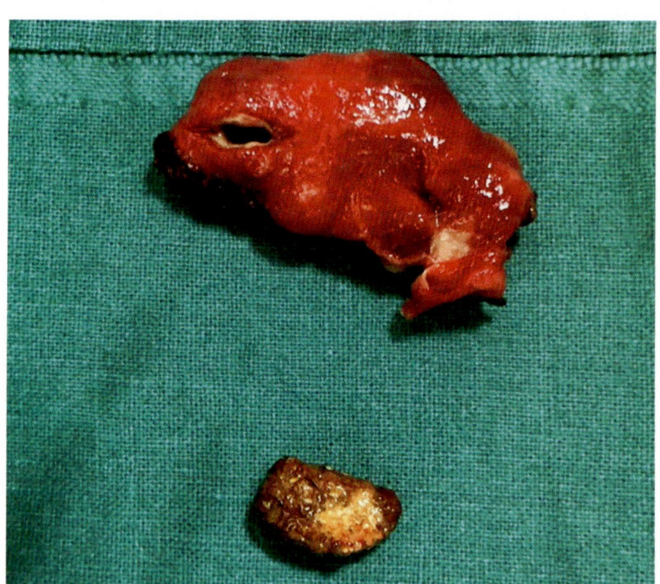

**Fig. 63.6:** Obstructive appendicitis due to large faecolith

## Pathogenesis (Fig. 63.7)

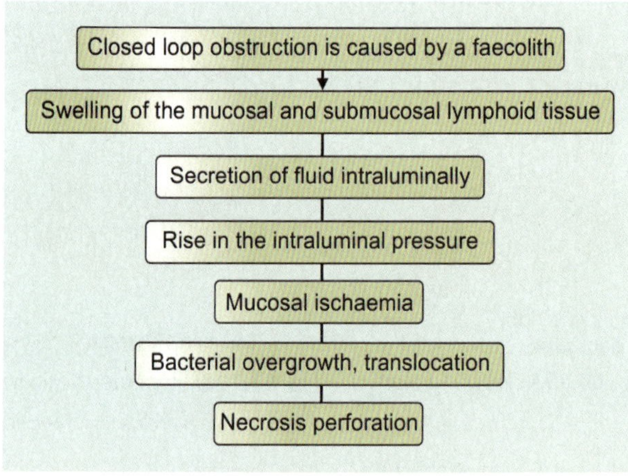


**Fig. 63.7:** Pathogenesis of appendicitis

## Pathology

### I. *In Non-Obstructive Cases (Catarrhal Appendicitis)*

- Process of inflammation is slow and gradual.
- A mild attack may completely resolve or mucosal and submucosal oedema can occur (Key Box 63.2).
- Ulceration of the appendix results in slow bacterial invasion of lymphoid tissue.
- Gangrene and perforation are rare.
- Rarely inflammation may resolve. But appendix is swollen with mucus—may result in **mucocele of the appendix.**

Key Box 63.2

**Nonobstructive Theory in Acute Appendicitis**

- This is seen in two-thirds of the cases. Hence, it is more common than obstructive theory.
- Bacterial or viral infection is the cause.
- It causes mucosal ulceration.
- This is followed by bacterial invasion.
- The decrease in the incidence of enteric fever in the Western world has decreased incidence of acute appendicitis—a support for infective theory.
- In many cases of appendicitis, the appendix is not dilated (against obstructive theory).

### II. *In Obstructive Cases*

- **Symptoms are abrupt, vomiting is more, pain is more and tenderness is more.**
- It is a more dangerous variety.
- Appendix looks inflamed, with congested blood vessels. The tip especially looks more inflamed. As the inflammation is more severe, the outer aspect looks dull and purulent exudates may be seen. Areas of blackening or green colour indicates gangrene or necrosis with perforation. In acute inflammation, neutrophils are dominant and in cases of gangrenous appendicitis, vascular thrombosis is a feature. The important pathological events can be summarized as follows—due to obstruction, the contents get infected fast and the tension increases. The appendix becomes a closed loop, which results in septic thrombosis of vessels. Gangrene of appendix, perforation, peritonitis, followed by a local abscess can occur (*see* Fig. 63.7).
- In **children, greater omentum is very thin**. Hence, it cannot localize the infection. In adults, omentum is like a fatty apron which localizes the infection.
- In **aged patients,** because of atherosclerosis, **gangrene** occurs **very fast** resulting in peritonitis. Obstruction is caused by faecoliths, worms and bands which cause tenting. ***Obstructed appendicitis is one of the examples for closed loop obstruction.*** Other causes are volvulus, carcinoma hepatic flexure with competent ileocaecal valve.

- **Common bacteria encountered in acute appendicitis are *Bacteroides fragilis, Escherichia coli, Clostridium perfringens, Streptococcus faecalis, Pseudomonas aeruginosa,* etc.**

## Clinical Features

The peak incidence is in the second and third decades. Very uncommon before the age of two.

### Symptoms

- **Pain** is severe, colicky type, initially felt in the umbilical region and it is due to ***distension of appendix.*** This is a visceral pain. After a few hours, the pain localizes to the right iliac fossa. It is a ***somatic pain*** which is due to ***inflammation of parietal peritoneum.*** This type of pain is called ***shifting pain of acute appendicitis*** (Fig. 63.8) or ***migratory pain—most reliable symptom of acute appendicitis.***
- Normal appendix is mobile. So, the site of maximum pain and tenderness can vary.
- **Vomiting** occurs once or twice due to reflex pylorospasm. It contains **stomach contents**. However, it is never frequent such as in intestinal obstruction.
- Appendicitis is unlikely in patients with normal appetite. Usually, patients have **anorexia.**
- **Fever** is of low grade (around 100°F) and indicates bacterial inflammation.

*Pearls of Wisdom*

Pain first, followed by vomiting and then by fever is called Murphy's[1] triad of symptoms of acute appendicitis (Murphy's syndrome).

- **Constipation** is the usual feature, except in pre- and post-ileal appendicitis, where they produce diarrhea due to irritation of ileum.

### Signs

1. ***Cough tenderness*** **(Dunphy's sign**—Fig. 63.9**)** indicates inflammation of parietal peritoneum. This is an important physical sign which differentiates acute appendicitis from right-sided ureteric colic.
2. ***Tenderness and rebound tenderness*** are present at McBurney's point. Rebound tenderness is called **Blumberg sign.** It is due to inflammation of the parietal peritoneum. This physical sign can be elicited in all cases of peritonitis.
3. ***Guarding and rigidity*** are present in the right iliac fossa **in complicated appendicitis**. However, guarding and rigidity of back muscles (erector spinae) indicates retrocaecal appendicitis.

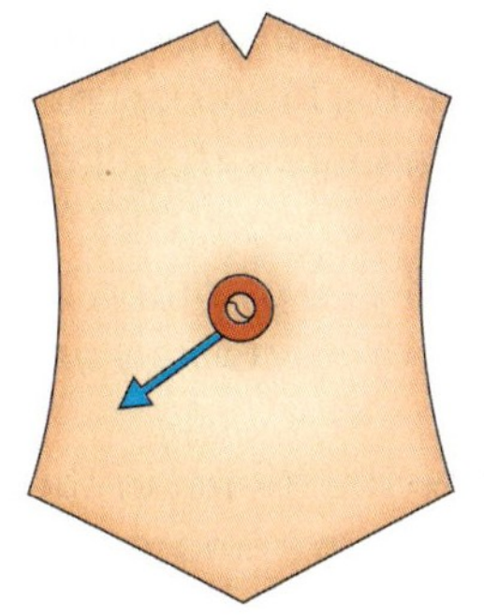

**Fig. 63.8:** Shifting pain (migratory pain)—most reliable symptom

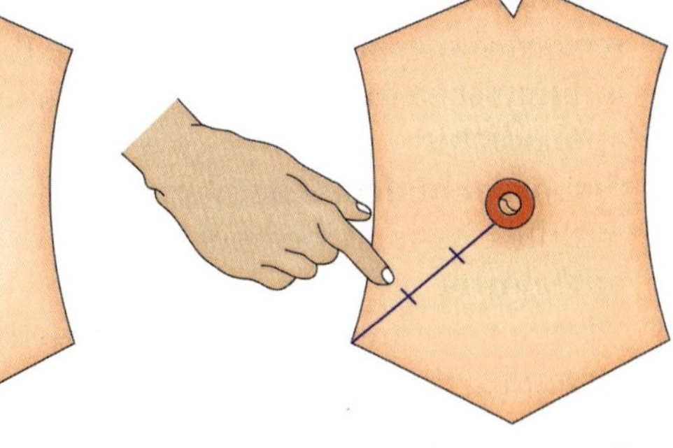

**Fig. 63.9:** Cough tenderness (Dunphy's sign)

4. ***Rovsing sign:*** Palpation of left iliac region of abdomen produces pain in the right iliac region. It is because of displacement of colonic gas and small bowel coils impinging upon the inflamed appendix (Fig. 63.10A).
5. ***Hyperaesthesia*** in the Sherren's triangle (Fig. 63.10B): Sherren's triangle is formed by anterior superior iliac spine, umbilicus and pubic symphysis. It is due to irritation of lower abdominal nerves.
6. ***Cope's psoas test:*** Seen in retrocaecal appendicitis. There will be irritation of psoas major which produces flexion at the hip. If any attempt is made to extend the hip, it produces pain.
7. ***Cope's obturator test:*** Seen in pelvic appendicitis due to irritation of the obturator muscle. Flexion and medial rotation produce pain.
8. ***Features of generalised peritonitis*** are seen only when there is a rupture. Gangrene and perforation is more common in elderly patients because of atherosclerosis. In infants, omentum is very thin without much of fat. Hence, diffuse peritonitis occurs very fast.
9. ***Rectal examination:*** There is tenderness in the right rectal wall—**differential tenderness.**

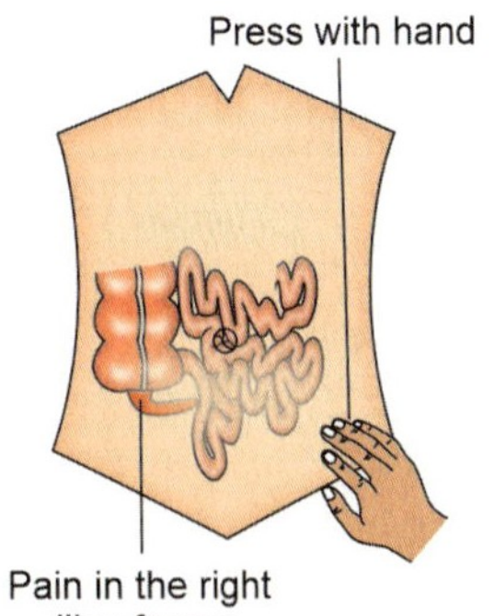


**Fig. 63.10A:** Rovsing sign

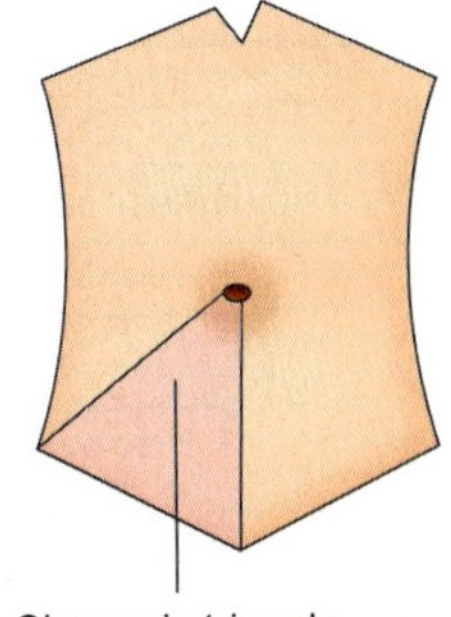


**Fig. 63.10B:** Hyperaesthesia in the Sherren's triangle

[1]Can you find out what is Murphy's sign and Murphy's punch test?

10. *Per vaginal examination:* Presence of ovarian mass, tenderness on **movement** of cervix, adnexal tenderness may suggest obstetric pathology.
    - Signs and symptoms vary depending upon the location (Key Box 63.3).

Key Box 63.3

**Variations in Acute Appendicitis**

1. **Retrocaecal:** Silent (no rigidity in the right iliac fossa).
2. **Pelvic:** Causes diarrhoea.
3. **Postileal:** Causes diarrhoea—called missed appendix.
4. **Subhepatic:** Manifests as pain in the right iliac fossa, very difficult to remove from gridiron incision.
5. **In pregnancy:** The location of the pain is shifted higher up and laterally.

*Pearls of Wisdom*

Pregnancy testing is mandatory in women of child-bearing age.

**SU28.15.3:** Describe complications and principles of management of acute appendicitis.

## Investigations

1. **Total WBC count** is almost always increased above 10,000 cells/mm$^3$, in most of the patients (95%).
    - A very high white blood cell count (>20,000/mm$^3$) suggests complicated appendicitis with gangrene or perforation.
2. **Urine examination** is mainly to rule out urinary tract infection, haematuria and sometimes pyuria. In suspected patients, pregnancy test can also be done.
3. **C-reactive protein** is elevated in any inflammatory condition such as appendicitis. Elevated in the first 12 hours of any acute inflammation and is very non-specific. **However, if total counts and CRP levels are not elevated, probability of acute appendicitis is almost nil.**
4. **Plain X-ray abdomen erect** is taken to rule out other causes of acute abdomen such as perforation of hollow viscus (free gas under the diaphragm) and intestinal obstruction (multiple air fluid levels). In appendicitis, one or two dilated small bowel loops may be seen in right lower region due to ileus. If a radio-opaque stone in the direction of ureter is found, it suggests ureteric colic. Presence of faecolith is highly suggestive of acute appendicitis in plain X-ray.
5. **Abdominal ultrasound** to rule out other causes including gynaecological causes. Ultrasound can demonstrate a non-compressible, aperistaltic tubular organ with a thick wall. It can be used to elicit probe tenderness (sensitivity of 85%, specificity of 90%).

***Advantages***

- It is a simple bedside investigation.
- Economical
- Can confirm acute appendicitis in about 50% of the patients.
- Appendicolith, pericaecal fluid collection or inflammation can be diagnosed—indirect features of acute appendicitis (Figs 63.11A and B).
- More sensitive and specific in children—thin abdominal wall.

***Disadvantages***

- It is operator-dependent
- It is not a choice in fatty obese patient
- Gas within the dilated intestine may obscure the appendix

6. **CECT: Contrast enhanced CT scan is the investigation of choice** (sensitivity of 90 to 100%, specificity of 90%), **especially** when diagnosis is not established or in atypical cases. All the findings mentioned in the ultrasound can also be defined by CT scan (Fig. 63.12).

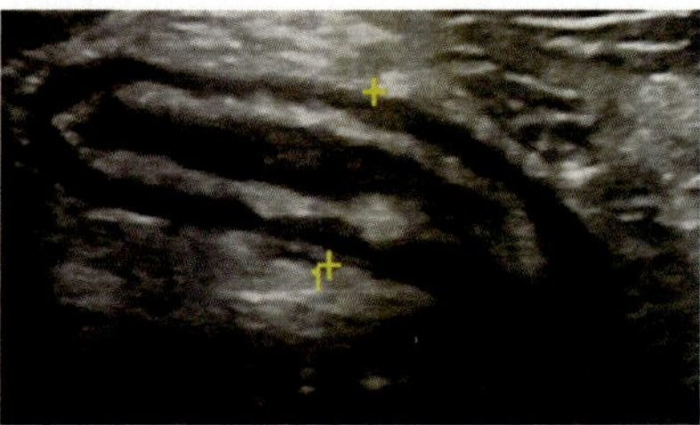

**Fig. 63.11A:** Ultrasound of appendix showing tubular, thickened, aperistaltic structure suggestive of acute appendicitis.

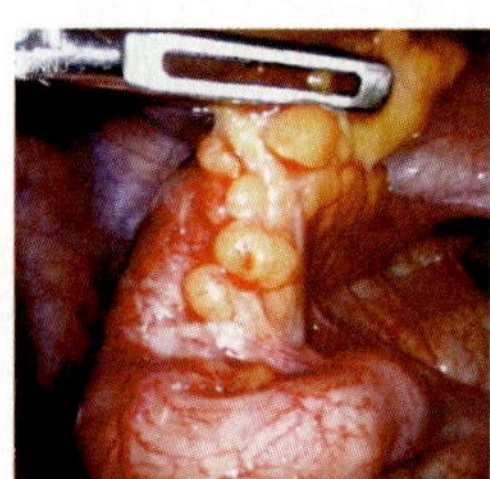

**Fig. 63.11B:** At Surgery, you can see inflamed and thickened appendix.

(*Courtesy*: Dr Naaz Jahan Shaikh, Consultant Surgeon; Hospapete, Karnataka)

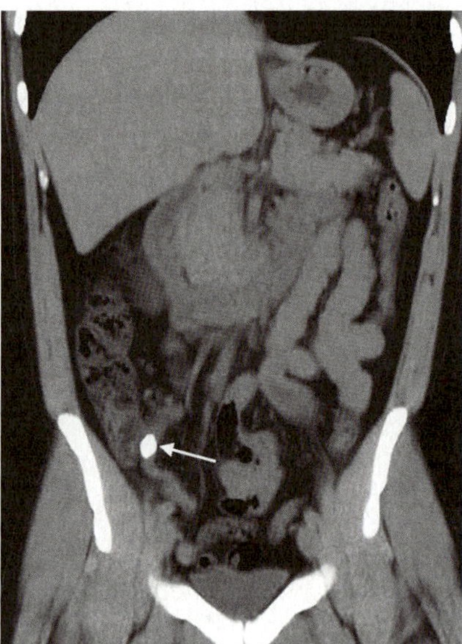

**Fig. 63.12:** CT scan in acute appendicitis—showing a faecolith

*Typical CT findings*

Appendix is more than 7 mm in diameter, thick inflamed wall, mural enhancement (target sign), and periappendicular fluid or air.

*Advantages*

More objective, sensitivity and specificity is almost about 95%, helps to rule out carcinoma caecum, duodenal perforation, acute pancreatitis, etc. Can detect anomaly as in subhepatic appendicitis.

*Disadvantages*

Pregnant woman—it is contraindicated. In children—better to avoid it for the fear of radiation exposure and risk of cancer developing at a later date, expensive, long time for the contrast to reach the site, low fat, sensitivity is less, allergy to contrast and contrast nephropathy (dehydration, high creatinine, diabetics precipitating factors). The importance of CT scan is highlighted in the clinical notes given later.

7. **MRI:** Ideal in pregnant women.

## SCORING SYSTEM

> **SU28.15.7:** Describe components, advantages and disadvantages of scoring systems applied in diagnosis of acute appendicitis.

To avoid negative appendicectomies, many scoring systems have been developed considering signs, symptoms and investigations. I have given 3 scoring systems.

1. **Alvarado scoring system** is given in Table 63.1.

   **Score less than 5** : Not sure
   **Score 5–6** : Compatible
   **Score 6–9** : Probable
   **Score more than 9** : Confirmed

- Even though Alvarado scoring is highly suggestive of appendicitis, it is only a simple and cost-effective scoring system. This can be applied when sophisticated investigations such as ultrasonography and CT scan are not available.

**TABLE 63.1:** Alvarado scoring system

| Features | Score |
|---|---|
| **Symptoms:** | |
| Migrating RIF pain | 1 |
| Anorexia | 1 |
| Nausea, vomiting | 1 |
| **Signs:** | |
| Tenderness RIF | 2 |
| Rebound tenderness | 1 |
| Elevated temperature | 1 |
| **Laboratory:** | |
| Leucocytosis | 2 |
| Shift to left | 1 |
| **Total** | **10** |

2. **Appendicitis inflammatory response (AIR) score:** It incorporates CRP ( C-reactive protein) and considers how right lower quadrant pain progresses. CRP is non-specific. It is not increased initially but raises after 8 to 10 hours following acute appendicitis. CRP is increased in several inflammatory conditions.
3. **The Tzanakis scoring system considers two clinical signs:** Right sided abdominal tenderness (four points) and rebound tenderness (three points). The only laboratory test is a white blood cell count (WBC) greater than 12,000 cells/mm$^3$ (two points). This score considers positive ultrasound scan findings (six points). So this is the big advantage of Tzanakis score. Positive score means increased diameter of appendix, probe tenderness, fecolith, etc.

> ***Surgical wisdom:*** Symptoms, signs (tenderness in McBurney point) and rebound tenderness with increased total counts, you often do not need any **sophisticated imaging** tests. In young women it is extremely useful investigation to rule out gynaecological and obstetric causes.

### Treatment of Acute Appendicitis

#### *Preoperative Resuscitation*

- Once diagnosis of acute appendicitis is suspected, the patient is admitted to the hospital.
- IV fluids—isotonic saline or Ringer lactate is given.
- Electrolytes are corrected especially in late cases of acute appendicitis/perforation peritonitis, etc.
- Ryle's tube is not necessary in simple appendicitis but is definitely required in complicated cases (peritonitis).
- Fluoroquinolones second generation cephalosporins along with metronidazole is given.
- Informed consent is taken.
- **Laparoscopic emergency appendicectomy:** Emergency appendicectomy is offered when patient comes within 24 to 48 hours of abdominal pain. It is very important to rule out or detect a mass, especially if a decision is made to operate around 2nd or 3rd day. If a mass is palpable, it is better not to operate at that time (please refer to operative surgery, appendicectomy). A few important steps are given here (Figs 63.13 to 63.15).
- The appendix is identified by tracing *Taenia coli* which converges onto the base of the appendix. Mesoappendix is divided in between ligatures. A purse-string suture is applied all around the appendix in the caecum. The appendix is divided in between ligatures, the stump is invaginated and the purse-string is tightened. The abdomen is closed in layers.
- **Laparoscopic appendicectomy** has become more popular nowadays because of less postoperative pain, speedy recovery. Benefit is maximum in obese, women and elderly patients. (*see* Chapter 70 Operative Surgery).

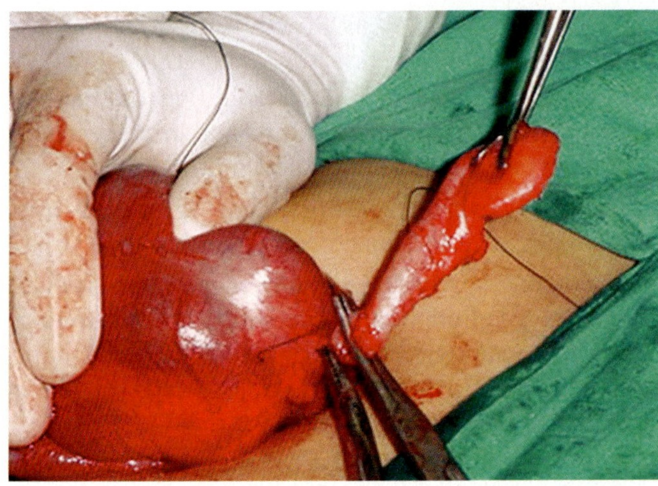

**Fig. 63.13:** Emergency appendicectomy—appendix is identified, isolated by dividing and freed till the base. The base is crushed and divided in between 2 artery forceps

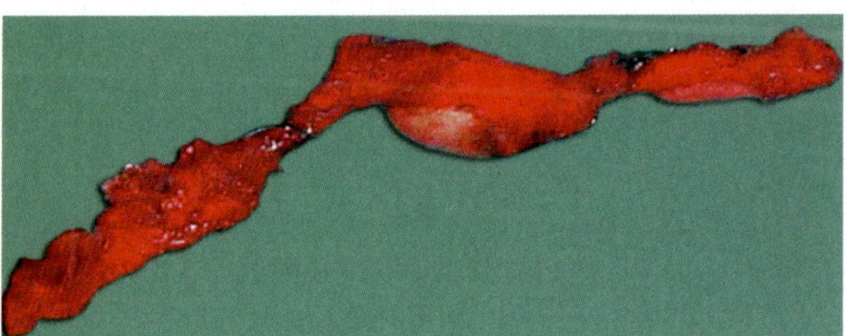

**Fig. 63.14:** Large faecolith resulting in acute appendicitis

*Pearls of Wisdom*

- Early uncomplicated appendicitis is increasingly being managed conservatively nowadays by some experts.
- When you trace Taenia coli and you do not find appendix, it means you are holding and tracing Taenia of the sigmoid colon. (It can be found on the right side sometimes).

Algorithm of treatment of appendicitis is shown in Fig. 63.15.

## COMPLICATIONS OF ACUTE APPENDICITIS

1. **Appendicular mass** (Figs 63.16A and B): Following an attack of acute appendicitis, infection is sealed off by greater omentum, caecum, terminal ileum, etc. which results in a tender, soft to firm mass in the right iliac fossa. **Presence of a mass** is a **contraindication for appendicectomy** because it is very difficult to remove appendix from such a mass. An attempt to remove it may result in a faecal fistula.

*Pearls of Wisdom*

If appendicitis is more than 2 days old and one cannot assess mass clinically due to guarding, always palpate right iliac fossa after general anaesthesia is given, to rule out mass. This can prevent unnecessary exploration.

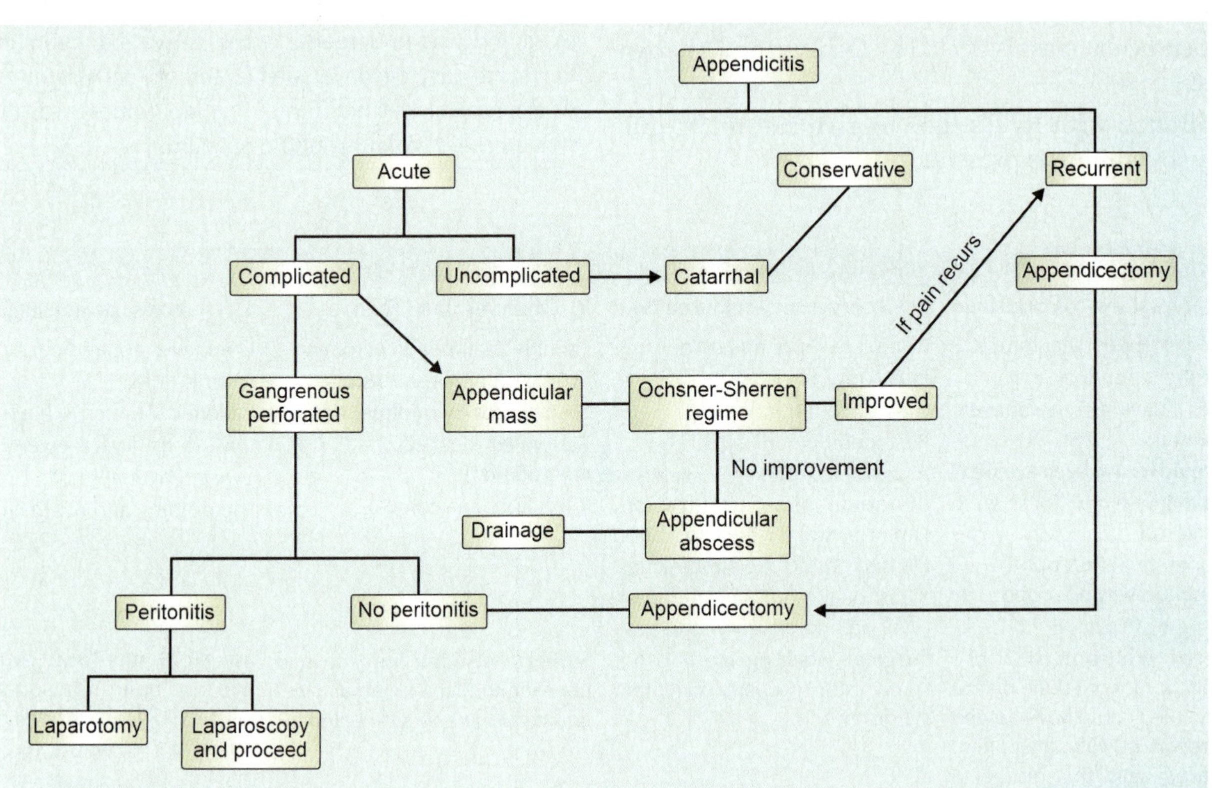


**Fig. 63.15:** Treatment of appendicitis (*Courtesy:* Dr Amith Jain, Professor of Surgery, SRR Medical College, Bengaluru, Karnataka)

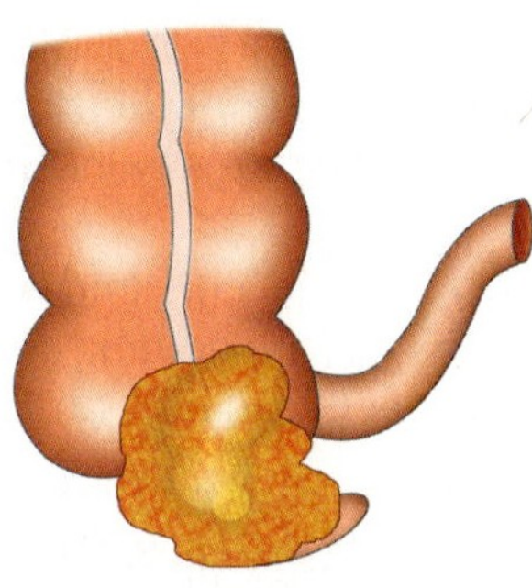

Fig. 63.16A: Appendicular mass—tender, diffuse mass

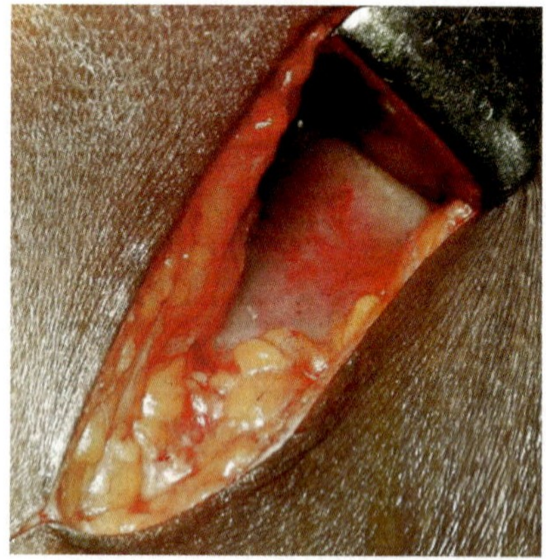

Fig. 63.16B: Appendicular mass: Laparotomy done for appendicectomy but could see the mass. Abandoned the procedure

**SU28.15.5:** Describe management of appendicular mass.

Appendicular mass is treated by **Ochsner and Sherren regime**.

- Aspiration with Ryle's tube to give rest to the gut, only if vomiting is present.
- Bowel care—purgatives should not be used (may cause perforation).
- Charts—temperature, pulse, respiration, diameter of the mass. Swinging temperature, and increase in size of mass indicates an appendicular abscess.
- Drugs to cover all the organisms—gram-positive, gram-negative and anaerobic organisms.
- Exploratory laparotomy should not be done. However, when the condition of the **patient is not improving,** there is a suspicion of an abscess (Fig. 63.17B) and when doubtful of the diagnosis, exploration is indicated (see the clinical notes).
- Fluids (Table 63.2): Patient is kept nil orally for one or two days. During this time, intravenous fluids are given to correct dehydration.
- After 3–4 days, the abdomen becomes soft, tenderness decreases and once stools are passed, Ryle's tube is removed. Clear oral fluids followed by soft diet is given. By one week, the patient is back to normal. **After 6–8 weeks,** patient is advised **elective appendicectomy**.
- Interval appendicectomy is not done nowadays until and unless patient has recurrent symptoms of appendicitis or there is faecolith.

**Clinical Notes**

A 60-year-old lady was diagnosed to have appendicular mass and was undergoing conservative management. On the fourth day, she developed features of early septic shock. As the patient was not improving, laparotomy was done. It was a case of volvulus of the caecum.

**TABLE 63.2:** Wisdom/mistakes/surprises for surgeon while conducting appendicectomy—4 scenarios

| 1. Observes straw-coloured fluid | 2. Observes bile-coloured fluid | 3. Observes 'foul' fluid | 4. Observes haemorrhagic fluid |
|---|---|---|---|
| Completes appendicectomy<br>Closes the wound<br>Realises 3 days later, it was acute pancreatitis<br>**How could it have been avoided?**<br>Serum amylase and lipase were not analysed<br>A preoperative ultrasound examination was not done | Completes appendicectomy<br>Puts a drain<br>Closes the wound<br>Postoperative biliary fistula<br>Asks for contrast CT, **realises duodenal ulcer perforation,** explores, sutures the perforation<br>He had not done a simple chest X-ray or plain X-ray abdomen erect preoperatively in this case | Completes appendicectomy<br>Postoperative faecal fistula<br>Re-explores by midline incision<br>Perforated Meckel's diverticulum<br>Resection, anastomosis | Completes appendicectomy<br>Ignores fluid<br>Patient continues to have pain<br>OBG consultation given<br>Twisted ovarian cyst<br>Laparotomy and ovariectomy |
| **Surgical wisdom:** If these investigations were done before surgery, they could have helped the surgeon. Luckily, the patient recovered from this unnecessary, avoidable surgery | **Surgical wisdom:** He had not taken history properly (Valentino syndrome) | **Surgical wisdom:** Surgeon had not examined the terminal 2 feet ileum during appendicectomy | **Surgical wisdom:** Surgeon had not done ultrasound and gynaecological consultation was not requested before surgery |

**2. Perforated appendicitis**

- Incidence is about 8–10%.
- More common in children and elderly patients.
- Delay in seeking medical treatment is the main factor.
- Other factors which precipitate perforation are diabetes mellitus, AIDS, faecolith.
- The pain usually localizes to the right lower quadrant, if the perforation has been walled off by surrounding intra-abdominal structures including the omentum.
- Perforated appendicitis can also give rise to generalised peritonitis and septic shock (Fig. 63.17).
- Rigors and chills with fever of 102°F (38.9°C) or above.
- As a complication of perforation peritonitis, portal pyaemia (pylephlebitis) can develop, it can be very dangerous.
- Emergency laparotomy, appendicectomy, drainage of pus, peritoneal lavage, and antibiotics are main principles.
- It causes generalised peritonitis with 10–20% mortality rate. Mortality depends upon various factors including age, performance status and delay in presentation to the hospital. Mortality is due to uncontrolled sepsis and multiorgan failure.

*Perforated appendicitis: Principles of surgery*

- Careful handling of appendix, gentle separation of bowel loops.
- Crushing of base is not required. Appendicectomy is done in the usual manner.
- Drainage of abscess cavity/pus. Always drain the peritoneal cavity.
- Wound is closed but skin is not closed (prevents wound infection).
- Continue antibiotics for 4 to 7 days. Enteral nutrition (oral) to be started once paralytic ileus settles down.

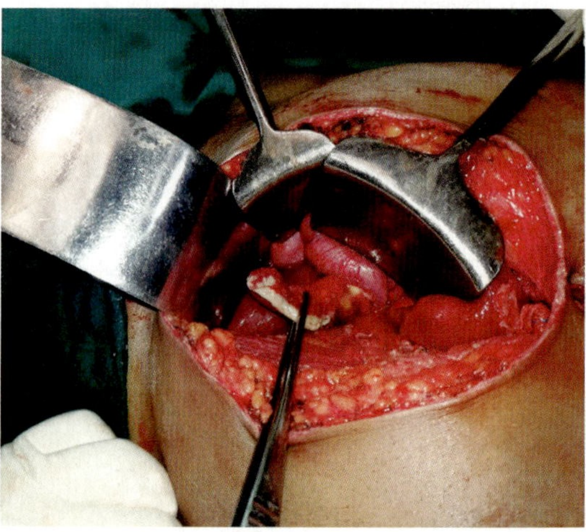

**Fig. 63.17:** Perforated appendicitis at surgery—22-year-old boy presented with septic shock

**3. Appendicular abscess** (Fig. 63.18A): If the infection is not controlled properly following an attack of appendicitis, an abscess can occur in relation to the appendix. They are (A) retrocaecal, (B) postileal and preileal, (C) pelvic, (D) subcaecal abscesses. Clinically, it presents with high-grade fever with chills and rigors and a tender boggy swelling in the right iliac fossa or in the right lumbar region. Pelvic abscess presents with diarrhoea. Diagnosis is by late presentation to the hospital (3–4 days) and high-grade fever with chills and rigors (Key Box 63.4).

Key Box 63.4

**Appendicular Abscess**

- Ultrasound/CT scan is done to assess the size and location of abscess.
- Abscess greater than 4–6 cm in size needs to be drained by guided percutaneous aspiration or drainage through rectum or vagina.
- Ongoing inflammation may force a surgeon to do appendicectomy (open/laparoscopic) at the same admission.
- Those who improve require appendicectomy after 6 weeks.

A. **Retrocaecal abscess** is drained by extraperitoneal approach. An incision of 5 to 6 cm is made in the right iliac fossa and all muscles are divided. However, peritoneum is not opened. It is swept medially and pus is drained outside. Appendicectomy is done at a later date (Figs 63.18B and C).
   - Most of abscesses of this type are drained by ultrasound guided pigtail catheter insertion.

B. **Preileal and postileal abscesses** also can be drained by a pigtail catheter.

C. **Pelvic abscess** is drained *via* the rectum (*see* page 882).

D. **Subcaecal:** May require extraperitoneal drainage.

4. Few cases can have spreading necrotizing fasciitis of the lateral abdominal wall including inguinal region and scrotum. They require more aggressive approach of treatment with antibiotics, debridement, appendicectomy, drainage of pus, etc.

**Clinical Notes**

A 65-year-old lady was examined for feature of acute appendicitis of 8 hours duration. On examination, she had McBurney tenderness but a vague mass was palpable. It is unusual for an appendicular mass to appear within 8 hours following appendicitis. Ovarian pathology was considered, and gynaecological opinion was requested. It was normal. CT scan was done. It revealed mucocoele of the appendix (8 cm size). CT scan gave a correct diagnosis, and it guided the treatment policy.

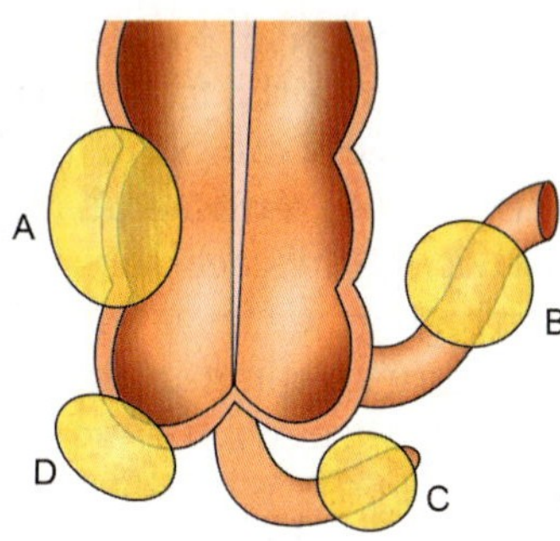


Fig. 63.18A: Appendicular abscess (*see* text for A to D)

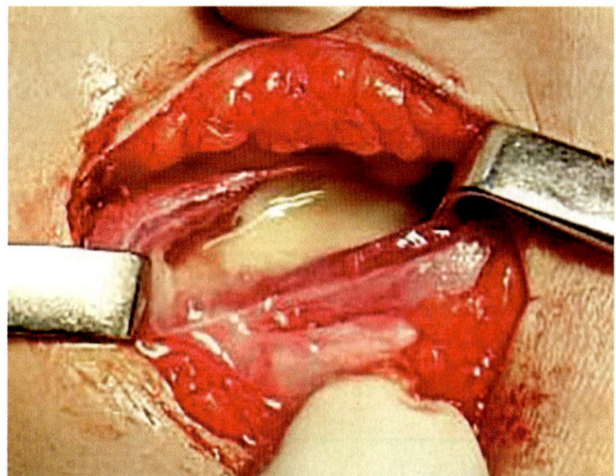

Fig. 63.18B: Appendicular abscess is drained by extraperitoneal route (*Courtesy:* Dr Jyothi, Head, Department of Surgery, GIMS, Gadag, Karnataka)

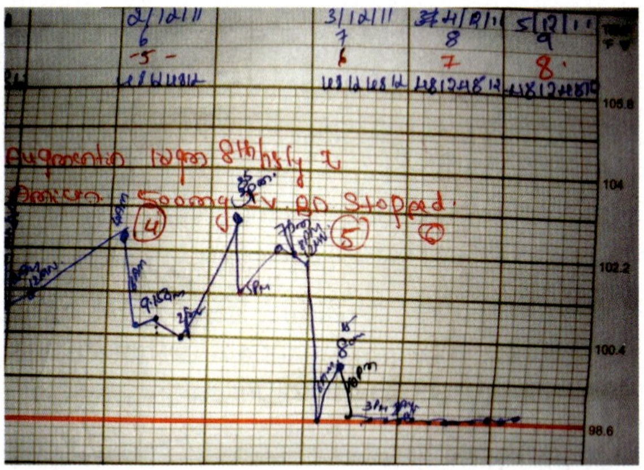

Fig. 63.18C: Appendicular abscess—once drained, fever touched the base

## DIFFERENTIAL DIAGNOSIS OF ACUTE APPENDICITIS

**SU28.15.4:** Describe the differential diagnosis of appendicitis in children, adult, and elderly individuals.

Innumerable conditions may mimic some signs of appendicitis. A few important conditions have been considered here.

### In Children (Figs 63.19A to D)

A. **Enterocolitis** is common in children. It presents with severe diarrhoea with blood and mucus in the stools.
B. **Meckel's diverticulitis** can present with abdominal pain, vomiting, fever—signs and symptoms are similar to acute appendicitis (difficult to differentiate clinically).
C. **Worm ball** is common in children in the developing countries. However, features of intestinal obstruction will be present.
D. **Acute iliac/mesenteric lymphadenitis**—non-shifting pain and rebound tenderness are absent. It is viral in origin and self-limiting. Neck nodes will give clue to the diagnosis.

### In Young Adults (Figs 63.20A to D)

A. **Right-sided ureteric colic:** Haematuria, severe pain from loin to groin, absence of cough tenderness help in excluding acute appendicitis.

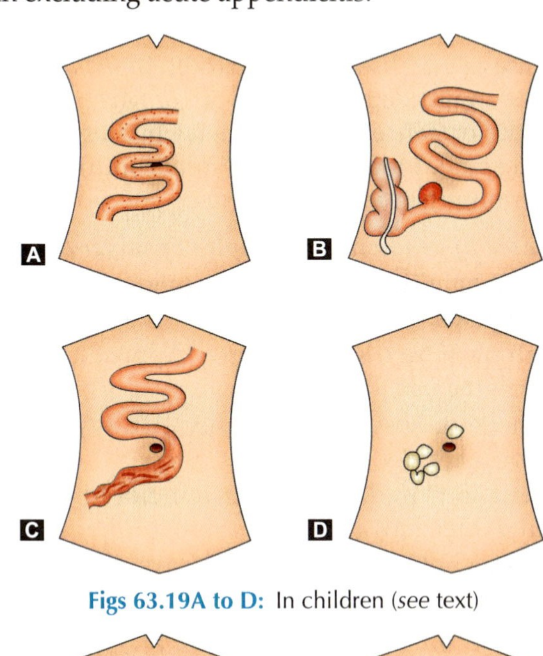


Figs 63.19A to D: In children (*see* text)

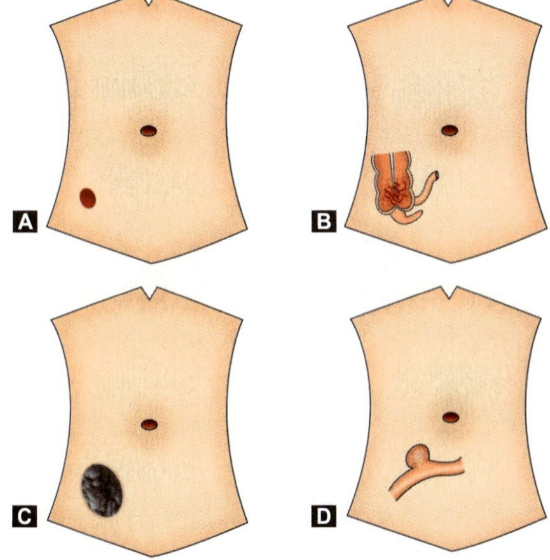


Figs 63.20A to D: In adults (*see* text)

**B. Amoebic typhlitis** is associated with diarrhoea, blood in the stools and tenderness in left iliac fossa (Manson Barr's amoebic point of tenderness).

**C. Torsion of undescended testis:** Absence of testis in the scrotum clinches the diagnosis.

**D. Meckel's diverticulitis**

**E. Yersinia ileitis:** Acute, self-limiting inflammation of the ileum caused by *Yersinia pseudotuberculosis*.

### In Middle Age (Figs 63.21A to D)

**A. Acute pancreatitis:** Inflammatory exudate collects and gravitates in the right iliac fossa resulting in pain, guarding and rigidity in the right iliac fossa. History of alcohol intake, severe backache and tenderness in the epigastrium help in diagnosing acute pancreatitis.

**B. Perforated duodenal ulcer** can present with pain in the right side of the abdomen due to similar causes mentioned above.

**C. Acute cholecystitis** can also present with features of acute appendicitis. However, it is common in elderly females.

**D. Pain** in the right iliac fossa and tenderness is due to dilated intestinal loop peristalsis as in ileocaecal tuberculosis or carcinoma caecum. Presence of an irregular and hard mass suggests carcinoma caecum.

### In Females (Figs 63.22A to D)

**A. Ruptured ectopic gestation:** Missed periods, features of haemorrhagic shock (pallor), and extreme tenderness on movement of cervix during *per vaginal* examination clinch the diagnosis.

**B. Pelvic inflammatory diseases:**

- These are group of inflammatory conditions affecting young women.

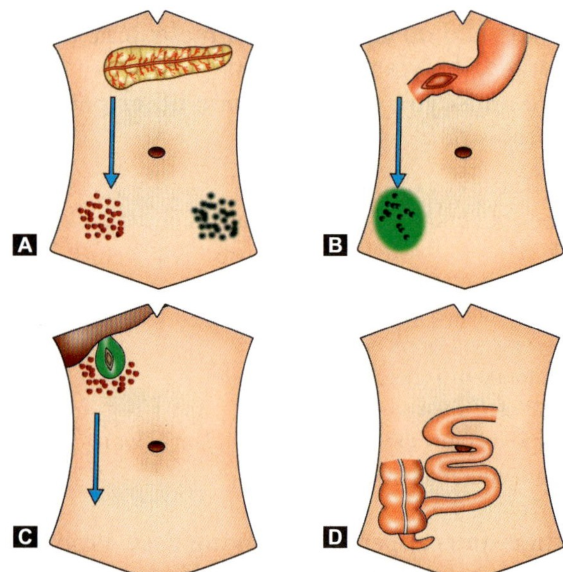


**Figs 63.21A to D:** In middle age (*see* text)

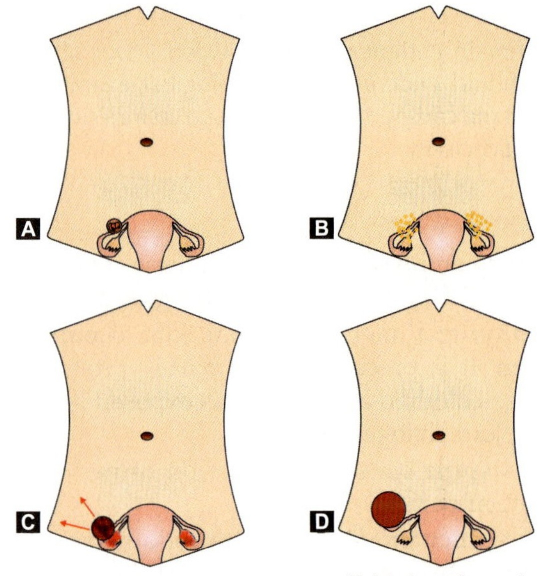


**Figs 63.22A to D:** In females (*see* text)

- Tubo-ovarian sepsis, salpingitis and endometriosis are grouped under this.
- Bilateral pelvic pain, high degree fever, and absence of anorexia are some of the features.
- Tenderness is present in both iliac fossae on deep palpation—no cough tenderness.
- Vaginal discharge helps in the diagnosis.
- Culture for *Chlamydia trachomatis* and *Neisseria gonorrhoeae* must be obtained.

**C. Midmenstrual** (mittelschmerz) rupture of ovarian follicle occurs about 14th to 16th day and can produce abdominal pain.

**D. Torsion of ovarian cyst** produces very severe abdominal pain with a mass.

#### Clinical Notes

- A 30-year-old lady was diagnosed to have acute appendicitis with classical features—pain, fever, vomiting and tenderness in the McBurney's point. A gynaecological examination revealed pelvic infection. An infected copper T was removed which was the cause of abdominal pain.
- A 22-year-old man underwent appendicectomy for right-sided abdominal pain. At laparotomy, appendix was normal. However, it was removed. He continued to have abdominal pain. An ultrasound of the abdomen revealed torsion of the undescended testis. Nobody had examined his external genitalia!
- A 36-year-old male who had previous history of abdominal pain underwent appendicectomy for tenderness and rebound tenderness in the right iliac fossa. Operative surgery notes said that the appendix was slightly inflamed and seropurulent fluid was present in the right iliac fossa. After 2–3 days, greenish fluid (bile) started draining out through the tube. The condition of the patient deteriorated and on reexploration this time, by midline incision revealed perforated chronic duodenal ulcer!!

*Pearls of Wisdom*

Any female patient with right-sided lower abdominal pain should undergo a gynaecological examination to rule out the causes mentioned above, before subjecting to appendicectomy.

## Systemic Diseases

1. **Pleurisy** and **pneumonia:** Both these conditions can have radiating pain and can have guarding.
2. **Porphyria:** Violent intestinal colic occurs due to spasm. It is precipitated by barbiturates. Urine is orange-coloured and when it is exposed to sunlight, the colour changes to amber.
3. **Pott's spine** causes compression of nerve roots—radicular pain.
4. **Preherpetic pain** of 10th and 11th dorsal nerves is located over the same area. Marked hyperesthesia is present.
5. **Purpura** and bleeding disorders.
6. **Polyserositis syndromes:** Dengue fever, leptospirosis, etc. can have peritoneal irritation and can secrete fluid in the peritoneal cavity. Ultrasound may even reveal probe tenderness. Doing an appendicectomy can be dangerous in these patients. It may worsen pre-existing condition including pneumonia, etc. may result in ARDS.

## A Few Special Situations

One should be careful and be firm in decision making of appendicectomy in these cases (Key Boxes 63.5 to 63.7).

## Problems Encountered during Appendicectomy

1. **The incision is small:** Location is higher up—one can extend the incision to about 2–3 cm in cases of slightly higher placed appendix. However, if it is sub-hepatic, never hesitate to close the incision and give a midline incision and do appendicectomy. An attempt to remove the appendix with McBurney incision, with traction and limited exposure may result in injury to ileum or colon and may result in faecal fistula.

Key Box 63.5

### Children and Acute Appendicitis

- Appendicitis is rare under 2 years of age because lymphatic tissue is not yet developed by that time.
- Signs are not very well located.
- Greater omentum is very thin. Perforation peritonitis is common.
- Hence, early surgery is recommended.
- Open or laparoscopic method is followed.
- Remember to rule out acute mesenteric lymphadenitis (viral), Yersinia ileitis and Meckel's diverticulitis.

Key Box 63.6

### Pregnancy and Acute Appendicitis

- Most common cause of abdominal pain and **non-obstetric** emergency in pregnancy is acute appendicitis.
- Incidence may be 1 to 1.5/1000 pregnancies.
- Symptoms of nausea and vomiting are confused for morning sickness.
- Migration of pain need not be present. Leukocytosis is seen in pregnancy cases—it is normal occurrence.
- Tenderness is shifted because appendix is displayed superiorly and laterally.
- Ultrasound is the investigation of choice. When in doubt MRI is useful investigation.
- Treatment is by laparotomy and appendicectomy.
- **Fetal loss** is 3% but with perforation, it is 30%.
- Maternal mortality rate in perforated appendicitis is 4%.

Key Box 63.7

### Acquired Immunodeficiency Syndrome (AIDS) and Appendicitis

- Incidence of acute appendicitis is more common in AIDS patients: 4-fold than non-AIDS patients
- Pain is chronic than acute
- Diarrhoea is more common
- Leukocytosis is not common
- Delay in the presentation may be present especially patients with low CD count
- Interestingly, outcome or results are surprisingly good after surgery

2. **Normal appendix is found:** Look for Meckel's diverticulitis, intestinal obstruction, stricture, etc. If bile is found, it means perforated duodenal ulcer—most common (Valentino appendix—page 1064). Close the incision and do laparotomy. If mesenteric nodes are enlarged, do lymph node biopsy.
3. **Sometimes you will find some other pathologies** (*see* Table 63.2).

*Pearls of Wisdom*

In cases of doubtful appendicitis, after appendicectomy look for:

1. Creeping fat: Crohn's disease
2. Ileum: Meckel's diverticulum
3. Mesentery: Lymph nodes
4. Peritoneum: Tubercles
5. Ovaries: Tubo-ovarian mass
6. Sigmoid colon: Diverticulitis (redundant colon)
7. Bile: Perforation of duodenal ulcer

4. **Gangrenous appendix involving base:** Problem one can face here is that the purse-string can be applied but invagination of the stump is not possible. Risk of

faecal fistula is also present. Appendicectomy, wash and a drain is kept.

5. **Difficult to isolate the appendix which is gangrenous but pus is present:** Limited ileocecectomy can be done.
6. **The appendix cannot be found:** First mobilise the caecum and look for subcaecal or retrocaecal sites. Look also into preileal or postileal sites. Then mobilise the ascending colon also. Agenesis of the appendix is very rare.
7. **Surprise findings of carcinoma caecum** (Fig. 63.23): If suspicion of a carcinoma is high, hemicolectomy should be done. Otherwise take a biopsy—do appendicectomy.

*Pearls of Wisdom*

Today because of imaging and laparoscopy majority of such wrong diagnosis/mistakes/problems encountered in an appendicectomy are largely eliminated or can be solved or treated with ease.

## Incidental Appendicectomy

It means removal of normal appendix at laparotomy for another condition. Examples: When you do laparotomy and ileal resection for stricture and anastomosis. (Can we do appendicectomy?)

Ovarian cyst: Torsion (right) ovary is removed. (Can we add appendicectomy?)

Since benefits of appendicitis/appendicectomy are more in young patients, if patient is under 30 years, it may be justifiable to do incidental appendicectomy provided it can be removed through same incision, without much difficulty. The patient should be stable to tolerate the procedure.

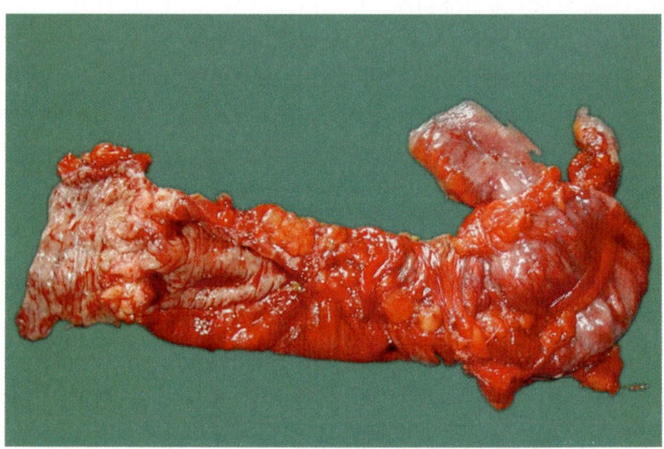

**Fig. 63.23:** Carcinoma colon with appendicitis

### Contraindications for Incidental Appendicectomy

- Crohn's of caecum
- Radiation treatment of caecum
- Immunosuppression
- Vascular grafted patient (aortoiliac, etc.)

Chances of infection are high in this group of patients. The result will be faecal fistula—difficult to treat.

**SU28.15.6:** Describe surgical management and postoperative complications of acute appendicitis. (For more details, refer to page 926 in operative surgery chapter.)

## Complications after Appendicectomy

A. **Postoperative fever** can be due to various factors. Thrombophlebitis, urinary tract infection and IV fluids are common causes. In the absence of these, wound infection, intraperitoneal abscess secondary to gangrenous appendicitis, may have to be considered.
   - Change of antibiotics according to culture and sensitivity reports of urine, pus and blood help in treating postoperative fever.
   - Elderly patients may have a pre-existing pulmonary disease. Respiratory tract infection also has to be considered.

B. **Wound infection:** It is the most common complication after appendicectomy. When in doubt open stitches and let out the pus.

C. **Intra-abdominal abscess** needs drainage.

D. **Faecal fistula—causes**
   a. Gangrene spreading into caecum
   b. Persistent infection
   c. Carcinoma caecum (elderly patients)
   d. Ileocaecal tuberculosis
   e. Crohn's disease (uncommon in India)
   f. Actinomycosis (rare)[1].

*Pearls of Wisdom*

Most of the faecal fistulae will heal by themselves provided there is no distal obstruction.

E. **Septicaemia,** portal pyaemia, gram-negative shock in late cases of peritonitis due to perforated appendicitis are uncommon but dangerous complications.
   - Mortality of appendicular perforation and peritonitis is around 2%.
   - It can occur after appendicectomy especially when gangrene of the appendix extends to base of the caecum. It can also occur, if purse-string suture is not properly applied, or injury to the terminal ileum or caecum, etc. Tuberculosis is one of the important causes of faecal fistula in Indian patients to be kept in

[1]In *viva voce* examination, when a question is asked as to what is the common cause of faecal fistula following appendicectomy, the usual answer by students is actinomycosis. Remember it is the answer to be told last.

mind. Actinomycosis is a rare cause of faecal fistula following appendicectomy, discharge of faeculent contents or faecal matter after appendicectomy suggests faecal fistula (Key Box 63.8).

- Usually discharge stops after a few days provided there is no distal obstruction.
- Cases which do not respond to conservative treatment: Fistula with long tracks, complex fistula, some diseases such as tuberculosis are managed by resection of the diseased portion of the caecum or ascending colon.

Key Box 63.8

**Faecal Fistula—can Occur**

- After drainage of appendicular abscess
- After appendicectomy—if purse-string sutures are not properly applied
- If the caecum is also involved by inflammation
- If the cause of appendicitis is carcinoma
- If chronic diseases develop or are present—tuberculosis, Crohn's disease or actinomycosis
- If appendicitis is associated with carcinoma caecum

*Pearls of Wisdom*

The important causes for faecal fistula are carcinoma caecum and ileocaecal tuberculosis in India and Crohn's disease in the West.

**Clinical Notes**

Post-appendicectomy faecal fistula—A case capsule

- A 23-year-old girl presented to the hospital with faecal fistula following appendicectomy of 6 months duration. It was a low output fistula. She had a colostomy bag applied to 4 × 2 cm oval opening at the incision site in the right iliac fossa.
- CT fistulogram showed two irregular contrast-filled tracts connected to caecum, ascending colon and retroperitoneum.
- Exploratory laparotomy and limited right colectomy were done. Tubercles were noted in the peritoneum. Biopsy was taken (Fig. 63.24).
- Final histopathology report was tuberculosis.
- She was put on ATT for 6 months. She recovered well.

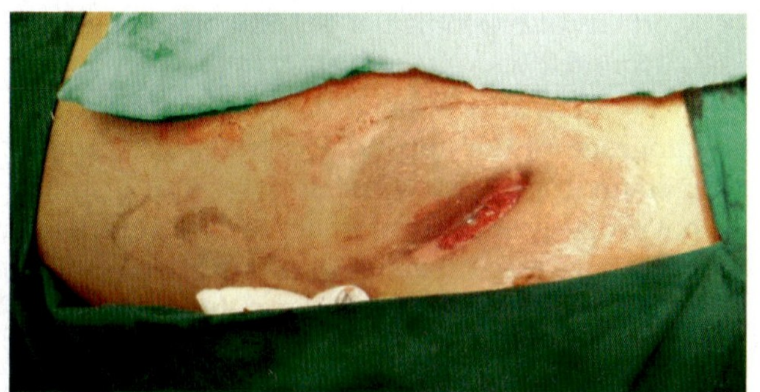

**Fig. 63.24:** Post-appendicectomy faecal fistula due to tuberculosis

## NEOPLASM OF THE APPENDIX

**SU28.15.8:** Describe tumours of appendix and clinical features, management of them.

### 1. Neuroendocrine Tumour

(more details on page 926)

- It is the most common neoplasm of the appendix (Fig. 63.25), less aggressive, majority are benign and cured with simple appendicectomy.
- Goblet cell carcinoid tumour—it is more aggressive, requires right hemicolectomy. If the tumour is more than 2 cm, has more than 2 mitosis per high power field and lymphovascular invasion, it is adenocarcinoma of the appendix.

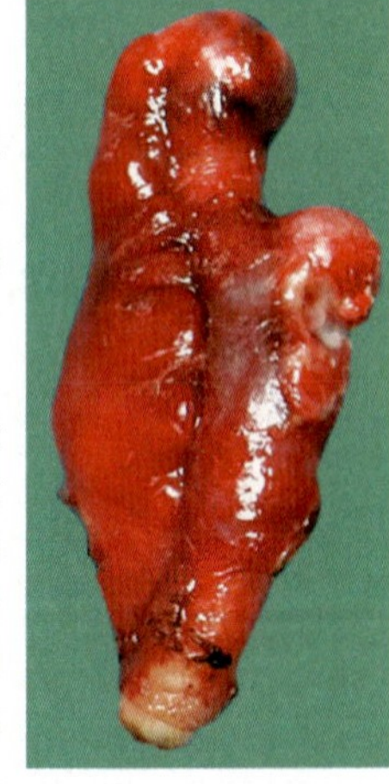

**Fig. 63.25:** Neuroendocrine tumour of the appendix

### 2. Carcinoma

- It is very rare.
- Often it is colonic type. Other type is mucinous adenocarcinoma.
- Can present as acute appendicitis due to obstruction caused by the tumour.
- Mucinous variety has better prognosis.
- Colonic variety should be treated by right hemicolectomy.

### 3. Cystic Neoplasm of the Appendix

- Rare occurrence.
- Simple cyst (non-neoplastic mucocoele) and mucinous cystadenoma (like pancreatic).
- Can attain large size.
- Diagnosis is by ultrasound/CT scan.
- Appendicectomy is the treatment of choice.
- It can rupture into peritoneal cavity resulting in pseudomyxoma peritonei.

## MUCOCOELE OF THE APPENDIX

**Definition:** It means accumulation of mucus within the lumen of the appendix.

**Causes:** It can be a simple retention cyst due to blockage by foreign body or mucosal hyperplasia. It can also be due to a mucinous adenocarcinoma (Fig. 63.26).

### Pathology (Figs 63.26 to 63.28)

- The majority of epithelial tumours of the appendix are mucin rich, thus results in gross distension.

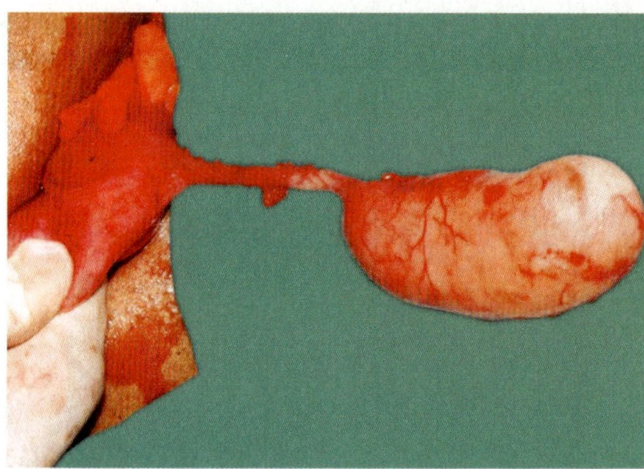

Fig. 63.26: Mucocoele of the appendix (*Courtesy:* Dr Raghunath Prabhu, KMC, Manipal)

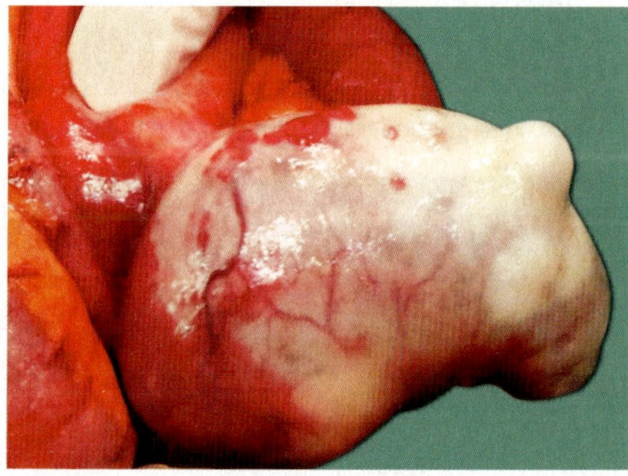

Fig. 63.27: Mucocoele (*Courtesy:* Dr Rajesh Sisodia, KMC, Manipal)

- Mucocoeles resulting from non-neoplastic occlusion (simple retention cysts) rarely exceed 2 cm in diameter.
- Mucinous neoplasms of the appendix are by far the most common cause of mucocoeles.
- Mucocoeles larger than 2 cm are more likely to represent benign neoplasms.

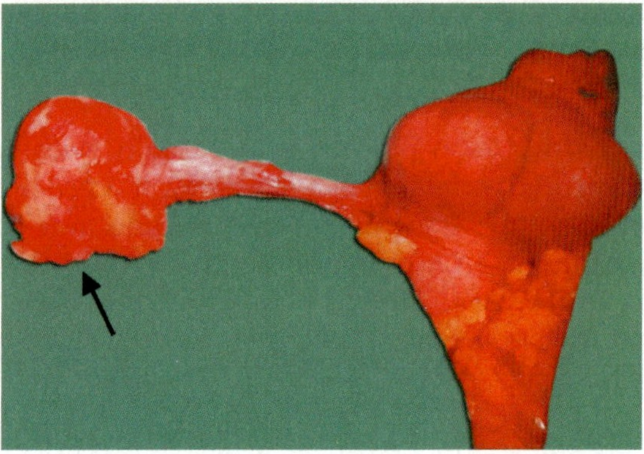

Fig. 63.28: Appendicular tumour arising from the tip has been removed—reported as carcinoid (*Courtesy:* Dr Raghunath Prabhu, KMC, Manipal)

## Diagnosis

- It is impossible to differentiate clinically mucocoele of the appendix and acute appendicitis when they present with abdominal pain. If a mass is palpable, it can be confused with appendicular mass.
- CT scan is the investigation of choice. The anatomic relationship between the elongated cystic mass and the caecum is usually more clear at CT scan than at ultrasound.

## Complications

1. **Gross enlargement** and can present as mass abdomen.
2. **Rupture** will result in pseudomyxoma peritonei (more details are given in Chapter 45, Peritonitis).
3. **Secondary infection:** Can result in 'empyema' of the appendix.

*Pearls of Wisdom*

Rule out adenocarcinoma of the base of the appendix causing mucocoele.

**Treatment:** Appendicectomy.

### INTERESTING 'MOST COMMON'

- Most common surgical emergency encountered by a general surgeon is acute appendicitis.
- Most common emergency surgery is appendicectomy.
- Most common non-obstetric surgical disease of the abdomen during pregnancy is acute appendicitis.
- Most significant symptom of acute appendicitis is migratory pain.
- Most significant sign of acute appendicitis is rebound tenderness in the McBurney's point.
- Most prominent scoring system to diagnose acute appendicitis is Alvarado score.
- Most common anaerobic bacteria in acute appendicitis is *Bacteroides fragilis* and aerobic bacteria is *Escherichia coli*.
- Most common complication after appendicectomy is wound infection.
- Most common age group for acute appendicitis is below 40 years.
- Most common neoplasm of the appendix is carcinoid tumour.

## CLINICAL CASE CAPSULE 9: Management Oriented Discussion in Surgery (MODS)

### POST-APPENDICECTOMY SEPSIS

A 32-year-old man presented to casualty with septic shock after 5 days after appendicectomy. It was a difficult appendicectomy. Gangrene of the appendix was almost involving the base. On examination, he was having paralytic ileus and jaundice. Abdomen was distended—guarding was present, more in the right iliac fossa. He was admitted to the hospital.

#### Investigations

- Total counts were 20,000 cells/cu mm: Indicate sepsis
- Urea: 51 mg%, creatinine 1.1 mg%—dehydration, pre-renal failure
- $[K^+]^-$ 3.2 mmol/L, $[Na^+]^-$ 129 mmol/L
- Total bilirubin: 19 mg%, direct bilirubin: 16.6 mg%
- AST: 189 IU/L, ALT: 100 IU/L, ALP: 167 IU/L
- ***Plain X-ray*** chest revealed free gas under the diaphragm (Fig. 63.29).

***Remarks:*** It showed he was in sepsis—counts were elevated, urea was high—renal failure set in slowly, increased bilirubin levels—sepsis with cholestasis.

***CT scan:*** Done after hydration—showed pneumoperitoneum and liver cyst (incidental) and free fluid in the peritoneal cavity (Fig. 63.30).

#### Conclusion

He was in sepsis. The probable reason was that the appendicular base (stump) had given way.

#### Exploratory Laparotomy

- Faecal peritonitis
- One litre of frank purulent pus in the peritoneal cavity.
- Gangrene of lateral wall of caecum with sloughing of caecal wall.
- Appendix not seen—post-appendicectomy
- Ileum normal

#### *Procedure*

- Limited resection of ileocaecal segment and end-to-end ileo-ascending colon single layer anastamosis
- Peritoneal lavage
- Drains in the pelvis and subhepatic space
- Skin not closed (wound infection is very common)

#### Postoperative

#### *6th Postoperative Day*

- Patient had greenish discharge from the right DT.
- Anastomotic leak and enterocutaneous fistula was suspected.
- Patient was passing flatus.
- RS: Basal crepitations
- Managed conservatively
- TPN was given for 5 days.
- Discharge subsided by 5 days.

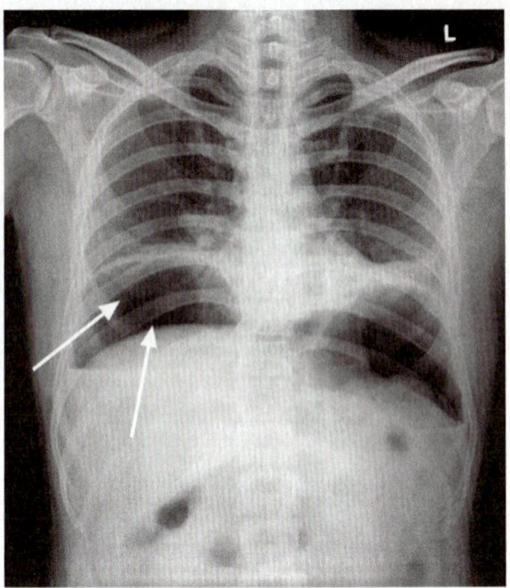


**Fig. 63.29:** Free gas under the right dome of the diaphragm

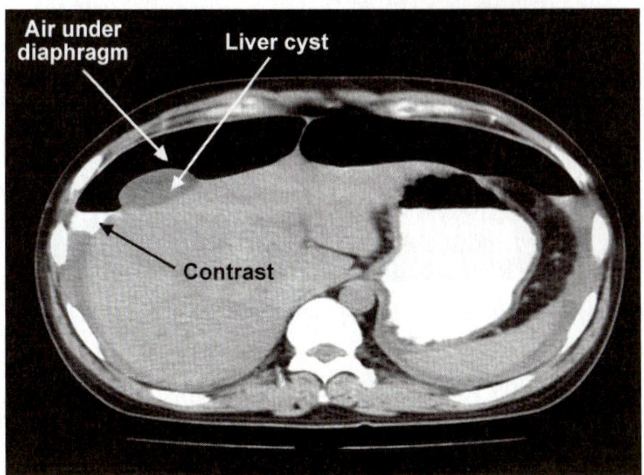


**Fig. 63.30:** Free gas under the right dome of the diaphragm pneumoperitoneum and liver cyst

#### *8th Postoperative Day*

- Breathlessness
- Fever
- Hypoxia: $SpO_2$: 85%
- Chest X-ray—pneumonia
- Intubated, ventilated for 5 days, appropriate antibiotics
- By 20th day, he was discharged from the hospital—leak had stopped.
- This case report has been given here for the following message:
  1. Acute appendicitis can be dangerous.
  2. Leak should be suspected, if a patient who underwent appendicectomy does not improve in the postoperative period.
  3. High total count, increased bilirubin, oliguria suggest sepsis.
  4. CT scan is the best investigation in such cases. When in doubt re explore. Danger lies in delay, not in resurgery.

## MULTIPLE CHOICE QUESTIONS

**1. The most common position of the appendix is:**
A. Subhepatic B. Subcaecal
C. Retrocaecal D. Pelvic

**2. The incidence of appendicitis is less after 30 years because:**
A. The appendix undergoes involution
B. The lymphatic tissue in the appendix decreases
C. Most people would have had their appendices removed
D. The vascularity reduces

**3. The name Seshachalam is associated with which of the following arteries?**
A. Accessory appendicular artery
B. Appendicular artery
C. Ileocolic artery
D. Posterior caecal artery

**4. Appendicular orifice is occasionally guarded by an indistinct semilunar fold of mucous membrane called:**
A. Valve of Gerlach
B. Valve of Heister
C. Valve of Kerckring
D. Valve of Houston

**5. The most common scoring system used for appendicitis is ____________ scoring system.**
A. Child-Pugh
B. Furtado
C. Murray
D. Alvarado

**6. Palpation of left iliac region of abdomen produces pain in the right iliac region in appendicitis because of:**
A. Sympathetic reaction
B. Displacement of colonic gas and small bowel coils
C. Sigmoid colon is also affected
D. Ileocolic reflex

**7. Cope's psoas test is positive in:**
A. Retrocaecal appendicitis
B. Pelvic appendicitis
C. Preileal appendicitis
D. Subcaecal appendicitis

**8. Rebound tenderness in acute appendicitis is called:**
A. McBurney's sign
B. Blumberg's sign
C. Rovsing's sign
D. Sherren's sign

**9. The most common cause of non-obstetric emergency with abdominal pain in pregnancy is due to:**
A. Acute appendicitis
B. Acute cholecystitis
C. Acute gastritis
D. Acute hepatitis

**10. Contraindications for incidental appendicectomy include all of the following, *except*:**
A. Crohn's of caecum
B. Radiation treatment of the rectum
C. Immunocompetent individuals
D. Previous vascular reconstruction in the abdomen

**11. The following statement is TRUE about appendicular abscess:**
A. Abscess greater than 4–6 cm in size needs to be drained by laparotomy
B. Appendicectomy must be done along with laparotomy for appendicular abscess
C. Can present with diarrhoea
D. Conservative management is advised till inflammation settles down.

**12. Most common aerobic bacterium involved in acute appendicitis is:**
A. *Salmonella typhi*
B. *Streptococcus*
C. *Escherichia coli*
D. *Clostridium perfringens*

**13. The following statement is FALSE about occurrence of faecal fistula following appendicectomy:**
A. Faecal fistula can occur if the cause of appendicitis is carcinoma caecum
B. Faecal fistula can occur if chronic diseases such as tuberculosis is present
C. Faecal fistula can occur if purse string sutures are not applied properly
D. It is always due to actinomycosis

**14. The most reliable symptom of acute appendicitis is:**
A. Fever
B. Migratory pain
C. Right iliac fossa pain
D. Vomiting

**15. Appendicular perforation is common because of the following reasons, *except*:**
A. Appendix is a cul-de-sac
B. It has blood supply with profuse collaterals
C. It has a narrow lumen
D. The muscle coat of appendix is thin

**16. Appendicular mucosa contains following, *except* (predominantly):**
A. Columnar epithelium
B. Neuroendocrine cells
C. Goblet cells
D. Paneth cells

**17. About Paneth cells following are true, *except*:**
A. They are found mainly in colon
B. Found just below crypts of Lieberkühn
C. Have antibacterial property
D. They produce lysozymes

**18. Following precautions have to be taken to treat appendicitis in a pregnant lady in the 2nd trimester, *except*:**
A. Initial evaluation should be by ultrasound imaging
B. MRI is the most ideal imaging
C. Gadolinium contrast should be used
D. Open (Hasson) technique is used in laparoscopic appendicectomy.

**Answers**

| | | | | | | | | | |
|---|---|---|---|---|---|---|---|---|---|
| **1.** C | **2.** B | **3.** A | **4.** A | **5.** D | **6.** B | **7.** A | **8.** B | **9.** A | **10.** C |
| **11.** C | **12.** C | **13.** D | **14.** B | **15.** B | **16.** D | **17.** A | **18.** C | | |

Chapter 64

# Hernia



## INTRODUCTION

- Hernia is not a disease but manifestation of a disease. Several factors may contribute to the development of a hernia. (They have been discussed later.)
- Hernia is a common condition affecting patients, especially inguinal hernia in males and incisional hernia in females. Even though several types of surgery have been described for hernias, mesh hernioplasty remains the gold standard treatment. Majority of the hernias require surgical treatment leaving apart small asymptomatic direct hernias in the elderly. Today, laparoscopic hernia is becoming gold standard. Obstructed hernia is an emergency and late cases carry significant mortality.
- Hernia means to bud, protrude or rupture (Latin).

## DEFINITION

Abnormal protrusion of a viscus or a part of it through a weak point in the body (opening) is known as a hernia. Inguinal hernia occurs either through the deep inguinal ring due to persistent processus vaginalis sac (indirect hernia) or through the posterior wall of the inguinal canal (direct hernia).

> **SU28.1.1,2,3,9,10:** Describe applied anatomy of abdominal wall and its weaknesses in pathophysiology of abdominal hernias.

It can be broadly classified into anatomy of the inguinal region, femoral region and abdominal wall. For better understanding of the etiopathogenesis of hernias, anatomy of the femoral region is discussed under femoral hernia and anatomy of the abdominal hernias are discussed under incisional hernias. So first we will study anatomy of the inguinal region.

## ANATOMY OF THE INGUINAL REGION (Fig. 64.1)

### Inguinal Ligament (Poupart's Ligament) (1)

- It is the ligamentous portion of the external oblique aponeurosis which folds inwards and extends from anterior superior iliac spine to the pubic tubercle.
- The midpoint between these two structures is called midpoint of the inguinal ligament.

### Lacunar Ligament (Gimbernat's Ligament)

- Some fibres of inguinal ligament pass posteriorly to attach to superior pubic ramus lateral to the tubercle and form lacunar ligament.
- The midpoint between the anterior superior iliac spine and pubic symphysis is called midinguinal point.

### Inguinal Canal (2)

It is 4 cm in length extending from the deep inguinal ring to the superficial inguinal ring.

### Deep Ring (Internal Ring) (3)

It is a U-shaped defect in the fascia transversalis which forms the posterior wall of the inguinal canal. It lies 1.25 cm above the midpoint of the inguinal ligament.

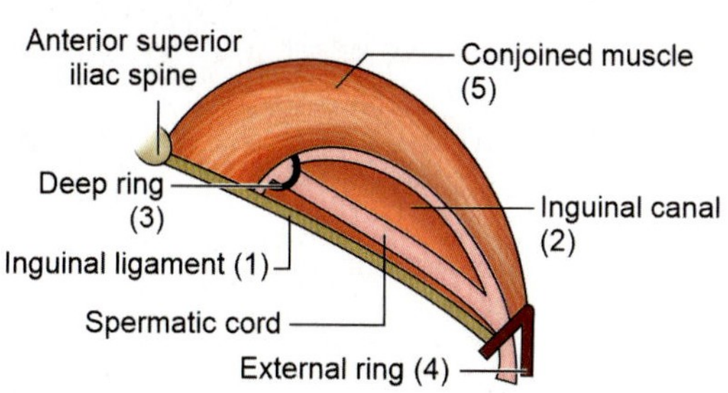


**Fig. 64.1:** Anatomy of the inguinal region

### External Ring (Superficial Ring) (4)

Superficial ring is a triangular defect in external oblique aponeurosis. It is bounded by the lateral and medial crura formed by the external oblique aponeurosis and the base of the triangle is formed by the pubic crest.

### Boundaries of Inguinal Canal

- **Anterior:** External oblique aponeurosis and a few fibres of the **conjoined muscle** (especially of internal oblique) laterally.
- **Superior:** Arched fibres of the **conjoined muscle** (5).
- **Inferior:** Inguinal ligament and the lacunar ligament on the medial side (Gimbernat's ligament).
- **Posterior:** Fascia transversalis and the conjoined tendon medially. Thus, the inguinal canal is strong in the lateral part anteriorly and the medial part posteriorly.

### Contents of Inguinal Canal

1. Spermatic cord (Key Box 64.1)
2. Ilioinguinal nerve (Key Box 64.2)
3. Genital branch of genitofemoral nerve
4. Round ligament in females
5. Vestigial remnant of processus vaginalis sac

Key Box 64.1

**Contents of the Spermatic Cord**

- Vas deferens
- Testicular artery
- Artery to the vas
- Cremasteric artery
- Pampiniform plexus of veins
- Lymphatics
- Sympathetic nerves
- Genital branch of genitofemoral nerve
- Processus vaginalis

Key Box 64.2

**Ilioinguinal Nerve**

- The ilioinguinal nerve is a branch of the first lumbar nerve (L1). It separates from the first lumbar nerve along with the larger iliohypogastric nerve.
  It pierces the transversus abdominis and internal oblique muscles to enter the inguinal canal from the side
- Ilioinguinal nerve does not pass through the deep inguinal ring. It only travels through part of the inguinal canal.
- After going through inguinal canal, it pierces the internal oblique muscle, distributes nerve fibres to it, and then accompanies the spermatic cord through the superficial inguinal ring.
- Divides into anterior scrotal nerve/anterior labial nerve.
- Supplies the skin of the upper and medial part of the thigh, scrotum/vulva.
- Entrapment or injury to the ilioinguinal nerve is one of the causes of post-herniorrhaphy pain.
- Hence, a few recommend division of ilioinguinal nerve during hernia surgery.

### Myopectineal Orifice of Fruchaud[1] (Fig. 64.2)

- This weak area is the site of all groin hernias according to Fruchaud.
- It is the area between inguinal ligament anteriorly and iliopubic tract posteriorly.
- **Iliopubic tract:** It is the thickened inferior margin of the transversalis fascia which appears as a fibrous band running parallel and posterior (deep) to inguinal ligament. It inserts into superior pubic ramus to form lacunar ligament.
- **Boundaries of myopectineal orifice of Fruchaud:**
  *Superiorly:* Arched fibres of internal oblique
  *Laterally:* Iliopsoas muscle

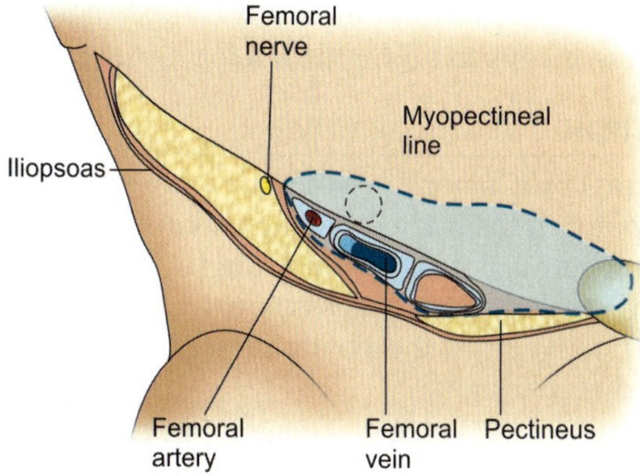


**Fig. 64.2:** Myopectineal line and anatomy

[1]Henri R Fruchaud, 1956: The surgical treatment of inguinal or femoral hernia must not be closure of inguinal canal or femoral ring but deep reconstruction of abdominal wall in the whole groin region

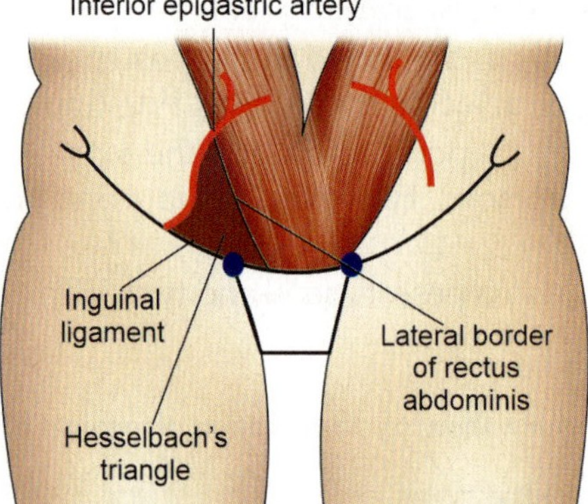


**Fig. 64.3:** Hesselbach's triangle

*Medially:* Lateral border of rectus abdominis muscle
*Inferiorly:* Pubic pecten—Cooper's ligament—bony margin of the pelvis

- **Surgical importance of iliopubic tract:** Recognition of this is a part of laparoscopic repair (initial step)—visualising from within. This structure reinforces posterior wall and floor of inguinal canal as it bridges structures traversing subinguinal space. Hesselbach's triangle (Fig. 64.3).
- It is bounded medially by lateral border of rectus abdominis muscle, laterally by inferior epigastric artery and inferiorly by inguinal ligament.
- Direct hernias occur commonly through Hesselbach's triangle (medial), indirect hernia lateral to inferior epigastric artery.

## INGUINAL DEFENCE MECHANISMS

1. Obliquity of inguinal canal (in children, it is straight).
2. During straining or coughing, the conjoined tendon contracts, and since it forms the anterior, superior and posterior boundaries, it closes the inguinal canal—**shutter or sphincter-like effect**.
3. Increased intra-abdominal pressure produces plugging effect at the external ring. The deep ring is pulled upwards and laterally because it is adherent to the posterior surface of **transversalis muscle**. This occludes the ring and prevents herniation—**Ball valve** effect.

## AETIOLOGY OF HERNIA: WHAT CAUSES HERNIA?

- **Indirect hernia occurs largely due to persistent processus vaginalis sac.** Manifestations of this can be seen in elderly patients in whom an indirect hernia can be triggered by some factors which increase intra-abdominal pressure.
- **Direct hernia occurs mainly due to weakness of transversalis fascia in Hesselbach's area.** However, increase in abdominal pressure due to chronic cough, constipation or difficulty in passing urine, development of ascites (portal hypertension, nephrotic syndrome), etc. can precipitate development of hernia.
- Collagen and hernia: Few studies involving studying fibres of transversalis fascia have proved that few cases of primary inguinal hernias and recurrent hernias occur due to intrinsic and inherent weakness in the tissue. Type I Collagen: It is characteristic for mature scars or fascial tissues. Type III Collagen: It is mechanically unstable, less cross-linked collagen synthesized during the early days of wound healing. For adequate strength and function of transversalis fascia, presence of collagen in adequate amount is important. The decreased tensile strength of collagen type III plays a key role in the development of incisional hernias.
- Collagen disorder: In prune-belly syndrome, collagen fibre disorder causes development of not only hernias but also interstitial hernias, bilateral hernias, etc. Hernia occurs due to inherited imbalance in the types of collagens.

### RISK FACTORS

It can be classified as patient related and external factors.

**I. Patient related:** A patent processus vaginalis sac. Chance of developing a hernia in males about 20–25%.

- Some other factors responsible are failed obliteration of the processus vaginalis (PV) sac, persistent smooth cells and insufficient calcitonin gene-related peptide from spinal nucleus of genitofemoral nerve. Smooth cells help in propelling testis into scrotum.
- Hernias are more common on right side in children because right PV sac is obliterated later than left PV sac.

**II. External factors:**

- Smoking causes increased collagen degradation and decreased synthesis. This is due to the effect of nicotine, which weakens the abdominal wall.
- Increased abdominal pressure caused by coughing, jumping, lifting of the load have been mentioned.
- Constipation has a doubtful relationship.

Summary of various factors for development of hernia has been summarized in Key Box 64.3.

## CLASSIFICATION OF HERNIA

**I. Anatomical classification:** (1) Indirect hernia, (2) direct hernia.

**II. Nyhus classification:** This classification is based **primarily on the defect**, which helps in planning an appropriate repair.

Key Box 64.3

**Aetiology/Causes of Hernia**

1. **Congenital:**
   Persistent processus vaginalis sac: Chief cause of indirect hernia.
2. **Collagen fibre disorder**
   - Prune-belly disorder—congenital
   - Smoking: Acquired collagen deficiency
3. Corpulence obesity
4. Chronic causes of increased intra-abdominal pressure
   - Chronic cough, chronic constipation, straining at micturition, ascites
5. Conjoined tendon weakness/rupture of a few fibres following:
   - Lifting heavy weight
   - Postappendicectomy—injury to ilioinguinal nerve.
   - Chronic illness/debilitating disease causing weakness of transversalis fascia in the Hesselbach's area.

**Type 1:** Indirect hernia with normal deep ring—normal posterior wall

**Type 2:** Indirect hernia with dilated deep ring—normal posterior wall

**Type 3:** Based on posterior wall defect: (a) Direct hernia, (b) pantaloon, sliding—enlarged deep ring, (c) femoral

**Type 4:** Recurrent hernia—direct, indirect femoral, combined.

### III. The European Hernia Society classification:

- Primary (P), Recurrent (R)
- Lateral (L), Medial (M), Femoral (F)
- Defect size assumed to be 1.5 cm

  Thus, primary direct hernia with 3 cm defect size is written as PM2.

### IV. Gilbert's classification (Table 64.1)

- It is based on the defect in the posterior wall (direct hernia) or defect in the internal ring (indirect).
- Depending upon the defect, the suggested repair is given below. However, basic principles are the same.
- The last two types—type VI and type VII are modifications by Robbin.

**Algorithm showing classification of inguinal hernia**

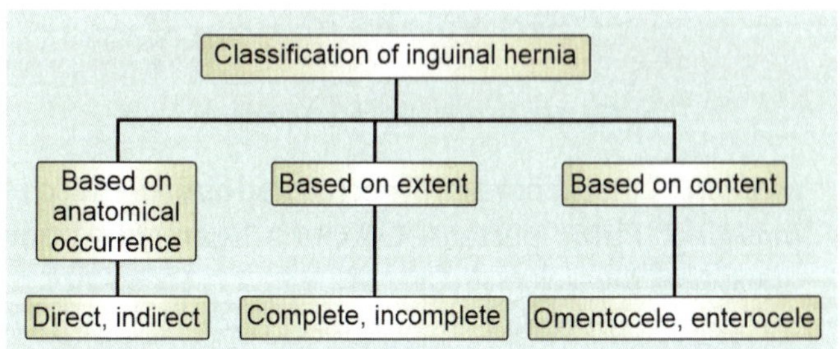


## INDIRECT HERNIA

It is a herniation of abdominal contents through the deep ring into the inguinal canal. **Indirect hernia occurs due to persistent processus vaginalis sac.** It is the most common type of hernia in the body. The preformed sac passes through the deep ring, traverses the inguinal canal and may extend into the scrotum through the external ring. As it comes into the inguinal canal, it is invested by the following coverings:

1. External spermatic fascia derived from external oblique aponeurosis.
2. Cremasteric fascia derived from internal oblique.
3. Internal spermatic fascia from fascia transversalis.

**TABLE 64.1:** Gilbert's classification and suggested repair

| Types | Classification | Repair |
|---|---|---|
| I. | Snug internal ring<br>Preperitoneal indirect sac<br>Does not admit one finger | Herniorrhaphy or hernioplasty |
| II. | Moderately enlarged internal ring<br>Bubonocoele<br>Admits one finger | Herniorrhaphy or hernioplasty |
| III. | Large defect—2 or 3 finger-breadths internal ring. May be sliding hernia | Preperitoneal mesh by slitting transversalis fascia |
| IV. | Large direct hernia with full blow out defect | Mesh repair |
| | Internal ring is normal | |
| V. | Direct hernia with punched out hole/defect in the transversalis fascia<br>The internal ring is intact | Plug the defect or purse-string closure of the defect followed by mesh repair |
| VI. | Pantaloon hernia | Mesh repair |
| VII. | Femoral hernia | Femoral hernia repair |

### Parts of the Hernia (Fig. 64.4)

Hernial sac is part of the peritoneum which is dragged into the inguinal canal. The mouth of the sac is in the peritoneal cavity. The neck is the narrowest portion (deep ring). The actual hernial sac has a body and a fundus. Depending upon the contents, it can be named as follows: Omentum—omentocoele, intestine— enterocoele.

When both direct and indirect hernias present it is called as Pantaloon hernia.
Littre's hernia—hernia containing Meckel's diverticulum. It may also contain ovary or appendix. **When part of the wall of the gut is involved, it is known as Richter's hernia.**

### Types of Indirect Hernia

1. **Complete hernia** (scrotal): When the sac is patent up to the bottom of the scrotum, it is a **complete scrotal hernia** (Fig. 64.5A).
2. **Funicular:** The processus vaginalis sac is patent up to the root of scrotum, it is an **incomplete indirect hernia** (Fig. 64.5B and Fig. 64.6).
3. **Bubonocoele:** Processus vaginalis sac is confined to the inguinal region or the inguinal canal only. Such hernias are seen in young patients (Fig. 64.5C).

### Coverings of the Indirect Inguinal Hernia from Outside to Inside

1. Skin
2. Two layers of superficial fascia: Fatty and membranous (Camper's and Scarpa's fascia respectively).

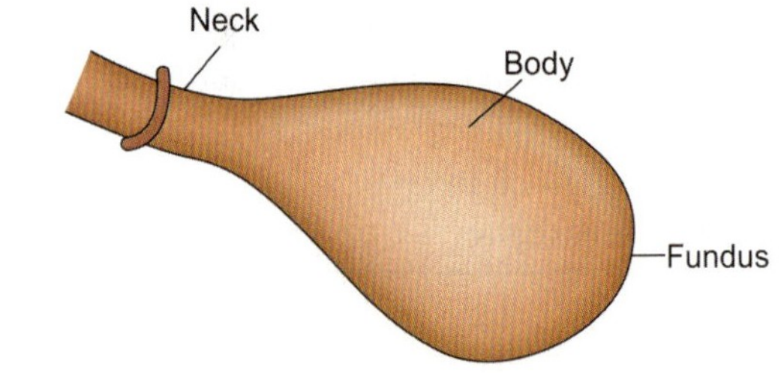


**Fig. 64.4:** Parts of the hernial sac

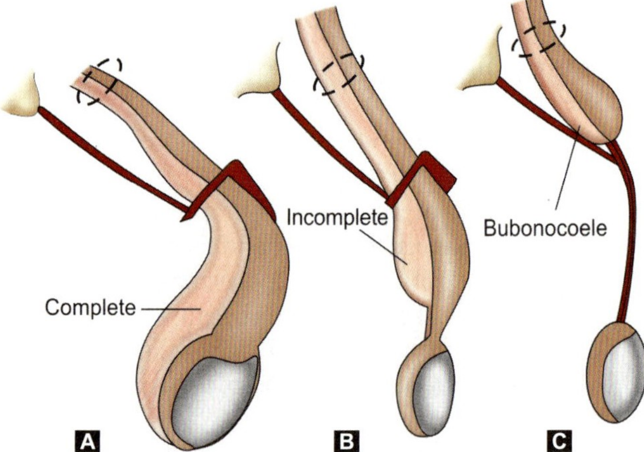


**Figs 64.5A to C:** Three types of indirect hernia

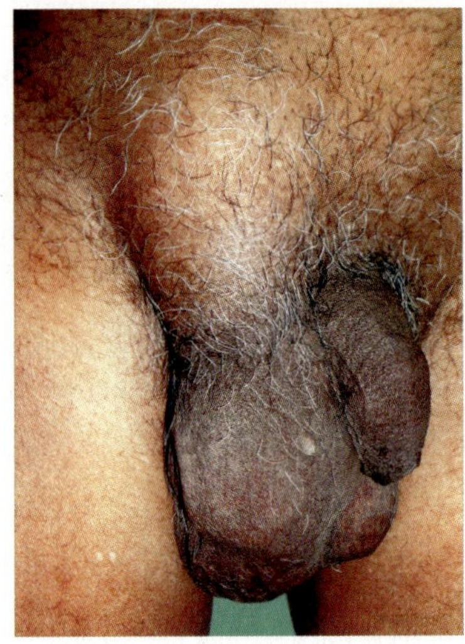

**Fig. 64.6:** Incomplete hernia bulge is seen

3. External spermatic fascia, a continuation of the external oblique aponeurosis.
4. Cremaster muscle and fascia, a continuation of the internal oblique.
5. Internal spermatic fascia: Derived from the fascia transversalis.
6. Extraperitoneal fat
7. Peritoneum

## DIRECT HERNIA

It is always acquired (Fig. 64.7). It occurs through ***Hesselbach's triangle,*** a weakness in the ***posterior wall*** of the inguinal canal (transversalis fascia). Chronic cough and benign prostatic hypertrophy (BPH) are the common risk factors. Other risk factors mentioned earlier such as smoking also apply here.

Boundaries of ***Hesselbach's triangle***

- Medially: Lateral border of the rectus abdominis
- Laterally: Inferior epigastric artery
- Below: Inguinal ligament

### Coverings of the Direct Inguinal Hernia from Outside to Inside

1. Skin
2. Two layers of superficial fascia
3. External oblique aponeurosis
4. Conjoined tendon
5. Fascia transversalis
6. Peritoneum

*Pearls of Wisdom*

As the direct hernia pushes through the posterior wall, it is very unusual for it to descend into the scrotum. It can descend into the scrotum if few fibres of transversalis fascia are missing (congenital).

### Ogilvie Hernia

This is a type of direct hernia wherein the hernial sac appears through a circular defect (congenital) in the conjoined tendon.

## CLINICAL EXAMINATION OF A CASE OF HERNIA

> **SU28.1.4:** Describe clinical presentation, examination findings, and role of radiological investigations in diagnosis and management of hernia.

### History

- Swelling in the inguinal region which is gradually increasing in size. To start with, the swelling disappears on lying down and increases on straining, walking, etc. Later it cannot be reduced (due to adhesions).
- History of dragging pain indicates omentocoele.
- Since the omentum is attached to the stomach above and supplied by T10, the pain is referred to the umbilical region.
- Sudden, severe pain in the hernia, vomiting and irreducibility indicates 'obstructed hernia'.
- History of chronic cough, constipation, difficulty in passing urine should be asked. If present, it may suggest the cause of hernia.
- **History of appendicectomy:** Division of ilioinguinal nerve during appendicectomy may cause denervation of fibres of the right transversus abdominis, which forms U-shaped ring, resulting in weakness of the abdominal wall.

### Clinical Examination: In the standing position

#### *Inspection (a Model Case of Incomplete Hernia)* (Figs 64.7 to 64.9)

Direct hernia pops out as soon as patient stands (Fig. 64.9).

- There is a swelling in the inguinal region extending to the root of the scrotum measuring about 6 × 3 cm.

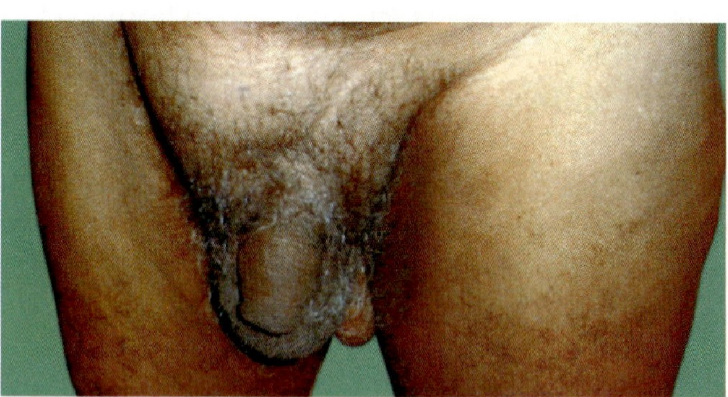

Fig. 64.7: Direct hernia pops out when patient stands

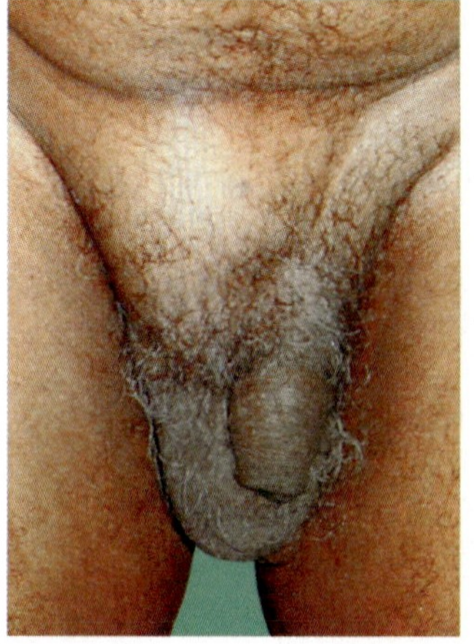

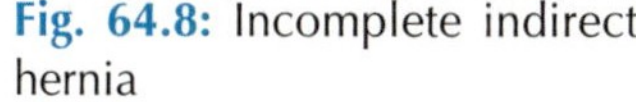

Fig. 64.8: Incomplete indirect hernia

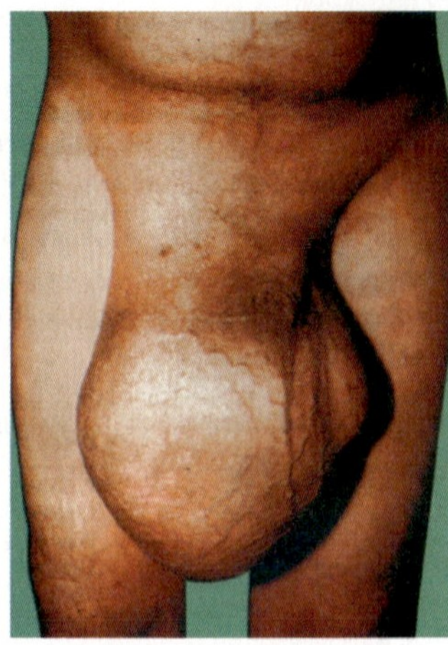

Fig. 64.9: Complete indirect hernia—scrotal hernia

**Its surface is smooth, borders are round, skin over the swelling is normal** and it is pyriform in shape.

- Ask the patient to cough—**expansile impulse on cough is present**. If peristalsis is present, it indicates an enterocoele. Expansile impulse on cough is diagnostic of hernia (Key Box 64.4).
- Presence of scar indicates a recurrent hernia. Ragged scar indicates infection.
- Direct hernia pops out as soon as the patient stands and often it is bilateral.

> Key Box 64.4
>
> **Expansile Impulse on Cough**
>
> - Hernia
> - Meningocoele
> - Dermoid cyst with intracranial communication
> - Laryngocoele
> - Lymphatic cyst in children
> - Empyema necessitans

#### *Palpation*

- Inspectory findings should be confirmed. Swelling is soft, and gurgles, if it is an enterocoele.
- It may be firm or granular, if it is an omentocoele.

1. **Ask the patient to cough**—expansile impulse is felt at the root of scrotum.
2. **Getting above the swelling**[1] should be done in the standing position (Fig. 64.10).
   - At the root of scrotum, the spermatic cord is palpated between the finger and the thumb. In cases of complete indirect hernia, spermatic cord cannot be felt as a naked structure because it is covered anterolaterally by the sac. This is called as **getting above the swelling not possible** (negative).

[1]This test has no meaning or usefulness in bubonocoele. It is a test to differentiate scrotal swelling from inguinoscrotal swelling and assumes significance in complete hernias.

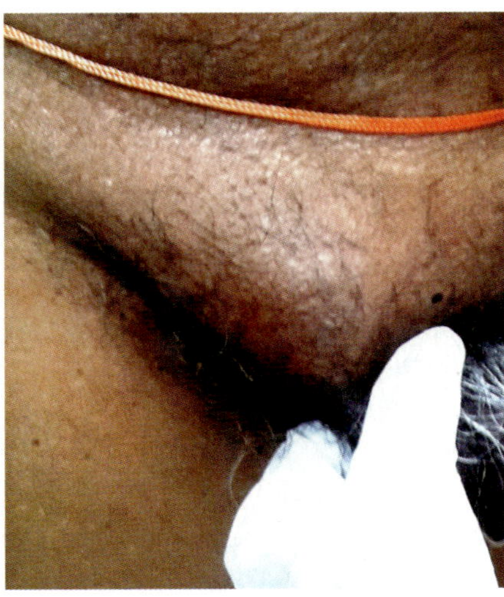

**Fig. 64.10:** The swelling is palpated at the root of the scrotum. Getting above the swelling is not possible. A case of incomplete hernia

*Pearls of Wisdom*

Getting above the swelling is a test to differentiate scrotal swellings from inguinoscrotal swellings.

3. **Reducibility**—ask the patient to lie down.
   - If the swelling becomes smaller or disappears, it is a hernia (hydrocoele is not reducible).
   - **Omentocoele:** Initially, reduction is easy but later, becomes difficult (due to adhesions). If it is difficult to reduce, ask the patient to reduce it. Otherwise, flex and medially rotate the hip and try to reduce it, a method called ***taxis***.
   - If in spite of this, the swelling is not reduced, it is called an irreducible hernia.
4. **Deep ring or internal ring occlusion test:** Reduce the swelling first (Fig. 64.11).

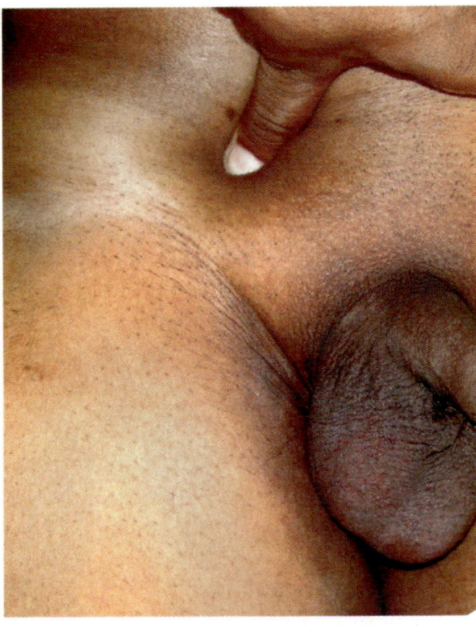

**Fig. 64.11:** Deep ring occlusion test

Locate the deep ring above the midpoint between anterior superior iliac spine and symphysis pubis. Occlude the deep ring with the thumb and ask the patient to cough.
   a. If impulse and the swelling are seen, it is a direct hernia because it occurs in the Hesselbach's triangle (medial to deep ring).
   b. If the swelling is not seen, it is an indirect hernia. Deep ring occlusion test can be done with the patient in standing and supine position.

   Problems of deep ring occlusion test:
   a. If occlusion is not done properly, results may vary.
   b. Pantaloon hernia (Romberg hernia, saddlebag hernia, dual hernia). It is a direct hernia having indirect component.
5. **Zieman's method** (Figs 64.12A and B): Three-finger method.

   Keep index finger at deep ring, middle finger on the posterior wall above and lateral to the external ring and ring finger at femoral ring. Now ask the patient to cough. Depending upon the type of hernia,

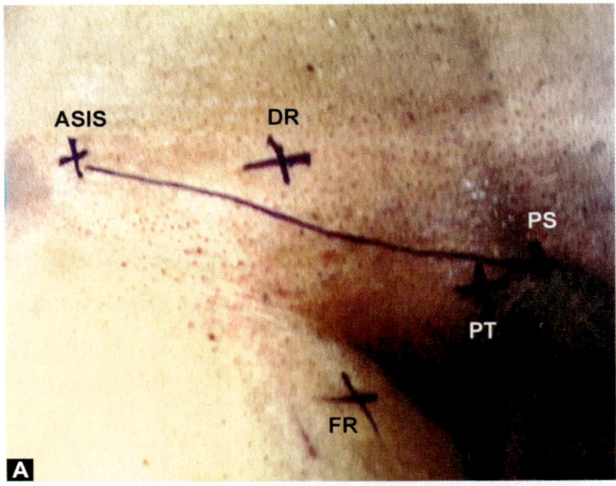


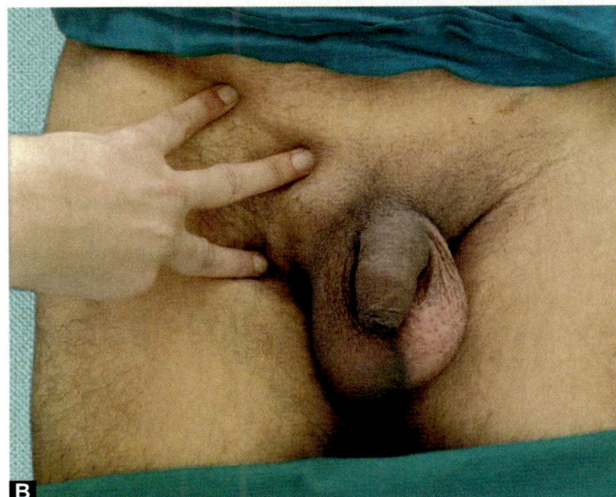


**Figs 64.12A and B:** Zieman's method: Anterior superior iliac spine (ASIS), deep ring (DR), pubic symphysis (PS), pubic tubercle (PT) and femoral ring (FR) have been marked for doing Zieman's test

impulse is felt. It is not necessary to perform this test in incomplete or complete indirect hernias.

6. **Leg raising test** or head raising test (Fig. 64.13):
   - Weakness of oblique muscles is manifested by Malgaigne's bulgings above the medial half of inguinal ligament. ***It is an absolute indication for hernioplasty.***
   - **Malgaigne's bulgings indicate weakness of the oblique muscles of the abdominal wall.**
7. **Per abdomen:** To rule out any mass (colonic).
8. **Look for phimosis/stricture urethra:** Young patients having urinary complaints with hernia may be suffering from stricture urethra. Lift the scrotum and feel for any strictures in the bulbar urethra. Retract skin of prepuce and rule out phimosis.
9. **Per rectal examination** should be done in elderly patients to rule out prostatic enlargement.
10. **Examination of respiratory system** is done to rule out chronic bronchitis, tuberculosis, etc.

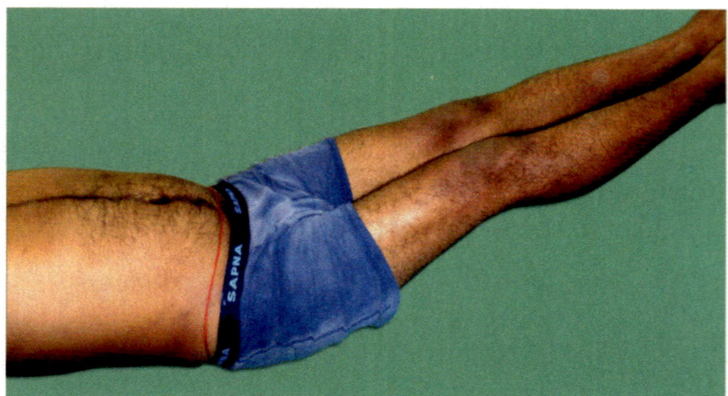


**Fig. 64.13:** Leg raising test

*Pearls of Wisdom*

Examine the opposite side and all hernial sites such as femoral, umbilical and incisional hernia sites.

### Clinical Examination of a Hernia in a Child

- Swelling may not be visible at first as it may be covered by thick pad of fat. Examine when a child strains (cry), or after child's play (jumping, etc.). Examine the root of scrotum—may find hernial sac (thickening).
- **Gornall's test:** By gentle compression on child's abdomen (hold the child on its back), hernia may become apparent.
- Invagination test is almost impossible. Hence, it is better not to do it.

### Diagnosis *(One Example)*

Right sided, indirect, incomplete, uncomplicated, reducible omentocoele. Table 64.2 for differences between direct and indirect hernia and Table 64.3 for differences between hernia and hydrocoele.

**TABLE 64.2:** Differences between direct and indirect hernia

| | Direct hernia | Indirect hernia |
|---|---|---|
| 1. Age | Common in elderly | Can occur in any age group |
| 2. Aetiology | Weakness of posterior wall of inguinal canal | Preformed sac |
| 3. Precipitating factors | Chronic bronchitis, enlarged prostate | — |
| 4. On standing | Pops out | Does not pop out |
| 5. Side | Usually bilateral | Unilateral (30% bilateral) |
| 6. Internal ring occlusion test | Swelling is seen | Swelling is not seen |
| 7. Malgaigne's bulgings | May be present | Absent |
| 8. Complications | Not common because neck is wide | Common, neck is narrow—obstruction and strangulation |
| 9. Relationship of sac to the cord | Sac is posterior to the cord | Sac is anterolateral to the cord |
| 10. Direction of the sac | It comes out of Hesselbach's triangle | Sac comes through the deep ring |

**TABLE 64.3:** Clinical differences between indirect complete hernia and vaginal hydrocoele

| | Indirect complete hernia | Vaginal hydrocoele |
|---|---|---|
| 1. Standing position | Swelling of scrotum and inguinal region | Swelling confined only to scrotum |
| 2. Impulse on coughing | Present | Absent |
| 3. Getting above swelling | Not possible | Possible |
| 4. Reducibility | Usually present unless complicated | Not reducible |
| 5. Consistency and transillumination | Soft, gurgling, no transillumination | Soft, fluctuant, transillumination is present |

## DIFFERENTIAL DIAGNOSIS OF A GROIN SWELLING

**SU28.1.11:** Describe differential diagnosis of inguinal and inguinoscrotal swellings.

Groin refers to the junction of lower abdomen with the thigh. Hence, swellings in the inguinal region and upper thigh (femoral region) close to the inguinal ligament are included under groin swellings.

1. **Inguinal hernia** (Fig. 64.14).
2. **Femoral hernia:** The main sac is below and lateral to pubic tubercle (Fig. 64.15).
3. **Vaginal hydrocoele:** Fluctuation and transillumination tests are usually positive and getting above swelling is possible. (Please note that in infantile hydrocoele and hydrocoele en bisac, getting above swelling is not possible) (Fig. 64.16).
4. **Retractile testis:** It can present as a firm swelling in the inguinal region. Scrotum is empty (Fig. 64.17).
5. **Saphena varix:** The patient can present with a swelling in the thigh. Swelling is usually about 2.5 cm below the pubic tubercle. **A swelling that disappears on elevation of the leg is characteristic of a swelling of venous origin** (Fig. 64.18).
6. **Funiculitis:** A funiculitis can occur with or without acute epididymo-orchitis. Severe pain in the inguinal region, tender swelling, high grade fever with chills and rigors are characteristic. Spermatic cord is thickened and swelling is not reducible (Fig. 64.19).
7. **Inguinal lymphadenitis:** Pain and nodular swelling below inguinal ligament is a feature. It is not reducible and some source of infection in the lower limb is usually present (Fig. 64.20).
8. **Lipoma of the cord:** It presents as a soft, lobulated but irreducible swelling in the inguinal region (Figs 64.21A and B).

### Investigations

Hernia is a clinical diagnosis. Except for small direct hernia in very elderly patients who have asymptomatic hernias and who are candidates for high cardiac risk, almost all inguinal hernias should be treated. In the vast majority of the cases, no investigations are required specific to the diagnosis of hernia. However, in appropriate cases imaging can be done.

- First advice in a smoker with hernia is to stop smoking at least four weeks before surgery. If a patient is high-risk patient, he should stop smoking at least 6 months before surgery.

1. **Ultrasound:** In apparently occult cases wherein patient has groin pain but clinically not evident, ultrasound can detect a sac—however it is operator dependent. In large hernias including sliding hernias, ultrasound can identify structures such as urinary bladder or colon, thus giving useful information to the surgeon. Ultrasound is also useful in cases of postoperative swelling in the groin to rule out haematoma/seroma/recurrence.

*Pearls of Wisdom*

Hernia is a clinical diagnosis. If you are asked to give one investigation to confirm hernia (may be in early cases), it is ultrasound.

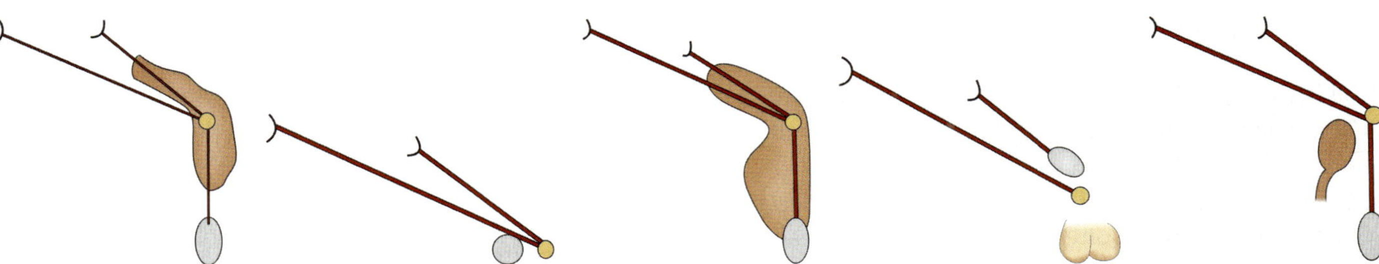

**Fig. 64.14:** Inguinal hernia

**Fig. 64.15:** Femoral hernia

**Fig. 64.16:** Infantile hydrocoele

**Fig. 64.17:** Retractile testis

**Fig. 64.18:** Saphena varix

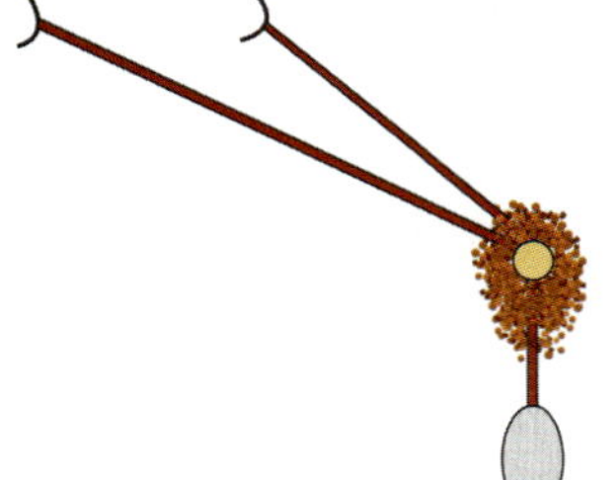

**Fig. 64.19:** Funiculitis

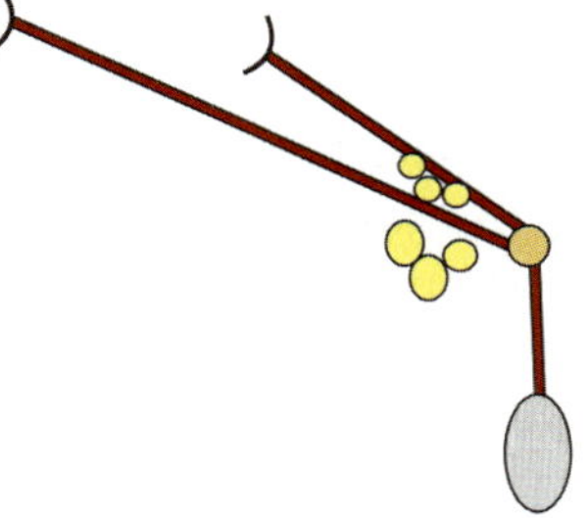

**Fig. 64.20:** Inguinal lymphadenitis

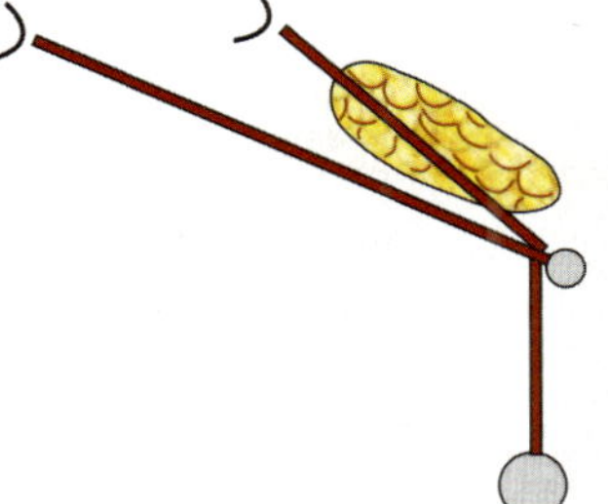

**Fig. 64.21A:** Lipoma of the cord

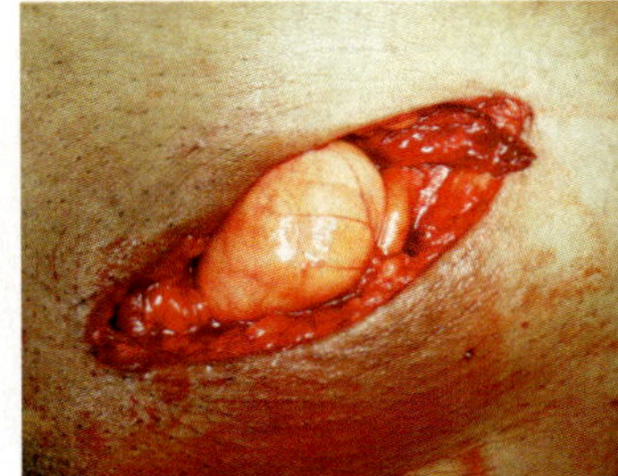

**Fig. 64.21B:** Left inguinal lipoma of the cord

2. **Computed tomography (CT)** scan is ideal in cases of giant hernias, sliding hernias or special types such as spigelian hernia, obturator hernia, perineal hernia, etc.
3. **Routine investigations** such as complete blood picture (CBP) and urine examination are done. In elderly patients, chest X-ray, electrocardiography or even pulmonary function tests may be necessary. Patients with urinary complaints are evaluated for prostatic enlargement and stricture urethra.
4. **Magnetic resonance imaging (MRI):** Ideal in sportsmen who complain of groin pain, to differentiate between hernia, to rule out muscle sprain or any other orthopaedic disorders.

## Preoperative Preparation

- A patient with chronic bronchitis and bronchial asthma should be properly treated with bronchodilators, antibiotics, mucolytic agents, etc. Cigarette smoking should be stopped at least 4 weeks.
- Elderly patients with bilateral hernia mostly suffer from benign prostatic hypertrophy. **Prostatectomy should be considered first followed** by repair of hernia, in such cases. Recent history of constipation and appearance of a hernia should arouse the suspicion of carcinoma colon. Investigate by colonoscopy/fibre-optic sigmoidoscopy before the treatment of hernia.
- Young adults with difficulty in passing urine may have a stricture urethra due to gonococcal urethritis. They should undergo proper treatment for the stricture. Now it is rare to find a patient with hernia having a stricture urethra.

## Treatment (Flowchart 64.1)

**SU28.1.6:** Describe general principles of management of abdominal wall hernias and the basic operative approach.

1. **Herniotomy:** Excision of hernial sac. No repair is required. It is done only in children.

**Flowchart 64.1:** Algorithm showing type of hernia surgeries

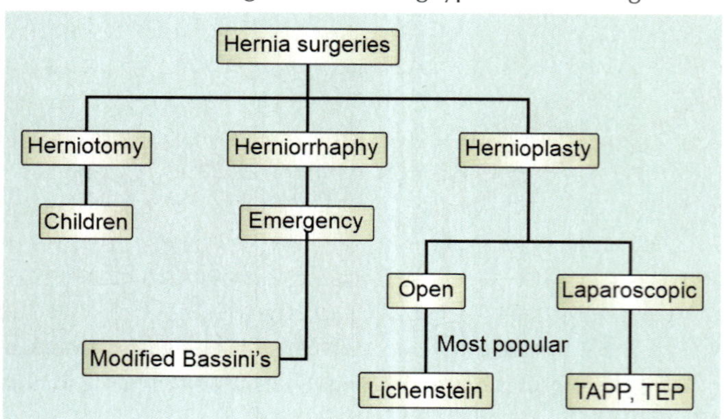


2. **Hernioplasty:** Strengthening of posterior wall—mostly by prolene mesh is the most popular surgery called **Lichtenstein repair**. Details of hernioplasty are given below. It can be done by open or laparoscopic method. Details are also available in the operative surgery chapter.
3. **Herniorrhaphy:** Approximation of conjoined tendon to inguinal ligament by using nonabsorbable sutures is called Bassini's herniorrhaphy. It is not done nowadays because of high chances of recurrence. Hence, it is not discussed here. However, in strangulated hernias, repair with mesh may result in infection due to foreign body reaction to mesh. In such cases, tissue repair like Bassini can be considered as it is a simple operation to perform.

*Pearls of Wisdom*

Herniotomy, herniorrhaphy and hernioplasty are the three fundamental principles for the repair of inguinal hernia. Mesh hernioplasty is the gold standard for inguinal hernias.

## HERNIOPLASTY

Today most popular hernia repair which is increasingly used is TEP (Total Extra Peritoneal repair) and TAPP (Trans Abdominal Pre Peritoneal repair). Desarda Technique, wherein undetached, incised external oblique aponeurosis is used. These have been discussed in the operative surgery chapter in page 1208. The most popular open method of tissue repair, Lichenstein repair is discussed here.

There are two types of hernioplasties.

A. **Lichtenstein repair:** The posterior wall **(Lichtenstein repair)** (Fig. 64.22, Key Boxes 64.5 and 64.6) of inguinal canal is strengthened by a prolene mesh or Marlex mesh. The fibroblasts and capillaries grow over the mesh, converting it into a thick fibrous sheath and strengthening the posterior wall. The mesh is fixed inferiorly to lacunar and inguinal ligaments, medially to overlap rectus sheath and fixed to fascia over the pubic bone. A few interrupted sutures are put to fix it to the transversalis fascia. **Laterally, an artificial deep ring is created by crossing of both upper and lower leaves of the mesh.** To attain this, a slit is given on one side of mesh. (Lacunar ligament is that portion of the inguinal ligament which extends backwards and upwards to the pectineal line and forms the medial margin of the femoral ring).

*Characteristics of the ideal mesh*

- Biocompatibility means it should not do any harm, should be chemically and physically inert.
- Risk of infection should not be there.
- Handling should be good.
- Economical
- Longevity (also refer to biological mesh given in next page).

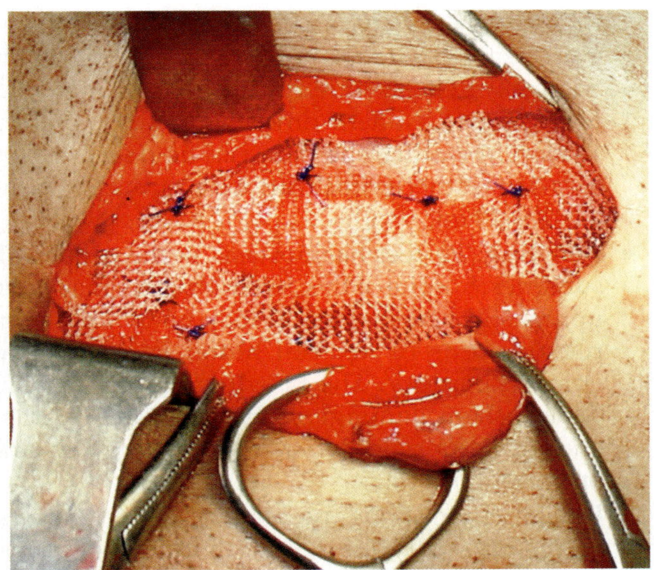

**Fig. 64.22:** Lichtenstein repair is the most popular type of open hernia repair

Key Box 64.5

**Lichtenstein Repair***

- Polypropylene mesh is used (Fig. 64.24).
- 8 × 16 cm mesh is tailored to patient's requirement.
- **Preparation of mesh:** Corners can be cut so as to give a round shape. A slit is given on the lateral border of the mesh at the junction of lower one-third and upper two-thirds, to allow spermatic cord to pass through. The two tails (slit-ends) are overlapped.
- **Suturing:** Medially, the mesh overlaps the pubic tubercle and is sutured over the tissue of symphysis (avoid pubic bone to prevent osteitis pubis). Laterally, the two tails are placed beyond deep ring and sutured. Inferiorly, it is sutured to inguinal and lacunar ligaments and superiorly to conjoined tendon.

****Dr Irving Lichtenstein—Lichtenstein repair: The tension-free repair 1989. Los-Angeles***

Key Box 64.6

**Advantages of Polypropylene Mesh**

- High tensile strength
- Biocompatible, nonabsorbable
- Monofilament strong, elastic and transparent mesh
- Ideal porosity for high visibility and colonisation
- Strong mechanical reinforcement
- Encourages rapid ingrowth of connective tissue
- Cheaper
- Flexible for any anatomic placement

**Advantages of Light Weight and Large Pores Mesh**

- Less shrinkage of mesh, more flexible, better tissue integration, better comfort.

B. **Prolene (polypropylene) nylon darning:** Suturing the conjoined tendon to the inguinal ligament without tension in a criss-cross manner by using prolene suture material (handmade mesh). This is preferred in direct and indirect hernias described by Maloney.

**Biological Mesh**

These are sterilised sheets of connective tissue derived from human or animal dermis or porcine intestinal submucosa:
- They are decellularised
- Like the mesh, they provide scaffold for connective tissue to grow and collagen deposition.
- Enzymatic reaction takes place in the host followed by fibrous tissue formation.
- Advantages: Chronic inflammation and foreign body reaction, stiffness and fibrosis, and mesh infection are uncommon—usually do not occur.
- They can be used in presence of infection.
- They are very expensive.

## Other Surgeries for Inguinal Hernia

1. **Shouldice repair**
   - It is the most popular tensionless method wherein only local tissues are used.
   - After opening the inguinal canal, herniotomy is done.
   - Transversalis fascia, which forms the posterior wall, is incised from the internal ring till pubic tubercles.
   - Then, upper and lower flaps of transversalis fascia are sutured in a double-breasting manner by using nonabsorbable sutures such as 34 gauge stainless steel wire, polyamide or polypropylene. This is the **first layer** of Shouldice repair.
   - The **second layer** is like Bassini's, wherein conjoined tendon is sutured to the inguinal ligament by using nonabsorbable sutures.
   - The **third layer** is completed by suturing upper flap of external oblique aponeurosis to the inguinal ligament.
   - The results have been good in Shouldice's hands. The operation needs **expertise**.
2. **Nyhus repair:** Ideally indicated in bilateral direct hernia or recurrent hernia, wherein a broad mesh is kept in the preperitoneal space. It requires a single large incision covering both groins. However, same surgery now can be done by laparoscopically by keeping a mesh in the extraperitoneal space.
3. **Dasarda technique:** In this operation, a strip of external oblique aponeurosis is prepared isolated but still connected medially and laterally to the external oblique muscle, and sutured to conjoined tendon and inguinal ligament below. *More details are given in operative surgery section on page 1291.*

**Rare/uncommon surgeries**

1. **Kuntz operation** (Fig. 64.23): In this operation, the spermatic cord is divided at the deep ring and it is removed along with the testis, so that the deep ring can be permanently closed, and hernia never recurs. It is indicated in elderly patients with recurrent hernia and poor abdominal muscle tone. Hamilton Bailey's operation—cord is divided but testis is retained.
2. **Stoppa repair**[1]**:The Stoppa repair is a tension-free type** of hernia repair. It is performed by wrapping the lower part of the parietal peritoneum with prosthetic mesh and placing it at a preperitoneal level over Fruchaud's myopectineal orifice. This operation is also known as giant prosthetic reinforcement of the visceral sac (GPRVS).

## COMPLICATIONS OF HERNIA SURGERY

These are common complications after surgery. Often they are mild and not so worrisome. However, some of the complications can be serious which require immediate attention and treatment.

1. **Complications during surgery**
   - **Injury to the iliac vessels:** The most serious but rare complication is injury to iliac vessels. It can happen in thin patients when suturing of the inguinal ligament is done from lateral to medial side. The sudden jet of fresh red blood indicates that the bite has been taken through the artery. It is better to call the vascular surgeon, extend the incision, have a proximal control, suture directly or do a resection and end to end anastomosis. They have to be anticoagulated with low molecular weight heparin followed by oral anticoagulants.
   - **Injury to the urinary bladder:** This can happen when anatomy is not clear as in few giant or scrotal hernias, perineal hernias or distortion due to previous surgery. Sudden finding of clear fluid with urinary smell means bladder injury. Immediate repair with 2–0 vicryl followed by urinary catheter placement for 3 weeks is the treatment.

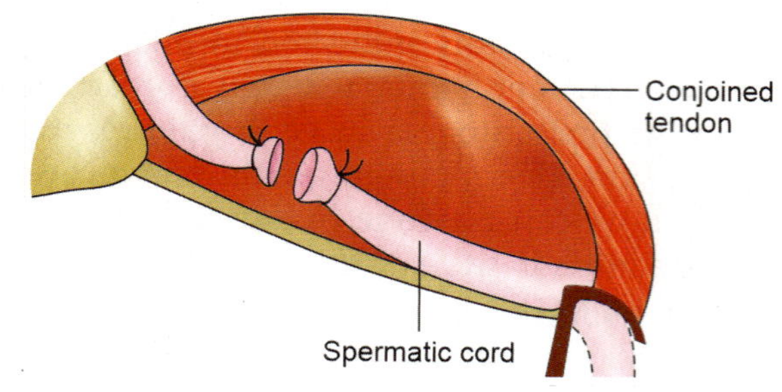

**Fig. 64.23:** Kuntz operation

2. **Early postoperative period**
   - **Pain:** Pain is common due to the incision in the skin and some degrees of retraction of structures such as inguinal ligament downwards and conjoint tendon upwards. The pain can be decreased by local anaesthetic infiltration, e.g. bupivacaine 0.25%—20 ml.
   - **Bleeding:** Perfect haemostasis is the aim of all surgeries. In spite of this, a few bleeders may open up, mostly venous blood—may be pampiniform plexus veins or arterial blood from inferior epigastric artery. The bleeding may stop with compression bandage. Otherwise, exploration and ligation of bleeders needs to be done in the operation theatre.
   - **Urinary retention is common, more so in males:** Pain, spinal or epidural anaesthesia, sedatives, lack of privacy are contributing factors. Provide analgesia, privacy and hot fomentation to suprapubic region. If all of these fail, catheterise bladder as a last step.
   - **Abdominal distension:** This is not common. It can happen when large intestinal contents of the hernia sac are reduced or handled as in scrotal hernias or sliding hernias. It is also important to realise that omentum is attached to stomach and colon above. One should see that bleeders from injured arteries of the omentum are ligated properly. Some intraperitoneal blood may add to paralytic ileus.
3. **Intermediate—between 3 and 7 days**
   - **Seroma** is due to inflammatory response to mesh or suture materials. It causes swelling and anxiety that it may be a recurrence. When in doubt, get an ultrasound examination first. Seroma needs to be aspirated. Seroma is more common after laparoscopic hernia repairs.
   - **Surgical site infection:** Hernia is a clean surgery. Infection should not occur. However, poor handling of the tissues, haematoma, seroma and diabetes may precipitate wound infection. Patients with skin disease or co-morbid factors are given injection cefazolin 1–2 g intravenously 30 minutes before the incision or clindamycin, if patient is allergic to cefazolin. If infection is suspected, open the sutures, drain the pus and use appropriate antibiotics. Persistent wound infection may prompt removal of the mesh. A few cases of tuberculosis have been reported. This is due to improper sterilisation of the mesh used.
4. **Late:** Late complications are not all that common. One complication which bothers a few patients is chronic

[1]It was first described in 1975 by Rene Stoppa.

pain called inguinodynia. It is seen in about 10% of post-hernioplasty pain. It is defined as persisting pain more than 3 months after surgery.

- **Inguinodynia:** The chief factor is injury to the following nerves: Iliohypogastric, ilioinguinal and genital branch of genitofemoral nerve. Injury can be in the form of entrapment of the nerves, traction injury, cauterisation, transection, etc. These are more common after mesh repair because of entrapment of the nerves or perineural fibrosis and adhesions between mesh and the nerves. Clinical features include dull aching or dragging pain in the groin, genitalia, suprapubic region. Some may complain of diminished sensation or even hyperaesthesia. Treatment usually includes reassurance, simple analgesics, nerve blocks with anaesthetic agents and injection of steroids. Neurolysis by inguinal exploration or neurectomy may be required in appropriate cases.

**Ischaemic orchitis and testicular atrophy**

- It occurs due to thrombosis of veins of pampiniform plexus within spermatic cord. It is more common in direct hernias where handling of the spermatic cord while separating it from the long-standing sac may result in thrombosis.
- It can also be due to injury to testicular artery.
- Venous congestion results in ischaemic orchitis causing pain in the testis.
- It is treated with anti-inflammatory drugs.
- Ischaemic orchitis is more common after recurrent hernia surgeries.

## COMPLICATIONS OF HERNIA

**SU28.1.5:** Describe complications of abdominal hernias.

### 1. Irreducibility (Key Box 64.7)

It occurs due to adhesions formed between omentum, sac and the contents. Irreducibility produces dull aching pain.

Key Box 64.7

**Diagnosis of Irreducible Hernia**

- Hernia is tense
- Tender
- Irreducible
- No impulse on cough
- Recent increase in size of swelling

### 2. Obstructed Hernia (Key Box 64.8 and Fig. 64.24)

Irreducible hernia + obstruction to the lumen of the gut gives rise to obstructed hernia. Clinically, it produces severe colicky abdominal pain, abdominal distension, vomiting and step ladder peristalsis.

#### *Treatment*

Urgent division of the neck of the sac followed by hernioplasty.

Key Box 64.8

**Factors Responsible for Obstructed Hernia**

- Narrow neck
- Irreducibility
- Sudden straining
- Too many contents
- Long duration of hernia
- Sliding hernia

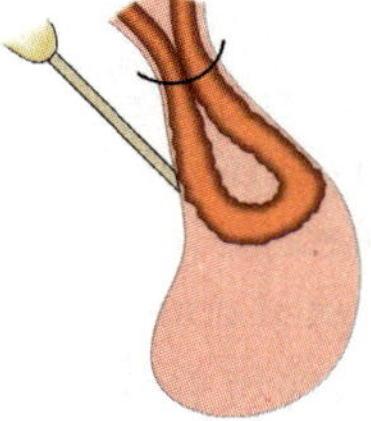

**Fig. 64.24:** Obstructed hernia

### 3. Strangulated Hernia

Irreducibility + obstruction + impairment of blood supply to intestine.

#### *Pathology*

- Strangulation commonly occurs in femoral hernia, obturator hernia and in indirect hernia.
- Initially the venous return is occluded, the part gets congested, and mucosal ulceration and haemorrhage occurs into the gut wall. It also results in oedema due to capillary exudation.
- If the obstruction is not relieved, constriction of the artery takes place resulting in gangrene of bowel. If this happens, there is a proliferation of bacteria.
- Gangrene appears at the ring of constriction first. Later it develops in the antimesenteric border (Fig. 64.25).
- Such a gangrenous segment contains decomposed blood in which gram-negative organisms multiply.

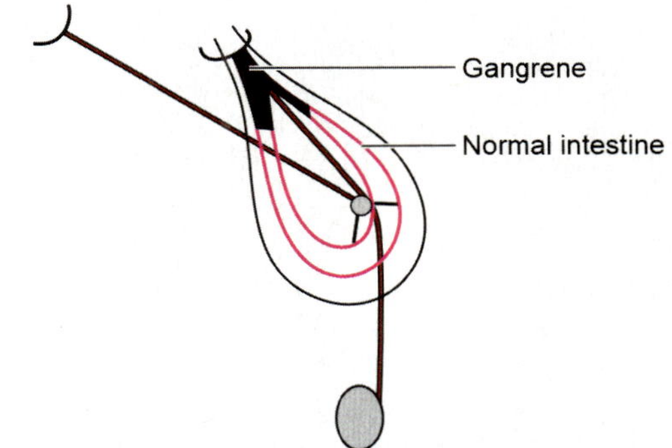


**Fig. 64.25:** Gangrene appears at ring of constriction first and then progresses

They produce endotoxins resulting in endotoxic shock. If the gangrene extends into the intra-abdominal segment of the bowel, peritonitis can occur.

- The deep ring and the external ring are the common constricting sites.

### Clinical Features

- Sudden, severe, prolonged pain with some features of shock are indicative of strangulation.
- **Clinical examination of such hernia reveals** (Fig. 64.26A to C):
  - Tense (hernial sac is tense—differentiates it from obstructed hernia)
  - Tender
  - No impulse on cough
  - Irreducible
  - Recent increase in size of the swelling
- General condition of the patient is poor:
  - Feeble pulse, hypotension, rebound tenderness, absent bowel sounds, toxic look.

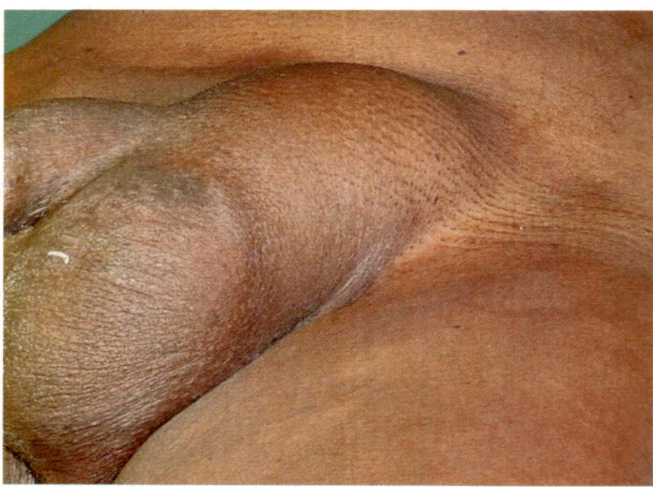

**Fig. 64.26A:** Strangulated hernia

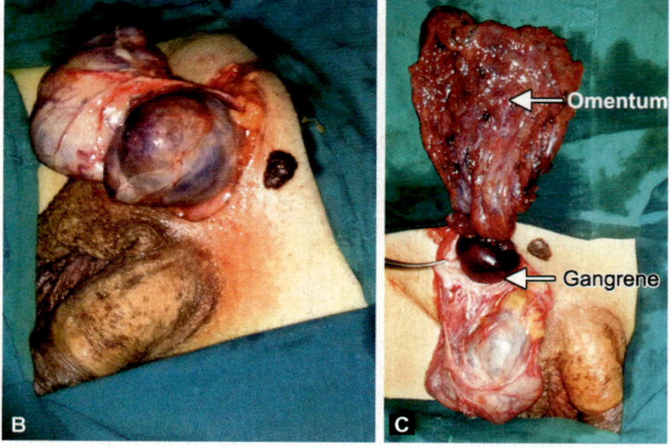


**Figs 64.26B and C:** Strangulated hernia with gangrene

### Treatment

*I. General measures*

- The patient is hospitalised. The foot end of the bed is raised so that an irreducible hernia may reduce by gravity. However, if there is a suspicion of gangrene, this step is not recommended.
- A Ryle's tube is introduced to decompress the stomach, thus preventing vomiting and reducing abdominal distension.
- Intravenous fluids are given to correct dehydration and to prevent renal failure.
- Narcotic analgesics are required to reduce the pain.
- An attempt should be made to reduce the swelling when there is no gangrene by the following measures:
  A. Good sedation
  B. Patient's thigh is flexed, adducted and medially rotated.
  C. With the right hand, the sac is gently squeezed by applying pressure over the scrotum. At the same time with the left hand, the proximal portion of the sac is guided into the inguinal canal. This procedure is described as taxis. **Taxis is contraindicated, if there is gangrene.**
  D. **Complications of forced reduction** include contusion of intestinal wall, rupture of the sac at the neck and reduction en masse, i.e. the entire sac with the contents are reduced into the abdominal cavity but the intestine still remains strangulated.
- The patient is prepared for surgery and blood is grouped and cross-matched.

*II. Surgery* (Key Box 64.9)

- With broad-spectrum antibiotic coverage, the hernia is explored by an inguinoscrotal incision and hernia sac is defined. At this stage, ***the constricting ring should not be divided.*** First all the toxic fluid from the sac is aspirated. The constriction is then divided using a grooved director or hernia bistoury. **While dividing the constricting ring, the inferior epigastric vessels which are situated medially may be damaged**. Therefore, care has to be taken to protect these vessels. High ligation of the sac should be done (Figs 64.27 and

Key Box 64.9

**Surgery for Strangulation**

- Generous inguinal incision, identify the sac
- First aspirate toxic fluid
- Divide constricting agent
- Check for viability
- Resection of gangrene
- Repair of hernia—without mesh
- Broad-spectrum antibiotics

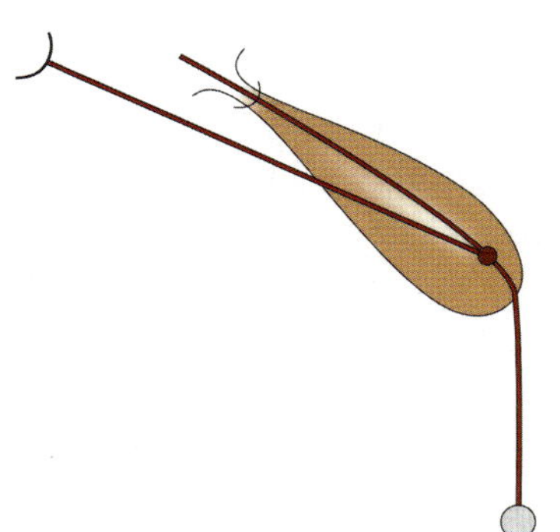
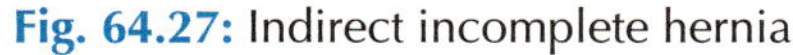

**Fig. 64.27:** Indirect incomplete hernia

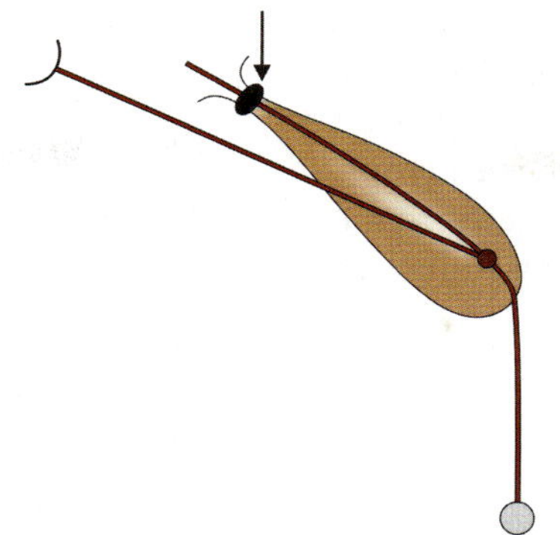

**Fig. 64.28:** High ligation—sac is ligated as close to the deep ring as possible

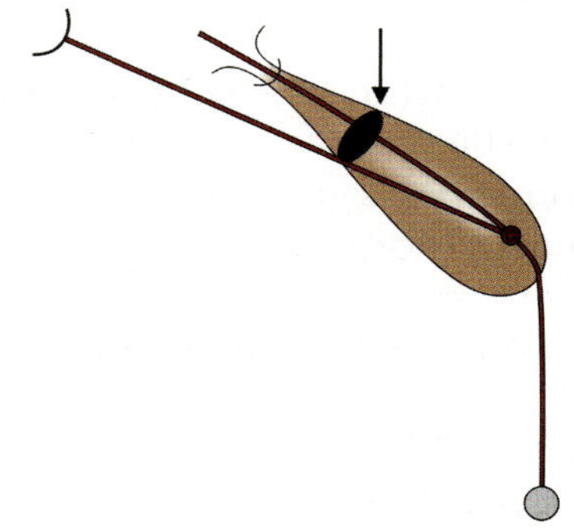

**Fig. 64.29:** Low ligation—cause for recurrence

64.28). Low ligation (Fig. 64.29) should not be done because it causes recurrence.

- If the bowel is gangrenous, resection of gangrenous segment and anastomosis is done. Closure of incision includes placement of tube drain, which is brought out through a separate incision.
- Mesh should not be used in this situation. A simple darning or herniorrhaphy can be done.
- If viability of the bowel is doubtful, the intestinal loops are covered with warm wet mops for a period of 5–10 minutes and 100% oxygen is given to the patient (request the anaesthetist). Return to pink colour, peristalsis of bowel and pulsations in the mesentery indicate viability.
- If the general condition of the patient permits, repair of the hernia may also be done.
- If evidence of peritonitis is present or if gangrene is spreading within, laparotomy should be done.

### 4. Incarcerated Hernia

It is an obstructed hernia due to obstruction caused by faecal matter. It generally occurs in a sliding hernia. ***(Nowadays incarcerated hernia has been renamed as obstructed hernia).***

### 5. Inflamed Hernia

It occurs when the contents of hernia get inflamed, e.g. appendicitis in a hernial sac, Meckel's diverticulitis in hernial sac. Thus, complications of hernia can be dangerous (Key Box 64.10). It may range from a simple obstruction to a life-threatening strangulation. Hence, early diagnosis and early treatment are necessary in all cases of indirect hernia. In a few selected cases of direct hernia, wherein the defect is big, the chances of strangulation are less. However, if there are no medical contraindications, surgery has to be advised.

- Following are a few examples of strangulations without obstruction. They have diarrhoea and bleeding per rectum rather than constipation (Key Box 64.11).

Key Box 64.10

**Summary of Complications of Hernia**

- Irreducibility
- Obstructed hernia
- Strangulation
- Incarcerated hernia
- Inflamed hernia

Key Box 64.11

**Strangulation without Obstruction**

- Omentocoele
- Richter's hernia page 1099
- Littre's hernia page 1100

## RECURRENT HERNIA

Incidence of recurrence is 10% and commonly occurs medially.

### Causes

#### *I. Preoperative*

- Chronic cough
- Weak muscle tone
- Straining while passing urine, constipation
- Obesity, ascites, anaemia.

#### *II. Intraoperative*

- **Improper excision of the sac: The sac should be ligated at the level of deep ring (neck).** This is called **high ligation of the sac**. Very often, the sac is seen as soon as the inguinal canal is opened. If it is ligated at the fundus or body (low ligation), it invariably results in recurrence. A missed indirect sac can be a cause of recurrence.
- **Absorbable sutures** such as catgut have lifespan of 2–3 weeks. 2-0 prolene, non-absorbable suture is used nowadays.

- **Bleeding:** At the end of the surgery, small bleeding points should be coagulated by using diathermy or ligatures. Haematoma formation predisposes to infection, which can be the cause of recurrence.
- **Tension** between suture lines can cause strangulation and fibrosis of muscle fibres. Hence, care and gentleness are important while suturing conjoined tendon to the inguinal ligament.

### *III. Postoperative*

Postoperative necrosis of midline incision due to vascularity which results in infection, tissue loss and incisional hernia (Fig. 64.30). Wound infection following hernioplasty is also one of the causes for recurrence.

- **Persistent postoperative cough** weakens the suture line.
- **Haematoma** can get secondarily infected resulting in pus formation. The sutures give way leading to recurrence. Hence, if there is a significant haematoma, it should be drained.
- **Infection:** Even though hernia is a clean surgery, chances of infection are present specially in diabetics, alcoholics and immunocompromised patients. Prophylactic antibiotics such as 2nd generation cephalosporin should be given. If infection occurs, it should be treated accordingly.
- **Exertion:** Too much exertion in the postoperative period, in the form of lifting heavy weights or carrying heavy weights on the shoulder, may weaken the suture line, resulting in hernia.

  Most of the recurrences occur within one year. Incidence of recurrent hernia may vary from 2 to 8% even in experienced hands. In a case of recurrent hernia, it is difficult to say whether it is a direct hernia or indirect hernia. From the management point of view, it does not matter.

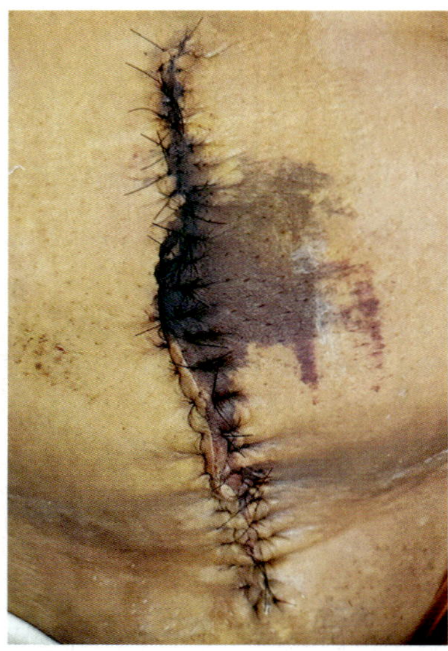

**Fig. 64.30:** Skin necrosis following incisional hernia

### Treatment

- If the sac is present due to incomplete excision at the previous surgery, it should be completely excised up to the level of deep ring, followed by hernioplasty.
- Meshplasty is the surgical treatment for a recurrent hernia. However, if mesh cannot be placed either due to infection or due to nonavailability, prolene darning can be done.
- Tuberculosis must be ruled out in cases of persisting infection.
- In all these cases, precipitating factors if any, should be treated first.
- The only way to totally prevent recurrence is by closure of the deep ring. This can be done only after dividing the spermatic cord (Kuntz procedure). It is indicated in elderly patients who have multiple recurrences.

## SPECIAL HERNIAS

1. **Giant hernia:** Sac extends up to mid-thigh (Fig. 64.31).

*Definition:* A giant inguino-scrotal hernia is defined as a hernia that extends below the midpoint of the inner thigh in the standing position.

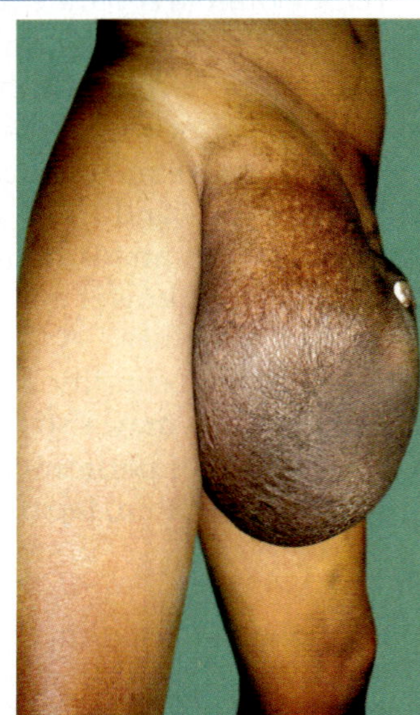

**Fig. 64.31:** Giant hernia

#### *Clinical features*

- Most patients would have had their hernia for several years.
- The contents often include colon, small intestines and bladder.
- A few of these are also sliding inguinal hernias.
- Hence, more prone for complications such as incarceration, intestinal obstruction and scrotal ulceration. The last complication is due to pressure necrosis or due to friction while walking or moving.
- Differential diagnosis includes scrotal elephantiasis.
- A few precautions to be taken during surgery are:
  - Preoperative chest physiotherapy.
  - Catheterise the bladder. This will decrease the incidence of urinary bladder injury.
  - Bowel wash before surgery.
  - Dissect the sac carefully all around.
  - Perfect haemostasis.
  - Omentectomy and rarely colectomy may be required (*see* Fig. 64.29) omentectomy.

- If bowel is not resected, mesh can be placed safely.
- In cases of emergency and patient with co-morbid factors including cardiac problems, take consent for orchidectomy—the best option will be to divide the cord at the level of deep ring and close the deep ring during orchidectomy.

2. **Dual hernia:** It has two sacs, one direct and another indirect, connected by an isthmus which is behind the inferior epigastric artery. It is also known as saddlebag hernia, **pantaloon hernia**, dual hernia or Romberg hernia.

   **Significance**
   - Deep ring occlusion test: The inference of the test may not be correct.
   - It is the cause of recurrence, if one sac is not treated properly.

3. **Prevesical hernia:** It is also called **funicular direct hernia**. It is a hernia containing portion of the bladder with prevesical fat through the defect in the conjoined tendon on the medial side. History of the swelling becoming less prominent after micturition may be present. Due to narrow neck, it is prone for strangulation.

4. **Maydl's hernia (Hernia-en-W)** (Fig. 64.32)
   - It is a **W** hernia wherein the intra-abdominal bowel loop segment becomes gangrenous very early but in the scrotum, there are no signs of gangrene.
   - The patient presents with obstructed hernia and at operation, the inguinoscrotal segment has no gangrene. The intra-abdominal segment must be examined and the gangrenous portion should be excised. It can also be called retrograde strangulation. Clinically, there is tenderness above the inguinal ligament.

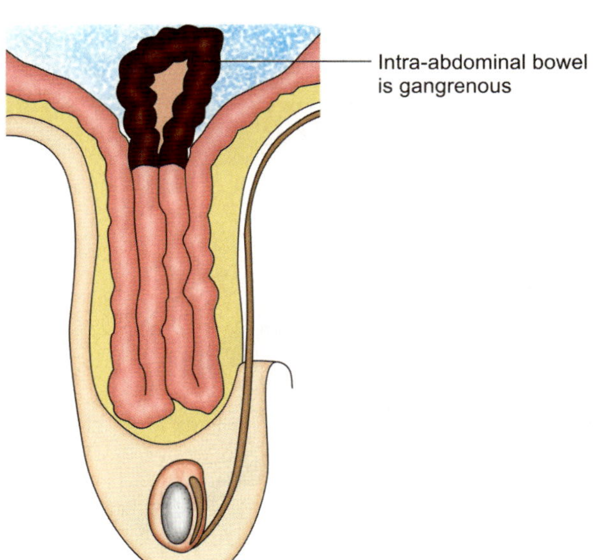


**Fig. 64.32:** Maydl's hernia

5. **Richter's hernia** (Fig. 64.33)
   - When only part of circumference of bowel becomes strangulated, it is called Richter's hernia.
   - It may spontaneously reduce
   - Thus, gangrene may be overlooked at operation
   - Even though the patient has features of intestinal obstruction, there will be diarrhoea and often blood in stools.

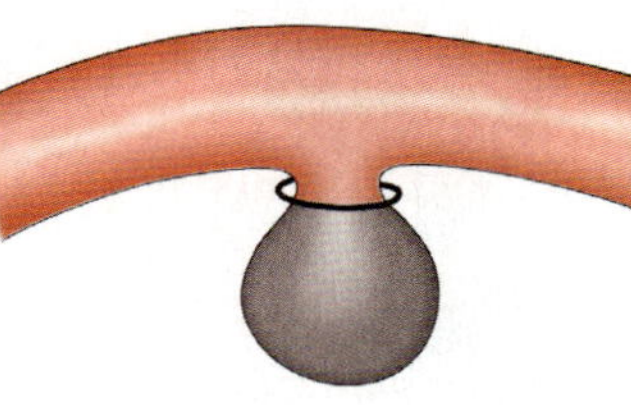

**Fig. 64.33:** Richter's hernia

   - Femoral hernia and obturator hernia are a few examples of hernia which can sometimes present as **Richter's hernia**.

6. **Sliding hernia** (Hernia-en-glissade) (Figs 64.34A to C)
   - Incidence: 1–3%
   - Always acquired hernia

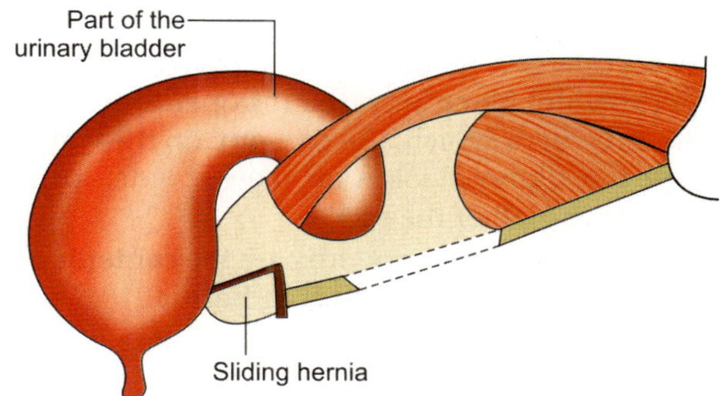


**Fig. 64.34A:** Sliding hernia

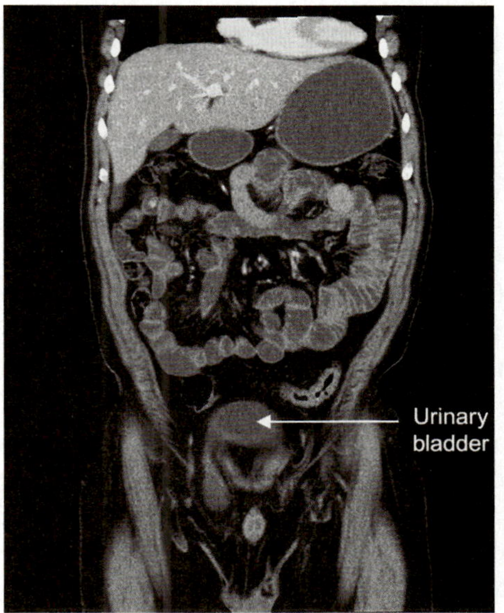


**Fig. 64.34B:** CECT scan: Sliding hernia showing part of the urinary bladder. (*Courtesy:* Prof. SS Prasad, Dr Rajendra, Dr Vijayendra, Associate Professors, Department of Surgery, KMC, Manipal)

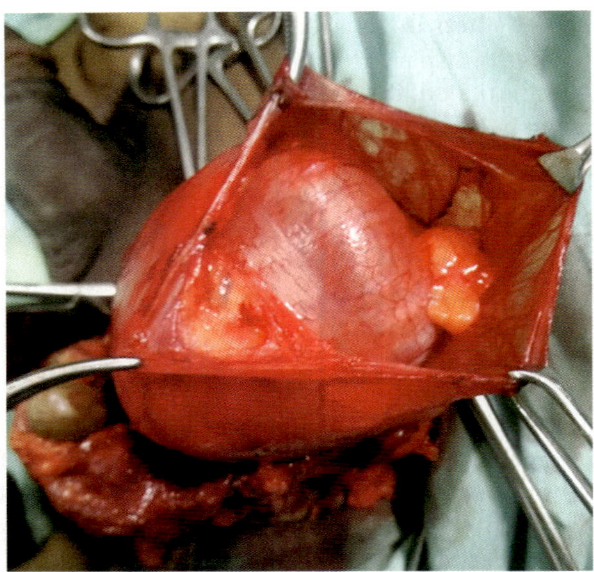

Fig. 64.34C: Sliding hernia. Note that sigmoid colon is forming wall of the sac. (*Courtesy:* Dr Amit Jain, Brindhavvan Areion Hospital, Bengaluru)

- It occurs as a result of the slipping of posterior peritoneum along with the retroperitoneal viscus. As a result of which, the caecum, on the right side and the sigmoid colon on the left side, form the posterior wall of the sac.
- **If the caecum and appendix are the contents of the hernial sac, it is not a sliding hernia.**
- However, a true hernial sac containing omentum or intestines exists.
- Weakness of the abdominal wall at the deep ring lateral to inferior epigastric vessels is also a contributing factor.
- Urinary bladder can also be the content of the hernial sac (*see* Fig. 64.34A).

### Clinical features

- It almost always occurs in males.
- It commonly affects elderly patients.
- It can be suspected when there is a large hernia descending down into the scrotum.
- Left-sided is more common than right-sided hernia.
- It practically always occurs in long-standing cases of inguinal hernia.
- They are not completely reducible.
- It can be direct hernia and indirect hernia also.

**Complications:** These hernias can easily strangulate and since its wall contents include the large intestine, the mortality and morbidity increases.

### Treatment

- Truss is absolutely contraindicated.
- Once the hernial sac is opened, the sac **should not be twisted**.
- A purse-string suture is applied within to avoid injury to caecum/sigmoid colon.
- The sac is removed and the repair of the hernia done.
- In elderly patients, orchidectomy is advised to give a permanent cure for hernia.

**SLIDING HERNIA—KEY POINTS**

- Always acquired
- Always (almost) in males
- Always occur in long-standing hernias
- Always irreducible
- Always colon or urinary bladder forms the wall of the sac
- Always requires a repair
- Always technical difficulties are encountered by junior surgeons while operating on these patients

**7. Sportsman's hernia**

- This is common in men who play rugby or football wherein injury due to the ball may occur.
- Pain is in the groin radiating to scrotum and upper thigh.
- On examination, there may be tenderness in the inguinal region.
- Orthopaedic disorders must be ruled out first by MRI or CT scan. They are soft tissue injury in the groin, pubic bone diastasis, adductor spasm, etc.
- If hernia is due to tearing of muscles **(Gilmore's groin)**—it should be repaired in the usual manner.

**8. Littre's hernia** (Fig. 64.35): It is referred to a hernia containing Meckel's diverticulum. When the diverticulum gets infected, such hernias are called inflamed hernias. Infection may be precipitated by partial obstruction to the diverticulum by constricting agents.

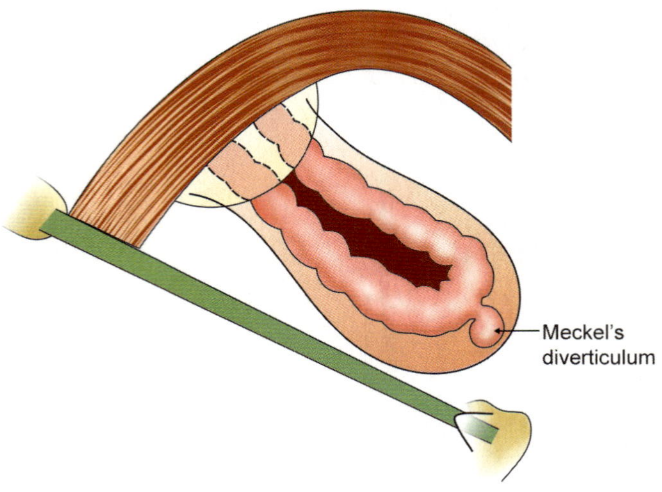


Fig. 64.35: Littre's hernia

## FEMORAL HERNIA

**SU28.1.15:** Describe anatomy, pathophysiology, required investigations for diagnosis of femoral hernia and the surgical techniques in management of femoral hernia.

Herniation of intra-abdominal contents through the femoral canal is described as femoral hernia. Women are more often involved, as compared to men with the ratio being 2:1, which is doubled in parous women. However, it should be remembered that **in women, inguinal hernias are the most common type of hernia, followed by incisional hernia.** Femoral hernia is the third most common type of hernia.

Commonly the hernia is unilateral, the right side being affected more often than the left side. It is bilateral in about 15–20% of the patients.

### Anatomy of Femoral Canal and Femoral Ring

(Fig. 64.36)

- The femoral canal extends from the femoral ring to the saphenous ring. It is 1½ inches below and lateral to the pubic tubercle. It is the innermost compartment of femoral sheath.
- It is similar to a truncated cone **which is narrow at the femoral ring**.
- **Contents of femoral canal are:**
  - Fat
  - Fascia
  - Lymphatics: Lymph node of Cloquet
- Femoral vein is in the middle compartment of the femoral sheath and femoral artery is in the lateral compartment.
- Femoral nerve is outside the femoral sheath.
- Femoral sheath: Fascia transversalis is continued downwards behind the inguinal ligament as the anterior layer of the femoral sheath. Fascia iliaca continues behind the femoral vessels as the posterior layer of the femoral sheath.

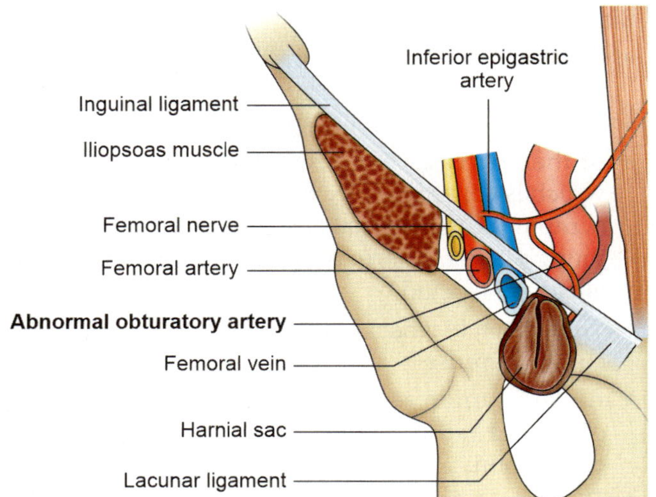


**Fig. 64.36:** Femoral hernia: Anatomy

### Boundaries of Femoral Ring

- ***Anterior:*** Inguinal ligament.
- ***Posterior:*** Ligament of Cooper, iliopectineal ligament.
- ***Medial:*** Lacunar ligament (Gimbernat's ligament).
- ***Lateral:*** Thin septum which separates the femoral canal from femoral vein (silver fascia).

### Causes for Femoral Hernia

1. **Pregnancy:** As the gravid uterus compresses the external iliac vein, the empty femoral sheath on the medial side allows the femoral vein to expand within femoral sheath. Thus, increased abdominal pressure due to repeated pregnancies is one of the chief factors responsible for femoral hernias. The maximum incidence is around 30–40 years of age.
2. **Wide femoral canal:** This is due to the narrow insertion of iliopubic tract into the pectineal line of the pubis and may be responsible for a few cases of femoral hernia.

*Pearls of Wisdom*

Femoral hernia is never congenital.

### Course of the Hernial Sac

As the hernia comes into the femoral canal, it is an oblong swelling due to the rigid femoral canal. When it comes out through the saphenous opening, it expands and becomes retort shaped because Scarpa's fascia is attached to the deep fascia of thigh below the saphenous opening. Hernia will be covered with following layers (Key Box 64.12).

Key Box 64.12

**Femoral Hernia: Coverings**

- Sac
- Fat and lymphoid tissue
- Transversalis fascia
- Cribriform fascia
- Superficial fascia
- Skin

### Clinical Features of Femoral Hernia

- Females between the age of 20 and 40 years are commonly affected.
- **Gaur sign: Dilatation of superficial epigastric/circumflex iliac veins due to compression.**
- Right side is more commonly affected because of the dominant nature of right side of the body.

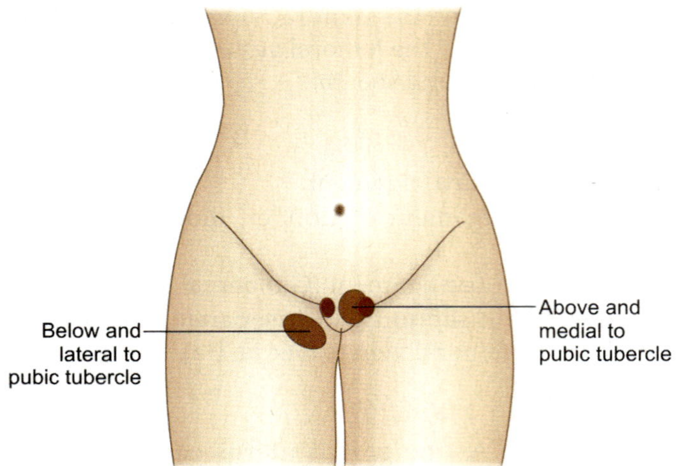


**Fig. 64.37:** Femoral hernia (R) and indirect hernia (L)

- To start with, there is a small swelling below the inguinal ligament, which goes unnoticed very often.
- Expansile impulse is often not present due to the narrow canal.
- Reducibility may be present.
- Typically, the swelling is below and lateral to the pubic tubercle (inguinal hernia is above and medial to pubic tubercle) (Fig. 64.37).
- Many (30–80%) present with strangulation.

### Treatment (Key Box 64.13)

1. **Low operation of Lockwood:** Incision is placed directly over the swelling in the thigh. The sac is carefully dissected out without damaging the femoral vein. The sac is ligated at the neck, excised and the hernia is repaired—the **inguinal ligament is sutured to Cooper's ligament** (iliopectineal ligament) thus obliterating the femoral ring. Nonabsorbable suture such as prolene or ethilon is ideal. Low approach is indicated in uncomplicated hernia. It is very difficult to manage a gangrenous loop of bowel with this approach.

Key Box 64.13

**Surgery of Femoral Hernia**

- Should be done as early as possible, once the diagnosis is made.
- For elective repair, low (femoral) approach: Incision directly over the swelling is ideal. Injury to abdominal obturator artery can occur in this route (found on lateral side in 20% of cases).
- Transinguinal (Lothiessen): Can use it when there is gangrene. However, it may weaken inguinal canal.
- Combined: High approach is the choice for strangulated femoral hernias. Approximate inguinal ligament and pectineal ligament.

**ABNORMAL OBTURATOR ARTERY**

Normal obturator artery is a branch of the internal iliac artery. It gives a pubic branch which anastomoses with pubic branch of the inferior epigastric artery. Occasionally, this anastomosis is large and obturator artery then appears to be a branch of the inferior epigastric artery. Usually, it passes lateral to the femoral canal in contact with the femoral vein. Occasionally, the abnormal artery may lie along the medial margin of the femoral ring, i.e. along the free margin of the lacunar ligament. This artery is in danger during surgery for obstructed femoral hernia.

2. **Inguinal operation**
   - Through an **inguinal incision,** the inguinal canal is opened. The transversalis fascia is incised. Hernial sac is visualised. This is followed by excision of the sac. The high approach is preferred when there is a strangulated femoral hernia. This offers a very good view of the abnormal obturator artery from above, if it is present.
   - Repair is done by suturing the conjoined tendon to iliopectineal line.
3. **Combined approach: High operation of McEvedy:** Inguinofemoral approach: A vertical incision is made over the swelling and extended above the inguinal ligament, and the sac can be dissected from both above and below (look for abnormal obturator artery—see below). This approach has the advantages of both operations mentioned above.
4. **Henry's approach:** Lower midline for bilateral hernia.

### Complications of Femoral Hernia

1. As the femoral ring and the neck of the sac are narrow, obstruction and strangulation are very common.
2. Richter's hernia
   - Commonly seen in femoral hernias and obturator hernias, which have narrow necks.
   - This occurs when a **portion of the circumference of the bowel** is caught within the hernial sac and which is constricted by the narrow ring. Signs and symptoms of intestinal obstruction are absent, even though it is an obstructed hernia, because the lumen is not obstructed.
   - The hernia is tense, tender, irreducible and has no cough impulse.
   - As the lumen is patent, there may be bloody diarrhoea rather than constipation. Gangrene can occur soon.
   - **Treatment:** Combined or inguinal approach to deal with gangrene.

## Summary of Femoral Hernia (Key Box 64.14)

### *Rare Types of Femoral Hernia*

1. **Lacunar hernia (Laugier's hernia):** In this case, the hernia passes through a small defect in the lacunar ligament.
2. **Prevascular hernia (Narath's femoral hernia):** In this case, the hernial sac is located behind the femoral vessels and the inguinal ligament. It may be associated with congenital dislocation of the hip (Narath's hernia).
3. **Pectineal hernia:** In this case, the hernia passes between the pectineus muscle and its fascia, behind the femoral vessels. It is also called Cloquet's hernia.
4. **External femoral hernia:** It is a hernia lateral to the femoral artery (Hesselbach's hernia).

Key Box 64.14

**Femoral Hernia**

- Rarely occurs in males (5–10%)
- Commonly associated with Richter's hernia
- Fatty female with small swelling under a big belly usually goes undetected
- Dangerous because of early strangulation
- Cannot be controlled by a truss
- Surgical repair is a must

## Differential Diagnosis of Femoral Hernia

1. **Inguinal hernia:** An inguinal hernia is above and medial to pubic tubercle. The femoral hernia is below and lateral to pubic tubercle.
2. **Saphena varix:** It is the dilated, saccular, upper end of long saphenous vein with varicosity. It disappears on lying down because of gravity. Thrill may be felt on coughing (Fig. 64.38).
3. **Lipoma:** Soft and lobular, slips under palpating fingers (Fig. 64.39).
4. **Femoral artery aneurysm** is rare. It presents as a pulsatile swelling in the groin with a continuous murmur. Peripheral pulses are often weak (Fig. 64.40).
5. **Enlarged femoral lymph nodes** are firm and round. They can be enlarged in lower limb infections, abrasions, wounds in the perineum and also in carcinoma penis (Fig. 64.41).
6. **Psoas bursa:** Osteoarthritis of the hip can produce distension of psoas bursa, which disappears on flexing the hip. Tuberculosis spine can present as iliopsoas abscess (Fig. 64.42).
7. **Psoas abscess:** It is an iliopsoas abscess due to tuberculosis of spine. There are two swellings, one above and one below the inguinal ligament. Cross fluctuation can be elicited between these two swellings. Tenderness over the spine and X-ray of the spine help in arriving at a diagnosis (Fig. 64.43).

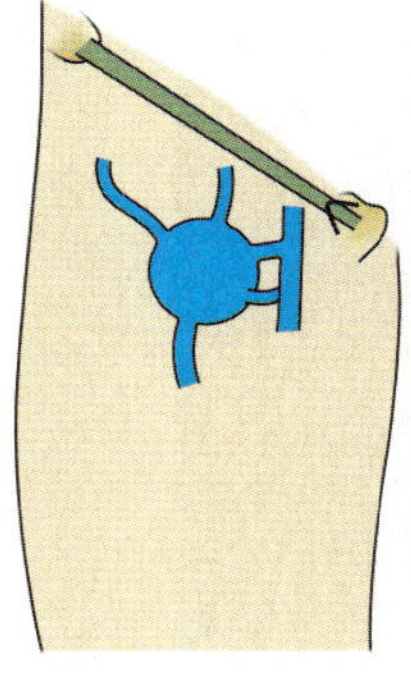
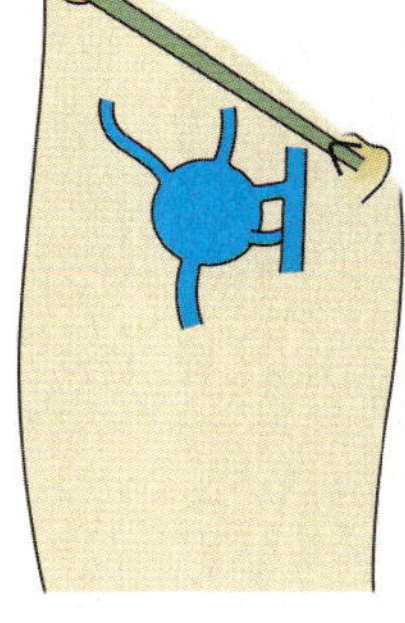

**Fig. 64.38:** Saphena varix

**Fig. 64.39:** Left inguinal lipoma of the cord

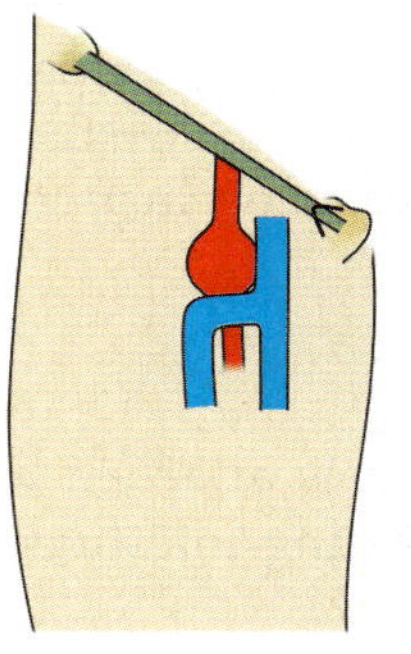

**Fig. 64.40:** Femoral artery aneurysm

**Fig. 64.41:** Lymphadenitis

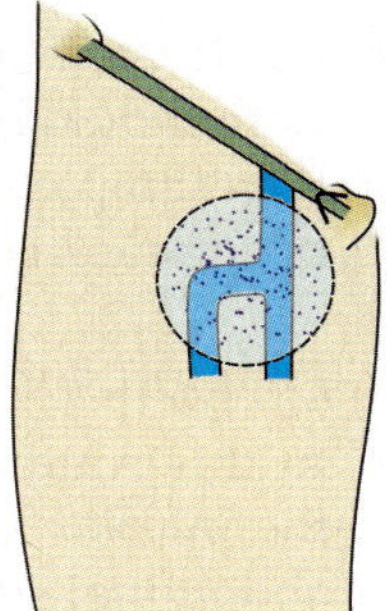

**Fig. 64.42:** Psoas bursa

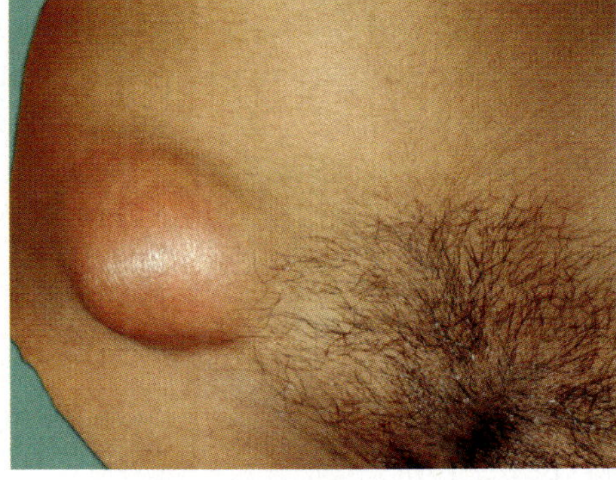

**Fig. 64.43:** Iliopsoas abscess

## VENTRAL HERNIAS

All hernias which occur in the ventral part of the abdomen are called as ventral hernias. They include umbilical hernia, epigastric hernia, postoperative incisional hernia and rare hernia, such as Spigelian hernia, interparietal hernia, etc. They are discussed below:

### UMBILICAL HERNIA

It can be discussed under three headings:

I. Umbilical hernia of newborn
II. Umbilical hernia of infants and children
III. Umbilical hernia of adults.

## Umbilical Hernia of Newborn

- It is called omphalocoele—exomphalos.
- It is found 1 in 6000 live births.
- Failure of midgut as a **whole or part** to return into coelomic cavity during embryonic life results in exomphalos.
- It is also associated with weakness of abdominal musculature (few fibres may be absent). Two types have been recognised.

### 1. *Exomphalos Minor* (Fig. 64.44A)

- In this condition, the umbilical cord is attached to the summit of the sac.
- Sac is small and defect less than 5 cm.
- It is treated by twisting the cord and ligating the sac. Care should be taken to avoid damage to the intestine. For example, nursing the child preoperatively in prone position can damage intestines.

### 2. *Exomphalos Major* (Fig. 64.44B)

- In this condition, the umbilical cord is attached to the inferior aspect of the sac, containing intestines, abdominal structures, e.g. liver, bowel.
- Many children are stillborn.
- This type of hernia is usually associated with absent abdominal musculature.
- The operation should be done before the rupture of the sac as the morbidity increases greatly in the event of a rupture of the sac.
- During the operation, skin flaps are raised on both sides to cover the defect. A true repair is necessary and is done at a later date.
- *See* also Figs 64.45 and 64.46.

## Umbilical Hernia of Infants and Children

- It occurs as a complication of umbilical sepsis, which weakens the umbilical scar.
- It is a true umbilical hernia containing either omentum/intestines.

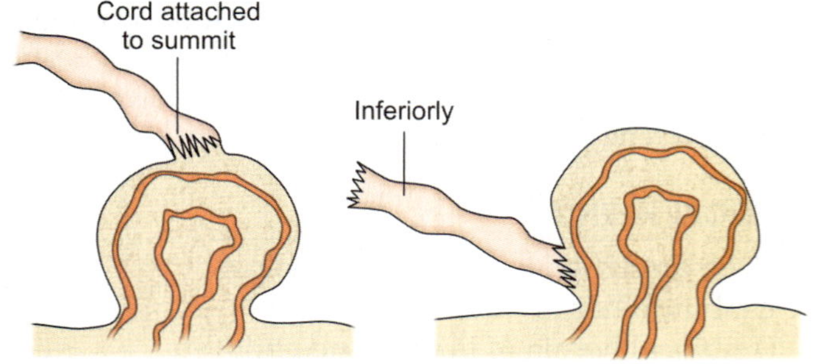


**Fig. 64.44A:** Exomphalos minor **Fig. 64.44B:** Exomphalos major

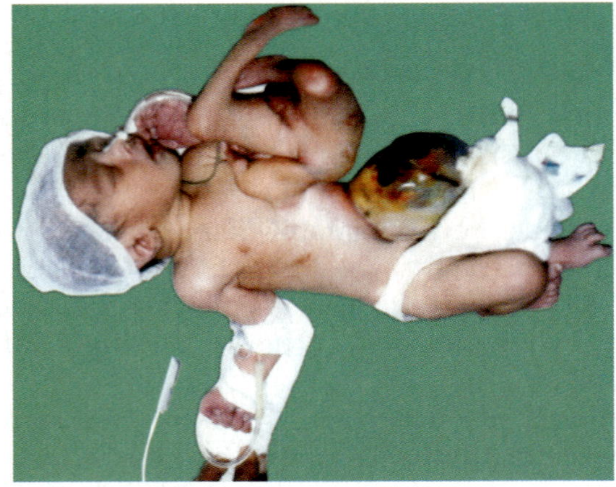

**Fig. 64.45:** Epigastric heterophagus with exomphalos major

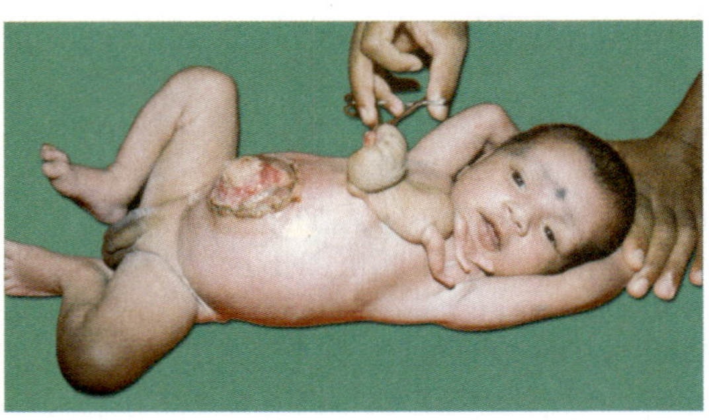

**Fig. 64.46:** Same child on the 21st postoperative day. The repair is done by rotating flaps from gluteal region of the parasitic baby. (*Courtesy:* Prof Vidyadhar Kinhal, Late Prof RS Channagiri, Dr Channanna, Department of Surgery, Vijayanagar Institute of Medical Sciences, Bellary, Karnataka)

### *Clinical Features*

- Common in male children
- The child is brought with the complaint of swelling in the umbilical region whenever the child cries.
- Most of the cases are symptomless. Parents are anxious about the swelling.
- Strangulation is rare (Fig. 64.47).

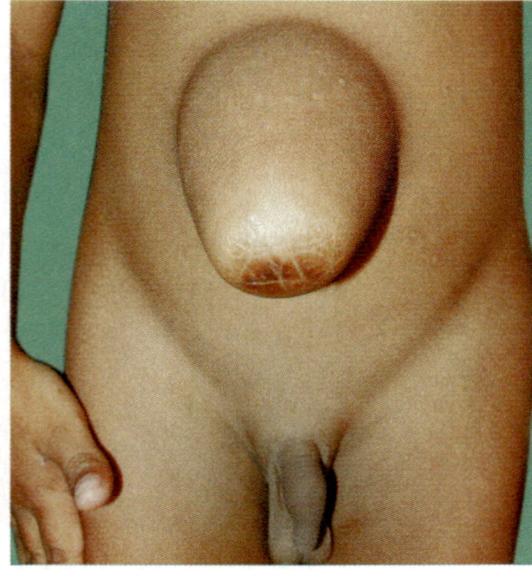

**Fig. 64.47:** Umbilical hernia in a child

### Treatment

- **Reassurance** is the most important advice given to the parents.
- **No treatment is required** other than **strapping** the abdominal wall by keeping a pad in front of umbilicus.
- Majority of the hernias get corrected by 2 years of age (90%).
- If the hernia does not correct itself, repair is necessary to close the defect in the linea alba.

## Umbilical Hernia of Adults

- It is not a true umbilical hernia but it is a paraumbilical hernia in which the hernia occurs either above, below or to the side of the umbilicus, through the linea alba.
- The contents are the greater omentum, transverse colon or small bowel. Due to adhesion, it is often irreducible.

### Aetiology

- Females in the 5th decade are commonly affected. Male:female ratio is 1:5.
- **Obesity** with flabby abdominal muscle predisposes to paraumbilical hernia.
- Repeated **pregnancies** also weaken the abdominal wall.
- Ascites may precipitate hernia especially in cirrhotic patients.

### Clinical Features

- Patient presents with a swelling in the umbilical region, which increases on straining or coughing.
- On asking the patient to cough, **expansile impulse** is present (Fig. 64.48).
- They may also have inguinal hernia.
- **Reducibility can be present.**
- **Dragging pain** is usually due to omentum which is felt as a firm or granular mass. If gurgling is present, it is indicative of small intestines in the hernial sac.
- After reducing the swelling, the **defect** can be felt in the linea alba.

***Refer to Table 64.4 for comparison between umbilical hernia in infants and adults.***

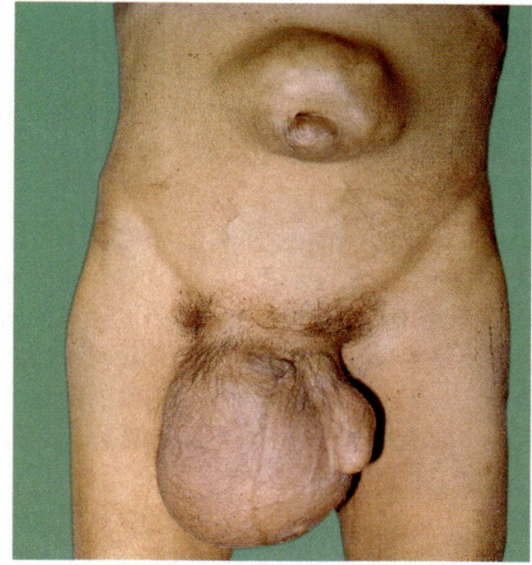

**Fig. 64.48:** Large direct hernia with umbilical hernia

### Complications

1. **Irreducibility** is common due to adhesions between omentum and the sac.
2. **Obstruction** presents with colicky abdominal pain and vomiting. Distension follows soon. Untreated cases develop strangulation. Very often, these patients present with **incarcerated** hernia due to the presence of transverse colon in the sac. They require urgent intervention, failing which gangrene will set in.
3. As the sac enlarges, due to its weight and gravity, it sags down resulting in friction of the skin and this causes **intertrigo** (Fig. 64.49).

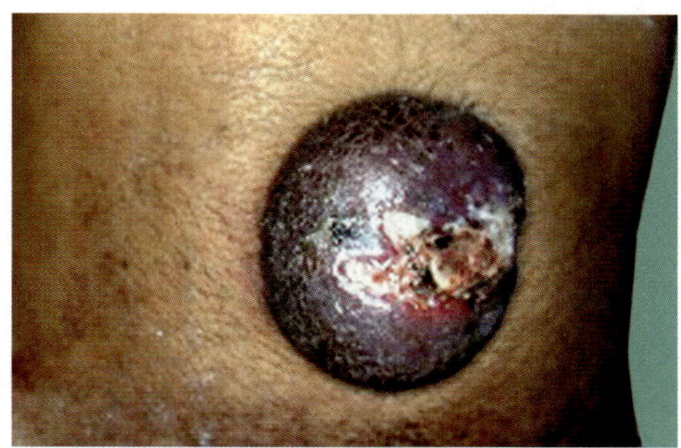

**Fig. 64.49:** Umbilical hernia in a cirrhotic patient with skin changes and ulceration

**TABLE 64.4:** Comparison between umbilical hernia in infants and adults

| Features | Infants | Adults |
|---|---|---|
| Age in years | 0–3 | 50–60 |
| Sex | Common in male child | Common in females |
| Causes | Neonatal sepsis | Obesity, weak muscles, pregnancy |
| Defect | A small defect in the umbilical scar | Above or below the umbilicus |
| Symptoms | Symptomless | Symptoms are present |
| Strangulation | Rare | Very common |
| Treatment | Conservative (strapping), surgery (rare) | Mayo's repair |

### Treatment

1. Reduction of weight.
2. **Anatomical repair:** Small defects can be closed with nonabsorbable sutures such as nylon or prolene (Fig. 64.50).
3. **Most favoured** surgery for umbilical hernia is laparoscopic **mesh repair**—IPOM (intraperitoneal onlay mesh repair). It is a tensionless repair. It is the gold standard surgery for umbilical and incisional hernia in suitable cases. When the defect is closed and mesh repair is done, it is called as IPOM plus (Figs 64.51 to 64.56).

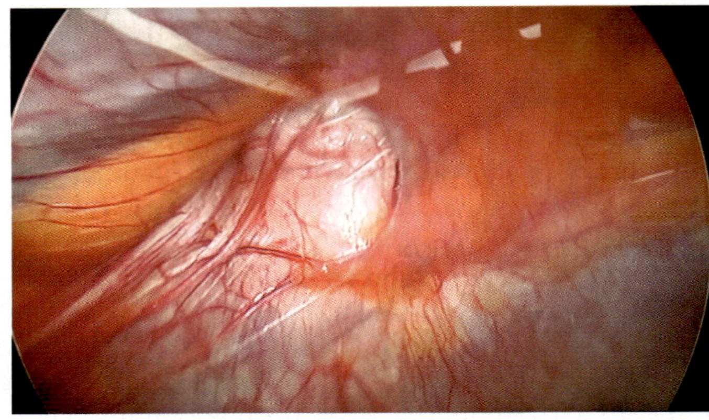

**Fig. 64.52:** Laparoscopic view of the defect

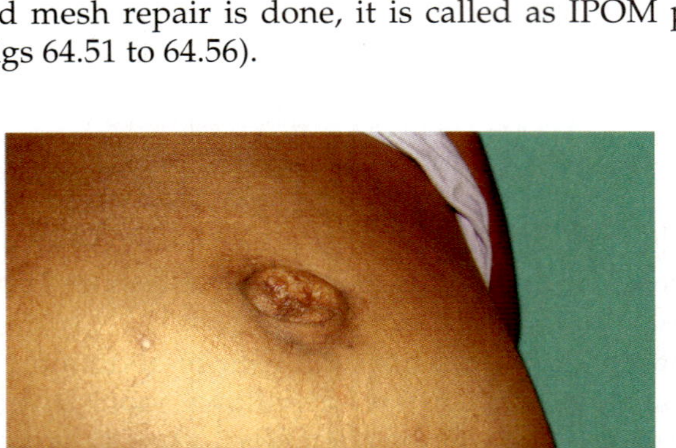

**Fig. 64.50:** True congenital umbilical hernia in an adult can be repaired by simple closure of the defect by non-absorbable sutures

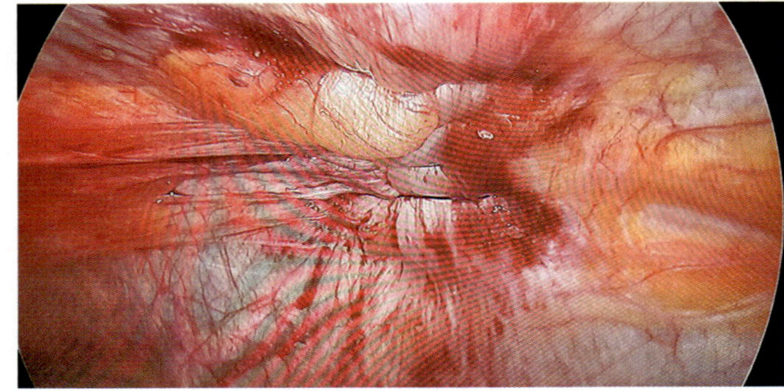

**Fig. 64.53:** Defect is closed

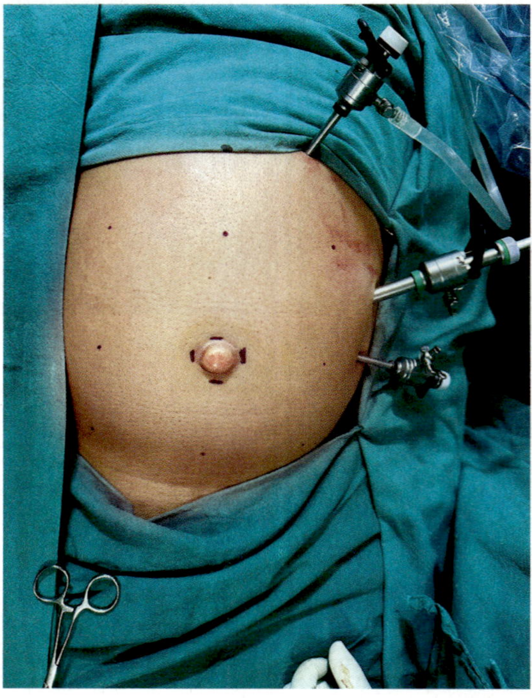

**Fig. 64.51:** External view showing umbilical hernia and markings of the umbilical defect and mesh coverage

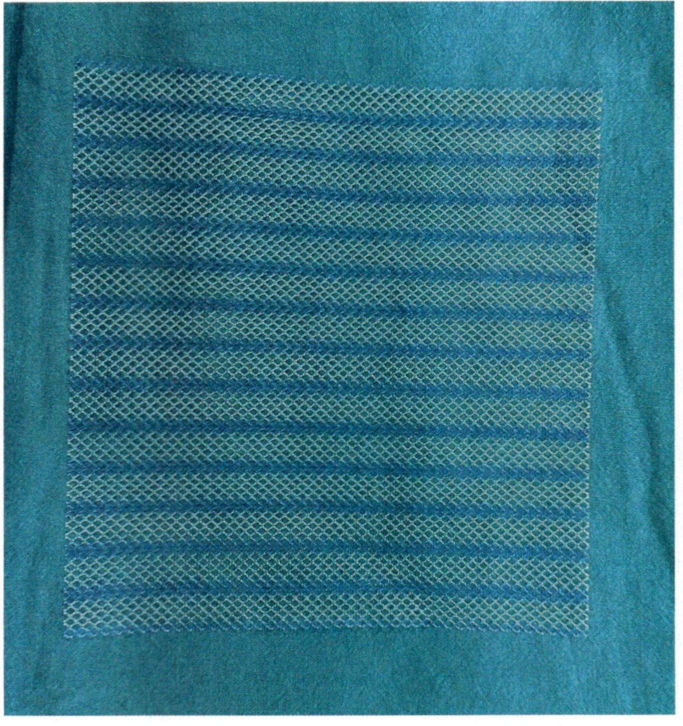

**Fig. 64.54:** 15 × 15 cm prolene mesh

Fig. 64.55: Mesh is rolled and long sutures applied and it is ready to be inserted into the peritoneal cavity

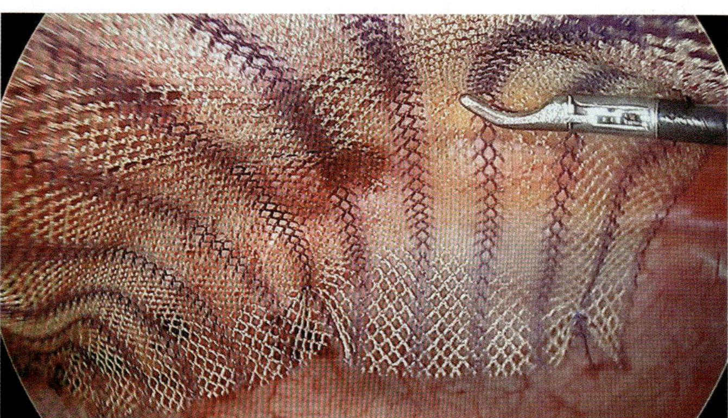

Fig. 64.56: Intraperitoneal mesh covering defect

4. ***Mayo's repair*** (surgical treatment, Fig. 64.57 and Key Box 64.15). Not done nowadays. In case of obstruction or strangulation, some surgeons may do this whereas others prefer anatomical closure.

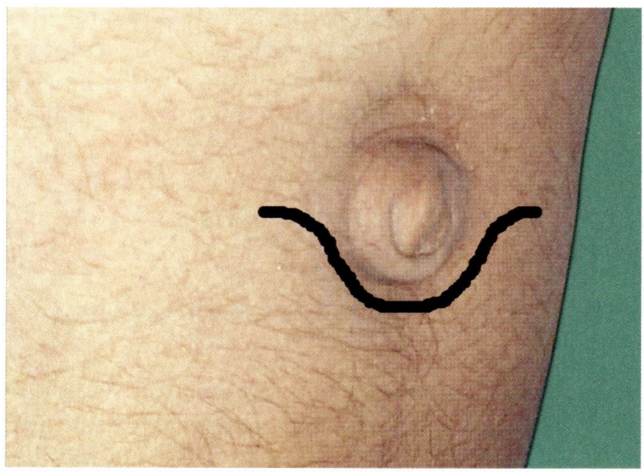

Fig. 64.57: Curvilinear incision

Key Box 64.15

**Mayo's Umbilical Herniorrhaphy**

- Excision of umbilicus
- Reduction of contents and excision of the sac
- Double breasting of the fibrous aponeurotic layer
- Haemostasis, suction and obliteration of dead space
- Additional lipectomy and umbilicoplasty

## INCISIONAL HERNIA

**SU28.1.16:** Describe classification of ventral hernias and clinical presentation and indications for surgical management of various ventral hernias.

It is also called **ventral hernia** or postoperative hernia. It is a hernia that occurs through a weak scar. Very common in females.

### ABDOMINAL WALL—SURGICAL ANATOMY

#### Contents

It consists of **skin, muscles, aponeurosis, linea alba, sheaths, ligaments, openings—rings**, blood vessels and nerves. Anatomically weak areas are the rings, junctions, empty spaces and where blood vessels pierce abdominal wall.

#### Formation of Rectus Sheath (Figs 64.58A to C)

A. Above the costal margin, only external oblique with aponeurosis contributes for rectus sheath.
B. Between xiphisternum and umbilicus, external oblique is in front. Internal oblique splits to enclose the rectus muscles. The transverse abdominis is behind the internal oblique. All fuse to form linea alba in the midline. Hence, this is the strong midline area.

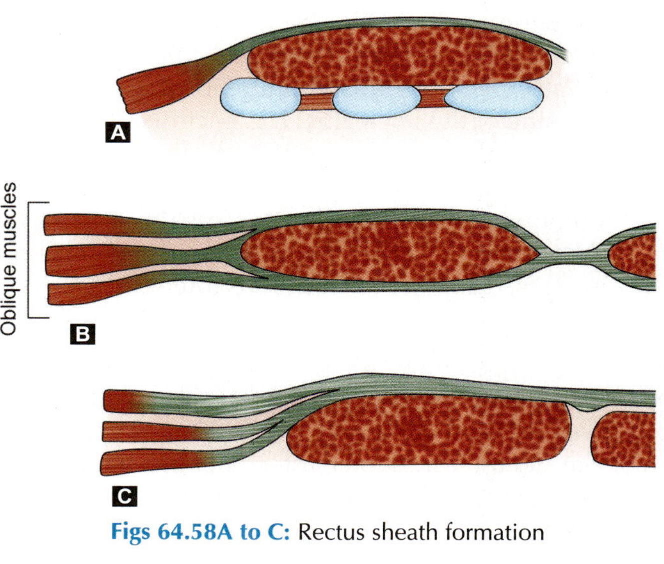


Figs 64.58A to C: Rectus sheath formation

C. Below semilunar line: All 3 aponeuroses are anterior to the muscles and fuse in the midline to form linea alba.

D. **Boundaries:** Roof is formed by diaphragm. Pelvis forms the inferior boundary with perineum which is the central muscular portion. Laterally, 3 abdominal muscles each having separate sheath run across towards midline and form rectus sheath (details later). Rectus sheath covers strong rectus abdominis muscles that extend from ribs to pelvis.

### Significance

- Rectus sheath—posterior rectus sheath is absent below semilunar line. Incisional hernia and spigelian hernia are common below the umbilicus.
- Linea alba—white, relatively avascular, broad above and narrow below. It is the strongest layer of the abdominal wall. Hence, during the closure of the midline incisions, it is important to include good bites through linea alba.
- Umbilicus—strong fibrous ring. Umbilical hernias are common in children due to childhood umbilical infections, in obese patients due to weak muscles and in multiparous woman due to stretching of the muscles due to repeated pregnancies.

## MUSCLES OF THE ANTEROLATERAL ABDOMINAL WALL—OBLIQUE MUSCLES

- The anterolateral abdominal wall is made up mainly of muscles. On either side of the midline, there are four large muscles. These are the external oblique, the internal oblique, the transversus abdominis and the rectus abdominis. Two small muscles, the cremaster and the pyramidalis are also present. The external oblique, the internal oblique and the transversus abdominis are large flat muscles placed in the anterolateral part of the abdominal wall. Each of them ends in an extensive aponeurosis that reaches the midline. Here the aponeuroses of the right and left sides decussate to form a median band called linea alba. The rectus abdominis runs vertically on either side of the linea alba. It is enclosed in a sheath formed by the aponeuroses of the flat muscles named above.
- Tendinous intersections—rectus sheath haematoma will be confined within the sheaths as it is prevented from spreading due to tendinous intersections.

### Precautions during Surgery

- Nerve supply—lower six thoracic and first lumbar nerves. They enter the rectus sheath laterally. In cases of paramedian incisions, after opening the anterior rectus sheath, rectus should be retracted laterally to define and incise the posterior rectus sheath.
- Blood vessels run within the rectus sheath. Rupture of inferior epigastric artery is a known entity resulting in a haematoma below the umbilicus (*see* page 1120). Differential diagnosis includes Spigelian hernia.
- Weak muscles—interstitial hernias—prune-belly syndrome: A partial or complete lack of abdominal muscles. There may be wrinkly folds of skin covering the abdomen. An undescended testicle in males can also be the problem.
- Weakness of muscles can also be due to damage to nerves, e.g. as in surgeries such as appendicectomy wherein ilioinguinal nerve may get damaged resulting in inguinal hernia. Empty spaces next to arteries are for expansion of veins but that may cause hernia. Example: Femoral hernia through medial empty space in femoral sheath.

### Anatomical Significance

- **Rectus sheath:** Posterior rectus sheath is absent below semilunar line. More chances of hernia.
- **Linea alba:** White, relatively avascular, broad above and narrow below—surgical incision in the midline can be made without any blood loss. Hernia of the linea alba occurs through the opening pierced by blood vessel.
- **Umbilicus:** Strong fibrous ring can also be the site of infections and weakness causing umbilical hernias.
- Tendinous intersections in the rectus sheath and branches of superior and inferior epigastric arteries run within rectus sheath, posteriorly—rectus sheath haematomas are always confined within.
- Nerve supply comes from lateral side. Hence, traction or retraction of rectus should be done laterally so as to avoid traction injuries to nerve fibres.
- Blood vessels like superior and inferior epigastric arteries run within the rectus sheath, posteriorly. Haematoma can occur due to rupture but it is confined within the rectus sheath.
- Weak muscles—interstitial hernias—Prune-Belly syndrome—a partial or complete lack of abdominal muscles. There may be wrinkly folds of skin covering the abdomen and undescended testicles in males.
- Ramirez component separation or slide operation is based on making relaxing incisions over the lateral muscles and slide them medially so as to cover large abdominal wall defects.

## FACTORS WHICH PRECIPITATE INCISIONAL HERNIA (Key Box 64.16)

1. **Infection:** Cases operated for peritonitis such as perforated duodenal ulcer, gangrene of the intestines, etc. usually develop incisional hernia. The drainage tubes which are placed inside the peritoneal cavity

Key Box 64.16

**Causes of Incisional Hernia**

- Infection uncontrolled
- Incision wrongly placed
- Improper suture material
- Increased intra-abdominal pressure

help in reducing the postoperative incisional hernias, by draining peritoneal contents outside.

2. **Anatomical site:** The midline[1] is especially weak in the lower abdomen because of absence of posterior rectus sheath below the arcuate line or semilunar line.
3. **Obesity with weak muscle tone** predisposes to incisional hernia.
4. **Faulty technique** of closure of the abdomen or **faulty sutures** are also responsible for incisional hernia.
5. **Ascites, distension and persistent postoperative cough** further weakens the incision.
6. **Wrongly placed incisions** wherein nerves of the abdominal muscles are cut, precipitate incisional hernia. Lumbar incisions, lower midline incisions and large transverse incisions often give rise to incisional hernias (Figs 64.59 to 64.61).
7. **Incisions** wherein nerves are cut, the chances of incisional hernias are more. Examples: Subcostal incision for removal of gallbladder.

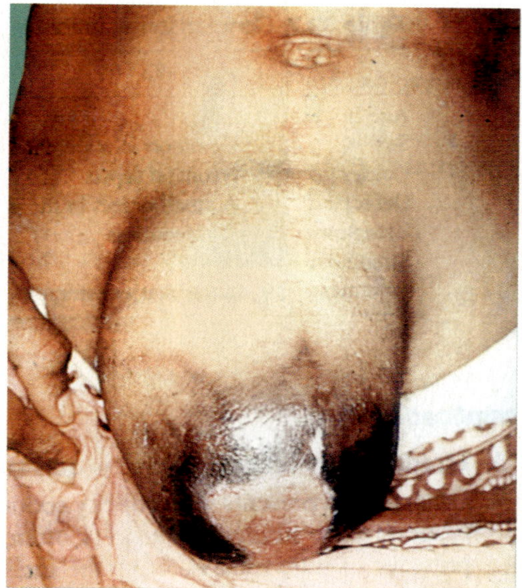

**Fig. 64.59:** Incisional hernia with decubitus ulcer due to obesity and weak muscle tone

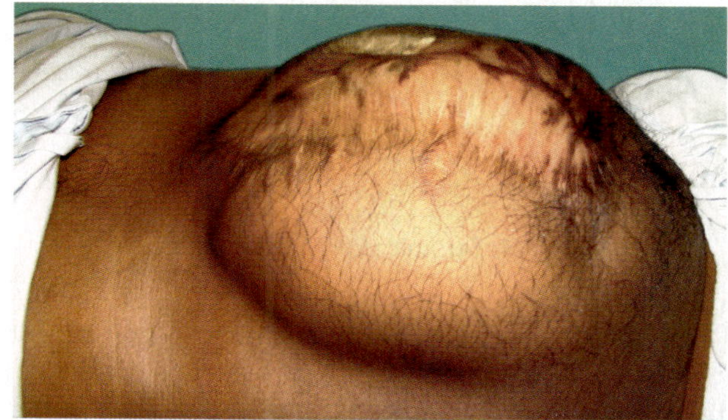

**Fig. 64.60:** Incisional hernia following laparotomy for perforated duodenal ulcer. He had stormy postoperative period

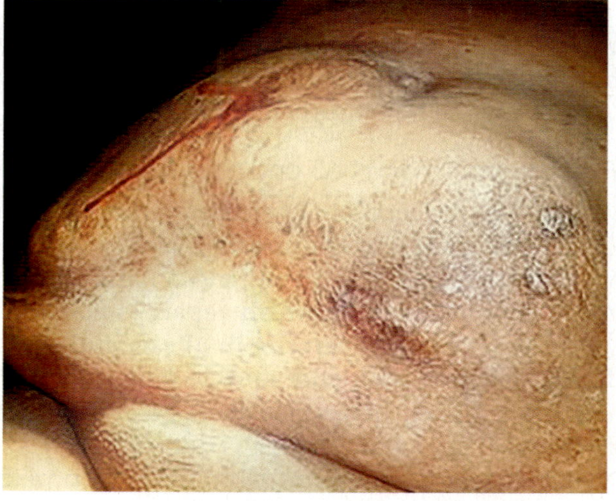

**Fig. 64.61:** Large obstructed incisional hernia

## Clinical Features

- Serosanguinous discharge on the 4th postoperative day through the main suture line is a signal of development of partial or total wound dehiscence. Such cases later develop an incisional hernia.
- History of infection during the first surgery, post-operative cough is usually present.
- There is a bulge/swelling in relation to the scar.
- Scar is thin and evidence of secondary healing in the form of irregular scar may be present.
- Expansile impulse on cough and reducibility may be present.
- After reduction of the contents, a defect can be palpated through the scar. Defect depends upon number of stitches that have given way.

## Treatment

- Surgical treatment is necessary if the **defect is narrow,** if there is **discomfort** to the patient or if there is a **danger** of obstruction (Figs 64.62 to 64.64).
- Preoperative preparation includes reduction of weight, control of cough, etc.

[1]Is that the reason why we see many cases of incisional hernia after gynaecological operations?

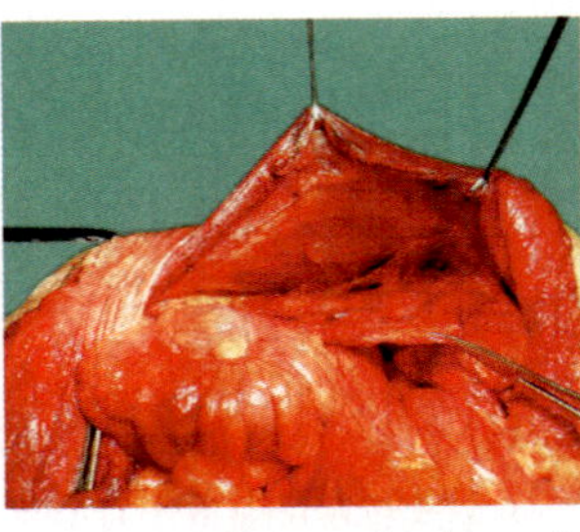
Fig. 64.62: Anatomical repair

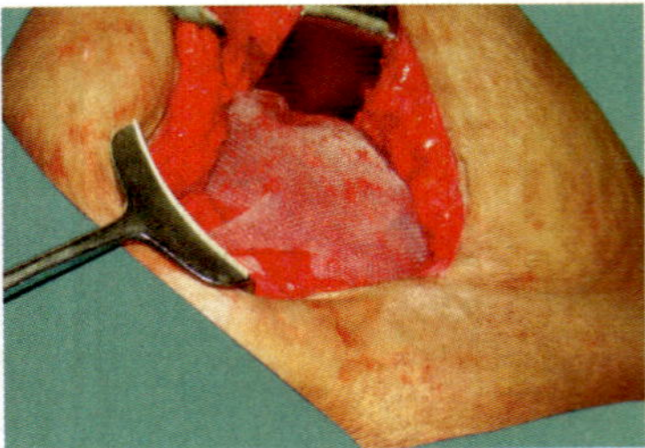
Fig. 64.63: Incisional hernia mesh repair

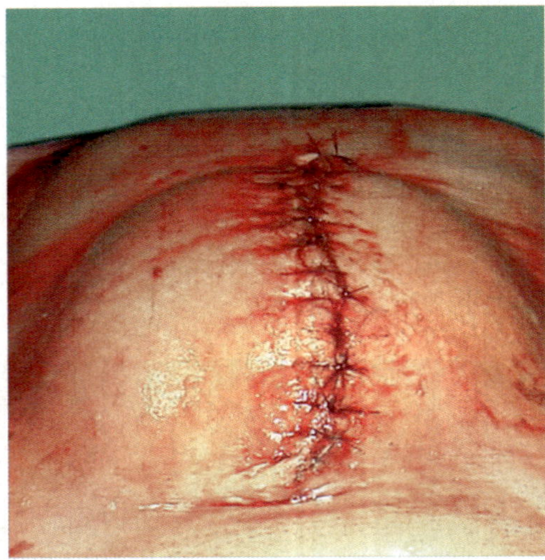
Fig. 64.64: Seroma after incisional hernia

- There are various operations for the treatment of incisional hernia depending upon the size of the defect, anatomical location of the incision and presence of precipitating factors.

### 1. Anatomical Repair

In this operation, all the anatomical layers such as peritoneum, posterior rectus sheath, linea alba and the subcutaneous tissue are identified. Closure is done layer by layer by using nonabsorbable suture material.

### 2. Mesh Repair (Fig. 64.63 and refer to Principles also)

- As most of the incisional hernias are due to a large defect in the main incision and the majority of it occurs in obese women, repair using mesh has become the most popular method. **Mesh repair is considered as the best repair, especially in obese, multiparous female patients with poor muscle tone.**
- In this operation, the sac is opened, greater omentum is excised, the contents are reduced followed by closure of the peritoneum. A mesh is then placed. Prolene mesh or Marlex mesh is commonly used. **In all these repairs, tensionless, nonabsorbable suture repairs are done.** Seroma is a common complication (Fig. 64.64).

#### PRINCIPLES

- Previous incision is opened to full length and the scar is excised
- Flaps are raised on both sides
- The edges of rectus abdominis muscles are defined
- The sac is identified, dissected, freed from surrounding structures
- It is opened, contents reduced, may have to excise omentum
- Redundant sac is excised
- Peritoneum is closed
- Placement of the mesh: Onlay means subcutaneous. It is a simple procedure. Mesh should overlap at least 5 cm all around the defect. Alternately, a plane is created between posterior rectus sheath and rectus muscle, mesh is placed in that location and anterior rectus sheath is sutured. This is called retromuscular sublay mesh repair. This may not be possible below the arcuate line because there is no posterior rectus sheath there.

### 3. Laparoscopic Mesh Repair

**This is the procedure of choice today.**

- It is increasingly used nowadays.
- Major advantage is minimal scars, minimal pain, early recovery.
- It gives an excellent exposure from within.
- One can define all the defects properly.
- Reduce all the contents and a broad sac.
- Defect can be sutured and broad mesh is placed.
- Mesh which has absorbable surface will face the peritoneal cavity and nonabsorbable surface will face abdominal wall.
- Transfascial sutures are placed to fix the mesh (Figs 64.65 to 64.68).

***Major disadvantage is cost of mesh and tackers***

**Following advice or techniques are followed before taking up these cases:**

1. Fitness for surgery
2. Chest physiotherapy
3. Reduction of weight

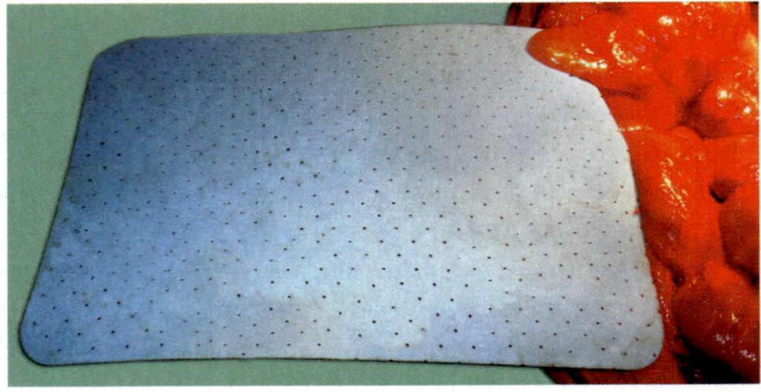
Fig. 64.65: Dual mesh

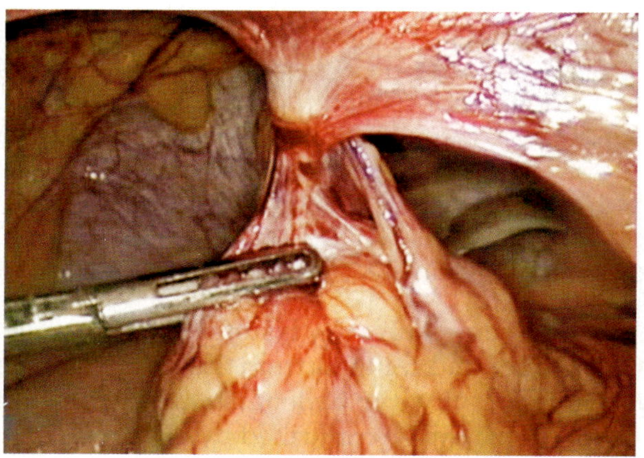

**Fig. 64.66:** Laparoscopic release of omentum from the hernial sac

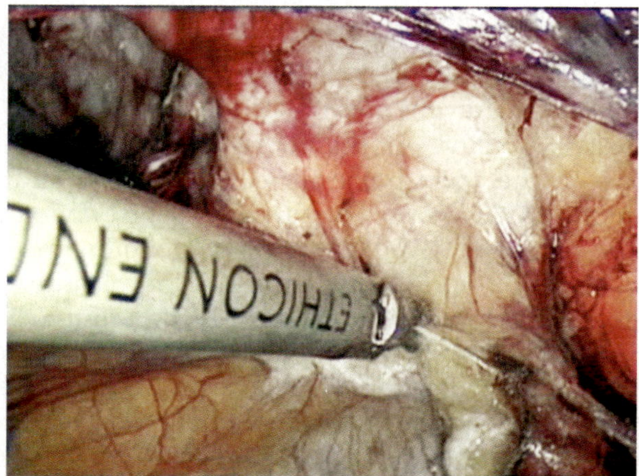


**Fig. 64.67:** Laparoscopic mobilisation of the sac

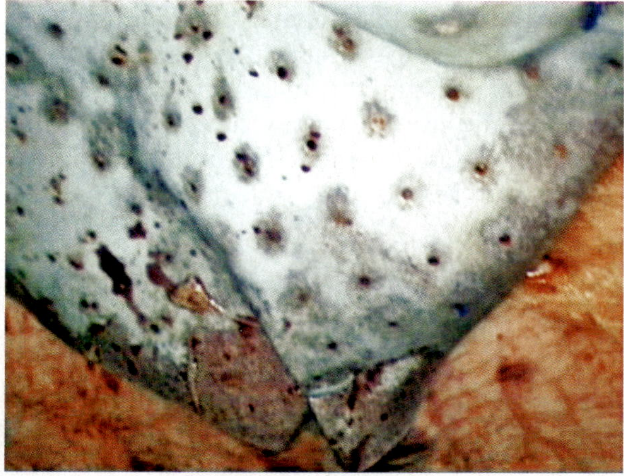

**Fig. 64.68:** Laparoscopic dual mesh has been kept in place and sutured

4. Deep vein thrombosis prophylaxis by using low molecular weight heparin.
5. Progressive pneumoperitoneum over weeks.
6. Additional lipectomy, removal of colon, omentectomy may have to be done.
7. *Ramirez component separation technique:* In this, relaxing incisions are given in the external oblique aponeurosis or rectus sheath so that they can be brought together and stitched together because in these cases, muscles are widely separated.

## MANAGEMENT OF MASSIVE ABDOMINAL WALL HERNIAS

Massive or giant ventral hernia poses a challenge to the surgeon in appropriate management and to the patient by incapacitating him to live with poor quality of life. There is no consensus on standard definition but most surgeons agree that giant or massive ventral hernias are those having more than 10 cm defect size with loss of domain. Giant ventral hernias can arise due to:

1. Primary hernias which are left unattended for a long time.
2. Recurrence after one or more failed hernia repairs.
3. Result of open abdomen or laparostomy. The contents in such cases may be multiple bowel loops or other viscera which protrude outside the abdominal cavity causing "second abdomen" due to muscle retraction on either side of the defect.

In such a clinical scenario, the standard repair becomes an impossible proposition. Closing the abdomen with tension is not an option because it causes cardiorespiratory embarrassment and later, lateral recurrence of hernia due to disruption of linea semilunaris.

The most critical issue in the management is to optimize these patients before posting them for surgery and to do a good counselling about the difficulties involved in such cases. The patient needs a thorough clinical examination not only of the hernia but rest of the abdomen and the whole body. Putting the abdominal muscles into contraction by head raising and leg raising test, asking the patient to cough in lying down position and again examination in standing position will give a fair knowledge of the loss of domain, reducibility and defect size. Loss of domain (LOD) means a significant amount of viscera has herniated through the abdominal wall into the sac and more viscera may be outside than inside the abdominal cavity. Imaging by CT scan is essential to assess the defect size, status of viscera, abdominal wall musculature and any other intra-abdominal pathology. If the surgeon is inexperienced or the center is not well equipped to manage such patients, then the patient needs to be referred to a higher centre (Fig. 64.69).

Such patients should stop smoking for at least 3 months prior to surgery and any remote infections should be treated. Diabetic patients need good glycemic control with HbA1c around 6.5% and they should not have any chronic liver disease. If there are any precipitating factors such as chronic cough, constipa-

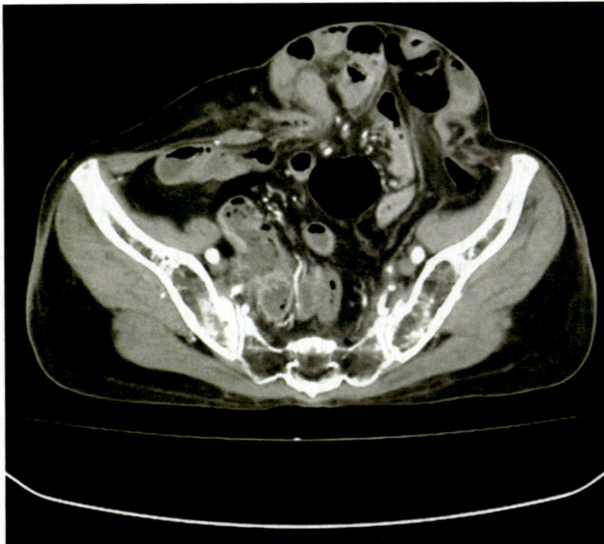

**Fig. 64.69:** CECT scan showing significant bowel has herniated outside. This is called as loss of domain.

tion or difficulty in passing urine, they should be corrected before surgery. Incentive spirometry and breathing exercises must be commenced prior to planned surgery.

If the patient is morbidly obese, the BMI needs to be reduced to around 35 kg/m$^2$. Some patients will require bariatric surgery (e.g. sleeve gastrectomy) as a first step and later definitive surgery for ventral hernia once the patient attains acceptable BMI.

There are two methods to optimize patients with loss of domain so that the capacity of the abdominal cavity increases and they do not develop cardiorespiratory embarrassment when the contents are pushed in during repair of ventral hernia.

1. Botulinum toxin (type A) injection to abdominal wall muscles.
2. Preoperative progressive pneumoperitoneum.

Botulinum toxin injected 4 weeks prior to surgery under ultrasound guidance on either side to abdominal wall muscles in anterior axillary line will cause temporary flaccid paralysis making midline closure possible. Similarly, progressively distending the abdomen with air for 10 to 14 days through an indwelling catheter inserted to abdominal cavity will facilitate reinsertion of bowel loops into abdominal cavity.

Once the abdominal cavity is sufficiently expanded by above methods and contents from the sac have returned to abdominal cavity, the patient is ready for definitive procedure. This can be confirmed by CT scan.

The aim of surgery is to correct the abdominal wall weakness by moving tissues medially by redistributing the abdominal muscles. A dynamic and durable repair is obtained with midline closure and reinforcement of abdominal wall with a large polypropylene mesh. Every precaution to prevent mesh infection is mandatory.

Most commonly performed surgery in massive ventral hernias is the open posterior component separation technique (PCST) or also known as transverse abdominal muscle release (TAR) which may be done on one side or on both sides for a tension-free midline closure. This can also be performed by robotic or laparoscopic (eTEP-TAR) method. Anterior component separation technique (ACST) is another way to achieve midline closure in massive ventral hernias. During emergency situations such as obstruction or gangrene, a staged repair strategy is adopted to deal with the emergency in first surgery and plan for hernia repair after a few months (Figs 64.70 to 64.72).

To conclude, the management of massive or giant ventral hernia requires a carefully planned approach with adequate optimization prior to surgery and a tension-free midline closure by component separation technique with reinforcement by a nonabsorbable mesh to achieve good results.

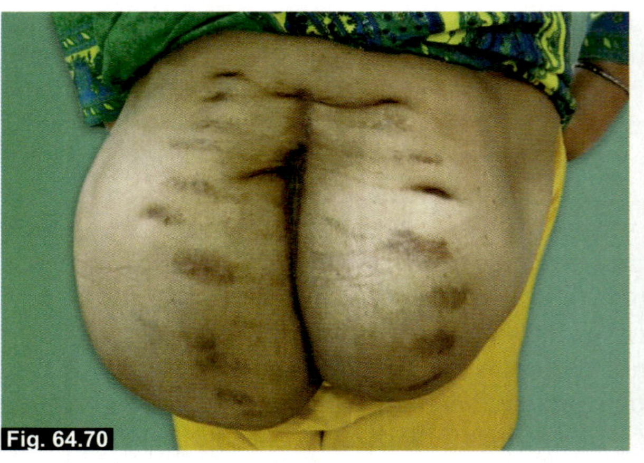


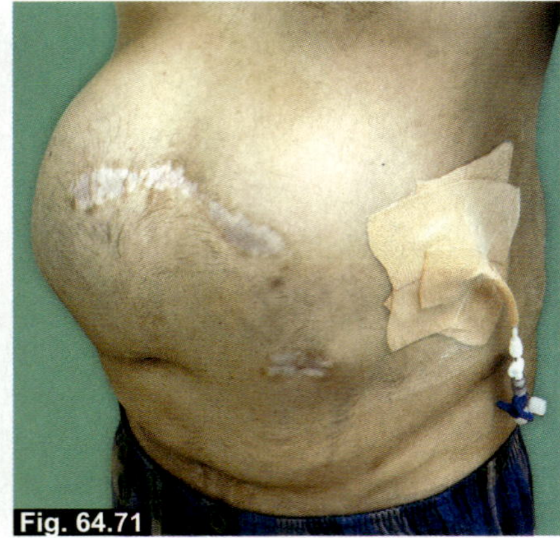


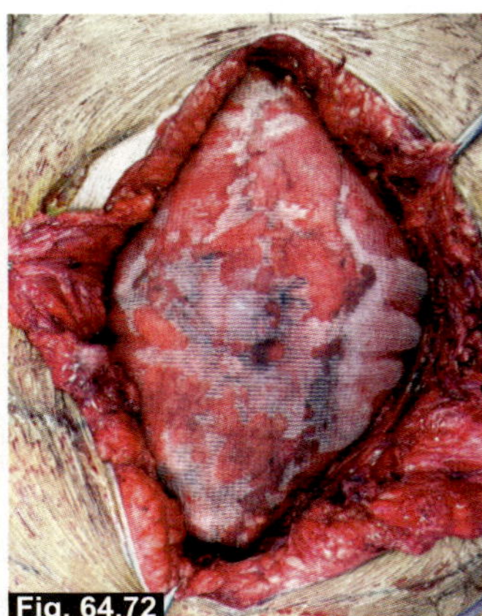


**Figs 64.70 to 64.72:** Massive incisional hernia repaired by component separation and mesh repair. (*Courtesy:* Dr HV Shivaram, Consultant Surgeon, Aster Hospital, Bengaluru, Karnataka)

## EPIGASTRIC HERNIA

- It is also called **fatty** hernia of the linea alba.
- This type of hernia occurs in the epigastrium through the linea alba which extends between the xiphoid process and umbilicus.

### Precipitating Factors

Sudden straining or heavy exercise results in the tearing of a few fibres of linea alba and is responsible for precipitating an epigastric hernia. Initially there is a small protrusion of extraperitoneal pad of fat. Rarely, if it enlarges, it is due to the dragging of the peritoneal sac. The opening is very narrow. Hence, the hollow viscus cannot enter the sac. Diastasis of rectus muscles which results in a wide linea alba can also precipitate an epigastric hernia.

### Clinical Features

- Common in muscular men, manual labourers.
- Typically the swelling is situated in the upper abdomen midway between xiphoid process and umbilicus. Often, it contains only an extraperitoneal protrusion of fat (Fig. 64.73).
- An expansile impulse on cough is rare.
- Dull aching pain is due to the fatty contents which are partially strangulated. However, tenderness is an important feature of epigastric hernia (Key Box 64.17).

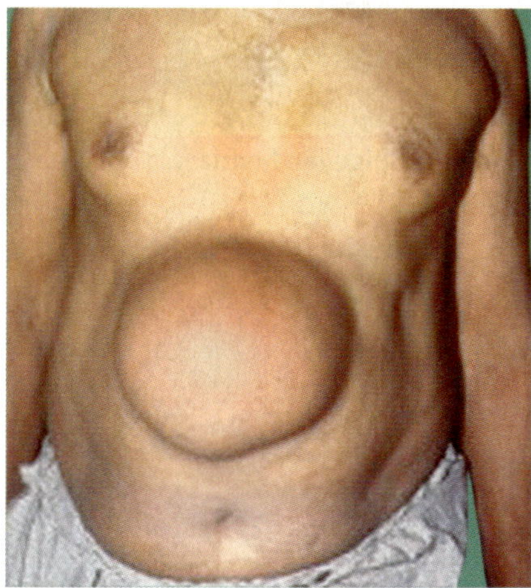

**Fig. 64.73:** Epigastric hernia

Key Box 64.17

**Peculiarities of epigastric hernia**

- Common in muscular men
- Hernial sac is uncommon
- Hollow viscus in the sac is rare
- Impulse on cough is rare
- Reducibility is rare
- Tenderness is an important feature

- Many cases are associated with peptic ulcer disease.
- On head-raising, it becomes more prominent (Fig. 64.74).

### Treatment

A small incision is made over the swelling and the fatty tissue is isolated. It is ligated and excised because usually a tiny blood vessel enters the pad of fat. If a hernial sac is present, it is opened, the contents are reduced and the defect is closed using nonabsorbable sutures (Fig. 64.75).

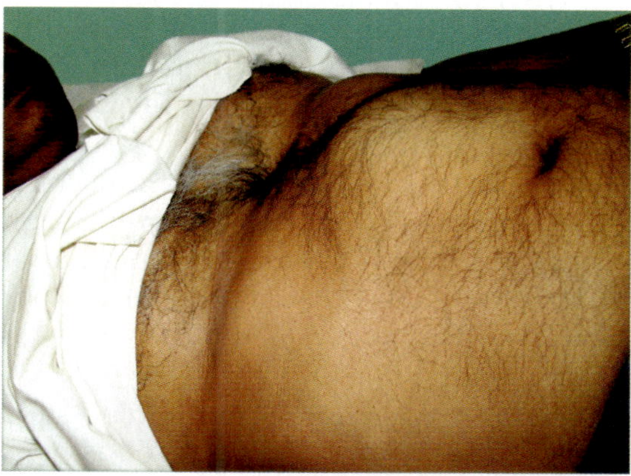

**Fig. 64.74:** Epigastric hernia: On head-raising, it becomes more prominent (head-raising test)

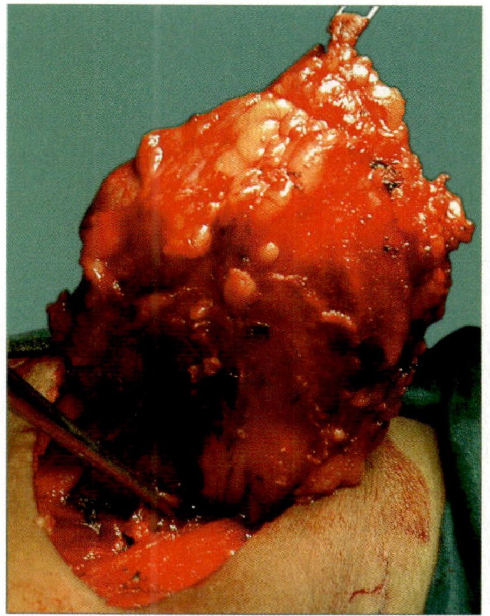

**Fig. 64.75:** Epigastric hernia sac

## RARE EXTERNAL HERNIAS

**SU28.1.17:** Describe special hernias—Spigelian, lumbar, obturator, perineal, sciatic and paranormal hernias and aetiology, clinical presentation, various surgical approaches and techniques in their management.

## INTERPARIETAL HERNIA

- It is also known as interstitial hernia.
- Basically, they are inguinal hernias. However, the processus vaginalis sac instead of following the normal route into the scrotum, traverses between various layers of the abdominal wall (parietes) resulting in interstitial hernias.
- Patients with Down's syndrome and prune-belly syndrome are commonly affected.

### Types

1. **Preperitoneal:** In this variety, the hernial sac lies between the transversalis fascia and peritoneum. It is seen in about 20% of patients. The sac is like a small diverticulum.
2. **Interparietal:** It is also called intermuscular type. It is the commonest variety wherein the sac passes between the external oblique and internal oblique muscles. The swelling caused by the hernial sac causes discomfort to the patient. Sometimes, this can be a bilocular sac.
3. **Extraparietal:** It is also known as inguino-superficial variety. In this variety, the hernial sac passes exterior (superficial) to the external oblique aponeurosis beneath superficial fascia of the abdominal wall. It is commonly associated with undescended testis or ectopic testis.
    - Majority of such cases present with features of intestinal obstruction.
    - They are treated by identifying the sac, excision followed by closure of the defect or repair by using nonabsorbable sutures.

## SPIGELIAN HERNIA[1]

- It is an interstitial hernia which occurs through the Spigelian fascia. This is a thin strip of fascia which runs parallel to the outer border of rectus sheath from the tip of the 9th costal cartilage to the pubic tubercle.
- Since, it is very wide in the region of umbilicus/ arcuate line, Spigelian hernias occur commonly at this level.
- Spigelian fascia contributes a few fibres to form rectus sheath.

### Spigelian belt

- It is a 6 cm horizontal transverse zone located within umbilicus and the two anterior superior iliac spines.
- Starts as a direct protrusion behind rectus abdominis.
- They are intramural; sac penetrates across transverse muscles and lies behind external oblique muscles.

### Precipitating Factors

Repeated pregnancies, advancing age, obesity, muscular degeneration, sudden strain due to coughing, weight lifting, etc. give rise to Spigelian hernias.

### Clinical Features

- Seen in both sexes equally around 50 years of age.
- A round, soft, reducible swelling situated just below and lateral to the umbilicus—located typically at the junction of the arcuate line and lateral border of rectus abdominis. Sometimes, it is tender.
- The swelling gives rise to an expansile impulse on cough.
- As the hernia enlarges, it insinuates between external and internal oblique muscle. Hence, it is an example for interparietal hernia (Figs 64.76 to 64.79).

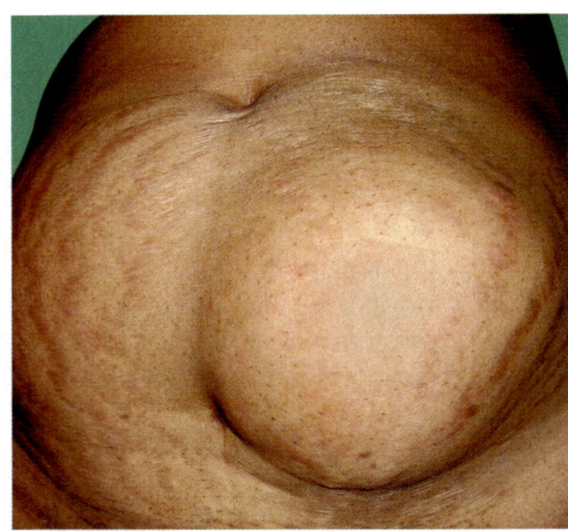

**Fig. 64.76:** Obstructed Spigelian hernia in a 70-year-old lady— first presentation to the hospital

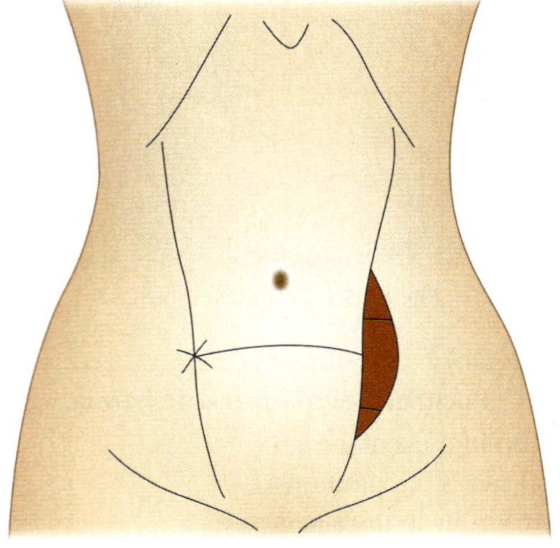

**Fig. 64.77:** Spigelian fascia and the site of hernia

[1]Prof Spigel, Professor of Anatomy and Surgery, not only described Spigelian fascia but also the caudate lobe of the liver.

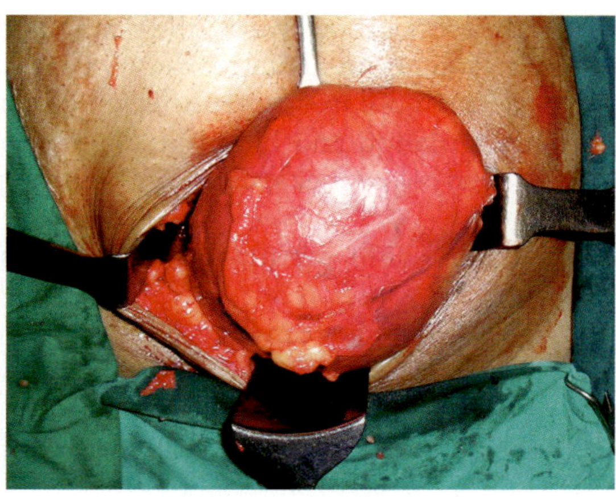

Fig. 64.78: Delivery of the sac

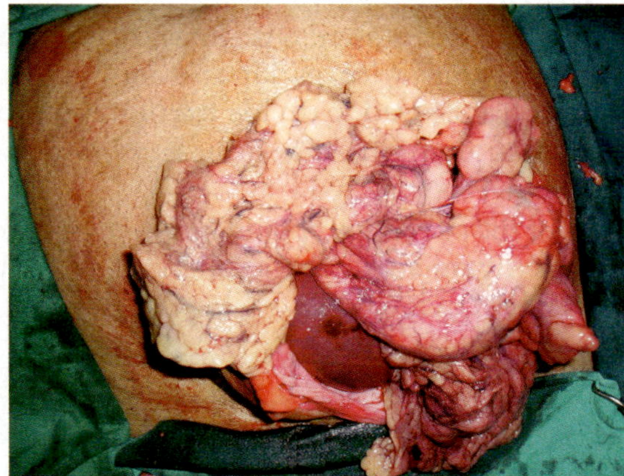

Fig. 64.79: Contents of the sac (*Courtesy:* Figs 64.78 and 64.79 Prof MG Shenoy and Dr Prasad, KMC, Manipal)

### Investigations

1. An ultrasound can define the defect in the semilunar line.
2. X-ray abdomen, lateral view shows coils of bowel outside the peritoneal cavity.

### Differential Diagnosis

- Haematoma within the rectus sheath. However, it will not give rise to impulse on cough. It occurs suddenly and it will be a tender swelling.
- Pyogenic or pyaemic abscess can occur in the abdominal wall, more so, in diabetic patients. Tenderness and high temperature clinches the diagnosis.

### Complication

Strangulation is common due to the rigid fascial ring surrounding the hernial sac. Richter's hernia also can occur here.

### Treatment

An incision of about 5 to 6 cm is made over the swelling and abdominal wall muscles are split or cut. The sac is excised after reducing the contents and the defect is repaired. Recurrence occurs in about 5% of the patients.

## LUMBAR HERNIA

Two types of lumbar hernia are well-recognised. They are as follows:

1. **Primary** which occurs through an anatomical defect:
   - **Through the inferior lumbar triangle of Petit (Fig. 64.80).** Its boundaries are:
     *Inferiorly:* Iliac crest
     *Laterally:* External oblique
     *Medially:* Latissimus dorsi
   - **Through the superior lumbar triangle of Grynfeltt.** Its boundaries are (Fig. 64.80)
     *Above:* 12th rib
     *Medially:* Sacrospinalis
     *Laterally:* Internal oblique
2. **Secondary** to a renal operation done through a loin incision. It is an example of a lumbar incisional hernia, which occurs due to either infection or weakness of loin muscles. The operation done for tuberculosis of spine through a loin incision, very often gives rise to a secondary lumbar hernia (it is an incisional hernia) (Fig. 64.81).

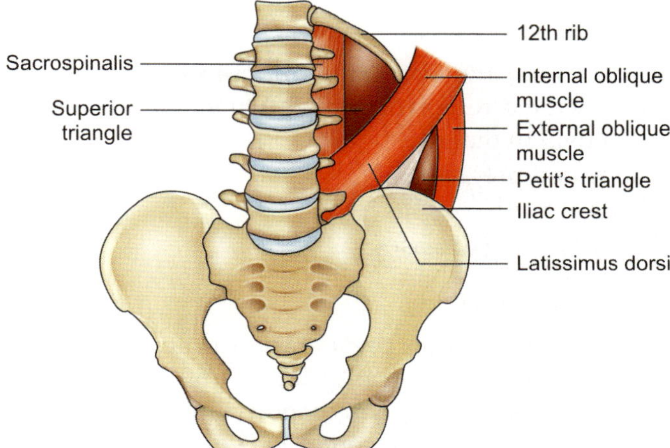


Fig. 64.80: Petit's triangle

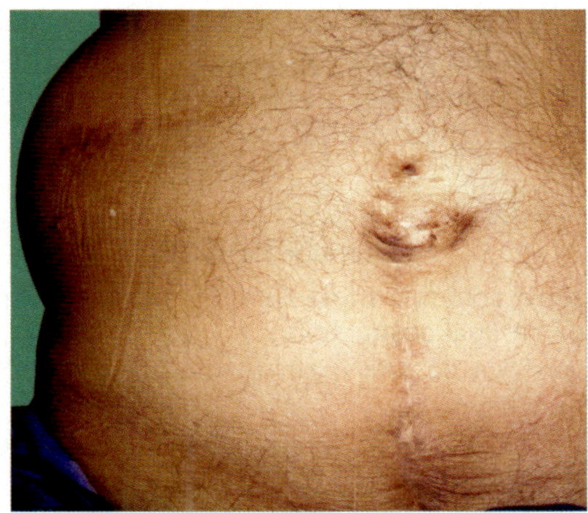

Fig. 64.81: Lumbar hernia

### Differential Diagnosis

1. **Lipoma** is common in the lumbar region (loin). It is soft, lobular, and slips under the palpating fingers.
2. **Cold abscess** secondary to tuberculosis of the spine gives rise to a nontender swelling in the paravertebral space. Tenderness is present over the spine which gives a clue to the diagnosis. Patients may have deformity of the spine in the form of gibbus.

### Treatment

Small defects can be closed with simple sutures. Large defects need to be closed with or without mesh.

*Pearls of Wisdom*

Primary lumbar hernias are very rare.

## OBTURATOR HERNIA

- This hernia occurs through the obturator canal which is bounded above by the superior ramus of pubis and below by the sharp edge of the obturator membrane.
- As the hernia is covered by the pectineus muscle, it is often overlooked.

### Precipitating Factors

- In females, the **obturator foramen** is wider in the transverse direction (it is triangular in shape in females and oval in males).
- Repeated pregnancies
- Loss of body weight
- Chronic lung diseases

### Clinical Features

- The **most common presentation** is acute intestinal obstruction **with strangulation** (80%). Recurrent attacks of intestinal obstruction which get resolved spontaneously is also common (Key Box 64.18).
- This hernia causes more pain than any other type of hernia. Pain often radiates along the obturator nerve and may even be referred to the knee via its geniculate branch called ***Howship-Romberg sign.*** The leg is usually kept in the semiflexed position and movement of the limb gives rise to pain. If the limb is flexed, abducted and rotated outwards, the hernia becomes prominent. Patients are usually over 60 years of age and women are more frequently affected than men.
- Due to strangulation and blood in the hernial sac, bruising is seen below the medial edge of the inguinal ligament.
- A few patients (20%) complain of palpable ***hernia mass*** in the groin.
- Per vaginal examination can reveal a tender lump on the lateral side of the vault.

Key Box 64.18

**Obturator Hernia**

- The most common presentation is not a swelling but acute intestinal obstruction
- Can present as only pain in the knee—(Howship-Romberg sign)
- Vaginal examination: Tender mass can be felt on the lateral side
- Very high chance of strangulation

### Treatment

The constricting agent in case of obstruction is the **obturator fascia**, which needs to be divided. Nerves and vessels are posterolateral to the hernial sac. Since majority of the cases present with intestinal obstruction and strangulation, a lower laparotomy is done. A grooved director is used to divide the obturator fascia.

- The contents are reduced or if there is gangrene, the affected bowel is resected.
- Closure of the obturator opening is done by stitching the broad ligament over the opening or by using monofilament nylon.

## PERINEAL HERNIA

These are very rare hernias which confuse many clinicians and present in different varieties. Hernia protrudes through muscles and fascia of the perineal floor.

1. **Anterolateral perineal hernia:** This occurs in women and presents as a swelling of the labium majus. Often, the patient is examined by a gynaecologist and Bartholin's cyst is diagnosed (Figs 64.82 and 64.83).
2. **Posterolateral perineal hernia:** This type of hernia passes through levator ani and enters ischiorectal fossa.
3. **Median sliding hernia** is nothing but complete prolapse of rectum.
4. **Postoperative hernia** through perineal scar, e.g. after abdominoperineal resection wherein rectum is removed. It is also used to occur following perineal prostatectomy.

### Clinical Features

They can present as asymptomatic swelling, pain, dysuria, bowel obstruction or perineal ulceration and bleeding.

### Diagnosis

- Ultrasound can detect loops of bowel/fluid.
- CT scan/MRI can clearly define the course of hernia, its relationship with urinary bladder/ureter and its descent into the pelvis.

### Repair

It can be very difficult in large hernias. Often a combined approach, both perineal and abdominal, may

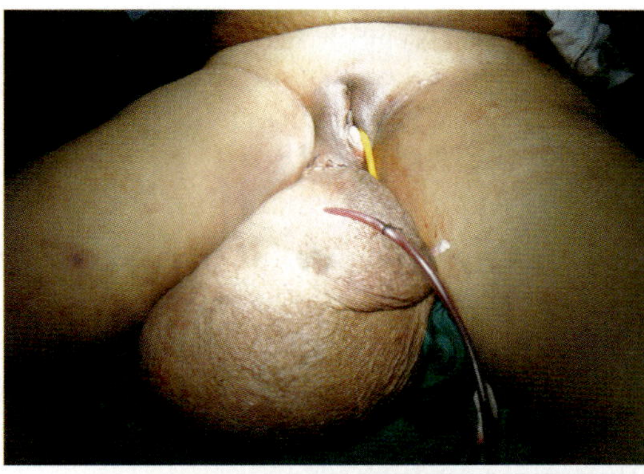

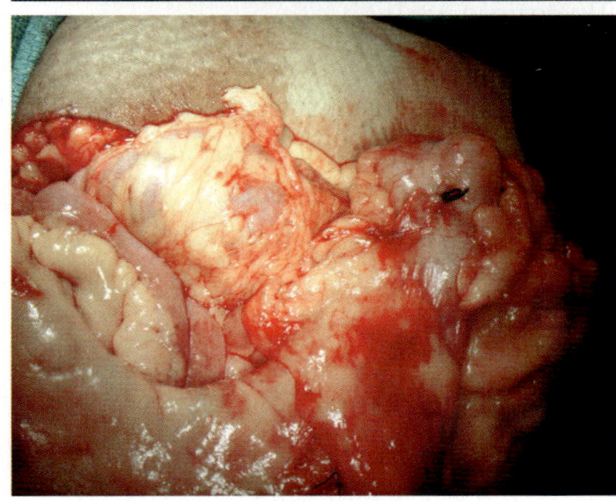

**Figs 64.82 and 64.83:** A 40-year-old lady with large perineal hernia was diagnosed to have a Bartholin's cyst and was explored by a gynaecologist. To his surprise, it had 3 feet of small intestine and portions of large intestines. It started bleeding and he kept a drain and referred the patient to our hospital

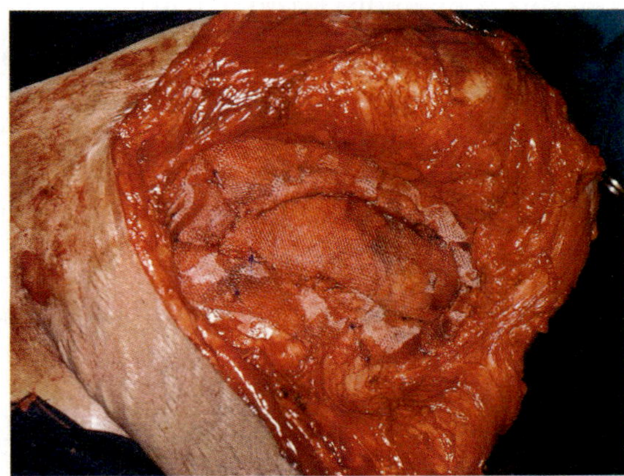

**Fig. 64.84:** Contents were reduced, sac was excised, a large mesh could be placed in the defect and sutured all around. Postoperatively she had urinary fistula. CT cystogram revealed bladder injury. It healed after two weeks

be necessary. Mesh repair with adequate fascial and muscular perineal repair is required (Fig. 64.84).

## PARASTOMAL HERNIA (Fig. 64.85)

- It is an acquired condition/iatrogenic
- It is a complication of ileostomy/colostomy

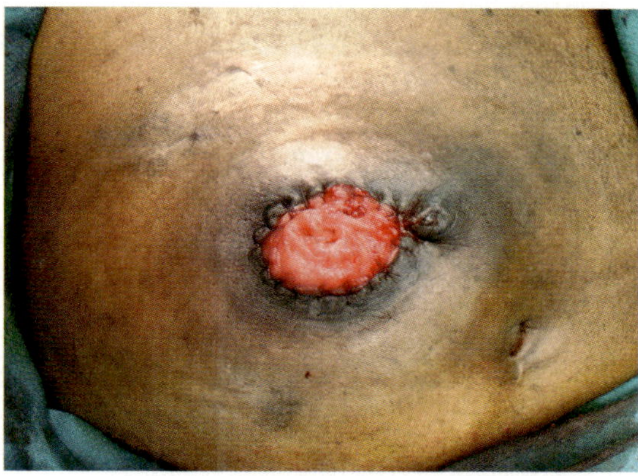

**Fig. 64.85:** Parastomal hernia. (*Courtesy:* Dr Vipin Goel, Surgical Oncologist Indo-American Cancer Hospital, Hyderabad)

- Herniation occurs from the side of colostomy/ileostomy and hence called parastomal hernia.

### Devlin's Classification

1. **Subcutaneous:** It is the most common variety. It takes more time for obstruction.
2. **Interstital:** In this variety, herniation happens through intermuscular plane—between transversus abdominis and internal oblique muscles, etc.
3. **Intrastomal:** Here, the herniation occurs between emerging and everting part of the stoma.
4. **Perstomal:** In this variety, herniation occurs between layers of prolapsed stoma.

### Clinical Features

- Patient complains of swelling on her side of ostomy, which increases/prolapses on coughing/straining, decreases at rest.
- Pain, irreducibility indicates obstruction.
- Tense and tender abdomen, pain indicates obstruction.

### Diagnosis

CECT abdomen provides accurate diagnosis of the type of hernia.

### Treatment

Contents are reduced, defects identified, broad mesh is placed over the intraperitoneal and parastomal defects and sutured by nonabsorbable sutures, and extra-peritoneal meshes applied.

## INTERNAL HERNIAS

These hernias occur intra-abdominally wherein the bowel protrudes through peritoneal or mesenteric aperture or foramen. They may cause obstruction. Examples are hiatus hernia and Petersen's hernia (occurs in space posterior to gastrojejunostomy).

## MULTIPLE CHOICE QUESTIONS

1. **Length of inguinal canal is:**
   A. 4 cm B. 6 cm
   C. 8 cm D. 10 cm
2. **Which of the following is not a boundary of the Hesselbach's triangle?**
   A. Rectus abdominis
   B. Inguinal ligament
   C. Inferior epigastric artery
   D. Testicular artery
3. **Following are true about external ring, *except*:**
   A. It is not a ring
   B. It is a defect in the internal oblique aponeurosis
   C. Invagination test is done through external ring
   D. It transmits spermatic cord
4. **About deep inguinal ring, which one of the following is true?**
   A. It is a defect in the external oblique aponeurosis
   B. It is a defect in the internal oblique aponeurosis
   C. It is a defect in the transversalis fascia
   D. It is a defect in the cremasteric fascia
5. **Following are true for deep inguinal ring, *except*:**
   A. Deep ring is a defect in the transversalis fascia
   B. Indirect hernial sac comes out lateral to the deep ring
   C. Pantaloon hernia can be on both sides of deep ring
   D. It is closed at the end of hernia repair to prevent recurrence
6. **The ideal surgical treatment for sliding inguinal hernia will be:**
   A. Herniotomy B. Bassini's herniorrhaphy
   C. Marsey's repair D. Lichtenstein's repair
7. **Following are contents of the spermatic cord, *except*:**
   A. Vas deferens
   B. Testicular artery
   C. Genital branch of genitofemoral nerve
   D. Ilioinguinal nerve
8. **About sliding inguinal hernia following are true, *except*:**
   A. Urinary bladder can be the part of hernial sac
   B. It can be both direct or indirect type
   C. The hernial sac should be twisted as in indirect hernia treatment
   D. Often it is irreducible
9. **Richter's hernia refers to:**
   A. Hernia containing intestines
   B. Strangulated hernia
   C. Only a part of circumference of the intestine is caught in a hernial sac
   D. Hernia containing urinary bladder
10. **Immediate structure anterior to direct hernial sac is:**
    A. External oblique aponeurosis
    B. Internal oblique aponeurosis
    C. Transversalis facia
    D. Posterior rectus sheath
11. **Femoral hernia has following features, *except*:**
    A. It is more common in women
    B. It is below and lateral to pubic tubercle
    C. It is known for strangulation
    D. It can be managed by hernia truss
12. **Diagnostic feature of a saphena varix is:**
    A. It is transilluminant
    B. It is soft and reducible
    C. It is below the pubic tubercle
    D. Disappears on elevation of the leg
13. **Which one of the following hernias is called Littre's hernia?**
    A. Hernia containing Meckel's diverticulum
    B. Hernia containing urinary bladder
    C. Hernia containing sigmoid colon
    D. Hernia containing ovary
14. **Which one of the following is the most important step in preventing recurrence of hernia?**
    A. Complete excision of cremasteric muscle
    B. Reconstruction of the external ring
    C. Reconstruction of the internal ring
    D. High ligation of the sac
15. **Following are true for strangulated inguinal hernia, *except*:**
    A. It will be tense
    B. Tender
    C. Irreducible
    D. Impulse on cough is present
16. **Following are true for anatomy of the femoral canal, *except*:**
    A. Femoral canal is the outermost compartment of femoral sheath
    B. Femoral canal extends from femoral ring to saphenous ring
    C. Femoral canal is below and lateral to pubic tubercle
    D. Femoral canal contains lymph node of Cloquet

**17. In obstructed femoral hernia, at surgery which of the following steps should not be done?**
   A. Best done with low approach through incision directly over the swelling
   B. Closure of the ring is done by prolene suture material
   C. Abnormal obturator artery should be looked for
   D. Urinary bladder may be in danger

**18. Following hernias are known for high chances of strangulation, *except*:**
   A. Femoral hernia B. Obturator hernia
   C. Spigelian hernia D. Direct hernia

**19. In which condition femoral hernia occurs behind the femoral vessels?**
   A. Prune-belly syndrome
   B. Poliomyelitis
   C. Congenital dislocation of the hip
   D. Defect in the lacunar ligament

**20. In cases of epigastric hernia, all are true, *except*:**
   A. It is more common in muscular men
   B. Impulse on cough is common
   C. Sac is uncommon
   D. It is tender

**21. Spigelian hernia, is an example for:**
   A. Direct hernia B. Indirect hernia
   C. Interstitial hernia D. Type of femoral hernia

**22. In Spigelian hernia swelling is seen:**
   A. Below and lateral to umbilicus
   B. Below the umbilicus
   C. Around the umbilicus
   D. Just above the umbilicus

**23. Differential diagnosis of lumbar hernia includes the following, *except*:**
   A. Lipoma B. Cold abscess
   C. Haematoma D. Meningocoele

**24. Following are true for obturator hernia, *except*:**
   A. Hernia is covered by pectineus muscle
   B. Pain is radiated to the knee
   C. Cannot be felt by vaginal examination
   D. Patients keep their leg semiflexed

**25. The most common presentation of obturator hernia is:**
   A. Groin swelling
   B. Intestinal obstruction
   C. Bruising below inguinal ligament
   D. Tender mass on vaginal examination

**Answers**

| | | | | | | | | | |
|---|---|---|---|---|---|---|---|---|---|
| **1.** A | **2.** D | **3.** B | **4.** C | **5.** D | **6.** D | **7.** D | **8.** C | **9.** C | **10.** C |
| **11.** D | **12.** D | **13.** A | **14.** D | **15.** D | **16.** A | **17.** A | **18.** D | **19.** C | **20.** B |
| **21.** C | **22.** A | **23.** D | **24.** A | **25.** B | | | | | |

# Chapter 65 Umbilicus, Wound Dehiscence, Wound Closure and Abdominal Wall Swellings

- Classification of umbilical diseases
- Umbilical inflammation
- Umbilical fistulae
- Umbilical neoplasms
- Umbilical hernia
- Abdominal dehiscence
- Wound closure
- Divarication of recti
- Desmoid tumour
- Endometriosis

## UMBILICUS—SURGICAL ANATOMY AND EMBRYOLOGY

**Definition:** The umbilicus is the normal scar in the anterior abdominal wall formed by the remnants of the root of the *umbilical cord*.

The position of the umbilicus is variable. In healthy adults, it lies in the anterior median line, at the level of the disc between the third and fourth lumbar vertebrae. It is lower in infants and **in persons with a pendulous abdomen (Fig. 65.1, Tanyol's sign).** It can be displaced upwards as in ovarian tumours (Fig. 65.2).

Apart from its embryological importance, there are several facts of interest about the umbilicus. These are given below:

### Anatomical Importance

1. With reference to the lymphatic and venous drainage, the level of the umbilicus is a *watershed*. Lymph and venous blood flow upwards above the plane of the umbilicus; and downwards below this plane. These do not normally cross umbilical plane.
2. The skin around the umbilicus is supplied by segment T10 of the spinal cord.
3. The umbilicus is one of the important sites at which tributaries of the portal vein anastomose with systemic veins (*portocaval anastomoses*). In portal hypertension, these anastomoses open up to form dilated veins radiating from the umbilicus called the *caput medusae*. However, the blood flow in the dilated veins is normal, and does not break the barrier of the watershed line.

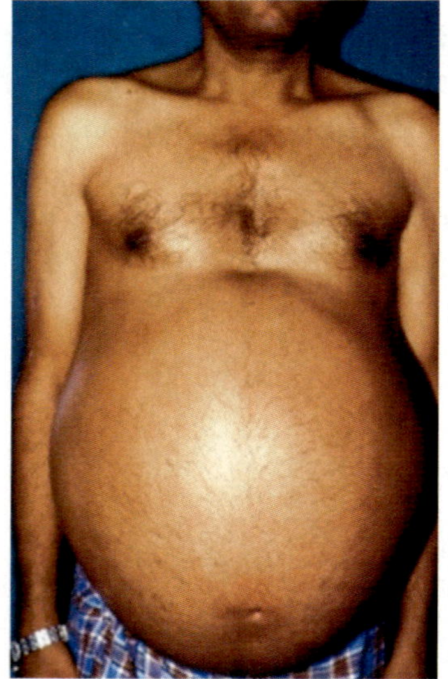

**Fig. 65.1:** Tanyol's sign

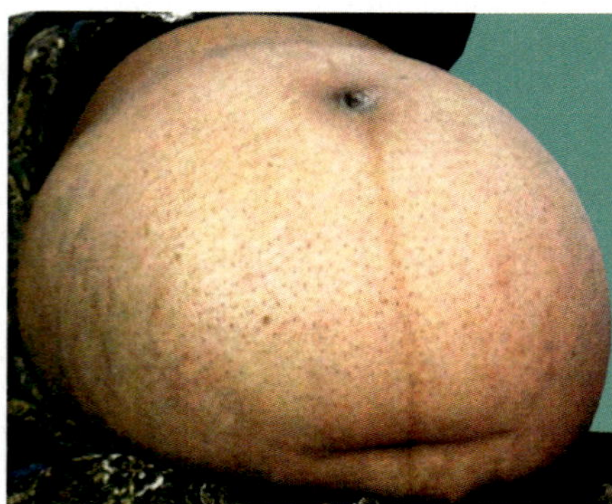

**Fig. 65.2:** Large ovarian tumour displacing umbilicus upwards

### Embryological Importance

1. Umbilicus is the meeting point of the four (two lateral, head and tail) folds of embryonic plate.
2. This is also the meeting point of three systems, namely the digestive (vitellointestinal duct), the excretory (urachus), and vascular (umbilical vessels).

## CLASSIFICATION OF UMBILICAL DISEASES

I. Inflammation
  A. Omphalitis
  B. Granuloma
  C. Dermatitis
  D. Pilonidal sinus
II. Fistulae
  **A. Faecal**
    1. Patent vitellointestinal duct (Key Box 65.1)
    2. Carcinoma transverse colon
    3. Tuberculous peritonitis
  **B. Urinary:** Patent urachus
  **C. Biliary**
III. Neoplasms
  **A. Benign**
    1. Adenoma: Raspberry tumour
    2. Endometrioma
  **B. Malignant**
    1. Primary carcinoma
    2. Secondary carcinoma from: Stomach, colon, ovary, and breast
IV. Umbilical hernia
V. Umbilical calculus (umbolith).

Key Box 65.1

**Umbilical Cord Structures**

**In foetal life**
- Umbilical vein
- Right and left umbilical arteries
- Urachus

**In embryonic life**
Vitellointestinal duct and structures mentioned above

## UMBILICAL INFLAMMATION

### A. Omphalitis

- Inflammation of the umbilical cord due to *Staphylococcus aureus* and streptococci occurs in the neonatal period 3–4 days after birth. The incidence is increased in hospital births.
- Rarely, gram-negative organisms and *Clostridium tetani* can cause omphalitis, if strict aseptic precautions are not taken. If infection is not controlled, it can result in further complications.
  1. **Abscess of the abdominal wall:** Pus can be seen coming out of umbilicus. It may need drainage with antibiotic cover. Gentle squeezing will help, followed by antiseptic dressings and systemic antibiotics.
  2. **Extensive ulceration of the abdominal wall,** similar to Meleney's ulcer, is a rare complication (subcutaneous synergistic gangrene) of omphalitis.
  3. **Septicaemia** can occur due to organisms entering the umbilical vein and then into portal vein. This results in pylephlebitis with jaundice, fever, chills and rigors.
  4. **Neonatal jaundice** due to intrahepatic cholangitis.
  5. **Portal vein thrombosis** resulting in extrahepatic portal hypertension (prehepatic).
  6. **Umbilical hernia** can occur due to a weak scar produced by sepsis.

### B. Granuloma

Granuloma indicates persisting inflammation underneath. It is a cause of great concern and worry to the patients. This can be destroyed by **application of copper sulphate or silver nitrate solution.**

### C. Dermatitis

Dermatitis more often occurs in adults wherein chronic infection of the umbilicus sets in with foul smelling discharge.

### D. Pilonidal Sinus

Umbilicus is a low area compared to the surface of abdominal wall. Hence, hairy men may shed their hair which accumulates in the umbilicus and may result in pilonidal sinus. It may need removal of sinus along with tuft of hair or rarely the umbilicus itself.

### E. Umbolith

- It is composed of desquamated epithelium which becomes inspissated and gets collected in the umbilicus. With secondary infection, there will be blood-stained discharge. It is treated by controlling infection, debridement and, if necessary, removal of umbilicus.
- This umbolith or umbilical calculus is black in colour.

## UMBILICAL FISTULAE

### A. Faecal

1. **Persistent vitellointestinal duct** is an uncommon congenital anomaly. Many a time the intestinal opening is so small that only mucoid contents come out of umbilicus. Rarely, if the opening is big, omphaloenteric faecal fistula results.
2. **Internal hollow viscus malignancies,** especially carcinoma of the transverse colon can erode through umbilicus resulting in a faecal fistula.
3. **Tuberculous peritonitis** induces dense adhesions, strictures and perforations. A perforation which is sealed off by coils of matted bowel and omentum

results in local abscess which may perforate through a weak point, i.e. umbilicus resulting in a faecobiliary fistula. If a diagnosis can be proved by wall biopsy of the sinus/fistula, antituberculous treatment can cure the disease. Laparotomy is extremely difficult in such cases. One may end up creating more holes in the bowel and is better avoided.

*Pearls of Wisdom*

One innocent disease (VI DUCT), one prevalent disease (TB) and one malignant disease (carcinoma bowel) are the causes of umbilical faecal fistula.

### B. Patent Urachus (Fig. 65.3 and Key Box 65.2)

- The ventral urogenital sinus which forms the urinary bladder is continued cranially as urachus which extends into the umbilical cord—allantoic stalk. If this portion persists, patent urachus forms which connect umbilicus with urinary bladder. If it is fibrosed, as it occurs normally, it is called **median umbilical ligament**.

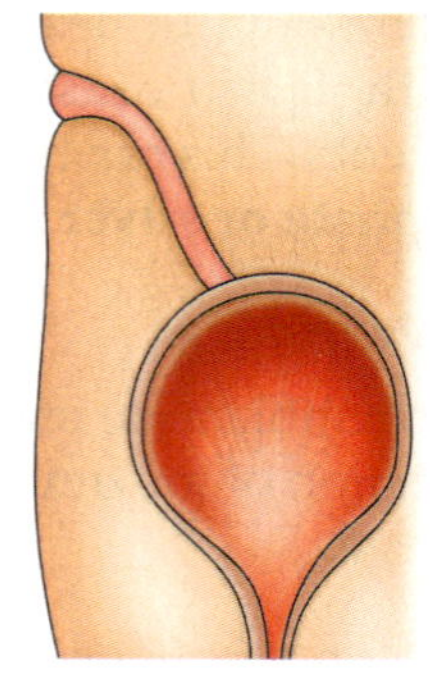

**Fig. 65.3:** Patent urachus

- A patent urachus may manifest as urinary discharge from umbilicus. It manifests usually in childhood and early adult life. In most cases, there will be some kind of obstruction to the normal passage of urine. Entire urachus is excised after correcting distal obstruction.

Key Box 65.2

**Abnormalities of Urachus**

- Patent urachus
- Urachal sinus
- Urachal cyst
- Urachal diverticulum

### C. Biliary Fistula

Rarely, perforation of gallbladder due to severe form of cholecystitis may result in local abscess which may rupture through umbilicus resulting in biliary fistula. Instances are recorded wherein stones have come out of umbilicus.

## UMBILICAL NEOPLASMS

1. **Umbilical adenoma** is a pedunculated swelling having raspberry colour. Hence, the name **Raspberry tumour**.
   - It is due to unobliterated vitellointestinal duct.
   - Mucosa of the persistent duct prolapses through umbilicus and produces this adenoma.
   - It is moist with mucus and tends to bleed (columnar epithelium rich in goblet cells).

   ***Treatment***
   - If the tumour is pedunculated, a ligature is tied around it and by a few days, the adenoma drops off.
   - If tumour reappears, excision of umbilicus is advised.
2. **Endometrioma** of umbilicus is rare but patients have a typical history to tell, i.e. it bleeds during menstruation.
3. **Malignant:** Secondary carcinomatous nodule in and around umbilicus reflects advanced malignancy commonly from stomach and colon. Ovary, uterus, breast are other causes. The nodule is tender, fixed and reddish in colour (*Refer* Sister Mary Joseph Nodule, page 739).

## UMBILICAL HERNIA

Umbilicus is one of the weak points in the body. Hence, it is one of the sites of hernia. All the details of umbilical hernia have been discussed on page 1103.

## ABDOMINAL WALL

Common diseases of abdominal wall can be infective or inflammatory such as abdominal wall abscess and Meleney's gangrene. Tumours or swellings of abdominal wall are desmoid tumours, endometriosis, rectus sheath hematoma, multiple lipomas, etc. Common diseases are discussed here.

### RECTUS SHEATH HAEMATOMA

Collection of blood in relation to rectus sheath and muscles occurs due to tearing of one of the branches of inferior epigastric artery. A parietal haematoma occurs usually at the level of the arcuate line. It is an uncommon condition. However, the causes can be as follows:

1. **Trauma:** A sudden blow to the abdominal wall.
2. **Straining:** Sudden straining such as violent cough or vigorous exercise in a muscular man can cause haematoma.
3. **Pregnancy:** Rarely, the cause of haematoma can be pregnancy, in late trimester. The exact cause is not known.

### Clinical Features

- History of sudden straining or coughing, etc.
- A tender lump develops just below and to the side of umbilicus at the level of arcuate line where posterior rectus sheath is absent.
- Nausea, vomiting, and pyrexia are the other features.

### Differential Diagnosis

Spigelian hernia (it is rare).

### Treatment

- The condition is self-limiting. With antibiotics and analgesics, a haematoma subsides within 5–7 days.
- If it persists or progresses or if there is a doubt about the diagnosis, exploration and evacuation of haematoma should be done and the bleeding vessels are ligated. The results and recovery are excellent.

## MELENEY'S PROGRESSIVE POSTOPERATIVE SYNERGISTIC GANGRENE

This dangerous complication is rare nowadays, thanks to the good pre- and postoperative antibiotics.

### Aetiopathogenesis

- It is caused by synergistic action of microaerophilic non-haemolytic *Streptococcus* and *Staphylococcus aureus*.
- Surgical operations which have increased risk of Meleney's gangrene include perforated appendix, biliary tract surgery, colectomy, etc.
- Atherosclerosis, and diabetes are the other precipitating factors.
- Starts as cellulitis with reddish skin and postoperative fever.
- The spread may occur within 3–5 days, with extensive gangrene and sloughing of the skin of the abdominal wall with purulent discharge.

### Clinical Features

- Postoperative patient with cellulitis of abdominal wall.
- Fever of moderate degree, an extremely tender abdominal wall and purulent discharge.
- Toxicity and deterioration of general health may follow soon.

### Treatment

1. **At the stage of cellulitis:** Broad-spectrum antibiotics to cover not only the organisms mentioned above but to cover anaerobic organisms also. Thus, a combination of benzylpenicillin, gentamicin and metronidazole is used.
2. **At the stage of gangrene:** Emergency aggressive debridement is the treatment. Dead skin and subcutaneous tissue are excised, pus drained and the slough is removed.
3. **Hyperbaric oxygen** may be very useful.
4. Skin grafting is done, once the wound is healed with granulation tissue.

## PYOGENIC ABSCESS (Fig. 65.4)

Abdominal wall is one of the sites of pyogenic abscess especially in diabetic patients. It is a part of pyaemia. Localised tenderness suggests an abscess. Diagnosis can be confirmed by ultrasound and it is treated by incision and drainage.

**Clinical Notes**

A 60-year-old diabetic male patient had a large pyaemic abscess on the abdominal wall below and to the right of umbilicus. An incision and drainage of the abscess was done. Within 2 hours of surgery, the surgeon was called to see this patient who had hypotension and blood was pouring out of the incision. Exploration of the wound revealed large 'clots' and bleeding from inferior epigastric artery, which was ligated. Probably, while breaking all the loculi of the abscess cavity, the vessel was injured.

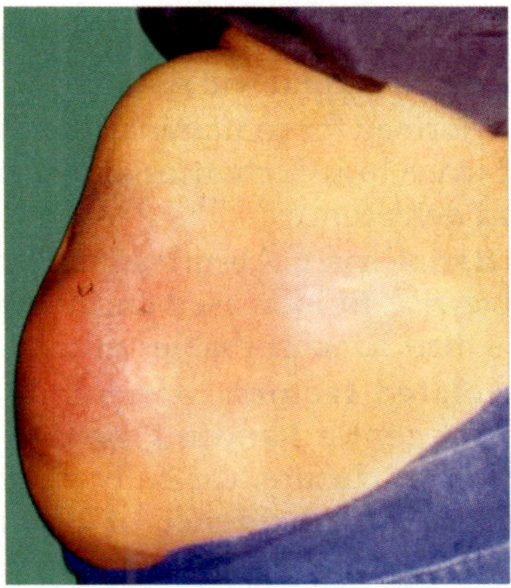

**Fig. 65.4:** Abdominal wall abscess in a diabetic patient (*see* clinical notes)

## BURST ABDOMEN: ABDOMINAL DEHISCENCE

A soundly healed abdominal scar can withstand any amount of intra-abdominal pressure. However, 1–2% of the abdominal wounds (incisions) give way resulting in prolapse of intra-abdominal contents outside.

This causes great concern, or anxiety to the patient, and more so for relatives. It is said that the anxiety and worry caused by the intestines prolapsing out is much more than that is caused by emergency re-explorations for open cardiac surgery. It is not possible to prevent wound dehiscence totally because causative agents are multifactorial.

### Factors Responsible for Wound Dehiscence (Key Box 65.3)

1. **Surgery:** It depends upon the type of surgery done. Surgery done for grossly contaminated cases such as peritonitis, biliary fistula or faecal fistula have a high incidence of wound dehiscence (Fig. 65.5).

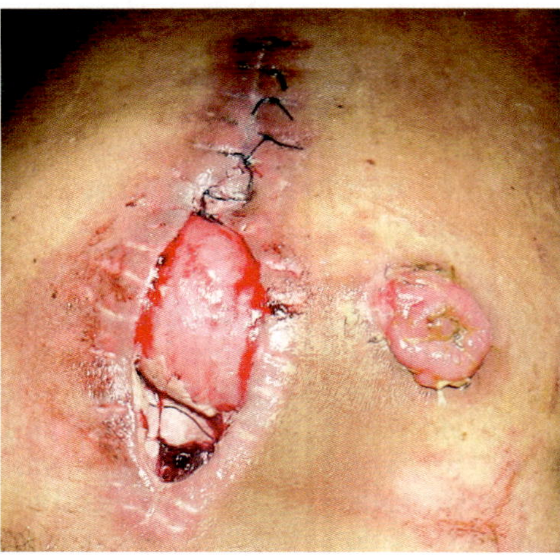

Fig. 65.5: Wound dehiscence in a case of APR (abdomino-perineal resection)—probably due to placement of colostomy closer to the suture line

2. **Sepsis:** Uncontrolled infection (sepsis) can digest the suture material used and will result in burst abdomen. Surgery performed for contamination cases (Figs 65.6 and 65.7) have 8 to 10% chances of incisional hernias and wound dehiscence.
3. **Suture material used:** Absorbable sutures, such as catgut, give rise to increased incidence of wound dehiscence than nonabsorbable sutures.
4. **Surgeon-related factors:** Meticulous dissection, haemostasis, gentle handling of tissues, a good tensionless tight closure, carefully judged incisions will have reduced incidence of burst abdomen. Midline vertical incisions have decreased chance of wound dehiscence than paramedian incision.
5. **Sick patient:** Patients with malignancy, jaundice, obesity, anaemia, hypoproteinaemia, uraemia have poor wound healing.

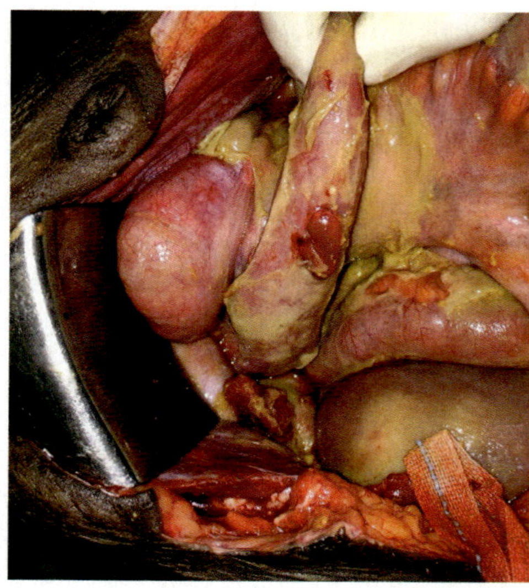

Fig. 65.6: Injury to ileum–faecal peritonitis

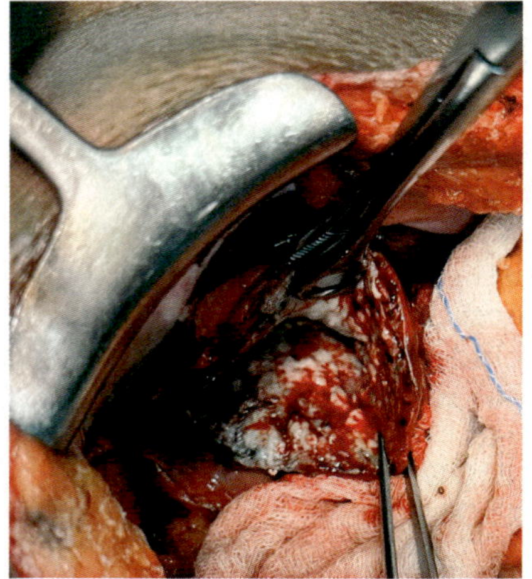

Fig. 65.7: Empyema gallbladder

6. **Straining:** In the postoperative period, violent cough, persistent vomiting, abdominal distension due to paralytic ileus predispose to burst abdomen.

Key Box 65.3

**Burst Abdomen: Factors**

- **S**urgery → Peritonitis
- **S**epsis → Uncontrolled infection
- **S**utures → Absorbable—catgut
- **S**urgeon → Poor quality
- **S**ick patient → Malignancy, diabetes, uraemia, jaundice
- **S**training → Coughing, vomiting

*Remember the causes of burst abdomen as* **6 Ss**

## Clinical Features

- Patients who are recovering reasonably well in the postoperative period suddenly complain of pink- or brownish-coloured serosanguineous discharge. It is the pathognomonic sign of burst abdomen.
- It usually occurs on the 6th to 8th postoperative day.
- If skin sutures are removed, omentum or small bowel coils will be seen outside (Figs 65.8 and 65.9).

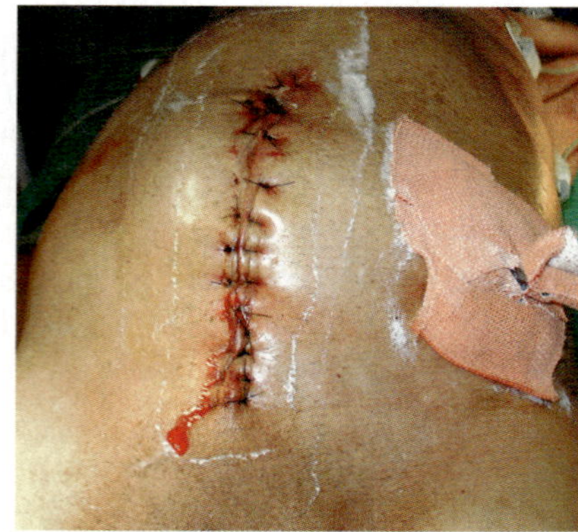

Fig. 65.8: Wound dehiscence—pink discharge

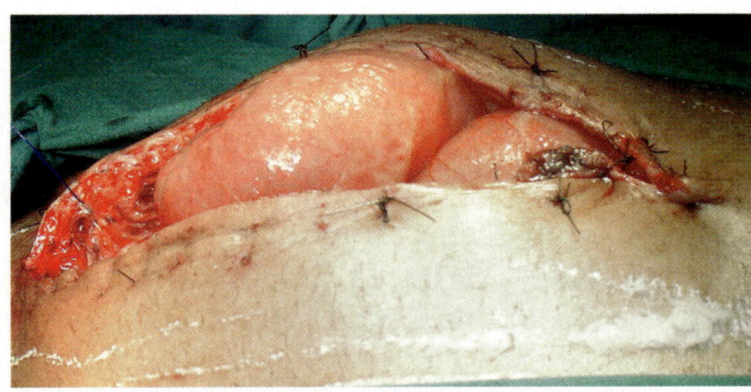

**Fig. 65.9:** Sutures opened. Distended bowels are seen

*Pearls of Wisdom*

Interestingly, it is a painless, shockless disruption (with) full of apprehension.

## Treatment

- Reassurance
- The bowel or the contents are covered with pads and bandage.
- Emergency surgery and closure is done.

## Principles of Surgery

1. Adequate exposure
2. Bowel is washed with saline and gently replaced into the peritoneal cavity.
3. Edges of the wound/incision are trimmed.
4. A single layer closure of the abdominal layer, by taking suture bites through whole thickness of the abdominal wall is done.
   - A few tension sutures (Figs 65.10 and 65.11) tied over a rubber or a plastic tube are placed and are removed after 2 weeks.
   - It should be remembered that **secondary wound healing is better than primary wound healing** and infection rarely occurs.

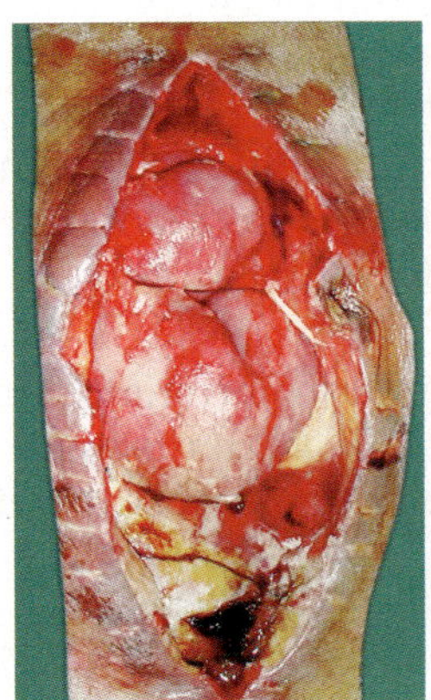

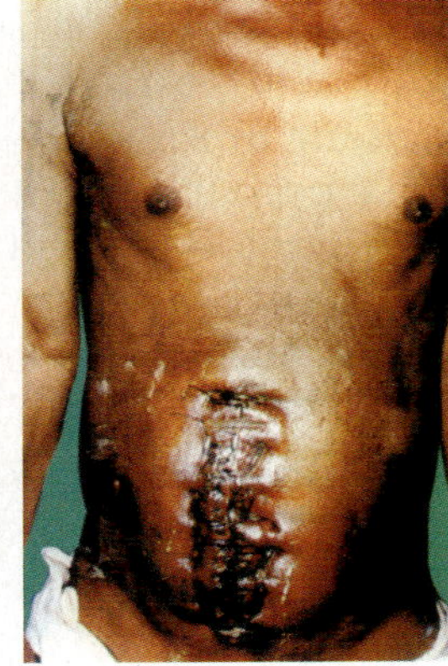

**Figs 65.10 and 65.11:** Wound dehiscence due to gangrene of the intestine—laparotomy was done, resection followed by closure of the abdomen with tension sutures. Many such patients require VAC dressings (*see* page 163)

5. **Closer of midline incision:** In all cases of midline incision, it is the linea alba with or without anterior fascial layer is approximated to the corresponding fascia on the other side.
   - 'Fascia' usually refers to the anterior rectus fascia, the fascia above the rectus muscles. This fascia holds the abdomen together and is the most important layer of closure.
   - The fascia can extend beyond the muscles and bind to other fascia.
   - An extension of the fascia is called an aponeurosis.

## Complications of Wound Closure

**I. Early complications:**
- Infection
- Dehiscence

**II. Late complications:**
- Incisional hernia
- Suture sinus
- Wound pain

## Prevention of Incisional Hernia

**SU14.3:** Describe the materials and methods used for surgical wound closure.

**Suturing techniques** (Key Boxes 65.4 and 65.5):

- There should be 1 cm interval between 2 suture bites.
- Length of suture material and length of wound should be 4:1 or more (Jenkins rule)[1], definitely not less.

Key Box 65.4

**Surgeon's Role in Preventing Incisional Hernia**

- Continuous *vs* interrupted sutures
- Knotting technique—secure knots
- Suture length/wound length ratio
- Bite size
- Mass closure *vs* aponeurosis only
- Tensionless sutures
- Suture material—nonabsorbable
- Anti-SSI (surgical site infection) measures—prophylactic antibiotics

Key Box 65.5

**Continuous Sutures**

- Continuous suturing is faster
- Accommodates wound lengthening due to distension
- Bursting strength of wound is significantly higher
- Minimises number of knots—equivalent or lower incidence of incisional hernia
- Disadvantages (theoretical): Wound security depends on single strand of suture and limited number of knots

[1]Jenkins rule refers to a surgical guideline, particularly in abdominal wound closure, attributed to a surgeon named Dr Evan Meredith Jenkins.

**A. Interrupted *vs* continuous technique:**

- Continuous is faster, accommodates wound lengthening due to distension, bursting strength of wound is significantly higher. It minimizes number of knots and thus lower incidence of incisional hernia has been found. **A continuous suture also provides** more type 1 collagen and thus has higher wound strength. Thus continuous sutures are better than interrupted.
- **Disadvantages:** Wound security depends on single strand of suture and limited number of knots.

**B. Mass closure:**

- Incorporate all layers of abdominal wall (except skin) as 1 structure and suturing is called mass suture. However, increased chances of hernia and dehiscence can occur following mass closure.
- Layered: Peritoneum, musculo-aponeurotic layer, skin. Adhesions, longer surgery time, compromises adequacy of subsequent layer closure.

**C. Aponeurosis only:**

- Good approximation of the edges of aponeurosis. No separation of wound edges. No soft tissue necrosis.
- Not necessary to suture peritoneum in midline incisions. A good closure of linea alba is all that is required. Peritoneum heals on its own by epithelialisation of mesothelium.

**Suture materials: A. Non-absorbable, B. Absorbable. (details are given in page 1192)**

- Non-absorbable sutures are associated with more pain and suture sinuses but less chances of incisional hernias. Example: Polypropylene.
- Equally good results are found with slowly absorbable sutures—**slowly absorbing like polydioxanone (PDS) sutures.**
- Fast absorbing sutures are related to higher rate of incisional hernias. Examples: Catgut or polygalactin (Vicryl).

**Antibacterial (PLUS) sutures to prevent SSI:**

- Presence of suture material may increase the risk of infection.
- Bacterial growth on suture material appeared to have the characteristics of biofilm formation. Suture with antiseptic may help in reducing complications related to infection of the suture material such as inflammation, pus discharge, etc.
- Technical details about sutures and measures to prevent incisional hernia are given in Key Boxes 65.3 and 65.6.

## FIBROMATOSES: DESMOID TUMOUR

### Classification

- *Superficial or deep.* **Deep** fibromatoses, also called ***aggressive fibromatoses and desmoid tumours,*** are **uncapsulated fibromas** which occur in the abdominal wall.
- They arise from muscles and aponeurotic layer of the abdominal wall.

### Incidence

- In children, most desmoid tumours are extra-abdominal with a female predominance.
- In young adults, desmoid tumours almost always occur in the abdominal wall (of women). ***Hormonal effects and pregnancy*** are believed to influence the growth of this tumour.
- Some tumours express hormone receptors (oestrogen and progesterone), and therefore ***tamoxifen*** and other hormonal modulators are among the adjuvant therapies for this tumour.

### Aetiopathogenesis

- Childbirth, trauma or operative scars are the possible aetiological factors.
- Desmoid tumour is one of the components of Gardner's syndrome.
- It is benign but has a tendency to infiltrate the muscles. Some fibromas exhibit dysplastic changes. The cut surface is compared to an onion—whorled fibroma with spindle-shaped cells.
- Sarcomatous changes and metastasis do not occur.

### Clinical Features

- **Abdominal fibromatosis** is far less prone to recurrences than desmoid tumours in other sites.
- It usually occurs in the abdominal wall of women of childbearing age during or after pregnancy.
- Clinically, the lesions present as deep-seated, firm, nonencapsulated, slow-growing, locally invasive and painless masses.
- It typically manifests as a slow-growing, progressive mass that becomes more prominent on abdominal muscle contraction. Mass is in the abdominal wall and is firm to hard in consistency.
- **Mesenteric fibromatosis**, probably the commonest among the group, usually presents as a slow-growing mass that involves small bowel mesentery or retroperitoneum.
- The recurrence rate of mesenteric fibromatosis seems to be substantially higher in patients who have Gardner's syndrome than in patients who do not have this syndrome.

### Treatment

- Simple excision results in recurrence. Hence, **wide excision with 2–3 cm** of normal **healthy margins** is necessary with reconstruction of the abdominal wall (Figs 65.12 and 65.13).
- In spite of adequate surgery, 10–20% chances of recurrence occur (Key Box 65.3).

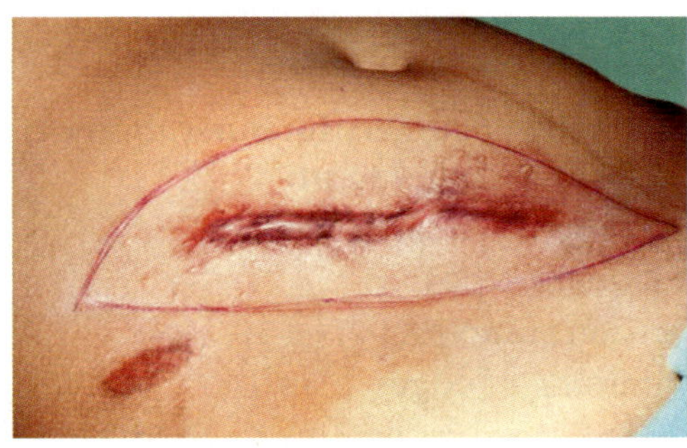

**Fig. 65.12:** Wide excision of recurrent desmoid tumour in the abdominal wall

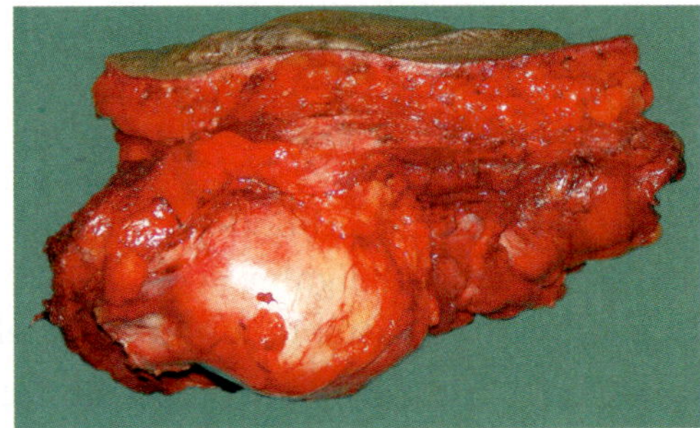

**Fig. 65.13:** Specimen of desmoid tumour which is removed along with normal tissue

Key Box 65.6

**Peculiarities of Desmoid Tumour**

- Uncapsulated fibroma
- Infiltrates muscles, even though benign
- Does not change into sarcoma
- It may be a part of Gardner's syndrome
- Simple excision results in recurrence
- Wide excision is recommended

## DIVARICATION OF RECTI

- In this condition, the two rectus abdominis muscles are widely separated (not in the midline).
- Repeated pregnancy in quick succession is the most important cause. Chronic constipation or overstraining may be another factor. Obviously women are commonly affected.
- Exercises and abdominal corset are helpful.
- Symptomatic cases are operated—divaricated recti are brought towards midline (Fig. 65.14).
- Mesh repair may be required.

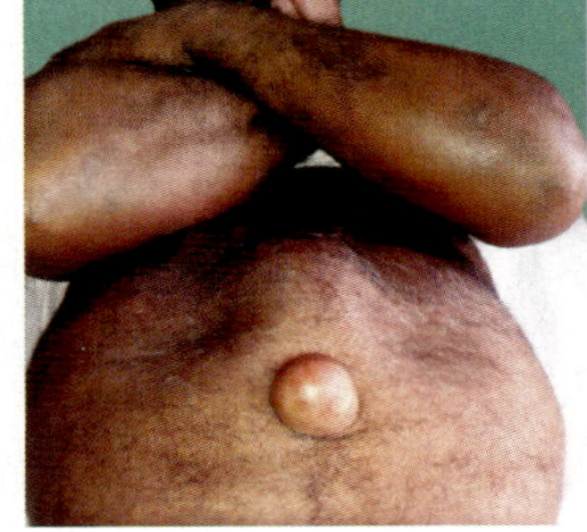

**Fig. 65.14:** Divarication of recti with umbilical hernia

## ENDOMETRIOSIS OF THE ABDOMINAL WALL

Drugs like sulindac and tamoxifen have also been used here, with some success.

- It occurs due to mechanical implantation of endometrial cells during surgery (sites—Key Box 65.7 and Fig. 65.15).
- Painful, palpable swelling, more symptomatic at the time of menstruation are characteristic features.
  - Perimenstrual cyclical bleeding can occur.
- Oral contraceptive pills may control the symptoms.
- Otherwise, excision of the nodule has to be done (Fig. 65.16).

Key Box 65.7

**Sites of Endometriosis**

- Laparoscopic port – Umbilicus
- Gynaecological surgery – Abdominal incision
- Episiotomy – Perineum

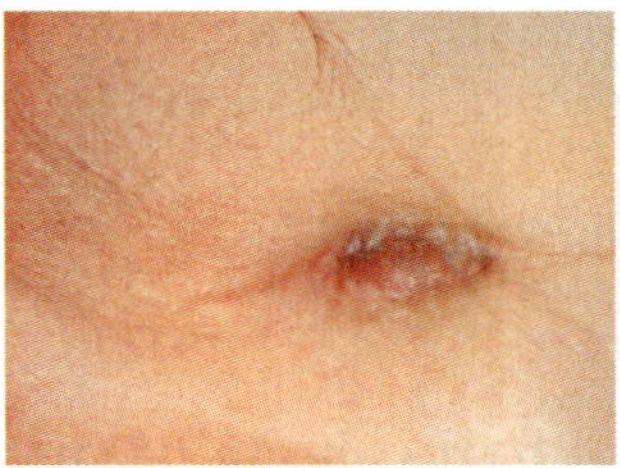

**Fig. 65.15:** Scar endometriosis

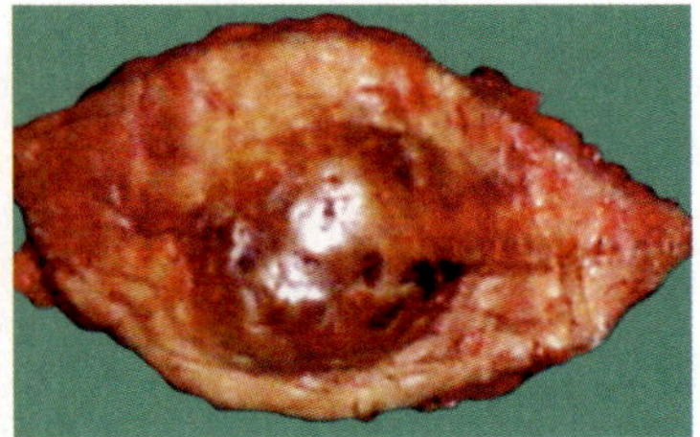

**Fig. 65.16:** Wide excision of scar endometriosis

## MISCELLANEOUS

### ABDOMINAL WALL VEINS

- Veins are seen in portal hypertension. In relation to umbilicus, they are called **caput medusae**. Direction of the veins are important which can be demonstrated by emptying the vein and filling (Fig. 65.17).
- In cases of inferior vena caval obstruction, veins are seen on the flank. These veins are called inguino-axillary veins (Fig. 65.18).

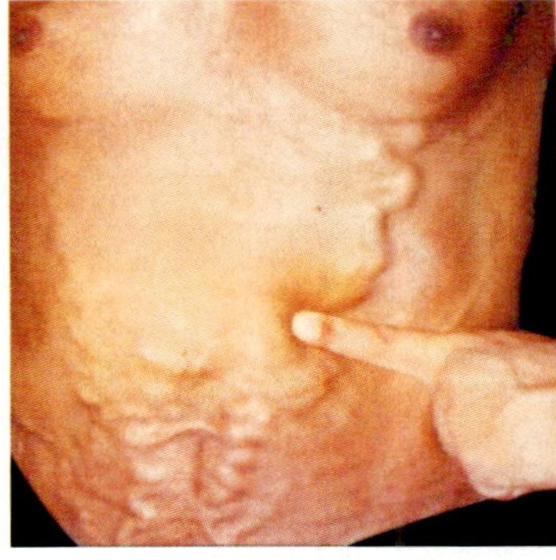

**Fig. 65.17:** Dilated tortuous veins due to portal hypertension—caput medusae

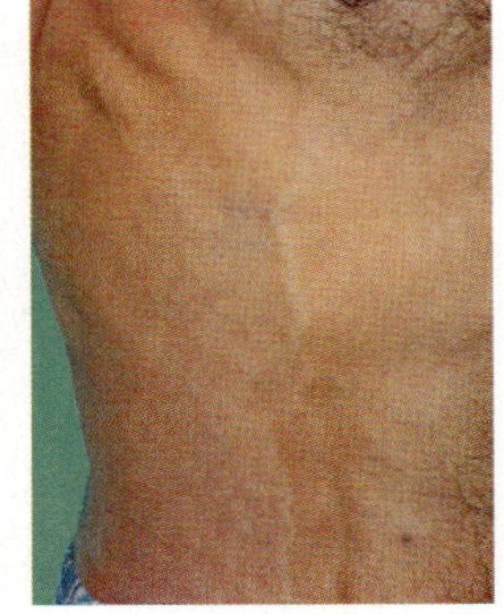

**Fig. 65.18:** Veins on the lateral abdominal wall suggestive of inferior vena caval obstruction

## MULTIPLE CHOICE QUESTIONS

**1. The following is not a cause of umbilical faecal fistula:**
   A. Persistent vitellointestinal duct
   B. Tuberculosis
   C. Carcinoma
   D. Raspberry adenoma

**2. The following statement is true about burst abdomen:**
   A. It is very painful
   B. It is associated with shock
   C. Straining can produce it
   D. Conservative management is the choice

**3. About desmoid tumour:**
   A. Is a capsulated fibroma
   B. Infiltrates muscles
   C. Often changes to sarcoma
   D. Simple excision is recommended

**4. The following is true of Meleney's postoperative synergistic gangrene, *except*:**
   A. Is progressive
   B. Can occur after appendicectomy
   C. Starts as cellulitis
   D. Is painless

**5. The following is true about rectus sheath haematoma, *except*:**
   A. It can occur with pregnancy
   B. Sudden straining can precipitate it
   C. Presents as painless lump above umbilicus
   D. Nausea, vomiting and fever are other features

**6. The principles of surgery for burst abdomen include all of the following, *except*:**
   A. Layer by layer careful suture
   B. Adequate exposure
   C. Tension sutures
   D. Trimming of edges

**7. The pathognomonic sign of burst abdomen is:**
   A. Shock
   B. Pink or brown serosanguinous discharge
   C. Pain
   D. Occurs on the second postoperative day

**8. Umbilical adenoma:**
   A. Sessile swelling
   B. Is a premalignant condition
   C. Can be treated with ligature
   D. Occurs due to persistent umbilical vessels

**9. Pilonidal sinus is known to occur in the following places, *except*:**
   A. Internatal cleft B. Umbilicus
   C. Interdigital cleft D. Axilla

**10. Meleney's gangrene is a synergistic gangrene caused by:**
   A. *Streptococcus* and *Staphylococcus*
   B. *E. coli* and *Klebsiella*
   C. *Clostridium* and *Pseudomonas*
   D. *Salmonella typhi* and *paratyphi*

**Answers**

**1.** D **2.** C **3.** B **4.** D **5.** C **6.** A **7.** B **8.** C **9.** D **10.** A

Chapter 66

# Trauma—Initial Management, Blunt Abdominal Trauma, War and Blast Injuries and Triage

- Initial management of trauma victims
- Blast injuries
- Warfare injuries
- Missile wounds of abdomen
- Gunshot wounds
- Blunt abdominal trauma
- Triage
- Liver injuries
- Small bowel injuries
- Colonic injuries
- Duodenal injuries
- Pancreatic injuries
- Renal injuries
- Retroperitoneal haematoma
- Vascular trauma

## INITIAL MANAGEMENT OF TRAUMA VICTIMS

### INTRODUCTION

*Trauma* originates from the Greek word meaning ***wound.*** This occurs due to physical force exerted on a person. Trauma constitutes a large proportion of the number of lives lost, especially in the productive age group. The most effective way of reducing trauma-related deaths is by prevention which involves building safer roads and educating the masses on observation of road discipline. Wearing of protective gear such as helmets for two-wheeler drivers and riders, seat belts for four-wheeler drivers and passenger must be made mandatory. Trauma can also be due to earthquakes, wars, major accidents involving trains, etc. So much has been learnt from various wars including World War I and II, Korean wars, Vietnam wars, etc. It is said—*those who cannot remember the past are condemned to repeat it (George Santayana)*—really holds good for trauma.

Once trauma occurs, all efforts will need to be made to reduce morbidity and mortality. Trauma-related deaths have a trimodal distribution: First, mortality that occurs at site or on transfer due to severity of trauma injuries. These deaths cannot be prevented and only a behavioural change can reduce them. The victim's injuries are so severe resulting in massive exsanguination or severe head injuries such that saving the life of that trauma victim is impossible. The second phase of deaths, usually due to hypovolaemia and other trauma-related injuries, are often avoidable and treatable. Timely and appropriate intervention at this stage can reduce the effects of trauma and prevent morbidity secondary to the injury. The third phase includes those patients who die of complications of trauma such as infection, embolism, sepsis, acute respiratory distress syndrome and septic shock. A well-managed second phase is likely to reduce the incidence of the third phase.

When a patient/patients sustain trauma, it is a natural tendency in India for onlookers, police or fire personnel to load them into the first available vehicle and transfer them to the nearest available hospital. Although their intentions are good, they may actually cause more harm. Many of these patients may have sustained cervical spine injuries which may be undisplaced at first but get displaced, if careful attention to prevention of neck movements is not given during transfer. In view of this, the salient features of trauma care must be widely publicised among the lay public.

Doctors and other medical personnel get involved in patient care only after the patient reaches the hospital. They too may not be trained to deal with trauma and it is common to find trauma care area in chaos, especially when multiple patients arrive in a short span. A systematic approach to victim/victims of trauma is very necessary to ensure best outcome.

### PREHOSPITAL PHASE

#### Scene Safety

Every rescuer must always ensure that the scene is safe for oneself before proceeding to help a trauma victim. A liquid petroleum leak, radiation exposure, floods, landslides are a few examples. When unsure, it may be more prudent to enquire from the fire personnel and then approach the victim.

### Trauma Triage

Modern medical triage was invented by Dominique Jean Larrey, a surgeon during the Napoleonic wars, **Triage** is derived from the French word ***trier***, meaning **to sort**. When there are multiple victims, the philosophy of trauma triage will need to be adopted. This is a method of sorting out injured patients, during mass casualties depending on the severity of injury. If you are the first on the scene, first priority is to get expert help (call up fire services, regional trauma centre, etc.).

Triage is a skilled activity by a trauma team, wherein there is a leader (usually senior-most doctor/surgeon) and there are many assistants. The leader sorts out patients (people) depending upon their severity of injury. The term ***'multiple casualties'*** is used when there are more than two trauma victims but the number does not overwhelm the facilities available at the treating centre. The term ***'mass casualties'*** is used when there are more than two trauma victims but the number overwhelms the facilities available at the treating centre.

### Colour Coding

When there are multiple or mass casualties, rescuers use universal colour codes to mark each victim based on the severity of injuries to help decide on the treatment priority to be given to each patient. The colour codes are as follows:

**CODE BLACK (EXPECTANT):** These patients have very severe injuries and may not be expected to survive very long with the available care.

**CODE RED (IMMEDIATE):** These patients may have life-threatening injuries to the airway, breathing or circulation which are potentially reversible with immediate care.

**CODE YELLOW (DELAYED):** These patients are relatively stable and would not be expected to become unstable in a few hours. They too can have a threat to life but not immediate.

**CODE GREEN (MINOR):** These patients have injuries but can be seen in due course. The 'walking wounded' belong to this group.

Thus, in the event of a large number of patients arriving at the trauma centre and they have been coded, all patients with 'red' code must be attended to immediately followed by the 'yellow' coded patients. The 'green' coded patients can be seen in the outpatient department, whereas the 'black' coded ones can be given attention when possible.

### Communication

All ambulance drivers must be instructed to store the telephone numbers of the contact person in the referral hospitals. It is essential that advance information is given to the trauma centre ahead of arrival of trauma victims to optimize care.

*Pearls of Wisdom*

The leader assesses the patient—flags and moves forward and it is his assistant who carries out the necessary resuscitation. The leader should not resuscitate any patient. There are others waiting for his expert help.

### *A Common Scheme or a Quick Assessment*

1. **Can the patient walk?**
   **Yes:** Delayed (green), No—check for breathing.
2. **Is the patient breathing?**
   **No:** Open the airway—Are they breathing (ventilating) him?
   **Yes:** Immediate (red), No—DEAD (white).
   **Yes:** Count or estimate respiratory rate (over 15 sec).
   <10 to >30 per minute—immediate (red).
   10–30 per minute—check the circulation.
3. **Check the circulation**
   Pulse >120/min (capillary refill >2s)—immediate (red).
   Pulse <120/min (capillary refill <2s)—urgent (yellow).

- If any regional trauma centre is well equipped and nearby, one has to transport all the injured patients to hospital (scoop and run), where expert help is available. Meanwhile trauma centre can be alerted about the arrival of casualties. If expert help is far away, then one may have to treat the patients at the accident site (stay and play). Resuscitation is done as per ATLS guidelines.
- During these exercises, do not forget to take care of your own safety, in burning vehicles, burning or falling buildings, etc.

*Pearls of Wisdom*

An initial quick evaluation of the patient for anaemia, level of consciousness, if necessary volume replacement, application of cervical (C) collar to the neck, etc. are done.

## TRAUMA CENTRE PREPARATION

### Plan in Advance

Every trauma centre must be in a state of constant preparedness to receive trauma victims. The trauma centre must be manned by dedicated personnel and must have the necessary equipment which is checked on a daily basis and rechecked after every use.

### Trauma Care Personnel

The core group responding to trauma cases include nurses, trauma technicians, qualified doctors (general surgeon, orthopaedician or emergency physician) and a set of doctors on call to deal with referrals (neurosurgeon, cardiothoracic vascular surgeon).

### Trauma Care Area

The trauma care area must be a dedicated area called the **'resuscitation bay'**. All personnel caring for the patient must wear **personal protective equipment** including goggles, gown, gloves and shoe covers. The patient must be received on a trolley bed and each bed must have a **multimodal monitor** including pulse oximeter, noninvasive blood pressure and electrocardiogram. An **oxygen source** and **suction apparatus** also must be available with each bed.

### Resuscitation Equipment

Resuscitation equipment will include **airway equipment** such as airways, endotracheal tubes, laryngoscopes, laryngeal mask airways, infraglottic airways, Magill's forceps and a stethoscope. *Cervical collar of different sizes must also be available.* **Equipment for circulatory resuscitation** include intravenous fluids (isotonic saline, Ringer lactate), intravenous cannulae, pressure bags, body and fluid warmers, syringes, **medications** including vasopressors, inotropes, anticholinergics, analgesics, etc.). An ultrasound machine must be available for focused abdominal sonography in trauma **(FAST)**. A portable X-ray machine must also be available to obtain the basic X-rays (neck, chest, pelvis).

> **SU17.1:** Describe the principles of first aid to trauma patients.

## APPROACH TO TRAUMA

The approach to trauma must be done in the following steps: **Primary survey and resuscitation, secondary survey and definitive care.**

### Primary Survey and Resuscitation

The purpose of this step is to very quickly evaluate for any life-threatening emergency and deal with it immediately. Often an obvious external trauma, such as fracture femur diverts the attention of the caregivers, but a life-threatening injury is missed. The evaluation must be performed in the following order: **A, B, C, D and E. However, when bleeding is obvious and external, it can be easily controlled. Thus, now it is being referred as cABCDE.**

> **A**—Airway with cervical spine control
> **B**—Adequate breathing
> **C**—Circulation with haemorrhage control
> **D**—Disability assessment, and
> **E**—Exposure and environment control.

**Control of bleeding:** When an external bleeding is visible and massive, control of bleeding is more important than airway. Often in a trauma, source of bleeding may be in the limbs—muscle or arterial bleeding. Immediate first aid involves **pressure packing principle. If an arterial bleeding is visible, a hemostat is used to control it. Hemostatic dressing is applied.**

If a tourniquet is available, rubber or pneumatic—should be used. Tourniquet time is noted and immediate transfer to referral centers should be done.

- **An obvious fracture lower limb due to a fall is common in elderly patients.** A posterior slab is given for immobilization.
- **Simple wounds which are bleeding and are thoroughly cleaned and sutured.**

#### *Survey*

A very quick way of evaluating airway, breathing and circulation is to address the patient and elicit a response (e.g. ask the patient's name). If he replies appropriately, it is evident that the patient's airway is patent, breathing is optimal and circulation to his brain is adequate. If the patient does not respond to call, a painful stimulus is given and the response is quickly graded on the *AVPU scale, where A = Alert, V = Responds to verbal commands, P = Responds to pain, and U = Unresponsive.* **Quick primary survey and actions are given below in the form of ABCDE of primary survey.**

**1. Airway with cervical spine immobilization:** *All patients sustaining trauma, especially to the head and who have an altered sensorium must be assumed to have cervical spine injury until proved otherwise.* The mechanism of injury would provide a clue to the possibility of cervical trauma. The neck must be immobilised in a rigid cervical collar (Philadelphia cervical collar or similar) as early as possible. Rapid assessment of signs of obstruction should be looked for—foreign body, laryngeal and faciomaxillary fracture, fallen back tongue (Fig. 66.1).

If the airway is not patent or the patient's ability to maintain his airway is questionable, the airway must be secured. Signs of compromised airway include snoring, stridor, agitation, active accessory muscles of ventilation/paradoxical chest movements and cyanosis.

*Open the airway first with a jaw thrust, **oral airway** or a **nasopharyngeal airway*** (Key Box 66.1). An oral

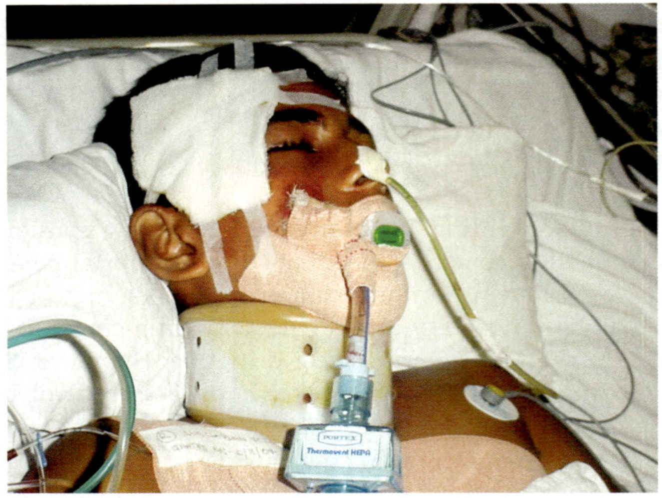

**Fig. 66.1:** Management of a polytrauma patient in an intensive care unit—cervical collar has been applied and patient is being ventilated

airway is preferred, if the patient is unconscious and is suspected to have sustained base of the skull fracture. A nasopharyngeal airway is chosen, if the gag reflex is intact and the patient is semiconscious. Insertion of a nasopharyngeal airway in a patient with base of skull fracture is risky as it can enter the brain through the fracture. Provide oxygen using face mask and ventilate as necessary.

Key Box 66.1

**Quick Reminder Mnemonic at Treatment Centre**

- **L**ift jaw
- **I**ntubation: Airway
- **F**allen tongue/foreign body to be checked
- **T**racheostomy/cricothyrotomy/oropharyngeal or nasopharyngeal throat suction
- **Jaw** fractures to be ruled out

*Remember as* **LIFTJAW**

Indications for **endotracheal intubation** or **tracheostomy** for securing the airway include obstructed airway, apnoea, hypoxia, severe head injury, maxillofacial injury, penetrating neck trauma with expanding haematoma and chest trauma.

Endotracheal intubation provides the most definitive airway. It is required in patients who are unconscious, not able to maintain their own airway, who have sustained extensive faciomaxillary injuries or airway burns. A rapid sequence induction and intubation is preferred. The level of sedation required for intubation would depend on the level of consciousness and haemodynamic stability. Generally, midazolam or etomidate is used for sedation and succinyl choline as the muscle relaxant for intubation.

The cervical collar is used to limit neck movements but it often also limits mouth opening and increases the difficulty of securing airway. Hence, it is recommended that *the cervical collar is removed during endotracheal intubation and the neck immobilized manually.* The collar is reapplied after airway is secured.

**If endotracheal intubation is difficult,** the airway can be maintained using **supraglottic airway** adjuncts such as laryngeal mask airway or laryngeal tube. If these are inadequate, a **cricothyrotomy** (infraglottic airway) may need to be performed. This should be followed by a regular **tracheostomy.** Cricothyrotomy is advocated as the initial choice as it can be done very quickly. Time is of essence in a hypoxic emergency.

**2. Breathing—look, listen and feel: Inspect** (look) at the chest for the respiratory rate, depth and pattern. If the patient's breathing is inadequate as evidenced clinically (rate and depth) or if the patient is cyanosed/oxygen saturation is low (<93%), breathing must be assisted and oxygen supplementation given as required. Look for presence of flail chest, open chest wounds and use of accessory muscles of respirations.

**Palpate** (feel) for tracheal shift, broken ribs and subcutaneous emphysema. **Percuss** for diagnosis of haemothorax and pneumothorax.

**Auscultate** both sides of the chest for equality of breath sounds and for any added sounds. Rule out endobronchial intubation, if an endotracheal tube is already in place.

If breath sounds are unequal, inspect the neck for any distended veins, tracheal position and then percuss the chest. If neck veins are distended, trachea is deviated and the chest is resonant to percuss on the side of reduced air entry, **suspect tension pneumothorax**. The patient may require needle thoracostomy. A large bore (16–18 G cannula) is inserted in the fifth intercostal space slightly anterior to the anterior axillary line (ATLS 10th edition). In children, an appropriately large bore needle or cannula must be placed in the second intercostal space in the midclavicular line. If air hisses out, decompression of chest would have been achieved. Chest tube insertion can follow later during secondary survey (Key Box 66.2).

*Pearls of Wisdom*

Tension pneumothorax is a clinical diagnosis. Do not delay the treatment while waiting for chest X-ray. More details are given in page 592, chapter 47.

**Cardiac tamponade:** It is a serious condition which results due to collection of blood/fluid in the pericardial cavity.

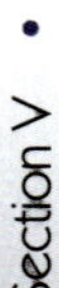

Key Box 66.2

**Tension Pneumothorax: Clinical Features**

- **T**achypnoea
- **T**achycardia
- **T**ympanic note on percussion
- **T**otal absence of breath sounds
- **T**racheal shift

*Observe* **5 Ts**

***Causes:*** Gunshot injuries, penetrating injuries, ruptured aortic aneurysms, invasive and interventional procedures including central venous catheter insertions, angiograms can also cause cardiac tamponade.

***Pathophysiology:*** **The distended pericardial cavity compresses all chambers of the heart.** As a result of this, venous return is impeded, ventricular filling is impaired resulting in hypotension, and hypoperfusion. **Ventricles cannot contract effectively and leads to cardiovascular collapse and cardiac arrest.**

***Clinical features:*** **Hypotension, tachycardia, low volume pulse, cold peripheries, chest pain, breathlessness, syncope and cardiovascular collapse.** The neck veins may be distended. **The Beck's triad** includes hypotension, **elevated systemic venous pressure**, often with jugular venous distention; muffled heart sounds. This can occur with sudden intrapericardial haemorrhage. The Kussmaul sign—a paradoxical elevation in jugular venous pulse (JVP) during inspiration is sometimes seen in cardiac tamponade.

***Diagnosis:*** **It is a medical emergency.** The gold standard investigation is ultrasound examination. The extended focussed abdominal sonography in trauma (E-FAST) obtained in patients with trauma includes evaluation for presence of cardiac tamponade. Echocardiography can confirm the presence of pericardial effusion and determine its size. It can also reveal compromise of cardiac function (right ventricular diastolic collapse, right atrial systolic collapse, plethoric IVC). A chest X-ray may show an enlarged heart. CT chest can diagnose pericardial effusion. However, if the cardiac tamponade is significant, one should not wait for chest X-ray or CT chest but proceed with pericardiocentesis using point-of-care ultrasound.

***Treatment:*** In case of urgency, a needle pericardiocentesis is performed at the bedside using ultrasound-guided needle placement from a subxiphoid window. If ultrasound is not available, the patient is on the verge of collapse and there is a strong suspicion of cardiac tamponade, the traditional landmark technique may need to be adopted. A large bore needle is inserted from the subxiphoid point into the pericardial cavity by directing it inwards, superiorly and towards the left shoulder with continuous aspiration. Support airway, breathing and circulation as necessary. Supplementing oxygen, positive pressure ventilation and leg elevation also will help these patients depending upon the severity of the tamponade. Standard cardiac life support measures (ACLS) will need to be provided, if the patient develops cardiac arrest.

**3. Circulation with haemorrhage control:** Feel the radial pulse for its rate, rhythm, quality (strong, feeble and thready) and equality with opposite side. Check blood pressure. *The commonest cause of shock in trauma is hypovolaemia.* Neurogenic shock is a possibility in cases of spinal injury. Obstructive shock can occur in tension pneumothorax and cardiac tamponade. Septic shock is unlikely but not impossible in early trauma.

If the pulse is feeble, irregular and the patient is hypotensive, rule out the possibility of a pericardial tamponade by looking at neck veins. If the neck veins are distended, radial pulse is not felt, heart sounds are faint and needle thoracostomy has not treated the condition, perform a pericardiocentesis. Ultrasound of the heart (FAST) is very useful to confirm the diagnosis and guide the procedure. If ultrasound is not available, it is reasonable to proceed with landmark-guided drainage of the pericardium.

*The possible sites of bleeding can be remembered as* ***blood on the floor and four more****. The blood on the floor refers to external and obvious bleeding. The four other sites are the thorax, abdomen, pelvis and long bones.* Look very quickly for any obvious bleeding from any part of the body. If present, apply pressure and stop the bleeding. Application of a tourniquet is not advisable unless absolutely necessary. If applied, it should be removed as early as possible to avoid injury to tissues.

An intravenous line should be secured and intravenous fluids, preferably around 40°C (crystalloids—saline, Ringer lactate or plasmalyte), infused very quickly to restore volume. Initial bolus of 2 litres of crystalloid solutions.

**Dextrose containing solutions are not recommended. Two large peripheral lines are preferred for the initial resuscitation.** Insertion of central lines is not recommended (unless done by skilled personnel) as it takes much longer to insert, requires expertise and can be associated with complications. If a peripheral intravenous access is not available, intraosseous needle can be inserted and fluids infused into the bone marrow. *All infusions that can be given intravenously can also be given intraosseously. External jugular venous access is another option for quick transfusion of large amounts of fluids and blood products.*

Obvious bleeding sites in the upper limb or lower limb in cases of soft tissue injuries with or without fractures should be inspected, if necessary, immediate tourniquet to be applied and even can be stopped by an artery forceps depending upon the severity.

**Pearls of Wisdom**

The immediate goal is to arrest bleeding rather than replacing the blood.

Check the abdomen and pelvis. Abdominal trauma can be penetrating or nonpenetrating. Inspect and then palpate the abdomen for any distension, abrasion or contusion. Spring the pelvis to rule out pelvic instability due to fracture. Perform a focused abdominal sonography in trauma **(FAST)** to rule out liver and splenic injuries. If any abdominal injury with haemorrhage is suspected, the patient will need an urgent life-saving laparotomy.

**'Damage control surgery/laparotomy'** should be done as soon as possible in patients with evidence of abdominal trauma and maintaining a systolic BP at 80–90 mmHg with fluid resuscitation is unsuccessful. The aim of this laparotomy is to stop the bleeding, often only packing, after which the mid-line incision is temporarily closed within 30 minutes with towel clamps. *This laparotomy is described as not a surgery, but a resuscitative procedure.* In polytrauma, when multiple organs are involved, to conduct the complete repair of all the injuries will require many hours. These patients develop coagulopathy, hypothermia, acidosis and thus they succumb. In such situations, packs are used to stop the bleeding and these packs need to be removed after 48 hours. Thus, laparotomy wound is closed only at the skin level. If intestine is transected, staple the intestine to avoid contamination. One can go in after 48 hours for a definitive repair. In presence of sepsis, instead of doing an anastomosis, it is better to exteriorize and definitive repair is done at a later date.

**The American College of Surgeons Classification** of hypovolemic shock can be used as a quick guide to gauge the amount of blood lost. If the patient is tachycardic (heart rate >120/min) and hypotensive (systolic blood pressure is <90 mmHg), the patient has Class III shock or higher where the patient has lost >30–40% blood volume. Such patients will also require transfusion of blood products (packed cells and fresh frozen plasma). It may be necessary to activate massive transfusion protocol (when available at the hospital) if the patient is bleeding profusely. Replacing the lost volume along with hemorrhage control is important to restore perfusion and prevent tissue damage.

In cases where the hemostasis is insecure or not definitive, volumes should be controlled to maintain systolic BP at 80–90 mmHg till the bleeding can be stopped. This is called *'hypotensive fluid resuscitation' or 'permissive hypotension'*. Small boluses of IV fluids—250 ml of O negative blood or normal saline can be given till blood is available. It is important to maintain the patient warm through the resuscitation as hypothermia impairs coagulation, increases bleeding, depresses respiration and circulation as well as increases chances of infection.

The pelvis should be examined by springing the pelvis. This should be done only once and if any instability is noted, the pelvis should be immobilized by application of pelvic binder and later on with an external fixator to stop bleeding.

**Role of tranexamic acid in trauma:**

- It is an anti-fibrinolytic drug to be used in trauma patients bleeding with.
- Given 1 g IV over 10 minutes followed by next dose of 1 g over 8 hours.
  - Tachycardia with pulse rate more than 110/minute or systolic blood pressure less than 110 mmHg.
- Ideally should be administered within 3 hours of trauma.

### Special Patient Groups

Trauma can affect a person of any age. Older patients on multiple medications may not manifest blood loss. Often, they may not show a tachycardia or hypertension. Children tend to have high heart rates, whereas trained athletes may have low heart rates making these signs unreliable in these patients.

### Disability

The patient's Glasgow Coma Scale (GCS) must be assessed as also the pupillary response to light must be recorded. Observe for neurologic deterioration. The patient must be turned to lateral position using log rolling technique and the spine is examined (Key Box 66.3).

Key Box 66.3

**Disability: AVPU system**

- **A**wake
- Open eyes to **V**oice
- Open eyes to **P**ainful stimulus
- **U**narousable

### Exposure

The patient's whole body must be exposed and every orifice must be examined. Quick examination of all orifices. Examples: Look for bleeding from the ear, nose, oral cavity, rectum, vagina, and urethra. A per rectal examination must be done after examination of the spine to rule out urethral injuries. Hypothermia must be avoided. A pregnancy test must be obtained in every female patient in the reproductive age group.

### Adjuncts to Primary Survey

**Monitors:** The patient's vitals are monitored using a pulse oximeter, noninvasive blood pressure and electrocardiogram. Arterial blood gases and capnography are extremely useful and must be made available in dedicated trauma centres.

**Tubes and catheters:** The patient is then placed supine. Tubes and catheters are inserted and X-rays obtained. A nasogastric tube and urinary catheter are inserted, X-rays of the neck, chest and pelvis and ultrasound abdomen are obtained at this stage.

### Secondary Survey and Definitive Care

Once the life-threatening emergencies are ruled out or dealt with, secondary survey involving a more detailed head-to-toe examination of the patient is performed. All through the secondary survey, if there is any change in patient condition the primary survey starting with A, B and C will need to be performed. If the patient is being treated in a smaller hospital without facility to treat that trauma, the patient must be transferred to a higher centre after stabilization of vital signs. The transfer itself must be well-planned with well-delegated tasks for each personnel and the transfer communicated to the referral hospital. More details are given under abdominal trauma.

## BLAST INJURIES

- Bursting of bombs or shells rupture their casing and impart high velocity to resulting fragments. These fragments cause more devastating injuries than blast wave.
- **The two main components are: Blast pressure wave** (dynamic overpressure) with positive and negative phase and mass **movement of air (blast wind).**
- Positive phase of blast wave lasts few milliseconds (close to the explosion it may be over 7000 kN/m$^2$) (tympanic membrane ruptures at 150 kN/m$^2$).
- Like sound waves blast, pressure waves flow over and around an obstruction and affect persons sheltering behind a wall. The pressure affecting such a person is known as incident pressure (pressure at 90° to direction of travel of blast shock front).
- Person standing in front of a wall facing an explosion is subject to added effect of reflected pressure. Mass movement of air displaces air at supersonic speed. This disrupts environment, hurting debris and people. Blast wave under the water travels at great speed and to greater distance. Injuries tend to be complex and severe.

*Pearls of Wisdom*

Structures injured by primary blast wave are ears, lungs, heart and gastrointestinal system.

- Most will have combination of blunt, blast and thermal injuries. Deafness, lung contusion, capillary leakage and haemorrhage into alveoli and ARDS precipitated by over transfusion are the features. Perforation of the intestines and penetration injuries to the eye are the other features.
- Management consists of resuscitation in a well-equipped trauma unit, blood transfusions, intensive care monitoring, antibiotics and appropriate surgical procedures.

## WARFARE INJURIES

Penetrating missile wounds, injuries from blast phenomena and burns are typical features of modern conventional war. The most common wounding agent in surviving casualties is a fragment wound and not a bullet wound as many erroneously believe. The aim in modern war is to incapacitate and **not to kill**. Hence, a large number of surviving casualties is a major financial and logistic burden on a nation engaged in war.

### Wound Ballistics and Mechanisms of Injury

Bullets fired from handguns are propelled at low velocity, have low available energy and result in low velocity transfer wounds (100–500 J), whereas those from assault rifle have high velocity and have high available energy (2000–3000 J) and they cause high energy transfer wounds. **Low energy** transfer wounds leave injury confined to wound tract. **High energy** transfer wounds cause local laceration, crush injury and also cause remote injury from wound tract due to temporary cavitation phenomena.

### Management

- Entrance and exit wounds do not indicate considerable damage that may have occurred to deeper structures.
- Resuscitate as per ATLS guidelines.
- Record the wounds in case sheets, take photographs, if necessary.
- Under anaesthesia, excise skin around entry and exit wounds, give liberal longitudinal incision through skin and deep fascia, which allows proper visualisation of underlying structures.
- Debride (cut till healthy tissues are seen) all dead tissues—dead muscle does not bleed or contract, looks dusky.
- Identify neurovascular bundles and examine them.
- Dissect and mark injured nerves for possible future repair.

- Repair arteries and veins, if injured.
- Give thorough wash and let out all the dirt.
- Injured tendons are trimmed and tied for easy identification at future surgery.
- Fix bones by appropriate methods.
- Cover the wound with absorbable dressing.
- Appropriate antibiotics and injection tetanus toxoid are given.
- Amputation may be necessary, if limb is grossly mutilated.
- Delayed primary closure is done (4–6 days later) once the wound starts healing.

## MISSILE WOUNDS OF ABDOMEN

- Every penetrating and perforating missile wound of the abdomen should be explored by laparotomy. A full midline incision from xiphisternum to pubis is recommended and it may be extended to thorax, if necessary.
- The rest of the treatment depends on the nature of injury. Bleeding mesenteric vessels are ligated, injured small bowel is repaired by suturing or by resection and anastomosis. In colonic injuries, simple closure or closure with protective colostomy is necessary depending upon the nature of the colonic injury and contamination.
- Liver, splenic, pancreatic and renal injuries have been discussed in respective chapters.

## GUNSHOT WOUNDS

Gunshot wounds are high energy injuries that can result in extensive damage to soft tissues, viscera, bone, etc. Depending upon the site of entry and exit points, damage can occur. Lucky are a few where on bullet enters and exists missing major vascular structure or viscera as it may happen in the abdomen.

Damage caused by a bullet is directly related to its kinetic energy. It is due to various factors such as passage of missile, cavitation and secondary shock wave. Cavitation refers to the damage caused by bullet to the surrounding tissue due to fragmentation, shearing forces and turbulence.

Kinetic energy is mass and velocity to the power of 2 divided by 2.

The basic principles of the management of gunshot wounds are control of haemorrhage, preventing infection, and reconstruction. The extent to which a gunshot wound needs to be surgically explored can be difficult to determine sometimes. The aim is not to remove the bullet which may be visible in an X-ray or CT scan but to see the effects of tissue destruction such as bleeding, intestinal perforations, mesenteric tear or soft tissue and vascular injuries in the neck.

If fractures occur and fragmentation of bullet occur means wound severity is more and, therefore, a requirement for more surgical exploration, followed by debridement of dead and crushed tissues.

Gunshot wounds should never be closed primarily; the full range of reconstruction from secondary intention to free tissue transfer may be required.

### *Treatment*

As an urgent measure, if active bleeding is visible, apply pressure and try to stop the bleeders. Bleeders can be from vessels or from muscles. Temporary tourniquet can be applied to buy some time and proceed to shift the patient to the operation theatre for corrective measures. Dressings are applied and antibiotics to be started. Tetanus toxoid injections are given. Wound debridement should be thorough with saline irrigation. Fractures are treated initially by immobilisation/stabilisation. Patient may require one more debridement or delayed exploration depending upon the situation.

Exploratory laparotomy is done in abdominal gunshot wounds—perforations are sutures, transacted intestines are resected, and anastomosis is done. Bleeding liver and spleen are sutured to stop the bleeding. Shattered spleen requires splenectomy. Bleeding mesenteric vessels are ligated. Look for intestinal ischaemia in such cases. Non-viable intestines need to be respected.

**SU5.4:** Describe medicolegal aspects of wound healing and gunshot wounds.

The process of wound healing will have following medicolegal implications:

1. **Formation of scar tissue:** Scar tissue over specific areas like face may cause disfigurement. If that scar formation is due to injury sustained as a result of trauma, then it is an example for grievous hurt as per section 320 IPC. Scar formation may result in contractures. If it involves a joint, then there will be restriction of movements leading to disability. Then the injury caused may be classified as grievous as per section 320 IPC.
2. **Child abuse (battered baby syndrome):** Presence of healing wounds of different duration indicates the possibility of repeated physical abuse of the child. This has to be kept in mind while examining a child with injury in paediatric outpatient department (OPD).
3. **Elder (geriatric) abuse:** Presence of healing wounds of different duration indicates the possibility of repeated physical abuse of the elderly. This has to be kept in mind while examining a geriatric age group person with injury in outpatient department (OPD).

## Penetrating Trauma of the Abdomen

Today all penetrating injuries of the abdomen need not be explored by laparotomy. Good physical examination of the patient, entry and exit point, and haemodynamic status of the patient followed by investigations such as ultrasonogram and CT scan will guide the decision for laparotomy (Key Box 66.4).

Advanced trauma life support—ATLS is essential in the early hour of trauma. It is ideal that every surgeon/ doctor has studied ATLS manual.

Key Box 66.4

**Indications for Laparotomy**

- Tenderness, guarding, rigidity
- Unexplained shock
- Evisceration of contents
- Positive investigations
  - Positive DPL
  - Gas under diaphragm
  - IVP, cystoscopy, cystogram
  - Ultrasonogram
  - CT scan

### Management

Primary survey cABCDE and resuscitation is done as described earlier.

**SU17.3:** Describe principles in management of mass casualities.

## Management of Mass Casualities

**Introduction:** In this modern world, terrorist attacks and bombings are largely responsible for mass casualties. When hundreds of patients are brought to the casualty, we need to quickly triage them in such a way that attention first should be given to treat moderate to severe injures patients who are likely to survive than severely injured patients who are unlikely to survive.

**Definition:** Any number of casualties that exceed the resources normally available from local resources has been described as mass casualties. Examples of mass casualties are terrorist attacks, bombings, railway accidents, etc. In cases of multiple casualties, full resources can be brought to treat each individual patient.

**Mass casualty level:** Depending upon number of patients who are brought to the casualty, a classification has been developed which is given below.

- Level 1—mass casualty incident resulting in less than 10 surviving victims.
- Level 2—mass casualty incident resulting in 10 to 25 surviving victims.
- Level 3—mass casualty incident resulting in more than 25 surviving victims.
- Level 4—mass casualty incident resulting in a number of surviving victims that could necessitate an inter-region response and/get ready for an additional disaster plan.

*Four steps in mass casualties*

1. **Mitigation:** Mitigation includes variety of measures which are taken before an event that occurs which may result in illness or loss of lives or property. Basically, in hospital in anticipation of a mass casualty or disaster, certain beds are year marked or a team of doctors are made available with the help of group messages or to arrange for many ventilators, etc.
2. **Preparedness:** This may vary from place to place depending upon resources available including staffing. Few important considerations are given for safety measures, security of the hospital and to treating doctors, arranging for quick radiological investigations, etc.
3. Response
4. Recovery.

*Health risk in mass casualty:* In the year 2001, earthquake happened in Gujarat. Around 20000 people died and about few thousands were injured. The organs which most commonly injured were lower extremity (56%), spinal and pelvic (17%), upper extremity (13%), and chest and/or abdomen (<2%). What one can observe here is many of such patients can be saved provided a good triaging is done and treatment is started immediately before shock and multiorgan failure develops.

*Responsibilities of a surgeon*

- Surgeons must be prepared for especially complex and difficult wounding patterns that are not typically seen in routine practice, and that greatly increase morbidity and mortality, such as blast lung, and multiple penetrating injuries from both destructive shrapnel increasingly used in bombs and from automatic firearms.
- Surgeon should be trained in managing mass casualties, disasters at local and community level.
- Surgeon should avoid over triaging—means patients who are likely to die should not be treated.
- We also should recognize small minority of patients with urgent and salvageable life-threatening injuries at immediate risk of death (undertriage).
- Ideally triage should be done outside the hospital.
- At operation theatre, damage control should be the principle till the influx to the operation theatre ends.
- All intensive care unit beds should be made available for accommodating these patients whenever it is possible.
- Every attempt is made to decrease mortality rate.

## BLUNT ABDOMINAL TRAUMA

### INTRODUCTION

Blunt abdominal trauma (BAT) is one of the common surgical emergencies encountered by general surgeons. Blunt injury abdomen with polytrauma is one of the commonest causes of death in the younger population. Thus, it is important for a house officer to recognise a polytrauma patient, to diagnose and to suspect intra-abdominal injury, so that urgent resuscitation and treatment can be offered to the patient at the proper time, at the proper hospital and by a proper surgeon. Major systems involved are given in Key Box 66.5.

Craniospinal and chest injuries are discussed in their respective chapters. Pelvic and skeletal injury is beyond the limits of this book. In this chapter, blunt injury of the abdomen is discussed.

Key Box 66.5

**Common Viscera Involved in Blunt Injury**

| | |
|---|---|
| Spleen | Significant bleeding |
| Liver | Significant bleeding |
| Kidney | Significant bleeding |
| Intestines | Perforation—peritonitis |
| Mesentery | Bleeding |
| Pancreaticoduodenal injuries | Usually missed—bleeding |
| Diaphragm | Missed—tachypnoea |
| Urinary bladder | Urinary peritonitis |

### Causes of Blunt Injury Abdomen

1. Rail and road traffic accidents (most common)
2. Fall from a height and dashing against an object
3. Seat belt syndrome
4. Assault

### Regions/Anatomy of the Abdomen (Fig. 66.2)

1. **Anterior abdomen** means it involves 9 regions, namely right and left hypochondrium, epigastrium, right and left lumbar regions, umbilical region, right and left iliac fossa and hypogastrium.
2. **Thoraco-abdomen:** This area is inferior to nipple line anteriorly and infrascapular line posteriorly and superior to costal margins. Liver, spleen and diaphragm are the important organs here.
3. **Flank:** It is between the anterior and posterior axillary lines from the 6th intercostals space to the iliac crest. Covered by thick muscles which often protects renal injuries from penetrating wounds.
4. **Back:** Again there are thick muscles such as erector spinae, quadratus lumborum, etc. Back is an area from the tip of the scapulae to the iliac crests, posterior to posterior axillary lines. These areas contain retroperitoneal structures which are usually missed sites in trauma of the abdomen. The organs include duodenum, posterior parts of the descending and ascending colons, pancreas, kidney and ureters, vascular structures such as aorta and inferior vena cava. Diagnostic laparoscopy, focussed assessment sonography in trauma (FAST), diagnostic peritoneal lavage will not be of help. CT is the best investigation of choice.
5. **Pelvic cavity:** It contains some very important structures such as rectum, urinary bladder, reproductive organs, iliac vessels, etc. It is also the extension of retroperitoneal and intraperitoneal spaces. Pelvic fractures and injuries may result in significant bleeding which can be life-threatening.

### Mechanisms of Injury/Pathophysiology

They can be broadly classified into blunt abdominal trauma (BAT) or penetrating abdominal trauma. Following are various mechanisms of abdominal trauma.

- **Direct blow or crush:** This can be from lower rim of steering wheel or from the door of a motor vehicle results in crushing injuries of both solid and hollow viscera. Transverse colon is one of the hollow viscera in this type of injuries.

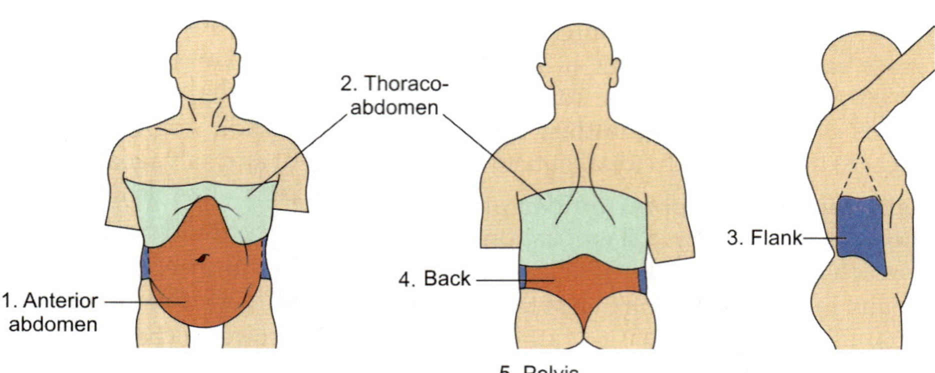


**Fig. 66.2:** Regions of abdomen for trauma assessment

**Crushing effect:** Here solid viscera are crushed between anterior abdominal wall and vertebral column or posterior thoracic cage.

- **Shearing:** These injuries will occur when a restraint device is worn improperly, e.g. lap belt.
- **Deceleration injuries** are the one in which differential movement of fixed and nonfixed parts of the body occurs. Examples being liver, spleen and small bowel injuries. It causes differential movement among adjacent structures. Shearing forces are created; they cause solid, visceral organs and vascular pedicles to tear at relatively fixed points of attachment. Examples:
  - Renal pedicle injury
  - Injury to distal aorta than proximal mobile aorta as former is attached to thoracic spine.
- **Bursting:** Acute tracheoaesophageal burst injuries are reported from blunt chest trauma.

  **Sudden dramatic rise in the intra-abdominal pressure** due to external compression.
  - Hollow viscus ruptures (in accordance with principles of **Boyle's law**).
- **Penetration:** Penetrating injuries are the result of stab wounds, gunshot wounds or due to pellets (used to shoot wild bore). Most commonly involved structures are liver, small bowel, diaphragm and colon. In cases of gunshots and pellets, injuries depend upon the speed of the shot, cavitation effect and bullet fragmentation.
- Vehicular trauma is by far the leading cause of blunt abdominal trauma.

## ASSESSMENT HISTORY—AT CASUALTY/TRIAGE

- *Exact nature of the accident*—collision, penetrating trauma, fall from height, shotgun, pellet injuries explosion. In addition to high-speed vehicle accidents, polytrauma is also common in India due to fall form height due to coconut plucking from coconut tree or from construction site fall.
- History of loss of consciousness initially followed by recovery may be the indication of extradural haemorrhage—to be kept in mind.
- History of medications especially beta-blockers and anticoagulants should be elicited, if present to be recorded. Even if a patient is not in hypovolaemia, there can be bradycardia, if patient is taking propranolol.

### Physical Examination—Primary Survey

| ABCDE (ATLS protocol) | AMPLE (History) |
|---|---|
| Airway | Allergy |
| Breathing | Medication |
| Circulation | Past medical illness |
| Disability | Last meal |
| Exposure | Events leading to incident |

### Secondary Survey and Definitive Care

- Inspection, palpation, percussion and auscultation should be done in the usual manner. Patient should be exposed full length—entire chest, abdomen and pelvis—both anterior and posterior.
- Tachycardia and hypotension are the early features of ongoing bleeding. Patient who is lying down without any pain but anxious may be having bleeding and one who is not moving but with pain may be having hollow viscus perforation. ***Restless patients have often head injuries.***
- Abdominal distension (Fig. 66.3) is quite often due to solid viscus bleed from liver or spleen. It is also due to perforation of a viscus and retroperitoneal injuries resulting in paralytic ileus.
- Abrasions, ecchymosis, lacerations over the abdominal wall, stab injuries, foreign bodies, evisceration of omentum or intestines to be recorded.
- Lap belt injuries sign: If these are present they indicate underlying injuries.
- Saree sign: *See* page 1149.

**Indian women—vulnerability:** The Saree and Churidar are traditional Indian dresses. One end of the Saree is tied around the waist and the other draped freely along the shoulder. If care is not taken, the free end often gets caught in the mill belt and causes injuries around the waist (blunt abdominal trauma) due to the drag created. The impression created on the abdomen is by the Saree and not the mill belt. The Shawl of the Churidar (has two free ends) can get caught in a belt or a wheel to cause injuries around the neck. The drag may be sufficient to cause even strangulation. The author remembers a case of scalp avulsion due to long hair of a woman getting caught in a mill belt.

- **Cullen sign, Grey Turner sign:** Discolouration around umbilicus and flanks respectively indicate retroperitoneal bleeding.

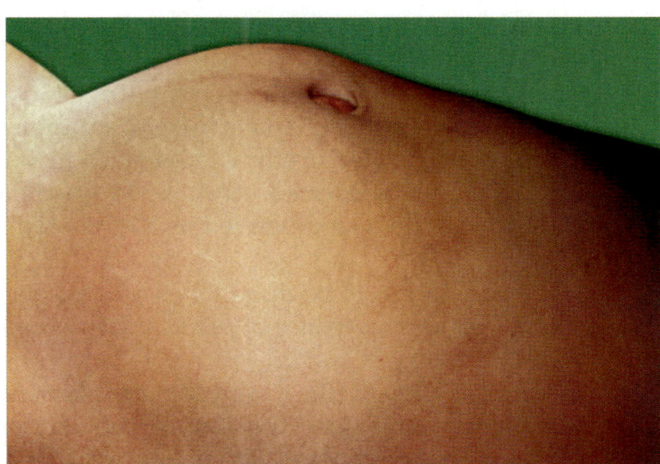

**Fig. 66.3:** Abdominal distension

- **London sign:** If you see some pattern of the tyre, seatbelt, it indicates a severe compression and invariably there will be underlying intra-abdominal injury.
- Entry- and exit-bullet wounds.

## PALPATION, PERCUSSION, AUSCULTATION

- Tenderness is a feature of peritonitis. It may be minimal in cases of bleeding. Superficial tenderness results due to abdominal wall muscle injures and deep tenderness is the sign of peritonitis. Palpation of high riding prostate is the sign of significant pelvic fracture.
- Percussion is done to elicit peritoneal irritation.
- Bowel sounds are absent in cases of peritonitis.

*Pearls of Wisdom*

**No time should be wasted in doing unnecessary percussion to find out the fluid because it will be detected later by FAST.** Once examination is completed, patient should be covered with warm blankets to **prevent** hypothermia. Because hypothermia results in coagulopathy and ongoing bleeding.

## ASSESSMENT OF PELVIC STABILITY

- **Pelvic fracture** should be suspected when hypotension is present in a conscious patient who has no obvious injuries. Blood at the urinary meatus, high riding prostate, scrotal haematoma (rupture urethra), limb length discrepancy suggest pelvic fracture.
- Gentle pressure over iliac bone in a downward and medial direction is applied. Laxity and instability suggests pelvic fracture. Only one attempt to test the pelvis should be done. Frequent tests may result in more bleeding and even dislodge the clot.
- **It is better to avoid this test in patients with hypotension.**

### Examination of Pelvic Organs and Gluteal Region

- **Urethra:** Blood at meatus and scrotal a haematoma suggests urethral injury. Catheterisation should not be done in such cases.
- **Rectal examination** to look for bleeding, loose sphincter and high riding prostate. In cases of rupture of membranous part of urethra, prostate will not be palpable as it is displaced upwards. It is called high riding prostate also described as **Vermooten's sign.**
- **Vaginal examination** to be done when you suspect vaginal injuries as in presence of perineal lacerations and pelvic fractures.

  **Gently turn the patient like a logwood** and examine the back and gluteal region. Gunshots or stab injuries may cause gluteal injuries. It may involve intra-abdominal injuries and rectum also.

**Signs of pelvic fracture can be remembered as PELVIS**

- **P**rostate—high riding
- **E**xternal meatus—drop of blood
- **L**imb discrepancy
- **V**aginal tear
- **I**liac vessels—hypotension
- **S**crotal haematoma

### Tertiary Survey

Repeat primary survey, secondary survey and repeat laboratory/imaging studies for wisdom lines in blunt abdominal trauma.

## ADJUNCTS TO PHYSICAL EXAMINATION—TUBES AND CATHETERS

- **Nasogastric (Ryle's) tube:** Vast majority of cases, tube is passed through nose—nasogastric. Confirm it is in place by auscultation of the abdomen and by pushing air. In cases of skull base fractures, the tube may enter the cranial cavity hence better to pass the tube through oral cavity, orogastric. When in doubt an X-ray abdomen can confirm the tube in the stomach. Blood in the aspirate suggests esophagogastric injuries. Nasogastric tube insertion will decrease the abdominal distension, prevents vomiting and thus aspiration. **One of the life-saving uses of nasogastric aspiration is for acute gastric dilatation (AGD) which is a potentially dangerous condition often seen following blunt trauma abdomen.** Passive air sucking by negative intragastric pressure and a flaccid lower oesophageal sphincter have been proposed as causes of AGD in trauma patients. Aerophagia in confused, agitated trauma patients, reflex gastric ileus due to visceral and somatic nerve stimulation and gastric atony due to excessive potassium and chloride losses have also been suggested as causes of AGD in trauma patients.
- **Urinary catheter:** Firstly, one should not introduce a Foley catheter, if you suspect urethral injuries. For example: Blood at the urinary meatus. Once urethral injury is ruled out, catheterization is done by using all aseptic measures and a proper lubrication. It will help in relieving retention—distended bladder (may help for DPL later), help in monitoring urinary output. Significant bleeding will indicate renal tract injuries, namely kidney and urinary bladder.

### *Investigations*

FAST is the most important and first investigation to be done in emergency department. Simultaneously blood tests and resuscitation should take place.

1. **Complete blood count,** coagulation studies, grouping and cross-matching. Fall in haemoglobin is an indication of on-going haemorrhage—especially while managing a patient with liver/splenic injury on conservative line of management.
2. **Serum electrolyte** analysis
3. **Serum amylase/lipase**
   - May be elevated because of **pancreatic ischaemia due to hypotension**
   - **Persistent elevation** may be indication of **pancreatic injury.**
4. **Plain X-rays** (Fig. 66.4)
   - **Chest X-ray:** If it shows pneumoperitoneum, crescenteric air shadow under the right dome of the diaphragm, it suggests perforation of the hollow viscus. Look for pneumothorax (Fig. 66.5). Fundic, stomach (air bubble in thorax as in diaphragmatic injury, retroperitoneal air—duodenal perforation).
   - Pelvic fractures.
5. **Role of ultrasound** (Fig. 66.6)

   **FAST:** Focused assessment with sonography for trauma.
6. **Diagnostic peritoneal lavage (DPL)**

   It is indicated in BAT in the following situations:
   - Multiple injuries and shock
   - Spinal cord injury
   - Obtunded patient with possible abdominal injury
   - Intoxicated patient

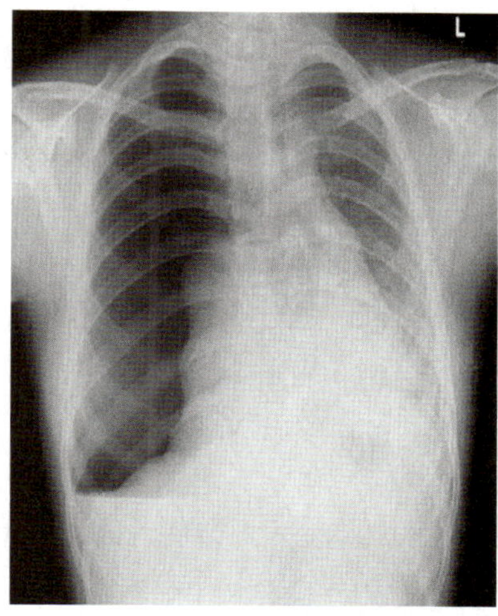


**Fig. 66.4:** Chest X-ray showing diaphragmatic hernia on the left side

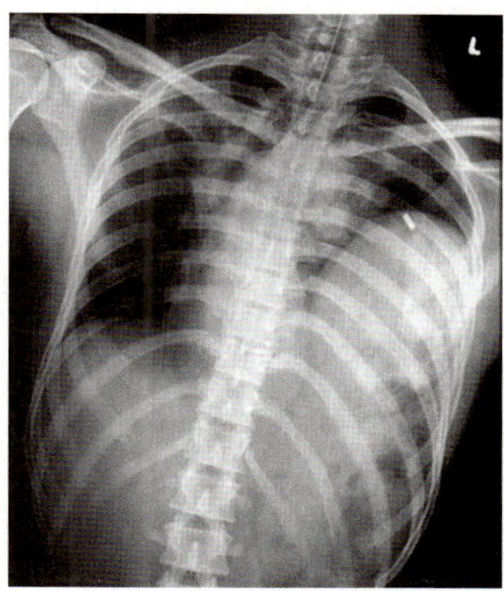


**Fig. 66.5:** Pneumothorax

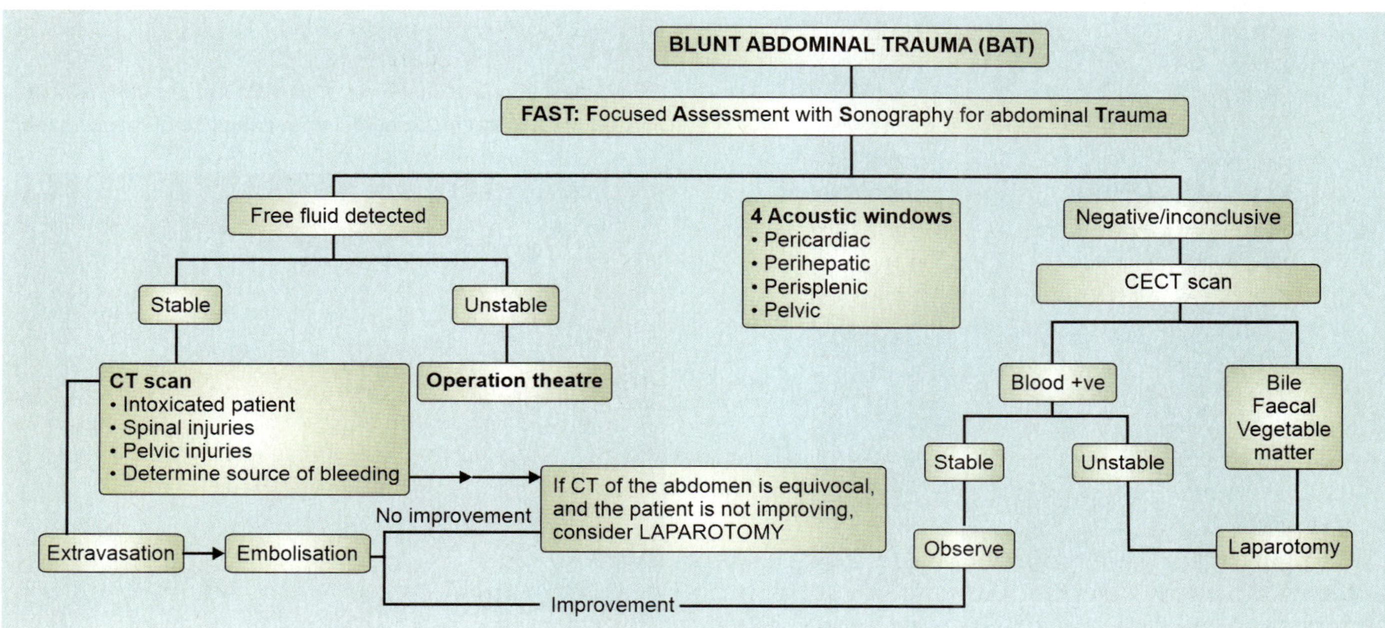


**Fig. 66.6:** Algorithm of investigations in BAT (*see* FAST)

*Types*

- **Open:** Infraumbilical skin incision and open peritoneum.
- **Semiopen:** Infraumbilical skin incision deepen up to linea alba.
- **Closed:** Blind insertion of needle.

*Precautions*

- Foley's catheter to empty bladder
- Ryle's tube to empty stomach
- X-ray pelvis to detect pelvic fracture.

*Positive DPL*

- 10 ml of gross blood aspirate before infusion of lavage fluid.
- More than 100,000 RBC/ml
- More than 500 WBC/ml
- Bile and bacteria are demonstrated
- Vegetable matter

*Pearls of Wisdom*

Positive DPL means intraperitoneal injury is present. It does not mean that the patient should be shifted to operation theatre immediately.

7. **CT scan** (Fig. 66.7)
   - Gold standard for solid organ injuries
   - CT also can reveal other associated injuries such as vertebral or pelvic fractures.
   - CT can also pick up **diaphragmatic injury** (CT chest).
   - It can detect **source of haemorrhage**.
   - CT is an excellent scan for pancreas, duodenum, etc.

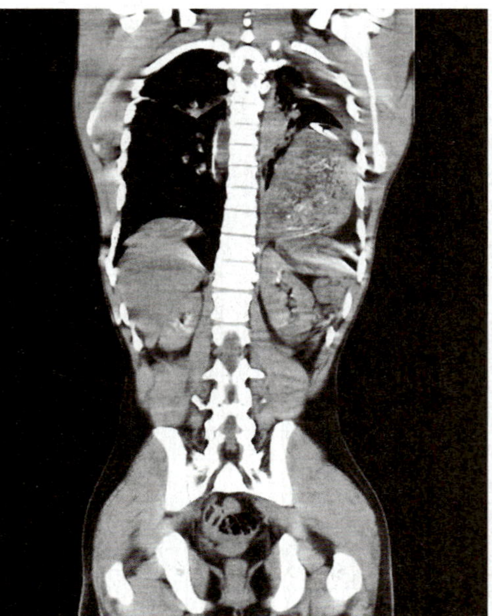

**Fig. 66.7:** Diaphragmatic hernia—CT scan (*Courtesy:* Dr Yashdeep Sharma, Associate Professor, KMC, Manipal)

8. **Diagnostic laparoscopy:** Done when CT scan is negative, suspicion of diaphragmatic injury is present (Fig. 66.8).

*Pearls of Wisdom*

Stable patients with solid organ injuries are managed more often by nonsurgical methods with close monitoring.

## Remarks

With the availability of FAST and CT scan, role of DPL is now limited to unstable patients whose FAST results are negative or inconclusive.

## Indications for Laparotomy

- BAT with hypotension and intraperitoneal bleeding and positive FAST
- Hypotension following stab injuries or penetrating wounds
- Evisceration (Fig. 66.9)

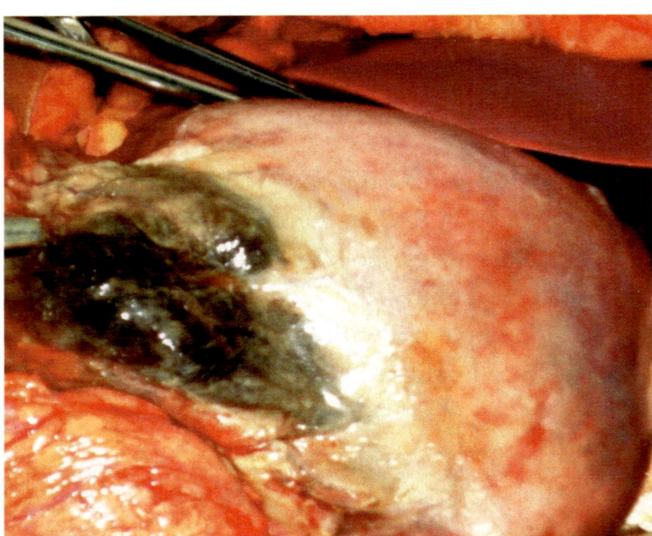

**Fig. 66.8:** Diaphragmatic hernia with gangrene of the stomach

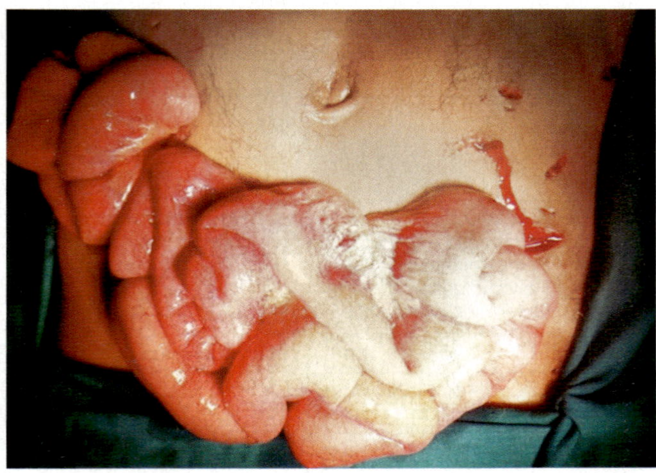

**Fig. 66.9:** Evisceration following stab injury

- Peritonitis—diffuse tenderness and rebound tenderness
- Free air, diaphragmatic rupture, retroperitoneal air
- Contrast CT with evidence of hollow viscous perforation, renal pedicle or splenic pedicle injury, intraperitoneal bladder injury.

> **SU28.10:** Describe the applied anatomy of liver. Describe the clinical features, investigations and principles of management of liver abscess, hydatid disease, injuries and tumours of the liver. *See* page 827 in liver chapter.

## LIVER INJURIES

Liver injury should be suspected when a patient with suspected blunt injury abdomen is brought with the following features:

- Right lower ribs fracture.
- Injury marks on the lower chest or upper abdomen.
- Patient with persistent hypotension or patient who had shock following blunt injury abdomen.
- A child can have liver injury without fracture of ribs because of elastic nature of the rib cage.

### Clinical Presentation

- The most common presentation is features of intraperitoneal haemorrhage, which includes hypotension, thready pulse, abdominal distension. Peritoneal signs are minimal as early bleeding does not produce much peritoneal irritation.
- However, massive lacerations of the liver including stellate fractures present with rapidly developing hypotension and shock, which are life-threatening.

### Investigations

- Ultrasonography and more precisely CT scan should be done in all patients who are haemodynamically stable with or without support (Figs 66.10 to 66.13 and Key Box 66.6).
- Also liver injury scale (Table 66.1).

Key Box 66.6

**CT Scan with IV Contrast**

- It can grade the liver injury.
- It can guide a conservative or operative treatment.
- It also rules out other injuries.
- Grade I and Grade II injuries can be managed by non-operative treatment.
- Free contrast in and around the liver is indicative of active bleeding.

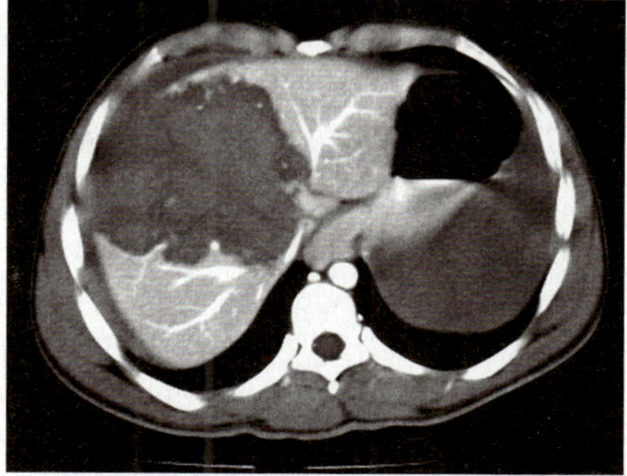

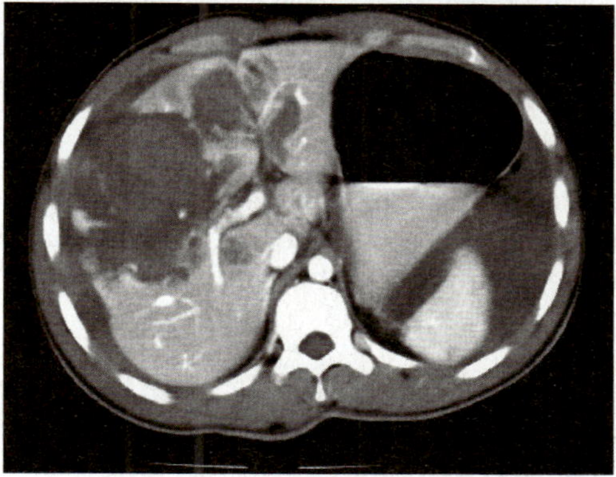

**Figs 66.10 and 66.11:** CECT arterial phase—Grade IV laceration of the liver with haemoperitoneum—interestingly patient was stable, managed conservatively, got discharged on 10th day

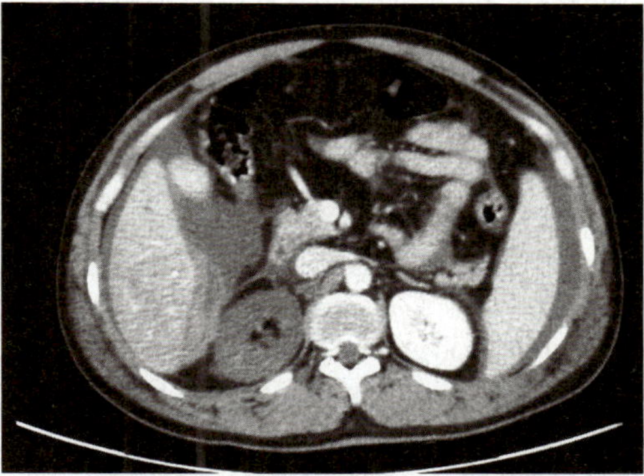

**Fig. 66.12:** Coronal section liver and kidney injury

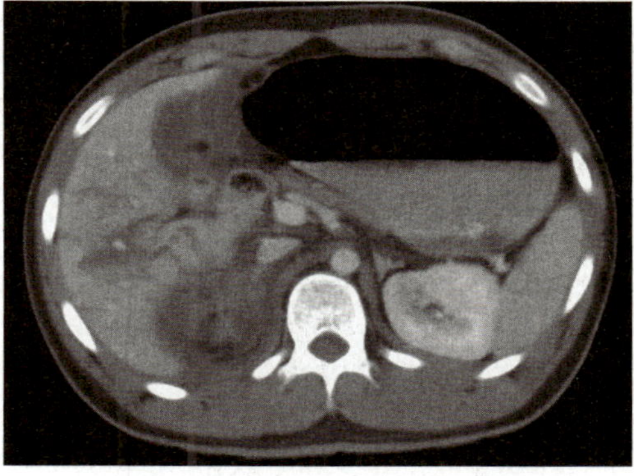

**Fig. 66.13:** Liver injury Grade II

**TABLE 66.1:** Liver injury scale

| Grade | Injury | Description |
|---|---|---|
| I | Haematoma<br>Laceration | Subcapsular haematoma; <10% surface area<br>Capsular tear, <1 cm parenchymal depth |
| II | Haematoma<br>Laceration | Subcapsular, 10–50% surface area; intraparenchymal extension <10 cm diameter<br><10 cm long; 1–3 cm parenchymal depth |
| III | Haematoma<br>Laceration | Subcapsular, >50% surface area; expanding intraparenchymal haematoma of >10 cm or expanding >3 cm, intraparenchymal depth |
| IV | Laceration | Parenchymal disruption of 1–3 Couinaud's segments within a single lobe |
| V | Laceration<br>Vascular | Parenchymal disruption >3 Couinaud's segments within a single lobe<br>Retrohepatic vena cava/central major hepatic veins |
| VI | Vascular | Hepatic avulsion |

## Treatment (Key Boxes 66.7 and 66.8)

1. **Simple lacerations which are not bleeding at laparotomy:** A drain is kept in the liver bed, blood and clots are sucked out and peritoneal wash is given.

Key Box 66.7

**Haemostatic Techniques at Surgery**

- Liver suture
- Perihepatic packing
- Resection
- Argon beam coagulator followed by fibrin glue and sheet of Surgicel (haemostatic agent)
- Selective arteriography and embolisation in arteriovenous fistula or haemobilia

Key Box 66.8

**Summary of Management of Liver Injuries**

| | |
|---|---|
| Laceration | Suturing |
| Expanding subcapsular haematoma | Evacuation |
| Deep laceration | Suturing biliary radicles and portal radicles, packing, etc. |
| Severe laceration | Debridement |
| Stellate fracture | Tractotomy; hepatic artery ligation |
| Complex injuries | Ligation of hepatic vein, portal vein branches or lobectomy, etc. |

2. **Simple laceration with bleeding:** It is sutured by interlocking horizontal mattress sutures by using special liver suturing needle. If too much tension is applied while suturing, cutting through can occur. Omentum can be used as a **Plug** in between the laceration (Fig. 66.14). Absorbable sutures are used.
3. **Subcapsular haematoma:** If present, should be evacuated.
4. **Deep laceration with bleeding:** In such situations, wound should be opened. Dead liver parenchyma is removed, bleeding vessel at depth and biliary radicle are ligated. It is described as **tractotomy**.
5. **Severe lacerations:** These injuries present with massive bleeding (Fig. 66.15). Temporary control is obtained by compression of portal vein and hepatic

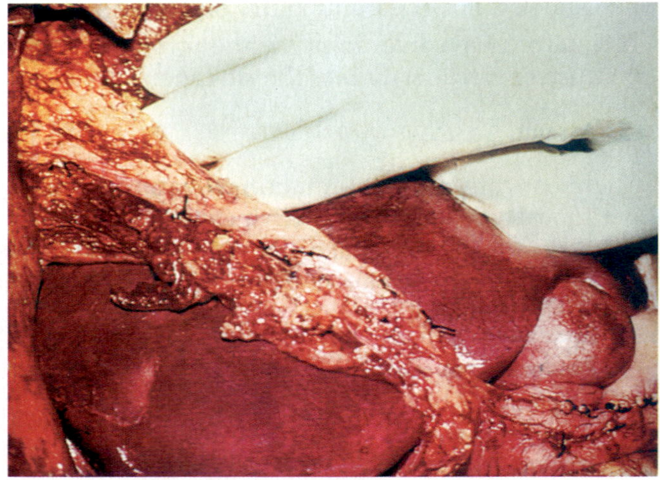

**Fig. 66.14:** Liver injury—use of omentum

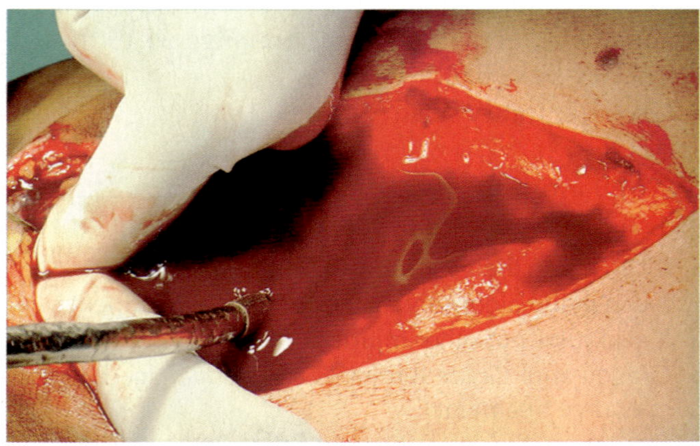

**Fig. 66.15:** Massive bleeding—challenging task (*Courtesy:* Dr Sunil Krishna, Associate Professor, KMC, Manipal)

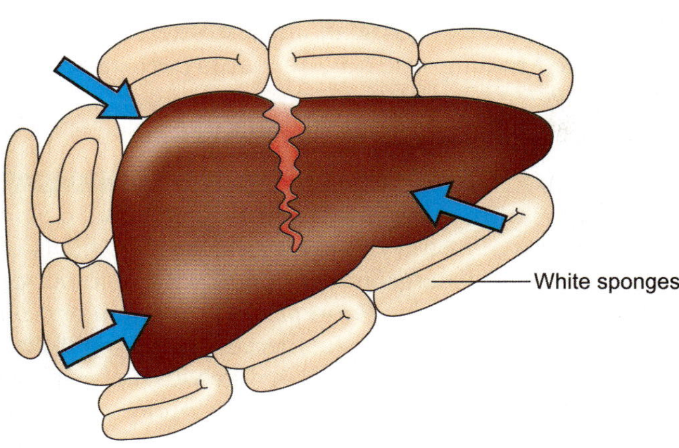


**Fig. 66.16:** Perihepatic packing

artery in gastrohepatic omentum in front of **foramen of Winslow (Pringle manoeuvre)**. If bleeding stops, portal veins or branches of hepatic artery are damaged. If bleeding continues, hepatic veins are the source of bleeding. Visualisation of source of bleeding with debridement of avascular liver tissue is done by finger fracture method. **Perihepatic packing can be used to compress the liver as a temporary measure to buy time for resuscitation, to explore rest of the abdomen or as a definitive treatment when other measures fail.** Pack is usually removed after 24–48 hours (Fig. 66.16).

- Nonanatomical resection may have to be done, in a few cases.

6. **Complex liver injuries:** These injuries involve hepatic veins, retrohepatic vena cava or branches of portal vein resulting in massive haemorrhage. This type of massive injury can be managed by a large thoraco-abdominal incision or abdominosternal incision by doing sternotomy. Division of the right triangular ligament helps in visualising bleeding from hepatic veins.
   - **Schrock shunt:** Failure of Pringle manoeuvre means juxtahepatic and retrohepatic vena caval injuries. In such cases, Heaney manoeuvre clamping both infra- and suprahepatic vena cava followed by atriocaval shunt or venovenous bypass can be done.

### Complications of Liver Injuries

1. Massive bleeding, hypovolaemia and cardiac arrest.
2. Haematoma can get infected resulting in an **abscess**.
3. Haematoma can rupture into the peritoneal cavity resulting in leakage of bile—biliary peritonitis.
4. **Haemobilia** refers to rupture of the haematoma into the bile duct—it may result in massive haematemesis or melaena.

**Clinical Notes**

- A 24-year-old male patient was operated for blunt injury abdomen by laparotomy. Liver laceration was found. It was sutured (Fig. 66.17).
- After 15 days, he came to our hospital with haematemesis. Initially it was diagnosed as erosive gastritis. Ultrasonography revealed a pseudoaneurysm of one of the branches of middle hepatic artery. CT angiography and embolisation was tried but not successful. He had another bout of haematemesis. He underwent exploratory laparotomy and ligation of branches of middle hepatic artery. Bleeding stopped. Now since 6 months, no further attacks of haematemesis.
- It was a case of haemobilia.

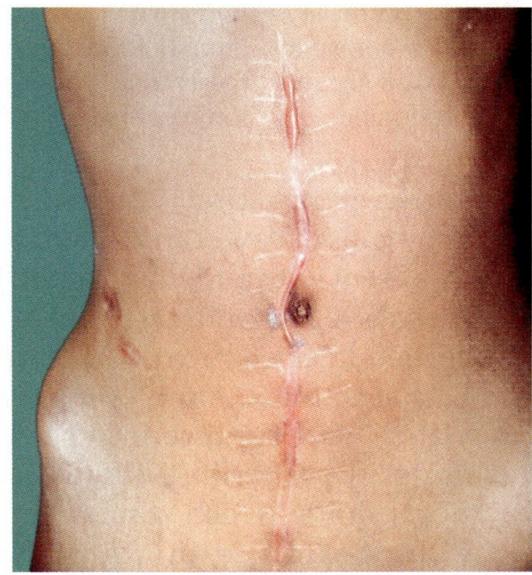

**Fig. 66.17:** Laparotomy scar in a patient who had liver laceration that was sutured. He presented with massive haematemesis late—**a case of haemobilia**

## SMALL BOWEL INJURIES

- The shearing injuries produce either disruption or laceration of the bowel between fixed and mobile points, i.e. at the **duodenojejunal flexure or at ileo-caecal junction**. These are the most common sites of small bowel injuries.
- Injury to the small bowel can also occur due to crush injury between spine and a steering wheel or handle bars, etc.
- Bruising on the abdominal wall may suggest perforation (Fig. 66.18).
- Mesentery and its vessels also get damaged and bleeding can be sufficient to produce hypovolaemia and shock (Fig. 66.19).

### Clinical Presentation

1. **Acute abdominal pain:** Features are like that of any perforation peritonitis with guarding and rigidity. Erect abdominal X-ray shows gas under the diaphragm.
2. **Features of peritonitis** with haemoperitoneum are the result of bowel injury with bleeding from the mesentery.

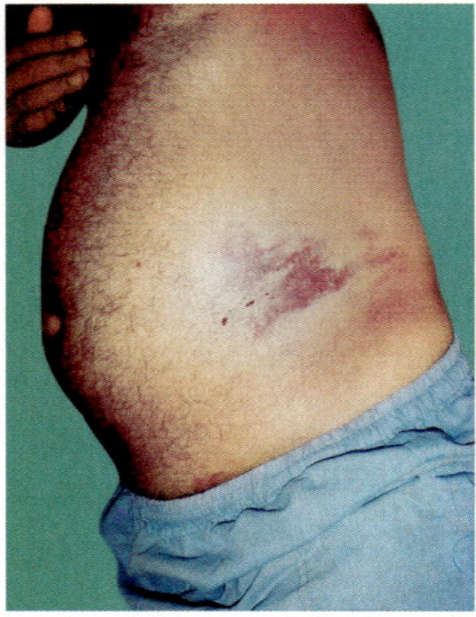

Fig. 66.18: Observe London's sign: Bruising (imprint abrasion) over the abdominal wall signifying hollow viscus perforation

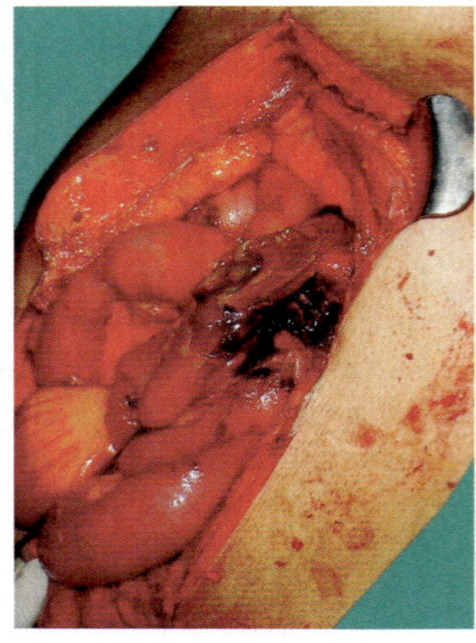

Fig. 66.19: Gangrene of the jejunal loop due to injury to mesenteric blood vessels in the same patient as in Fig. 66.18

3. **Occult or hidden perforation:** A small perforation gets sealed off by coils of bowel and omentum. Most of these patients present with abdominal pain. However, very often, features of peritonitis are missed as a result of other associated injuries such as fracture pelvis or retroperitoneal haematoma. After 3–4 days, a localised abscess may form and rupture into the peritoneal cavity, resulting in peritonitis. This is aggravated by intake of oral fluids which stimulate peristalsis. **Repeated examination is the most honoured, most fruitful investigation in blunt injuries of the abdomen** (*see* clinical notes).

## Investigation

- X-ray abdomen, erect or lateral decubitus (Fig. 66.20), demonstrates free gas under the right dome of the diaphragm in majority of cases. Four-quadrant tap or diagnostic peritoneal lavage is also useful.

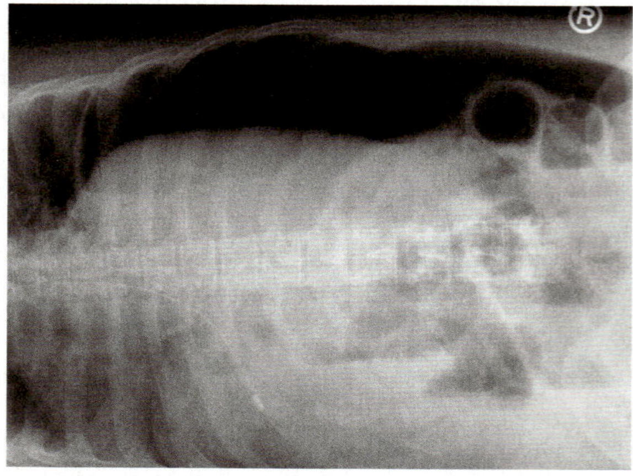

Fig. 66.20: Lateral decubitus picture is extremely useful in polytrauma cases when patient is unable to stand due to fractured limbs. However, **CT scan is the best investigation in blunt abdominal trauma** because it not only detects pneumoperitoneum but also other injuries

- When in doubt, CT scan of abdomen should be requested to diagnose hollow viscus perforation and bleeding.

### Clinical Notes

- A 23-year-old male with fracture femur and pelvic fracture was admitted to the hospital after 12 hours of injury. A general surgeon was consulted to rule out an intra-abdominal injury. Pulse rate was 100/min and on deep palpation, there was tenderness in the right iliac fossa. Keeping in mind associated pelvic injury, it was decided to treat him conservatively. X-ray abdomen left lateral decubitus (Fig. 66.20) (erect film could not be taken as patient could not stand) film did not show free intraperitoneal air (gas). Ultrasound revealed a retroperitoneal haematoma of 8 cm × 3 cm.
- The patient was treated conservatively with Ryle's tube for 3 days. On the 4th day, oral fluids were started, as patient passed stools once. On 7th day morning, patient had tachypnoea. Pulse was 120/min, BP was 90/60 mmHg. Previous 24 hours urine output was only 450 ml. Abdominal examination revealed guarding and rigidity in the right iliac fossa. It was decided to do a laparotomy. At laparotomy, there was a small 2 cm perforation in the ileum with bilioma surrounded by intestinal loops and gross contamination of peritoneal cavity. The perforation was closed and the peritoneal cavity was drained. The patient made a good recovery from septicaemia, thanks to early antibiotics and surgery.

## Treatment

**Golden time to operate is within 6 hours.**

- **Perforation:** Single or multiple, have to be closed, after trimming the edges by using non-absorbable sutures such as silk (Fig. 66.21).
- A **lacerated** or a macerated bowel has to be resected.
- Bleeding mesenteric vessels have to be ligated, haematoma must be evacuated and bowel should be inspected for any ischaemia. Food particles and bile should be evacuated (Figs 66.22 and 66.27).
- A perforation of ileum **close to the ileocaecal junction** is treated by **ileocolectomy** rather than simple closure for the fear of enterocutaneous fistula, due to suture line leakage.

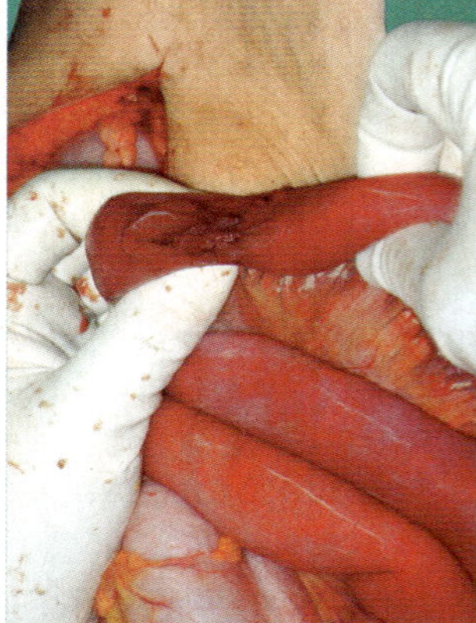

Fig. 66.21: Peritonitis following ileal perforation. Golden time to operate is within 6 hours of perforation

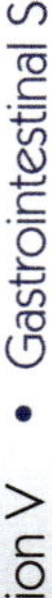

## PHOTOGRAPHS OF SMALL INTESTINAL PERFORATION (Figs 66.22 to 66.26)

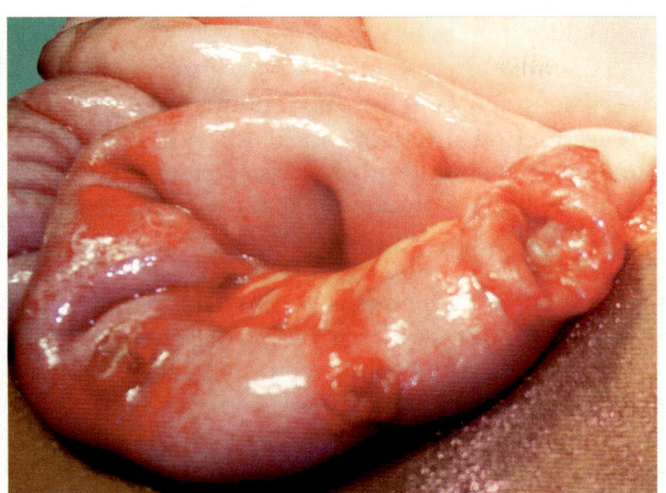

**Fig. 66.22:** Jejunal transection—6 cm away from DJ flexure. It is better to resect and anastomose in this type of cases (*Courtesy:* Dr Saurabh Aggarwal, Associate Prof, KMC, Manipal)

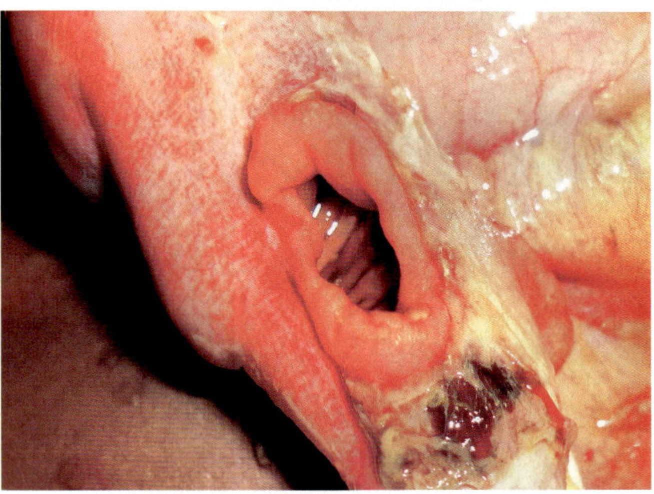

**Fig. 66.23:** 72 hours old perforation close to ileocaecal junction. Limited colectomy done

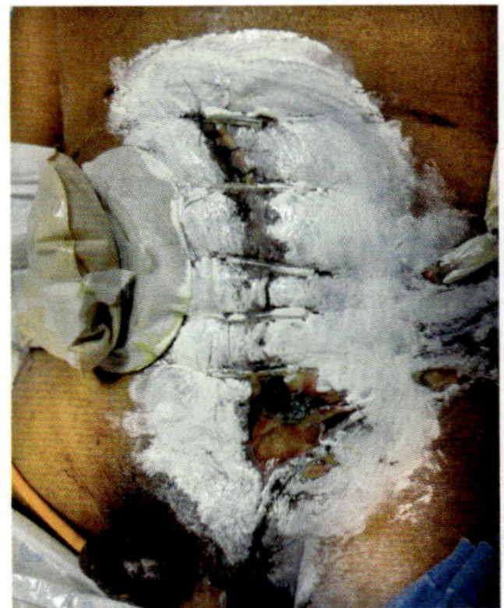

**Fig. 66.24:** Anastomotic leak following limited colectomy. Ileostomy done. It was closed after 8 weeks. You can see the wound infection

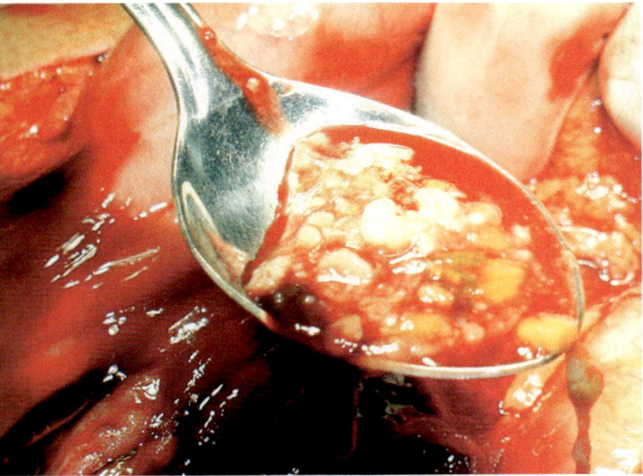

**Fig. 66.25:** Food particles—definite indication, if found in DPL for laparotomy

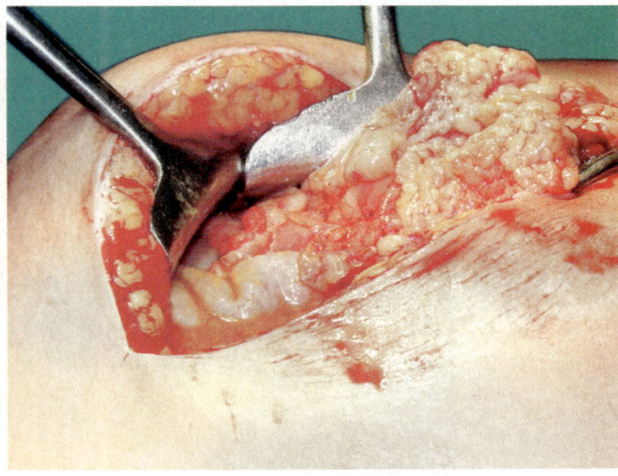

**Fig. 66.26:** Bile and blood in the peritoneal cavity

## COLONIC INJURIES

- Blunt injury of the colon is not uncommon.
- Mobile sigmoid is more prone to injury than fixed parts.
- Steering wheel injury can directly crush the transverse colon and can cause perforation.
- Bruise or laceration of the colon can undergo ischaemic necrosis and it can present after 5–7 days with signs of peritonitis/sepsis (Figs 66.27 and 66.28).
- Diagnosis is by clinical examination/contrast enhanced CT scan.
- Depending upon the contamination, contusion or laceration and duration of injury, treatment can be resection and anastomosis within 6–8 hours of the

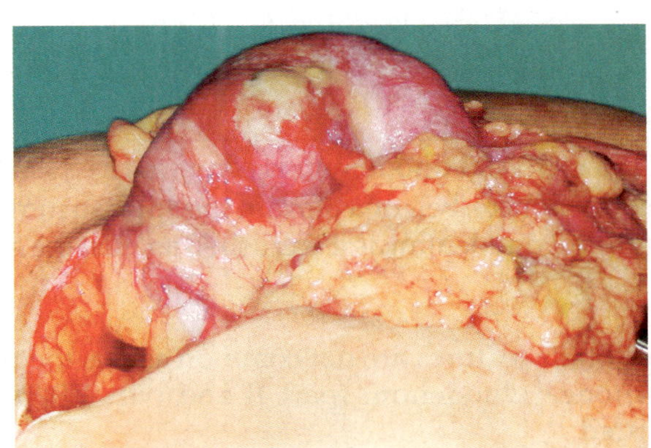

**Fig. 66.27:** Colonic perforations. The patient presented 7 days later with abdominal distension and early sepsis—steering wheel injury to the transverse colon

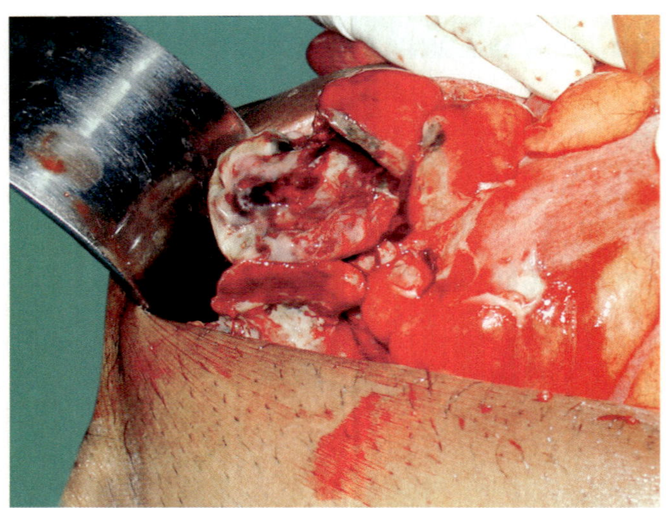

Fig. 66.28: Sigmoid perforation

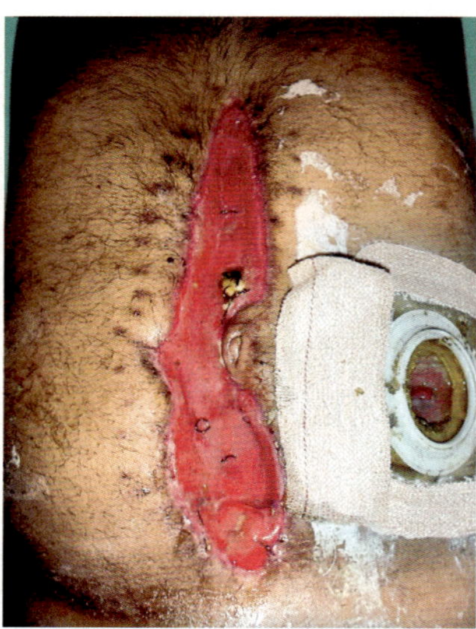

Fig. 66.29: Traumatic faecal fistula

injury or simple suturing or diversion colostomy, if gross contamination is present (Fig. 66.29).

- Even in penetrating injury, primary closure can be done.

## DUODENAL INJURIES

- Retroperitoneal duodenum is commonly injured.
- Steering wheel, belt or a blow in the epigastrium may injure the duodenum as it is crushed against the spine.

### Clinical Features

- Peritonitis features are not common as it is the retroperitoneal duodenum (part II and part III) that is injured.
- Tenderness is present on deep palpation.
- Being retroperitoneal, these injuries manifest late with abscess formation or fluid in lesser sac, etc.

### Investigations

- X-ray abdomen
  - Obliteration of psoas shadow
  - Air outlining the kidney—Chilaiditi's sign (Fig. 66.30)
  - Absence of air in the duodenum
- Raised serum amylase is one of the biochemical parameters that should arouse a suspicion of pancreatic injuries along with duodenal injury.

### Treatment

- Golden time to operate is within 6 hours.
- When in doubt, about narrowing of lumen, duodenojejunostomy may be indicated.
- When in doubt regarding duodenal fistula, tube duodenostomy is done.
- Duodenal haematoma is managed conservatively.
- Better to add a feeding jejunostomy.

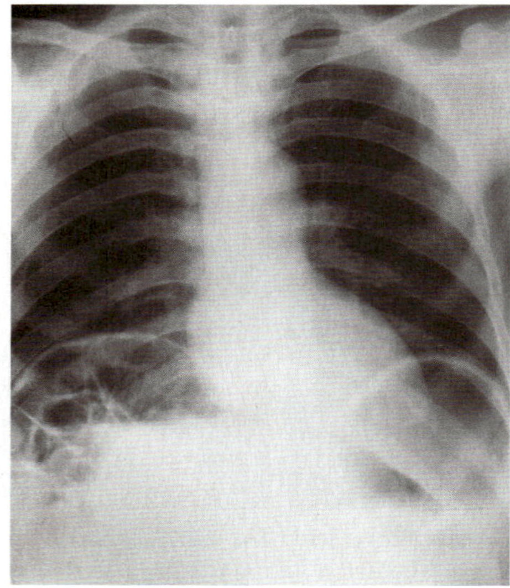

Fig. 66.30: Air outlining small portion of the kidney and air pockets under the diaphragm—Chilaiditi's sign

## PANCREATIC INJURIES

Because of anatomical close approximation of pancreas with vertebral column, blunt injury abdomen in the epigastrium, kicks or **seat belt injuries** crush the pancreas against **the vertebral column** (Key Boxes 66.9 and 66.10).

Key Box 66.9

**Pancreatic Injuries**

- Anatomically hidden
- Very often, injuries missed
- Peritonitis features are not seen
- Dangerous because of enzymatic activation
- Can manifest as pleural effusion

Key Box 66.10

**Pancreaticoduodenal Injuries**

- Diagnosed late
- Peritonitis features are minimal
- Shock is very rare
- At laparotomy, they are missed
- Surgical treatment needs more skill and experience
- Feeding jejunostomy is very useful
- Mortality and morbidity around 50%

**Mill belt:** Saree or *churidar* cloth may be caught in the belt of a running conveyor belt and result in compression force in the centre of the abdomen (Figs 66.31 to 66.34 and clinical notes).

## Diagnosis

- Pancreatic injury alone is diagnosed when patient presents with a pseudocyst of the pancreas 2–3 weeks following an injury.
  CECT is the gold standard investigation. 5 grades have been described. When ductal injuries are suspected ERCP also can be done.

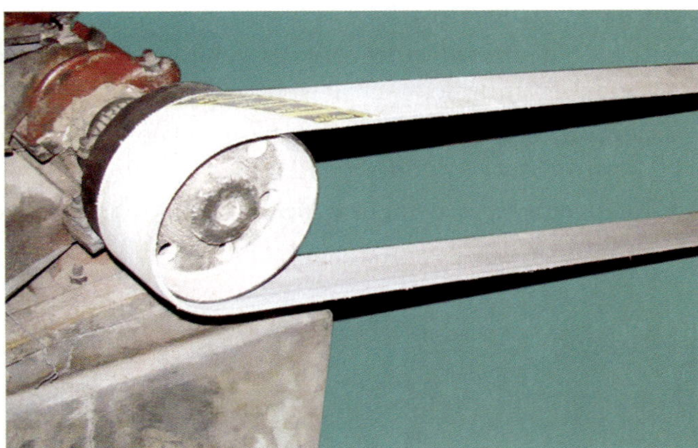

**Fig. 66.31:** Grinding mill having a conveyor belt (*Courtesy:* Dr Rakesh Hegde, Associate Professor, Department of Surgery, KMC, Manipal, 2006–2009)

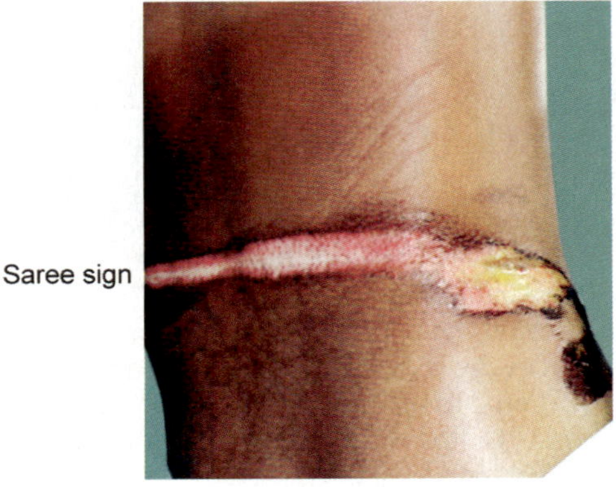


**Fig. 66.32:** Impression of the saree all around waist in a lady who was dragged by the conveyor belt when her saree got caught

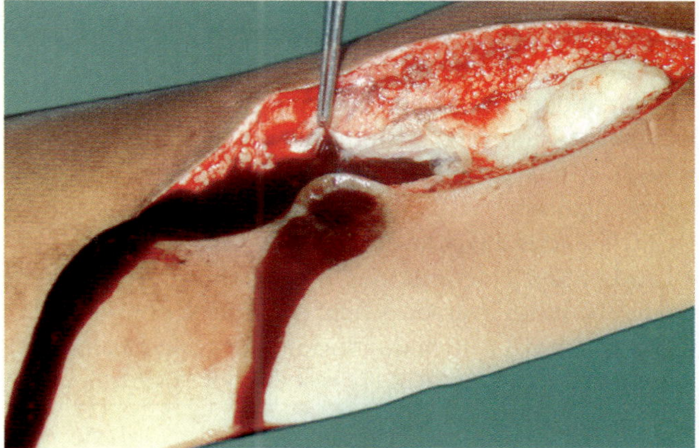

**Fig. 66.33:** On laparotomy, blood gushing out (*Courtesy:* Dr Raghunath Prabhu, Associate Prof, KMC, Manipal)

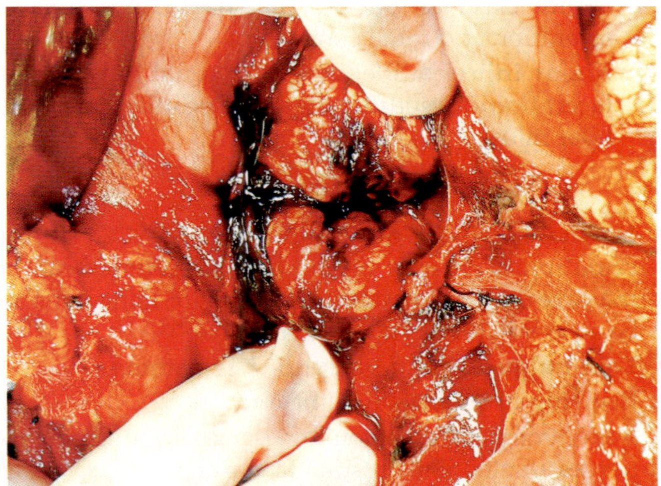

**Fig. 66.34:** Pancreas split into 2 parts

- Very often, laparotomy is done for haemorrhage or perforation. In such situations, retroperitoneal bleeding, collection of bile or collection of fluid in the lesser sac arouses suspicion of pancreatic injuries.

## Treatment

- **Pseudocyst** following blunt injury abdomen invariably requires **surgical drainage,** e.g. **cystogastrostomy** because of injury to pancreatic duct, fistula will remove for a long period.
- Injury to body and tail require **subtotal pancreatectomy** with splenectomy.
- Rarely, **pancreaticoduodenectomy** may be required for significant injury to the head of pancreas with injury to the duodenum.

## Complications

- Pancreatic fistula
- Pancreatic pseudocyst
- Pleural effusion.

Clinical Notes

**Summary of the pancreatic injury**

- Blunt abdominal trauma is common cause
- Pancreas is crushed against vertebral column
- Abdominal pain, distension, bleeding are clinical presentations
- CECT scan is the gold standard investigation
- Grade 1 and 2—contusions, haematoma and even minor ductal injuries in grade 3 can be managed conservatively
- Grade 4 and 5 with major ductal injuries and lacerations are managed by pancreatic resection and lavage, etc.

## RENAL INJURIES

### Types (Fig. 66.35)

I. **Minor injuries:** Subcapsular haematoma, minor laceration and renal contusions.

II. **Major injuries:** Bleeding into renal pelvis from laceration of medulla, corticomedullary rupture, hilar injury.

### Clinical Features

- **Haematuria** is the most important (80–90%) sign of renal injury. It may be mild, or sometimes can be massive depending upon the extent of injury. It may be absent in renal pedicle avulsion.
- **Loin bulge** due to perinephric haematoma
- **Bruising** of soft tissue in the loin
- Retroperitoneal haematoma compressing on splanchnic nerves (meteorism) results in paralytic ileus, which causes **abdominal distension.**
- Associated injuries such as fractures of the transverse process of lumbar spine may be present.

### Investigations

1. **Intravenous pyelography can demonstrate:**
   - Intrarenal extravasation
   - Extrarenal extravasation (pararenal pseudohydronephrosis due to extravasated blood and urine, slowly occluding pelviureteric junction).
   - Function of injured kidney
   - Function of opposite kidney
2. **Ultrasound and CT scan** are other investigations which are useful when there is an expanding haematoma (Figs 66.36 and 66.37).

### Treatment

1. **Conservative:** Minor injuries are managed conservatively with close monitoring of vital signs such as pulse, blood pressure, temperature and respiration, Hb% and PCV.
   - Sedation and analgesics are also given.
2. **Surgical exploration**
   - **Small laceration** sutured over gel foam or by using detached muscle.
   - **Major laceration** involving one pole—a partial nephrectomy is done.
   - **Major multiple lacerations**, avulsions, require nephrectomy.

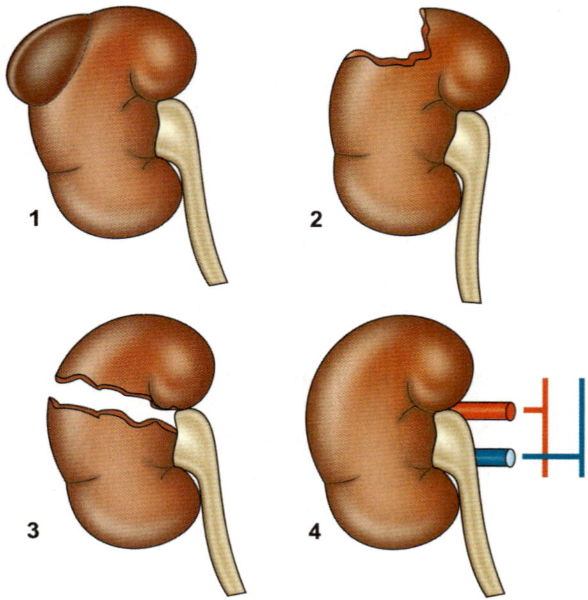


**Fig. 66.35:** Closed renal trauma: 1. Subcapsular haematoma, 2. laceration, 3. avulsion of one of the poles, and 4. avulsion of renal pedicle

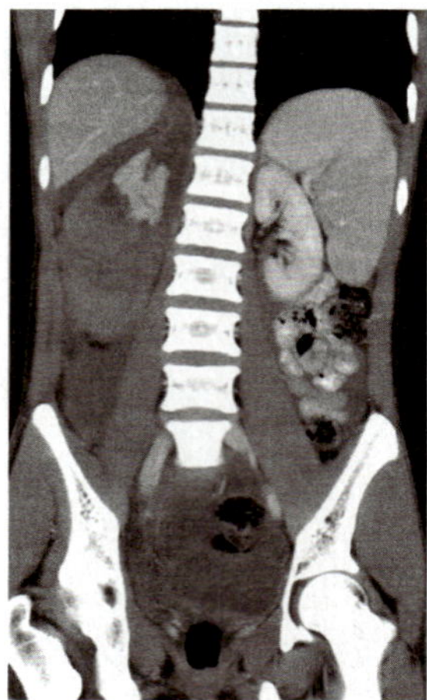

**Fig. 66.36:** Renal trauma: Right kidney is transected and upper pole is displaced by a large haematoma. Left kidney is normal (*Courtesy:* Dr Padmaraj Hedge, Professor and Head, Department of Urology, KMC, Manipal)

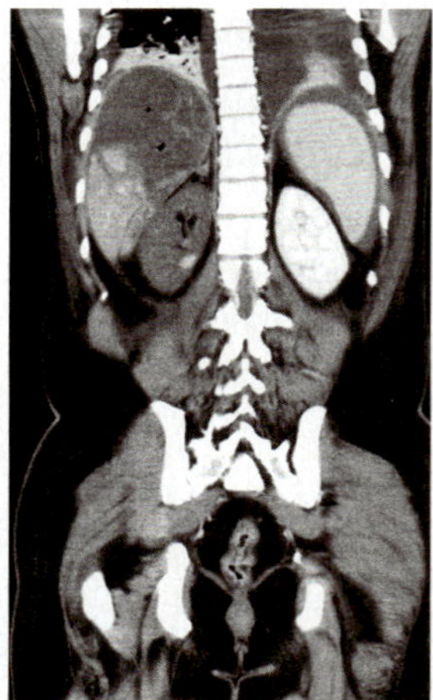

**Fig. 66.37:** Liver and kidney injury. It is not uncommon to get liver and kidney injuries in a blunt abdominal trauma. Always look for urine microscopy/haematuria while treating liver injury cases

## RETROPERITONEAL HAEMATOMA

- It is quite common because of accidents, fall from height.
- Fracture vertebrae, fracture pelvis, injury to retroperitoneal veins give risk to RPH.
- Bleeding from vena cava and aorta can be fatal.
- Haematomas which are not expanding should not be disturbed.

  Diagnosis and management of retroperitoneal haematoma as shown in Fig. 66.38.

### Pelvic Fractures and Retroperitoneal Haematoma

- Pelvic fractures are also an important cause of retroperitoneal haematoma.
- The most frequent mechanisms causing pelvic fractures are motor vehicle accidents, motorcycle accidents, falls and accidents involving pedestrians. Associated injuries to urethra in males should be ruled out first. Per rectal examination should be done to evaluate the position of the prostate. CT scan is done to assess pelvic fracture and also to assess retroperitoneal haematoma.
- Retroperitoneal bleeding can be arterial, venous, or osseous in origin. Unstable pelvic fractures are generally associated with increased blood loss. Posterior fractures with involvement of the sacroiliac joint are frequently associated with arterial bleeding, which can be controlled by embolisation of the bleeding vessel, usually branches of the internal iliac artery. Unstable fractures should be fixed by external fixation. Expanding haematoma should be explored. Control the bleeders, otherwise pack the pelvis. Nonexpanding haematoma should not be explored. Wait and watch.

## GENERAL PRINCIPLES IN A BLUNT INJURY ABDOMEN

- A patient should be admitted to the hospital and carefully monitored if there is a slight doubt regarding blunt injury abdomen.
- **Repeated examination,** careful monitoring of pulse rate, temperature and blood pressure, chest X-ray, estimation of Hb%, frequently help in many cases of silent blunt injuries.
- Most of the cases today are **polytrauma** cases, hence all systems should be examined. Among all these, priority should be given to life-threatening, salvageable injuries such as **extradural haematoma, haemothorax, splenic injuries, liver injuries**.
- It is easier to make a diagnosis of fracture (revealed injuries) which can be treated later. FRACTURE CAN WAIT BUT NOT RUPTURE. Concealed injuries should be carefully looked for.
- Undoubtedly, **diagnostic peritoneal lavage, ultrasound** (CT scan is the immediate noninvasive investigation) help in diagnosis of more than 90% of cases of blunt injury abdomen.
- Adequate blood, appropriate antibiotics, aggressive resuscitation before surgery to treat hypovolaemia and shock are the major factors which decide the outcome of surgery.
- In a major accident involving many patients and limited resources, quick decision should be taken regarding **triage**—who can be saved, who cannot be saved (Fig. 66.39).

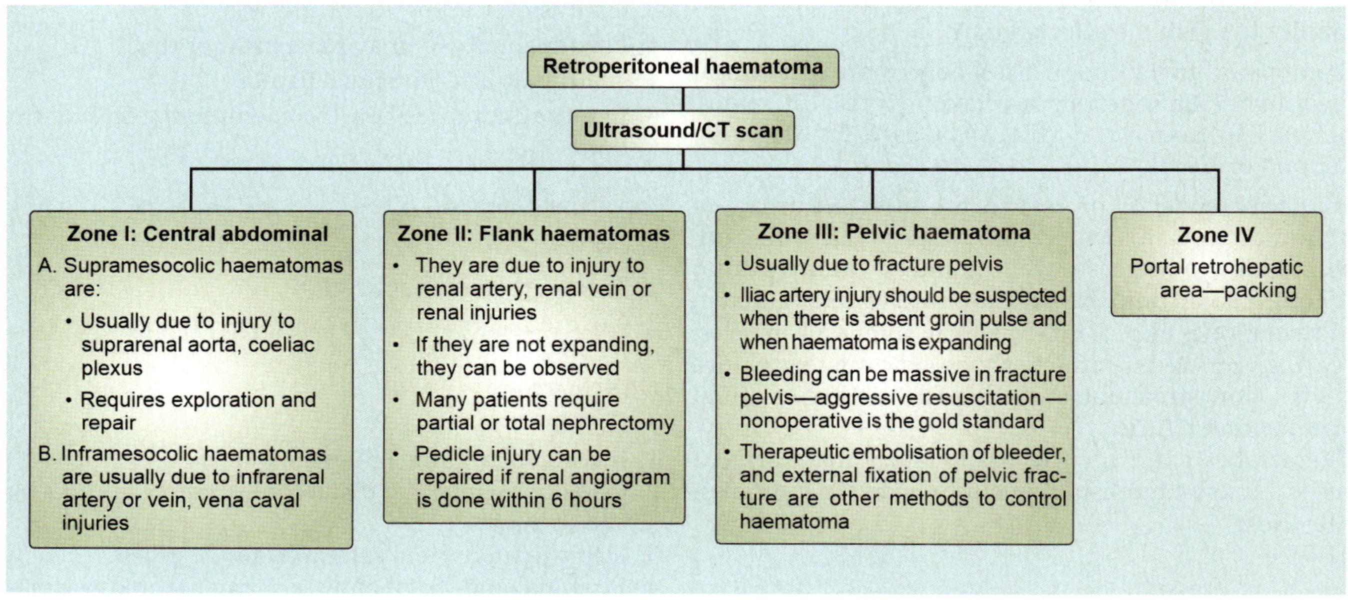


**Fig. 66.38:** Diagnosis and management of retroperitoneal haematoma

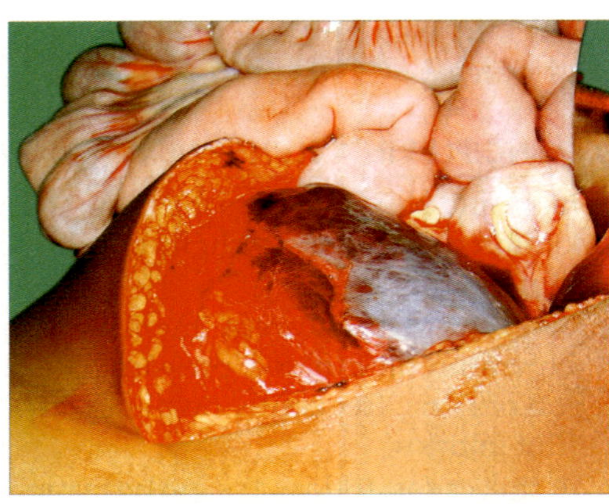

**Fig. 66.39:** Splenic haematoma—initially managed by conservative method. However, patient was developing hypotension—importance of careful monitoring of the patient in intensive care unit

## SOFT TISSUE INJURIES

> **SU17.7:** Describe the clinical features of soft tissue injuries. Chose appropriate investigations and discuss the principles of management.

Soft tissue injury term is used to describe injuries occurring to muscle, tendons or ligaments. They are common in clinical practice especially in sport events (like football, cricket or rugby), falls/slips or during exercises. One of the most commonly involved joint is the knee joint that gets affected.

Strains, sprains and contusion are examples of soft tissue injuries. Other types include tendinitis and bursitis.

Injury to muscle or tendon is referred to as strain whereas injury to ligament is referred to as sprain. Common areas for strain are ankle, knee and wrist.

**Common symptoms** include swelling, pain and weakness. Examination often reveals oedema, tenderness, inability to move the affected part.

**Diagnosis** is often through history and thorough clinical assessment. Radiographs are taken to rule out bony injuries. Ultrasound and MRI can be used for diagnosis of sprain or strain.

**Treatment** consists of rest to the affected area, ice application that aims to decrease pain and inflammation, compression to decrease swelling and elevation to drain the accumulated fluid. NSAIDs are used to decrease pain.

Prevention is important strategy in soft tissue injuries. Wearing appropriate athlete shoes, warming up before activity, slow stretching and adequate rest are essential in preventing injuries.

Remember **RICE** for soft tissue injury management (this is a known published pneumonic in old journals)

**R**—Rest
**I**—Ice
**C**—Compression
**E**—Elevation

## VASCULAR TRAUMA

Although any blood vessel can be injured in a traumatic event, injuries of extremities account for 80% of cases. Traumatic event can be blunt trauma or penetrating injury.

### Mechanism of Injury

1. **Blunt trauma:** Compression and crushing of blood vessels.
2. **Penetrating trauma:** Compression and direct tissue separation by sharp object.

### Clinical Presentation

1. Tissue ischaemia distal to site of injury
2. External bleeding
3. Occult bleeding in body cavities or tissue planes with or without hypovolaemic shock
4. Pulsatile haematoma

Clinical features are divided into soft and hard signs to triage and guide further treatment of patients in accident and emergency department.

| Soft signs | Hard signs |
|---|---|
| 1. History of significant haemorrhage<br>2. Diminished distal pulses<br>3. Neurologic deficit in affected limb<br>4. Injury near area of major vessel | 1. Pulsatile external haemorrhage<br>2. Absence of distal pulses<br>3. Ischaemic limb<br>4. Pulsatile haematoma<br>5. Bruit or thrill |

**Types of arterial injuries**

1. Partial laceration
2. Complete transection
3. Contusion leading to thrombosis
4. Pseudoaneurysm may have bruit or thrill
5. Traumatic arteriovenous fistula
6. External compression by haematoma or fractured bone

### Treatment (Fig. 66.40)

#### *Endovascular*

1. Transcatheter embolization
2. Covered stents

#### *Operative*

***Principle***

1. Incision along line of vessel
2. Obtain proximal and distal control before approaching site of injury
3. Debride till normal arterial wall
4. Proximal and distal embolectomy to remove clot
5. Heparinization

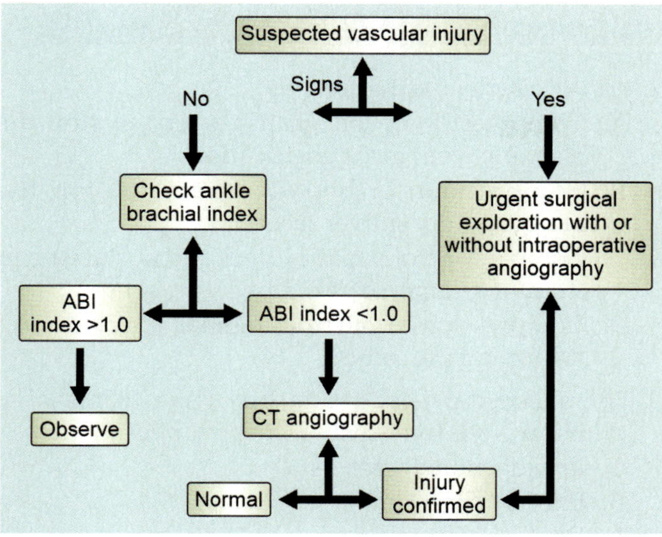


**Fig. 66.40:** Algorithm of management of vascular trauma

***Type of repair:*** Repair depends upon extent of vascular damage.

1. Ligation of injured vessel can be considered at sites where good collateral flow is present, e.g. forearm and leg.
2. End-to-end anastomosis, if vessel can be sufficiently mobilized to ensure tension free anastomosis.
3. Interposition graft is used in majority of cases.

## Vascular Grafts

**1. Autologus saphenous vein**
- Harvested from uninjured leg
- Used in reverse direction because of venous valves
- Best patency rates
- Small vein can lead to size discrepancy with injured artery

**2. Prosthetic graft**
- Used, if autologous vein is not sufficient or poor quality.
- Various sizes are available, so can be used for most of vessels.

***A. Expended polytetrafluoroethylene (ePTFE)***
- Inferior to autologous vein but better than Dacron for infrainguinal or upper limb revascularization.
- More needle hole bleeding during surgery.
- Resistant to infection compared to Dacron.

***B. Dacron***
- It can be woven or knitted depending on textile technique used.
- Woven graft has less porosity and less bleeding.
- Knitted grafts are more porous and need preclotting before implantation.
- Mainly used for thoracic or abdominal aortic surgeries, rarely used for limb vascularization.

## Complications

- Irreversible limb ischaemia and necrosis, if repair delayed beyond 6–8 hours
- Infection
- Pseudoaneurysm
- Graft thrombosis
- Reperfusion injury
- Rhabdomyolysis and myoglobinuria leading to renal failure

## Miscellaneous

*Please Note:*

Remember following mnemonics in blunt injury abdomen:

- AMPLE : *See* page 1139
- ABCDE : *See* page 1139
- FAST : *See* page 1141
- LIFT JAW : *See* page 1132
- AVPU : *See* page 1131
- PELVIS : *See* page 1134

## CLINICAL CASE CAPSULE 10: Management Oriented Discussion in Surgery (MODS)

**Wisdom in Polytrauma Patient**

This 37 years old patient who had blunt abdominal trauma–polytrauma involving head injury (comatose patient but no indications for craniotomy), multiple long bone fractures, rib fractures, pelvic trauma was admitted after all the investigations. Every department said no intervention and CT scan abdomen was also normal. Patient's condition worsened. There is always an element of suspicion on bowel injury even though scans can be normal. Tachycardia, tenderness, ileus can be confusing. In this patient, normal bowel sounds were heard on auscultation. His worsening was due to lung contusion. We, the authors, would like to stress again that a complete, thorough and repeated clinical examination is essential in a patient with trauma (Fig. 66.41).

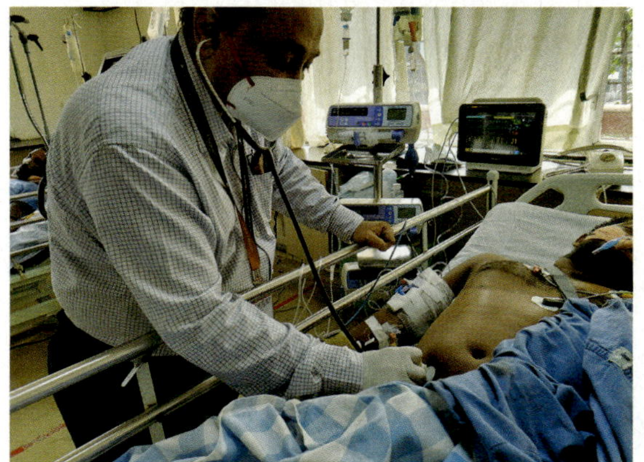

**Fig. 66.41:** Auscultation in a comatose polytrauma patient

## MULTIPLE CHOICE QUESTIONS

**1. The most common bedside investigation done for suspected blunt abdominal trauma for bleeding is:**
A. CT scan
B. MRI scan
C. Diagnostic peritoneal lavage
D. Ultrasound

**2. Which one of the following is a definite indication for laparotomy in blunt injury abdomen?**
A. Splenic injury
B. Pancreatic injury
C. Liver injury
D. Aspiration of bile in the peritoneal aspirate

**3. If air bubble like picture is found within the thorax following blunt injury abdomen what do you suspect?**
A. Splenic rupture
B. Liver injury
C. Injury to the stomach
D. Diaphragmatic injury

**4. How do you rule out a head injury with factors given below?**
A. Hypotension responding to fluid
B. CSF rhinorrhoea
C. Fracture skull
D. Hypertension and bradycardia

**5. Which is an important sign of hollow viscus perforation?**
A. Cullen's sign B. Grey Turner's sign
C. Mallet Guy sign D. London sign

**6. The following are true for conservative management of liver injury, *except*:**
A. Hollow viscus injury should not be there
B. Free contrast in and around liver in CT scan
C. Grade I and Grade II injury
D. Haemodynamically stable patient

**7. Pringle manoeuvre refers to:**
A. Compression of left gastric artery to stop the bleeding from giant gastric ulcer
B. Compression of hepatic artery to stop the bleeding during liver resection
C. Compression of hepatic artery and portal vein in front of foramen of Winslow
D. Compression of gastroduodenal artery during Whipple's procedure

**8. The salvage procedure to buy time in massive bleeding from liver include following:**
A. Pringle manoeuvre
B. Plug by omentum
C. Perihepatic packing
D. Portovenous shunt

**9. Perforation within 4 cm of the ileocaecal junction following blunt injury is better treated by:**
A. Suturing and drainage
B. Resection and anastomosis and drainage
C. Suture and bypass
D. Exteriorisation

**10. Which of the following is not a feature of retroperitoneal duodenal perforation?**
A. Can occur with steering wheel injury
B. Chilaiditi sign may be present
C. Free gas under diaphragm
D. Guarding and rigidity is minimal

**11. Initial third of resuscitation in haemorrhagic shock in blunt abdominal trauma is:**
A. Ringer lactate B. Saline
C. Dextrose D. Plasma

**12. Death triad in blunt abdominal trauma is:**
A. Hyperthermia, acidosis, coagulopathy
B. Hypothermia, acidosis, coagulopathy
C. Hypothermia, alkalosis, coagulopathy
D. Hyperthermia, alkalosis, coagulopathy

**Answers**

**1.** D **2.** D **3.** D **4.** D **5.** D **6.** B **7.** C **8.** C **9.** B **10.** C
**11.** A **12.** B

Section

VI

# *Viva Voce* Examination

Chapter 67

# Principles of Radiology and Imaging

- Plain X-rays
- Barium swallow
- Barium meal
- Enteroclysis
- Barium enema
- Angiography
- Ultrasonography
- Computed tomography
- Virtual colonoscopy
- Cholangiogram/ERCP/MRCP
- Magnetic resonance imaging
- PET scan
- Interventional radiology

## Introduction

One of the sessions in the undergraduate and post-graduate examinations is questions on plain X-rays and images. More and more images such as ultrasound, CT scan, MRI, PET scan, etc. have been used in the evaluation of the patients. These investigations are done to achieve evidence based science and surgery. Several CT images have been included in the book. Students are requested to study the principles behind these investigations so as to understand the investigations properly. This is only an exercise for you to perform better in the final examination.

## PLAIN X-RAYS

- When a plain X-ray is projected look carefully and identify the side—right or left. To give an example, if fundic air bubble is seen and cardiac shadow is seen it is on the left side. Similarly, because of the liver, diaphragm on the right side is usually elevated compared to the left side.
- Look at the bony cage—clavicle, ribs, sternum, vertebrae.
- Chest X-ray is taken always PA view so as to avoid sternal shadow.
- Then look at the soft tissue shadows—in the lungs, oesophageal shadow, cardiac shadow for any cardiomegaly and aortic shadow for any prominence.
- A Few examples are given below which are commonly asked questions.

### I. PLAIN X-RAY CHEST PA VIEW SHOWING COLLECTION OF FREE GAS UNDER THE RIGHT DOME OF THE DIAPHRAGM

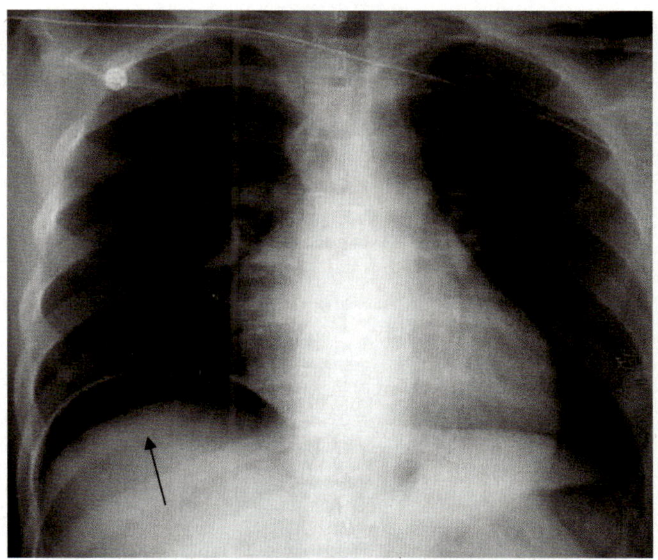

**Fig. 67.1:** X-ray chest PA view showing free gas under the right dome of the diaphragm

Normally, fundic air bubble is present on the left side. Hence, importance is given to the gas on the right side.

1. **What are the causes of free gas under the right dome of the diaphragm?**
   - Perforation of hollow viscus. Examples: Duodenal ulcer, gastric ulcer, enteric ulcer, Meckel's diverticulum, malignant ulcers—colonic, gastric, perforation of the tuberculous ulcer—ileum

- Abdominal stab injury, laparotomy
- Tubal insufflation test done for tubal patency—not done nowadays

2. **Is there any other finding in the X-ray?**
   - Ground glass appearance indicates significant fluid in the peritoneal cavity.
3. **How do you manage a case of perforated duodenal ulcer?**
   - With antibiotic coverage, Ryle's tube aspiration and early resuscitation with intravenous fluids, exploratory laparotomy is done. The site of perforation is identified which is in the first part of the duodenum. The perforation is closed by using nonabsorbable sutures. Omentum can be used to reinforce the suture line. This is called Roscoe Graham operation. Tube drain is used to drain peritoneal cavity.
4. **What are the common complications which can occur in the postoperative period?**
   - Basal atelectasis, oliguria, wound infections and wound dehiscence are a few common complications.
5. **What are the stages of duodenal ulcer perforation?**
   - Stage of chemical peritonitis
   - Stage of illusion or delusion
   - Stage of bacterial peritonitis

## II. PLAIN X-RAY ABDOMEN SHOWING MULTIPLE GAS AND FLUID LEVELS

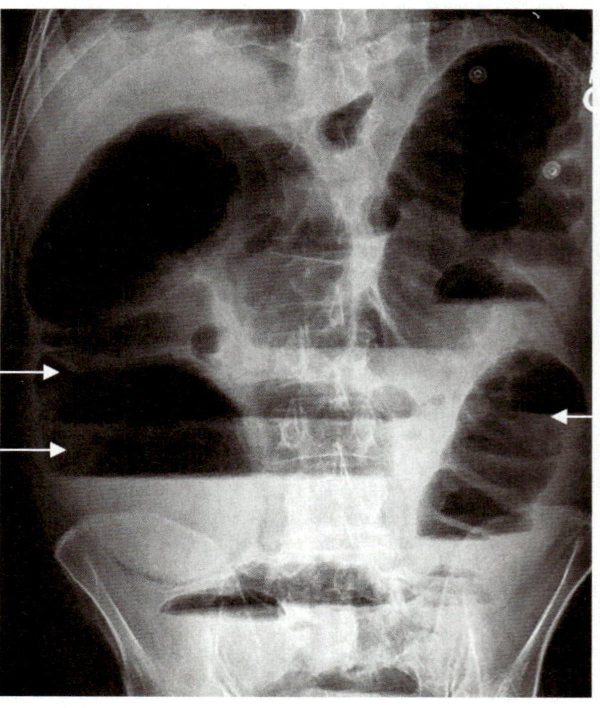

Fig. 67.2: Plain X-ray abdomen showing multiple gas and fluid levels with prominent valvulae conniventes

1. **What is the diagnosis?**
   - Since jejunal loops are prominently seen and loops are centrally located, it is probably terminal ileal obstruction.
2. **What are the common causes of terminal ileal obstruction?**
   - Tuberculous stricture
   - Bands—congenital
   - Adhesions
   - 'Worm ball' in children
   - Obstructed hernia
3. **How do you identify jejunum, ileum and colon in a plain X-ray?**
   - Jejunum—valvulae conniventes—regularly placed mucosal folds placed opposite to each other.
   - Ileum—no character—characterless loop of Wangensteen.
   - Colon—haustrations—a large incomplete mucosal folds not placed opposite to each other.
4. **How do you treat tuberculous strictures?**
   - Resection and end-to-end anastomosis.
5. **Can any other surgical procedure be done?**
   - Stricturoplasty (like pyloroplasty), if there is a single stricture.

## III. PLAIN X-RAY ABDOMEN SHOWING RADIO-OPAQUE SHADOW IN THE RIGHT UPPER ABDOMEN

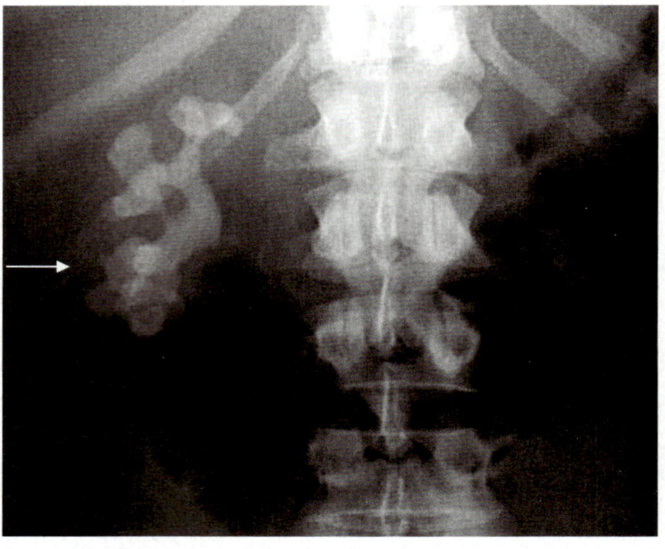

Fig. 67.3: Plain X-ray abdomen showing staghorn calculi right kidney region

1. **What is the diagnosis?**
   - Probably renal stone
2. **Why is it not a gallstone?**
   - The location of the stone is at lower level when compared to gallstone.

- The shape of the stone suggests that it is a stone in the pelvis growing within calyces.

3. **What do you call such a stone?**
   - Staghorn calculus
4. **What type of X-ray is ideal to distinguish renal stone from gallbladder stone?**
   - Lateral view
5. **What will be the findings in case of renal stones in a lateral picture?**
   - Renal stones are found superimposed on vertebral bodies. On the other hand, gallstones are found anterior to it.

## IV. PLAIN X-RAY ABDOMEN SHOWING RADIO-OPAQUE SHADOW IN THE REGION OF GALLBLADDER

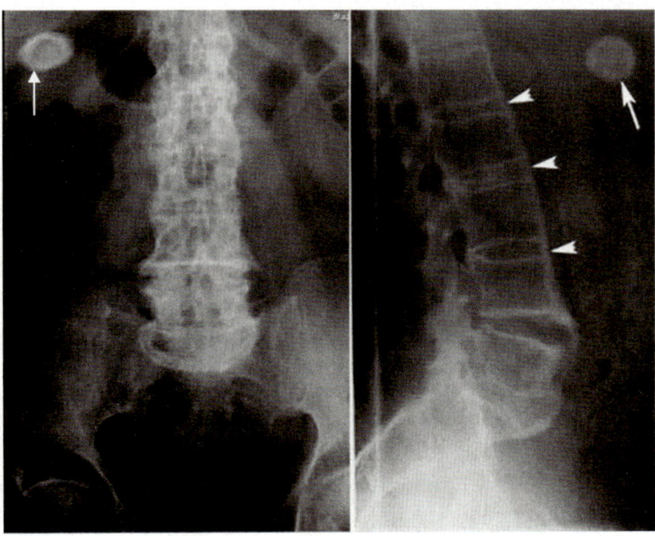

**Fig. 67.4:** Plain X-ray abdomen AP and lateral view, showing gallstone

1. **What is the diagnosis?**
   - It is gallstone because in the lateral picture it is in front of vertebral column
2. **What percentage of gallstones are visible in a plain X-ray?**
   - Only 10%
3. **What is the reason for that?**
   - The calcium content in gallstones is very less.
4. **What are the causes of radio-opaque shadow in the abdomen?**
   - Gallstones
   - Renal stones
   - Pancreatic stones
   - Renal tuberculosis
   - 'Chip' fracture of the transverse process of the vertebrae
   - Calcified lymph nodes—tuberculosis
   - Faecoliths
   - Phleboliths
5. **What is the treatment of symptomatic gallstones?**
   - Cholecystectomy

## V. X-RAY CHEST PA VIEW SHOWING MULTIPLE ROUND SHADOW IN BOTH LUNG FIELDS

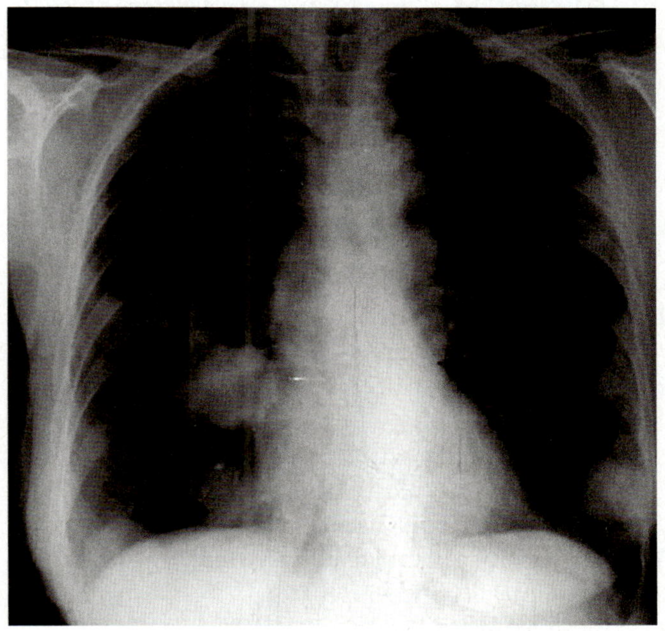

**Fig. 67.5:** Chest X-ray PA view showing cannonball secondaries

1. **What is the diagnosis?**
   - Bilateral chest secondaries
2. **What are they called?**
   - Cannonball secondaries
3. **Why are secondaries in the lung round?**
   - Lung is an elastic tissue, it has resilience. Hence, during the act of inspiration and expiration, equal amount of pressure is exerted on secondaries, which are growing. Hence, they tend to become round.
4. **What are the common causes of chest secondaries?**
   - Carcinoma breast
   - Carcinoma testis
   - Malignant melanoma
   - Hepatoma
   - Renal cell carcinoma
   - Sarcoma
5. **Is there any other differential diagnosis?**
   - Miliary tuberculosis: The shadows will be very small and numerous.

## VI. X-RAY CERVICAL VERTEBRAE WITH UPPER RIBS SHOWING BILATERAL CERVICAL RIBS

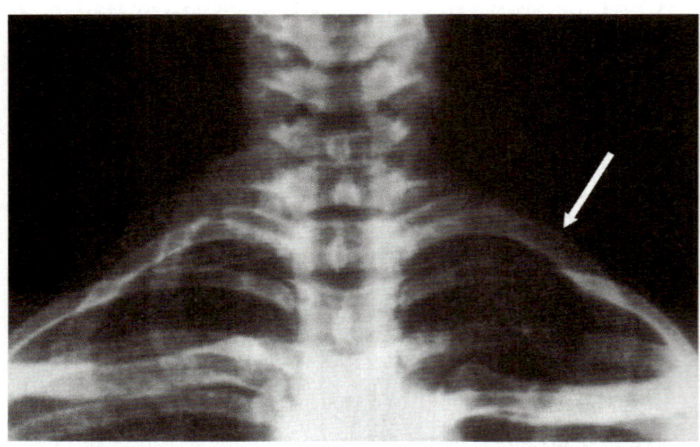

**Fig. 67.6:** X-ray cervical vertebrae with upper ribs showing bilateral cervical ribs

1. **What is a cervical rib?**
   - It is an extra rib arising from 7th cervical vertebra.
2. **What are 4 types of cervical rib?**
   - Incomplete bony
   - Complete bony with anterior expanded bony end.
   - Partly fibrous, partly bony
   - Complete fibrous band
3. **What variety gives rise to vascular symptoms?**
   - The fibrous band variety
4. **What is your finding here?**
   - On the right side, it is complete variety and on the left side, it is incomplete.
5. **If cervical rib is symptomatic, what is the treatment?**
   - Extraperiosteal excision of cervical rib which means removal of the rib along with the periosteum. Some surgeons also do cervical sympathectomy to decrease vasomotor tone of vessels.

## VII. X-RAY LATERAL VIEW OF THE SKULL SHOWING A LARGE SWELLING WITH EROSION IN THE PERICRANIUM

1. **What is the diagnosis?**
   - Rapidly growing secondary deposits in the skull bone. It is a flat bone which is rich in red marrow. Also, secondaries produce few vascular growth factors, hence they grow more rapidly than primary.
2. **Why is it not a lipoma or neurofibroma?**
   - Erosion of the bone is seen in malignancy, not in benign tumours.

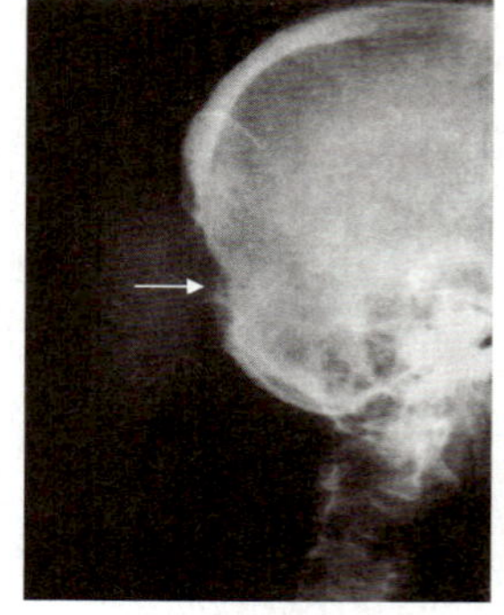

**Fig. 67.7:** X-ray lateral view of the skull showing a large swelling with erosion in the pericranium

3. **If this patient is a female aged 40 years, what are the causes?**
   - Follicular carcinoma thyroid
   - Carcinoma of the breast
   - Renal cell carcinoma
4. **What is the treatment if this is follicular carcinoma thyroid?**
   - Total thyroidectomy followed by radioiodine therapy and external radiotherapy for metastasis in bones.
5. **How do you diagnose follicular carcinoma thyroid histologically?**
   - Angioinvasion and capsular invasion (lobectomy–total thyroidectomy).

## VIII. PLAIN X-RAY ABDOMEN SHOWING EXTENSIVE CALCIFICATION IN THE REGION OF PANCREAS

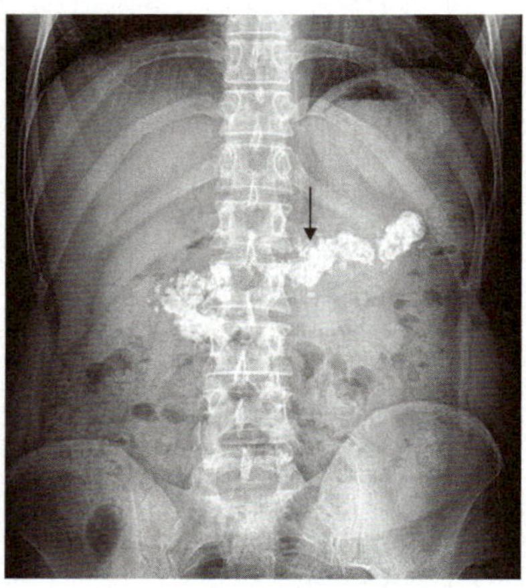

**Fig. 67.8:** Plain X-ray abdomen showing extensive calcification in the center of the abdomen

1. **What is the diagnosis?**
   - Chronic pancreatitis
2. **Why do you say so?**
   - Extensive calcification involving head, body and tail of pancreas.
3. **What other investigation can be done here, which is used for therapeutic purpose?**
   - ERCP-stent can be placed-one of the methods of treatment of chronic pancreatitis.
4. **What are the manifestations of chronic pancreatitis?**
   - Severe abdominal pain, diabetes, steatorrhoea, multiple strictures.
5. **If pancreatic duct is dilated more than 8 mm in a patient with severe abdominal pain with chronic pancreatitis, what is the treatment?**
   - Longitudinal pancreaticojejunostomy—Puestow's operation. In this operation, pancreatic duct is laid open, strictures are divided, and the duct is anastomosed to jejunum. Coring the head mass (Frey's) also need to be done.

## BARIUM STUDIES

This is the study of the gastrointestinal tract by instillation/ingestion of barium suspension made up of/made from pure **barium sulphate**.

### BARIUM SWALLOW

It is the contrast study from the oral cavity up to the fundus of the stomach.

#### Indications

Dysphagia and obstruction, odynophagia, assessment of mediastinal masses, motility disorders of oesophagus—achalasia, scleroderma.

#### Relative Contraindications

- Tracheo-oesophageal fistula, perforation.

#### Procedure

One mouthful of contrast media is given and the act of deglutition is observed fluoroscopically. After a mouthful of barium, films are exposed to the region of interest.

#### Interpretation of Study

1. Malignant obstructions are seen as annular constrictions, shouldering cranial and caudal to the lesion, mucosal destruction, ulceration and fistulae formation.
2. Benign strictures are long segment narrowings with no mucosal abnormalities.
3. Achalasia cardia is evident as 'rat tail' appearance of the lower end of the oesophagus, with gross dilatation of the oesophagus proximally and thin streaks of contrast entering the stomach.
4. Scleroderma shows dilatation, atonicity, poor or absent peristalsis and free gastro-oesophageal reflux.

**A few examples of barium swallow X-rays**

### 1. BARIUM SWALLOW SHOWING INTRINSIC, IRREGULAR, AND PERSISTENT FILLING DEFECT IN THE LOWER OESOPHAGUS

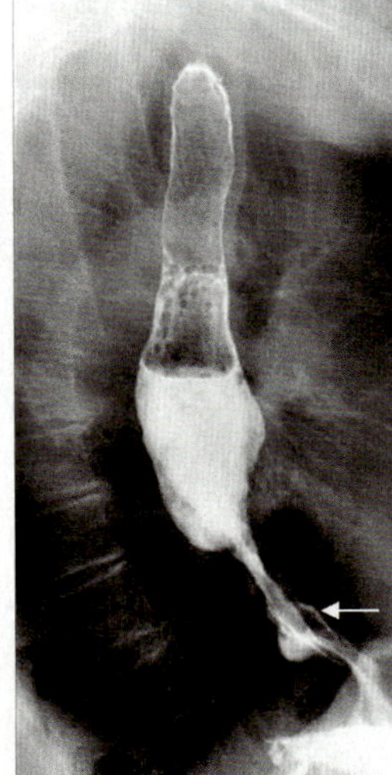

Fig. 67.9: Barium swallow showing filling defect in the lower oesophagus

1. **What is the diagnosis?**
   - Carcinoma lower one-third of oesophagus.
2. **What are the other findings?**
   - Proximal shouldering is very characteristic of malignancy.
3. **How do you confirm the diagnosis?**
   - Oesophagoscopy and biopsy
4. **If biopsy report is adenocarcinoma, what is the treatment?**
   - Operable—oesophagogastrectomy
   - Inoperable—to relieve Dysphagia, Self Expandable Metallic stents (SEMS) can be introduced. Thus, surgery can be avoided.
5. **What are the premalignant conditions?**
   - Achalasia cardia
   - Reflux oesophagitis
   - Corrosive stricture
   - Plummer-Vinson syndrome

### 2. BARIUM SWALLOW SHOWING EXTENSIVE AND IRREGULAR FILLING DEFECT INVOLVING MIDDLE ONE-THIRD OF OESOPHAGUS

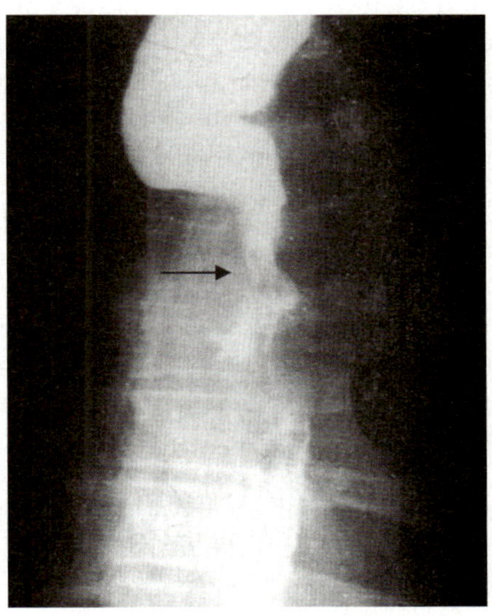

Fig. 67.10: Barium swallow showing extensive and irregular filling defect involving middle one-third of oesophagus

1. **What is the diagnosis?**
   - Carcinoma middle one-third of oesophagus
2. **How do you confirm the diagnosis?**
   - Oesophagoscopy and biopsy
3. **What will be the biopsy report?**
   - Squamous cell carcinoma
4. **What other investigations are necessary in such case?**
   - Bronchoscopy, CT scan of the chest and endosonography are important investigations.
5. **Looking at this advanced lesion, what is probably the best treatment for this patient?**
   - Chemotherapy and radiotherapy followed by dilatation of the oesophagus, since chances of fibrosis and narrowing of the lumen following radiotherapy are high.

## BARIUM MEAL

This is the radiological study of oesophagus, stomach, duodenum and proximal jejunum.

### Indications

- Symptoms of vomiting, epigastric pain, heart burn, dyspepsia
- Upper abdominal mass
- Gastric or duodenal obstruction
- Malignancies

### Contraindications

- Suspected perforation
- Suspicion of aspiration
- Large bowel obstruction

### Procedure

An undiluted barium suspension is given and deglutition is seen under fluoroscopy. Once barium reaches the stomach, the patient is rotated so as to coat the entire stomach and filming is done. More barium is given to distend the stomach wall. Filming is done as contrast enters the duodenum and opacifies proximal jejunum.

### Interpretation of Study

1. **Hiatus hernia** is evident as presence of the stomach above the oesophageal hiatus. In addition, gastroesophageal reflux will be evident. Mucosal ulceration and strictures may be demonstrable in long-standing cases.
2. **Gastric and duodenal ulcers** appear as projections from the normal contour with pooling of contrast. Benign **ulcers** usually **project out** and have the mucosal folds radiating up to the edge of the ulcer. Deformity of the stomach and duodenal cap are seen in chronic stages.
3. **Bezoars of stomach** are seen as radiolucent masses in the stomach and the barium fills the crevices between the particles forming a characteristic appearance.
4. **Infantile hypertrophic pyloric stenosis:** Thin **streak** of barium is seen extending across pylorus—indentation of barium-filled antrum is seen.
5. **Persistent, irregular filling defect** is seen in carcinoma of the stomach.

**Few examples of barium meal X-rays**

## 1. BARIUM MEAL: CONTRAST OPACIFIED STOMACH DEMONSTRATING A PROJECTION FROM LESSER CURVATURE

1. **What is the diagnosis?**
   - Benign gastric ulcer

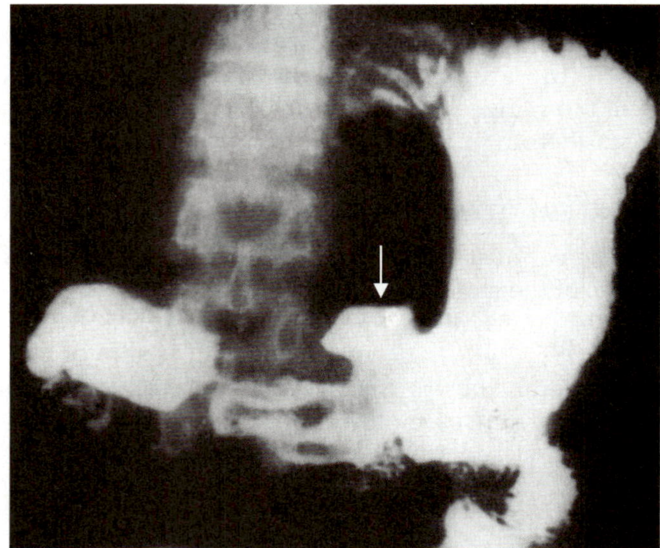

Fig. 67.11: Barium meal: Contrast opacified stomach demonstrating a projection from lesser curvature due to a benign gastric ulcer (niche)

2. **What is the finding called?**
   - Niche
3. **Will you do a biopsy?**
   - Yes because 1–2% of gastric ulcers can turn into malignancy.
4. **What is the treatment of benign gastric ulcer?**
   - Avoid irritants such as smoking, spicy food, alcohol and drugs such as nonsteroidal anti-inflammatory drugs.
5. **Mention complications of gastric ulcer.**
   - Bleeding, tea pot deformity, hour glass contracture, perforation and carcinoma.

## 2. BARIUM MEAL SHOWING INTRINSIC, IRREGULAR, AND PERSISTENT FILLING DEFECT INVOLVING PYLORIC ANTRUM

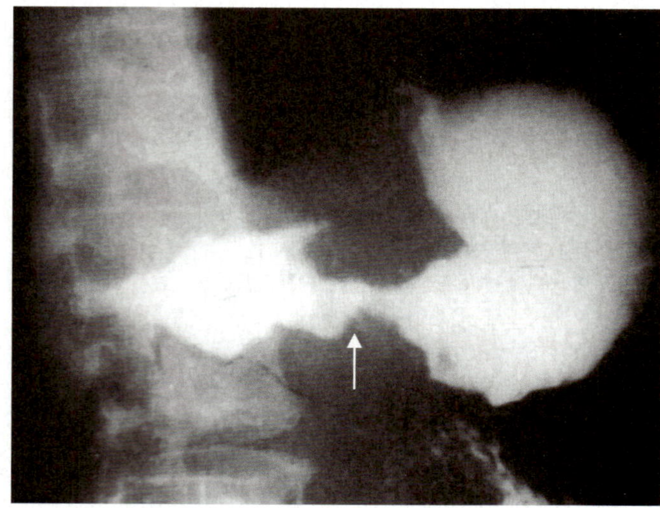

Fig. 67.12: Barium meal showing intrinsic, irregular and persistent filling defect involving pyloric antrum

1. **What is the diagnosis?**
   - Carcinoma pyloric antrum
2. **How do you confirm diagnosis?**
   - Gastroscopic biopsy
3. **What will be the biopsy report?**
   - Adenocarcinoma
4. **What is the treatment, if it is operable?**
   - Subtotal gastrectomy
5. **What structures are removed in the operation?**
   - Growth along with 60–70% of distal stomach, omentum, removal of primary of group of lymph nodes along the lesser and greater curvature, and in the vicinity of major blood vessels followed by gastrojejunal anastomosis—D2 gastrectomy.

## 3. BARIUM MEAL X-RAY SHOWING ENORMOUS DILATATION OF THE STOMACH AND FAILURE OF BARIUM TO FILL INTO THE DISTAL INTESTINE

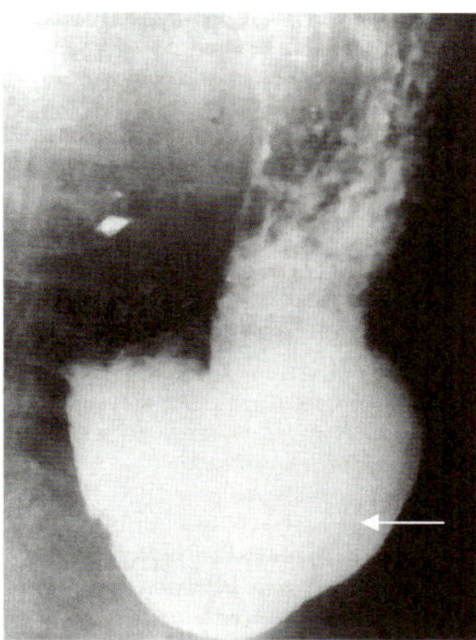

**Fig. 67.13:** Barium meal X-ray showing enormous dilatation of the stomach and failure of barium to fill into the distal intestine

1. **What is the diagnosis?**
   - Gastric outlet obstruction due to chronic cicatrized duodenal ulcer (pyloric stenosis is an old terminology).
2. **Why is it not due to carcinoma pyloric antrum?**
   - There is no filling defect in the pyloric antrum.
3. **How do you treat this case?**
   - With a preoperative stomach wash, adequate intravenous fluids, total truncal vagotomy with GJ is the treatment of choice.
4. **Why GJ and vagotomy?**
   - After vagotomy, motility of the stomach is lost and in pyloric stenosis, there is already obstruction at the pyloric antrum. Hence, gastrojejunostomy is the drainage procedure of choice.
5. **Why not pyloroplasty or highly selective vagotomy?**
   - Pylorus is scarred and deformed. Hence, it is not safe to do pyloroplasty. HSV is contraindicated in the presence of pyloric obstruction.

## SMALL BOWEL ENEMA OR ENTEROCLYSIS

This is the radiological study of the small bowel (from jejunum to the ileocecal junction) by intubation of the jejunum and instillation of contrast media through the tube. This investigation has replaced barium meal follow through. *Refer* to Key Boxes 67.1 and 67.2.

Key Box 67.1

**Indications**

- Mechanical obstruction
- GIT bleeding
- Tumours of small intestine
- Unexplained abdominal pain
- Diarrhoea

Key Box 67.2

**Contraindications**

- Complete obstruction
- Suspected perforation
- Massive dilatation of small bowel
- Duodenal obstruction
- Gastrojejunostomy

### Procedure

- Bilbao Dotter tube is inserted with the guide wire through one of the nostrils and advanced caudally with the swallowing action till the tip reaches the stomach. The tube is then advanced through the antrum of the stomach to the pyloric canal. Then it is advanced under fluoroscopic guidance to about 4–5 cm distal to the Treitz ligament (duodenojejunal junction).
- 200 ml barium suspension is injected at a rate of 75 ml/min followed by 5% of methylcellulose at a rate of 100 ml/min. The head of the barium column is followed with intermittent fluoroscopy and films exposed wherever necessary.
- Ileocaecal spot films are taken when the junction is opacified and distended.

### Interpretation of Study

1. Normal small bowel shows a decrease in calibre from jejunum to ileum and the change of prominent valvulae conniventes to featureless ileum is evident.
2. Malignancies and lymphomas show evidence of strictures, proximal dilatations and mucosal abnormality. Large mesenteric nodal masses displace the bowel loops.

3. Strictures and ulceration of terminal ileum: Dilatation of the segment proximal to the narrowed segment and conical shrunken caecum are seen in ileocaecal tuberculosis. In later stages, ileal strictures, fistulae, etc. may be seen.

### Complications

Perforation, inspissation of barium, transient bacteraemia.

**One example of small bowel enteroclysis or small bowel enema**

## 1. SMALL BOWEL ENEMA SHOWING STRICTURE TERMINAL ILEUM

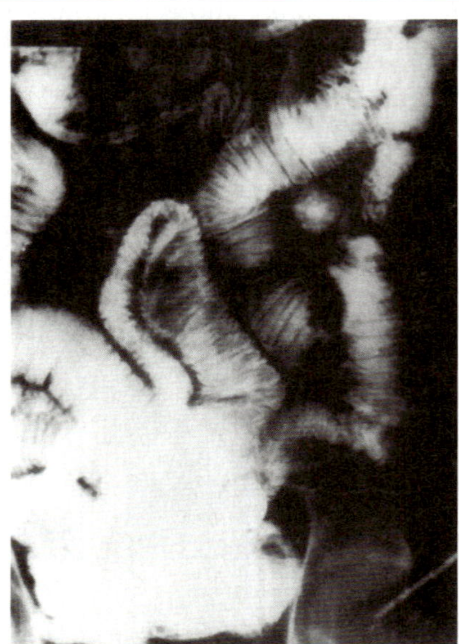

**Fig. 67.14:** Small bowel enema showing stricture terminal ileum

1. **What is the diagnosis?**
   - Most probably intestinal tuberculosis.
2. **What are the nature of the strictures in tuberculosis?**
   - Transverse
3. **How do you confirm the diagnosis?**
   - CT enterography can be done. Later balloon enteroscopy is done and biopsy can be taken.
4. **What is the treatment?**
   - Single stricture can be treated by stricturoplasty and multiple strictures are treated by resection anastomosis.
5. **What are the complications of tubercular stricture?**
   - Intestinal obstruction, perforation peritonitis.

## BARIUM ENEMA

This is the radiographic study of the large bowel by administration of contrast media through the rectum.

### Types

Single contrast barium enema and double contrast barium enema.

### Indications

Change in bowel habit, melaena, mass suspected to be arising from colon.

### Contraindications

Toxic megacolon, pseudomembranous colitis, rectal biopsy done recently (procedure withheld for 7 days).

### Procedure

- Bowel is prepared with low residue diet, purgation and cleansing water enema. High density barium suspension is allowed to flow up to the ileocaecal junction and reflux into the terminal ileum. Single contrast filming is done. The patient is asked to evacuate the barium and a post-evacuation film is taken. Once barium is evacuated properly, air insufflation is carried out so as to distend colon up to the ileocaecal junction.
- Filming is done to demonstrate the double contrast of large bowel with additional spots of hepatic, splenic flexures and rectosigmoid junction in oblique positions so as to open up these regions.

### Interpretation of Study

A few examples are:

1. **Ulcerative colitis**
   - Loss of haustral pattern, fine granularity of mucosa
   - Strictures, pipe stem colon, increase in presacral space
2. **Malignant lesions**
   - Circumferential/eccentric growth narrowing the lumen
   - Hold up of barium proximal to the lesion, mucosal abnormality—ulcerations
3. **Tuberculosis:** Ileocaecal region is the commonest site. Deformed, elevated caecum, stricture and ulceration involving ascending colon and ileum.
4. **Crohn's disease:** Multiple ulcerations, thickening and distortion of valvulae conniventes, short or long strictures, cobblestone pattern and separation of bowel loops are the features.
5. **Malabsorption:** Dilution of barium, segmentation of the column of barium, 'Moulage sign' (barium in a featureless tube) and jejunal dilatation are the findings.

## A few examples of barium enema studies

### 1. BARIUM ENEMA SHOWING THE LEFT COLON, TRANSVERSE COLON AND A PART OF ASCENDING COLON

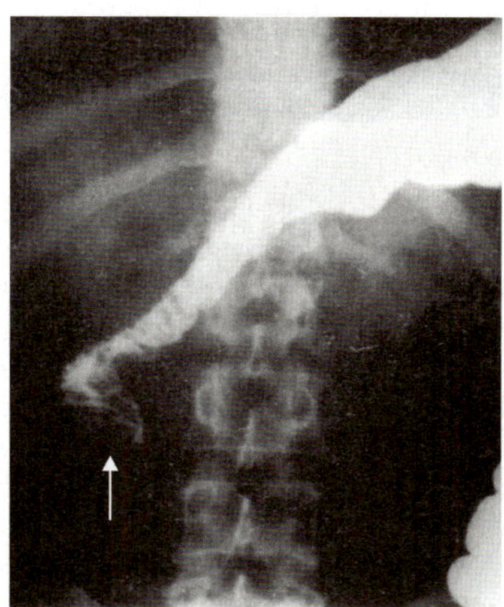

**Fig. 67.15:** Barium enema showing the left colon, transverse colon and a part of ascending colon with pincer ending

1. **What is the diagnosis?**
   - Ileocolic intussusception
2. **Why do you say so?**
   - The 'claw' like ending or pincer ending is typical of intussusception.
3. **What are the causes of intussusception in adults?**
   - Submucous lipoma, or polyps
   - Meckel's diverticulum
   - Growth in the caecum
   - Leiomyoma of the ileum
4. **In a child, what are the causes?**
   - Weaning of the diet or viral infection.
5. **What is the treatment of adult intussusception?**
   - Resection because there is a precipitating cause.

### 2. BARIUM ENEMA SHOWING INTRINSIC, IRREGULAR AND PERSISTENT FILLING DEFECT IN THE ASCENDING COLON

1. **What is the diagnosis?**
   - Carcinoma ascending colon
2. **What is the confirmatory investigation?**
   - Colonoscopy and biopsy
3. **What is the report, if it is carcinoma?**
   - Adenocarcinoma
4. **What is the treatment?**
   - Right radical hemicolectomy, if it is operable. Structures removed in this operation include terminal ileum (6–8 cm), caecum including appendix, ascending colon and 1/3rd of right transverse colon. If it is inoperable, part of ileum is anastomosed to the transverse colon to prevent or relieve intestinal obstruction (side to side). One need not remove two feet of ileum.

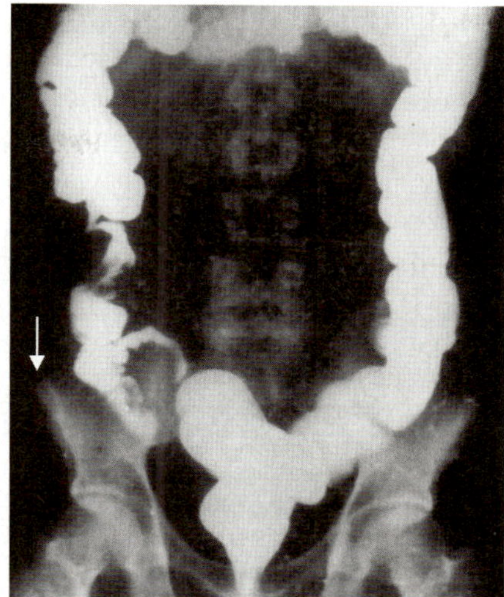

**Fig. 67.16:** Barium enema showing intrinsic, irregular and persistent filling defect in the ascending colon

5. **What is the differential diagnosis?**

   Ileocaecal tuberculosis: In this condition:

   A. Irregular filling defect is not seen.

   B. Caecum is usually pulled up and then ileocaecal angle becomes obtuse.

### 3. BARIUM ENEMA SHOWING LOSS OF HAUSTRATIONS IN THE LEFT COLON, SMALL AND MULTIPLE, REGULAR FILLING DEFECTS DUE TO PSEUDOPOLYPOSIS

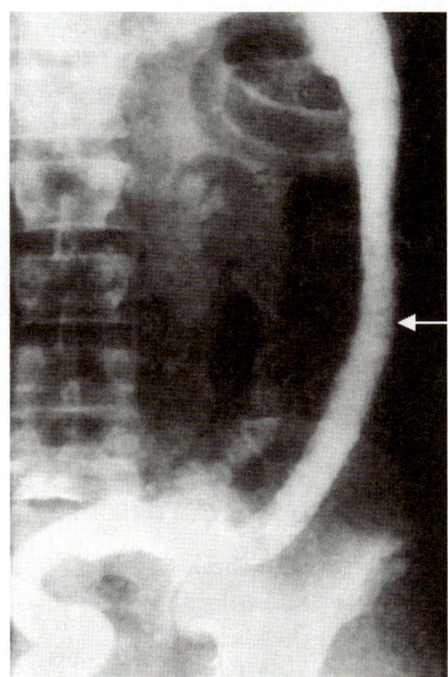

**Fig. 67.17:** Barium enema showing loss of haustrations in the left colon, small and multiple, and regular filling defects due to pseudopolyposis

1. **What is the diagnosis?**
   - Ulcerative colitis.
2. **What is pseudopolyposis?**
   - An attempt at healing in between the ulcers produces granulation tissues which have the appearance of polyps. Hence, pseudopolyposis.
3. **What are the dangerous complications of ulcerative colitis?**
   - Haemorrhage, toxic megacolon, perforation and malignancy.
4. **What are the drugs used in the treatment of ulcerative colitis?**
   - Salazopyrines and corticosteroids
5. **What are the surgical treatments?**
   - Total colectomy with permanent ileostomy, OR
   - Total colectomy, creation of a pouch with anastomosis of the pouch to the anal canal.

## 4. BARIUM ENEMA SHOWING PULLED UP CAECUM

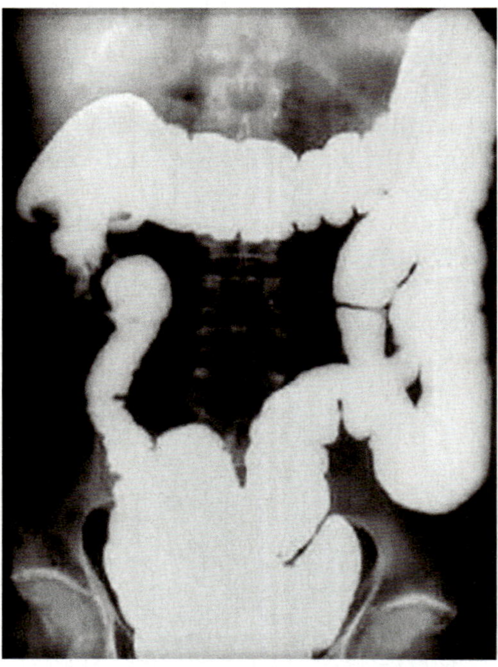

**Fig. 67.18:** Barium enema showing pulled up caecum—an increase in the ileocaecal angle from acute to obtuse

1. **What is the diagnosis?**
   - Ileocaecal tuberculosis
2. **Why caecum is pulled up?**
   - Involved caecum and ascending colon are contracted and fibrosed resulting in caecum in a higher position.
3. **What are the other signs you will look for in this case?**
   - Narrowing of terminal ileum (Fleischner's sign), fibrotic terminal ileum opening into the contracted caecum (Stierlin's sign).
4. **What about ileocaecal angle?**
   - Normal angle is acute. In this case, it becomes obtuse.
5. **What are the surgical treatments?**
   - If obstruction is present, better to do limited colectomy followed by anti-tuberculous treatment.

## ANGIOGRAPHY

### Definition

This is the study of blood vessels by injection of a contrast medium containing iodine into the vessel. For lower limbs, femoral artery is selected because it is superficial and easily palpable. It is punctured under local anaesthesia. Today majority of the cases undergo CT angiogram. In CT angiogram, iodine-based contrast is injected through the intravenous line, thus avoiding a direct puncture of artery, thus avoiding complications such as pseudoaneurysm formation, bleeding, etc. Investigation is designed to increase the absorption of X-ray photons and thereby enhancing the image contrast of blood vessels and well-perfused tissues.

### Indications

1. Primary vascular diseases such as vaso-occlusive disease, aneurysm, arteriovenous malformation (AVM).
2. Vascularity assessment of a tumour.
3. Congenital vascular conditions such as coarctation.
4. Percutaneous interventional vascular procedures.

### Contraindications

1. Bleeding tendencies
2. Skin infections at site of entry
3. Cardiovascular disease such as recent myocardial infarction, overt congestive cardiac failure
4. Hepatic failure

### Procedure

- Local anaesthesia at site of puncture is preferred except in children or restless patients, wherein general anaesthesia is preferred. Using a Seldinger needle the artery is punctured.
- The catheter of appropriate dimension is placed into the artery and negotiated into the desired vessel to be studied. Contrast is injected and filming is done (Figs 67.19 and 67.20).

### Puncture Sites

Femoral artery, axillary artery and brachial artery.

### Interpretation of Study

1. Aneurysms are seen as focal dilatations of vessel or projecting from the main vessel through a neck.

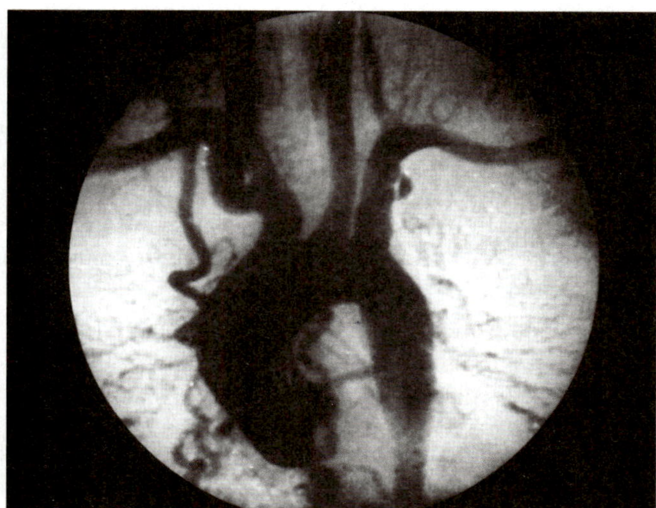

Fig. 67.19: **Arch aortogram:** Contrast in the arch of aorta demonstrating the major vessels arising from it

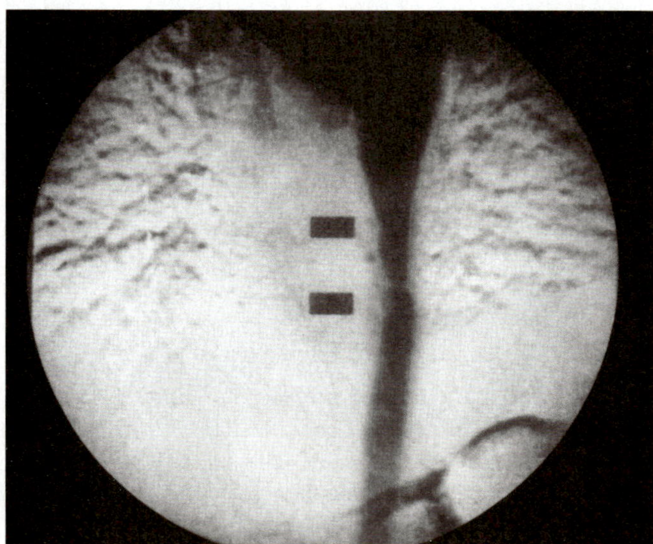

Fig. 67.20: **Aortogram:** Contrast in the thoracic aorta showing narrowing

2. Tumour vessels show abnormal branching pattern, vascular encasement, displacement, arteriovenous shunting and pooling of contrast in the lesion.
3. AVM shows evidence of a dilated feeding artery/ abnormal blush and early draining vein.
4. Vascular occlusions are seen as abrupt or gradual tapering of vessel with collateral supply distally.

## Complications

- Damage to arterial walls at the site of puncture
- Severe hypotensive reactions
- Thrombosis of arteries, catheter clot embolus, haematoma at puncture site
- Vagal inhibition
- Allergic reactions to contrast
- Damage to nerves and to organs

*A few examples:*

## 1. RETROGRADE ANGIOGRAPHY SHOWING OCCLUSION OF FEMORAL ARTERY ON THE LEFT SIDE

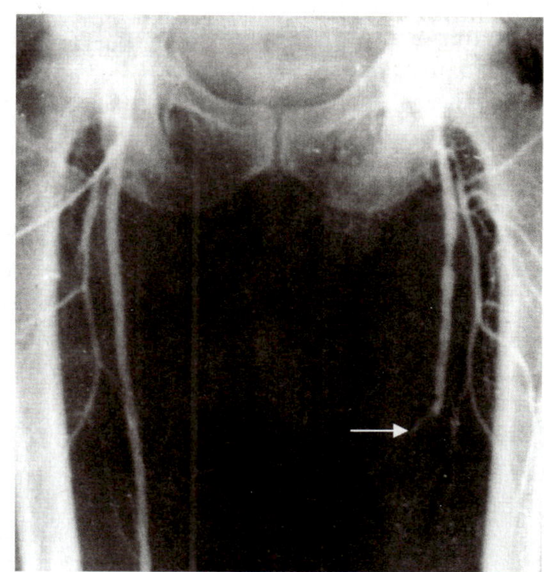

Fig. 67.21: Retrograde angiography showing occlusion of femoral artery on the left side

1. **What is the technique employed in this angiography?**
   - Seldinger's technique—percutaneous, transfemoral, retrograde.
2. **What is the probable cause in our country?**
   - Buerger's disease (thromboangiitis obliterans).
3. **Why do you say so?**
   - Buerger's disease affects medium-sized vessels and narrowing of femoral artery is segmental in this radiograph.
4. **What is the surgical treatment for Buerger's disease?**
   - Lumbar sympathectomy
5. **How does lumbar sympathectomy help these patients?**
   - By reducing the sympathetic tone of the lower limb, arterioles and capillaries get dilated allowing cutaneous ulcers to heal.
6. **If patient is 65 years old, what diagnosis you would have considered? What is the treatment in such cases?**
   - Atherosclerosis. Femoropopliteal bypass.

## 2. CT ANGIOGRAM SHOWING FEMORAL ARTERY AND ITS BRANCHES

1. **What is the technique employed in this angiography?**
   - It is CT angiogram.

**2. What is the indication?**

- Patient with severe claudication with or without ulcers as in atherosclerotic disease.

**3. What are the findings?**

- In the first film (Fig. 67.22A), superficial femoral artery is narrowed and in the second picture (Fig. 67.22B), you can see dye flowing freely after dilatation—angioplasty. It is done by a balloon dilatation using 6 or 7 mm and stent of the same size is used. Stents used are nitinol stents (Key Box 67.3).

**4. How angioplasty is done?**

- Under local anaesthesia, thin catheter is advanced into the femoral artery and with help of balloon it is dilated followed by a small stent is placed.

**5. What is the usual site of obstruction of femoral artery?**

- It is in the hiatus of adductor magnus—Hunterian canal.

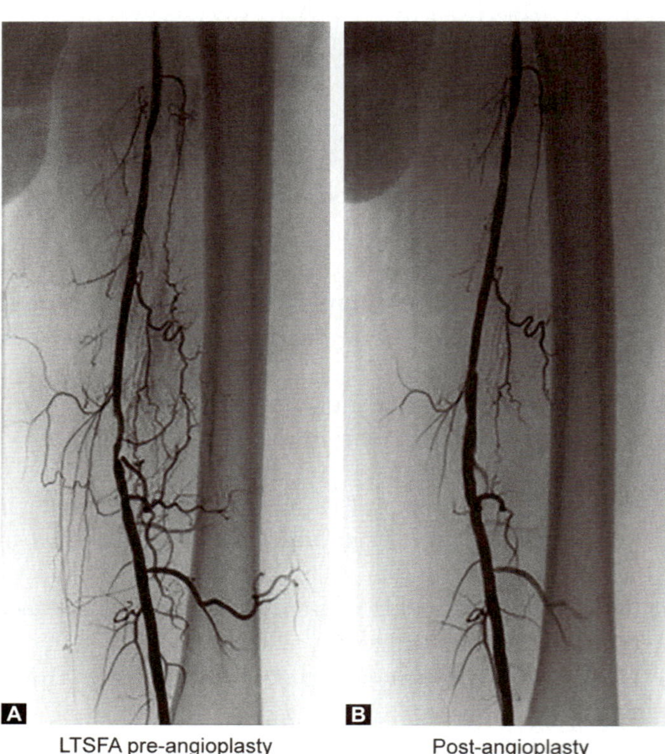


**Fig. 67.22:** (A) CT angiogram showing narrowing of superficial femoral artery; (B) Balloon angioplasty is done

Key Box 67.3

**Nitinol Stents**

1. These are combination of nickel-titanium alloys
2. Self-expanding stents
3. Good memory and good elasticity of these stents
4. Resistant to corrosion
5. Biocompatible

## ULTRASONOGRAPHY (Figs 67.23 and 67.24)

### Principle

This imaging modality is based on the **piezoelectric effect** which is the property of certain substances to convert **electrical energy to sound energy.** These are the active portions of the ultrasonic transducers. **The commonly used substance in the transducer is lead zirconate titanate (PZT).**

### Applications (Key Box 67.4)

- Ultrasonic beam of **high frequency** gives excellent resolution images of only superficial structures. This is used for study of musculoskeletal system, joints, thyroid, scrotum, etc. For imaging **deeper structures of abdomen, a low frequency** probe with greater **penetrancy** is used.

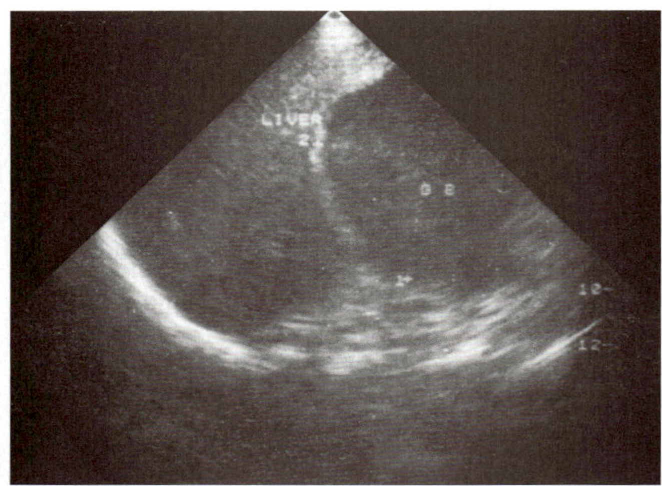


**Fig. 67.23:** Ultrasound of liver and gallbladder demonstrating an isoechoic mass lesion occupying the lumen of gallbladder which was due to malignancy

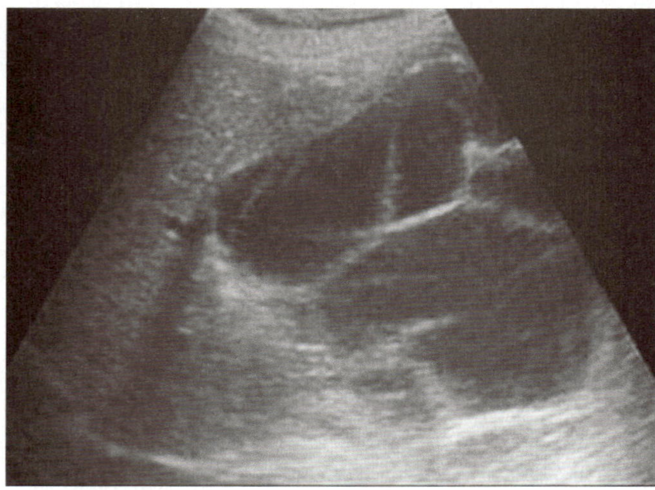

**Fig. 67.24:** Ultrasound of liver shows hydatid cyst which is anechoic with multiple daughter cysts

Key Box 67.4

**Frequency of Various Ultrasound Beams**

- 2.5 to 3.5 MHz: Deep abdomen, obstetric and gynaecological imaging
- 5.0 MHz: Vascular, breast, pelvic imaging
- 7.5 MHz: Breast, thyroid
- 10.0 MHz: Breast, thyroid, superficial veins, superficial masses such as parotid swelling, musculoskeletal imaging
- 15.0 MHz: Superficial structures such as lipoma, musculoskeletal imaging including soft tissue sarcoma

### Interpretation of Images

- Images are dependent on the **intensity of echoes** received back by the transducer.
- Structures which reflect all the sound waves back are depicted as **bright echoes** and **termed hyperechoic**.
- Structures which reflect **moderate** level of sound waves appear as uniform grains and are **termed isoechoic.**
- Fluid-filled structures which transmit all the sound waves, **do not reflect any echoes and are termed hypoechoic.**
- The reflection of sound waves in the form of echoes depends on the density of the organ and the transmission of sound through the same.

### Advantages of Ultrasonography

1. It is a cost-effective investigation.
2. It is widely available.
3. Noninvasive.
4. Owing to the relatively small size of the apparatus, it is fairly portable, and can thus be brought to the bedside of the moribund patient.
5. It does not involve the use of ionising radiation, and can, therefore, be safely used in a pregnant patient and can be repeatedly used as a follow-up modality.

### Limitations of Ultrasonography

1. Its use is limited in thorax.
2. Limited use in the abdomen when there is gaseous distension.
3. Operator expertise is all important.
4. It cannot image bone.

## COMPUTED TOMOGRAPHY (CT)

This is an imaging procedure where detailed information is obtained from thin sections in collimated X-rays.

### Indications

- Structural evaluation of intracranial lesions (Fig. 67.25)
- Detailed evaluation of lung, mediastinal pathologies
- Intra-abdominal and pelvic masses where exact site of origin and relation to adjacent structures can be evaluated.

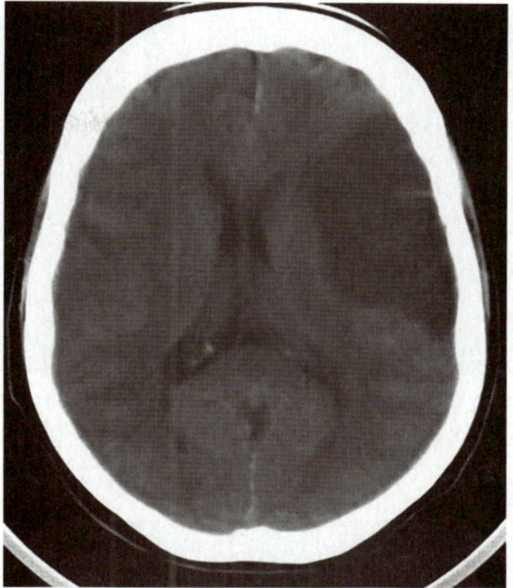

**Fig. 67.25: Cranial CT:** Hypodensity of the left (L) frontoparietal cerebral parenchyma suggestive of a (L) middle cerebral artery territory infarct

- Extra-osseous and soft tissue extension of bone tumours.
- Vascularity of the normal organ and the abnormal tissue can be evaluated and compared.

### Contraindications (Relative)

- Pregnancy
- Restless patients

### Interpretation of Images

- Structures imaged appear densely white to densely black depending on the absorption of X-rays and the emerging resultant X-rays which are detected. **The composite picture is actually a collection of Hounsfield numbers.** Each Hounsfield number being assigned a specific shade of grey, thus producing a picture that might be easily understood. Some of the common densities to be encountered in practice are as follows (Hounsfield units = HU):

| | |
|---|---|
| Air | –1000 HU |
| Fat | –50 to –100 HU |
| Water | 0 HU |
| CSF | 0 to +3 HU |
| White matter | +22 to +32 HU |
| Grey matter | +36 to +46 HU |
| Clotted blood | +60 to +80 HU |
| Calcification bone | +80 to +1000 HU |

- In order to increase the contrast that may exist between the structures in the body, **intravenous contrast (iodine containing) is administered.** Certain tissues show enhancement of their density and various pathologies also show fairly characteristic contrast uptake patterns (Figs 67.26 to 67.29).

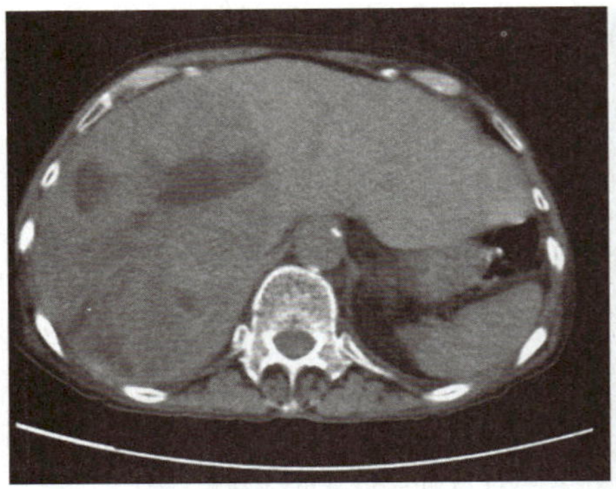
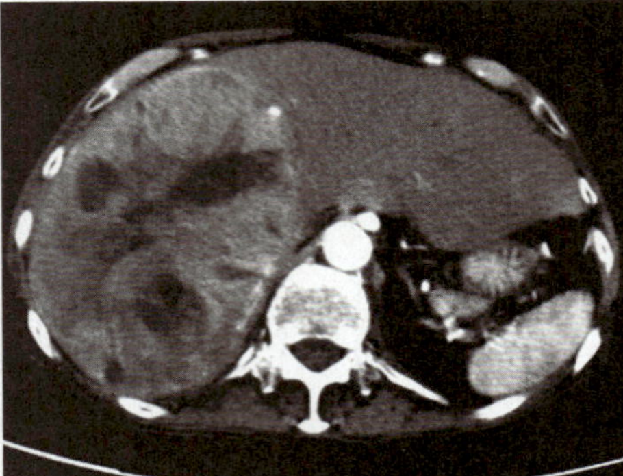
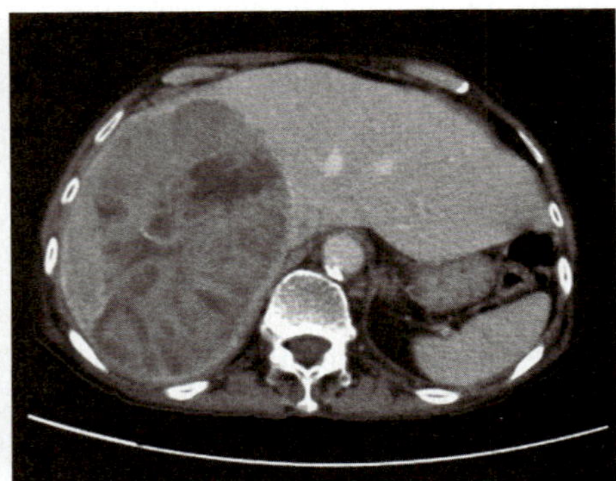

**Figs 67.26 to 67.28:** CT scan axial section through liver shows large mass in plain scan. Brightly enhancing in arterial phase of contrast study. Finally wash-out of contrast in portovenous phase which is a classical feature of hepatocellular carcinoma in multiphase contrast CT scan

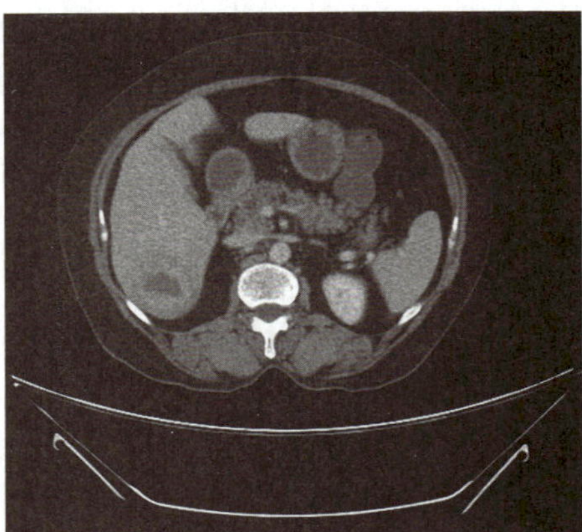

**Fig. 67.29: CT scan of abdomen:** Contrast-enhanced scan demonstrating a hypodense lesion in right lobe of liver posteriorly due to an abscess

- In abdominal scanning, **oral contrast** is administered to the patient before the procedure, to enable the operator to accurately separate the bowel loops from the other intra-abdominal structures.
- The advantages of CT over conventional radiology are that it can visualise extremely small pathology, not evident on conventional films, is cost-effective as multiple X-ray films and procedures can be avoided. It is noninvasive and the radiation levels applied to the patient are extremely low.

## VIRTUAL COLONOSCOPY

- It is a recently developed technique that uses a CT scanner and computer virtual reality software to look inside the body without having to insert a long tube (conventional colonoscopy) into the colon or without having to fill the colon with liquid barium (barium enema).
- More formally known as three-dimensional CT colonography, the virtual procedure allows radiologists to obtain 3D images from different angles, providing a sort of movie of the colon's interior without having to insert an endoscope into the bowel.

### Advantages

- Noninvasive procedure, well-tolerated by patient
- Requires no sedation, less time-consuming
- Useful in elderly who are frail and infirm
- Useful when a tumour is large enough to block passage of scope (Figs 67.30 and 67.31).

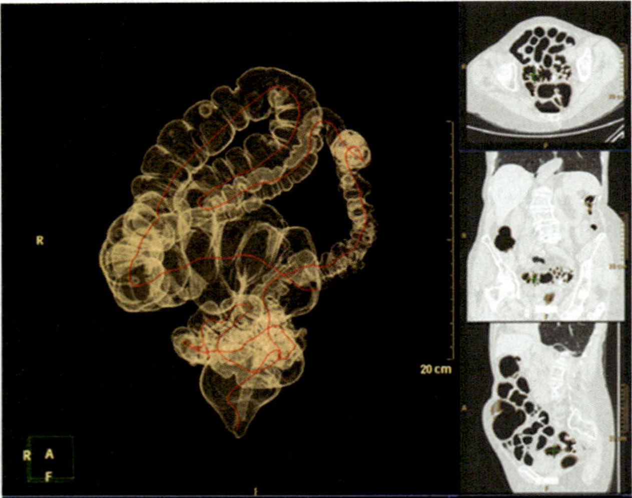

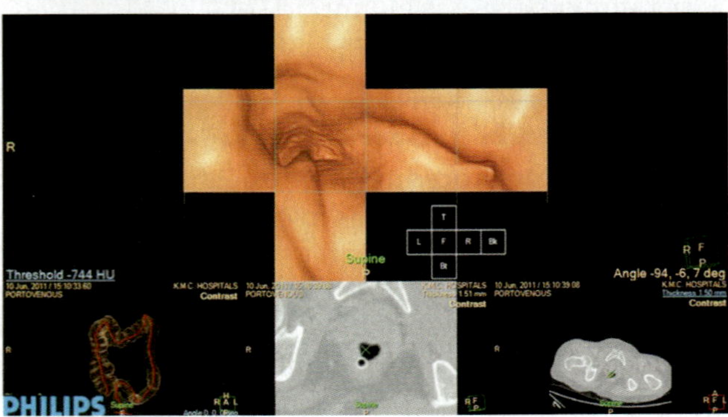


**Figs 67.30 and 67.31:** Virtual colonoscopy shows opened-up view to look for small mass or polyp

### Disadvantages

- Exposure to radiation, less detail of inner lining of colon
- Small polyps are located more reliably by colonoscopy
- Strictly a diagnostic procedure (unlike colonoscopy).

**A few examples are given below.**

## 1. CONTRAST ENHANCED (CE) CT ABDOMEN SHOWING MASS IN THE RIGHT ILIAC FOSSA

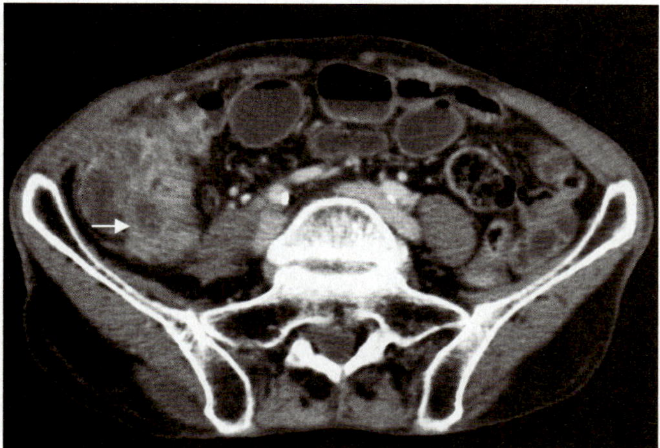

**Fig. 67.32:** A hypodense mass in the right iliac fossa involving caecum

1. **What is this investigation?**
   - Contrast-enhanced CT scan
2. **How to interpret the CT scan?**
   - Structures imaged appear as densely white or black.
3. **What is the name used to the picture in terms of number of units?**
   - Hounsfield units
4. **Why do you give contrast?**
   - This is to increase the density between various structures. *Example:* Aorta appears bright with contrast.
5. **What are the precautions?**
   - Pregnancy is a contraindication. Iodine containing contrast can give rise to nephropathy. Allergy to contrast can happen. Hence, dehydration should be corrected. Serum creatinine should be checked before contrast.
6. **When do you use oral contrast?**
   - While studying abdominal viscera, e.g. if leak is suspected.
7. **What is the finding here?**
   - It is showing a hypodense lesion in the right iliac fossa.
8. **What is the diagnosis?**
   - Mostly carcinoma caecum
9. **Why do you say so?**
   - Anatomically it is a lesion occupying the right iliac fossa involving caecum.
10. **How do you describe this?**
    - It is a hypodense mass with solid and cystic areas. Cystic areas represent tumour degeneration.
11. **What else is seen in this picture?**
    - Fat planes between the mass and the abdominal wall are obliterated.
12. **What is the importance of that?**
    - Probably it is infiltrating the abdominal wall.
13. **Why do you want to know this information?**
    - At surgery, the involved portion of the abdominal wall has to be removed.
14. **How do you confirm the diagnosis?**
    - Colonoscopy and biopsy
15. **What will be the report expected?**
    - In majority of the cases it is adenocarcinoma
16. **What is the treatment, if it is operable?**
    - Right radical hemicolectomy
17. **If it is inoperable, what is the treatment?**
    - Palliative ileo-transverse anastomosis

## 2. CECT SHOWING HYPODENSE LESION WITH AIR POCKETS IN THE LEFT SUBPHRENIC SPACE

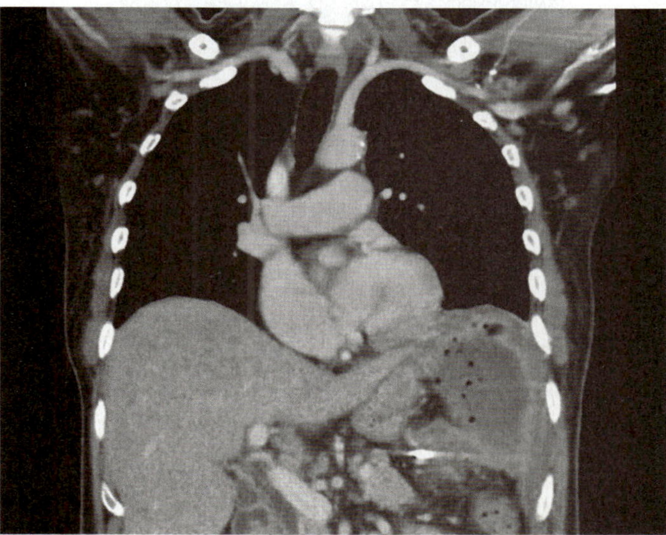

**Fig. 67.33:** CECT showing left subphrenic abscess

1. **What are the findings in this film?**
   - About 5 cm sized hypodense lesion with air-filled lesion.
2. **What is the most likely diagnosis?**
   - Abscess
3. **What are causes of abscess in that location?**
   - Pancreatic necrosis, posterior gastric perforations, ruptures liver abscess

4. **Left posterior subphrenic space is called as what?**
   - Lesser sac
5. **What is the treatment?**
   - Ultrasound-guided percutaneous aspiration of pus.

## CHOLANGIOGRAM/ERCP/MRCP

**Introduction:** These are used in the evaluation of biliary tract and pancreas. Details have been given in the gallbladder and pancreas chapter. T-tube cholangiogram is used following open choledochotomy. ERCP is preferred for evaluation of lower biliary obstructions, classical example being stones in the CBD. MRCP is used in the evaluation of high bile duct strictures or obstructions. A few examples are given below.

### 1. T-TUBE CHOLANGIOGRAPHY SHOWING A FILLING DEFECT IN THE LOWER END OF THE COMMON BILE DUCT (CBD)

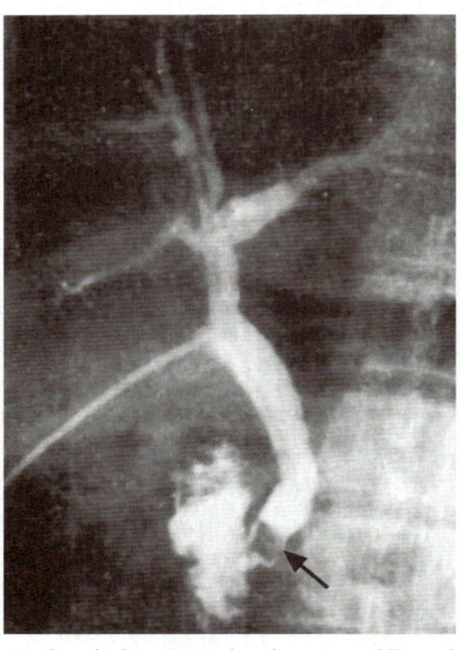

**Fig. 67.34:** T-tube cholangiography showing a filling defect in the lower end of the common bile duct (CBD)

1. **What is the diagnosis?**
   - Postcholecystectomy—residual stone in the CBD.
2. **What is the surgery done for this patient?**
   - Cholecystectomy and choledocholithotomy.
3. **Why do you insert a T-tube after CBD exploration?**
   - In case of distal obstruction by a residual stone, the bile starts leaking from the suture line on the CBD and may result in biliary peritonitis. In such situations, T-tube helps in drainage of the bile.
4. **What material is T-tube made of?**
   - Latex
5. **How do you treat this patient in order to extract the stone?**
   - Endoscopic sphincterotomy and extraction of the stone.

### 2. ERCP SHOWING FILLING OF THE DYE IN THE DUODENUM LOWER CBD AND PARTIAL FILLING OF INTRAHEPATIC BILE DUCT RADICALS. ALSO 3 CLIPS ARE VISIBLE ALONG THE LENGTH OF COMMON HEPATIC DUCT. GALLBLADDER IS NOT VISUALIZED

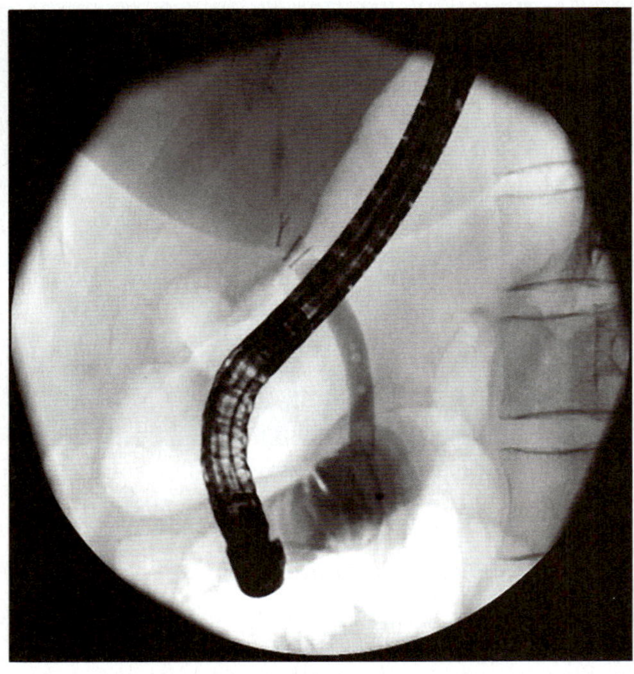

**Fig. 67.35:** ERCP showing partial obstruction of CBD/CHD caused by clips. Gallbladder is not seen.

1. **What is the diagnosis?**
   - Postcholecystectomy—stricture common hepatic duct/common hepatic duct.
2. **What is the type of injury is this?**
   - Strasberg D—probably a lateral injury due to partial clips.
3. **What is the next investigation?**
   - CET is done to know any significant bile collection/biloma—if present and if sepsis is present, better to explore.
4. **How do you treat this patient in order to eliminate sepsis?**
   - Explore, drain the bile, remove clips, if possible insert T-tube drain, Morrison's pouch and come out
5. **In cases of complete transections, how do you treat?**
   - If detected on table, do primary repair—hepaticojejunostomy. If detected later, assess for sepsis—treat it, improve nutrition and surgery can be done 4 to 6 weeks later.

## MAGNETIC RESONANCE IMAGING (MRI)

### Principle

Certain atomic nuclei, which possess unpaired protons or neutrons, have an inherent spin. The nucleus is positively charged and therefore creates a small magnetic field around itself, when it spins. The human body contains in abundance such spinning nuclei in the atoms of hydrogen which is found in water and lipids (Figs 67.36 to 67.40).

When the tissues containing these nuclei are within a strong magnetic field, the nuclei tend to align themselves along the lines of the force. The spinning protons now tend to precess, i.e. wobble about the axis of the main magnetic field. Now a radiofrequency (RF) is applied, being of the same frequency as the processing but at right angles to the main magnetic field. This excites the protons at low energy states into higher energy states. Thus, an absorption of energy takes place, which is used, as the excited protons 'relax' back to their original energy level when the radiofrequency is switched off. The relaxation of protons back to equilibrium and lower energy state is termed **spin-lattice relaxation** or **longitudinal relaxation**. It is exponential and referred to by the time **constant** T1. When the RF pulse is applied the protons process together in synchronism or in phase with each other. During relaxation, however, they go quickly out of phase due to small variations in local magnetic fields. This loss of phase is termed **spin-spin relaxation** or **transverse relaxation**. It is also an exponential and referred to by the time constant T2. Depending on the type of tissue under study, the T1 and T2 relaxation times will differ, thus giving rise to differences in the image.

The MRI image depends upon four main factors:

1. The T1 relaxation time
2. The T2 relaxation time
3. The proton density
4. The blood flow

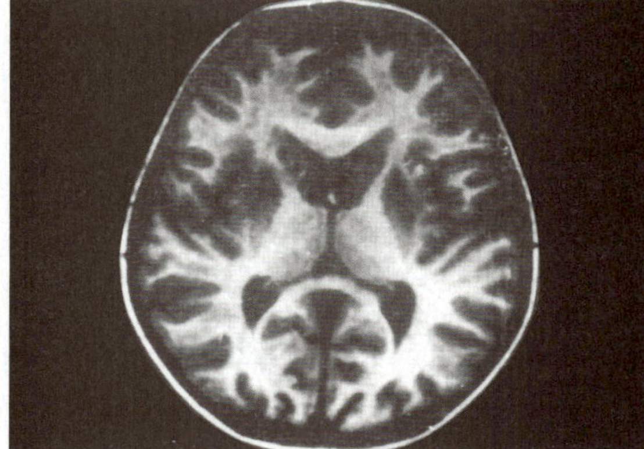

**Fig. 67.36:** MRI: T1- and T2-weighted axial and coronal scans of normal brain

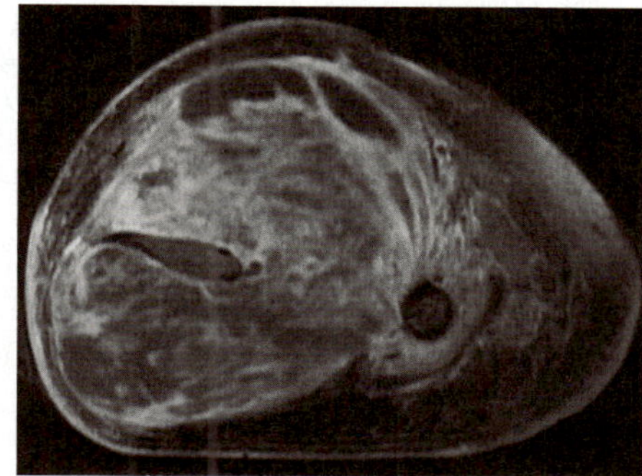

**Fig. 67.37:** Soft tissue sarcoma involving the muscle of thigh. The lesion is hyperintense in appearance

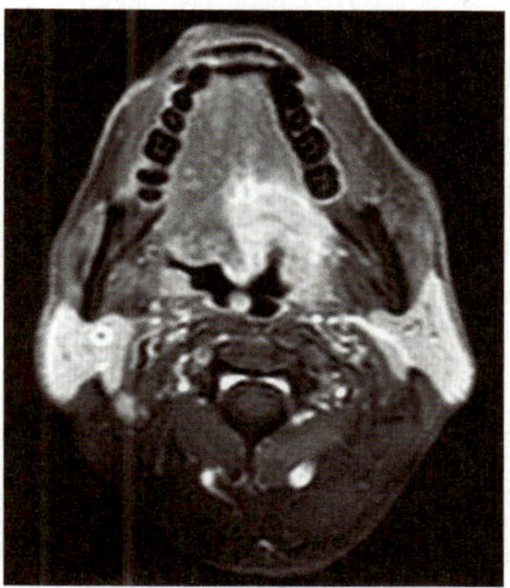

**Fig. 67.38:** Carcinoma tongue. MRI image shows hyperintense lesion is involving the posterior and base of the tongue on the left side. The other bright structures seen bilaterally are parotid glands

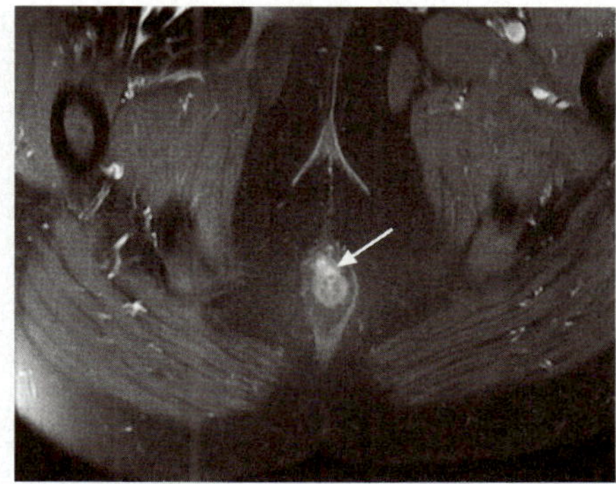

**Fig. 67.39:** Intersphincteric fistula—axial section of MRI pelvis showing hyperintense fistula (arrow)

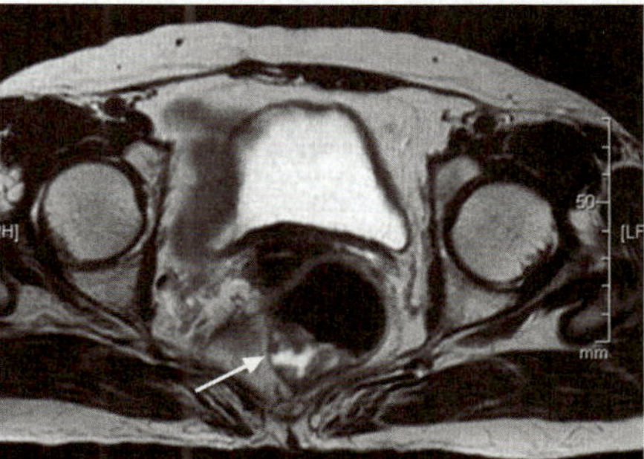

**Fig. 67.40:** Axial section of pelvis shows wall thickening of the rectal wall (arrow)

Depending on the characteristics of the above four parameters, the signal intensity of the image will vary, thus deciding the appearance that any given tissue will finally cast.

### Advantages of MRI

1. It is noninvasive.
2. It does not involve the use of ionising radiation. Hence, it is safe in that respect.
3. It gives high intrinsic contrast.
4. Direct transverse, sagittal and normal imaging possible.
5. No bone/air artefact.
6. It has no known biological hazard.

### Disadvantages of MRI

1. The imaging time is long. Hence, movement of the patients may produce artefacts.
2. Due to variety of protocol options during scanning, the final image is highly operator-dependent and this requires expert technical staff.
3. Expensive
4. Poor bone and calcium detail
5. **Patients with pacemakers, metallic implants and critically ill patients cannot be scanned.**

**A few examples are given below.**

## 1. MRI SHOWING STONES IN THE CBD

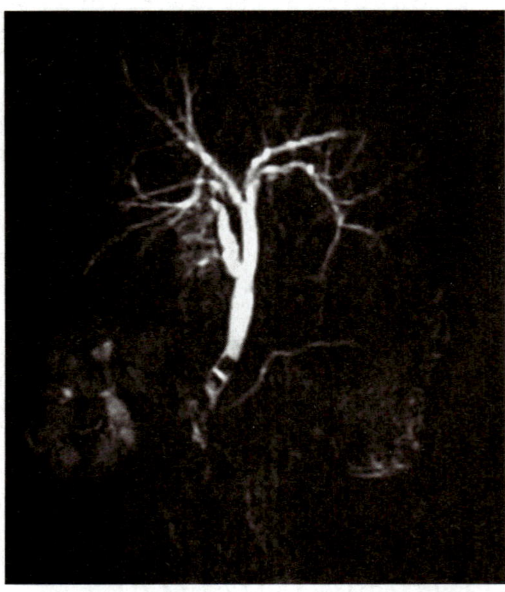

**Fig. 67.41:** MRI showing stones in the CBD

1. **What structures are seen here?**
   - Intrahepatic radicles, common bile duct and duodenum.
2. **What are the findings?**
   - Filling defects are seen as dark shadows in the CBD.
3. **What is the final diagnosis?**
   - Choledocholithiasis
4. **What are the advantages of MRI?**
   - It is non-ionizing and no contrast is used.
5. **How do you treat this condition?**
   - ERCP, basketting of stones followed by laparoscopic cholecystectomy.

## 2. MRI OF THE THIGH

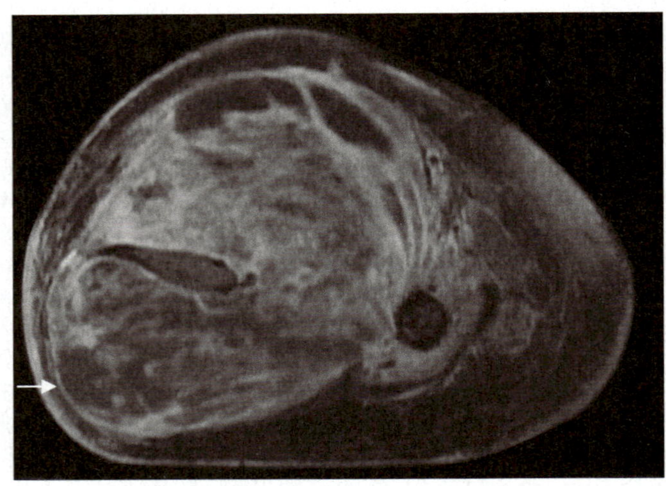

**Fig. 67.42:** MRI of the thigh

1. **Name this investigation.**
   - Magnetic resonance imaging
2. **What are the principles of MRI?**
   - Certain atomic nuclei, which possess unpaired protons or neutrons, possess an inherent spin. The nucleus is positively charged and, therefore, creates a small magnetic field around itself, when it spins. The human body contains in abundance such spinning nuclei in the atoms of hydrogen, which is found in water and lipids.
3. **What are the chief advantages of MRI over CT scan?**
   - It is noninvasive and does not involve the use of ionising radiation. Hence, it is safe.
4. **What are the disadvantages of MRI?**
   - The imaging time is long. Hence, movement of the patients may produce artefacts.
   - Expensive
   - Patients with pacemakers, metallic implant and critically ill patients cannot be scanned.
   - Claustrophobia
5. **What does this picture show?**
   - A hyperintense mass occupying the thigh region.
6. **What is the diagnosis?**
   - Soft tissue sarcoma
7. **How do you confirm the diagnosis?**
   - Tru-cut biopsy

**8. Why not FNAC?**

- FNAC cannot diagnose the type of sarcoma.

**9. What are common tumours in this location?**

- Malignant fibrous histiocytoma (MFH) and liposarcoma.

**10. What is the treatment?**

- Wide excision with 2–3 cm margin.

**Few MRI images:**

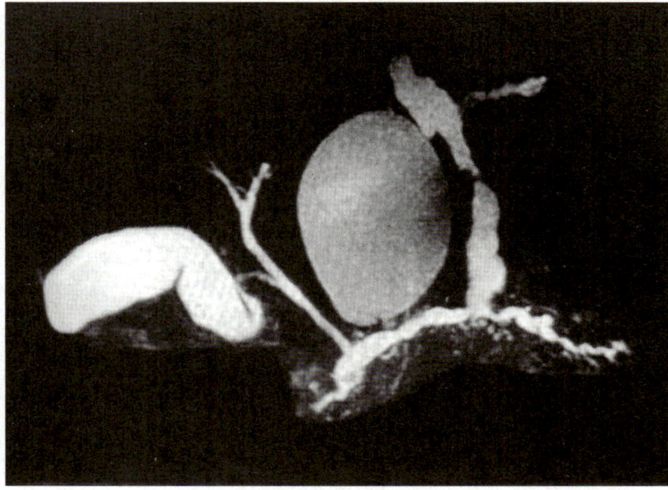

**Fig. 67.43:** MRI showing pancreaticopleural fistula

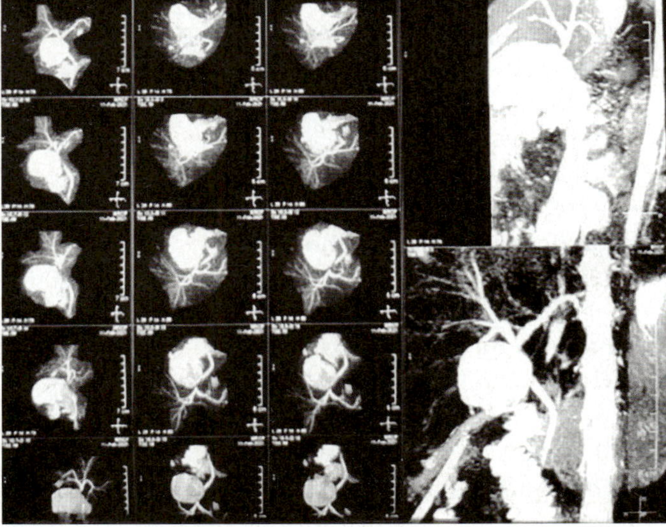

**Fig. 67.44:** MRI showing leak from bile duct after cholecystectomy

## POSITRON EMISSION TOMOGRAPHY (PET SCAN)

- PET scan is a medical imaging technique that combines computed tomography (CT) and nuclear scanning. It is used to determine the metabolic or biochemical activity in the brain, heart and other organs by tracking the movement and concentration of a radioactive tracer injected into the blood stream.
- A camera records the tracer's signal as it travels through the body and collects information about the organs. A computer then converts the signals into 3D images of the examined organ, which provide a clear view of an abnormality.
- One of the main differences between PET scan and other imaging tests like CT or MRI is that the PET scan reveals the cellular level metabolic changes occurring in an organ and functional changes at cellular level. A PET scan often detects these changes very early, whereas CT or MRI detect changes a little later as the disease begins to cause structural changes in organs or tissues.
- Positron emission tomography (PET-CT) constitutes major progress in management of cancer patients for the initial diagnosis, staging and follow-up of various malignancies. PET-CT is also useful in the follow-up of patients following chemotherapy or surgical resection of tumour, since, most of them have a confusing appearance at CT or MR imaging due to postoperative changes or scar tissue (Figs 67.45 to 67.50).

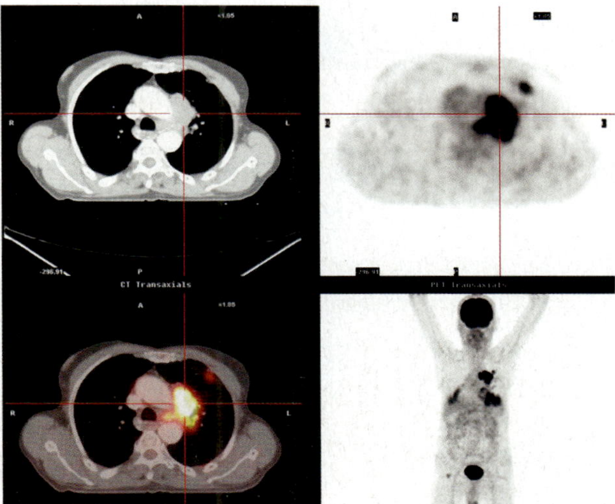


**Fig. 67.45:** Carcinoma breast with metastasis

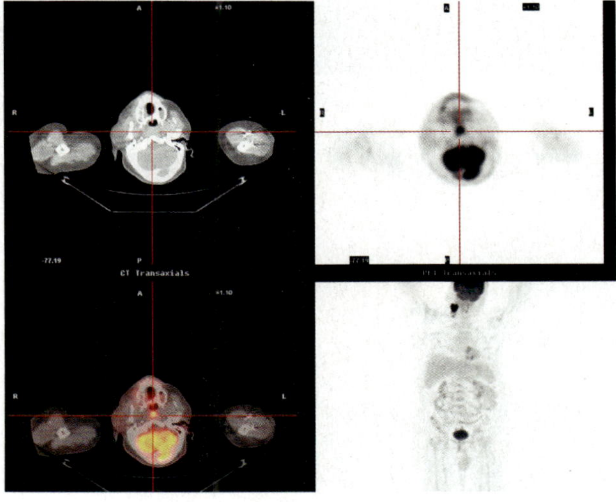


**Fig. 67.46:** Carcinoma oesophagus

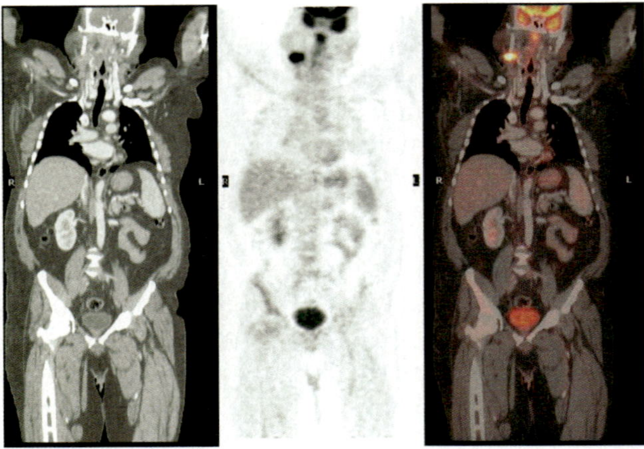
Fig. 67.47: Carcinoma lung—PET-CT scan

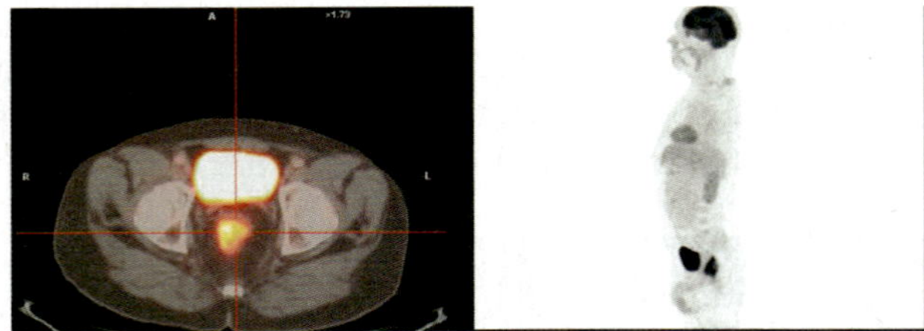
Fig. 67.48: Carcinoma nasopharynx—PET-CT scan

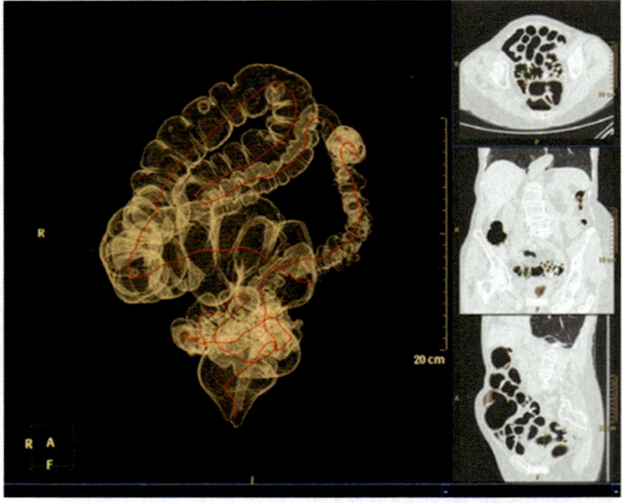
Fig. 67.49: Another case of carcinoma nasopharynx

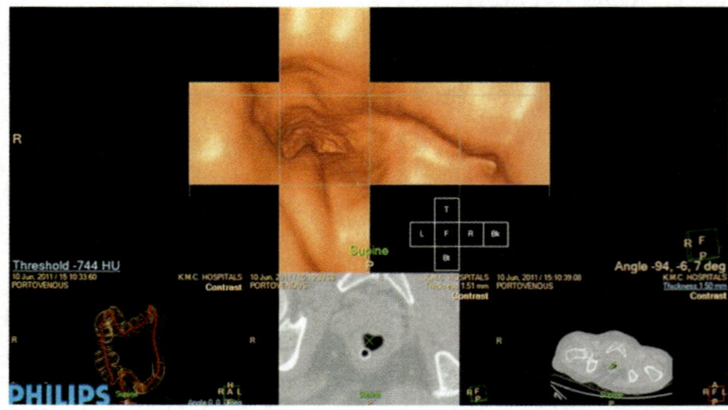

Fig. 67.50: Carcinoma rectum—PET-CT scan

## 1. POSITRON EMISSION TOMOGRAPHY (PET) SCAN

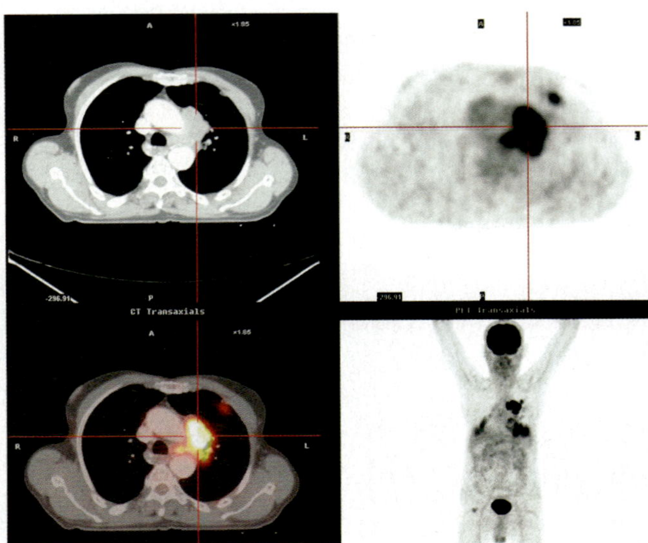

Fig. 67.51: CT and PET of lung

1. **Name this investigation.**
   - PET-CT scan
2. **What is PET scan?**
   - Positron emission tomography
3. **What is the most commonly used positron emitting radionuclide?**
   - Fluorodeoxyglucose (FDG).
4. **What are the chief uses of PET scan?**
   - For myocardial perfusion and viability, detection of metastasis from cancer—carcinoma lung, colon, nasopharynx, etc.
5. **What are the disadvantages?**
   - Very expensive and limited availability.
6. **What does this picture show?**
   - Hilar mass with a nodule anteriorly on the left side of pleura
7. **What may be the diagnosis?**
   - Carcinoma lung
8. **How do you confirm the diagnosis?**
   - Bronchoscopy and biopsy
9. **If the report is adenocarcinoma lung, what is the next step?**
   - To stage the disease by whole body bone scan, PET scan, and CT scan.
10. **If confined to lung, what is the treatment?**
    - Lobectomy/pneumonectomy.

## INTERVENTIONAL RADIOLOGY

The role of radiology was limited as only a diagnostic art until mid-1970s. However, now radiology has taken on an exciting new aspect and has entered the field of interventional radiology. Two main types of interventional procedures: Vascular and nonvascular.

### Vascular

1. **Angioplasty:** This is performed by the use of intraluminal balloon catheters and may be performed for almost any diseased vessel in the body. The more commonly treated vessels are the coronaries, renal arteries, peripheral limb vessels, etc.
2. **Embolisation:** This procedure is performed either preoperatively to reduce the vascularity of certain tumours, or as a curative treatment for vascular malformations, aneurysms, GI bleeding, etc. Temporary embolisation may be achieved by using gel foam or autologous clots and permanent embolisation by using balloons, steel coils, ethanol, etc. Inferior vena cava (IVC) umbrella placement, IVC membranotomy are also done.
3. **Intravascular ultrasound:** The use of ultrasound inside a blood vessel to visualise the interior of the vessel in order to detect problems inside the blood vessel.
4. **Stent placement:** A tiny, expandable coil, called a stent, is placed inside a blood vessel at the site of a blockage. The stent is expanded to open up the blockage.
   - **Important types of stents and stent selection: Self-expanding stents** are compressed within a catheter device and released by removing a constraining sheath or membrane. The final diameter of the stent is a function of the outward elastic load of the stent and the inward recoil of the elastic wall.
   - **Balloon expandable stents** are mounted on angioplasty balloons in a compressed state and then deployed by balloon inflation. These stents retain the diameter imposed by angioplasty balloon unless externally compressed.
5. **Foreign body extraction:** The use of a catheter inserted into a blood vessel to retrieve a foreign body in the vessel.
6. **Needle biopsy:** A small needle is inserted into the abnormal area in almost any part of the body, guided by imaging techniques, to obtain a tissue biopsy. This type of biopsy can provide a diagnosis without surgical intervention.
7. **Blood clot filters:** A small filter is inserted into a blood clot to catch and break up blood clots.
8. **Injection of clot-lysing agents:** Clot-lysing agents, such as tissue plasminogen activator (tPA) are injected into the body to dissolve blood clots, thereby increasing blood flow to the heart or brain.
9. **Catheter insertions:** A catheter is inserted into large veins for giving chemotherapy drugs, nutritional support, and haemodialysis. A catheter may also be inserted prior to bone marrow transplantation.
10. **Cancer treatment:** Administering cancer medications directly to the tumour site.

### Nonvascular

1. **Hepatobiliary:** Percutaneous transhepatic biliary drainage (PTBD) is widely accepted in cases of biliary obstruction, along with percutaneous biliary calculus removal. Biliary stent placement across a malignant lesion is widely being done in inoperable cases as a palliative procedure.
2. **Urinary:** Percutaneous nephrostomy, percutaneous stenting and percutaneous nephrolithotomy are being performed.
3. **Guided biopsy:** Fluoroscopy, ultrasound or CT-guided biopsy of various lesions are now part of routine technique.
4. **Other interventional procedures:** Percutaneous gastrostomy, catheter drainage of abscesses, pseudocysts, ultrasound-guided intrauterine foetal surgeries, etc.

### Advantages of Interventional Procedures

1. Patient compliance is high as surgery is avoided.
2. Cost-effectiveness is high.
3. Infection rates are low.
4. Can be repeated as it is relatively noninvasive.
5. Certain untreatable conditions are treated palliatively with interventional procedures.

> ***Please Note:*** X-rays discussed here are the common X-rays which are asked in the MBBS examination. However, modern investigations such as mammogram, ultrasound, CT scan and MRI also may be asked. You are requested to read the chapters on radiology and breast for more details about these investigations.

## MULTIPLE CHOICE QUESTIONS

**1. Niche and a notch mark is an absolute contra-indication for myelography:**
A. Chronic duodenal ulcer
B. Chronic gastric ulcer
C. Carcinoma stomach
D. Stromal tumour

**2. Trifoliate/clover deformity is diagnostic of:**
A. Chronic duodenal ulcer
B. Chronic gastric ulcer
C. Carcinoma stomach
D. Stromal tumour

**3. The substance used in barium studies is:**
A. Barium chloride B. Barium sulphate
C. Barium carbonate D. Barium sulphide

**4. Barium follow through extends up to:**
A. Proximal duodenum
B. Fundus of the stomach
C. Ileocaecal junction
D. Proximal jejunum

**5. Which of the following is a contraindication for barium study?**
A. Dysphagia and odynophagia
B. Motility disorders of the GIT
C. Perforation of gastric mucosa
D. Assessing mediastinal masses

**6. Achalasia cardia shows the following findings on barium swallow, *except*:**
A. Shouldering effect cranial and caudal to the lesion
B. Rat tail appearance of lower end of the oesophagus
C. Gross dilatation of the proximal oesophagus
D. Thin streaks of contrast entering the stomach

**7. 'Moulage' sign (barium in a featureless tube) is a feature of:**
A. Crohn's disease B. Intestinal TB
C. Ulcerative colitis D. Malabsorption

**8. Which of the following statements is false?**
A. Angiographic studies use $^{123}$I as contrast substance
B. Enteroclysis is done for mechanical obstruction of the intestine
C. Peripheral venography done for deep vein thrombosis uses $^{125}$I
D. Papilloedema is an absolute contraindication for myelography

**9. Which of the following statements is false?**
A. Ultrasound is based on the principle of piezo-electric effect, the most common substance used in ultrasonic transducers being lead zirconate titanate (PZT)
B. MRI uses ionising radiation, hence it is unsafe
C. Patients with pacemakers and critically ill patients cannot be scanned using MRI
D. CT scan gives good bone and calcium detail

**10. The most common side effect of peripheral venography is:**
A. Complications due to contrast
B. Tissue necrosis
C. Thrombophlebitis
D. Pulmonary embolism due to dislodged clot

**11. Which of the following statements is false about PET scan?**
A. PET scan uses protons for radiological examination
B. It combines CT and nuclear scanning
C. It detects changes at the cellular level
D. It helps in early detection of changes in various pathologies.

**12. BI-RADS score of 5 indicates which of the following?**
A. Normal mammogram, no evidence of cancer
B. Mammogram normal, some evidence of cancer present
C. Suspicious findings on mammogram, 20–35% chance of cancer
D. Mammogram findings highly suspicious, 95% chance of cancer

**13. The following statements about virtual colonoscopy are true, *except*:**
A. It is also called CT pneumocolon, purely diagnostic
B. It is invasive, requires sedation and contra-indicated in elderly
C. It involves exposure to radiation
D. It cannot identify polyps measuring between 2 and 10 mm

**14. Which of the following in future may be a gold standard test for screening of colorectal cancer?**
A. PET scan
B. Sigmoidoscopy and colonoscopy
C. MRI
D. Virtual colonoscopy

**15. The following is true about MRI, *except*:**
A. It is noninvasive
B. Gives high intrinsic contrast
C. Imaging possible in transverse, sagittal and normal views
D. Bone/air artefact can be a problem

### Answers

**1.** B **2.** A **3.** B **4.** C **5.** C **6.** A **7.** D **8.** A **9.** B **10.** A
**11.** A **12.** D **13.** B **14.** D **15.** D

Chapter 68

# Instruments, Sutures, Needles, Skin and Anastomosis

- Forceps
- Retractors
- Occlusion clamps
- Dilators
- Tracheostomy tube
- Rubber tubes
- Catheters
- Sengstaken tube
- Needles
- Suture
- Skin closure techniques
- Intestinal resection and anastomosis

## ARTERY FORCEPS (HAEMOSTAT)

- It is also called **Spencer Well's artery forceps**. It has a ratchet and two blades with uniform serrations.
- It is used to control bleeding, not only from arteries but also from veins and capillaries. Once the bleeding points are caught, they are coagulated or ligature is applied.
- The smaller version of this is called mosquito forceps (Fig. 68.1A). This is extremely useful in repair of harelip, cleft palate or other plastic surgery operations.
- The curved artery is commonly used (Fig. 68.1B).
- It is also available as straight artery which is used to hold the stay sutures (Fig. 68.1C).

## ALLIS TISSUE HOLDING FORCEPS (Fig. 68.2)

- It has a ratchet and triangular expansion at the tip, where serrations are present.
- It can be used to **hold tough structures** such as fascia, aponeurosis, etc.

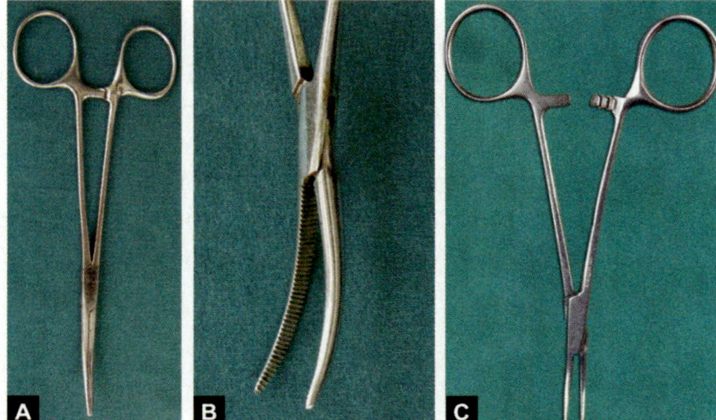


**Figs 68.1A to C:** (A) Mosquito forceps; (B) Curved artery forceps; (C) Straight artery forceps

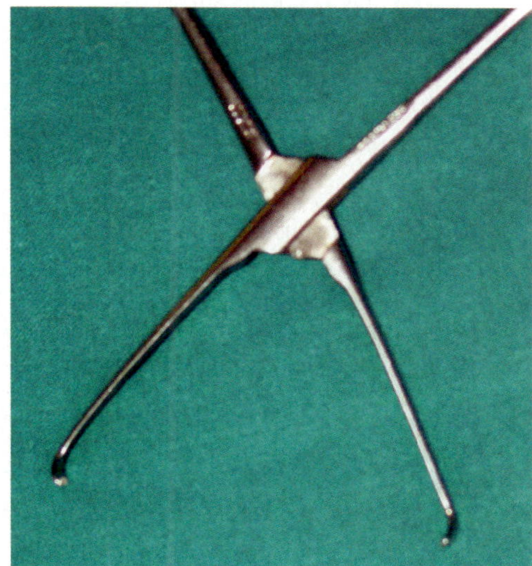

**Fig. 68.2:** Allis forceps

- Even though it can cause trauma, because of its better grip, it can be used to hold the duodenum for duodenal closure during gastrectomy.

## KOCHER'S FORCEPS (Fig. 68.3 and Key Box 68.1)

- This is similar to an artery forceps with serrations. It is available as curved and straight.
- There is a sharp tooth at the tip of the instrument. Hence, it has a better grip.
- Kocher's forceps can be used to **hold tough structures** like **aponeurosis, fascia**, etc.
- During thyroidectomy, it can be used to hold the strap muscles for dividing them.
- Theodor Kocher, a Swiss surgeon, got the Nobel prize for his contribution to thyroid surgery.

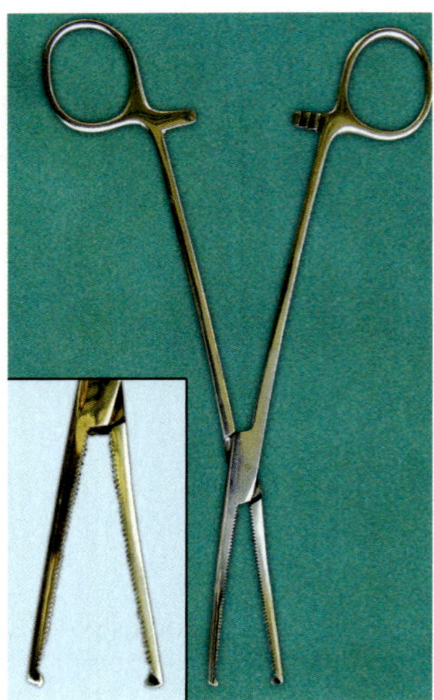

Fig. 68.3: Kocher's forceps

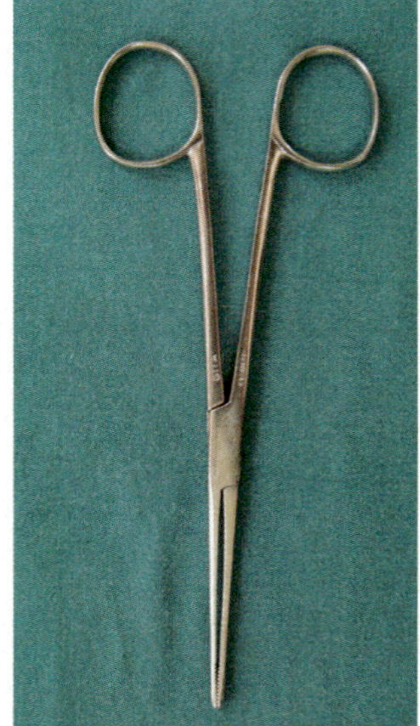

Fig. 68.4: Sinus forceps

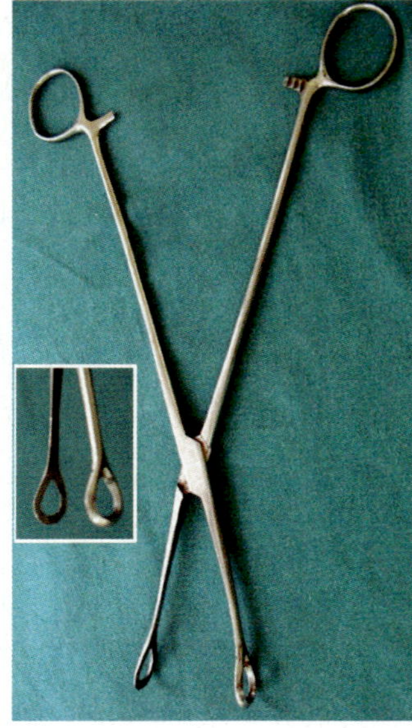

Fig. 68.5: Swab holding forceps

Key Box 68.1

**Remember**

- Kocher's forceps
- Kocher's test
- Kocher's collar incision for thyroidectomy
- Kocher's sign—eyelid phenomenon in hyperthyroidism-staring and frightened look
- Kocher's thyroid dissector
- Kocher's vein
- Kocher's subcostal incision
- Kocher's gland holding forceps

## SINUS FORCEPS (Fig. 68.4)

- This is like an artery forceps which has **No ratchet**.
- Serrations are confined to the tip so as to hold the wall of an abscess cavity, for biopsy.
- In ***Hilton's method*** of drainage of an abscess, once the incision is made, the sinus forceps is thrust into the abscess cavity and by opening the blades in all directions, the loculi are broken. To facilitate free opening of the blades, sinus forceps has no ratchet.

## SWAB HOLDING FORCEPS (Fig. 68.5)

- This has a ratchet and two long blades
- Operating end is rounded with serrations
- It is used to hold the swab (gauze pieces) to prepare the parts with antiseptic agents at the time of surgery.
- This instrument can also be used as a blunt 'dissector' with the swab, while dissecting at a depth, e.g. lumbar sympathectomy, vagotomy.

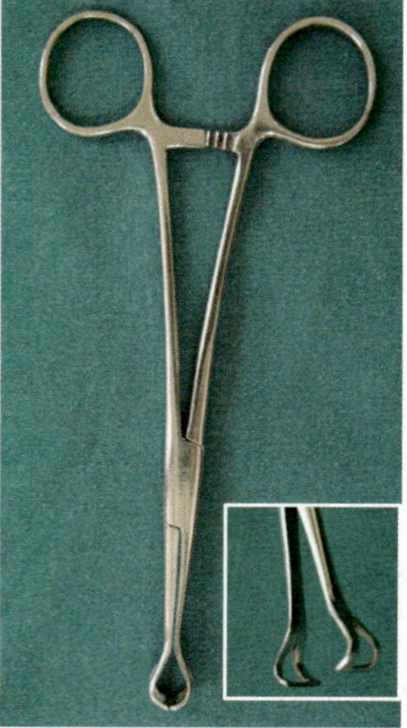

Fig. 68.6: Babcock's forceps

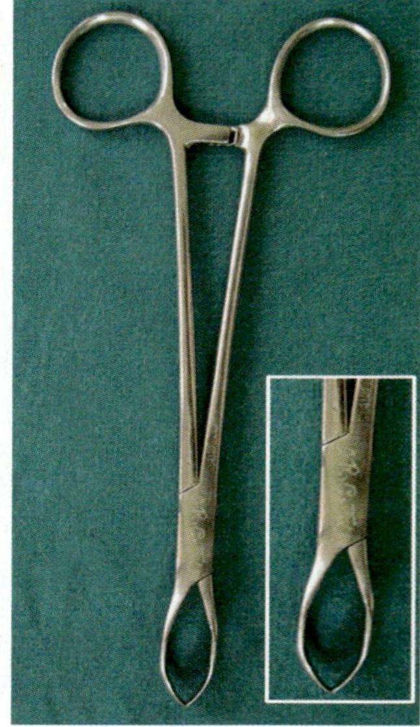

Fig. 68.7: Lane's forceps

## BABCOCK'S FORCEPS (Fig. 68.6)

- An instrument with a ratchet and a triangular expansion with fenestrations at the operating end. It does not have any teeth. Thus, it is used to hold intestines during anastomosis or resection.
- This instrument can also be used to hold many other structures such as thyroid gland, mesoappendix, uterine tubes, etc.

## LANE'S FORCEPS (Fig. 68.7)

- This is similar to Babcock's forceps but the tip is more broad, expanded with a bigger opening.
- It is used to hold the appendix

- However, it does not seem to have any additional advantage when compared to Babcock's forceps.

## DISSECTING FORCEPS (Fig. 68.8)

- This is a toothed forceps. It is also available as non-toothed forceps.
- Dissecting forceps with dissecting scissors makes good 'tool' for a surgeon to develop a tissue plane in majority of surgeries.
- The forceps is very useful to 'pick' individual layers such as serosa, seromuscular layers, mucosa, etc. during anastomosis.

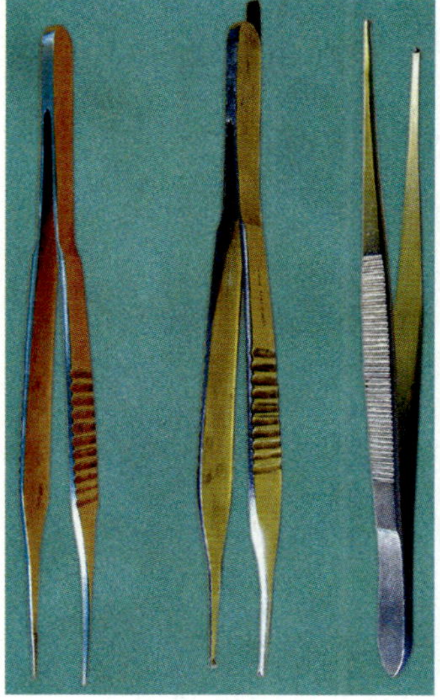

**Fig. 68.8:** Dissecting forceps

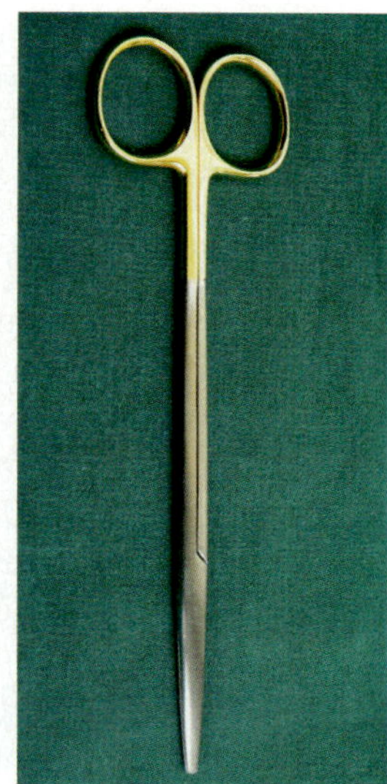

**Fig. 68.9:** Mayo's scissors

## DISSECTING SCISSORS

- This is also called **Mayo's scissors** (Fig. 68.9 and Key Box 68.2).
- It does not have ratchet and operating end is sharp
- This is used to dissect tissue planes during surgical operations and to cut or divide important structures.
- It is popularly called **tissue scissors**.

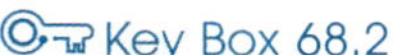

Key Box 68.2

**Remember**

- Mayo's scissors
- Mayo's herniorrhaphy
- Mayo's posterior GJ
- Mayo's vein
- Mayo's needle (used for hernia repair)

## STRAIGHT SCISSORS (Fig. 68.10)

It is used to cut the sutures or knots. Hence, called suture-cutting scissors.

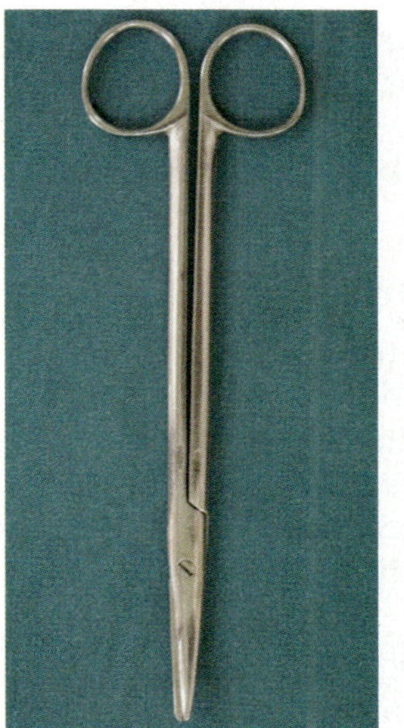

**Fig. 68.10:** Straight scissors

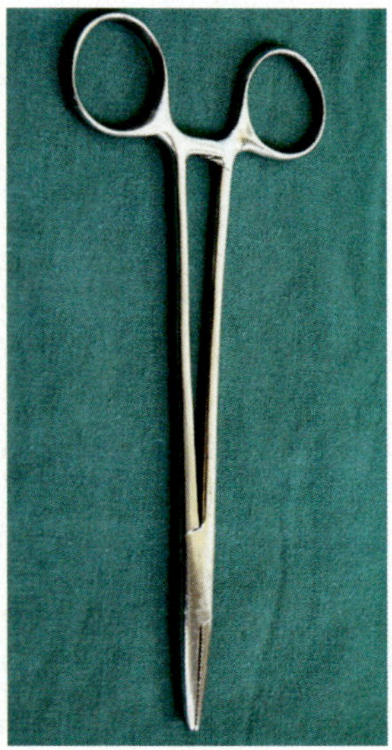

**Fig. 68.11:** Needle holder

## NEEDLE HOLDER (Fig. 68.11)

- This is a long instrument with a ratchet at non-operating end.
- The operating end has two small blades with serrations.
- The instrument is used to **hold the curved needles** which are used to suture the parts.
- A firm grip is essential to apply proper sutures.

## SCALPEL WITH BLADE (Fig. 68.12)

- This is popularly called **surgeon's knife.**
- This is used to incise the skin and subcutaneous tissue.
- Due to the sharp nature, it can be used to divide a major vascular pedicle once ligatures are applied.

## CHEATLES FORCEPS (Fig. 68.13)

- It is a long instrument having a curved shaft
- The **handle has no lock**

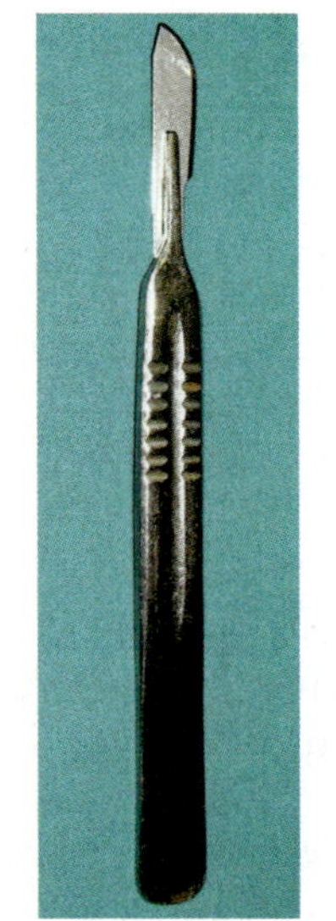

**Fig. 68.12:** Scalpel with blade

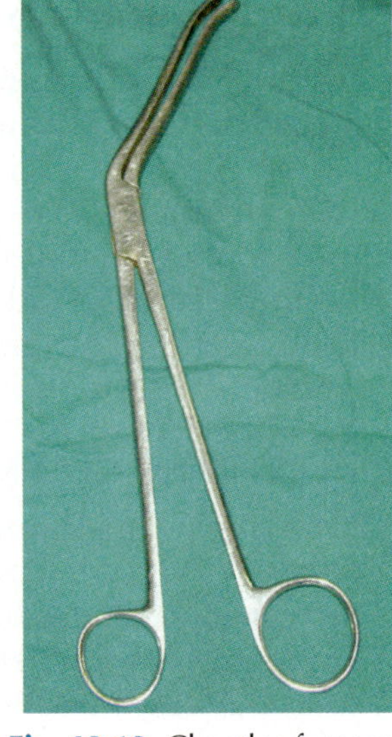

**Fig. 68.13:** Cheatles forceps

- It is kept dipped in antiseptic solutions
- This instrument is used to pick up sterilised articles such as sponges, gauze pieces or other instruments and to transfer to the instrument trolley.

## DEAVER RETRACTOR (Fig. 68.14)

- This is popularly called **Deaver liver retractor**
- It has a long blade and operating end is curved
- It can be used to retract the liver during vagotomy, cholecystectomy or gastrectomy, etc.
- Since, it has long blades, it can be used to retract the kidney upwards, during lumbar sympathectomy or to retract the urinary bladder during surgery on the rectum.

## MORRIS RETRACTOR (Fig. 68.15)

- This is a long instrument with broad operating end.
- This is used **to retract the abdominal wall**, once the peritoneum is opened.
- However, if a self-retaining retractor is used to widen the laparotomy wound, the use of Morris retractor gets limited.
- Fenestration (opening) makes an instrument lighter in weight.

## CZERNY RETRACTOR (Fig. 68.16)

- This is a double-hooked retractor on one side and a single blade on the other side.
- This is a **superficial retractor**, can be used to retract layers of the abdominal wall, muscles, etc. Thus, during appendicectomy, herniorrhaphy or thyroidectomy, this instrument is very useful.

## LANGENBECK RETRACTOR (Fig. 68.17)

- This instrument has only **one blade**
- The uses of this are similar to that of Czerny's retractor.

## MOYNIHAN'S STRAIGHT OCCLUSION CLAMP (Fig. 68.18)

- This is a long instrument with a ratchet. The operating end has two long blades with serrations in the line of blades.
- This instrument is used to **occlude the intestinal lumen** to prevent spillage of intestinal contents during intestinal resection or intestinal anastomosis.
- This does not interfere with the vascularity of the intestine.

## PAYR'S CRUSHING CLAMP (Fig. 68.19)

- This is a heavy instrument with **double lever system**, because of which it has a better grip
- The two short blades have uniform serrations
- During gastrectomy, when portion of the stomach is excised, this instrument is applied on the stomach side so that the stomach with this instrument is excised.

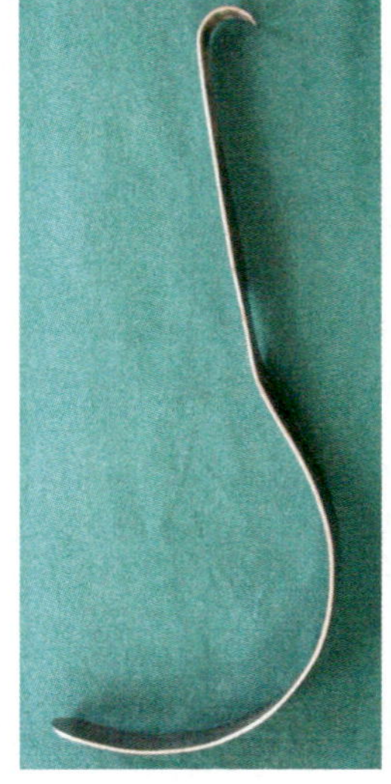

**Fig. 68.14:** Deaver retractor

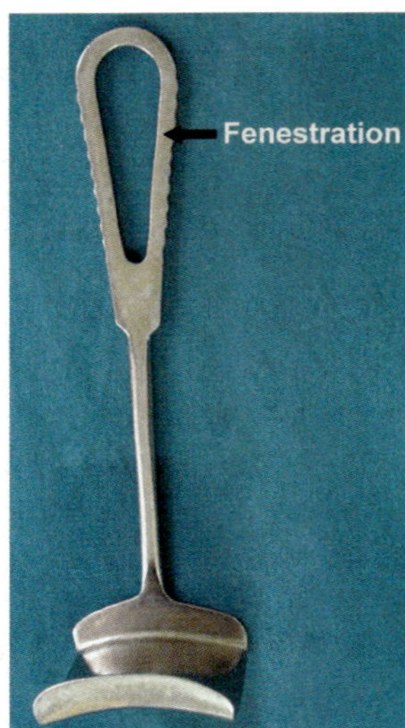


**Fig. 68.15:** Morris retractor

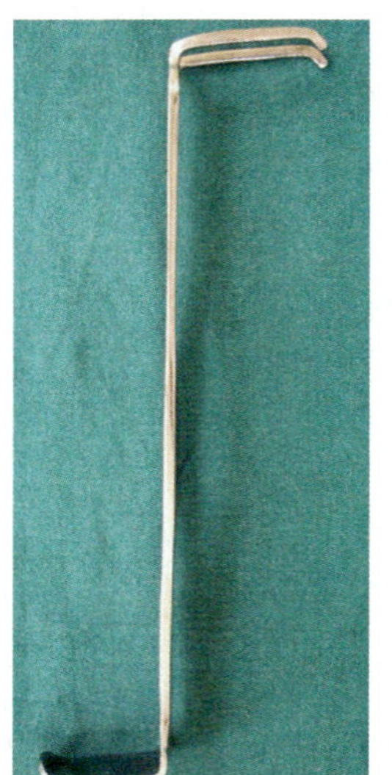

**Fig. 68.16:** Czerny retractor

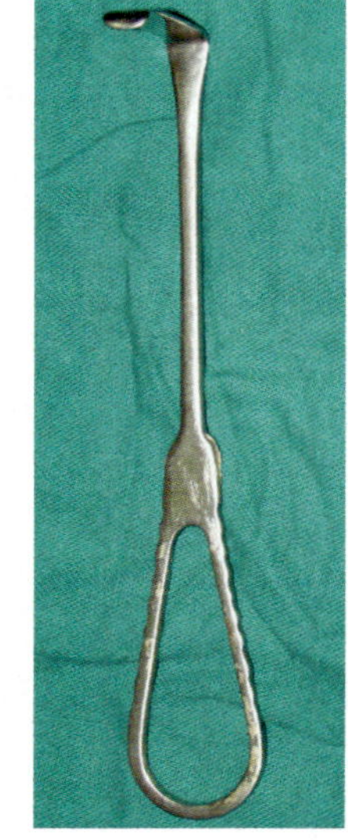

**Fig. 68.17:** Langenbeck retractor

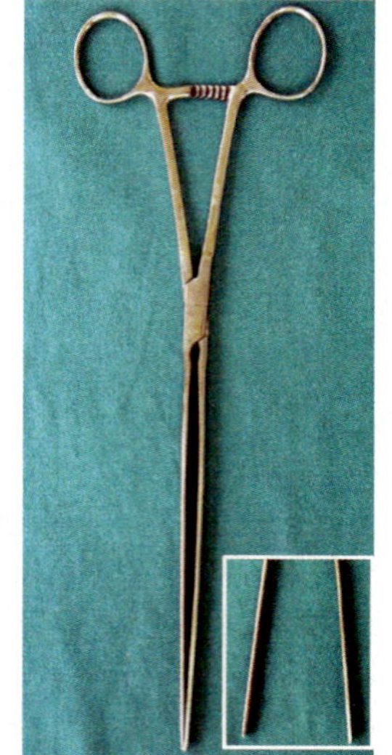

**Fig. 68.18:** Moynihan's occlusion clamp

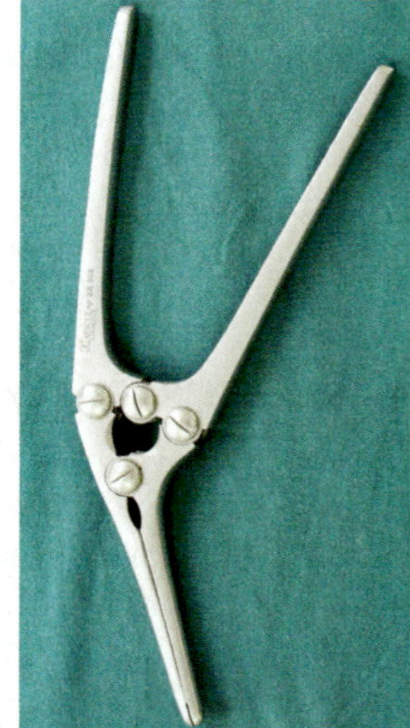

**Fig. 68.19:** Payr's crushing clamp

## DESJARDIN'S CHOLEDOCHOLITHOTOMY FORCEPS (Fig. 68.20)

- This is a long curved instrument with no **ratchet**
- The operating end is expanded with fenestrations
- The tip is blunt
- It is used to **extract stones from common bile duct**. It can also be used to extract stones from the ureter.
- Since there is no ratchet, free opening is possible, and the stones do not get crushed.

## BAKE'S DILATOR (Fig. 68.21)

- This is a long malleable instrument available in various diameters.
- It has a handle, long body and the tip is blunt.
- Once common bile duct exploration is completed, this dilator is passed, to assess for any distal obstruction.
- The free passage of Bake's dilators of different sizes indicate that there is no distal obstruction (however, to be confirmed by cholangiogram).

## KOCHER'S THYROID DISSECTOR (Fig. 68.22)

- This has a long handle and the operating end is small and blunt with an opening.
- A few longitudinal serrations are present at the tip.
- This was used to dissect the upper pole of thyroid gland.
- This instrument can also be used to dissect the isthmus of the thyroid gland from the trachea.
- **Silk thread can be fed** into the opening so as to ligate the vascular pedicle or isthmus.
- With the availability of the right-angled forceps, this instrument is not in routine use nowadays.

## ANEURYSM NEEDLE (Fig. 68.23)

- It is a long instrument with an ***eye*** at the operating end.
- It is called aneurysm needle because it was used to ligate the feeding artery in an aneurysm. However today, this instrument is of limited use.
- During **venesection or cut down**, the silk suture can be threaded within the ***eye***, passed round the vein and it is tied.

## TROCAR AND CANNULA (Fig. 68.24)

- This has two parts. The inner sharp part is the trocar and outer blunt part is cannula.
- It is used to drain hydrocoele fluid.
- Once hydrocoele sac is delivered, it is punctured with trocar and cannula, the trocar removed and the fluid drained.
- Make sure that trocar and cannula should match, otherwise injury to the deeper structures (testis) can occur.

## HUMBY'S KNIFE (Fig. 68.25)

- This instrument has a handle and a long sheath.
- When in use, a disposable blade can be attached to it.
- The instrument is used to take skin graft. Hence, it is also called skin grafting knife.
- To facilitate the exact thickness of the skin to be removed, there is a screw at the operating end, with which, prior adjustment should be done.

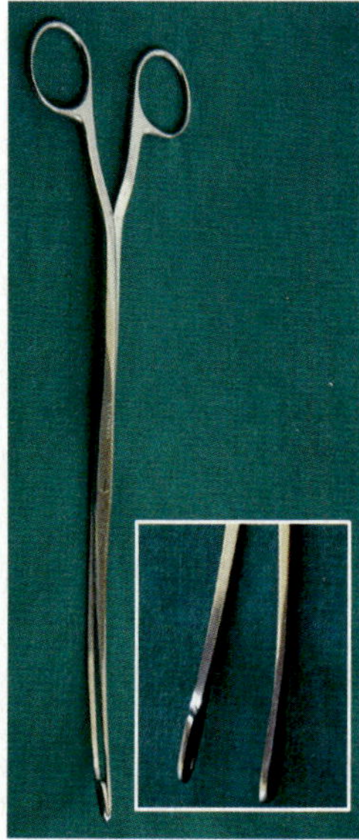

**Fig. 68.20:** Desjardin's forceps

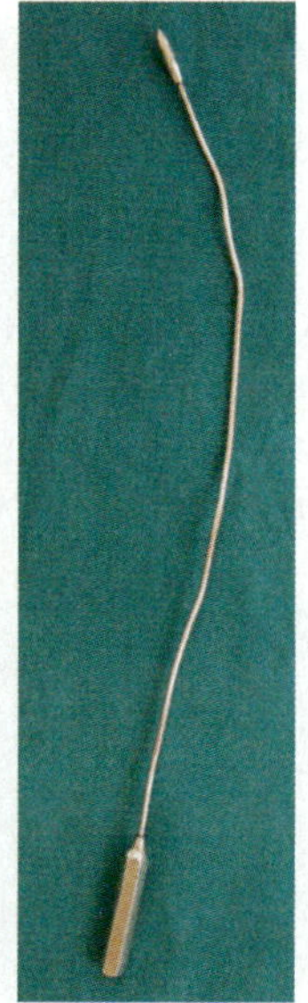

**Fig. 68.21:** Bake's dilator

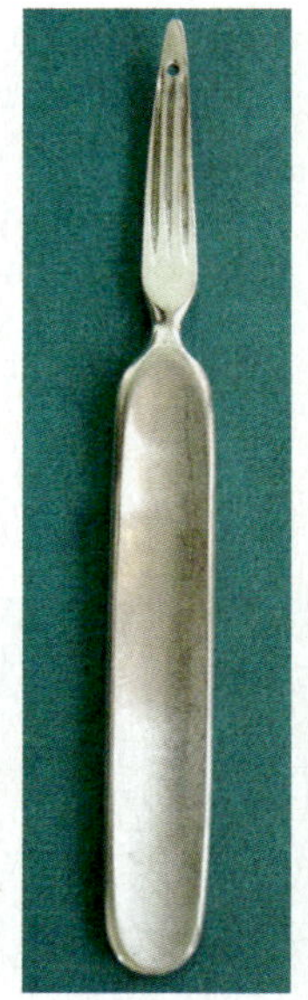

**Fig. 68.22:** Kocher's thyroid dissector

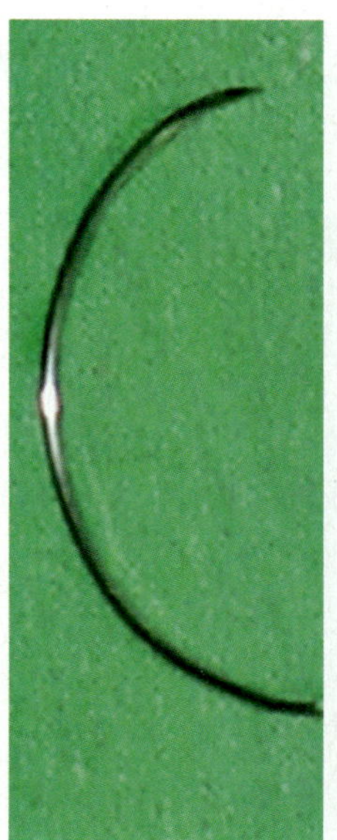

**Fig. 68.23:** Aneurysm needle

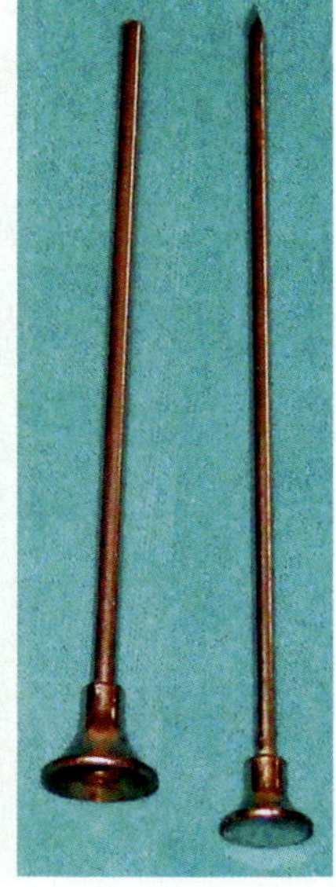

**Fig. 68.24:** Trocar and cannula

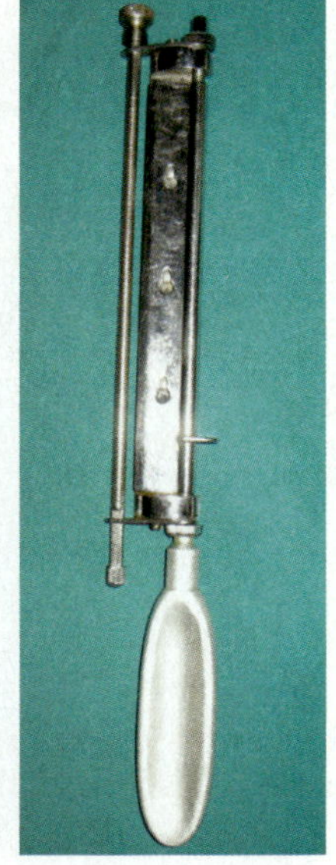

**Fig. 68.25:** Humby's knife

## MYER'S METAL STRIPPER (Fig. 68.26)

- This is a long metallic chain or a stripper used in varicose vein surgery.
- It has a handle which is T-shaped and the 'advancing' end which enters the vein. This is blunt. Once this end comes out of the cut end of the vein, a medium-sized head is connected to it.
- With gentle force (traction) exerted on the handle, the varicose vein can be stripped.
- Hence, it is also called vein stripper.

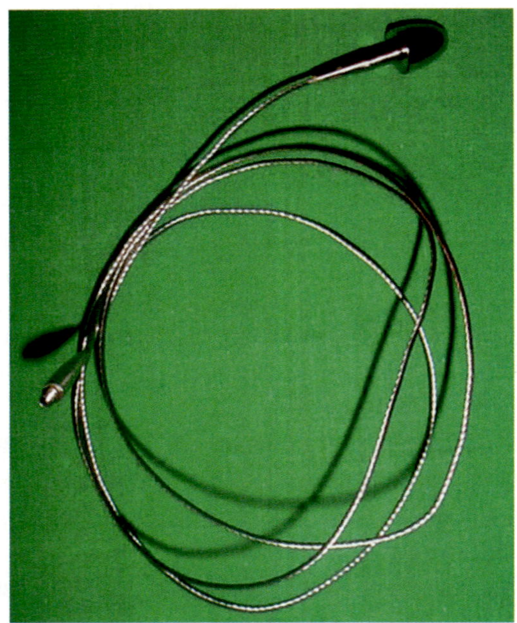

**Fig. 68.26:** Myer's metal stripper

## SELF-RETAINING RETRACTOR (Fig. 68.27)

- It is a strong, heavy instrument, with two blades.
- This is used to spread the laparotomy wound. Hence, it is called self-retaining retractor.

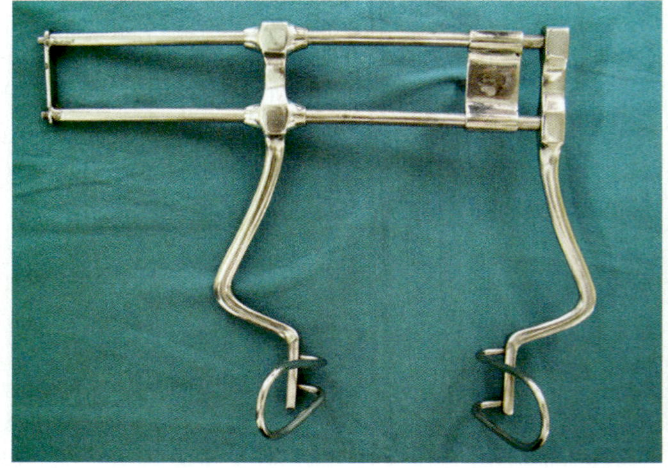

**Fig. 68.27:** Self-retaining retractor

## RIB SPREADER (Fig. 68.28)

- This is also a strong heavy instrument with two long blades.
- Once an incision is deepened through the intercostal spaces and the pleura is opened, the rib spreader is used and by rotating the latch handle, the ribs are spread apart.

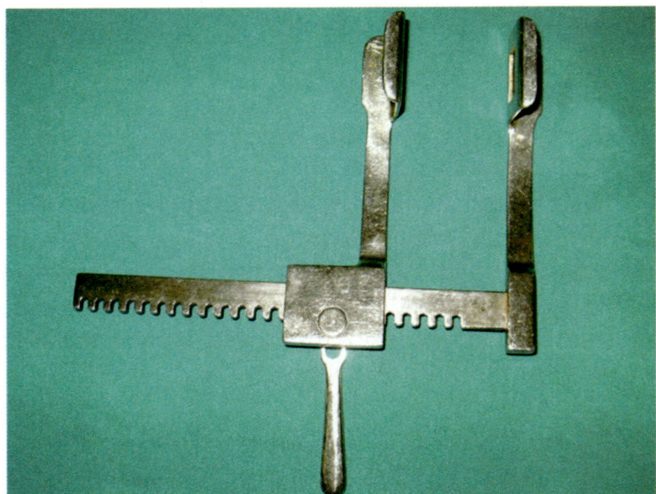

**Fig. 68.28:** Rib spreader

## PROCTOSCOPE (Fig. 68.29)

- This is an instrument used to visualise the rectum and the anal canal.
- It has an outer sheath with the handle (A).
- An inner blunt part is called obturator (B).
- Before introducing the proctoscope one must make sure that obturator and the outer sheath must match. Lubricate the instrument well before introducing.
- In painful conditions such as fissure *in ano*, proctoscopy is contraindicated.
- Once rectal examination is done, proctoscope is held firmly with the left hand (buttocks separated), the obturator is supported by the right hand. The instrument is slowly introduced inside. The obturator is removed and rectum is visualised using light source.
- Proctoscope is used to diagnose haemorrhoids, carcinoma rectum or rectal ulcers, etc. Biopsy can be

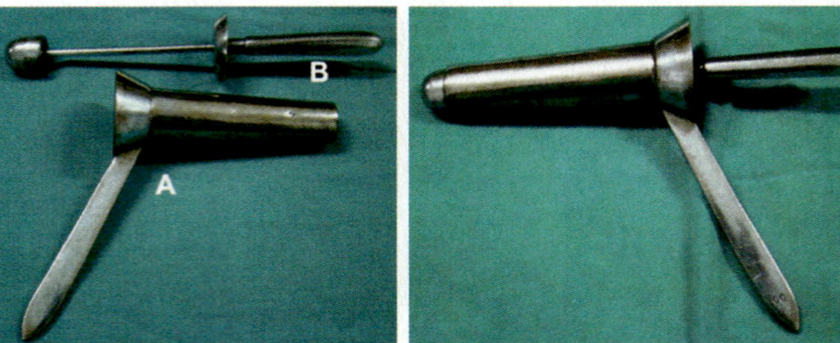


**Fig. 68.29:** Proctoscope

taken with a biopsy forceps in nonhealing ulcers of the rectum. Haemorrhoids can be injected and pelvic abscess can be drained into the rectum with the help of a proctoscope.

## LISTER'S METAL DILATOR (LISTER'S BOUGIE)

- This is a long instrument curved at the tip. Its diameter is written near the handle. It is available in various diameters. The difference between the two numbers is 3. The maximum size of the Lister's dilator is 9/12 (Fig. 68.30).
- The tip is olive-pointed and the end of the handle is round. The minimum and maximum diameter of the instrument is written on the handle. The other type of bougie is Glutton's bougie with a plain tip and the end of the handle is trapezoid. The maximum size of Glutton's bougie is 24/28 and difference between the two numbers is 4.

## MALE METALLIC CATHETER (Fig. 68.31A)

- These catheters are used to drain urine in cases of retention of urine when rubber catheter fails.
- It is a long instrument which is curved because the male urethra is long and curved.
- It has two eyes at the distal end which are situated laterally and at different levels so that the instrument does not become weak at that spot.
- Once the urine is drained, the catheter can be left in place by passing a thread through the two rings present at the proximal end and fixing them to patient's thigh.
- Due to the fear of false passage, injury to the urethra and introducing infection, this catheter is not used nowadays. It is replaced by trocar suprapubic cystostomy.

## FEMALE METALLIC CATHETER (Fig. 68.31B)

- Used to drain urine in females
- This is a short and straight instrument because the urethra is short and straight in females.
- It has multiple holes at the tip
- Indications for usage of this catheter are very rare because acute retention of urine is rare in females and even if it occurs, a red rubber catheter can be passed.
- It is used to empty bladder before vaginal hysterectomy and other gynaecologic surgeries.
- Emptying the bladder is mandatory before any gynaecological examination of a patient.

## TOWEL CLIP (Fig. 68.32)

- This instrument has a ratchet and the operating end is sharp.
- This is available in different sizes.
- Once the part is cleaned and draped the clips are used to hold the towels in place.

## RIGHT-ANGLED FORCEPS: LAHEY'S FORCEPS

- This is a long instrument with right angle at the operating end (Fig. 68.33).
- This instrument is extremely useful in **ligating the major vascular pedicles**, e.g. superior thyroid pedicle—thyroidectomy.
- Cystic artery: Cholecystectomy
- Lumbar veins: Lumbar sympathectomy

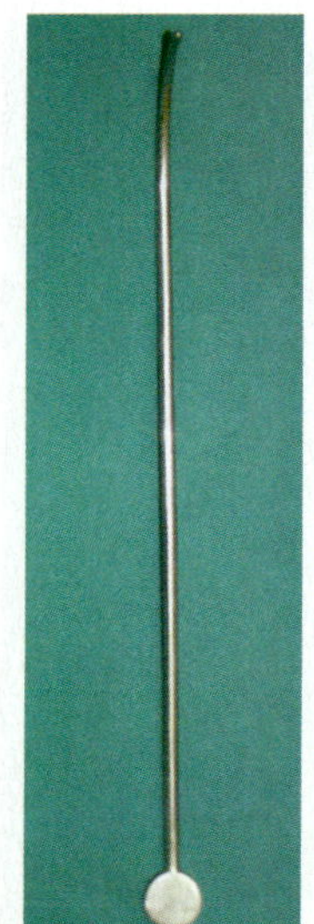

**Fig. 68.30:** Lister's dilator

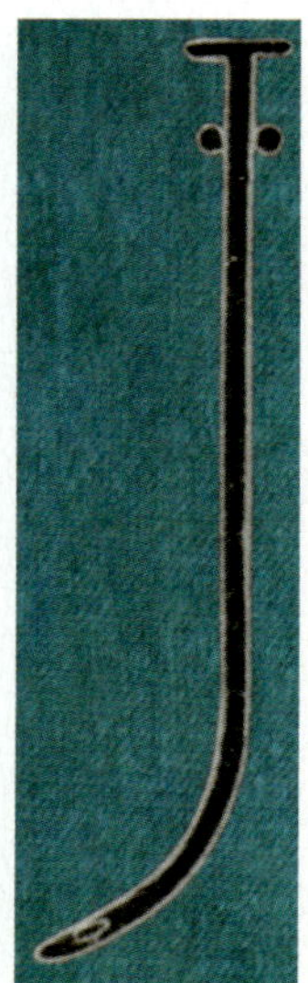

**Fig. 68.31A:** Male metallic catheter

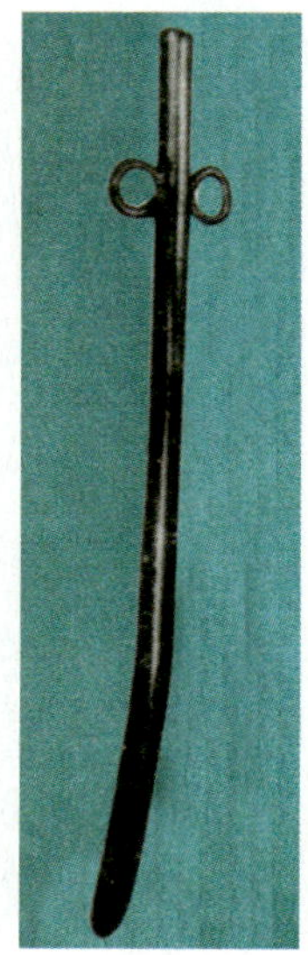

**Fig. 68.31B:** Female metallic catheter

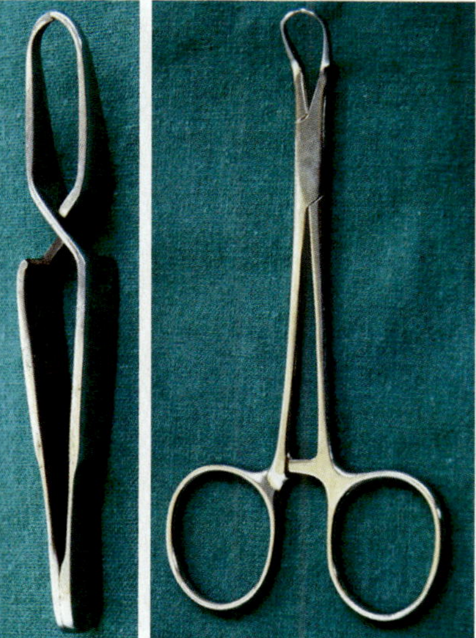

**Fig. 68.32:** Towel clip

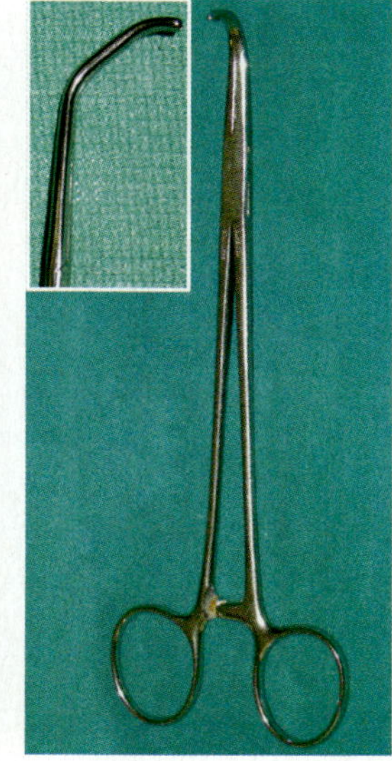

**Fig. 68.33:** Right-angled forceps

## HUDSON'S BRACE AND THE BURR (Fig. 68.34)

- This is a heavy instrument with a brace and the burr (drill).
- This is used to create **openings into the cranium** so as to get an access to the structures within.
- Thus once a 'burr' is made, drainage of blood, fluid or pus can be done.

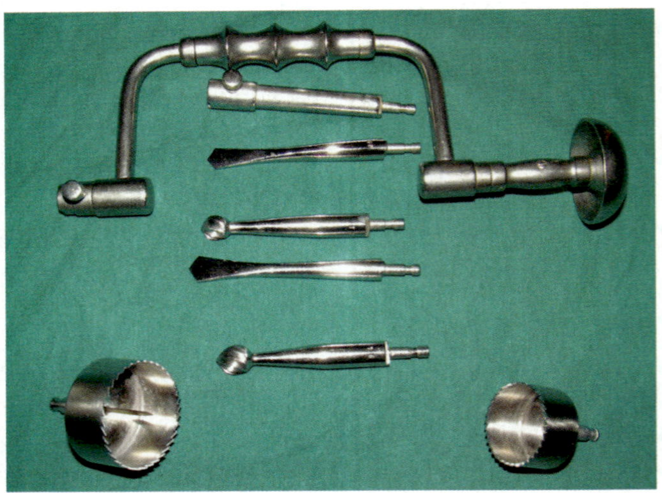

**Fig. 68.34:** Hudson's brace and the burr

## CRICOID HOOK (Fig. 68.35)

- This has a broad handle and a thin shaft with a hook at the operating end.
- This is used to stabilise the trachea by hooking the cricoid cartilage 'up'.
- This step is essential in children wherein veins are very superficial and can get injured easily when child moves the head and neck. By stabilising the trachea, it is easy to incise the trachea, without injuring the vessels.

## TRACHEAL DILATOR (Fig. 68.36)

- This is an instrument with **no ratchet at** the non-operating end.
- The operating end is blunt and curved.
- The peculiarity of this instrument is that **when the handle is opened, operating end is closed** and **when the handle is closed, operating end is opened**.
- Tracheal dilator is used in the **post-tracheostomy period**, when the tube has to be changed due to blockage. In such situations, once the tube is removed, tracheal dilator is introduced, the opening in trachea is kept open, and the new tube is introduced. However, once the track is formed, tracheal dilator need not be used.

## FERGUSSON'S AMPUTATION SAW (Fig. 68.37)

Amputation saw has teeth on its cutting edge to facilitate cutting through the bone and is of different sizes. They are manufactured with one- or two-sided cutting edge for limb amputations.

**Uses:** In lower limb, amputations commonly—above knee (AK) amputation and below knee (BK) amputation.

## BONE NIBBLER (Fig. 68.38)

It is also called double action bone nibbler, identified by long handle and small jaws, top jaw is used for cutting and lower jaw is used to hold the tissue firmly.

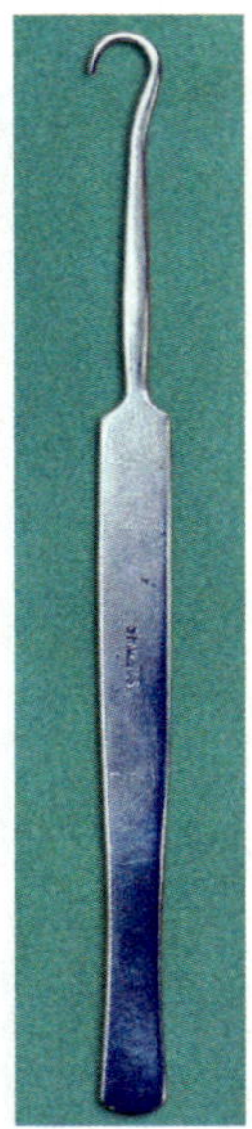

**Fig. 68.35:** Cricoid hook

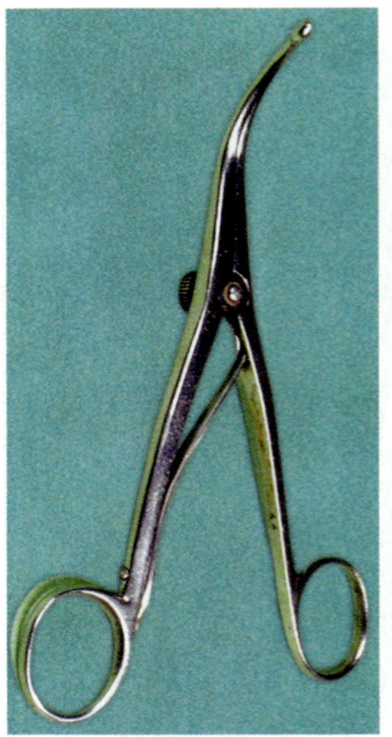

**Fig. 68.36:** Tracheal dilator

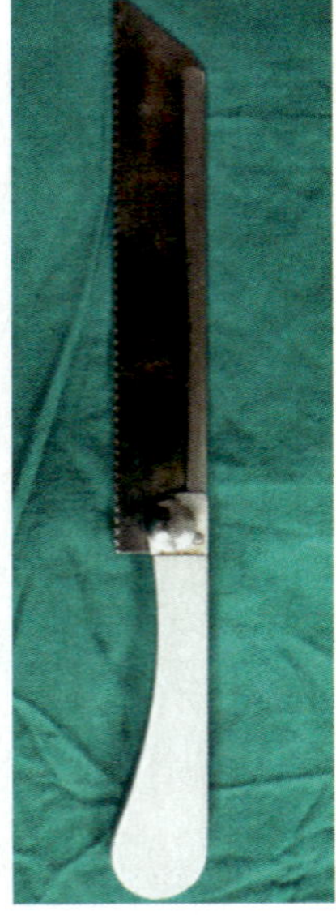

**Fig. 68.37:** Fergusson's amputation saw

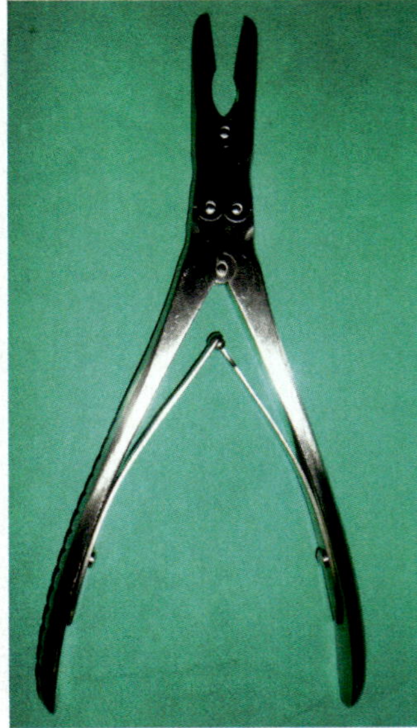

**Fig. 68.38:** Bone nibbler

**Uses:** To make cut end of the bone smooth after amputation rib cutting and to enlarge burr hole.

## BONE FILE/RASPATORY (Fig. 68.39)

One side of the raspatory is used to hold as a handle, while its other side has sharp projections with both fine and coarse teeth on both sides with a flat blade.

**Uses:** Blunt separation of the periosteum and connective tissue from the surface of the bone, smoothening of sharp bony edges after amputation and before fixing fractures.

## VOLKMANN CURETTE (Fig. 68.40)

The edges of the distal spoon-shaped part of this instrument are sharp which make it possible to remove the tissues.

**Uses:** Scoop the granulation tissue, to clean the base of the infected wound, and to remove the infected bone in the case of osteomyelitis.

## DEBAKEY FORCEPS (BAYONET STYLE) (Fig. 68.41)

They are typically large—some examples are upwards of 12 inches (36 cm) long, and have a distinct coarsely ribbed grip panel, as opposed to the finer ribbing on most other tissue forceps, a type of atraumatic tissue forceps.

**Uses:** In vascular procedures to avoid tissue damage during manipulation. Less traumatic manipulation of tissue and used during suturing.

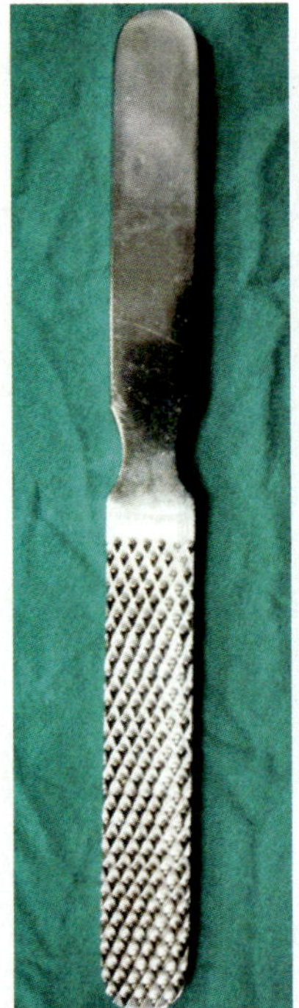

**Fig. 68.39:** Bone file

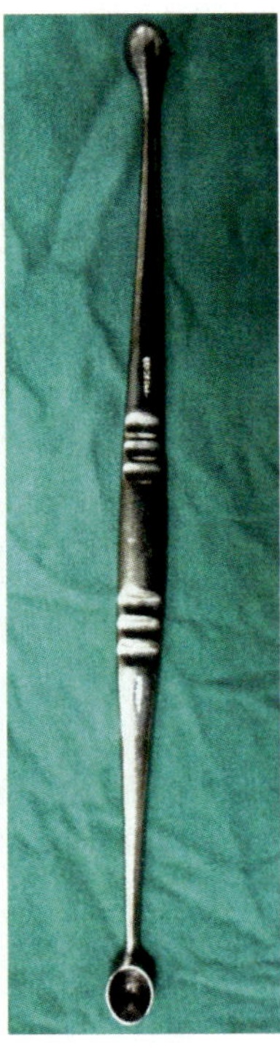

**Fig. 68.40:** Volkmann curette

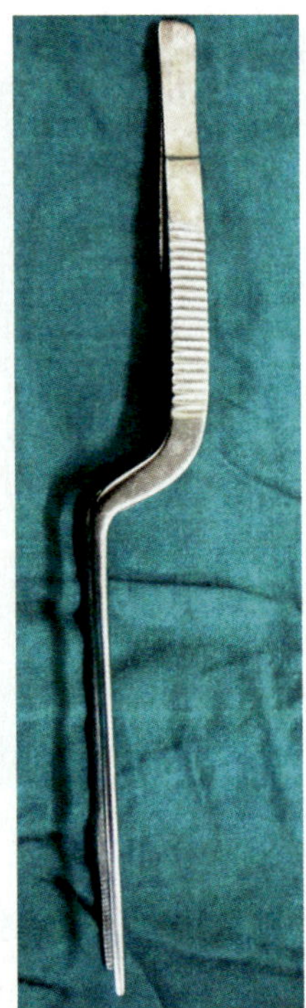

**Fig. 68.41:** Debakey forceps

## BECKMAN-ADSON LAMINECTOMY RETRACTOR (Fig. 68.42)

It has hinged blades with 4 × 4 prongs, an adjustable swivel arms and a ratchet to hold tissue apart.

**Uses:** Retraction in procedures involving deep tissues like in laminectomy for spinal surgeries.

## RIBBON MALLEABLE RETRACTOR (Fig. 68.43)

A malleable or ribbon retractor (manual) may be bent to various shapes.

**Uses:** It is used at the end of the case to keep the viscera away during the fascial closure and is also used to retract deep wounds.

## THE HARMONIC SCALPEL (Fig. 68.44)

The harmonic scalpel is a new device that has been introduced to surgery during the last decade. It is a device that uses high-frequency mechanical energy to cut and coagulate tissues at the same time.

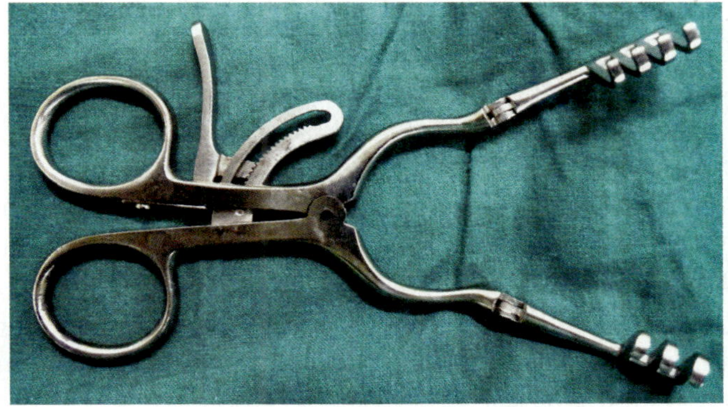

**Fig. 68.42:** Beckman-Adson laminectomy retractor

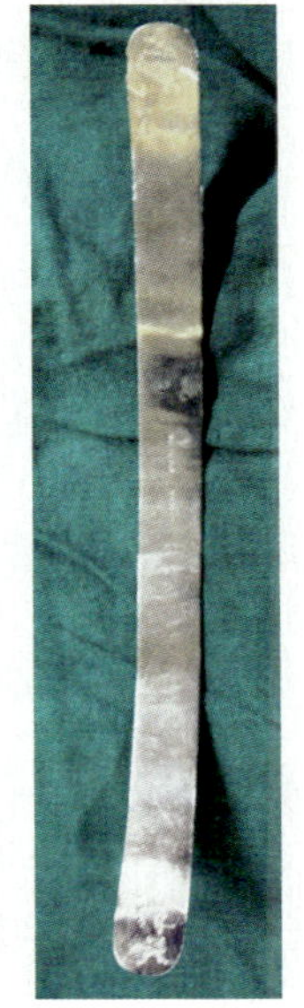

**Fig. 68.43:** Malleable retractor

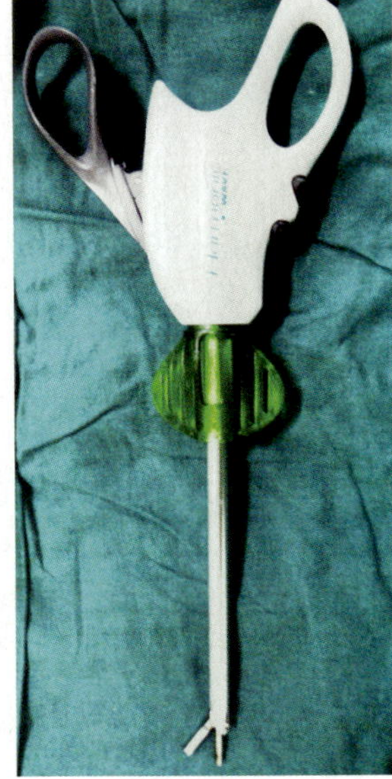

**Fig. 68.44:** Harmonic scalpel

It uses ultrasound technology to cut tissues while simultaneously sealing the edges of the cut. (More details on page 1244.)

Active tips of the harmonic scalpel employ a rigid active lower blade through which the vibrating energy is transmitted. The movable upper jaw is used to compress the vessel against the lower blade, thus allowing transfer of the vibrational energy.

The instrument is similar to an electrosurgery instrument and can be used in all open and laparoscopic surgeries, but superior in that it can cut through thicker tissue, creates less toxic surgical smoke and may offer greater precision especially during a laparoscopic surgery.

## BIPOLAR CAUTERY (Fig. 68.45)

When the electric current is passing between the two parts of the instrument, we call it the bipolar diathermy/cautery (e.g. bipolar forceps).

It makes possible to perform a more precise work and the size of the burned area is small and is more useful when haemostasis is required close to the nerves.

**Uses:** Thyroid surgery when close to RLN (recurrent laryngeal nerve) neurosurgery or spinal surgeries.

## ALLISON'S LUNG RETRACTOR (Fig. 68.46)

It is retractor with a special type of blade, made of wires, in the form of a net over one end and a handle at the other end.

**Uses:** For retraction of the lung in thoracotomy. It does not damage the lungs and the lungs can expand in between the wires.

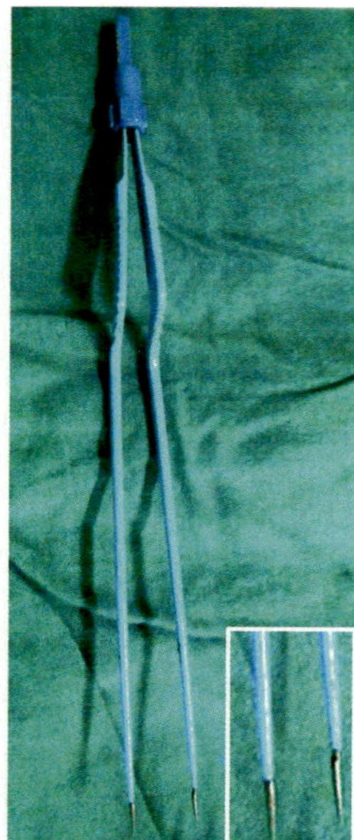

**Fig. 68.45:** Bipolar cautery

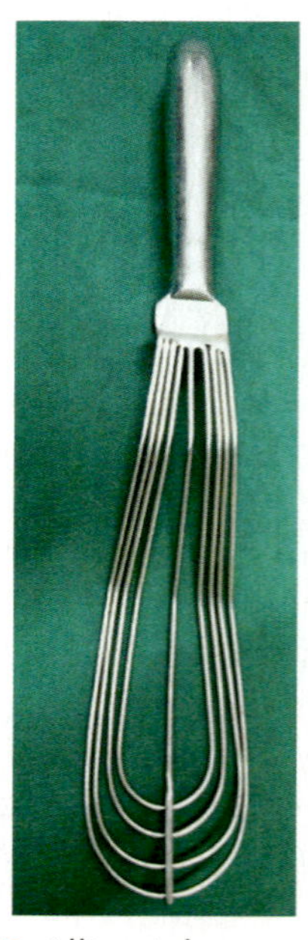

**Fig. 68.46:** Allison's lung retractor

## GIGLI SAW (Fig. 68.47)

Composed of a wire as a blade and two handles to hold the wire on either side.

**Uses:** For bone cutting in amputation surgeries similar to amputation saw such as below knee and above knee amputations commonly.

## JOLL'S THYROID RETRACTOR (Fig. 68.48)

It is a self-retaining retractor, which is held by the two towel clip like forceps on both sides to hold the flaps and can be adjusted using a screw in between.

**Uses:** To retract skin flaps during thyroid surgery.

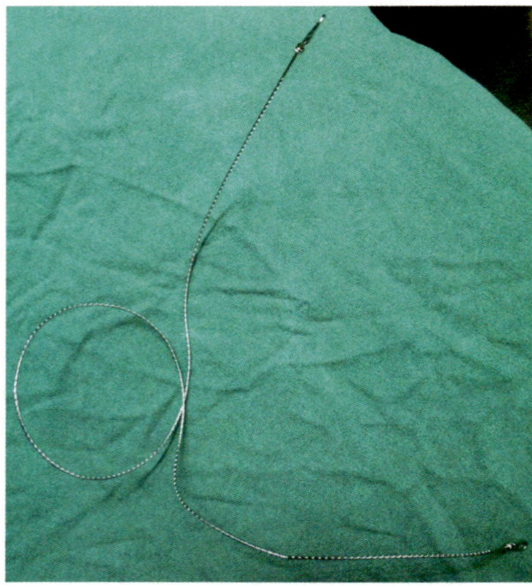

**Fig. 68.47:** Gigli saw

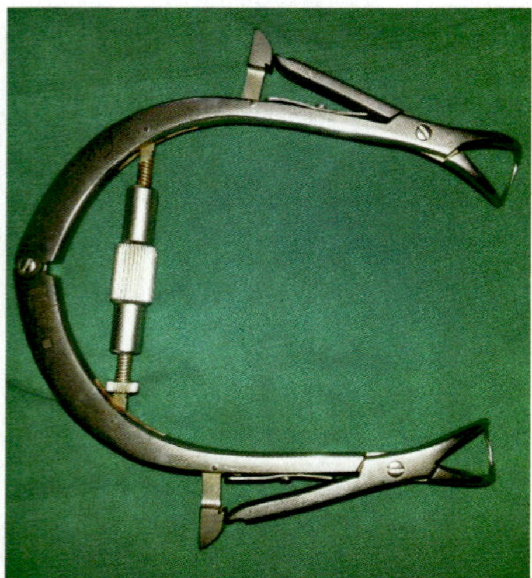

**Fig. 68.48:** Joll's retractor

## METAL TRACHEOSTOMY TUBE (Fig. 68.49)

- This has **two tubes**, the inner long and the outer short tube.
- This has no **cuff**.

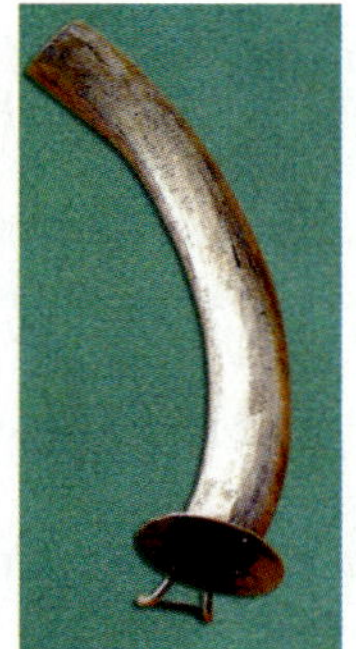

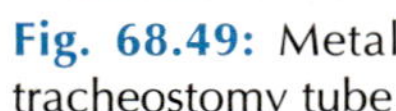

**Fig. 68.49:** Metal tracheostomy tube

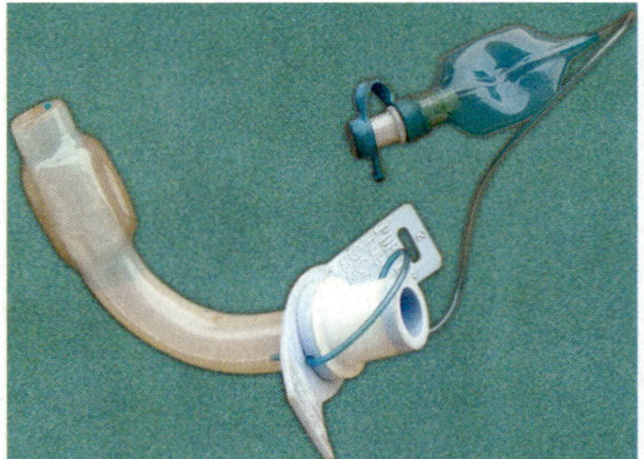

**Fig. 68.50:** Cuffed tracheostomy

- Once the tube is introduced, the tape is passed around the neck, passed through the opening and tied so as to keep the tube in place.
- If the tube is blocked, the inner tube can be removed, cleaned and reintroduced.
- Metal tracheostomy tubes are useful as permanent tracheostomy tube.

## CUFFED TRACHEOSTOMY TUBE (Fig. 68.50)

- This is made of polyvinyl chloride. It is a **single tube**.
- Once the tube is introduced within the trachea, the cuff is inflated by using 3–5 ml of air.
- The cuff prevents leakage of air and prevents **acid aspiration syndrome (Mendelson's syndrome)**.
- If this tube is blocked, it is an emergency. In such cases, the tube has to be cleaned and mucus plugs have to be removed. Otherwise, the tube is removed, the tracheal opening is kept open with the help of tracheal dilator and a new tube is introduced. Alternatively, endotracheal intubation may need to be done to ensure patency of the airway.

## CORRUGATED RED RUBBER DRAIN (Fig. 68.51)

- It is made of red rubber. It has corrugations on both sides. Whenever a major surgery is done, some amount of blood loss or anastomotic leakage is expected. This drain is used so that **fluid can escape freely outside**.
- Thus, it is used after thyroidectomy, gastrectomy, cholecystectomy, etc. The drain is removed after it stops draining. Usually it takes about 3–5 days.
- After laparotomy for peritonitis, these drains are used to prevent residual abscess in the postoperative period.

## MALECOT'S CATHETER (Fig. 68.52)

This is made of red rubber. It has flower-shaped end and has a wide diameter. It is used to drain amoebic liver abscess. It is straightened with the help of an introducer and left in cavity and brought outside. It is

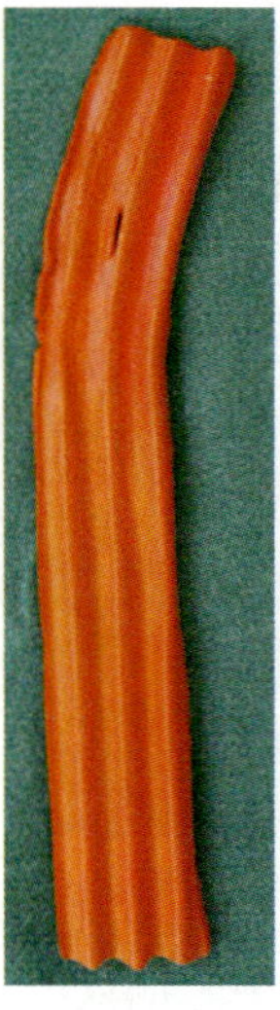

**Fig. 68.51:** Corrugated red rubber drain

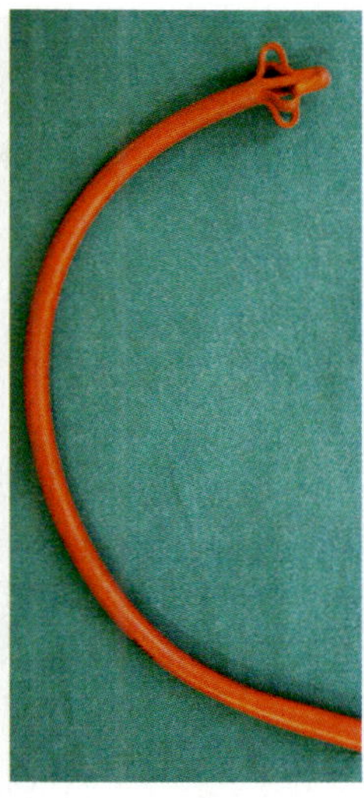

**Fig. 68.52:** Malecot's catheter

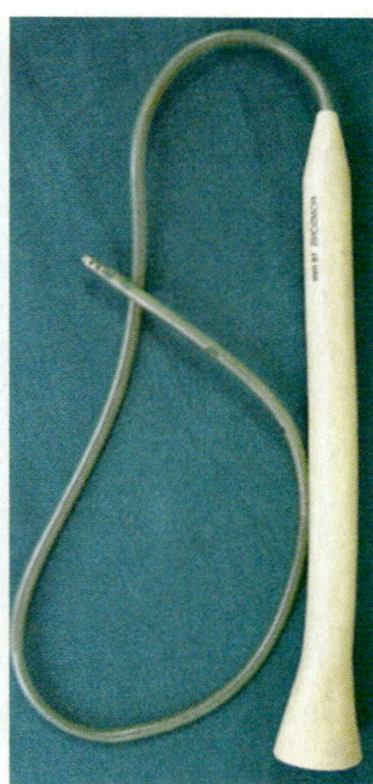

**Fig. 68.53:** Mousseau Barbin's tube

a self-retaining catheter. This is used to drain urinary bladder after transvesical prostatectomy or can be used as feeding gastrostomy tube. It can also be used to drain empyema thoracis.

## MOUSSEAU BARBIN'S TUBE (Fig. 68.53)

- This is also called MB tube. It is a funnel-shaped tube with Ryle's tube like attachment. It is used in inoperable cases of carcinoma oesophagus to palliate dysphagia. It is stitched to the Ryle's tube which is brought out through the mouth and it is slowly drawn in by pulling the other end of Ryle's tube which is in the stomach, after doing a gastrostomy.
- Once the tube is below the level of growth, it is cut at a sufficient distance and is stitched to the stomach wall.
- With the availability of laser coagulation of the growth, and considering discomfort caused by the tube including its migration, the MB tube is not popular and not preferred.

## FOLEY'S SELF-RETAINING URINARY CATHETER (Figs 68.54A and B)

- This is made of **latex with silicon coating**. At the tip, there is a bulb, capacity of which is written at the other end.
- Before inflating the bulb, one must make sure that **catheter is in the urinary bladder, not in the urethra**. This is assessed by free flow of urine.
- After introducing the catheter, the bulb is inflated using saline. Thus, it becomes self-retaining. After the usage, it is removed by deflating the bulb. It can also be used to drain peritoneal cavity as in biliary peritonitis. Inflated bulb compresses the prostatic bed and controls bleeding after prostatectomy.

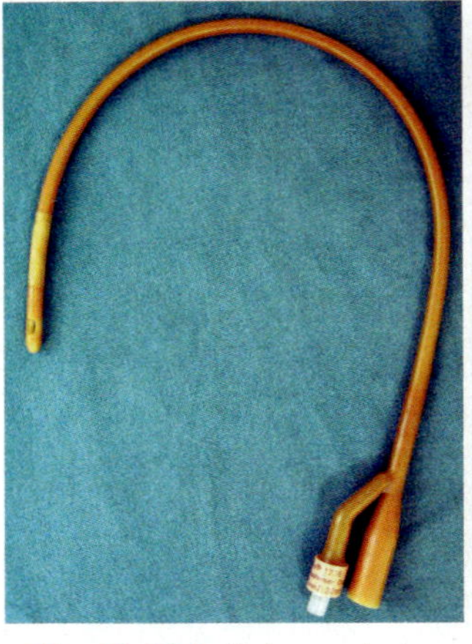

Fig. 68.54A: Foley catheter

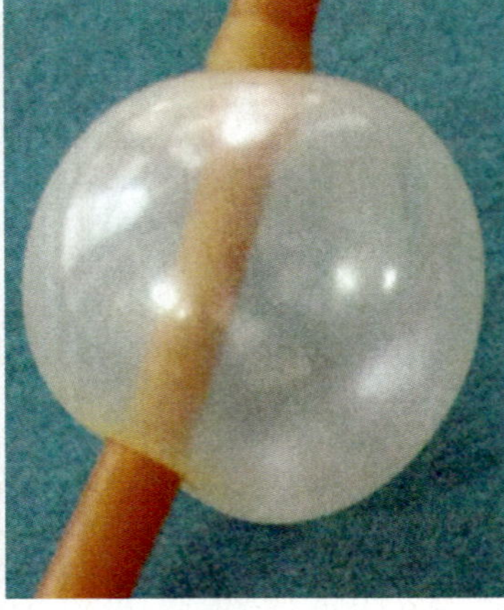

Fig. 68.54B: Distended bulb

## RED RUBBER CATHETER (Fig. 68.55)

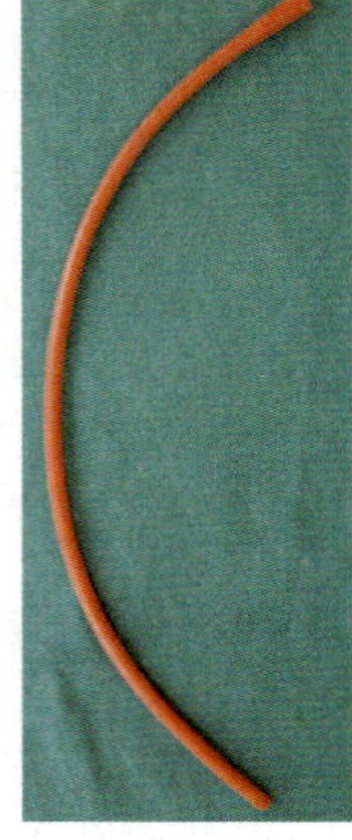

Fig. 68.55: Red rubber catheter

This is used to drain urine temporarily. It causes urethritis if it is left long in the urinary bladder. Once the urine is emptied, it is removed. It is not a self-retaining catheter. Not routinely used nowadays because of availability of Foley's catheter. It is more stiff than Foley catheter. Hence, **in cases of stricture urethra,** where **Foley's catheter cannot be passed, red rubber catheter may be used.**

## NASOGASTRIC TUBE/RYLE'S TUBE (Fig. 68.56)

- This is also called **nasogastric tube**. At the end of this tube there are **lead shots**. After introducing within the stomach, its position is confirmed by pushing 5–10 ml of air and auscultating in the epigastrium or aspirating gastric juice. It is a long tube having 3 marks. When the tube is passed up to the 1st mark, it enters the stomach. Usually it is passed up to 2nd mark. Life-saving use of **Ryle's tube** is in **acute gastric dilatation**.
- **In volvulus of the stomach, it is impossible to pass a Ryle's tube.**
- Ryle's tube is used to decompress the stomach as in intestinal obstruction or pyloric stenosis.
- It is used in the diagnosis of GI haemorrhage.
- It is also used to provide enteral nutrition to comatose patients or critically ill patients.

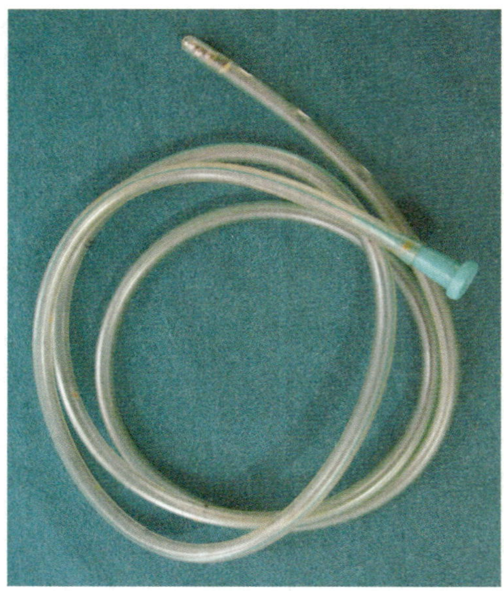

Fig. 68.56: Ryle's tube

## T-TUBE (KEHR'S) (Fig. 68.57)

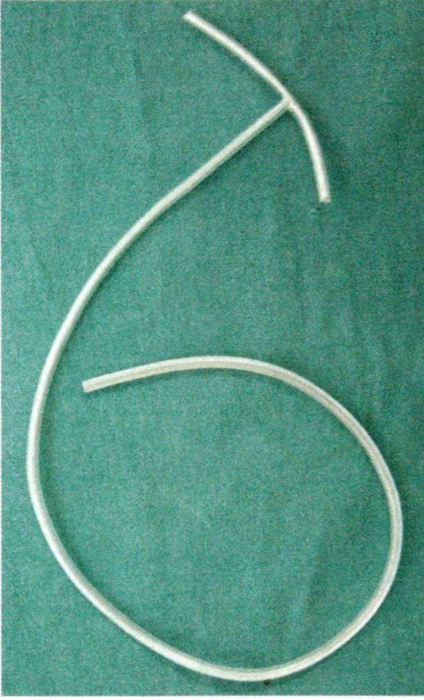

Fig. 68.57: T-tube (Kehr's)

- This is a flexible tube made of latex with a long vertical limb and a short horizontal limb.
- Whenever the **common bile duct (CBD) is incised**, it is sutured after inserting the T-tube. The short horizontal limb is placed vertically within the common bile duct after making 2–3 holes within. Some surgeons slit open the entire length of the short limb.
- The long limb is brought to the exterior from the most dependent part of the common bile duct and connected to a sterile container.
- Presence of the T-tube may prevent peritonitis due to biliary leakage in cases of residual stones blocking the lower end of the CBD.

## REMOVAL OF THE TUBE

About 7–10 days later, a T-tube cholangiography is done and the T-tube is removed with a gentle pull, provided following criteria are fulfilled.

1. The dye flows freely into the duodenum.
2. No filling defects in the CBD.
3. After clamping the tube for 24 hours, there is no abdominal pain or fever.
4. Patient is passing normal coloured stools.

Once the tube is withdrawn, some amount of biliary leak may persist for 2–3 days and it stops by itself provided there is no distal obstruction.

## SENGSTAKEN-BLAKEMORE DOUBLE BALLOON TRIPLE LUMEN TUBE (Fig. 68.58)

- It is used in controlling bleeding **oesophageal varices.** It has 3 lumens and 2 balloons, a gastric balloon and an oesophageal balloon.
- **Gastric balloon is inflated** with about **200–250 ml** of air and oesophageal balloon is inflated with about **40–60 ml of air**. It is pulled upwards so as to snugly fit at the oesophagogastric junction and thus it acts by internal tamponade.
- Sengstaken tube should not be kept in place for more than 48 hours because it can cause pressure necrosis of oesophagus.
- It should be deflated for a few minutes after 24 hours.
- Sengstaken tube should be used by an experienced physician. Oesophageal secretions and saliva cannot be aspirated while using this tube, and if gastric balloon is deflated suddenly, it slides up and causes choking. The oesophageal balloon should be immediately deflated in such situations.
- **Modification of Sengstaken tube is called Minnesota tube or 4 lumen tube.** It has 4 lumens. The 1st to inflate oesophageal balloon, the 2nd to inflate gastric balloon, the 3rd to aspirate like a Ryle's tube, and the 4th lumen is used to aspirate oesophageal secretions. If there is any difficulty in breathing while using Sengstaken tube or Minnesota tube, bulb should be deflated or tube should be cut.

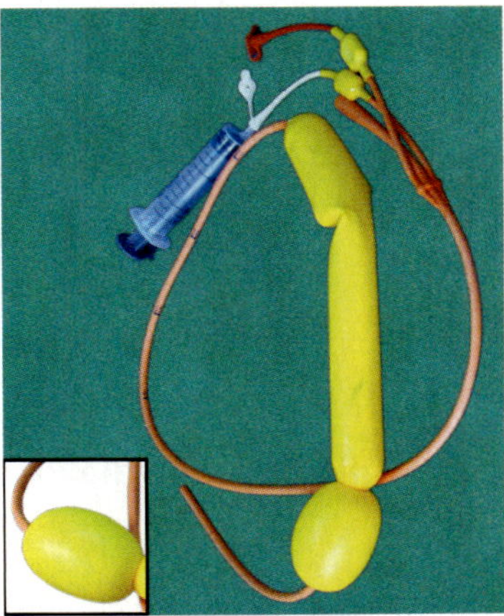

**Fig. 68.58:** Sengstaken-Blakemore double balloon triple lumen tube

> **SU14.3:** Describe the materials and methods used for surgical wound closure and anastomosis (sutures, knots, and needles).

## NEEDLES AND SUTURES

### INTRODUCTION

- Needles are very essential part of surgery. Every surgeon should know details about various types of needles, their diameter, their shape and their usefulness. Thus, it helps in conduct of surgery very well. Wrong usage of sutures may result in serious complications—such as tissue trauma, bleeding, sepsis, anastomotic leak, etc.

### CLASSIFICATION

- **Traumatic:** Needles with eye, suture material loaded into the eye. Needle holes in tissues are larger than suture material.
- **Atraumatic:** Eyeless needles, suture material embedded into the needle. When suture is attached to needle with a single, continuous unit of suture and needle, it is known as swaged needle.

> Scottish pharmacist George Merson, who runs a suture manufacturing company, developed eyeless needled sutures with a single strand of material pre-attached through the butt of the needle.

#### Parts of the Needle (Fig. 68.59)

- **Needle has three main parts:** Shank, body, point. The body of the needle is either round, triangular or flattened.
- **Round-bodied needles:** Uniformly round, gradually taper to a point designed to separate tissue fibres rather than cut through soft tissue. *Examples:* They are used in intestinal and cardiovascular surgery.
- Cutting needles are used for suturing tough or dense tissue, e.g. skin, fascia, aponeurosis, etc.

#### Point of the Needle (Fig. 68.60)

- Round with a tapered end.
- Reverse cutting in which the cutting edge is on the outside of the needle curvature.
- Conventional cutting—cutting edge faces the inside of the needle curvature.
- Taper cutting.

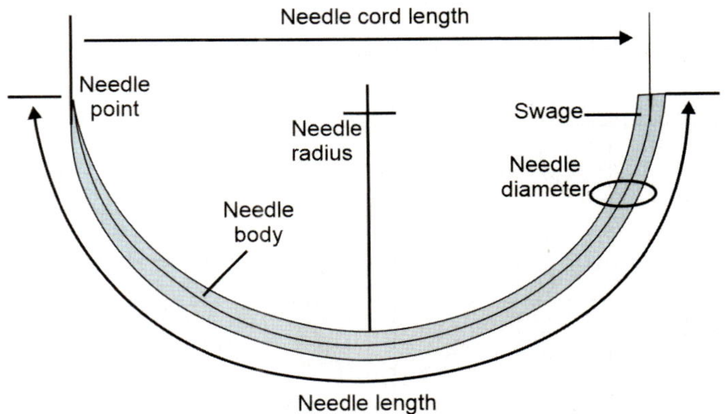


**Fig. 68.59:** Needle and parts

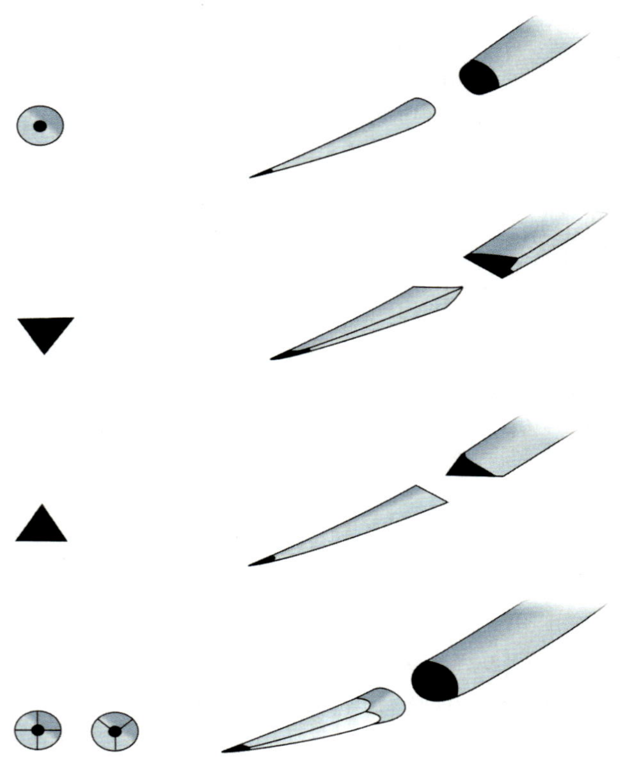

Fig. 68.60: Tip of needles and cross-section

## Choice of the Needle (Fig. 68.61)

- Choice of needle shape depends on accessibility of the tissue to be sutured—more confined the operative space, the more curved the needle. *Example:* Deep in the pelvis, stitches in and around gastro-oesophageal junction, etc.
- Half circle needles are commonly utilized in the gastrointestinal tract.
- **J-shaped needles,** quarter circle needles and compound curvature needles: Used in special situations, such as the **vagina, eye and oral cavity, respectively**.
- Size of needle corresponds with the gauge of the suture material.

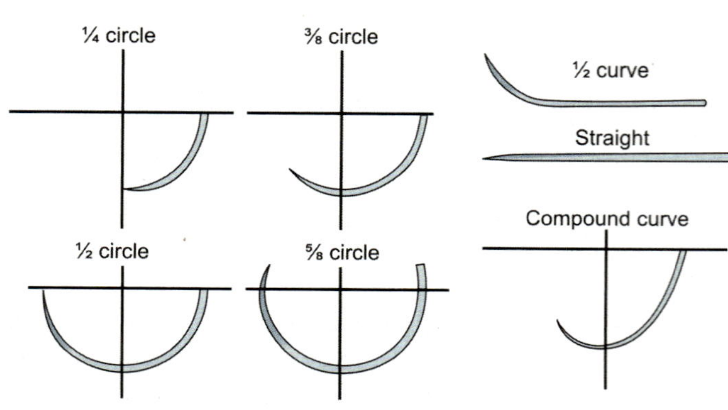


Fig. 68.61: Commonly used needles in surgical practice

## Special Needles

- Aneurysm needle is a blunt pointed curved needle with the eye at the point; used for passing ligatures around aneurysms or over the vessels.
- Aspirating needles: Long, hollow needle for removing fluid from a cavity.
- Menghini needle is a needle for liver biopsy, does not require rotation to cut loose the tissue specimen.
- Reverdin's needle is a surgical needle with an eye that can be opened and closed by sliding.
- Silverman needle is a biopsy needle for taking tissue specimens. It consists of an outer cannula and an inner split needle with a longitudinal groove in which tissue is retained when the needle is withdrawn.

| *Round body needle* | *Cutting needle* |
|---|---|
| • Uniformly round needle | • No uniform shape |
| • Tip is tapered | • Sharp end has a triangular shape on cross-section |
| • They separate the tissue | • They cut, penetrate fibres and tough structures |
| • Used to suture tissue fibres muscles, intestines, vessels | • Used to suture fascia aponeurosis, linea alba and skin |

# SUTURE MATERIALS

## INTRODUCTION

Selecting an appropriate suture material for surgery is equally important as selecting a needle. Suture materials are of different varieties, materials and properties. An understanding of properties of various suture materials will help in doing surgeries easily and effectively. A few common sutures and their uses have been given here.

## CLASSIFICATION

- **Absorbable:**
  - Natural: Catgut
  - Synthetic: Polyglactone, polydiaxonone
- **Non-absorbable:**
  - Natural: Silk
  - Synthetic: Polypropylene, polyamide monofilament

### Catgut

- The word **catgut is derived from kitgut means violin strings**.
- Natural absorbable suture, derived from submucosa of the sheep because of rich content of elastic fibres.
- It is easy to handle, knots well.
- Plain or chromicised (mixed with chromic salts).
- Tensile strength: 15 days for plain catgut and 28 days for chromic catgut.

- Absorbed in 60 days (plain) or 90 days (chromic)
- Plain catgut is used to suture subcutaneous tissue for closure, during circumcision, repair of wounds of lip or oral cavity.
- Chromic catgut is used to suture muscles, bowel anastomosis, closure of peritoneum, appendicectomy, etc.
- Chromic and plain catgut are preserved in 70% alcohol and it is kept soft due to 5% glycerine.

Synthetic absorbable suture polyglycolic acid and polyglactin has replaced catgut suture for most of the uses.

### Vicryl (Polyglactin 910)

- Made of polyglactin-synthetic absorbable polyfilament suture.
- **Co-polymer of 90% glycolide and 10% L-lactide**
- **Digested by hydrolysis,** not by enzymatic degradation, hence less tissue reaction when these sutures are used.
- Maintains **tensile strength in the tissues for about 28–30 days** and get absorbed in 80–90 days.
- Available in different sizes ranging from No. 1 to 8-0.
- The suture length may be 90 cm, 70 cm or 45 cm.
- Needles available with Vicryl are round bodied, cutting, taper cut or atraumatic.
- Size of needles can be 30 mm, 22 mm, 16 mm, etc.
- Available as undyed Vicryl and coated Vicryl.
- **Triclosan, a broad-spectrum antiseptic agent, which has been used to provide Vicryl sutures with antimicrobial activity—it is called Vicryl plus.**

#### *Uses of Vicryl*

- No. 1 or 1-0 suture may be used for closure of subcostal, paramedian, Pfannensteil, McBurney's incision.
- 3-0 or 4-0 sutures on atraumatic round bodied needles are used in biliary enteric anastomosis: Choledochoduodenostomy, choledochojejunostomy, hepaticojejunostomy.
- 4-0 sutures are also used in pancreaticojejunal anastomosis.
- 2-0 sutures used in intestinal anastomosis, suturing external oblique aponeurosis in inguinal hernia repairs.
- Also used for subcutaneous closure, transfixation of vessels, achieving haemostasis, etc.
- Finer polyglactin sutures 5–0 and 6–0 are used in vascular surgery—monofilament sutures
- **Reverse cutting endoport:** Used for closure of laparoscopic port incisions—the rectus or the umbilical port/camera port.

### Rapid Vicryl

- A variety of polyglactin 910 suture, with rapid absorption. Undyed Vicryl.
- Rapid absorption is due to exposure of coated Vicryl to gamma irradiation which leads to the material having a low molecular weight than coated Vicryl.
- Tensile strength: Maintained for 10–12 days.
- Gets absorbed in 42 days.
- Used for skin or mucosal closure.
- Sutures need not be removed, gets spontaneously absorbed.
- Used for circumcision.

### Monocryl

- Polyglecaperone is a synthetic absorbable monofilament suture
- Available as undyed or may be dyed violet
- Good handling properties: Very smooth surface, passes through tissues with ease
- Tensile strength: 21 days.
- Absorbed by hydrolysis in about 90–120 days.
- Used for closure of subcutaneous tissue apposition.
- Used for skin closure, subcuticular sutures.
- **Used in urological procedures—pyeloplasty, ureter repair.**

### Polydiaxonone (PDS)

- Polydiaxonone suture: Synthetic, delayed absorbable, monofilament suture. Dyed violet.
- PDS II sutures: Improved version of initial PDS suture.
- Suture characteristics: Soft, pliable and smooth; allows easy passage through the tissues. Knotting characteristics—best among the synthetic absorbable sutures.
- Available in various sizes with different types of needle and different suture lengths.
- Tensile strength: Maintained for longer periods (about 56 days)
- Suture is absorbed by hydrolysis, complete in about 180–210 days (6–7 months)
- No. 1 loop PDS is used for closure of paramedian or midline and other abdominal incisions.
- 3-0 and 4-0 sutures are used for intestinal or biliary enteric anastomosis.

### Silk

- Natural non-absorbable sutures
- Derived from cocoon of the silkworm larva
- It is braided and coated with wax to reduce capillary action
- Tensile strength: Maintained for a long time (2 years)
- In the tissues, it incites a polymorphonuclear reaction and a fibrous capsule formed around the silk in 14–21 days.

- *Available as:*
  - **Sutupak:** Sterile pack containing black braided silk, precut into different sizes. Suture thickness may be 6-0 to 3, 75 cm long.
  - **Silk reels:** Nonsterile, available in thickness from 6-0 to 4. Sterilized by autoclaving.
  - **With needles:** Different types of needles, and different sizes (No. 7-0 to 1) and different lengths (45 cm, 76 cm and 90 cm)
- 2-0 and 3-0 mersilk can be used for anterior and posterior seromuscular sutures in intestinal anastomosis and in gastrojejunostomy.
- 3-0 mersilk may be used for pancreaticojejunal anastomosis.
- 4-0 mersilk may be used for suturing nerve.

### *Uses of Silk*

- Cholecystectomy—to ligate the cystic duct and cystic artery.
- During intestinal resection—to ligate mesenteric vessels.
- Ligation of the pedicles—during nephrectomy, splenectomy, major amputations, etc.
- During Trendelenburg procedure and perforator ligation.

### Ethilon

- Synthetic monofilament nonabsorbable suture (made of polyamide, a variety of nylon). Very low coefficient of friction—readily passes through the tissues.
- Tensile strength: Maintained for a long time (tensile strength loss after 1 year is 25%).
- Available in different sizes.
  - **Suture:** Monofilament polyamide black, No. 2-0, 70 cm.
  - **Needle:** Reverse cut—used for closure of skin incision. (No.1, 1-0, 2-0, 3-0)
  - Also available as finer sutures 3–0, 4–0, 5–0 up to 10-0: Used in vascular surgery, reverse cutting, 45 mm, 3/8 circle

### Prolene

- Polypropylene is a synthetic monofilament nonabsorbable suture.
- It is inert, has extremely low tissue reactivity and is non-biodegradable.
- Low coefficient of friction, slides through the tissues readily.
- Tensile strength maintained for indefinite period.
- Demonstrates memory, requires 4–5 knots to secure.
- Available with a variety of needles in various sizes from 8-0 to 1, with different lengths.
- **Suture:** Monofilament polypropylene blue, No. 3-0, 70 cm.
- **Needle:** Round bodied, 25 mm, 1/2 circle.
- **Suture:** Monofilament polypropylene blue, No. 4-0, 90 cm.
- **Needle:** Taper cut needle, 26 mm, 1/2 circle
- Used in inguinal hernioplasty for closure of posterior wall defects, fixation of mesh, etc.
- Used during orchidopexy
- In vascular anastomosis 5 or 6-0 is selected. In microvascular surgery 8 or 10-0 sutures are used.

### Ethibond Excel

- Polyester—synthetic nonabsorbable braided sutures.
- Are dyed green for better visibility.
- Available along with pledgets.
- Used for cardiovascular surgery in valve replacements.
- **Suture:** Polyester, No. 3-0, 100 cm.
- **Needle:** Round bodied, 26 mm, 1/2 circle.

### V LOC

- Novel suture materials: Eliminates the need for knot tying in some situations, such as laparoscopic surgery.
- These sutures have unidirectional or bidirectional barbs that secure the suture in the tissues.
- Available as absorbable (polymer of glycolide, dioxanone and trimethylene carbonate) and non absorbable (polybutester).
- **Suture:** Absorbable, No. 3-0, 30 cm.
- **Needle:** Taper, 26 mm, 1/2 circle.

## SKIN CLOSURE TECHNIQUES

Good closure begins with a good incision:

- Incision should be made with scalpel at right angles to the skin.
- It should be made along the relaxed skin tension lines, this also results in minimal scarring on healing.
- Skin should be handled gently to avoid devitalising the margins.
- The skin edges should be everted and approximated without tension.
- Circular incisions should be converted to elliptical incisions that are at least three times as long as wide, to allow the wound to heal without tension.
- Tension on the skin sutures can be minimised by using deep dermal and subdermal sutures. It is better to leave the suture line lax than using too much tension, as postoperative oedema will often take up any slack in the suture material. Using too much tension can compromise the vascularity of the edges.

The commonly used suture techniques for skin closure are:

- Simple interrupted sutures.
- Mattress sutures (Fig. 68.62): Can be either vertical or horizontal mattress sutures. These produce accurate approximation of wound edges.
- Subcuticular sutures: Good cosmetic outcomes.

**Other skin closure techniques include:**

- Tissue glue which are composed of cyanoacrylate
- Skin adhesive strips, skin staples (Fig. 68.63)

### Knotting Principles

Tying a knot is one of the most fundamental skills that a surgeon has to acquire and perfect.

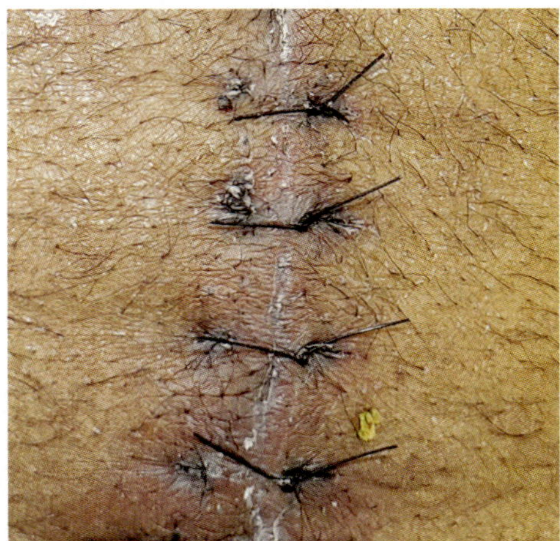

**Fig. 68.62:** Mattress sutures

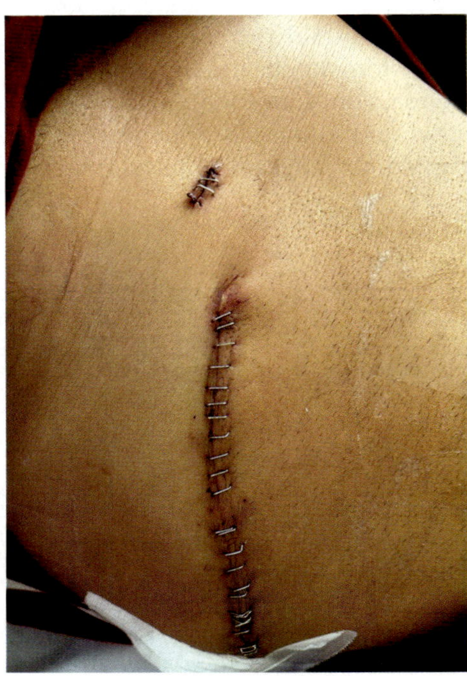

**Fig. 68.63:** Skin staplers

The important principles of knotting are:

- The knot should be tied firmly, not too tight, without exerting too much tension on the tissues.
- The knot should not slip. A few suture materials, such as prolene, require additional throws to secure the knot.
- The knot should be compact and small to minimise the foreign material.
- The standard surgical knot is the reef knot, and additional throws are added for security. All knots should be squared.
- The suture should be cut appropriately after knotting leaving the thread at 1–2 mm length.
- In cases of continuous suture technique, an Aberdeen knot is used at the end.

## INTESTINAL RESECTION AND ANASTOMOSIS

### Introduction

Bowel anastomosis involves the surgical join between two intestinal segments. Bowel anastomosis is usually done to restore bowel continuity as part of surgery for diseased bowel or to bypass unresectable bowel. It may be accomplished either by handsewn technique or by the use of stapler devices. It has been stated that the key to a successful anastomosis is the accurate union of two viable bowel ends with complete avoidance of tension (Key Box 68.3). If anastomosis is not successful, complications can be very, very disastrous as shown in Fig. 68.64.

Key Box 68.3

**Key Factors for Successful Intestinal Anastomosis**

- Good exposure in the operative field
- Gentle handling of the bowel
- Meticulous surgical technique
- Approximation of well vascularized bowel
- Avoid tension at anastomosis
- Minimize faecal contamination
- Good haemostasis

### Physiology of Anastomosis Healing

The healing process at the anastomotic site is divided into three phases:

1. **Inflammatory phase:** The inflammatory phase lasts for the first 4 days during which the anastomosis is dependent on the mechanical strength provided by the sutures or staples. Hence, any AL occurring during the first two postoperative days is likely to be due to technical factors.
2. **Proliferative or fibroplasia phase:** The second phase of proliferation starts from the 5th postoperative day

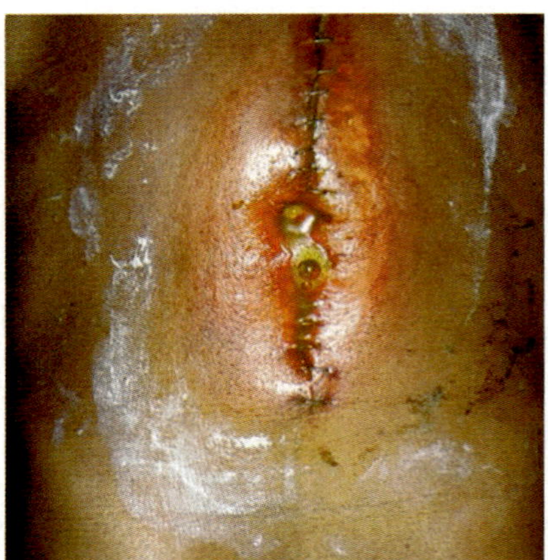

Fig. 68.64: Anastomotic leak

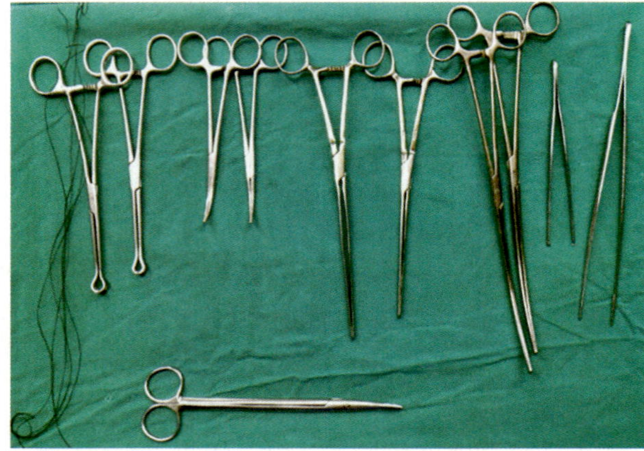

Fig. 68.66: Instruments used for intestinal anastomosis

and lasts up to the 14th postoperative day. There is an increased collagen deposition during this phase to give tensile strength to the anastomosis.

3. **Reparative or remodelling phase:** The last phase of remodelling occurs up to 1 year after the surgery. During this phase, rebuilding of the intestinal wall layers occurs at the anastomotic site.

## Blood Flow and Anastomosis

The blood supply to the bowel is derived from the mesentery with vessels travelling on either side of the bowel wall to reach antimesenteric border. Hence, the anastomosis is centred on the antimesenteric border when possible (Fig. 68.65).

## Instruments used for Intestinal Anastomosis (Fig. 68.66)

- Straight artery forceps for stay sutures, scissors to cut the intestines and forceps to hold the edge of the intestines to see carefully the layers taken while suturing.
- Curved small artery forceps for catching the bleeders followed by coagulation.
- Babcock's forceps for holding the intestines together, thus getting ready for anastomosis.

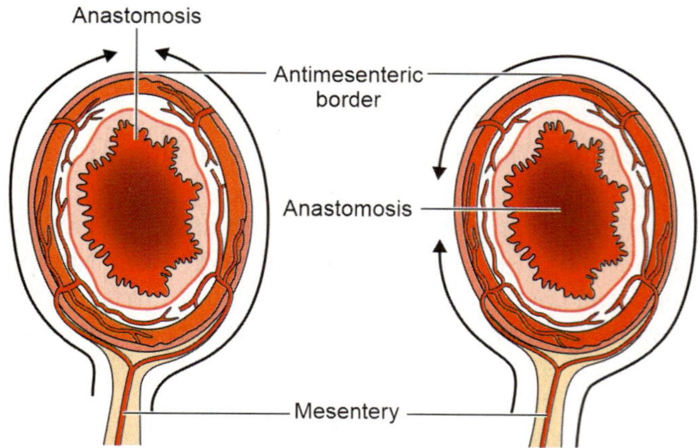


Fig. 68.65: Blood flow at anastomotic site

- Moynihan's occlusion clamps—straight and curved—are applied to occlude the lumen so that contents of the intestine are not spilled over and also to control bleeding.

## Suture Materials Used

Intestines: Inner absorbable such as 2–0 polyglactin (Vicryl) and outer 2–0 atraumatic silk.

## Handsewn Anastomosis

It can be performed in a single layer or double layer fashion. Single layer anastomosis usually employs full thickness bites of the bowel wall (Fig. 68.67). In a double-layered anastomosis, the inner layer consists of full thickness bites whilst the outer layer consists of seromuscular bites. There is no proven advantage regarding the type of suture material used. The ideal suture material should provide good tensile strength during the anastomotic site healing process with minimal local tissue reaction. Commonly used suture materials are 2–0 Vicryl continuous for inner mucosal sutures and 2–0 interrupted for outer seromuscular layer.

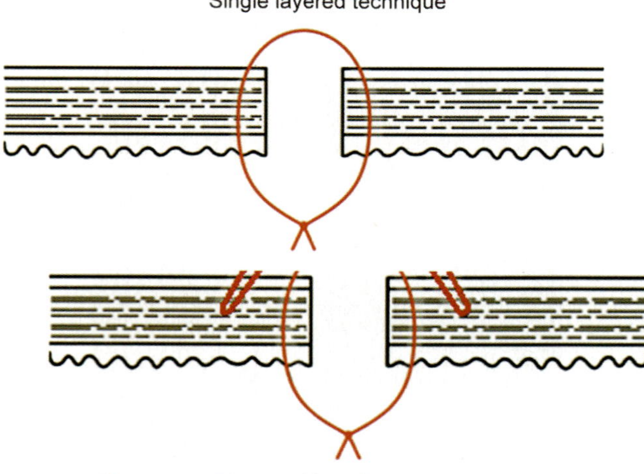


Fig. 68.67: Types of handsewn anastomosis

## Stapler Anastomosis

Stapler anastomosis drastically reduces the operating time, however, it requires the surgeon to be familiar with the stapling devices. They are usually not preferred, if the bowel is edematous due to high risk of anastomotic leak. There are different types of surgical staplers available for resection and anastomosis of bowel.

- **Transverse anastomosis (TA) staplers:** They are non-cutting staplers that require the specimen to be cut with scalpel or scissors after laying down the stapler rows.
- **Linear staplers:** They are popularly known as gastrointestinal anastomosis (GIA) staplers. They have a cutting mechanism for transection of bowel in addition to laying down stapler rows. These types are very commonly used for bowel resection and anastomosis in small and large bowel (Fig. 68.68).
- **End-to-end anastomosis (EEA) staplers:** These are circular cutting staplers that place several rows of staples. These are used in colorectal and oesophago-gastric anastomosis.

Staplers are available in different staple line lengths and configurations. The cartridges are colour coded to indicate the height of the staples which are used based on the thickness of bowel being anastomosed (Fig. 68.69). One example of using blue cartridge is shown in Fig. 68.70.

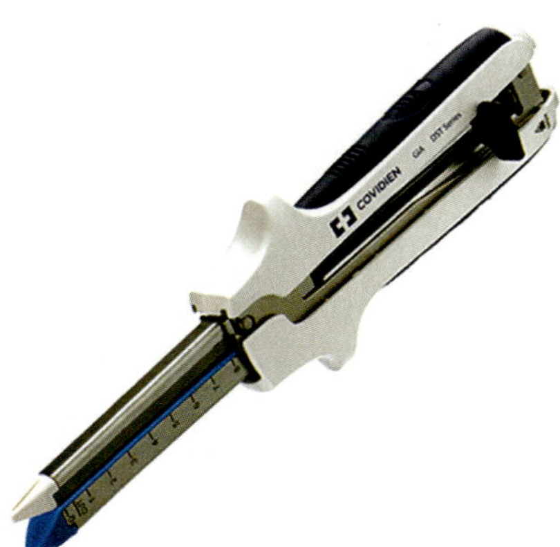


**Fig. 68.68:** GIA stapler device

| Colour | Tissue type | Open staple height | Closed staple height |
|---|---|---|---|
| Grey | Mesentery | 2.0 mm | 0.75 mm |
| White | Vascular | 2.5 mm | 1.0 mm |
| Blue | Standard | 3.5 mm | 1.5 mm |
| Gold | Standard/ thick | 3.8 mm | 1.8 mm |
| Green | Thick | 4.1 mm | 2.0 mm |

**Fig. 68.69:** Colour coding of the cartridge

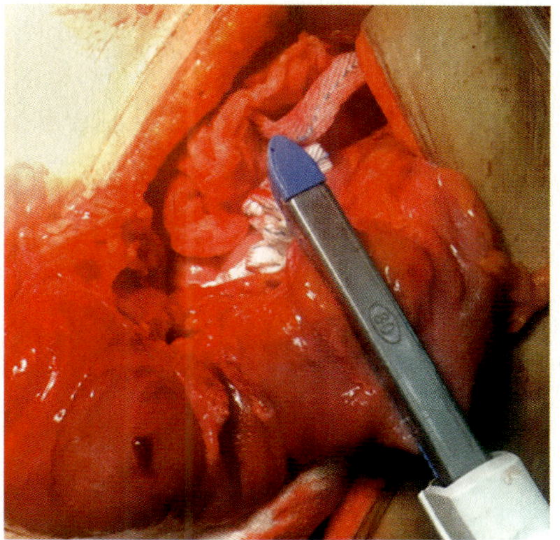

**Fig. 68.70:** Stapler resection of bowel

## Type of Anastomosis (Figs 68.71 to 68.73)

Anastomosis between two bowel segments can be created in various ways.

- **End-to-end:** This is performed when two bowel segments are of roughly equal caliber. In case of an unequal caliber, a Cheatle slit on the smaller caliber bowel will aid in anastomosis.
- **End-to-side:** This type is preferred when one bowel segment is wider than the other.
- **Side-to-side:** This type of anastomosis is carried out on the antimesenteric side of two bowel segments. It is the most commonly employed type of anastomosis.

## Complications of Bowel Anastomosis

- Anastomotic leak
- Bleeding
- Wound infection
- Prolonged ileus
- Anastomotic stricture

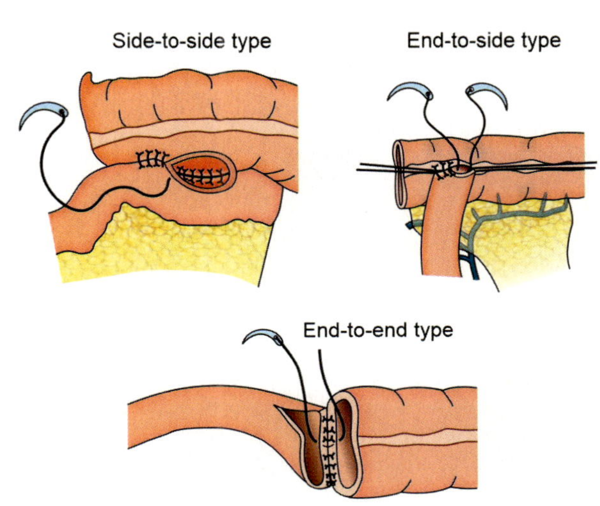


**Fig. 68.71:** Types of anastomosis

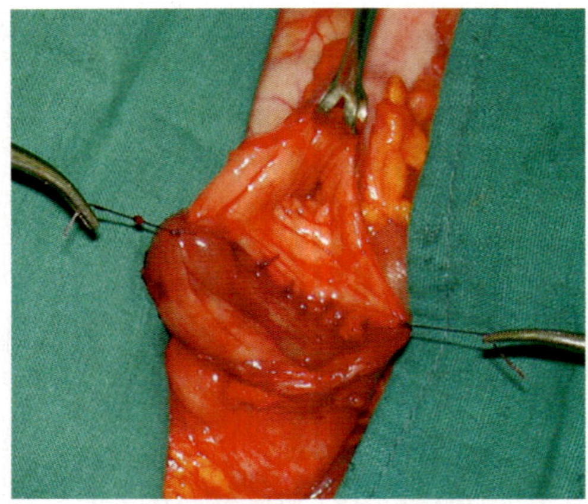

**Fig. 68.72:** End-to-end anastomosis

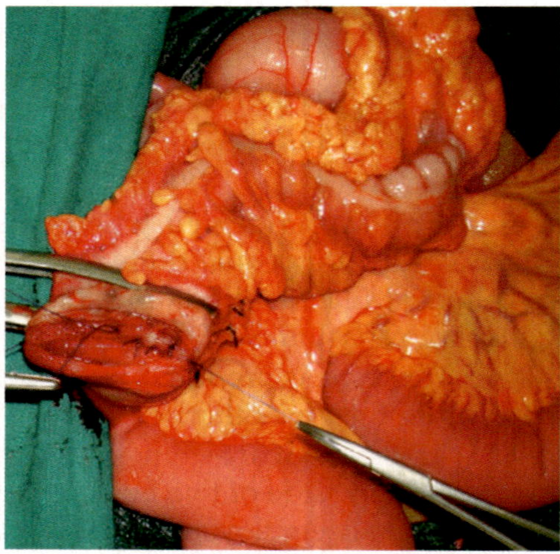

**Fig. 68.73:** Ileocolic anastomosis

### Anastomotic Leak

Anastomotic leak is the most dreaded complication following intestinal resection and leads to high morbidity and mortality. Anastomotic leaks are usually identifiable by postoperative days 3–5. It occurs due to the breakdown or insufficiency at the anastomotic line and is defined as the leak of luminal contents from a surgical join between two hollow viscera which is identified.

- Clinically by extravasation of bowel content through drain/wound.
- Radiologically by the presence of collection adjacent to anastomosis.
- Intraoperatively during re-exploration.

***Risk factors for anastomotic leak:*** They may be categorized into patient factors and technical factors. Some of the risk factors (Table 68.1) like smoking and consumption of alcohol may be modifiable.

**TABLE 68.1:** Risk factors for anastomotic leak

| Patient factors | Technical factors |
|---|---|
| • Old age (>60 years)<br>• Male gender<br>• High dose steroids<br>• Smoking<br>• Hypoalbuminaemia<br>• Preoperative radiotherapy<br>• High-risk site of anastomosis<br>• Diabetes mellitus<br>• Anaemia<br>• Uraemia | • Emergency surgery<br>• Poor surgical technique<br>• Faecal contamination<br>• Haematoma formation<br>• Prolonged operating time<br>• Intraoperative blood loss |

Chapter 69

# Specimens

- TB lymphadenitis
- Hodgkin's lymphoma
- Carcinoma tongue
- Chronic gastric ulcer
- Linitis plastica
- Intussusception
- Carcinoma rectum
- Gangrenous appendicitis
- Carcinoma colon
- Meckel's diverticulum
- Polycystic kidney
- Renal cell carcinoma
- Hydronephrosis
- Carcinoma penis
- Seminoma testis
- Cholecystectomy
- Hydatid cyst
- Carcinoma stomach
- Lipoma
- Malignant melanoma
- Thyroidectomy
- Wide excision of skin
- Whipple's pancreaticoduodenectomy
- Splenectomy

## I. TUBERCULOUS (TB) LYMPHADENITIS

**1. What is this specimen?**

- Specimen of lymph nodes which are matted. Cut surface shows caseation. Hence, it is tuberculous lymphadenitis.

**2. What is the microscopic picture?**

- Central caseation surrounded by epithelioid cells, Langhans' type of giant cells.

**3. What are the stages of TB lymphadenitis?**

- Stage of lymphadenitis
- Stage of matting
- Stage of cold abscess
- Stage of collar stud abscess
- Stage of sinus formation

**4. Why is matting seen in TB lymphadenitis?**

- It is because of periadenitis

**5. What is the treatment of cold abscess?**

- Nondependent aspiration by using wide bore needle, to avoid sinus formation.

## II. LYMPHOMA

**1. What is the diagnosis?**

- Multiple lymph nodes which are discrete and not matted. Cut surface does not show caseation. It is homogenous. Hence, this is a specimen of Hodgkin's lymphoma.

**2. How do you confirm the diagnosis?**

- Lymph node biopsy

**3. What is the microscopic picture?**

- Cellular pleomorphism: Lymphocytes, histiocytes, eosinophils, monocytes with giant cells containing mirror image nuclei—Reed-Sternberg cell.

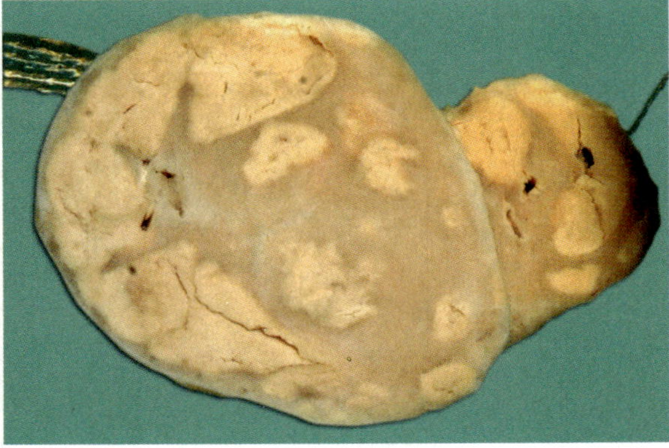

**Fig. 69.1:** Tuberculous (TB) lymphadenitis

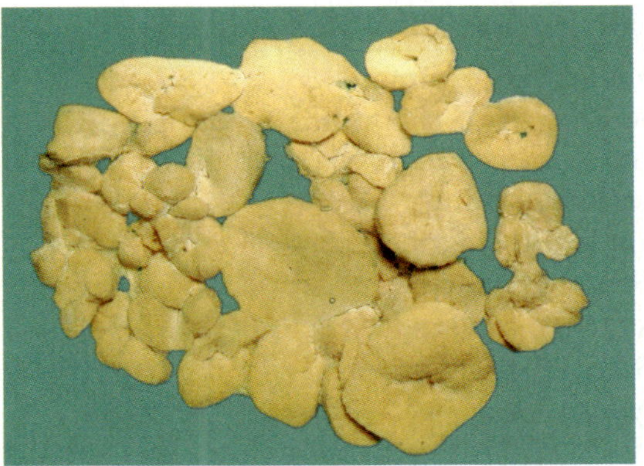

**Fig. 69.2:** Lymphoma

4. **What are the common lymph nodes involved in Hodgkin's lymphoma?**
   - Cervical, axillary, para-aortic, iliac and inguinal lymph nodes.
5. **Is Waldeyer's ring involvement seen in Hodgkin's lymphoma?**
   - No, it is usually seen in non-Hodgkin's lymphoma.

## III. SPECIMEN OF HEMIGLOSSECTOMY WITH HEMIMANDIBULECTOMY

1. **What is this specimen?**
   - Specimen showing growth arising from the tongue and infiltrating the mandible.
2. **What is the diagnosis?**
   - Advanced carcinoma tongue
3. **Is radiotherapy indicated in this situation?**
   - No, because chances of radionecrosis of the mandible are high.
4. **What type of X-ray is taken to look for involvement of the mandible?**
   - Orthopantomogram
5. **What is Commando's operation?**
   - Hemiglossectomy with excision of the floor of the mouth, hemimandibulectomy, with radical block dissection of the neck done in a single stage, with *en bloc* removal.

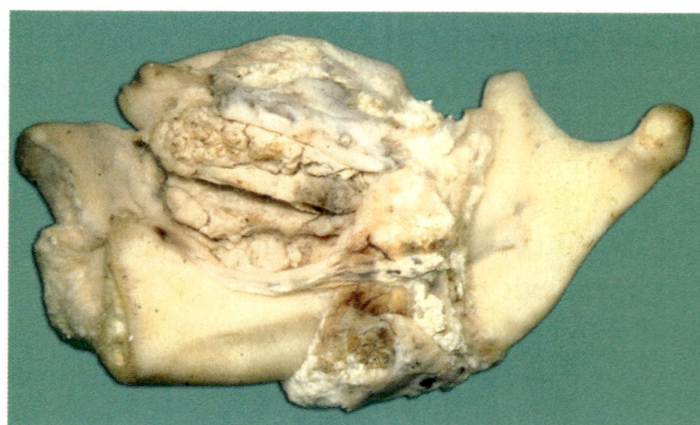

**Fig. 69.3:** Specimen of hemiglossectomy with hemimandibulectomy

## IV. CHRONIC GASTRIC ULCER

1. **What is this specimen?**
   - Specimen of the stomach showing rugosity of the stomach. There is a deep ulcer crater along the lesser curvature.
2. **What is the diagnosis?**
   - Benign gastric ulcer
3. **Why is it a benign gastric ulcer?**
   - Since the rugae are of converging type, it is a benign gastric ulcer.
4. **How do you rule out malignancy in a gastric ulcer?**
   - Endoscopic biopsy

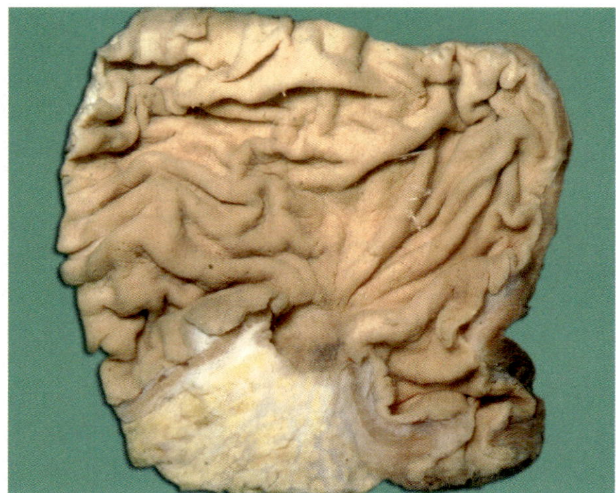

**Fig. 69.4:** Chronic gastric ulcer

5. **What is the incidence of gastric ulcer turning into malignancy?**
   - 0.5 to 2%

## V. LINITIS PLASTICA

1. **What is this specimen?**
   - Specimen of the stomach showing loss of normal rugosity. There is a nodular extensive infiltrating lesion along the entire length of the stomach.
2. **What is the diagnosis?**
   - Linitis plastica—leather bottle stomach.
3. **What is linitis plastica?**
   - It is an extensive fibrosis involving entire submucosa of the stomach initially and involves other layers also later.
4. **What is the treatment for linitis plastica?**
   - Radical total gastrectomy
5. **What is the D2 prognosis?**
   - Very poor

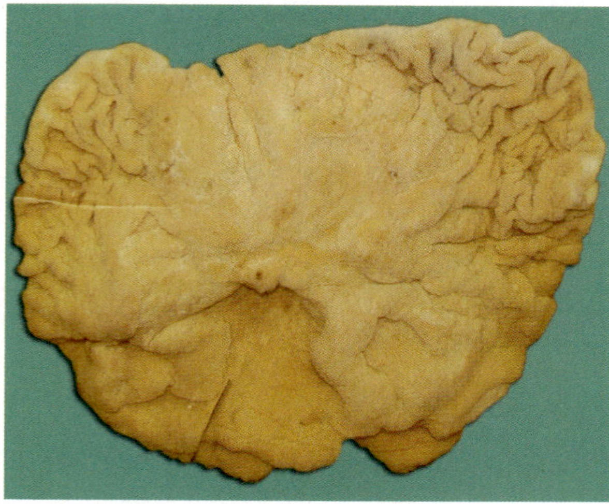

**Fig. 69.5:** Linitis plastica

## VI. INTUSSUSCEPTION

1. **What is this specimen?**
   - Specimen of intestine showing one portion of bowel invaginated within the other.
2. **What is the diagnosis?**
   - Intussusception
3. **What is the common type of intussusception?**
   - Ileocolic
4. **What are the parts of intussusception?**
   - Intussusceptum, intussuscipiens, neck and apex.
5. **What is the treatment in children?**
   - Hydrostatic reduction or operative reduction.
   - If there is gangrene—resection followed by end-to-end anastomosis.

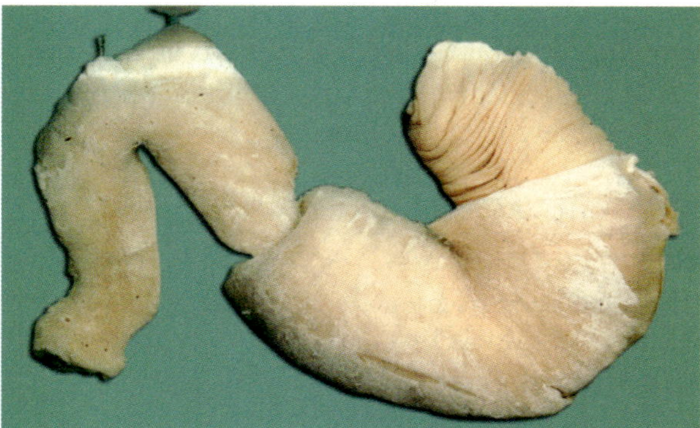

Fig. 69.6: Intussusception

## VII. CARCINOMA RECTUM

1. **What is this specimen?**
   - Specimen of rectum showing ulceroproliferative growth in the middle of the rectum. Specimen also shows entire rectum and anal canal.
2. **What is the diagnosis?**
   - Carcinoma rectum
3. **What is this surgery?**
   - Abdominoperineal resection (excision) (APR). In this operation, entire rectum, anal canal, part of the sigmoid colon, fat, fascia, lymphatics and regional nodes are removed *en bloc* followed by permanent colostomy in the left iliac fossa.

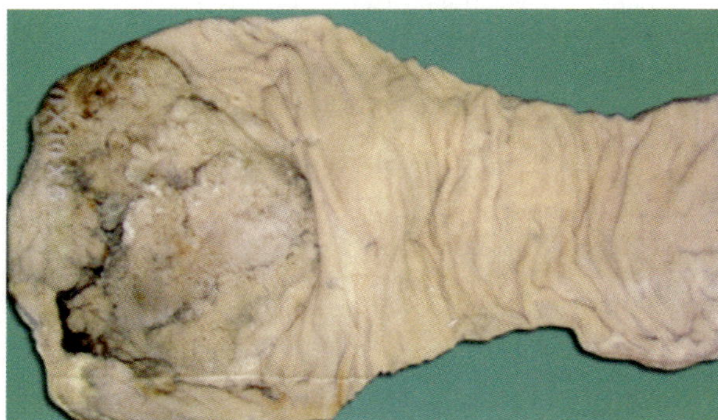

Fig. 69.7: Carcinoma rectum

4. **What are the indications for APR?**
   - Growth in lower rectum wherein sphincter cannot be saved.
5. **What is the position of the patient during APR?**
   - Supine with lithotomy called Lloyd Davis position.

## VIII. GANGRENOUS APPENDICITIS

1. **What is this specimen?**
   - It is an appendicectomy specimen showing blackish discolouration of the appendix.
2. **What factors cause gangrene of the appendix?**
   - Gangrenous appendicitis occurs usually in elderly patients, where there is decreased vascularity due to atherosclerosis. It can also occur when the lumen is blocked due to faecolith, thereby causing ischaemia.
3. **What is the one simple investigation which is useful in diagnosing appendicitis?**
   - Total WBC count. Above 10,000 cells/cu mm of blood with increased neutrophil count.
4. **What are the complications of acute appendicitis?**
   - Appendicular mass (in untreated cases)
   - Perforation with an abscess
   - Perforation with generalised peritonitis
   - Pylephlebitis, portal pyaemia
   - Septicaemia, gram-negative shock
5. **How do you treat an appendicular mass?**
   - Conservative line, Oschner-Sherren regime—liquid and semisolid diet, antibiotics, intravenous fluids, etc.

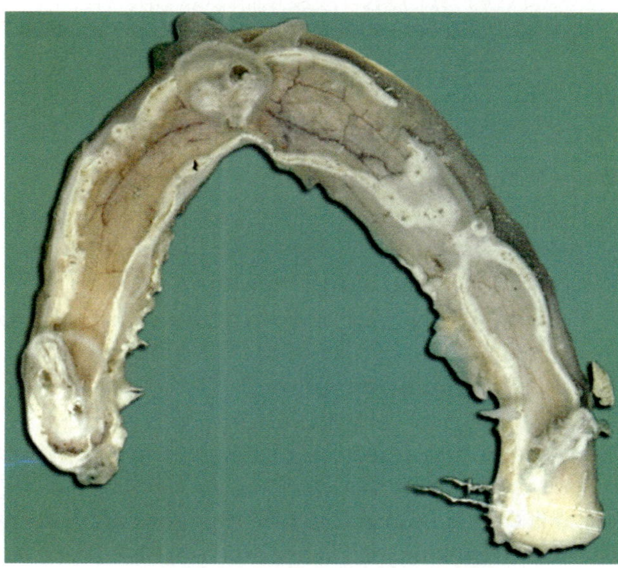

Fig. 69.8: Gangrenous appendicitis

## IX. CARCINOMA ASCENDING COLON

**1. What is this specimen?**

- Specimen of terminal ileum, caecum and right colon with removal of involved lymph nodes and fat fascia. Nowadays, only 4–6 cm of ileum is removed.

**2. What is the surgery?**

- Right radical hemicolectomy done for growth in the ascending colon.

**3. How do you identify colon?**

- *Taenia coli* and appendix are seen. The colon has a larger diameter compared to small intestine.

**4. What are the investigations?**

- Barium enema will show persistent filling defect. However, colonoscopy is the investigation because the growth can be visualised and biopsy can be taken.

**5. What do you mean by limited resection?**

- It is done for ileocaecal tuberculosis wherein diseased segment is removed.

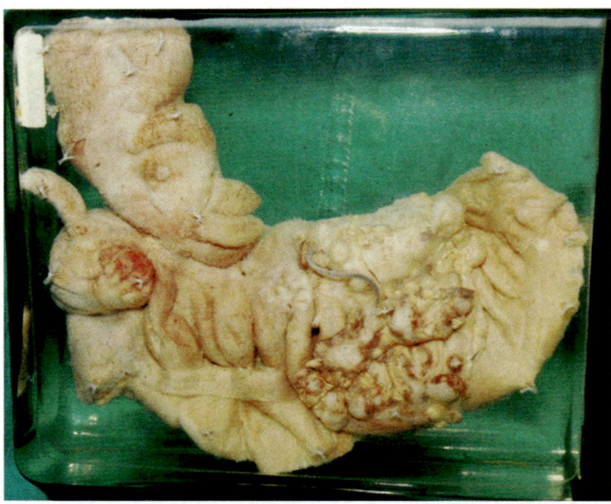

**Fig. 69.9:** Carcinoma ascending colon

## X. MECKEL'S DIVERTICULUM

**1. What is the specimen?**

- Resected specimen of intestine showing a diverticulum. Hence, it is a Meckel's diverticulum.

**2. Why is it a Meckel's diverticulum?**

- Because it is a single diverticulum arising from antimesenteric border of the intestine.

**3. What are common symptoms?**

- Bleeding per rectum, abdominal pain due to inflammation, intestinal obstruction and peritonitis due to perforation.

**4. What is the cause and what are the types of bleeding?**

- Ulcer in the ectopic gastric mucosa. Bleeding can be occult, in small quantities or rarely can be massive.

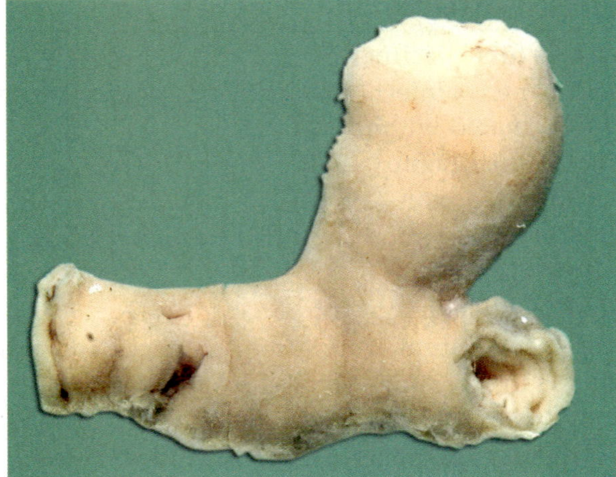

**Fig. 69.10:** Meckel's diverticulum

**5. How do you diagnose Meckel's diverticulum?**

- Radio-nuclear ($^{99m}$Tc pertechnetate) scan is helpful when there is active bleeding.

## XI. POLYCYSTIC KIDNEY

**1. What is this specimen?**

- Specimen of kidney with multiple cystic lesions. Entire kidney is involved.

**2. What is the diagnosis?**

- Polycystic kidney

**3. Why do you say it is polycystic kidney?**

- Kidney is grossly enlarged
- Outer surface is bosselated
- Multiple cysts are present

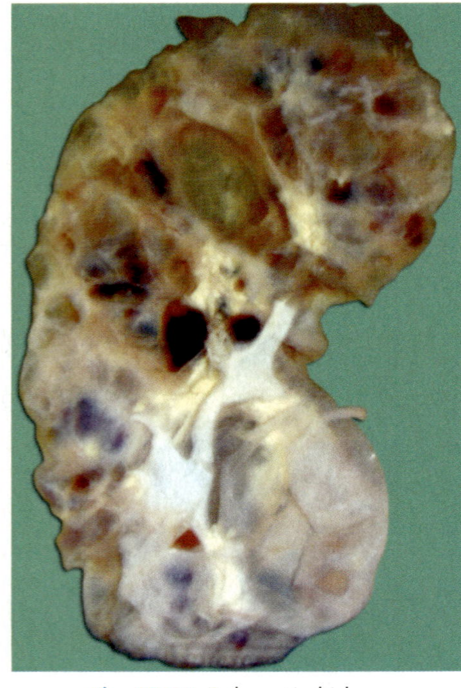

**Fig. 69.11:** Polycystic kidney

**4. What are clinical features of polycystic kidney?**
- Women: 30–50 years
- Bilateral renal mass
- Hypertension
- Haematuria
- Renal failure

**5. What is the treatment?**
- If there is no renal failure, control hypertension.
- If there is renal failure—dialysis followed by renal transplantation.

## XII. RENAL CELL CARCINOMA

**1. What is this specimen?**
- Specimen of the kidney because it is reniform shaped, ureter and calyces are seen.
- In the upper pole, there is destruction of the calyces with solid mass. Cut surface is smooth.

**2. What is the diagnosis?**
- Renal cell carcinoma.

**3. What is the microscopic picture?**
- Cuboidal or polyhedral clear cells with deeply stained rounded nuclei—clear cell carcinoma. Sometimes, dark cells can coexist. In some cases, walls of blood vessels are lined by tumour cells.

**4. How does it spread?**
- Lymphatic and blood spread

**5. What are the primary malignant tumours which spread by blood?**
- Renal cell carcinoma, follicular carcinoma thyroid, carcinoma prostate, carcinoma breast, bronchogenic carcinoma.

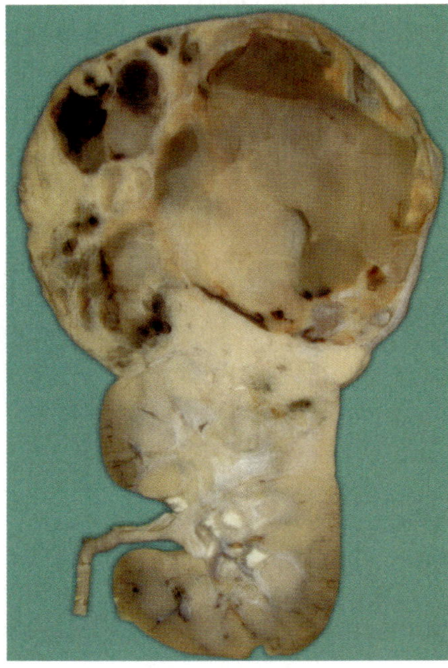

**Fig. 69.12:** Renal cell carcinoma

## XIII. HYDRONEPHROSIS

**1. What is this specimen?**
- Specimen of the kidney with ureter showing dilatation of pelvicalyceal system. Calyces are club-shaped.

**2. What is the diagnosis?**
- Hydronephrosis—probably due to pelvi-ureteric junction (PUJ) obstruction.

**3. Why PUJ obstruction?**
- Ureter is not dilated

**4. What are the common causes of obstruction at PUJ?**
- Stone in the pelvis
- Aberrant vessels—a lower polar artery or vein arising from the main vessels in an aberrant position obstructs the upper ureter.
- PUJ dyskinesia—occurs due to incoordination between neuromuscular impulses and pelvis.

**5. What is the treatment of PUJ dyskinesia?**
- Anderson-Hynes pyeloplasty.

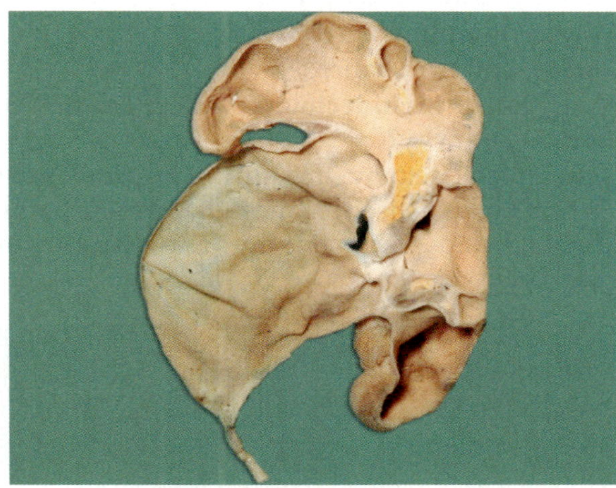

**Fig. 69.13:** Hydronephrosis

## XIV. CARCINOMA PENIS

**1. What is this specimen?**
- Specimen of penis, showing the glans. Prepuce is cut open showing the growth.

**2. What is the diagnosis?**
- Partial amputation done for carcinoma penis

**3. What are the indications for partial amputation of the penis?**
- Growth confined to the glans penis or to the prepuce.

**4. If shaft is involved, what is the treatment?**
- Total amputation of penis followed by perineal urethrostomy.

**5. What are the complications of perineal urethrostomy?**
- Bleeding, dermatitis and stenosis. The stenosis should be dilated by using Hegar's dilators.

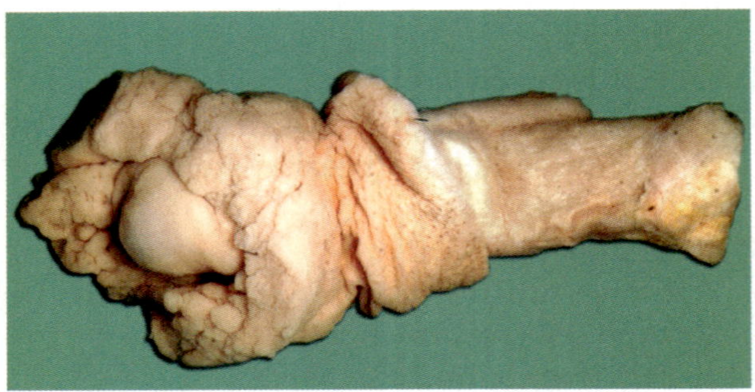

Fig. 69.14: Carcinoma penis

## XV. SEMINOMA TESTIS

1. **What is this specimen?**
   - Specimen of testis showing spermatic cord. Cut surface of the testis is smooth and homogenous with a tumour in the upper part.
2. **What is the diagnosis?**
   - Seminoma
3. **Why not a teratoma?**
   - In a teratoma, the cut surface is not homogenous.
4. **How does seminoma spread?**
   - Mainly by lymphatics.
5. **What type of orchidectomy is done for testicular tumours and why?**
   - High orchidectomy, through an inguinal incision. If scrotum is incised, chances of alternate pathway of lymphatics opening up are high. Hence, inguinal exploration is the choice.

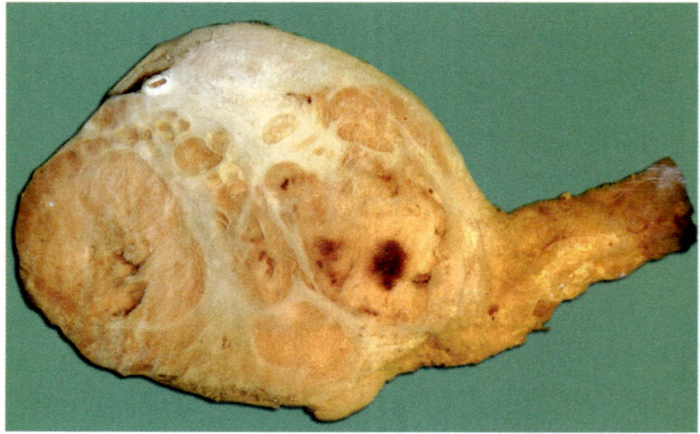

Fig. 69.15: Seminoma testis showing spermatic cord on the right side

## XVI. CHOLECYSTECTOMY FOR GALLSTONES

1. **What is this specimen?**
   - Cholecystectomy specimen.
2. **What is the diagnosis?**
   - Multiple stones are present within lumen—diagnosis is probably chronic cholecystitis.
3. **Why do you say it is a gallbladder?**
   - It is pear-shaped with fundus, body and a narrow portion—cystic area.

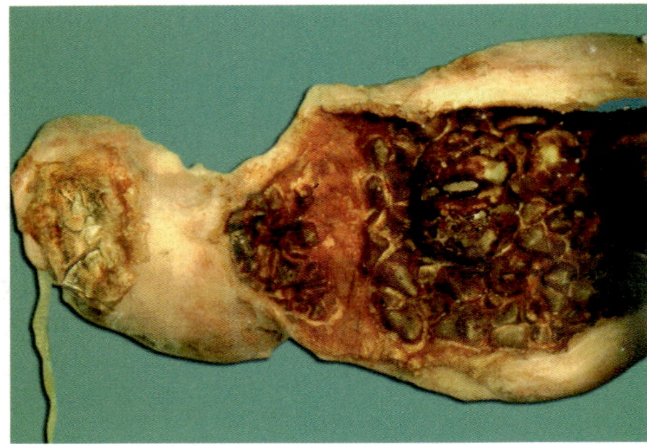

Fig. 69.16: Gallstones

4. **What is Hartmann's pouch?**
   - It is the distal angulated portion of gallbladder wherein a stone commonly lodges.
5. **What are the common symptoms of gallstones?**
   - Flatulent dyspepsia, gallstone colic, acute and chronic cholecystitis are common symptoms of gallstones. Mucocoele, empyema, perforation and gallstone pancreatitis are other complications.

## XVII. HYDATID CYST

1. **What is this specimen?**
   - Specimen of laminated membranes—this layer is also called ectocyst. It is thick and elastic resembling onion skin appearance.
2. **What is the diagnosis?**
   - Hydatid cyst—mostly liver
3. **What are the other layers of hydatid cyst?**
   - Outermost layer is called adventitial layer which blends firmly with liver tissue. The middle layer is ectocyst, also called laminated membrane. Inner layer is germinal epithelium, also called endocyst within which brood capsules and daughter cysts are present.

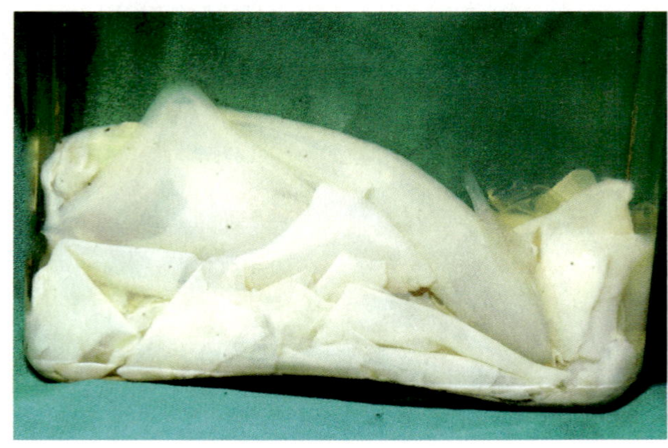

Fig. 69.17: Hydatid cyst

4. **What is the drug for hydatid disease?**
   - Albendazole 400 mg, a day for 15 days followed by no drug for 15 days. Then restart the cycle. Such treatment may have to continue for 6 months depending on the response rate.
5. **What are the common complications of hydatid cyst of the liver?**
   - Infection, rupture, calcification, cholangitis with jaundice are a few complications.

## XVIII. RADICAL GASTRECTOMY INCLUDING REMOVAL OF THE COLON

1. **What is the specimen?**
   - Specimen of stomach with transverse colon.
2. **Why stomach and colon?**
   - It has lesser curvature and greater curvature—pylorus, body and proximal stomach. Colon is the immediate structure below the stomach.
3. **What does it show?**
   - Exophytic growth infiltrating the colon
4. **What is the final diagnosis?**
   - Most probably it is carcinoma stomach infiltrating transverse colon.
5. **What is the best investigation in such cases to identify local infiltration?**
   - CT scan

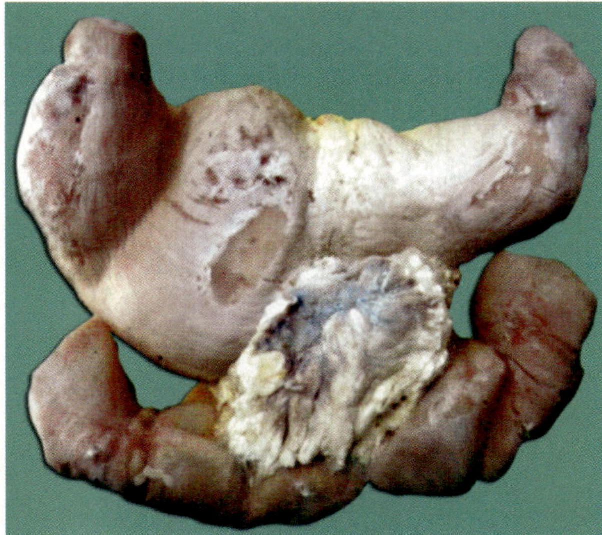

**Fig. 69.18:** Radical gastrectomy including removal of the colon

## XIX. LIPOMA

1. **What is this specimen?**
   - Specimen of lipoma
2. **Why do you say it is lipoma?**
   - It is lobular, yellow in colour

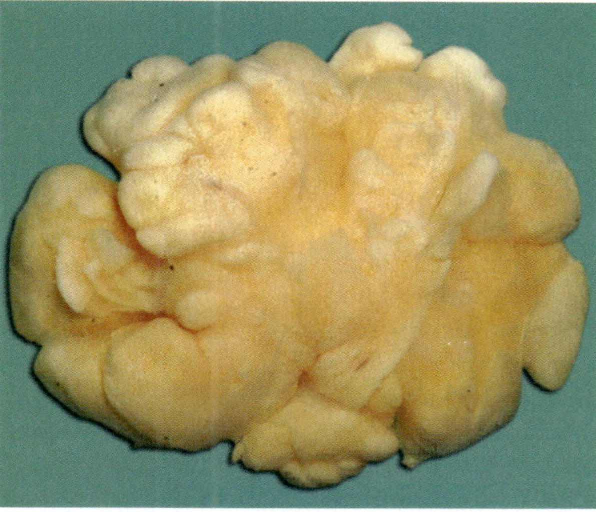

**Fig. 69.19:** Lipoma

3. **What is the commonest site and type of lipoma?**
   - Flank is the commonest site. Single and subcutaneous variety is the commonest type.
4. **What are the common complications of lipoma?**
   - Liposarcoma and intussusception
5. **Which type of lipoma gives rise to intussusception?**
   - Submucosal type

## XX. MALIGNANT MELANOMA

1. **What is this specimen?**
   - Specimen of foot showing a large ulcerated growth in the sole of the foot.
2. **What is the diagnosis and why do you say so?**
   - Malignant melanoma because the lesion is pigmented.
3. **What is the commonest type of malignant melanoma?**
   - Superficial spreading is the first followed by nodular variety.
4. **What are the staging systems available for this condition?**
   - Clark's level of invasion and Breslow's thickness are important staging systems in addition to TNM staging.

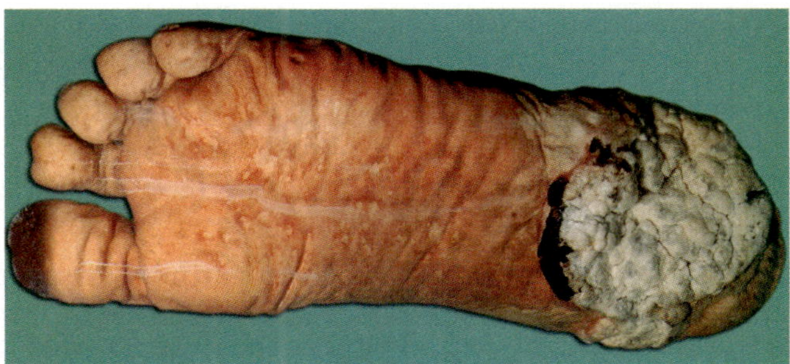

**Fig. 69.20:** Malignant melanoma

**5. What are the ABCDE of melanoma?**
- Asymmetry
- Border irregular
- Colour variegation
- Diameter >6 mm
- Elevation

## XXI. THYROIDECTOMY SPECIMEN

**1. What is this specimen?**
- Specimen of thyroid gland showing both lobes and isthmus.

**2. What is the diagnosis and why do you say so?**
- Probably it is a subtotal thyroidectomy specimen—surgery is done for multinodular goitre.

**3. What is the commonest type of malignancy of the thyroid gland?**
- Papillary carcinoma—63%. 2nd common type is follicular carcinoma thyroid.

**4. What is the surgical treatment for well-differentiated carcinoma thyroid gland?**
- Most centres follow total thyroidectomy. If the patient is in low-risk category, lobectomy can be done.

**5. What blood investigation is useful in the follow-up period of papillary carcinoma thyroid gland?**
- Thyroglobulin

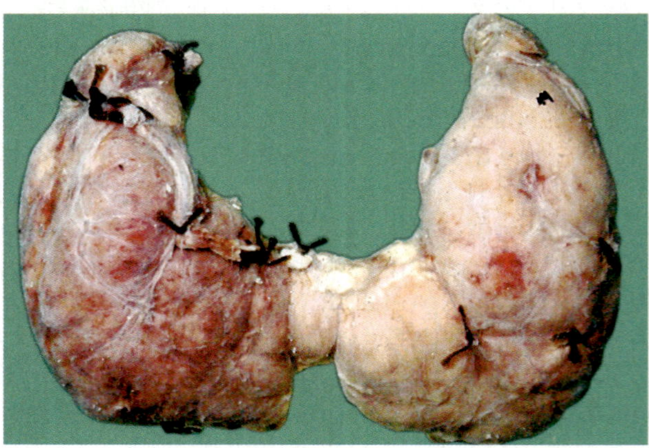

Fig. 69.21: Thyroidectomy specimen

## XXII. WIDE EXCISION SPECIMEN OF SKIN

**1. What is this specimen?**
- Specimen of skin which has been excised with normal skin. Hence, wide excision specimen.

**2. What is the diagnosis and why do you say so?**
- Probably it is a squamous cell carcinoma because edges are everted.

**3. What are the common sites of squamous cell carcinoma skin?**
- Areas with chronic irritation, e.g. Kangri cancer in the abdominal wall, chimney sweepers cancer, etc.

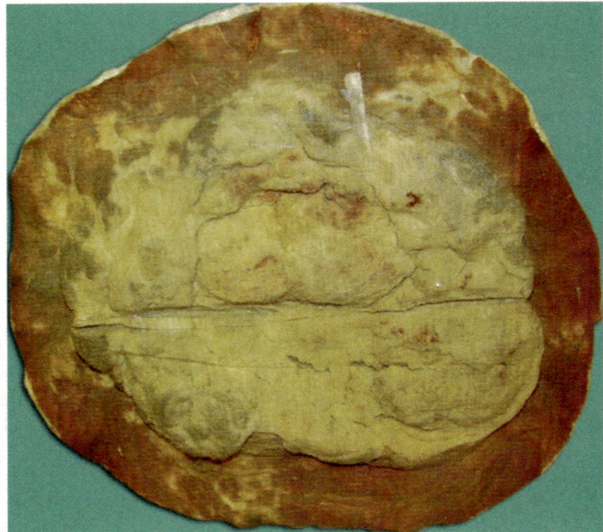

Fig. 69.22: Wide excision skin

**4. What are the common precancerous lesions for squamous cell carcinoma?**
- Leukoplakia, Bowen's disease, chronic irritation and scar tissues, etc.

**5. What do you call squamous cell carcinoma arising in a scar tissue?**
- Marjolin's ulcer

## XXIII. WHIPPLE'S PANCREATICODUODENECTOMY

**1. What is this specimen?**
- Specimen showing distal stomach, duodenum, proximal jejunum and pancreatic head.

**2. What is the name of this operation?**
- Whipple's pancreaticoduodenectomy

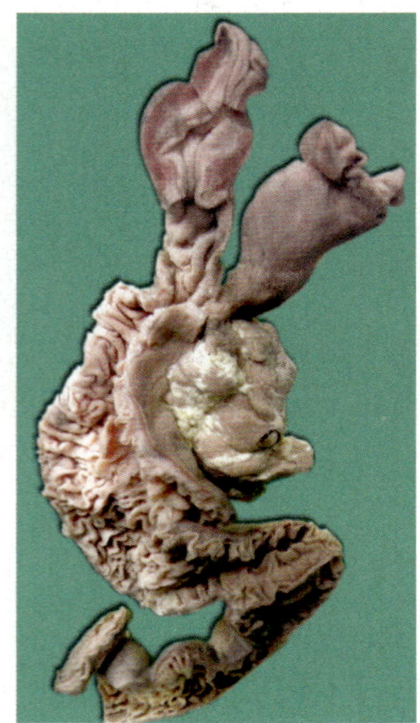

Fig. 69.23: Whipple's pancreaticoduodenectomy

3. **Why is it done?**
   - Mostly due to periampullary carcinoma
4. **How can you get histopathological diagnosis?**
   - Endoscopic biopsy
5. **Is there any other indication for Whipple's surgery?**
   - Pancreatic head mass—doubt exists between chronic pancreatitis and carcinoma head pancreas. Provided experience of the surgeon is good.

## XXIV. RIGHT HEMICOLECTOMY FOR CARCINOMA CAECUM

1. **What is this specimen?**
   - Specimen showing distal ileum, caecum, part of the ascending colon and a few lymph nodes
2. **What is the name of this operation?**
   - Limited colectomy

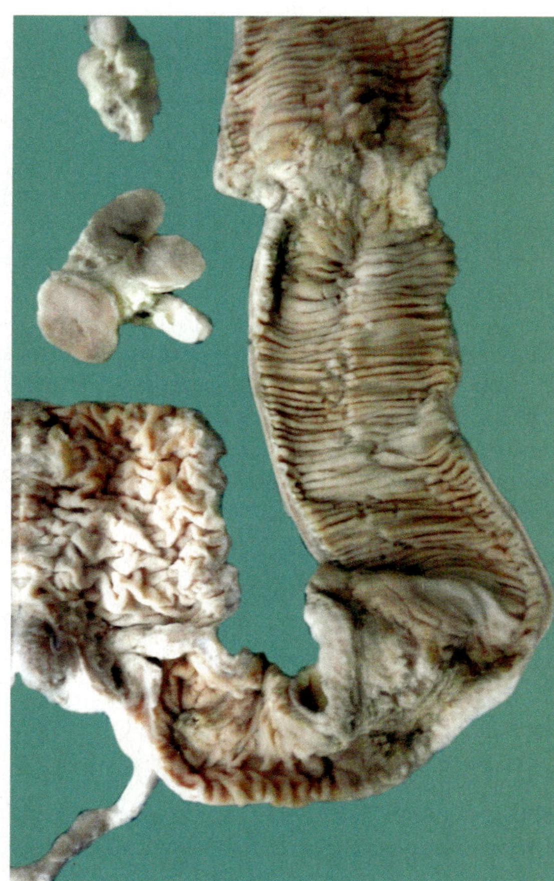

**Fig. 69.24:** Right hemicolectomy for carcinoma caecum

3. **Why is it done?**
   - Mostly due to ileo-caecal tuberculosis
4. **Why do you say so?**
   - Stricture is seen in the terminal ileum
5. **What was the indication for surgery?**
   - Acute intestinal obstruction

## XXV. SPLENECTOMY SPECIMEN

1. **What is this specimen?**
   - Specimen showing spleen with laceration of the diaphragmatic surface.
2. **Why laceration?**
   - Blunt injury is the most common cause of rupture spleen.
3. **What will be clinical manifestation?**
   - Bleeding
4. **What other surgery can be done for bleeding?**
   - Partial splenectomy or splenorrhaphy
5. **What is the dangerous complication after splenectomy?**
   - Opportunistic post-splenectomy infections.

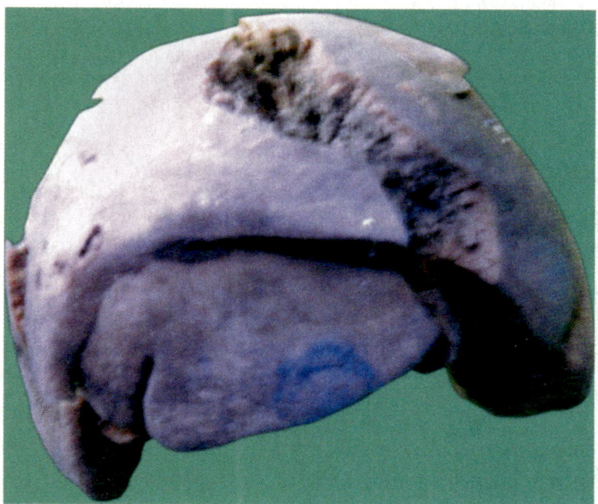

**Fig. 69.25:** Splenectomy specimen

***Useful Tips***
- Please look into the specimen carefully
- Please see both sides of the specimen
- Think which is the most likely organ involved
- Think what is the probable diagnosis.

Chapter 70

# Operative Surgery, Laparoscopic Surgery and Accessories

- History of surgery
- Operative surgery techniques
- Excision of swellings
- Surgery for hydrocoele
- Incision and drainage (I and D)
- Incision and drainage of breast abscess
- Circumcision
- Venesection or cut down
- Vasectomy
- Tracheostomy
- Thyroidectomy
- Amputations
- Amputations in leg
- Upper limb amputations
- Abdominal incisions
- Appendicectomy
- Bassini's herniorrhaphy
- Open cholecystectomy
- Vagotomy gastrojejunostomy (GJ)
- Colectomy
- Staplers in surgery
- Laparoscopic surgery/Minimal access surgery
- Hernia repair: TAPP (Transabdominal Preperitoneal Mesh Repair)
- TEP: Totally Extra Peritoneal Repair
- SILS
- Natural orifice transluminal endoscopic surgery (notes)
- VAAFT technique
- Robotic surgery
- Energy sources in surgery
- Harmonic scalpel
- Lasers in surgery

## Introduction

Over a period of time, the number of operations an undergraduate is expected to know has become less and less. Today no MBBS doctor is supposed to do a surgical procedure because qualified surgeons are available even in a village. Hence, I have discussed only some common surgical procedures that an undergraduate student is expected to know. Every operation has been discussed along a certain basic pattern as given in the next page and the key words used are given in Key Box 70.1. *Students should study surgical anatomy before reading this chapter.* Father of ancient surgery was an Indian, Sushruta. Under history of surgery, I have listed a few eminent surgeons who have contributed to surgery in the past. The most common surgeries done are appendicectomy hernioplasty, etc. Students should study these surgeries in more detail. In addition to these common operations, laparoscopic surgeries and few other accessories related to surgery are discussed.

## HISTORY OF SURGERY

- Surgery emerged as a specialty in the late 19th century.
- There are many eminent surgeons who have contributed significantly in the development of surgery. A few surgeons are uniquely associated with their work on a particular disease or specialty. There are numerous surgeons who have made distinct contribution in their respective specialty. Some of the commonly known works and the surgeons associated with them are listed below.

| Surgeons | Associated work |
|---|---|
| Ambroise Pare | Haemorrhage control |
| Joseph Lister | Asepsis/antisepsis |
| Theodor Kocher | Thyroid surgery |
| Theodor Billroth | Gastric surgery |
| William Halsted | Breast surgery |

**Theodor Kocher (1841–1917):** He was a student of Theodor Billroth and Bernhard von Langenbeck. He did extensive work on thyroid and excised the thyroid for goitre in 1876. Some of the contributions of Kocher are Kocher's transverse incision for thyroid surgery, kocherization of duodenum, Kocher's sign for Graves' disease, Kocher's forceps, etc. He is known to be the father of thyroid surgery. He won the Nobel prize in 1909.

**Theodor Billroth (1829–1894):** He was the first surgeon to remove a part of the oesophagus in 1872. In 1873, he performed the first complete excision of a larynx. He was the first surgeon to excise a rectal cancer. He is credited with distinct eponymous work named after him that includes Billroth's I operation, Billroth's II operation, Billroth's cord, etc. He is considered to be the father of abdominal surgery.

**Halsted (1852–1922):** He is well known for radical operation for breast cancer. He introduced surgical gloves to protect the hands of his scrub nurse, Caroline Hampton. He developed surgery for inguinal hernia. He also developed topical anaesthesia.

**Sushruta:** Ancient history showed Sushruta (600 BC) to be the pioneer in plastic surgery and his work is described in *Sushruta Samhita*. It describes various surgical procedures and instruments used. His famous surgery on ear lobe is believed to be a classical example of flap surgery used more than 2500 years ago in India. He is known to be "Father of Plastic Surgery".

## OPERATIVE SURGERY

**Introduction:** I have given in the section 1 of this manual about basic principles of the surgery, which includes various components such as Communication, Counselling, Ethics, Safety principles including WHO check list, Role of antibiotics, etc. Every surgeon must follow these guidelines so that our aim is achieved, be it is cure, prophylactic surgery, relief from pain or palliation. Again to remind an important component of surgery is—Do no harm. In the following pages you will come across commonly done surgeries.

**Commonly used abbreviations** are given in Key Box 70.1.

Key Box 70.1

**Commonly Used Abbreviations**

| | |
|---|---|
| SA | Spinal anaesthesia |
| GA | General anaesthesia |
| LA | Local anaesthesia |
| RA | Regional anaesthesia |
| OT | Operation theatre |
| NPO | Nil per oral |
| IV | Intravenous |
| RT | Ryle's tube |

**Steps of operative surgery**

1. Indications
2. Contraindications
3. Position of the patient
4. Anaesthesia
5. Preparation of parts
6. Procedure
7. Closure
8. Postoperative management
9. Postoperative complications
10. Advice at discharge

**Antiseptic agents**

- Povidone-iodine 7.5% to 10% as skin antiseptic and surgical scrub. It is a bactericidal/virucidal in reducing microorganisms prior to surgery.
- Spirit 70%
- Savlon

**Autoclave and sterilisation:** Table 70.1 and *see* Chapter 10 on sterilisation.

**TABLE 70.1:** Sterilisation

| Agents for sterilisation | Common of items |
|---|---|
| 1. Autoclaving | Linen, operative instruments, glass syringes |
| 2. Dettol or phenol | Sharp instruments (scissors, needles, blades) |
| 3. Glutaraldehyde | Endoscopy and laparoscopy equipment |
| 4. Ethylene oxide gamma radiation | Syringes |
| 5. Formaldehyde | Disinfect rooms like OT |
| 6. Skin | 70% spirit, povidone-iodine |

## EXCISION OF SWELLINGS

### A. LIPOMA

#### 1. Indications

- Large size (cosmesis/patient's wish)
- Recent rapid increase in size
- Symptomatic naevo-/neurolipomas
- Pressure symptoms based on site.

#### 2. Contraindications

Strictly speaking, there are no contraindications. Excision of lipoma is a simple procedure. However, small the surgery may be, safety is an important principle to be kept in mind.

#### 3. Position of the Patient

Supine/lateral/prone depending upon the location.

#### 4. Anaesthesia

If small, under LA; if large, regional anaesthesia or GA.

#### 5. Preparation of the Parts

Povidone-iodine and spirit

#### 6. Surgical Procedure

- **Incision:** A linear incision over the summit of the swelling is placed and flaps raised on both sides of the incision.

- **Layers opened:** Skin and some part of the subcutaneous tissue till the capsule of the swelling is encountered.
- **Dissection:** Using an artery forceps or a mosquito forceps (if a small swelling), a plane is created between the raised flaps and the capsule of the swelling. Pressure is applied at the base of the swelling to deliver out the lipoma. A small vessel may be encountered as the base is being dissected that should be identified and cauterised or ligated. The specimen should be sent for histopathological evaluation (Fig. 70.1).

### 7. Closure

If a large cavity is created due to excision of swelling, the excised skin flaps can be refreshed and excess skin can be removed.

- A few interrupted Vicryl sutures can be placed to close subcutaneous layer.
- The skin is closed with non-absorbable sutures. Sometimes, a drain may have to be kept in the cavity.

### 8. Postoperative Management

Nothing specific other than monitoring vitals and the operated area for bleeding. Majority of them can be done as day care surgery.

### 9. Postoperative Complications

- Infection, bleeding
- Injury to the structures in the vicinity
- Seroma formation, if large cavity remains

### 10. Advice at Discharge

Suture removal after 7–10 days, if non-absorbable sutures are used such as 3-0 silk. If absorbable sutures such as monocryl (3-0 Polyglactin) are used, there is no need to remove the sutures.

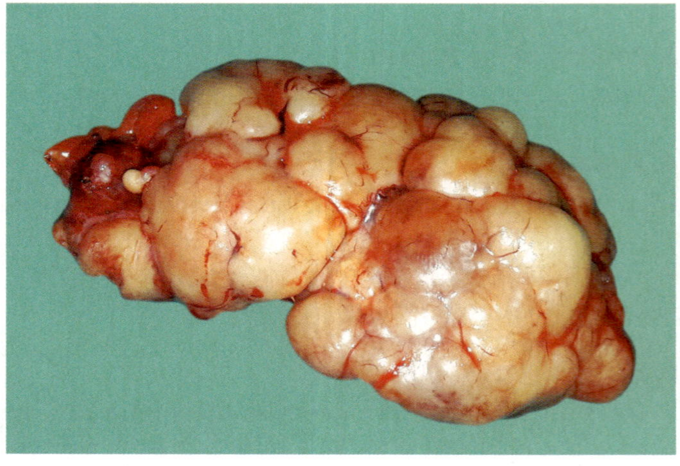

Fig. 70.1: Excised lipoma—watch lobularity

## B. SEBACEOUS CYST

### 1. Indications

- Infection—results in abscess
- Complications such as **Cock's peculiar tumour**, horn and calcification.

### 2. Contraindication

No specific contraindication.

### 3. Position of the Patient

Supine/lateral/prone depending upon the location.

### 4. Anaesthesia

Mostly LA. Multiple cysts over scalp and scrotum may require GA or regional anaesthesia.

### 5. Preparation of the Parts

Povidone-iodine and spirit.

### 6. Surgical Procedure

- **Incision: Elliptical incision** around the summit of the swelling encircling the punctum.
- **Layers opened**
  - Incision should be superficial. Care should be taken not to cut open the cyst wall.
  - The principle is to **completely excise the cyst** with its wall and the overlying punctum and a bit of the surrounding skin around the punctum (Fig. 70.2).
- **Dissection**
  - A plane is created between the skin and the cyst wall, carefully, preventing opening of the cyst wall.
  - An Allis forceps may be applied to the punctum and the elliptical skin to obtain traction. Flaps need to be raised gradually on either sides of the incision and then deliver the cyst *in toto.*
  - If the cyst wall opens up, the sebum is removed completely and an effort to remove all the cyst wall, in piecemeal, is made.

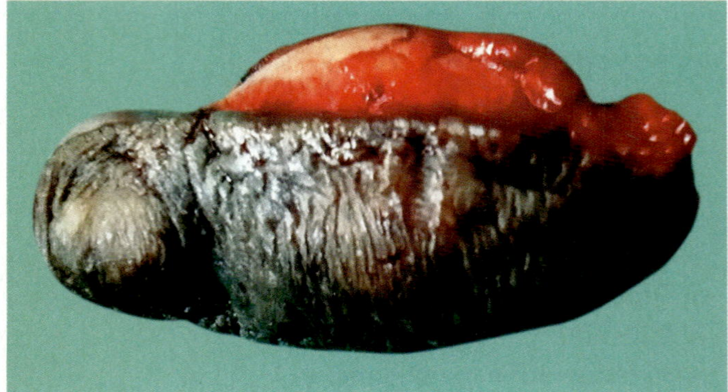

Fig. 70.2: Sebaceous cyst excised with punctum and central portion of the skin

### 7. Closure

Single layer closure of the skin.

### 8. Postoperative Management

Watch for haematoma especially after removal of cyst from the scalp. In infected cases, antibiotics are given.

### 9. Postoperative Complications

- Infection
- Recurrence, if cyst wall is not completely removed.

### 10. Advice at Discharge

Suture removal after 7–10 days.

## C. NEUROFIBROMA/NEURILEMMOMA

### 1. Indications

- Cosmesis
- Symptoms of pain on pressure
- Pressure effects causing neurological deficits
- Sarcomatous changes

### 2. Contraindication

In von Recklinghausen's disease, only symptomatic neurofibromas should be removed.

### 3. Position of the Patient

Supine/lateral/prone depending upon the location.

### 4. Anaesthesia

Mostly LA, sometimes GA.

### 5. Preparation of the Parts

Povidone-iodine and spirit.

### 6. Surgical Procedure

- **Incision:** A linear incision over the summit of the swelling is placed and flaps raised on both sides of the incision.
- **Layers opened:** Skin and some part of the subcutaneous tissue till the capsule of the swelling is encountered.
- **Dissection:** Using an artery forceps or a mosquito forceps (if a small swelling), a plane is created between the raised flaps and the capsule of the swelling. Pressure is applied at the base of the swelling to deliver out the neurofibroma. Care should be taken not to injure the underlying nerve while dissecting (Fig. 70.3).

### 7. Closure

It can be closed in two layers, subcutaneous—vicryl, interrupted and skin 2–0/3–0 sutures.

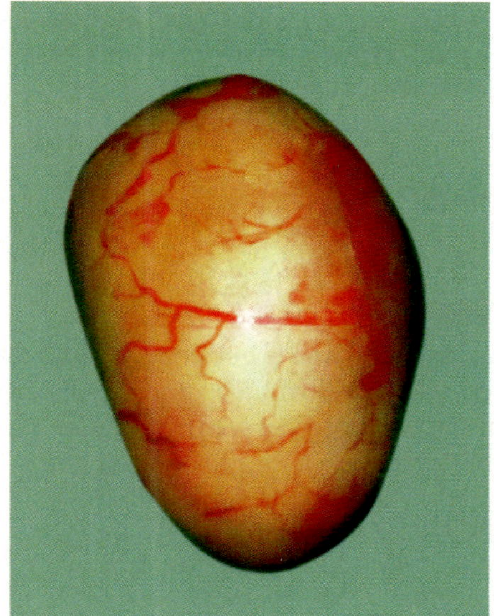

**Fig. 70.3:** Schwannoma/Neurilemmoma

### 8. Postoperative Management

Nothing specific other than monitoring vitals and the operated area for bleeding. Majority of them can be done as day care surgery.

### 9. Postoperative Complications

- Infection
- Injury to the nerve causing weakness, loss of sensations of the affected part.
- If partially left behind, recurrence and chance of sarcomatous changes.

### 10. Advice at Discharge

Suture removal after 7–10 days.

## SURGERY FOR HYDROCOELE

**This is done as a day care surgery.**

### 1. Indication

Vaginal hydrocoele. However, infantile and funicular hydrocoeles are also treated surgically in the same manner.

### 2. Contraindication

Secondary hydrocoele due to *testicular tumours*. They contain haemorrhagic fluid. It will be a big blunder to incise the scrotum mistaking it to be a vaginal hydrocoele. Suspect testicular tumours if the hydrocoele is recent and lax, if the testis is felt separately and is hard in consistency or transillumination is negative.

### 3. Position of the Patient

Supine

**Pearls of Wisdom**

Before incising scrotum for hydrocoele, palpate carefully testis and epididymis and rule out testicular tumour. When in doubt, get ultrasound examination of testis.

## 4. Anaesthesia

SA or LA.

## 5. Preparation of the Parts

Savlon and spirit (iodine is better avoided because it can cause severe scrotal dermatitis and excoriation of skin, which can cause more discomfort to the patient than hydrocoele surgery).

## 6. Procedure (Key Box 70.2)

### *Incision*

Hydrocoele is held tense by an assistant and 5–6 cm incision (depending upon size) is made over the most prominent part of the swelling parallel to the median raphe of the scrotum.

Key Box 70.2

**Hydrocoele Surgery**

- Aspiration: Not advised
- Lord's plication: Small hydrocoele
- Jaboulay's: Large hydrocoele

### *Layers Opened*

- Skin
- Dartos
- External spermatic fascia
- Cremasteric fascia
- Internal spermatic fascia

At this stage, hydrocoele sac is visible and is delivered outside the incision (Fig. 70.4).

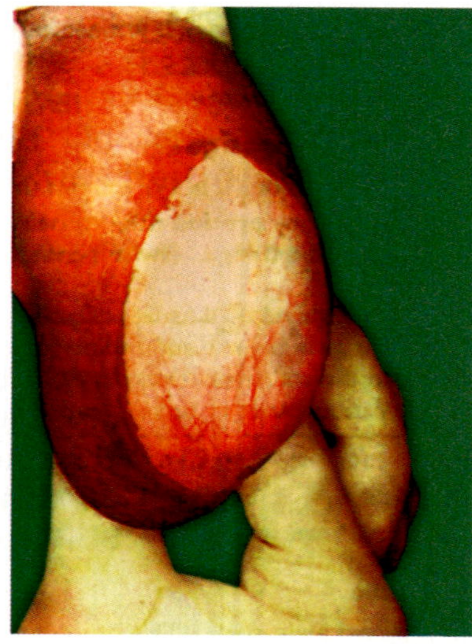

**Fig. 70.4:** Hydrocoele sac being delivered

Hydrocoele fluid is drained by using ***trocar and cannula.*** An opening is made in the tunica vaginalis sac and it is enlarged. All fluid is drained out. Testis and epididymis are inspected for any pathology, e.g. Craggy epididymis can be found in tuberculosis. Depending on the size of the hydrocoele and thickness of the wall of the sac, two types of surgery can be done.

a. **Small tunica vaginalis sac (TV sac):** The redundant tunica vaginalis is plicated by interrupted sutures. The sac gets crumpled up and surrounds the testis. This is called **Lord's plication** (Fig. 70.5). Advantage of this operation is minimal dissection, hence no complications.
b. **Sac is large and thick or multilocular hydrocoele:** Partial excision of the hydrocoele sac is done leaving a margin of 1–2 cm. After obtaining hemostasis, eversion of sac is done. Here cut edge of the sac is everted and sutured behind the testis. This is called **Jaboulay's operation. By eversion of the sac, the secreting surface of the testis becomes anterior and secretions are absorbed by subcutaneous lymphatics** (Fig. 70.6A and B).

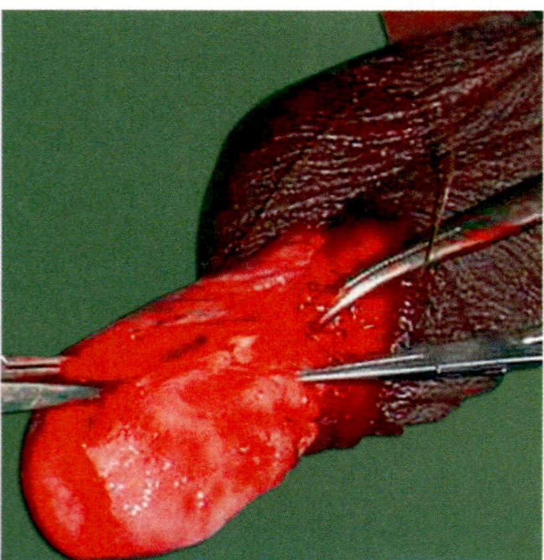

**Fig. 70.5:** The sac has been everted and edges of the sac sutured together

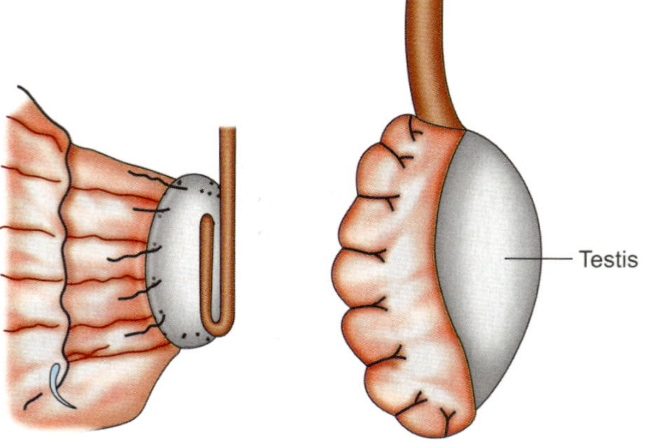


**Fig. 70.6A:** Lord's plication **Fig. 70.6B:** Jaboulay's operation

(*Courtesy:* DR Capt. Ramachandra L, Former Professor and Head, Department of Surgery, KMC, Manipal)

c. ***Sharma and Jhawer's technique:*** In this, minimum dissection of the sac is done to separate from surrounding region. This will avoid complications such as bleeding.

### 7. Closure

- In vast majority of the cases, if perfect hemostasis is obtained, draining the cavity is not required. A tube drain can be kept in the scrotum, if required. When kept brought out separately by making a stab incision and is anchored to the scrotal skin by white thread.
- Subcutaneous layer by using absorbable suture such as vicryl sutures.
- Skin—interrupted absorbable sutures (polyglactin—rapid vicryl). Silk is avoided for skin closure over the scrotum as black colour of the silk is not seen clearly over dark pigmented skin of the scrotum, making stitch removal difficult.
- Scrotal support is given to reduce oedema.

### 8. Postoperative Management

- NPO for 2 to 4 hours followed by soft diet.
- Prophylactic antibiotics are given. Postoperative antibiotics are not required.
- Use Monocryl which is a synthetic, absorbable suture—No need to remove sutures.

### 9. Postoperative Complications

- **Haematoma:** If it is large and increasing, wound should be reopened urgently and bleeders have to be ligated. It may be due to injury to the testicular artery, vein or pampiniform plexus of veins.
  Scrotal oedema can occur which resolves within 2–3 days.
- **Wound infection** can result in discharging pus.
- Testis can undergo necrosis. Such cases are treated with orchidectomy.
- **Injury to the spermatic cord**.

### 10. Advice at Discharge

Normal activity within 1 or 2 days.

> *Pearls of Wisdom*
> Even though surgery for hydrocoele is minor, it should be done meticulously to avoid complications.

## INCISION AND DRAINAGE (I AND D)

### 1. Indication

Pyogenic abscess, pyaemic abscesses.

### 2. Contraindication

Cold abscess.

### 3. Position of the Patient

Supine, prone or lateral depending upon site of abscess.

### 4. Anaesthesia

- Regional anaesthesia or GA is preferred because abscess is multiloculated and infiltration of lignocaine into the abscess cavity does not act because of the acidic pH of the pus.
- However, a superficial abscess which is pointing can be managed without GA.

### 5. Preparation of the Parts

Iodine and spirit.

### 6. Procedure

- **A stab incision** is made over the most prominent part of the swelling where skin is red, thinned out and is pointed.
- Pus that is drained is ***sent for culture and sensitivity.***
- A sinus forceps or finger is introduced within the abscess cavity and all the loculi are broken. When fresh blood oozes out, it indicates completion of the procedure.
- The cavity is irrigated with antiseptic agents such as iodine solution. It is followed by irrigation with normal saline.
- If the cavity is large, it is packed with roller gauze soaked in iodine and it is removed after 24–48 hours. Packing helps in controlling the bleeding, and keeps the abscess cavity open. By 7–10 days, the cavity collapses, granulation tissue fills up the cavity and healing takes place.

**Hilton's method of drainage:** When an abscess is located over a major vessel, as in axilla or neck, **do not make a stab incision**. An incision is made on the skin and subcutaneous tissue and sinus forceps is introduced. Later, it is treated like the treatment of an abscess. This method is followed to avoid injury to major vessels and nerves. It is also indicated in parotid abscess to avoid damage to facial nerve. Sinus forceps is selected because it is blunt tipped instrument without lock system so that opening and closing the blades are easy. It has a few serrations at the tip so that, if necessary, biopsy of the wall can be taken.

### 7. Closure

An abscess should not be closed, as it contains pus, bacteria (*see* also breast abscess drainage). However, in breast abscess, once all loculi are broken and after a thorough wash, the wound is closed with sutures, a drain is kept in the dependent position and brought out by a separate incision.

### 8. Postoperative Management

- Antibiotics
- Control of diabetes (if patient is diabetic)
- Regular dressings of the wound with antiseptic agents.

### 9. Postoperative Complications

- During the process of breaking the loculi, vessels underneath may be injured causing haematoma which requires drainage. Otherwise, there are no specific complications.
- Injury to vessels or nerves can occur, if basic principles of drainage of an abscess are not followed.

### 10. Advice at Discharge

Control of diabetes (if present).

## INCISION AND DRAINAGE OF BREAST ABSCESS

### 1. Indication

Breast abscess (Key Box 70.3)

Key Box 70.3

**Breast Abscess Drainage**

- GA is preferred
- Do not wait for fluctuation
- Throbbing pain is an indication for surgery
- Small curved incision
- Keep in mind, mastitis carcinomatosa
- Today ultrasound-guided aspiration of the pus is the first line of treatment.

### 2. Contraindication

None. However, ultrasound-guided aspiration of breast abscess should be done first especially in unilocular breast abscess and if pus recurs, aspiration can be repeated also.

### 3. Position of the Patient

Supine

### 4. Anaesthesia

GA

### 5. Preparation

Iodine and spirit.

### 6. Procedure (Figs 70.7 and 70.8)

About 3 to 4 cm semicircular incision is made over the swelling where there is maximum tenderness. It is drained just like pyogenic abscess. Another stab incision is made in the dependent position and tube drain is brought out through this incision.

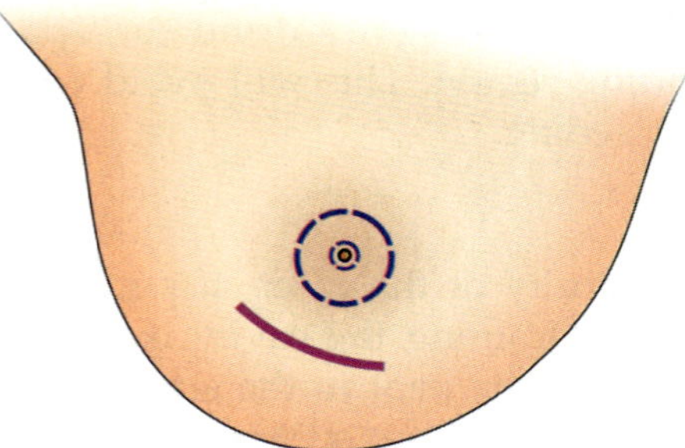

**Fig. 70.7:** Incision for breast abscess

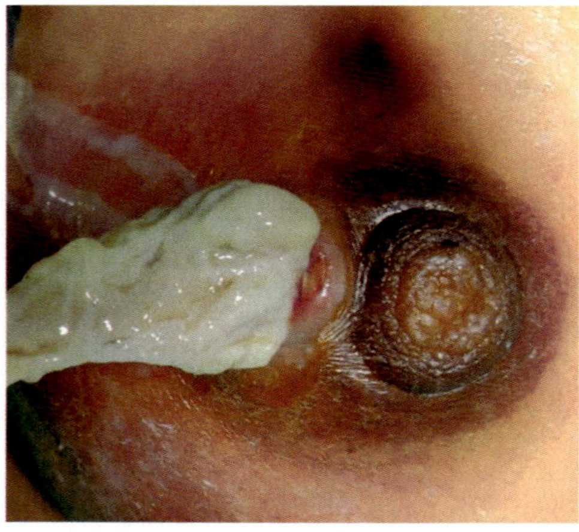

**Fig. 70.8:** Drainage of pus after a stab incision

*Pearls of Wisdom*

Radial incision can be given, if abscess is in the peripheral part of the breast.

### 7. Closure

- If infection is very severe, **do not close the incision**.
- Otherwise, main wound is sutured and tube drain is brought down at the dependent position. Once the drainage is minimal, the drain is removed.

*Pearls of Wisdom*

Minor breast abscess need not be drained. Ultrasound-guided one or two aspirations may be curative in many cases.

### 8. Postoperative Management

- NPO for about 6 hours
- Antibiotic of choice is **cloxacillin** 500 mg 6th hourly because the common organism is *Staphylococcus aureus*. Please refer to MRSA and breast abscess on page 483.
- It may take 7–15 days for complete healing.
- One should not wait for fluctuation to develop in a breast abscess. If pain and tenderness does not subside by 48 hours, breast abscess is incised. Otherwise, breast tissue gets damaged.

### 9. Postoperative Complications

Haematoma needs evacuation.

### 10. Advice at Discharge

Lactating women should clean the nipple after every breastfeed and keep it clean.

## CIRCUMCISION

Circumcision refers to removal of the preputial skin.

### 1. Indications

a. Ritual: Religious
b. Phimosis

### 2. Contraindication

Hypospadias

*Pearls of Wisdom*

Preputial skin is required for repair of hypospadias.

### 3. Position of the Patient

Supine

### 4. Anaesthesia

a. In children—GA
b. In adults—LA

### 5. Preparation of the Parts

Savlon and spirit

*Pearls of Wisdom*

Use plain lignocaine (without adrenaline) for LA during circumcision. Dose: 2% lignocaine 10–15 ml.

### 6. Procedure

***In Adults*** (Fig. 70.9)

- Skin of the tip of the penis is held in two places by using artery forceps, prepuce is separated from the glans and is slit up in mid-dorsal line to a point a little beyond the middle of the glans.
- Preputial layers are trimmed away in a line parallel to the corona. ***On the ventral surface, frenular artery needs to be ligated by using figure of 8 stitch.*** Two layers of prepuce are united by interrupted fine 3-0 or 4-0 absorbable sutures such as dexon or Vicryl. Dressings are applied.

***In Children*** (Fig. 70.10)

- Prepuce is held by two artery forceps and gentle traction is applied. A small artery clamp is applied distal to the glans and skin distal to the clamp is removed.
- Once clamp is removed, bleeding points are identified and ligated.

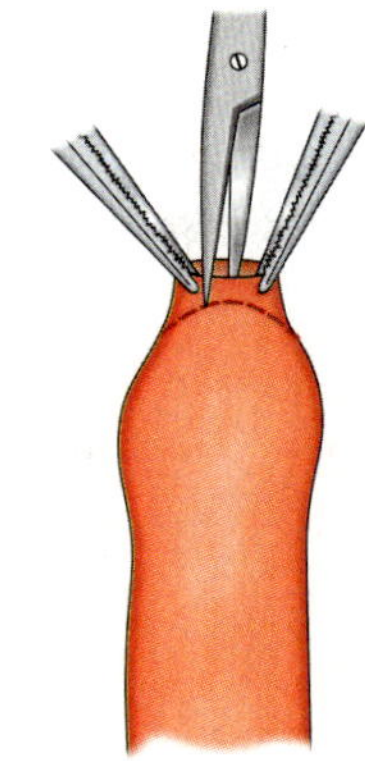

Fig. 70.9: Circumcision in adults

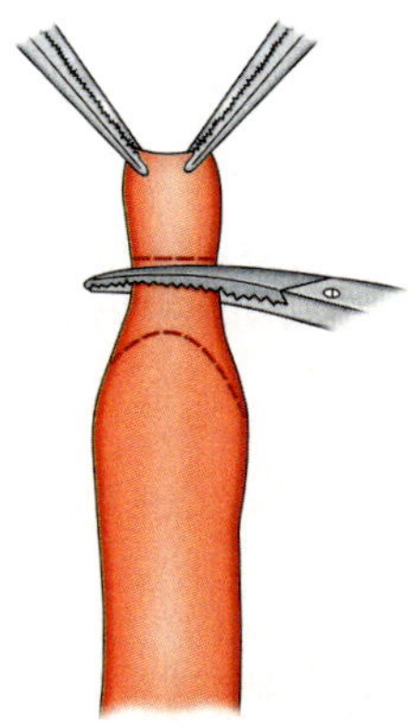

Fig. 70.10: Circumcision in children

- Two layers of prepuce are approximated by using 5–0 Vicryl.

### 7. Closure

Two layers of prepuce by using Vicryl sutures.

### 8. Postoperative Management

- Analgesics
- Antibiotics
- Removal of sutures is very painful. Hence, **do not use nonabsorbable sutures**.

### 9. Postoperative Complications

a. Injury to the glans penis can occur when there are extensive adhesions between prepuce and glans. It needs suturing.
b. **Haematoma:** Due to injury to the corpora cavernosa or due to the bleeding from cut edges.
c. **Tension at suture line,** if too much skin is removed. This may cause painful erection at a later date.

### 10. Advice at Discharge

This surgery in adults is done on an outpatient basis. Patients are discharged within a few hours. Hence, patients are advised to report, if there is bleeding and also not to wet the area for 2–3 days.

**What is sutureless circumcision?**

Instead of suturing, cyanoacrylate glue is used to approximate the two layers of the prepuce. The tissue glue has hemostatic and bacteriostatic properties. Procedure can be done more fast than conventional technique of circumcision.

## VENESECTION OR CUT DOWN

### 1. Indications

- Shock: Hypovolaemic, haemorrhagic, burns, etc.
- When peripheral veins are not visible due to shock, burns or massive haemorrhage, an incision is made in

the anatomical sites of the vein. The vein is identified, isolated and cannulated for transfusion of fluids. This procedure is called *venesection* or *cut down* (Fig. 70.11).

### 2. Contraindication

None

### 3. Position of the Patient

Supine

### 4. Anaesthesia

Local infiltration by using 2% lignocaine 3–5 ml.

### 5. Preparation

Iodine and spirit

### 6. Procedure

Cephalic vein cut down is the most popular and an ideal procedure. A transverse incision about 5 cm is made in the deltopectoral groove. The cephalic vein is isolated and the distal end of the vein is ligated so that venous blood does not leak. A nick is made in the vein, through which a sufficient sized cannula (infant feeding tube can be used) is introduced. A silk ligature is applied above, just tight enough to hold cannula in place. Free flow of venous blood in the cannula indicates that it is inside the vein. The cannula is advanced further for about 10–15 cm. It is connected to IV line containing fluid (Fig. 70.8).

#### *Precautions*

- Take care not to inject air bubbles. Remove all air bubbles present in the drip set also to avoid air embolism.
- **Upper ligature should not be tight.** It may obstruct the flow of fluids.
- **Strict antiseptic principles** must be followed to avoid septicaemia.

#### *Other Veins Selected for Cut Down*

- Basilic vein in arm.
- Cubital vein at the elbow.
- Long saphenous vein in the leg. Veins in the leg, as far as possible, should be avoided to prevent deep vein thrombosis.

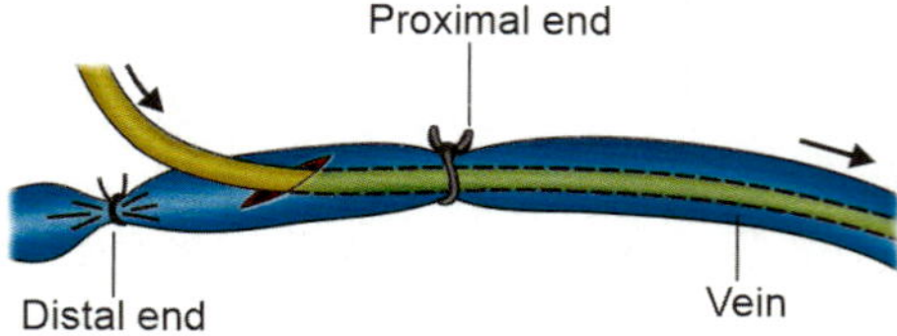


**Fig. 70.11:** Venesection

### 7. Closure

Skin—interrupted silk

### 8. Postoperative Management

- Care of wound by dressing
- To avoid air bubbles in the drip set

### 9. Postoperative Complications

- Infection, chills, rigors and septicaemia
- Air embolism

### 10. Advice at Discharge

Nil

### Advantages of Cephalic Vein Cut Down

- Reliable vein and easy to do.
- If cannula is advanced into the right heart, CVP can be measured.
- Mobility of the patient is not restricted.
- Substances which cannot be given in a peripheral vein, such as 50% dextrose, etc. can be given without risk of thrombosis of the vein, for hyperalimentation purposes.

*Pearls of Wisdom*

Cannulate vein, not an artery for venesection. Thin-walled nonpulsatile bluish structure is vein.

## VASECTOMY

Division and removal of a part of the vas deferens is vasectomy.

### 1. Indications

- Family planning
- To prevent epididymo-orchitis after prostatectomy. (Nowadays not routinely done.)

### 2. Contraindications

- **Relative:** Tuberculosis epididymo-orchitis. The incision may result in a nonhealing sinus. Hence, control of tuberculosis is done first followed by vasectomy.
- **Absolute:** Suspicion of testicular malignancy.

### 3. Position of the Patient

Supine

**Cleaning and draping:** Parts are cleaned and draped. Vas is palpated.

### 4. Anaesthesia

Local anaesthesia using 3–5 ml of 2% lignocaine.

### 5. Preparation of the Parts

- Savlon and spirit
- Iodine is better avoided.

### 6. Procedure

#### *Feeling the Vas Deferens*

After cleaning and draping, the vas is felt, at the root of scrotum between the index finger and thumb. It feels like a cord (Fig. 70.12). Lignocaine is infiltrated and wait for 1–2 minutes for lignocaine to act.

#### *Incision*

An incision of 2–4 cm is made in root of scrotum and it is deepened through layers of scrotum. An 'Allis forceps' is introduced within the incision and spermatic cord is held. During this step, fingers of the other hand help in guiding/locating/stabilising the cord. The coverings of the cord are incised.

#### *Precautions*

- Do not damage testicular vessels.
- Vas is separated. It is confirmed by its white colour, and it feels like a cord (Fig. 70.13).
- Division of vas by three clamp method (Fig. 70.14).

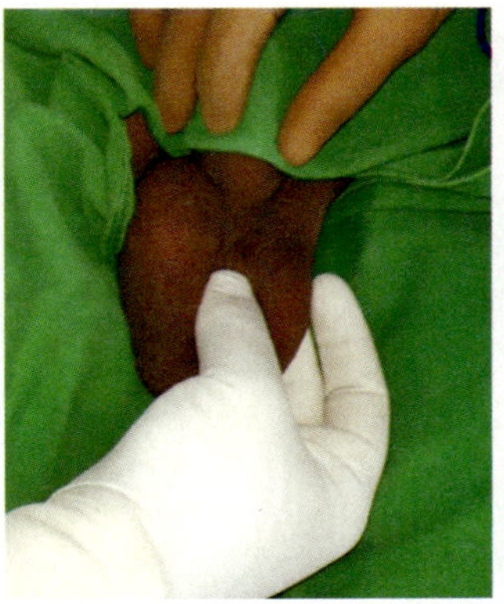

**Fig. 70.12:** Vas deferens is felt at the root of the scrotum

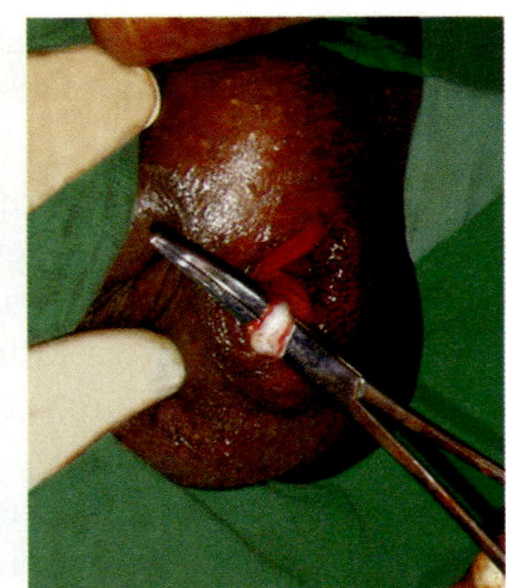

**Fig. 70.13:** Vas deferens is isolated from spermatic cord structures

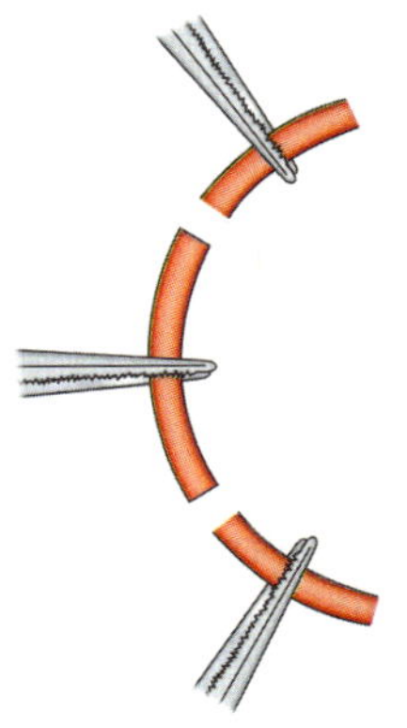

**Fig. 70.14:** Division of vas deferens by three-clamp method

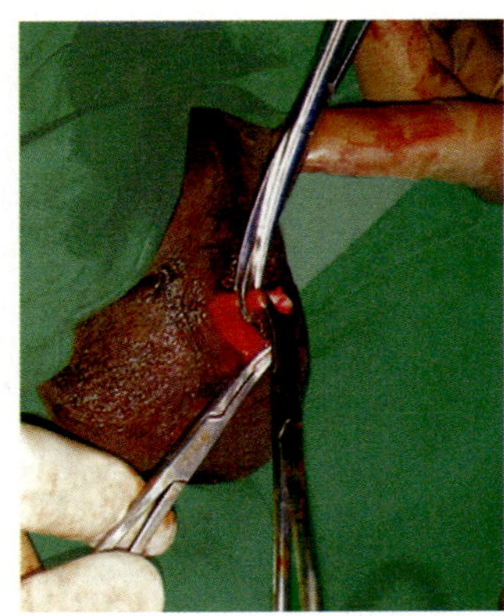

**Fig. 70.15:** Vas deferens is cut and a piece is sent for histopathology

- Vas is cut in two places A and B so that a piece of vas is removed, which can be sent for histopathology to confirm that it is vas (Fig. 70.15).
- Since a piece of vas is removed, reunion of the cut ends will not occur.
- The two cut ends of vas are doubly ligated by using silk.

### 7. Closure

The skin is closed by absorbable one or two sutures so that removal not required.

### 8. Postoperative Management

- Rest for a few hours
- Antibiotics and analgesics

> *Pearls of Wisdom*
>
> The procedure is repeated on the other side.

### 9. Postoperative Complications

- Injury to the vessels, resulting in a large haematoma.
- Infection
- Testicular atrophy can occur a few years later. It is due to immunological reaction rather than disuse atrophy.

### 10. Advice at Discharge

To use other methods of family planning for two months while having sexual intercourse, as some sperms may be present in the distal end of the vas and seminal vesicle.

> *Pearls of Wisdom*
>
> Vasectomy being a part of family planning project, every student should be familiar with this.

### No Scalpel Vasectomy

- It is a technique to do vasectomy through one single puncture which does not require any suturing. It is less traumatic than conventional vasectomy and shortens recovery time.
- The procedure is done with LA.
- A special instrument is used to puncture the scrotum and grasp the vas deferens. Vas is then cut and through the same puncture, the other side is also operated.

## TRACHEOSTOMY

An opening made in the trachea is tracheostomy.

### 1. Indications

**a. Emergency**

- Choking of the larynx due to dentures, foreign bodies, fish bones, etc.
- Stridor due to diphtheria, carcinoma larynx and bilateral recurrent laryngeal nerve paralysis after thyroidectomy.

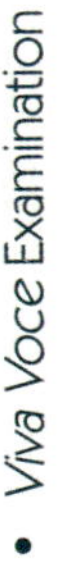

**b. Elective**
- Coma
- Tetanus
- Barbiturate poisoning
- Head injuries
- Prolonged respiratory failure

### 2. Contraindications

- Absence of any specific indication. In patients with anaplastic carcinoma of thyroid presenting with stridor due to infiltration of growth into trachea, it may not be possible to do a tracheostomy or an attempt to do tracheostomy may result in the growth fungating through the incision (which is best avoided). In such patients, **endotracheal intubation** is done, if possible. If not possible, no other intervention is done.
- In very urgent cases, needle cricothyrotomy can be done.

### 3. Position of the Patient

Supine with extension of the neck and head by keeping a sandbag or a pillow under the shoulders.

### 4. Anaesthesia

Local infiltration anaesthesia

### 5. Preparation of the Parts

Iodine and spirit

### 6. Procedure

- **Incision:** Transverse curved incision for about 3–4 cm is made at the level of 2nd tracheal ring.
- **Dissection:** Skin, subcutaneous tissue and deep fascia are incised. Isthmus of thyroid is separated.
- **Procedure:** A transverse cut is made in the 2nd tracheal cartilage, its edge is held with Allis forceps and a small cuff of cartilage is removed. 'Cricoid hook' can be used to stabilise the trachea (found more useful in children).
- A suitable-sized tracheostomy tube is introduced within.
- The cuff of tracheostomy tube is inflated by using 2–5 ml of air and is held in place by passing a tape around the neck.
- Confirm that the **tube** is in the **trachea**, not in the subcutaneous plane.
- Confirm **air entry** on both sides of lung.

### 7. Closure

A few interrupted skin sutures by the side of the tracheostomy tube and dressing is applied.

### 8. Postoperative Management

- Suction of tracheostomy tube, regular dressing
- Humidification of air
- Check for air entry

### 9. Postoperative Complications

- Wound infection
- Air leakage
- Improper air entry
- Cricoid stenosis (high tracheostomy).

#### *Closure of Tracheostomy*

- Once patient improves and is able to take care of his own airway, the tracheostomy tube is blocked. Observe for 24–48 hours.
- If there is **no respiratory distress**, the cuff is deflated and the tube is removed. A few skin sutures can be put or dressing is applied. It closes automatically.

### 10. Advice at Discharge

- Tracheostomy done after laryngectomy is permanent. Patients should learn to use metal tracheostomy, cleaning the tubes, etc.
- Percutaneous tracheostomy: This is done in ICU. A 2 to 3 cm vertical incision is given below the cricoid cartilage. Introducer, guidewire and and tracheostomy tube is intoduced through the 2nd or 3rd tracheal rings after dilating the tract. Appropriate sized tube is fixed with a purse string. Most important precaution is to palpate and check for any pulsating vessel (it may be high position of innominate artery).

## THYROIDECTOMY

### 1. Indications

- All goitres with symptoms—MNC, toxic goitre, colloid goitre, and malignant goitre.
- Goitre with compression symptoms
- Goitre with carcinoma proved
- Goitre with carcinoma suspected
- Goitre with toxicity
- Goitre with cosmetic reasons
- Any nodule more than 4 cm in size

*Pearls of Wisdom*

In all cases of toxic goitres, patients have to be optimised into normothyroid or euthyroid before surgery to avoid dangerous complications such as thyrotoxic storm or crisis.

### 2. Contraindications

Asymptomatic goitre, Hashimoto's thyroiditis, anaplastic carcinoma thyroid.

### 3. Position of the Patient

- Supine with extended neck by keeping a sandbag under the shoulders.
- Head end of the patient is elevated to about 15 degrees to reduce venous congestion. This position is called **anti-Trendelenburg position (Rose or Kocher's position)**.

### 4. Anaesthesia

GA.

### 5. Preparation of the Parts

Iodine and spirit

### 6. Procedure

***Incision*** (Figs 70.16A and B)

6–8 cm collar neck incision (Kocher's incision) or crease incision is given about 2 cm above the suprasternal notch along the natural crease of the neck or just above it.

#### *Layers Opened*

- Skin, platysma, subcutaneous tissue in the line of incision. Small bleeders are coagulated.
- Deep fascia is incised vertically after rising the flaps (Fig. 70.17).
- Strap muscles are separated (can be cut in very large goitres). Sternothyroid, thyrohyoid and sternohyoid muscles. Most superficial muscles are sternohyoid.
- Pretracheal fascia is incised.
- Thyroid gland is mobilised by using blunt dissection.

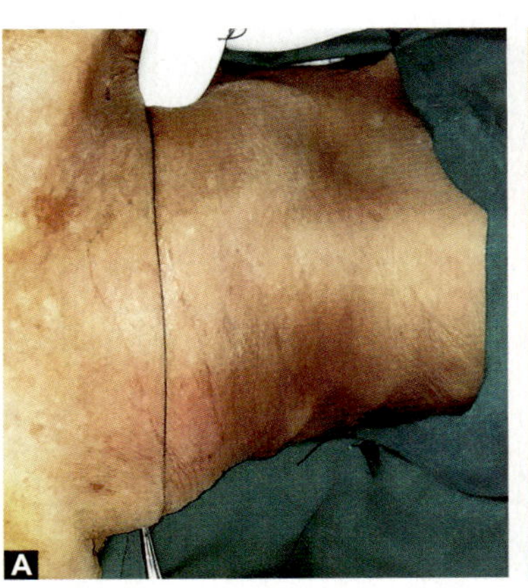

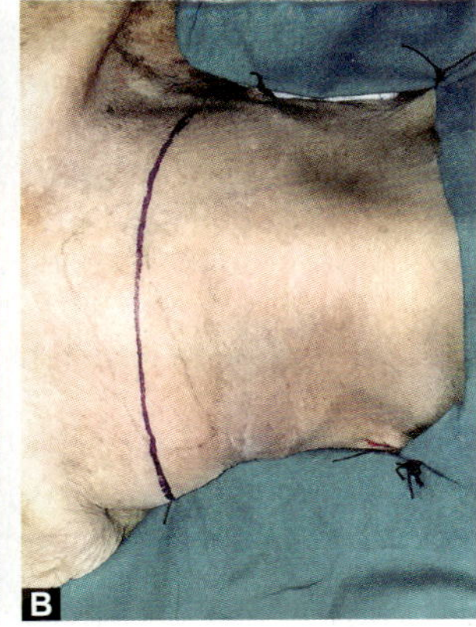

**Figs 70.16A and B:** Neck incision is marked by using silk, and marker pen. This incision is also called Kocher's collar neck incision

- Assess the entire gland to know whether it is a solitary nodule or multinodular goitre.
- One of the lobes is mobilised by dividing middle thyroid vein (single, short, thin, vein).
- Then, upper pole is dissected. This pedicle contains superior thyroid artery and veins. They are ligated and divided in between. Please apply double ligature proximally. Let the dissection be close to the gland. Dissection and retraction of the upper pole of the right thyroid lobe laterally will open up a space called **cricothyroid space of Reeves**. Here we can find the external branch of the superior laryngeal nerve.
- Upper pole should be ligated as close to the gland as possible to avoid damage to external laryngeal nerve.
- Inferior thyroid artery used to be ligated[1] well away from the gland. It has a horizontal course. It is thick and pulsatile. Nowadays, branches of inferior thyroid artery rather than the main artery are ligated. This will avoid injury to recurrent laryngeal nerve and it will prevent hypoparathyroidism also. Multiple veins, present in the lower pole, are ligated and divided.

*Pearls of Wisdom*

All major arteries should be ligated twice proximally. Example: Superior thyroid artery, facial artery, left gastric artery, cystic artery, renal artery.

- Isthmus is separated from trachea, both above and below.
- In subtotal thyroidectomy, the entire isthmus, parts of the right and left lobes are removed in flush with tracheal surface, leaving behind tissue in the tracheoesophageal groove to protect recurrent laryngeal nerve and parathyroid gland. Cut edges of thyroid gland are sutured by using Vicryl sutures. In total thyroidectomy, almost entire gland is removed (Fig. 70.18).

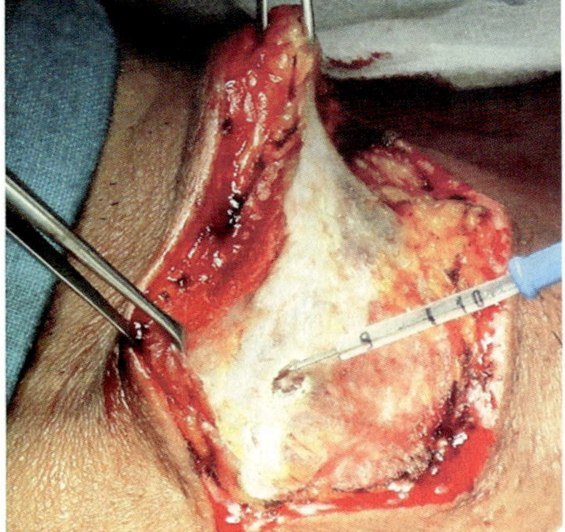

**Fig. 70.17:** Upper flap is raised. Plane of dissection is deep to platysma and superficial to pretracheal fascia

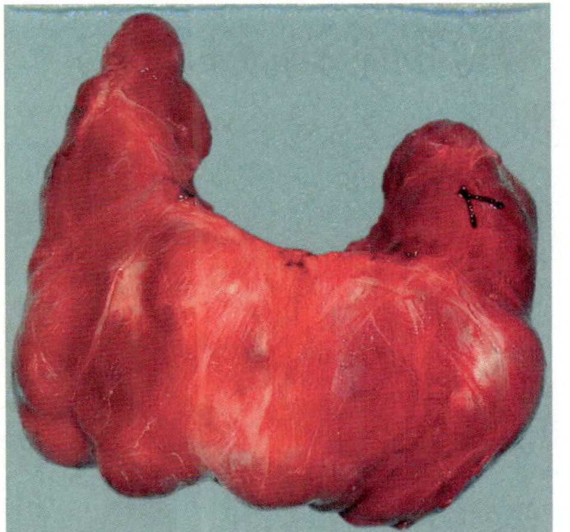

**Fig. 70.18:** Total thyroidectomy specimen for papillary carcinoma thyroid

[1]Today, branches of inferior thyroid artery are ligated—not the main artery so as to preserve blood supply to parathyroid gland.

### Precautions

- Any structure directly entering the gland is unlikely to be RLN and hence, can safely be divided.
- Always identify the RLN (*Refer* page 385). That is the best way to avoid injury to the nerve. Recurrent laryngeal nerve enters the thyrohyoid membrane, after running a vertical course, in the tracheoesophageal groove.

### 7. Closure

- A suction drain is kept in the thyroid bed (not always required).
- Deep fascia is sutured with 2-0 Vicryl
- Subcutaneous fat—Vicryl
- Skin—interrupted silk/subcuticular sutures or clips
- A bandage is applied.

### 8. Postoperative Management

- NPO for 6–8 hours followed by liquid diet.
- Antibiotics are not necessary.
- **Head end must be elevated** to reduce oedema of the wound.
- In toxic goitres, propranolol must be continued after surgery and slowly tapered over a week.
- Blood transfusion depending upon blood loss.
- Drain removal after 2–3 days (once it stops draining).
- Suture removal after 4–5 days.

### 9. Postoperative Complications

(for details see Chapter 37, page 419)

- **Haemorrhage: Tension haematoma.** Reactionary haemorrhage is due to slipping of ligature due to coughing, hypertension, etc. If it is alarming, deep fascial sutures have to be opened, haematoma drained and haemostasis has to be achieved.
- **Thyrotoxic crisis** in patients with toxic goitre
- **Tracheomalacia**—resulting in stridor
- Recurrent laryngeal nerve paralysis
- Hypothyroidism
- Hypoparathyroidism
- Wound infection

### 10. Advice at Discharge

This depends on the type of indication for thyroid surgery, e.g. those who undergo subtotal thyroidectomy for thyrotoxicosis have to be closely followed for recurrent thyrotoxicosis or hypothyroidism. If calcium levels are low, it has to be supplemented.

**TEN COMMANDMENTS: THYROIDECTOMY**

1. All thyroidectomies should be done in euthyroid patients. If there is any toxicity, it should be very well controlled.
2. Collar neck incision should be given properly.
3. Haemostasis should be perfect at every stage of surgery.
4. **Identify external laryngeal nerve at cricothyroid space of Reeves.**
5. **Identify recurrent laryngeal nerve in the tracheo-esophageal groove—Riddle's triangle.**
6. Identify and preserve all parathyroids by their location posterior to lobes and size of a small pea and yellow colour with a capsule. It has a separate blood supply from posterior branch of inferior thyroid artery.
7. Use bipolar cautery while coagulating a vessel near the RLN.
8. Upper pedicle is ligated—artery and vein are ligated separately.
9. Inferior thyroid artery branches are ligated.
10. When in doubt, keep a drain.

*Pearls of Wisdom*

Thyroidectomy is an operation which provides a surgeon to demonstrate his skills and meticulousness.

### *Different Types of Thyroidectomy* (Table 70.2)

**TABLE 70.2:** Different types of thyroidectomy

| Diseases | Before surgery | After surgery | Name of the operation |
|---|---|---|---|
| 1. Solitary nodule (benign) | | | Hemithyroidectomy means removal of one lobe with isthmus (*see* page 415) |
| 2. Multinodular goitre | | | Total thyroidectomy (*see* page 395) |
| 3. Toxic multinodular goitre | | | Total thyroidectomy (*see* page 396) |
| 4. Primary thyrotoxicosis | | | Total thyroidectomy (*see* page 401) |
| 5. Malignant neoplasm | | | Total thyroidectomy (*see* page 408) |

**What is Zuckerkandl's tubercle?**

- Zuckerkandl's tubercle is a pyramidal extension of the thyroid gland, located at the most posterior side of each lobe.
- The structure is important in thyroid surgery as it is closely related to the recurrent laryngeal nerve, the inferior thyroid artery, Berry's ligament and the parathyroid glands.
- It is also important to remove this *in toto* while doing thyroidectomy for malignancies.

## AMPUTATIONS

**SU27.4:** Describe the type of gangrene and principles of amputation (*Refer* page 198).

### Definitions/Terminologies of Amputation

- End bearing: Weight is taken by the body.
- Non-end bearing: Here weight is taken by the joint.
- *Guillotine* amputation: Here no flaps are raised, all the tissues are divided at the same level and the stump is kept open.
- Formal amputation: In this case depending upon the indications and the decisions taken by the surgeon, amputation is done with closure of the stump.

### Indications

1. Vitality of the part is destroyed by injury or disease—***dead limb.***
2. Life of patient is threatened by spread of a local condition—***deadly limb.*** *Examples:* Gas gangrene, extensive melanoma.
3. Patient may be better served by an artificial limb because of deformity or paralysis—***deformed limb. In such cases, better to amputate and fit in an artificial limb.***
4. Dying limb—acutely ischaemic limb, late presentation.

### Optimum Levels of Amputation

Level of amputation depends not only upon the extent of disease but also function desired in the remaining stump. This differs markedly in the upper and lower limbs.

### Ideal Stump

- Should have ideal length for proper fitting of prosthesis. Examples: Below knee: 8 to 12 cm from tibial tuberosity, above knee: 23 cm from greater trochanter and above and below elbow: 20 cm stump.
- Should be conical and rounded.
- Should not be tender.
- Should have adequate muscle padding so that its movements are adequate
- Should have adequate blood supply so that it heals with primary intention in the postoperative period.
- Should have a thin scar which should not interfere with prosthetic function.
- Should not have any redundant soft tissue hanging.
- Skin and scar should not be adhered to the underlying tissue.

### Incisions

Depending upon the site of the level of amputation and keeping in mind the blood supply of the part, different types of incision are given. They are as follows:

- *Racquet incision:* This is used in amputation for digits or toes.
- Elliptical or oval incision is given for metatarsal amputations.
- Circular incision is given especially in *Guillotine* amputation.
- U-shaped incisions: These are given to raise flaps—anterior and posterior flaps as in below knee or above knee. By convention equal flaps are used for above knee and a long posterior and short anterior flaps are used for below knee amputation. This is because, vascularity of the posterior flap is good below the knee due to bulky muscles with good blood supply when compared to the thin, muscle less anterior flap (*see* ten commandments).

## AMPUTATIONS IN LEG

**Skeleton of foot:** To have a better understanding of amputations kindly study Figs 70.19 and 70.20 first.

- One of the common indications for lower limb amputations is diabetic ulcer/gangrene foot. Various types and various levels of amputations are done with the main aim is to conserve as much as possible. However, when the limb is a useless limb, a below knee or an above knee amputation is done depending upon the seriousness of the problem.
  1. **Ray amputation:** It is amputation of the toe with head of metatarsal or metacarpals.
  2. **Transmetatarsal/metacarpal amputation:** It is called Gilles' amputation. When multiple toes are involved with gangrene as in vasculitis syndromes or in diabetic patients, amputation is done through metatarsal bones—proximal to the neck, distal to the base. Long volar flap is created and sutured to the dorsal skin.
  3. **Lisfranc's amputation (tarsometatarsal amputation):** Tarsometatarsal articulations are called Lisfranc joint. The bones forming these are the first, second, and third cuneiforms, and the cuboid, which articulate with the bases of the metatarsal

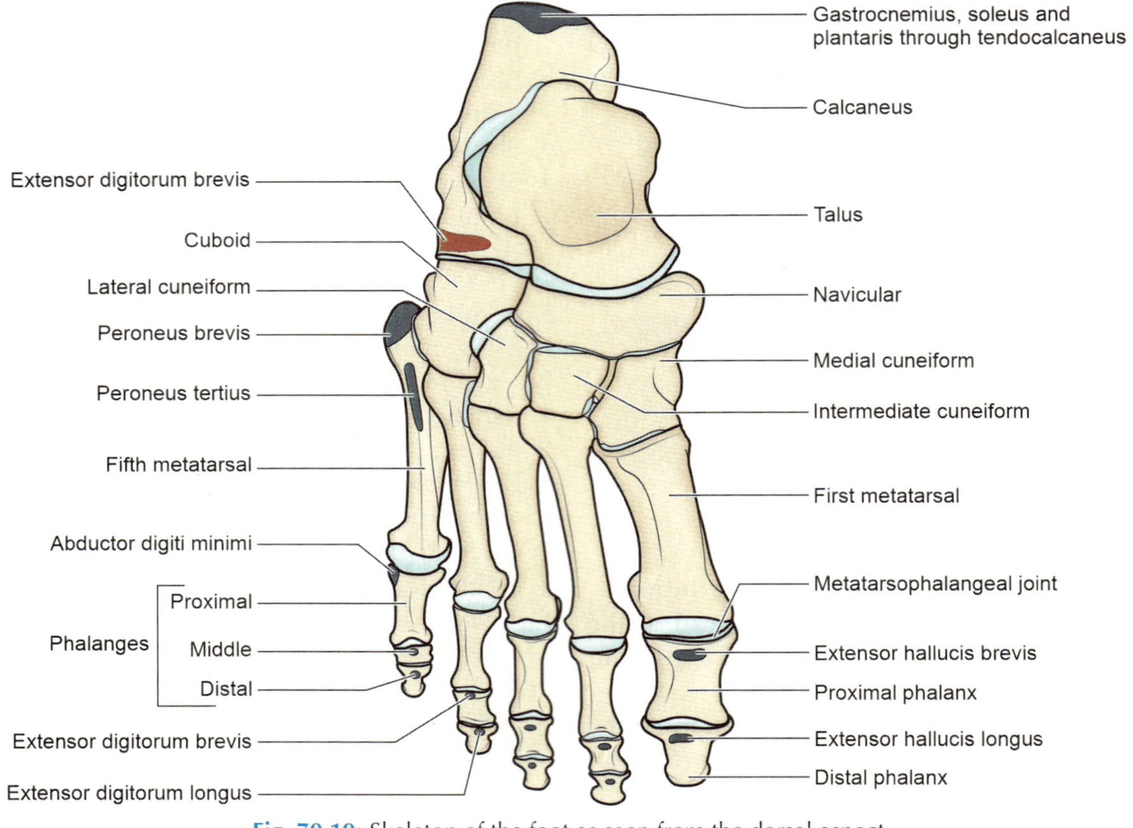


**Fig. 70.19:** Skeleton of the foot as seen from the dorsal aspect

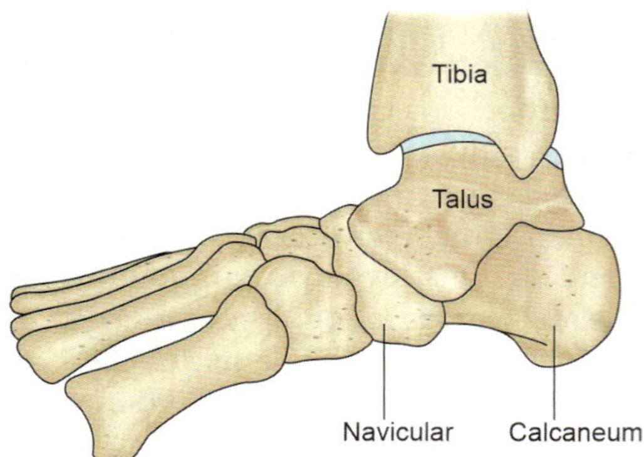


**Fig. 70.20:** Tarsal bones

bones. The bones are connected by dorsal, plantar, and interosseous ligaments. These ligaments have to be divided. A long volar flap is used. Patient needs a surgical boot.

4. **Chopart's amputation:** Francis Chopart first described disarticulation through midtarsal joint. It is midtarsal amputation. Disarticulation of the foot is completed through talonavicular joint and through calcaneocuboid joint. Thus, Chopart amputation removes the forefoot and midfoot, saving talus and calcaneus. Tibialis anterior muscle is sutured to the drilled talus bone.
   - **Contraindication:** Ischaemic feet as in atherosclerosis.
   - **Disadvantages:** It is a very unstable amputation, because most of the tendons supporting the foot will be removed. Thus, it will go for equinus and must usually be fitted with a prosthesis that extends up to the patellar tendon level.

5. **Syme's amputation:**
   - The tibia and fibula are divided at or immediately above the level of ankle joint and their ends are covered with a single flap obtained from heel.
   - The end of the stump is at a height of about 6–8 cm from the ground.
   - 50% of people will be able to walk on the stump without prosthesis.
   - It is of value in patients who do not have access to modern artificial limbs.
   - **Pirgroff's modification of Syme's amputation** retains a small portion of calcaneum in the flap obtained from heel (Fig. 70.21).
   - Heel flap is supplied by medial and lateral calcaneal vessels, both are branches of posterior tibial artery.
   - Those who will not be able to walk after this amputation, can be fitted with elephant boot.

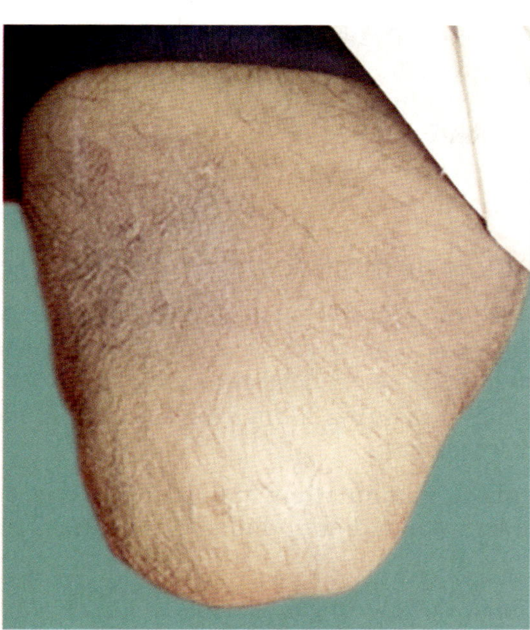

Fig. 70.21: Conical stump

**TEN COMMANDMENTS: GENERAL PRINCIPLES IN AMPUTATIONS**

1. Should mark the incision
2. Should give prophylactic antibiotics
3. Should avoid tourniquet in arterial occlusive diseases.
4. Should ensure adequate blood supply to the flaps—if raised as in below knee and above knee amputations.
5. Should ligate the blood vessels securely to avoid haematoma and then infection in the postoperative period.
6. Should not clamp the nerves but they are pulled down and transected as high as possible so that nerve ends are not caught in the suture line.
7. Should saw the anterior part of the bone obliquely to give a smooth anterior bevel which prevents pressure necrosis of the flap.
8. Should excise the bulky muscles so as to give a good conical stump (Fig. 70.21). Example: Excise soleus muscle in below knee amputations.
9. Should use absorbable sutures to unite the muscle ends.
10. Should drain the cavity with a suction drain which is brought out through the skin clear of the wound.

**6. Below knee amputation:**

- It is the operation of choice when it is not possible to preserve the foot or heel.
- The ideal length of the tibial stump is 14 cm.
- Minimum length required to fit an artificial leg is 8 cm. Stump shorter than this tends to slip out of the socket of an artificial limb.
- The stump is covered by creating long posterior flap.
- This is the amputation commonly done in patients who are in severe sepsis involving the leg with uncontrolled diabetes and life is in danger.
- All the rules mentioned above in ten commandments are followed here such as division of the nerve, flap vascularity, reduction of bulky muscles and the anterior scar, thus prosthesis will not cause discomfort while walking.
- Advantages of below knee amputation include greater range of movements without limp and without support.
- This amputation is also called Burgess amputation.
- POP cast should be put to prevent contractures (Fig. 70.22).

**7. Amputations through thigh**

- Ideal length is 25–30 cm as measured from tip of trochanter.
- It is done when it is not possible to save at least 8 cm of tibia as in some cases of diabetes or spreading infections of the leg and when muscles involved are not bleeding at surgery.
- When this amputation is done in children, as much length as possible should be preserved (growing epiphysis of femur is at lower end).
- Unlike, below knee amputation, equal flaps are raised—anterior and posterior.
- Any length less than 10 cm of femur will not help. In such cases, hip disarticulation is done.
- In peripheral arterial occlusive disease, an attempt is made first by raising below knee flaps. If edges of the skin flaps do not bleed, better to go ahead with above knee flaps because vascularity of above knee flaps are better. Above knee amputation stump healing is better than below knee.

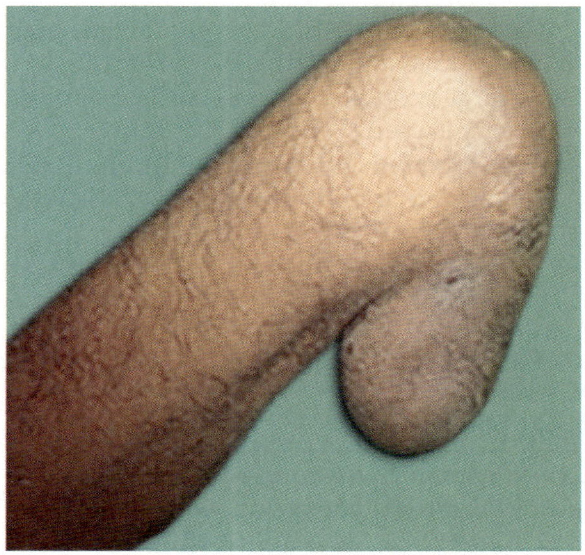

Fig. 70.22: Amputation contracture

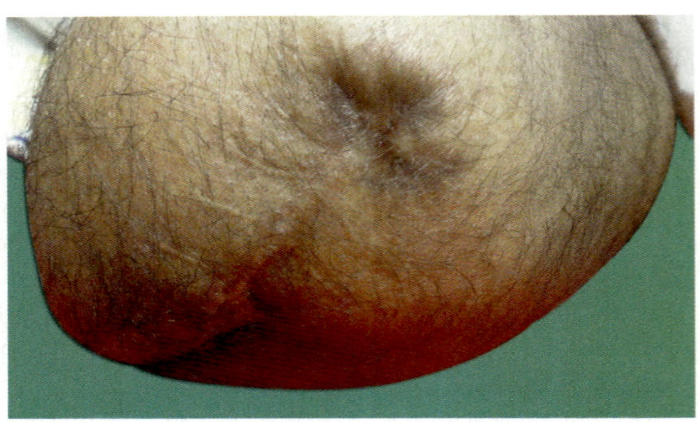

**Fig. 70.23:** Infected scar

- Disadvantages of this amputation are difficult rehabilitation (not easy), prosthesis fitting is not good, invariably patient needs one more support (Fig. 70.23).

**8. Hip disarticulation**

- When it is not possible to get minimum of 10 cm length of stump of the femur, hip disarticulation is done. This situation can occur in trauma or malignancies to get a wide clearance. Examples: Sarcomas or in cases of malignant melanomas.
- Usually a single posterior flap is raised—Solcum's approach.
- Anterior approach can also be used (2nd option)—Boyd's approach.

**9. Hindquarter amputation**

- In this amputation—one side of pelvis with innominate bone, pubis, muscles and vessels are removed. Hence, it is called hemipelvectomy today.
- Indications are trauma and tumour (malignancy).
- In the original description, common iliac artery used to be ligated. However, now the branches of external and internal iliac artery are ligated.
- A large posterior flap based on superior gluteal artery is used.
- Variations in this amputation are: Extended hemipelvectomy with removal of posterior part of the sacrum.
- Limb preserving hemipelvectomy: It is called internal hemipelvectomy.

## UPPER LIMB AMPUTATIONS

### GENERAL PRINCIPLES

- Conserve as much tissue as possible.
- Skin closure should not be under tension.
- Soft tissue cover over bony stump is desirable. Otherwise, painful adherent scar will result.
- Amputation through middle or terminal phalanx is preferred to disarticulation at interphalangeal joints since attachment of flexor tendons is thereby preserved.
- Every effort should be made to preserve as much of the thumb.

### AMPUTATION THROUGH FOREARM AND UPPER ARM

- Ideal stump is 16–20 cm measured from olecranon.
- Stump less than 8 cm is useless for transmitting movement to an artificial elbow joint.
- A stump measuring 20 cm from acromion is ideal for fitting prosthesis.

**Krukenberg's amputation:** In this amputation, a gap is created between radius and ulna like a claw. It helps in holding objects.

#### Interscapulothoracic Amputation (Forequarter Amputation)

- Indications are for malignancy involving axial skeleton such as sarcoma. Sepsis involving the upper limb is another indication such as gas gangrene.
- It is a very radical mutilating operation, hence all possible limb saving attempts should be done first.
- Entire upper limb with scapula and lateral 2/3rds of the clavicle with all the muscles attached to it are removed.

#### Complications following Amputation

1. **Wound infection:** Especially it is common in amputations done for diabetic gangrene cases. Stitches may have to be opened to release pus followed by secondary suturing at a later date.
2. **Flap necrosis:** It is a common complication because of several reasons, important one being decreased blood supply to the limb either due to arterial occlusive disease or due to diabetes. Necrotic skin and subcutaneous tissues should be removed followed by secondary suturing at a later date. Hence, blood supply of the flap has to be kept in mind when raising the flaps.
3. **Stump ulcers** are common in the initial stages of wearing artificial limbs.
4. **Contracture:** If the artificial limb is not fitted, the stump will develop flexion contracture.
5. **Amputation neuroma:** This is an end neuroma. The cut end of the nerve is entrapped in the scar tissue and gives rise to pain. To avoid this, nerve end is pulled and cut so that after division of the nerve, the end gets retracted.
6. **Phantom limb:** A **phantom limb** is the sensation that a missing limb is attached to the body. Approximately 60 to 80% of individuals with an amputation experience phantom sensations in their amputated

limb, and the majority of the sensations are painful. It is probably due to presence of a severe pain at the amputated site before surgery and the corresponding site in the brain has registered this sensation.

## ABDOMINAL INCISIONS

### Introduction

Incisions are given to approach an organ for removal or repair. The most important 3 criteria when incisions are given are: 1. Accessibility, 2. Extensibility, and 3. Safety. Many examples can be given for each one of these. However, one example for each one of the above 3 criteria has been given below.

#### *1. Accessibility*

When an incision is given, if a surgeon should be able to reach the organ without many difficulties. Classical example is: McBurney incision given at the site of maximum tenderness. As soon as peritoneum is opened, you can see appendix (More details later). Subcostal incision on the left side gives direct access to the spleen for splenectomy.

#### *2. Extensibility*

Surprises are known inside abdomen and hence it is called as Pandora's box. When a upper midline incision is given for perforation peritonitis, if a lesion is identified in the lower abdomen, incision can be extended easily till midline incisions are popular and have this great advantage. If a surgeon has given McBurney incision for suspected appendicitis, after opening the abdomen he finds that the appendix is normal but it is a case of perforation of Meckel's diverticulitis, often the McBurney incision has to be closed and midline incision given to facilitate removal of Meckel's diverticulum.

#### *3. Safety*

Midline incisions are safe during laparotomy because no important nerve or artery is present in the midline. If precautions are not properly taken in paramedian incisions, traction on the nerves while retracting the muscles can result in nerve injuries. This may weaken the rectus abdominis muscle.

### Various Incisions (Key Box 70.4)

Midline incisions, McBurney grid iron incision, Kocher's subcostal incision, Pfannenstiel incision are commonly used incisions. Left abdominothoracic—an oblique incision above the umbilicus crossing along the 7th or 8th intercostal space for removing large spleens or exposure of lower oesophagus and right midline incision with right posterolateral thoracotomy through 5th intercostal space for oesophageal cancer are other incisions used. Details are not required for undergraduate students. Those of you are interested can refer to operative surgery books.

**Key Box 70.4**

**Midline:** Upper and lower
**Paramedian:** Upper, lower, right and left
**Grid Iron:** McBurney's
**Kocher's:** Subcostal
**Pfannenstiel:** Used by gynaecologists
Roof top-incision—Chevron incision
Left thoracoabdominal
Midline with right posterolateral thoracotomy through 5th intercostal space—Ivor Lewis operation

### MIDLINE INCISIONS

Upper and lower midline and mid-midline are commonly used incisions which give exposure to every viscus in the abdominal cavity.

- To understand the formation of rectus sheath and linea alba which forms basis of midline incisions, *refer* page 1107 in Chapter 64.
- **Upper midline incision:** Layers opened are—skin, subcutaneous fat, linea alba, preperitoneal fat and peritoneum. Closure is done mainly by taking good bites from the linea alba and skin. Peritoneum heals with proliferation of mesothelial cells. A few surgeons also take bites through peritoneum with absorbable sutures such as 2–0 polyglactin, linea alba with 2–0 prolene/PDS and skin with silk sutures.
- **Lower midline incision:** Layers opened are—skin, subcutaneous fat, linea alba. However, linea alba is not present in the lower part of lower abdomen below linea semilunaris line. Then preperitoneal fat and peritoneum are incised. Closure is done mainly by taking good bites from the linea alba and skin. Closure is similar to that of upper midline incision.
- Principles of midline closure (Key Box 70.5).

**Key Box 70.5**

- Peritoneum need not be closed
- Linea alba is sutured from one side to the other by using small bites and small tissues.
- Small means it is less than 10 mm from the wound edge.
- Suture to wound length is more than or about 4:1 ratio (Jenkin's rule).
- Continuos closure with slowly absorbing (PDS) is better than inetrrupted sutures.

## APPENDICECTOMY

This is the most commonly done emergency surgery by general surgeons all over the world. Today almost every appendicectomy is done by laparoscopic approach. Basic concepts of laparoscopy have been given in the pages 1238.

*Pearls of Wisdom*

Appendicectomy can be one of the easiest and sometimes one of the most complicated surgeries.

## 1. Indications

- Acute appendicitis—emergency appendicectomy
- Recurrent appendicitis—elective appendicectomy

## 2. Contraindications

Appendicular mass

## 3. Position of the Patient

Supine

## 4. Anaesthesia of the Parts

This surgery can be done either under GA or regional anaesthesia (spinal or epidural).

## 5. Preparation

Parts are cleaned with iodine and spirit, from the level of umbilicus above to the upper part of thigh below.

## 6. Procedure

### *Incision*

1. McBurney's grid-iron incision is the most popular incision. It is at right angles to spinoumbilical line placed at McBurney's point. It is about 6–8 cm in length (Fig. 70.24).
2. **Lanz** incision is a curved transverse incision, placed at the McBurney's point. Cosmetically, it is a better incision (Fig. 70.25).
3. Midline incision is made when diagnosis is in doubt as a part of **exploratory laparotomy**. This is also preferred in females where there is a gynaecological pathology such as ovarian cyst which may be the cause of right iliac fossa pain (Fig. 70.26).

### *Layers Opened*

- Skin
- Two layers of subcutaneous tissue—superficial fatty (Camper's), deep membranous (Scarpa's). (C: comes first, S: later). There is no deep fascia in the abdomen.

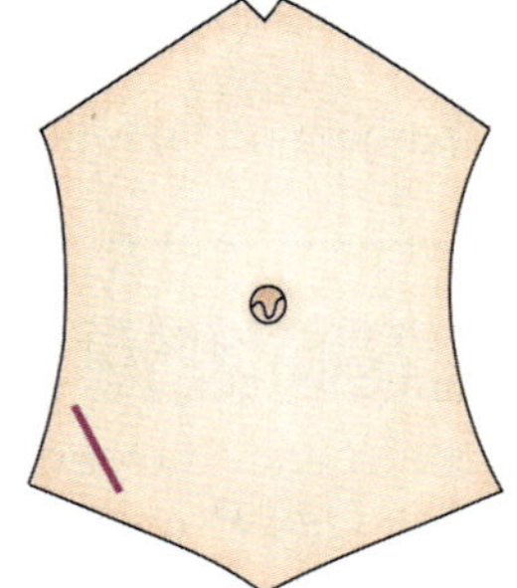

**Fig. 70.24:** Grid iron incision

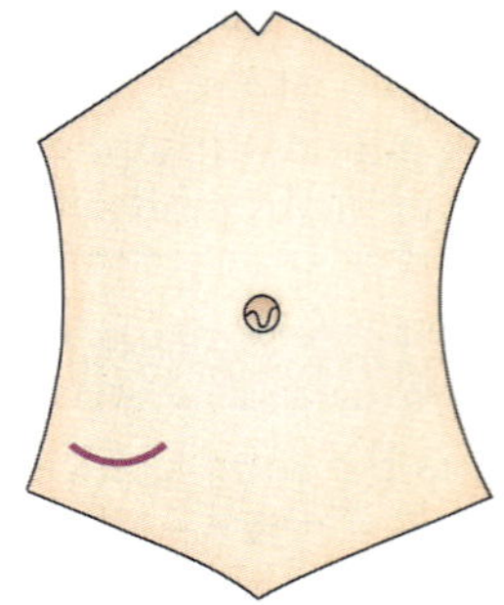

**Fig. 70.25:** Lanz incision

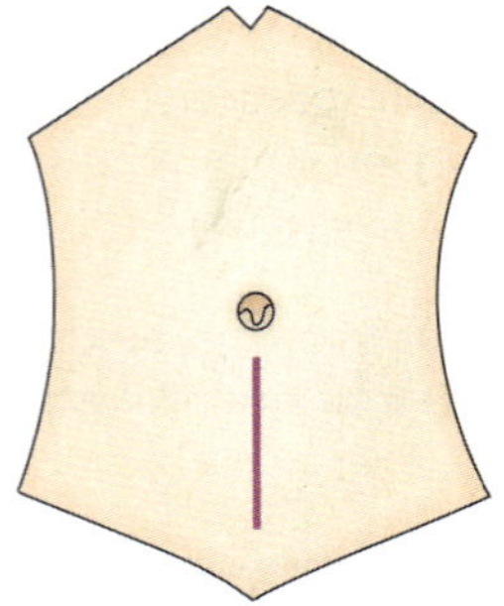

**Fig. 70.26:** Midline incision

- External oblique aponeurosis is seen running downwards and medially. It is incised in the direction of its fibres.
- Internal and transverse abdominal muscles are split (grid iron—right angle to each other).
- Peritoneum is incised.

### *Features of Acute Appendicitis at Operation*

- Inflamed, turgid appendix—send pus/inflammatory exudate for culture/sensitivity
- Pus in the right iliac fossa
- Presence of omentum in the right iliac fossa
- Black or green appendix (gangrenous)
- Faecolith

### *Identification of the Appendix*

- Trace taenia coli. They will lead to the base of appendix (**all roads lead to Rome**).
- Identify round structure—caecum and then look for appendix.
- Often it is retrocaecal. In such cases, you need to mobilise right paracolic space by incising posterior peritoneal reflection.
- When you are tracing taenia coli, if you are not able to identify the appendix, it means most probably you are tracing taenia coli of the sigmoid colon.
- It may be subhepatic in cases of undescended caecum.

### *Surgical Procedure*

- Appendix is gently held at mesoappendix by using Babcock's forceps and blood vessels in the mesoappendix are divided. These include appendicular artery, branch of ileocolic artery (accessory appendicular artery of Seshachalam, is a branch of posterior caecal artery). Once appendix is freed up to the base (caecum), a **purse string suture** is applied all round appendix, taking bites from caecum, using 2–0 atraumatic silk (Fig. 70.27).

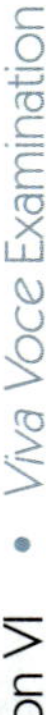

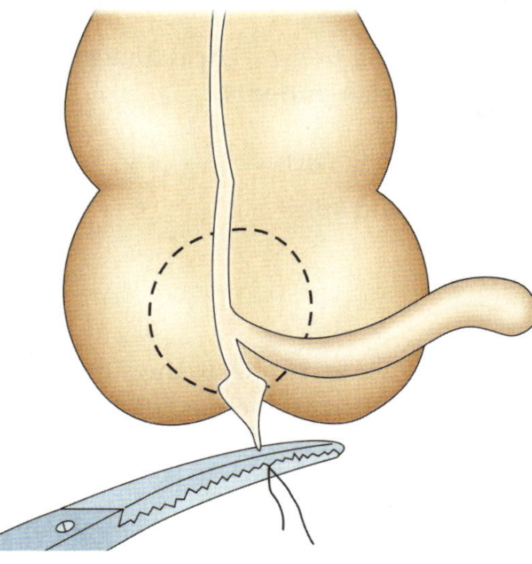

Fig. 70.27: Purse string suture

- Appendix is crushed at base and is held 1 cm above the crush. A tight silk ligature is applied at the crushed site and appendix is cut in between. Stump is cleaned with spirit, invaginated and purse string is tightened. This is called burial of the stump. Perfect haemostasis is obtained (Figs 70.28A to C).
- Look for Meckel's diverticulum and if found make a note of this in the operative surgery notes.

*Pearls of Wisdom*

Look for Meckel's diverticulum, which may be the cause of right iliac fossa pain. You may find Meckel's diverticulum with narrow lumen, inflammation with band—remove it.

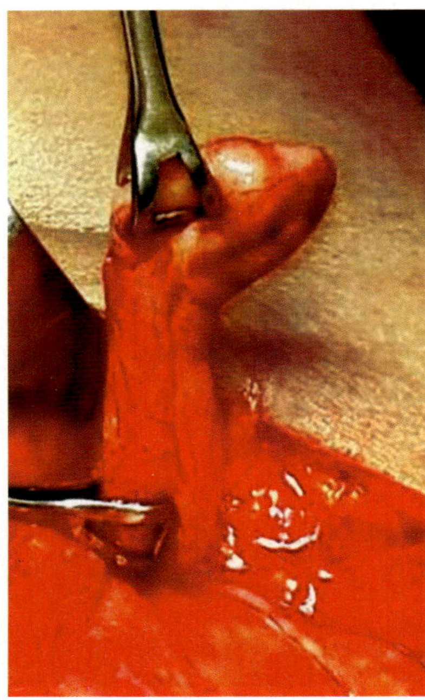

Fig. 70.28A: Acute appendicitis. Turgid swollen appendix. You can see Babcock's forceps used to hold the mesoappendix

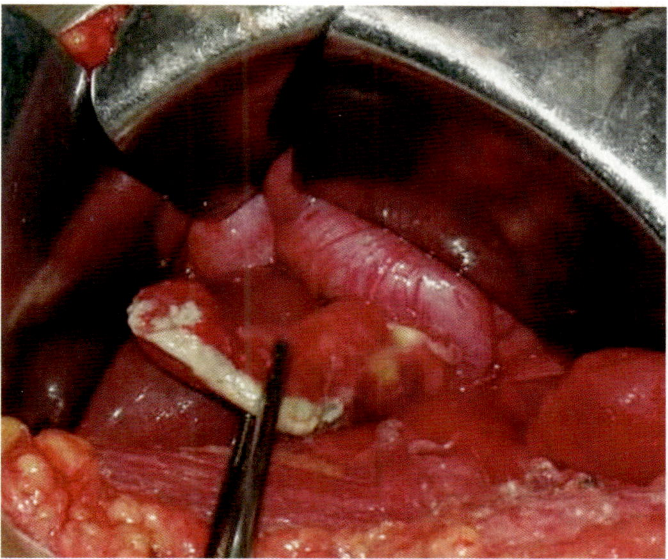

Fig. 70.28B: Perforated appendicitis at surgery due to a large faecolith

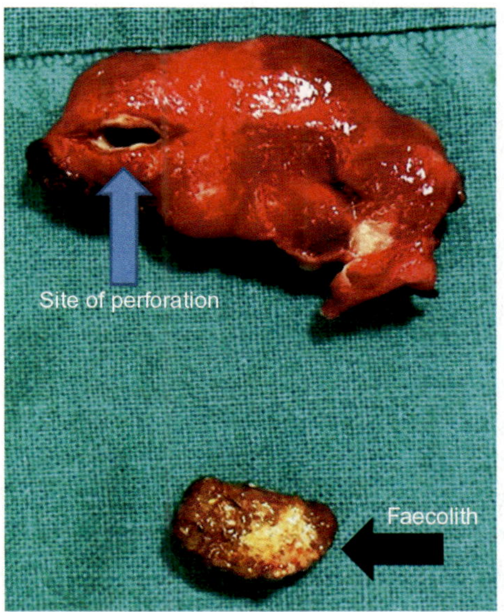


Fig. 70.28C: Specimen of appendix and a large faecolith

## 7. Closure

- Peritoneum—continuous 2–0 Vicryl
- Split muscles—sutured together by a few interrupted sutures using 2–0 Vicryl
- External oblique is sutured with silk
- Subcutaneous fat is sutured with Vicryl
- Skin with interrupted silk.
- Peritoneal wash with saline is given and the area is dried with mop.
- Tube drain is not kept routinely unless there is gangrenous appendicitis or a lot of pus in the peritoneal cavity.

### 8. Postoperative Management

- RT aspiration is only in cases of peritonitis or persistent vomiting. Otherwise, nasogastric aspiration is not required.
- IV fluids 100 ml DNS/day with or without Ringer lactate solution.
- Oral fluids are allowed within 6–8 hours or very next day once abdomen is soft and bowel sounds are heard.
- Appropriate antibiotics to cover gram-positive, gram-negative and anaerobic organisms.
- Suture removal by 7–10 days.

### 9. Complications after Appendicectomy

(see Page 1077)

**A. Postoperative fever**

**B. Wound infection**

**C. Intra-abdominal abscess**

**D. Faecal fistula—causes**

**E. Septicaemia**

### 10. Advice at Discharge

To report, if any fever or discharge from the wound.

## BASSINI'S HERNIORRHAPHY

- This means herniotomy and approximation of conjoined tendon to inguinal ligament to strengthen the posterior wall of the inguinal canal. With availability of the mesh, this surgery is not done. **However, in strangulated hernias, after resection of the bowel, one cannot repair with mesh. Bassini's herniorrhaphy is still a good option.**
- In large, long-standing hernias and in sliding hernias, especially in elderly patients, it is better to catheterise their bladder before surgery for two reasons. Firstly, to avoid injury to the urinary bladder and secondly, they invariably develop retention of urine in the postoperative period.

### 1. Indication

Strangulated hernias.

### 2. Contraindication (Relative)

Severe cardiopulmonary insufficiency

### 3. Position of the Patient

Supine

### 4. Anaesthesia

Regional anaesthesia or GA. **Local anaesthesia** can be preferred in **high-risk patients**.

### 5. Preparation of the Parts

Povidone-iodine and spirit.

### 6. Procedure

#### *Incision*

4–6 cm incision is made parallel to the inguinal ligament at the level of deep ring in the medial two-thirds of the inguinal ligament.

#### *Layers Opened*

- Skin
- Two layers of superficial fascia
- External oblique is incised in the line of direction of fibres, till external ring is slit open.
- Thin cremasteric box—thin covering is opened
- Identification of the sac—glistening white colour.
- Isolate the cord from the sac—by blunt and sharp dissection. The cord is held separately by using cord holding forceps.
- Mobilisation of the sac: The sac is mobilised up to the deep ring (Fig. 70.29). Mobilisation is complete when inferior epigastric artery pulsations and extraperitoneal pad of fat are seen.
- Opening of the sac: **The sac is opened and contents are examined.**

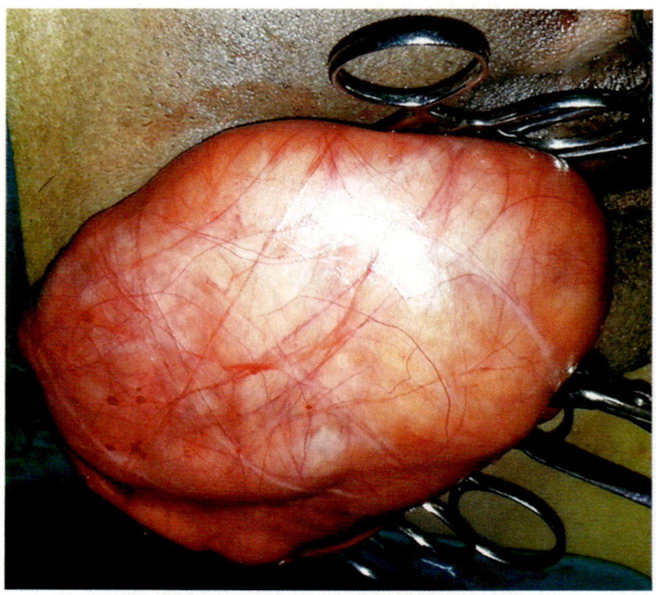

**Fig. 70.29:** Hernial sac is identified—glistening white in colour

- Reduction of contents: **The contents are reduced into the peritoneal cavity carefully by using blunt forceps. Check carefully in bleeding from omental vessels** (Fig. 70.30).
- **Twist the sac** so that contents get reduced completely so as to avoid injury to the contents of the sac later while excising the sac (Figs 70.31A and B).
- **Transfixation ligature: It means suture ligature is passed through the sac:** It is applied as high as possible at the neck of sac and it is tightened.
- **Excision of the sac: As a rule, after excision, the ligated end of the sac should disappear from the operative field (means it will go into the peritoneal cavity).** After excision, see the excised sac and see whether omentum or intestine have been injured. Up to this stage, it is called **herniotomy**.

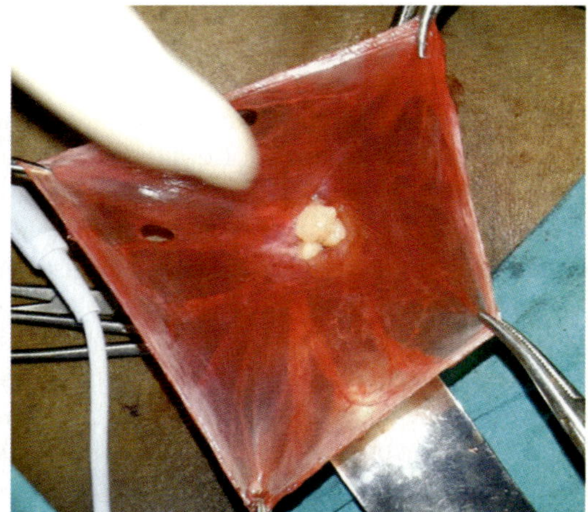

**Fig. 70.30:** Contents of the sac omentum—omentocele

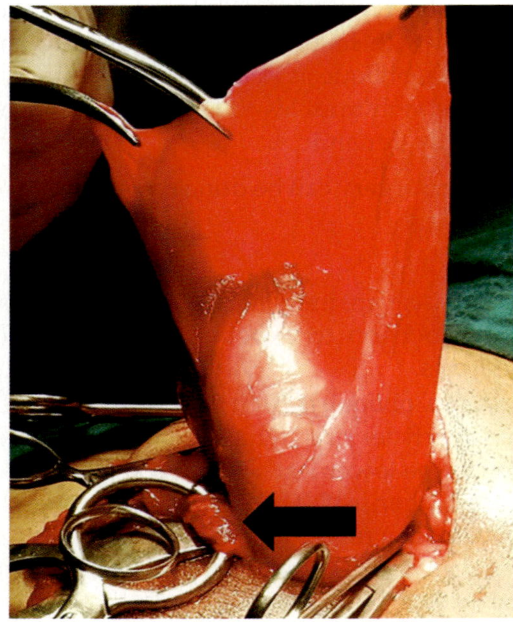

**Fig. 70.31A:** Sac is isolated and opened. You can see cord holding forceps with cord which is isolated and held separately

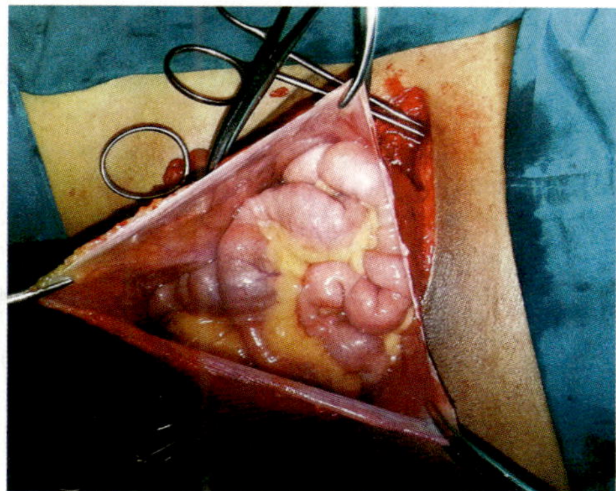

**Fig. 70.31B:** Contents of the sac—enterocele

- Conjoined tendon above is approximated to the inguinal ligament below by using nonabsorbable suture such as nylon or prolene. However, in strangulated hernias, PDS (polydioxanone)—a synthetic but absorbable sutures can be used. It gets absorbed between 130 and 180 days.
- Nonabsorbable suture is used so that its strength remains for a long time. This repair is called **Bassini's herniorrhaphy** (Key Box 70.6).

Key Box 70.6

**Herniorrhaphy**

- Identify the sac and identify the cord
- Isolate the sac and isolate the cord
- Mobilise the sac and open the sac
- Release adhesions, if any, and reduce the contents
- Twist the sac, transfix and ligate the sac

Excision of the sac and posterior wall repair

## 7. Closure

- External oblique is sutured with chromic catgut or silk (Fig. 70.32).
- Subcutaneous fat with absorbable catgut suture.
- Skin with silk.

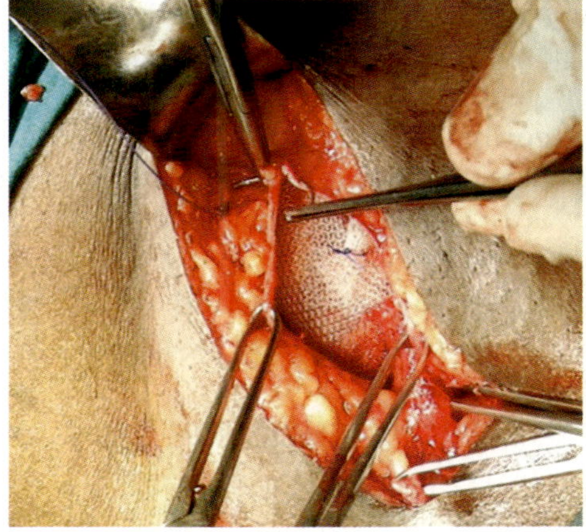

**Fig. 70.32:** You can see the mesh used here. So this is Lichenstein's hernioplasty (most popular procedure for hernia)

**Pearls of Wisdom**

Do not twist the sac in direct hernias and in sliding hernias.

***Precautions*** (Key Box 70.7)

1. Ilioinguinal nerve should not be caught in ligature.
2. Conjoined muscles should not be strangulated.
3. There should not be any tension in the suture lines.

**Key Box 70.7**

**Take Care of**

- 1 nerve—ilioinguinal nerve. Entrapment causes inguinal neuralgia (*see* page 1095)
- 1 bone—pubic bone do not take a stitch from the bone. It may cause periostitis pubis
- 1 cord—spermatic cord do not tighten the deep ring too tight
- 1 artery—inferior epigastric artery—see the pulsations near the deep ring and protect it
- 1 large artery—external iliac artery—while inguinal ligament being sutured to conjoined tendon on the lateral sides. Feel the pulse and protect
- 1 organ—urinary bladder—especially in elderly patients, large hernias and sliding hernias

### 8. Postoperative Management

- NPO for 6–8 hours, oral fluids and soft diet later.
- Analgesics.
- Prophylactic antibiotics, 1 dose is given 6 hours before surgery.
- Scrotal support, if the dissection is more (complete hernia).
- Suture removal after 7–10 days.

### 9. Postoperative Complications

1. **Immediate:** Haematoma due to injury to the pampiniform plexus of veins or improper haemostasis. It may need re-exploration.
2. **Wound infection** may result in discharging pus which is the cause of postoperative fever. Infection is the chief cause of recurrence.
3. **Severe periostitis pubis** (to avoid this nowadays, the repair is not done by taking bites through pubic bone). X-ray of the bone may have to be taken for diagnosis.
   - It is managed by analgesics and in intractable cases, injection of corticosteroids locally may reduce the pain.
4. **Nerve entrapment causing pain.**

### 10. Advice at Discharge

- Not to strain or lift heavyweights (e.g. bucketful of water) or to carry load on the shoulders for 3 months.
- If there is any precipitating cause such as chronic cough or difficulty in passing urine, etc. they have to be treated first. Otherwise, hernia will recur once again.

**Pearls of Wisdom**

Dissecting an inguinal canal and performing a good repair is a good exercise for a postgraduate because he has to dissect various anatomical layers, preserve nerves, vessels, vas deferens and do a good repair. Various steps of herniorrhaphy teach a postgraduate basic fundamental principle of surgery—**Prof. CR Ballal, *Former* Professor and Head, Kasturba Medical College and Hospital, Mangaluru.**

***Please note:*** Today, the procedure of choice for inguinal hernia is mesh repair—Lichtenstein's repair. It is given in hernia Chapter 64, page 1092). Please refer to hernia chapter on other repairs.

## DESARDA REPAIR

**Principle of Desarda repair:** In normal individuals, the transversus abdominis aponeurosis (aponeurotic extensions) in the posterior wall is strong and elastic because of its aponeurotic nature and healthy muscles around keep it physiologically dynamic to give lifelong protection against hernia formation. This transversus abdominis aponeurosis is absent or deficient in hernia patients. **The Desarda repair technique uses an undetached strip of nearby external oblique aponeurosis to replace those absent aponeurotic extensions. This gives again a strong and elastic posterior wall.** Another fact noted in hernia patients is weakness of the muscle arch muscles that fail to keep the posterior wall physiologically dynamic. In Desarda repair, the strip is continuous with its original strong muscle and this nearby external oblique muscle gives additional strength to the muscle arch muscles to keep this posterior wall physiologically dynamic.

**Anaesthesia:** Surgery can be done under local or spinal anesthesia.

**Surgery:**

1. Skin and fascia are incised through a regular oblique inguinal incision to expose the external oblique aponeurosis.
2. The external oblique is cut in line with the upper crux of the superficial ring, which leaves the thinned-out portion in the lower leaf so a good strip can be taken from the upper leaf. The external oblique, which is thinned out as a result of aging or long-standing large hernias, can also be used for repair if it is able to hold the sutures.
3. Upper and lower leaves are cleared from surrounding tissue by proper undermining.

4. Sac is excised protecting ilio-inguinal nerve.
5. The upper leaf of the external oblique aponeurosis (EOA) is sutured to the inguinal ligament from the pubic tubercle to the internal ring using PDSII no. 1 or '0' (Monofilament Polydioxanone violet, Ethicon) continuous sutures (*see* Fig. 70.33). The first suture is taken in the anterior rectus sheath part of the external oblique aponeurosis upper leaf above and the medial most part of the inguinal ligament below near the pubic tubercle. The last suture is taken so as to sufficiently narrow the new internal ring without constricting the spermatic cord by pushing the cord against the arching muscle fibres to its maximum extent (*see* Fig. 70.30). ***Here, we are creating a new internal ring in the EOA with the help of the strip while suturing strip's lower border to the inguinal ligament. The original internal ring becomes defunct.*** Lateral pushing of spermatic cord against the arching muscle fibres to maximum extent is necessary while this suturing is done. Each suture is passed first through the inguinal ligament and then the external oblique upper leaf. Needle bites are taken as close to the border of the EOA as possible (about 1–2 mm). The index finger of the left hand is used to protect the iliac vessels and retract the cord structures laterally while taking lateral sutures.
6. A splitting incision is made in this sutured upper leaf, partially separating a strip of 1–2 cm width but never more than 2 cm. Normally 1.5 cm wide strip is sufficient for most of the patients. This splitting incision is extended medially up to the pubic symphysis and laterally 2–3 cm beyond the internal ring. The medial insertion and lateral continuation of this strip is kept intact (Fig. 70.34).
7. A strip of the external oblique is now available, the lower border of which is already sutured to the inguinal ligament. The upper free border of the strip is now sutured to the internal oblique or conjoined muscle lying close to it with PDSII no. 1 or '0' (Monofilament Polydioxanone violet, Ethicon) continuous sutures throughout its length (Fig. 70.35). The aponeurotic portion of the internal oblique muscle is used for suturing to this strip wherever and whenever possible; otherwise, it is not essential for the success of the operation. This will result in the strip of the external oblique being placed behind the cord to form a new posterior wall of inguinal canal (Figs 70.35 to 70.37).
8. At this stage the patient is asked to cough and the increased tension (physiological tension) on the strip exerted by the external oblique to support the weakened internal oblique and transversus abdominis is clearly visible.
9. The spermatic cord is placed in the inguinal canal and the lower leaf of the external oblique is sutured to the newly formed upper leaf of the external oblique

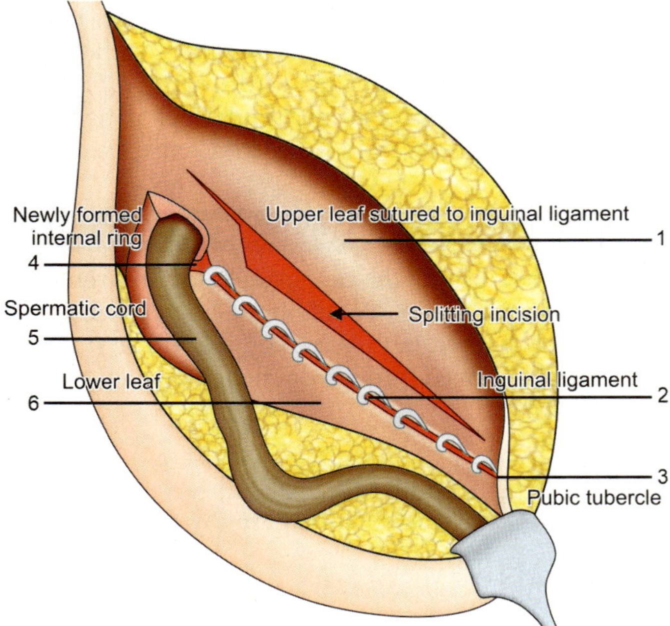


**Fig. 70.33:** The medial leaf of the external oblique aponeurosis is sutured to the inguinal ligament and a splitting incision is taken (*Courtesy:* Prof. Desarda Mohan Phulchand, Professor of Surgery and Chief of the Hernia Centre, Poona Hospital and Research Centre, Pune)

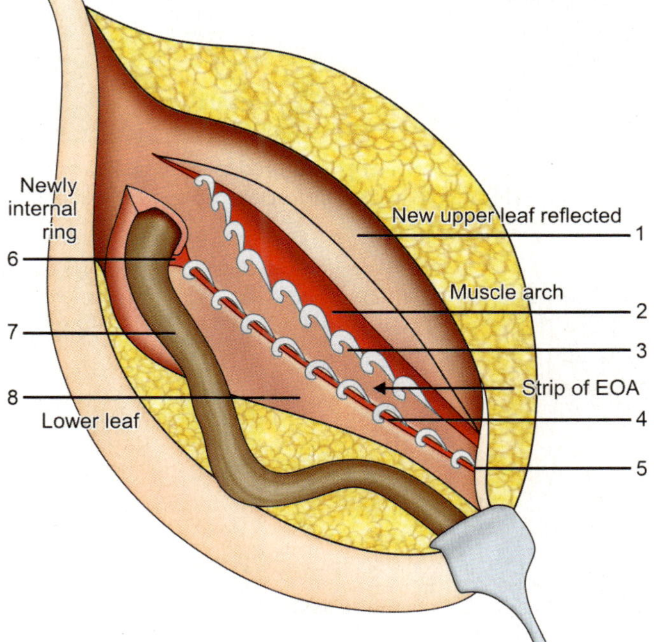


**Fig. 70.34:** Undetached strip of external oblique aponeurosis forming the posterior wall of inguinal canal. 1. New upper leaf, 2. Internal oblique muscle, 3. Sutures between the upper border of the strip and conjoined muscle, 4. Sutures between the lower border of the strip and the inguinal ligament, 5. Pubic tubercle, 6. Newly formed internal ring, 7. Spermatic cord, and 8. Lower leaf

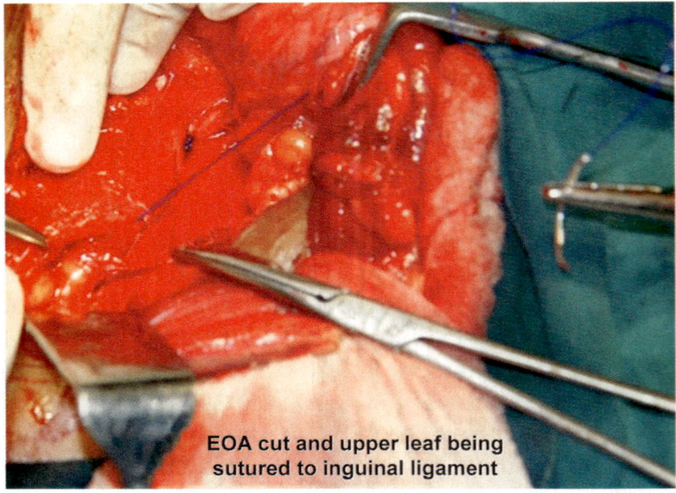


**Fig. 70.35:** Upper leaf of EOA being sutured to inguinal ligament

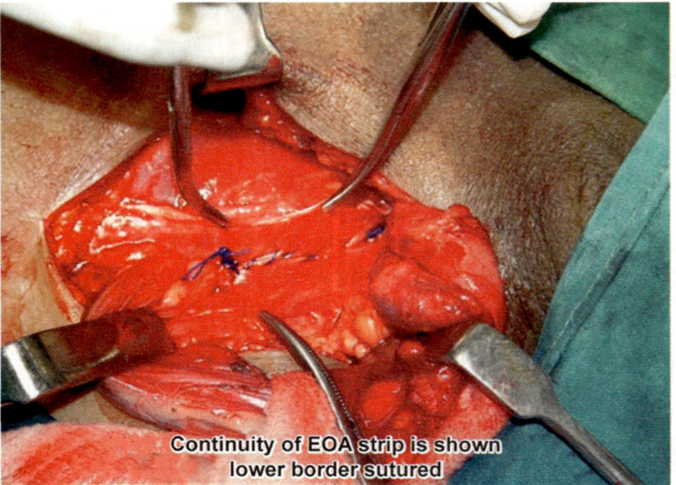


**Fig. 70.36:** Lower border of strip is sutured to inguinal ligament and upper border is lifted with two artery forceps. Continuity is kept intact

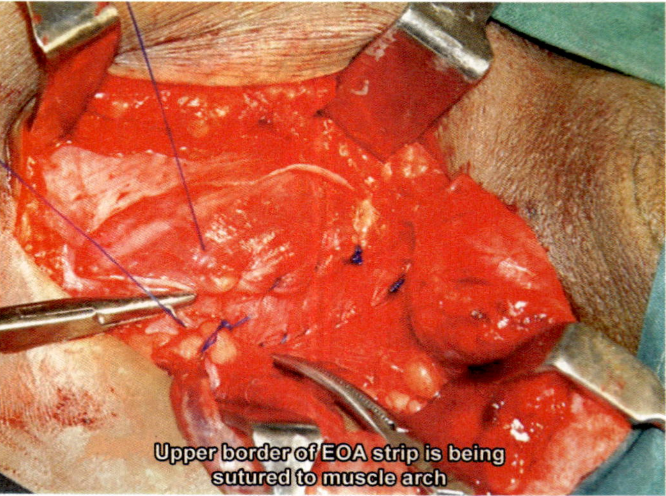


**Fig. 70.37:** Upper border of strip is sutured to the nearby internal oblique muscle with absorbable continuous sutures

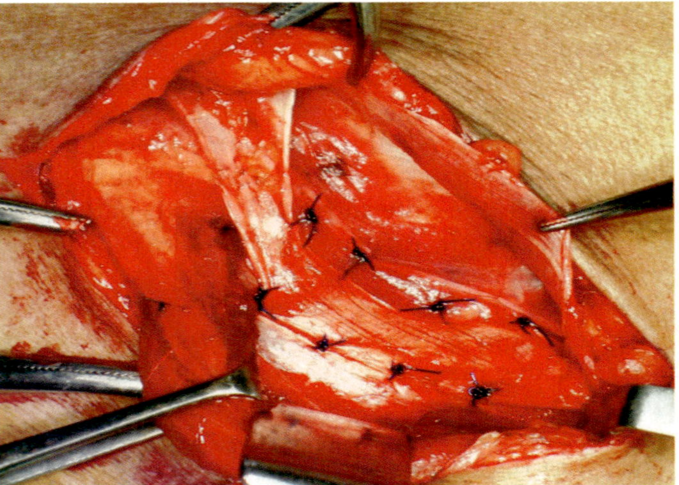

**Fig. 70.38:** Desarda repair completed

in front of the cord, as usual, again using PDSII no.1 or '0' (Monofilament Polydioxanone violet, Ethicon) continuous sutures. Undermining of the newly formed upper leaf on both of its surfaces facilitate its approximation to the lower leaf. The first stitch is taken between the lateral corner of the splitting incision and lower leaf of the external oblique. This is followed by closure of the superficial fascia and the skin as usual (Fig. 70.38). This repair is written by Prof. Desarda and has been edited by authors.

### Further Reading

A short handbook of Desarda Repair for inguinal hernia-published on electronic and print media—Author: Prof. (Dr) Desarda Mohan Phulchand (MB, MS, FICS, FICA), Professor, Department of Surgery and Chief of the Hernia Centre, Poona Hospital and Research Centre, Pune.

## OPEN CHOLECYSTECTOMY

In the vast majority of the cases, gallbladder is removed by laparoscopic route. Details have been given in the gallbladder chapter. In this chapter, we will be studying gallbladder removed through open method—after doing a laparotomy.

### DEFINITION

Removal of the diseased gallbladder by a laparotomy.

### 1. Indications

Laparoscopic cholecystectomy is now the gold standard for cholecystectomy. However, the role of open cholecystectomy is present when laparoscopic cholecystectomy fails due to extensive adhesions, **excessive bleeding**, CBD injury, impacted gallbladder, etc. (complications of laparoscopic cholecystectomy)

- Symptomatic gallstones
- Acute/chronic/acalculous cholecystitis
- Empyema gallbladder
- Mucocoele of gallbladder
- Asymptomatic gallstones—patients with high risk such as diabetes, haemolytic anaemias such as sickle cell anaemias and hereditary spherocytosis.

### 2. Contraindications

- Unfit for surgery
- Chronically debilitated patients

### 3. Position of the Patient

**Supine:** In laparoscopic cholecystectomy, the head end is elevated and a slight tilt is given to left side so that omentum and bowel fall away from the operating field.

### 4. Anaesthesia

GA.

### 5. Preparation of the Parts

From level of nipple to lower abdomen, parts are cleaned with povidone-iodine and spirit.

### 6. Surgical Procedure

- **Incision:** Right subcostal incision (**Kocher's incision**) preferred/right paramedian.
- **Layers opened:** Skin, subcutaneous tissue, muscles (external oblique, internal oblique and transversus abdominis), preperitoneal fat and peritoneum.
- **Dissection**
  - After opening the abdomen, colon and stomach are retracted away.
  - Fundus of the gallbladder is held with a sponge holding forceps and retracted.
  - Assistant retracts the liver using a Deaver retractor.
  - **Calot's triangle is identified.** The cystic artery is identified, doubly ligated with 2.0 silk sutures and cut.
  - Cystic duct is now identified, skeletonised, doubly ligated with silk or vicryl sutures and cut.
  - The gallbladder is dissected off the gallbladder fossa using electrocautery and haemostasis is achieved.
  - Rarely, fundus first approach: When Calot's triangle anatomy is not clear due to inflammation and adhesions, the dissection is started from the fundus and proceeded towards the cystic duct which is ligated in the end.
  - Intra-abdominal drain is placed.

### 7. Closure

- Inner muscle layer—No. 1 prolene continuous interlocking.
- Outer muscle (2nd layer of muscles)—same suture.
- Subcutaneous layer—2.0 Vicryl interrupted.
- Skin—2.0 ethilon/silk vertical mattress.

### 8. Postoperative Management

- Nil per oral till patient passes flatus
- To continue antibiotics in diabetic patients
- Watch for hypotension (bleeding), tachycardia, abdominal distension, pain (bile leak).
- If drain is kept, it is usually removed within 2–3 days.
- To avoid having oily foods

### 9. Postoperative Complications

- Infections and subphrenic abscess
- Bleeding from cystic artery
- Injury to CBD or hepatic duct—presents with jaundice in the postoperative period.
- Bile leak and fistulae
- Biliary stricture formations (late)
- Injuries to colon, duodenum and mesentery.

*Pearls of Wisdom*

If bile leak continues or CBD clipping is suspected, ask for ERCP and treat accordingly. Cystic duct stump leak is best treated by ERCP and stenting of CBD as early as possible.

### 10. Advice at Discharge

- Not to strain for 30 days—to prevent incisional hernia developing later.
- To report if jaundice develops (CBD injury or retained stone in CBD) or fever which may be due to subphrenic collection. (It can be treated with ultrasound-guided aspiration.)

*Pearls of Wisdom*

Identification of Y junction at open surgery and identification of cystic duct joining the infundibulum at laparoscopic surgery (dilated portion resembling elephant trunk) are the key points, which will help in avoiding bile duct injuries to a very large extent (*Refer* page 774, critical view of Strasberg).

## VAGOTOMY GASTROJEJUNOSTOMY (GJ)

Vagotomy GJ, as it was called, is a procedure that was commonly performed by surgeons for peptic ulcer disease with or without complications. With effective medical treatment for peptic ulcer disease including *H. pylori* eradication, vagotomy GJ procedure has significantly come down. Today, the only indication for this surgery is complication of peptic ulcer, namely gastric outlet obstruction. Until the invention of proton pump inhibitors increasing awareness and advent of upper GI endoscopies. Earlier, the incidence and complications of peptic ulcer were high and the commonly performed surgery for peptic ulcer was vagotomy GJ.

### 1. Indications

Gastric outlet obstruction.

### 2. Contraindication

Vagotomy needs a bit of dissection near the hiatus. Hence, a risk of mediastinitis is present, if vagotomy is done in cases of perforation. Often, many perforations are due to nonsteroidal anti-inflammatory drugs (NSAIDs). Simple closure of perforation is done.

### 3. Position of the Patient

Supine

### 4. Anaesthesia

GA

### 5. Preparation of the Parts

From level of nipple to lower abdomen, parts are cleaned with povidone iodine and spirit.

### 6. Surgical Procedure

- **Incision**—upper midline
- **Layers opened**—skin, subcutaneous tissue, linea alba, preperitoneal fat, peritoneum.
- **Dissection**
  - After opening the abdomen, the pathology in the stomach or duodenum is noted and confirmed.
  - Gentle traction is given at the anterior stomach wall. The stomach is delivered out of the wound.
  - The oesophagus is palpated with the *in situ* nasogastric tube between the thumb and the fingers.
  - The peritoneum over the overlying distal oesophagus is incised and the oesophagus is gently mobilised. The oesophagus is encircled with a Penrose drain and lifted to visualise the anterior vagus. Once identified, it is cut after ligating or applying clips. A 2 cm portion of the nerve may be excised.
  - Similarly, the posterior nerve is found as a taut band between the right crus of diaphragm and the oesophagus which is identified and cut.
  - The duodenogastric junction is identified after lifting the transverse colon and its mesentery.
  - The first loop of the jejunum (about 10 to 12 cm from duodenojejunal (DJ) flexure from the DJ) is taken and gastrojejunal anastomosis is performed in 2 layers—inner full thickness continuous suture with 3.0 Vicryl and outer seromuscular interrupted sutures with 3–0 silk. The loop is usually taken posterior to the transverse colon through a surgically made rent in the transverse mesocolon (retrocolic) and is isoperistaltic.

### 7. Closure

- Peritoneum along with linea alba is sutured with 1.0 prolene or loop ethilon continuous interlocking suture.
- Subcutaneous —2.0 Vicryl interrupted sutures.
- Skin —2.0 ethilon vertical mattress sutures.

### 8. Postoperative Management

- NPO for 2 days till patient passes flatus—indication that there is no anastomotic leak. Ryle's tube is removed, then followed by clear fluids by mouth for 2–3 days followed by soft diet.
- Suture removal by 10 days postoperatively.
- Fluid and electrolytes have to be checked in the postoperative period.

### 9. Postoperative Complications

- Postvagotomy diarrhoea, due to denervation of the gut.
- Afferent loop obstruction/stomal oedema.
- Gallstone formation due to denervation of gall-bladder.
- Stomal ulcers due to bile reflux
- Bile reflux gastritis

### 10. Advice at Discharge

- To avoid large heavy meals
- Small frequent feeds better
- Avoid spicy and oily foods

All details about complications of vagotomy and GJ are given on page 720.

## STAPLERS IN SURGERY

### Principle

They are used for apposition of tissues.

### Types

1. **Cutaneous staplers**
   - Used after thyroidectomy. It is quick and gives clean apposition.
   - Needs a special instrument for removal.
2. **Linear staplers**
   - Used to close the bowel partially or completely.

**3. Circular staplers**
- Are also called EEA stapler: End-to-end anastomosis.
- Uses in surgery:
  a. After low or high anterior resection done for carcinoma rectum
  b. After oesophagogastrectomy
  c. Any other intestinal resection

**4. GIA stapler** (Fig. 70.39)
- Gastrointestinal anastomosis stapler: Used for side-to-side anastomosis.

**5. Endostapler**
- With the increasing use of laparoscopy surgeries for facilitating a quick and safe anastomosis, endostaplers are used for intestinal anastomosis.
- Endovascular staplers are used to ligate vascular pedicles. Examples: **Renal pedicles** during laparoscopic nephrectomy, **adrenal veins** during laparoscopic adrenalectomy.

### *Advantages of Staplers*

- Saves operating time
- The low rectal and oesophageal anastomosis have higher incidence of leakage rates. However, it can be decreased by using staplers.

### *Disadvantages*

- Expensive
- Improper apposition results in leakage

### *Parts of the Stapler*

1. Handle
2. Shaft
3. Head, detachable anvil + a staple cartridge.

The staples (approximately 15 in number) are present in the cartridge. The cartridge also has a circular knife.

*Pearls of Wisdom*

The doughnuts (rings of excised tissue) should be complete after the stapled anastomosis. Incomplete doughnut means incomplete wound closure (Fig. 70.40).

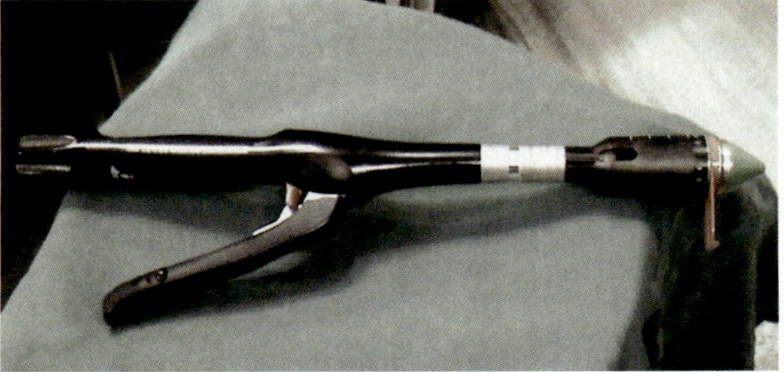

**Fig. 70.39:** GIA stapler

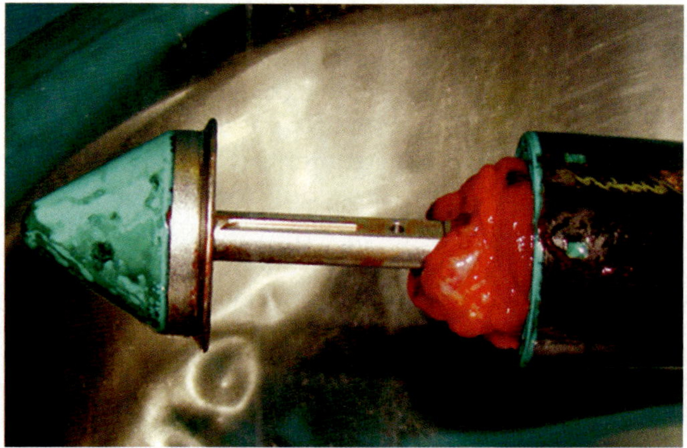

**Fig. 70.40:** Doughnut of stapler haemorrhoidopexy

### Contraindications

1. If the tissues which have to be approximated are under tension, they should not be stapled.
2. Different lumen diameters should not be stapled end-to-end.
3. If the circular head is of greater diameter than the lumen, it should not be used.

## LAPAROSCOPIC SURGERY

### Introduction and History

- Laparoscopy made marked advances in the 1990s.
- Although the term minimally invasive surgery (MIS) is relatively recent, the history of its component parts is nearly 100 years old. What is considered the newest and most popular variety of MIS, laparoscopy, is in fact the oldest.
- Primitive laparoscopy, placing a cystoscope within an inflated abdomen, was first performed by Kelling in 1901.
- In the late 1950s, Hopkins described the rod lens, a method of transmitting light through a solid quartz rod with no heat and a little light loss.
- Muhe in Germany began performing laparoscopic-assisted cholecystectomies in 1985.
- In 1987, Mouret and Dubious performed the first video-laparoscopy in France.
- The explosion of **video-assisted surgery** in the past 20 years was a result of the development of compact, high-resolution, charge-coupled devices (CCDs) that could be mounted on the internal end of flexible endoscopes or on the external end of a Hopkins telescope.
- Coupled with bright light sources, fibreoptic cables, and **high-resolution video monitors**, the video endoscope has changed our understanding of surgical anatomy and reshaped surgical practice.

## Basic Instrumentation

- **0° or 30° angled laparoscope** either 5 or 10 mm in diameter attached to camera connected to video source and monitor, ports for gas connection.
- **5 mm laparoscopic instruments** including Maryland dissector, blunt-tip dissecting forceps, cup-biopsy forceps, atraumatic grasping forceps, liver retractor, Babcocks forceps and scissors (Fig. 70.41).
- **5 or 10 mm suction/irrigation device**
- **Laparoscopic ultrasound probe** (optional)

## Equipment

1. **Telescope:** 30°, 0° or 45°
2. **Video camera:** A high-resolution video camera attached to the eyepiece of the telescope acquires the image for projection on the monitor. The video image is transmitted *via* a cable to a video unit, where it is processed into either an analog or a digital form (Fig. 70.42).
   - Analog is an electrical signal with a continuously varying wave or shift of intensity or frequency of voltage. Digital is a data signal with information represented by ones and zeros and is interpreted by a computer. These are the methods by which the picture is transmitted to the video monitor.
   - **The camera and cable are designed so that they can be sterilised in glutaraldehyde**.

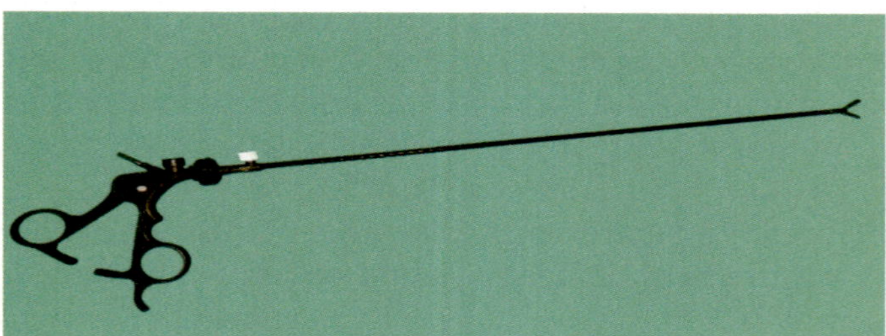

**Fig. 70.41:** Atraumatic grasper

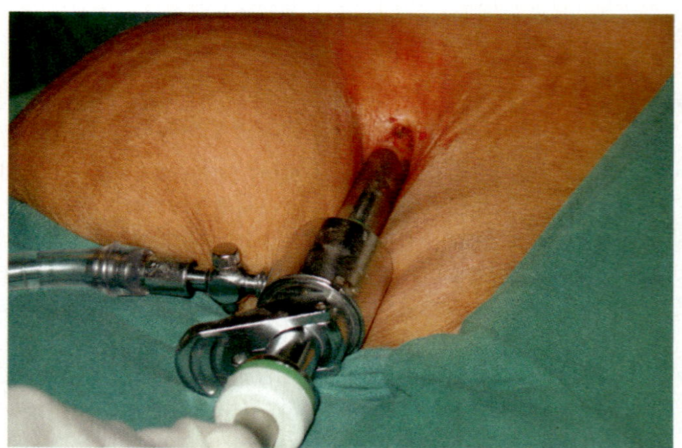

**Fig. 70.42:** Camera port (umbilical port)

3. **Light sources:** High-intensity light is created with bulbs of mercury, halogen vapour or xenon. Since light is absorbed by blood, any procedure in which bleeding is encountered may require more light. The light is carried to the fibreoptic bundles of the laparoscope *via* a fibreoptic cable. The current systems create even brightness across the field.
4. **Insufflators:** An insufflator delivers gas from a high pressure cylinder to the patient at a high rate with low and accurately controlled pressure (Fig. 70.43).
5. **Video monitors:** High-resolution video monitors are used to display the image. These monitors may be positioned optimally.

## Anaesthesia

- Usually done under general anaesthesia.
- Laparoscopic surgeon can influence cardiovascular performance by **reducing or removing the $CO_2$ pneumoperitoneum**.
- **Insensible fluid losses are negligible**, and therefore, IV fluid administration should not exceed that necessary to maintain circulating volume.
- Minimally invasive surgical procedures are often outpatient procedures. So, short-acting anaesthetic agents are preferable.
- Since, the factors that require hospitalisation after laparoscopic procedures include the management of nausea, pain and urinary retention, the anaesthesiologist should minimise the use of agents that provoke these conditions and maximise the use of medications that prevent such problems.
- Critical to the anaesthesia management of these patients is the **use of non-narcotic analgesics** (e.g. diclofenac) when haemostasis allows it, and the **liberal use of antiemetic** agents, such as **ondansetron and steroids.**

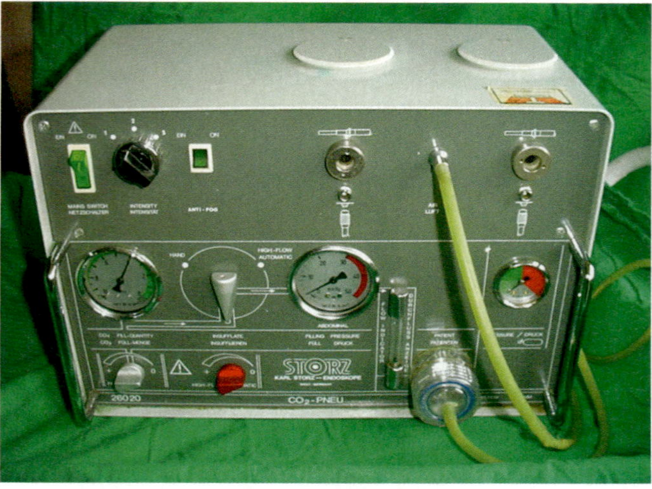


**Fig. 70.43:** Insufflator

## Procedure and Principles

The unique feature of laparoscopic surgery is the need to lift the abdominal wall from the abdominal organs by creating pneumoperitoneum.

## Gases Used

| Gases | Advantages | Disadvantages |
|---|---|---|
| Air | Historical importance | Poorly insoluble in blood<br>So lower absorption<br>More painful |
| $CO_2$ | Inert | Rapidly absorbable<br>Respiratory acidosis |
| $N_2O$ | Inert<br>Less painful<br>Reduced intraoperative end tidal $CO_2$ | Rapidly absorbable<br>Danger of combustion<br>Not safe in pregnancy |

## Laparoscopic Access (Fig. 70.44)

- The requirements for laparoscopy are more involved because the creation of a pneumoperitoneum requires that instruments of access (trocars) contain valves to maintain abdominal inflation (Key Box 70.8).
- Two methods are used for establishing abdominal access during laparoscopic procedures. The first, direct puncture laparoscopy, begins with the elevation of the relaxed abdominal wall with two towel clips or a well-placed hand. A small incision is made in the umbilicus, and a specialised springloaded (Veress) needle is placed in the abdominal cavity (Fig. 70.45). With the **Veress needle,** two distinct pops are felt as the surgeon passes the needle through the abdominal wall fascia and the peritoneum. The umbilicus usually is selected as the preferred point of access because, in this location, the abdominal wall is quite thin, even in obese patients. The abdomen is inflated with a pressure-limited insufflator. $CO_2$ gas is used usually with maximal pressures in the range of 14 to 15 mmHg. During the process of insufflation, it is essential that the surgeon observe the pressure and flow readings on the monitor to confirm an intraperitoneal location of the Veress needle tip (Key Box 70.9).
- Occasionally, the direct peritoneal access (Hasson) technique is advisable. With this technique, the surgeon makes a small incision just below the umbilicus and under direct vision locates the abdominal fascia.

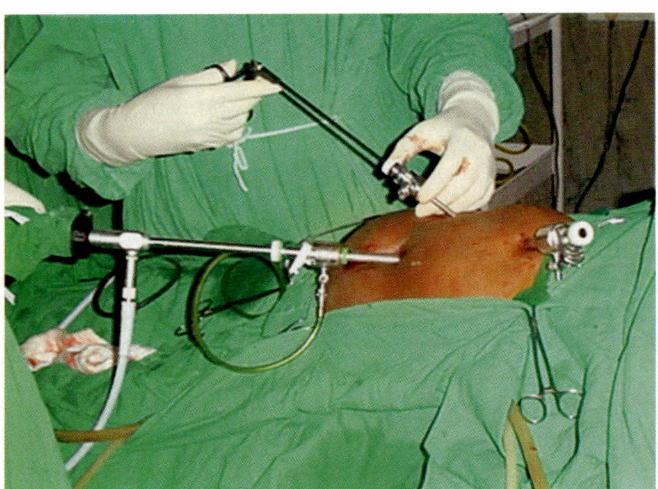

**Fig. 70.44:** 3 ports in place

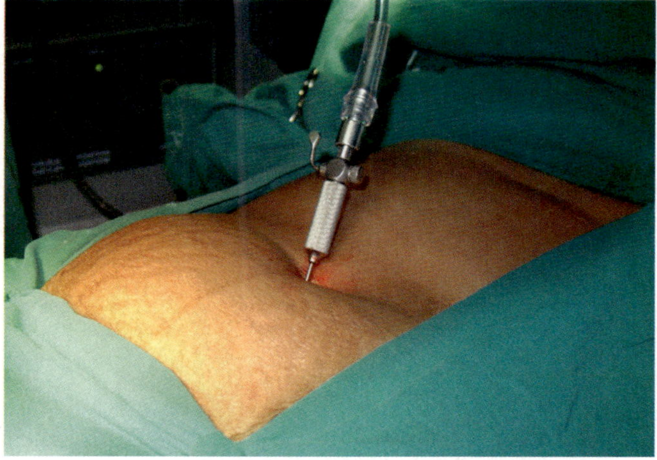

**Fig. 70.45:** Veress needle is used to create pneumoperitoneum

Key Box 70.8

**Laparoscopic Access**

1. Closed Veress needle technique
2. Open technique: Hasson's technique
3. Direct trocar insertion
4. Access using umbilical cicatrix tube
5. Disposable optical trocar

Key Box 70.9

**Veress Needle**

12–15 cm length with 2 mm external diameter. It has got outer and inner cannula. Outer cannula sharp cutting edge and inner cannula blunt edge with spring action.

Confirmation of Veress needle position

1. Hiss test
2. Aspiration test
3. Drop test
4. Percussion test
5. Reading of the insufflator

   Preferred position for Veress needle insertion is subumbilical or Palmer's point (3 cm below the middle of left subcostal margin).

## Utility and Scope of Laparoscopic Surgery

**I. Basic**

- Appendicectomy
- Cholecystectomy (Fig. 70.46)
- Hernia repair

**II. Advanced**

- Nissen fundoplication
- Heller's myotomy
- Gastrectomy
- Oesophagectomy
- Enteral access
- Bile duct exploration
- Colectomy (Fig. 70.47)
- Splenectomy
- Adrenalectomy
- Lymph node dissection
- Nephrectomy

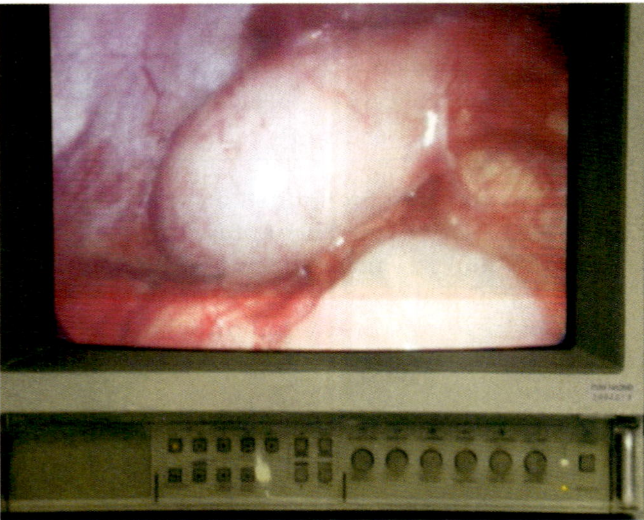

**Fig. 70.46:** Laparoscopic view of the gallbladder

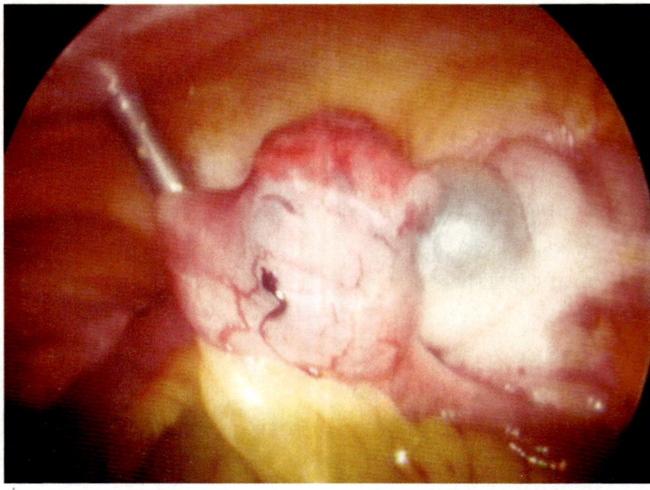

**Fig. 70.47:** Laparoscopic-assisted mobilisation of colon

- Robotics
- Stereo imaging
- Telemedicine

**III. Laparoscopy-assisted procedures**

- Hepatectomy
- Pancreatectomy
- Prostatectomy
- Hysterectomy

## The Physiologic Effects of Pneumoperitoneum

- The pneumoperitoneum has many effects that are only partially known despite years of study in humans and in animal models. There are effects resulting from the pressure within the abdomen and effects resulting from the composition of the gas used, generally carbon dioxide.
- The pressure within the abdomen from pneumoperitoneum decreases venous return by collapsing the intra-abdominal veins, especially in volume-depleted patients.
- This decrease in venous return may lead to decreased cardiac output.
- To compensate (Key Box 70.10), there is an elevation in the heart rate, which increases myocardial oxygen demand.

Key Box 70.10

**Absolute Contraindications**

- Advanced generalised peritonitis
- Massive abdominal distension secondary to obstruction
- Irreducible hernia
- Uncorrected coagulopathy, hypovolaemic shock
- Inability of the patient to tolerate a formal laparotomy
- Surgeon's lack of experience in performing laparoscopic procedures

**Relative Contraindications**

| | |
|---|---|
| Previous surgery | Adhesions leading to visceral injury |
| Ongoing intra-abdominal sepsis | Friable bowel prone to injury |
| Bowel obstruction | Friable bowel prone to injury |
| Morbid obesity | Difficult access, requirement for longer instruments |
| Pregnancy | Foetal distress, injury to gravid uterus |
| Aortic or iliac aneurysmal disease | Vascular injury |
| Cardiopulmonary compromise | Raised intra-abdominal pressure may significantly reduce cardiac preload. $CO_2$ insufflation may result in $CO_2$ retention |

- High-risk cardiopulmonary patients cannot always meet the demand and may not tolerate a laparoscopic procedure. In volume-expanded healthy patients with full intra-abdominal capacitance vessels (veins), the increased intra-abdominal pressure actually may serve as a pump that increases right atrial filling pressure.
- Urine output often is diminished during laparoscopic procedures and usually is the result of diminished renal blood flow owing to the cardiovascular effects of pneumoperitoneum and direct pressure on the renal veins.
- In addition to direct effects, elevated intra-abdominal pressure results in release of antidiuretic hormone (ADH) by the pituitary, resulting in oliguria that may last up to 60 minutes after the pneumoperitoneum is released.

### Complications of Laparoscopy

1. Injury to bowel/bladder
2. Injury to major vessels
3. $CO_2$ related complications
   a. **Hypercapnia:** Hypercapnia and acidosis are seen with pneumoperitoneum and are likely due to the absorption of carbon dioxide from the peritoneal cavity. Hypercapnia and acidosis that are difficult to control may follow, especially in elderly patients, those undergoing long operations and patients with pulmonary insufficiency.
   b. **Carbon dioxide embolus:** The incidence of clinically significant $CO_2$ embolism is very low, although recent reports using more sensitive tests suggest that tiny bubbles of gas are present commonly in the right side of the heart during laparoscopic procedures. Clinically important $CO_2$ embolism may be noted by unexplained hypotension and hypoxia during the operation.
   c. **Capnothorax/pneumothorax:** Capnothorax can be caused by carbon dioxide escaping into the chest through a defect in the diaphragm or tracking through fascial planes during dissection of the oesophageal hiatus. It can also be due to opening of pleuroperitoneal ducts most commonly seen on the right side.

## HERNIA REPAIR: TAPP
(Transabdominal Preperitoneal Mesh Repair)

### KEY POINTS IN LAPAROSCOPIC INGUINAL ANATOMY

### Space of Bogros

This 'preperitoneal space' is divided into two by the posterior lamina of the transversalis fascia. The posterior compartment of this space is called the 'Space of Bogros (proper)', described by French anatomist Bogros in 1923. The anterior space has been termed as the 'Vascular Space'. Medially it is continuous with the space of Retzius.

### Prevesical Space of Retzius

The preperitoneal space that lies deep to the supravesical fossa and the medial umbilical fossa is the prevesical space of Retzius (described in 1858, by Swedish anatomist Retzius). Dissection of this space during a laparoscopic hernia repair is mandatory to enable proper mesh overlap of the hernial defect to aid in proper mesh placement/fixation.

### Corona Mortis/Crown of Death/Circle of Death

- The pubic branch of the inferior epigastric artery courses in a vertical fashion inferiorly, crossing the Cooper's ligament and anastomosing with the obturator artery. In 25–30% of individuals (can be as high as 70–80%), the pubic branch is large and can replace the obturator artery.
- This large arterial branch is called aberrant obturator artery can partially encircle the neck of a hernia sac and be injured in a femoral hernia repair. It could also be injured while exposing the Cooper's ligament by freeing it of areolar adipose connective tissue.
- Because of this possibility an enlarged pubic branch of the inferior epigastric artery has in the past been known as the 'Corona Mortis'. The danger of injury in this area is more significant for obturator veins.

### Triangle of Doom

- It is a misnomer. It is not a triangle. It indicates an area where it is dangerous to place staples or sutures during laparoscopic hernia surgery.

The "triangle of doom" is an inverted "V"-shaped area with its apex at the internal (deep) inguinal ring. The "triangle of doom" is bound laterally by the gonadal vessels, and medially by the vas deferens in the male, or the round ligament of the uterus in the female.

- Within the boundaries of this area you can find the external iliac artery and vein.
- Injury to these vessels can be catastrophic.

### Triangle of Pain

Formed medially by gonadal vessels, laterally by iliopubic tract and inferiorly by peritoneal reflection. It contains lateral femoral cutaneous nerve, genital femoral nerve.

### Introduction

Novel method used for hernias wherein transabdominally (intraperitoneal) dissection is done through a laparoscope, and a mesh placed in the preperitoneal space.

### Indication

Large indirect hernias and irreducible hernias.

### Procedure

- **10 mm infraumbilical port** is used for the laparoscopic camera.
- **5 mm ports** are placed one on each side on pararectal point at or above the level of umbilicus, so as to achieve adequate triangulation.
- Once ports are inserted, the hernial sac is recognized and the contents are reduced by pulling it transabdominally using a dissector (laparoscopic).
- Hernial sac is dissected in the preperitoneal plane after incising at the upper part of the hernial sac opening.
- Once the sac is dissected and excised, a prolene mesh is placed in the preperitoneal space. It is fixed to the pubic bone using tacks. Peritoneum is closed with prolene sutures.

### Complications

- Mesh displacement
- Intestinal obstruction, if the mesh displaces into the peritoneum.
- Expensive
- Higher recurrence rates

## HERNIA REPAIR: TEP (TOTALLY EXTRAPERITONEAL REPAIR)

### Indications

1. Recurrent hernia
2. Bilateral inguinal hernias
3. Indirect/direct/femoral hernias

### Contraindications

1. Obstructed/strangulated hernias
2. Ascites
3. Bleeding disorders

**This surgery has surpassed the TAPP procedure and is turning out to be a promising procedure for management of hernias.**

### Procedure (Figs 70.48 to 70.50)

- Subumbilical incision (10 mm) placed
- **Extraperitoneal space** is created by passing the scope between the rectus muscle and the posterior rectus sheath medial to the muscle bundle edge.
- Initial dissection is carried out using laparoscope itself and **inflation of $CO_2$.**
- 2 more 5 mm ports are placed in the midline **4 cm and 8 cm below the 1st port respectively**.
- **Dissection** is carried out medially till the pubic tubercle, iliopectinate ligament and laterally till the iliac vessels and inferior epigastric vessels. Once adequate space is dissected, the sac is reduced by pulling it down from the inguinal canal (reduction of sac) and a 15 × 15 cm mesh is placed and spread.
- Mesh may be sutured, left as it is or fixed with tackers.
- Both sides can be done together through the same ports.

### Complications

1. Cord/vas injuries
2. Inadvertent opening of the sac/peritoneum and creation of pneumoperitoneum
3. Seroma formation
4. Infection

### Advantages of TEP

1. Approach is totally extraperitoneal
2. Smaller incisions
3. No need for fixing mesh
4. Peritoneum is intact

## SILS (LESS)

### Introduction

- Single port access (SPA) surgery, also known as laparoendoscopic single-site surgery (LESS), single incision laparoscopic surgery (SILS) or single port incision less conventional equipment-utilising surgery (SPICES) or embryonic natural orifice transluminal

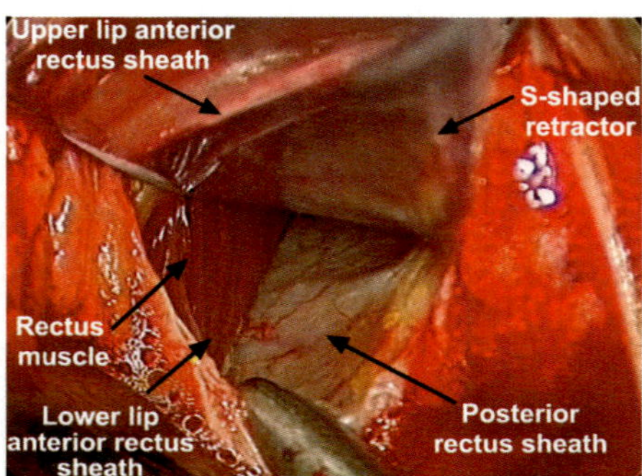


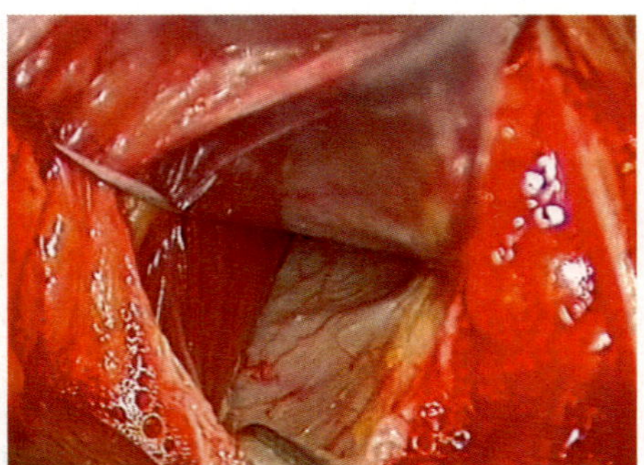

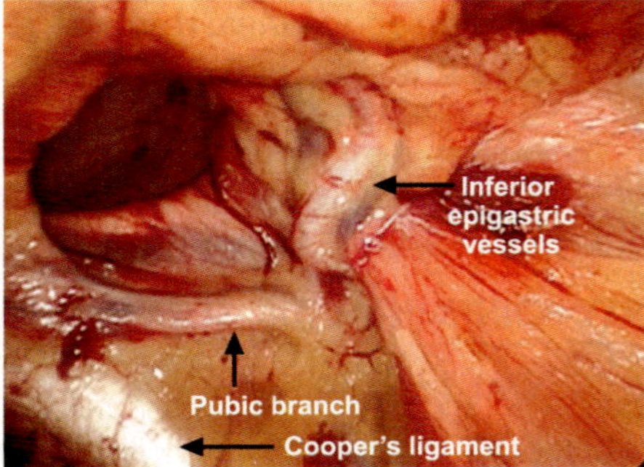


**Figs 70.48 to 70.50:** Totally extraperitoneal repair (TEP) (*Courtesy:* Dr Praveen Bhatia, Consultant Surgeon and Medical Director, Bhatia Global Hospital and Endosurgery Institute, New Delhi)

endoscopic surgery (E-NOTES) is an advanced minimally invasive surgical procedure in which the surgeon operates almost exclusively through a single entry point, typically the patient's navel.

- SPA surgical procedures are like many laparoscopic surgeries in that the patient is under general anaesthesia; insufflated and laparoscopic visualisation is utilised.
- In laparoendoscopic single-site surgery (LESS), a single small incision is used at the entry point rather than four to five small incisions.
- All surgical instruments are placed through this small incision and also the incision site is located in the left abdomen or umbilicus. In general, SILS techniques take the same amount of time to do as traditional laparoscopic surgeries.
- However, SILS is recognised as to be a more complicated procedure because it involves manipulating three articulating instruments through one access port.
- Obesity, severe adhesions, or scarring from previous surgeries are a few cases, SILS may not be possible. Failure rates are high.

### How SILS Differs from Traditional Laparoscopic Surgery?

- In single incision laparoscopic surgery, only one incision of around 1.5–2 cm is made just below the umbilicus to allow placement of three thin 5 mm port side by side parallel to each other.
- Port, a especially designed port is inserted into the abdomen; this port carries the telescope and laparoscopic instruments.
- Steps of surgical procedure are similar to the conventional laparoscopic surgery.
- As there is only one incision, pain is less as compared to traditional laparoscopic surgery and recovery is faster. The healed incision leaves practically no scar, thus making SILS cosmetically a superior option.
- In 5 to 10% patients, it may not be possible to complete the operation by SILS due to technical difficulties. One has to place one or two additional ports and completes the procedure in the traditional laparoscopic manner.

## NATURAL ORIFICE TRANSLUMINAL ENDOSCOPIC SURGERY (NOTES)

### Introduction

It means surgery performed endoscopically by initially passing the flexible endoscope through the body's natural orifices, like the mouth, anus, vagina, or urethra, to achieve access into areas that would not otherwise be accessible endoscopically, such as the abdomen and pelvis. Kalloo's did the first transgastric peritoneoscopy in 2004. In India, Dr GV Rao and Dr Nageshwar Reddy from Hyderabad, performed the first—NOTES in a patient who had appendicitis with extensive scars over the abdominal wall. The entry from abdomen was not possible. They performed transoral, transgastric appendicectomy.

### Advantages

- Less invasive
- No abdominal incision
- Reduction in postoperative pain
- Wound infection, hernia formation and adhesions are very less.

### Commonly Performed NOTES

- Transgastric appendectomy
- Transvaginal cholecystectomy

### Future Upcoming Technologies

- Magnetically anchored and guidance systems (MAGS) are designed to manoeuvre intra-abdominal instruments. They use the external handheld magnet.
- The fundus of the gallbladder can be retracted above the costal margin by coupling the interior aspect of an external magnet. The graspers are situated on the gallbladder with the help of endoscopic biopsy forceps.
- Magnets may become valuable, within the operating room.

## VAAFT TECHNIQUE

### Introduction

It is performed for the surgical treatment of complex anal fistulas and their recurrences. Key points are the exact localisation of the internal fistula opening under vision, the fistula treatment from inside, and the hermetic closure of the internal opening. No risk of faecal incontinence as no sphincter damage—one of the great advantages over the conventional treatment.

### Materials

- Fistuloscope, a unipolar electrode connected to a high frequency unit, a fistula brush and a forceps.
- A semicircular or linear stapler and 0.5 ml of synthetic cyanoacrylate with a tiny catheter are used as well.
- The fistuloscope is equipped with an optical channel, a working channel and an irrigation channel. The working length adds up to 18 cm; the use of a handle reduces it to an effective length of 14 cm.
- The optimal patient positioning is the lithotomy position. Spinal anaesthesia is required.
- The fistuloscope is connected to the Karl Storz equipment and to the washing solution bag (5000 cc glycine and mannitol 1% solution).

### The Technique

It comprises a diagnostic phase and an operative phase.

### The Diagnostic Phase

- The fistuloscope is inserted through the external fistula opening with the washing solution (glycine 1% and mannitol 1%) already running. Thus, it provides clear view of the fistula pathway which is seen on the screen.
- With right index finger in the rectum, fistuloscope is guided slowly into the fistula.
- Complete relaxation of the surrounding tissue induced by the spinal anaesthesia helps in gentle up and down movements to advance the fistuloscope.
- The continuous flow of the glycine-mannitol solution allows for an optimal view of the fistula's inside up to the internal opening.
- At this stage, insert an anal retractor in order to localise the internal fistula opening by looking for the light of the telescope in the rectum or anal canal.
- When the fistuloscope exits through the internal opening the rectal mucosa clearly appears on the screen. At this point, two or three stitches are put, in two opposite points of the internal opening margin in order to isolate those points and not to lose them.

### The Operative Phase

- First locate the internal opening. From the internal opening to external opening, the fistula wall and all granulation tissues are coagulated. Procedure is done slowly so that fistula is destroyed under vision using a unipolar electrode. All the necrotic material is removed. Abscess cavity is irrigated.
- Fistuloscope is removed at this stage. The assistant stretches the threads towards the internal rectal space or rather the anal canal using a straight forceps in order to lift the internal fistula opening at least 2 cm into the shape of a volcano.
- Subsequently, stitch is inserted at the volcano's base and complete the mechanical cutting and suturing by using a linear stapler. The hermetic closure of the internal fistula opening can also be accomplished. This also depends on the internal opening position. Using a semicircular stapler, the suture will be horizontal. Using a linear stapler, the suture will be vertical.
- Last step is insertion of 0.5 ml of synthetic cyanoacrylate after the suture/staple line via the fistula pathway to further reinforce the suture. It helps in perfect closure of the fistula opening.
- This procedure assures a perfect excision and a hermetic closure of the internal fistula opening, excluding the risk of stool passage. Since the suture is situated tangential to the sphincter, the postoperative pain is low even if the suture falls both in the anal canal and the rectum.

### Conclusion

- The advantages of the VAAFT technique are: No surgical wounds on the buttocks or in the perianal region, there is complete certainty in the localization of the internal fistula opening, and the fistula can be completely destroyed from the inside.
- Since operations are done from inside, no damage is caused to the anal sphincters. The risk of postoperative faecal incontinence is excluded.

## ROBOTIC SURGERY

The term **robots** was introduced and coined in 1921, ***"robota"*** meaning forced labour. The first documented use of robotic-assisted surgery was in 1985. PUMA 560 robotic surgical arm was used successfully in a delicate neurosurgical biopsy, a non-laparoscopic surgery. The first laparoscopic procedure involving a robotic system was a cholecystectomy done in 1987. The following year the same PUMA system was used to perform a transurethral resection. da Vinci Surgical System is the first robotic system approved by the FDA for general laparoscopic surgery. The da Vinci system's 3D magnification screen allows the surgeon to view the operative area with the clarity of high resolution. The "Endo-wrist" features of the operating arms precisely replicate the skilled movements of the surgeon at the controls and filter out any shaking, greatly improving accuracy in small operating spaces. da Vinci system has been approved by the FDA for use in: Urological surgeries, general laparoscopic surgeries, general non-cardiovascular thoracoscopic surgeries and thoracoscopically-assisted cardiotomy procedures.

There are three different types of robotic surgery systems currently in use. The main difference between each system is how involved a human is in the process.

1. **Supervisory controlled systems:** The surgeon inputs data into the robot and the robot does all of the following surgery.
2. **Tele-surgical systems:** Cutting and sewing is performed by a surgeon at a console remote from the patient. The surgeon can be miles away at another site while performing this type of surgery.
3. **Shared control systems:** Doctors perform the work with the assistance of the robot technology, simultaneously.

### Advantages

- Surgeons are able to perform more complex tasks (increases precision), physically easier, less awkward positioning for the surgeon. Procedures reduce the risk of death, complications, and hospital stay. It provides enhanced 3-D high-definition visualisation.

- For the patients: Reduced trauma to the body, less risk of infection along with faster recovery.

### Disadvantages

- More expensive than traditional surgery.
- Removal of physical contact with surgery surface.
- The procedure can take nearly twice as long, depending on how well the surgeon knows the equipment.
- The size of the actual equipment can take up a lot of space inside the operating room.
- All operating instruments are NOT compatible with the technology required for robotic surgery.

**Common procedures which can be done by da Vinci surgical system**

| | |
|---|---|
| Bladder cancer | Obesity |
| Colorectal cancer | Prostate cancer |
| Coronary artery disease | Throat cancer |
| Endometriosis | Uterine fibroids |
| Gynaecologic cancer | Uterine prolapse |
| Kidney cancer | Mitral valve prolapse |

**Please note:** For more details about robotic surgery, please refer to digital contents.

## ENERGY SOURCES IN SURGERY

### Introduction

In present-day surgery, energy-based devices and technologies have become indispensable tools to perform complicated surgical procedures with precision. Each modality of energy source offers unique advantages and operates through distinct mechanisms of action. They also have side effects.

Understanding the principles, applications, and safety considerations of various energy sources is fundamental for modern surgical practice.

### Classification of Surgical Energy Sources

1. Electrical energy: Electrosurgery involves the application of high frequency alternating electrical current to raise intra-cellular temperature to achieve vaporization of water or a combination of desiccation and protein or tissue coagulation. Thus one can cut, coagulate, desiccate, or fulgurate tissue. Monopolar electrosurgery, bipolar electrosurgery and advanced bipolar devices are a few examples:
2. Ultrasonic energy
3. Laser energy
4. Plasma energy
5. Hybrid energy systems

## 1. ELECTRICAL ENERGY (Figs 70.51 and 70.52)

### A. Monopolar Electrosurgery

#### Principle

- High-frequency electrical current passes through the patient's body.
- Current flows from the active electrode to the return electrode.
- The tissue effect occurs at the point of contact with the active electrode.

#### Uses

- Cutting and coagulation of tissues, fulguration of superficial lesions.
- Tissue dissection while achieving hemostasis simultaneously.

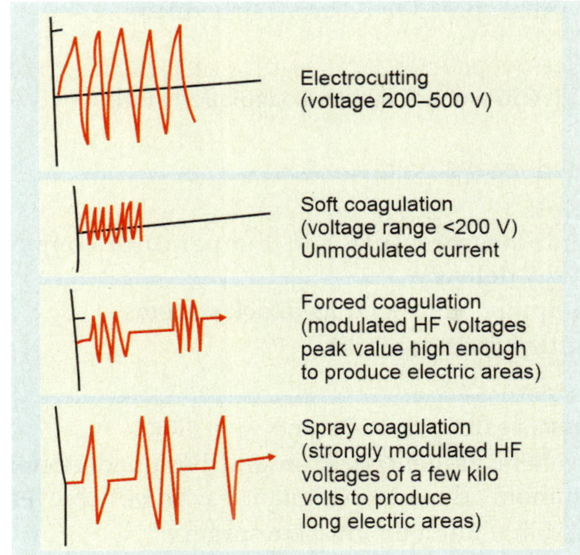


**Fig. 70.51:** Electrocautery

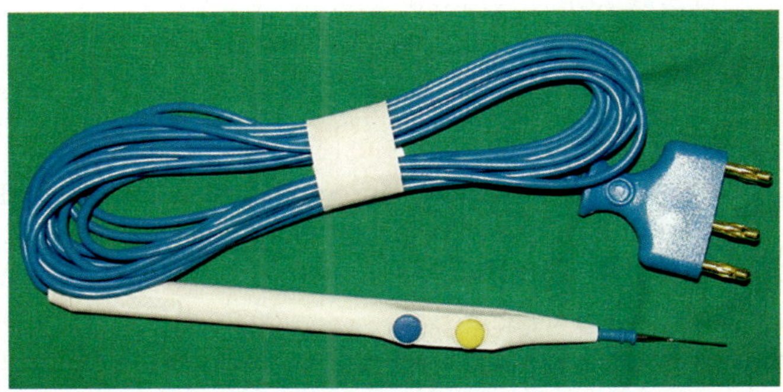

**Fig. 70.52:** Cautery cord: Yellow button is for cutting current and blue button is for coagulation

### Complications

- Burns at the return electrode site and capacitive coupling and direct coupling
- Interference with cardiac devices
- Fire hazards

## B. Bipolar Electrosurgery

### Principle

- Current flows between two electrodes of the instrument
- Limited tissue effect between forceps tips, thus small volume of tissue is injured. This principle is used often while coagulating vessels near facial nerve and recurrent laryngeal nerve.
- No return electrode is needed

### Uses

- Precise coagulation of vessels and delicate tissue dissection such as dissection in and around nerve.
- Neurosurgical procedures and microsurgery.

### Complications

- Thermal spread to adjacent structures

*Pearls of Wisdom*

Effective in wet fields, uses coagulation current only.

## C. Advanced Bipolar Devices

### Principle

- Combines pressure and temperature-controlled energy delivery
- Computer-controlled feedback systems
- Tissue fusion capability

### Uses

- Vessel sealing up to 7 mm
- Excellent tissue dissection and lymphadenectomy–commonly done in malignancies can be achieved.
- Used in minimally invasive surgery

### Complications

- Lateral thermal spread and delayed tissue separation
- Device failure

## 2. ULTRASONIC ENERGY

### Principle

- Converts electrical energy into mechanical energy and protein denaturation occurs.
- Mechanical vibration at 55,500 Hz and cavitation effect.

### Uses

- Tissue dissection, vessels sealing up to 5 mm and hence used widely in laparoscopic surgery.
- Precise dissection near vital structures thus the damage to the adjacent structures are minimized.

### Complications

- Aerosolization of tissue particles
- Lateral thermal spread
- Tip can get heated when activated in air
- Mist formation

## HARMONIC SCALPEL

It is an example for ultrasonic energy.

- It is a high frequency mechanical energy device which uses ultrasound technology. This instrument has a handheld ultrasound transducer and scalpel. While using by hand or foot pedal, scalpel vibrates in the range of 20,000–55,500 Hz. During this process it cuts the tissues and seals the tissues. Process of sealing is by protein denaturation. No ligatures are required, and perfect haemostasis is obtained. Scalpels have different sizes. It has three compatible probes that are the shear, blade and a hook. The shear can coagulate vessels up to 5 mm, whereas the hook and blade only 2 mm in diameter.
- Types of vessels which can be coagulated and sealed are up to 5 mm diameter. Newer instruments can coagulate vessel up to 7 mm diameter. However, to be on the safer side, 4–5 mm diameter arteries such as right colic artery and veins, superior thyroid arteries and veins and such many vessels can be sealed and cut.
- ***Advantages of harmonic scalpel:*** No smoke, no lateral thermal tissue injury, no ligatures and less operative time. Thus, it is the popular choice of energy sources in laparoscopic surgeries. It can also be used for open surgeries—a few examples are excision of pile masses (haemorrhoidectomy) and raising flaps for mastectomies.
- ***Disadvantages:*** More time for coagulation. A spurting artery can be ligated by a haemostat or coagulated by cautery than harmonic scalpel. It is costly.

## 3. LASERS IN SURGERY

- Light amplification by simulated emission of radiation.
- Molecules which are placed in a compact area are activated when power is passed through. as a result of this, they move in different directions, they hit each other, releasing energy. This energy is used as laser to the area whenever required.
- It is a focused light energy, with specific wavelengths for different applications and various tissue interactions (absorption, scatter, reflection) occur.
- Precise tissue ablation and less trauma
- Photocoagulation

### Types

- Argon laser
- Neodymium: Yttrium-aluminium-garnet laser (Nd:YAG laser)
- $CO_2$ laser
- Neon laser

### Advantages and disadvantages

- Most important advantage is a bloodless field—especially useful in head and neck surgeries and ENT surgeries.
- It is quick and there is less tissue trauma and expensive.

### Precaution

- To avoid injuries to normal tissues, all reflecting instruments should be avoided so that the laser does not get reflected.
- All theatre personnel should wear special protective goggles.

### Clinical applications

- Vascular malformation of the GIT.
- Endoscopic laser for advanced carcinoma oesophagus to relieve obstruction and dysphagia.
- Obstructed colorectal cancer.
- Liver resections: Nd:YAG laser combined with CUSA can be used for liver resections.
- $CO_2$ laser and Nd:YAG laser can be used for haemorrhoidectomy.

## 4. PLASMA ENERGY

### Principle

- Plasma energy is used in surgery through various devices like plasma scalpel, argon beam coagulator (ABC), and J-Plasma.
- Ionized gas creates a plasma field at low-temperature atmospheric plasma
- Controlled tissue effect

### Uses

- Surface ablation—it uses gas discharge to treat tissue
- Used in sterilization of tubes and catheters
- Wound treatment
- Soft tissue modification—plasma scalpel is used to conduct splenectomy

### Complications

- Tissue desiccation
- Equipment malfunction

## 5. HYBRID ENERGY SYSTEMS

### Principle

- A combination of different energy modalities are used here. They work on synergistic effects
- Computer-controlled delivery

### Uses

- Complex tissue dissection and advanced vessel sealing
- Minimally invasive procedures—laparoscopic surgeries

### Complications

- Combined risk factors
- Equipment complexity

### Prevention

- Comprehensive training
- Regular maintenance
- Following manufacturer guidelines
- Proper system checks

## PLEASE READ THESE INSTRUCTIONS

Students are requested to confirm the list of operations which will be asked in the examination with their teachers in their respective medical colleges and be prepared for exams. You should realise that what operation an undergraduate student is expected to know in more detail is not stated clearly in the syllabus. Nevertheless, you do not lose anything trying to understand more operations. Rather, it may help you in your postgraduate entrance examinations.

- The last four chapters are important for *viva voce* examination in general surgery. The questions given in these chapters are most commonly asked. This does not mean, however, that they are the only questions asked. As the subject is vast, the number of questions that can be asked can be unlimited. The purpose of *viva voce* section is to see how much the student knows as well as the depth and understanding of the subject.

*Our best wishes to you once again. Enjoy reading Manipal Manual of Surgery, 7th edition—Authors*

*Please enjoy watching digital contents including videos for better learning.*

# Index

This Index consists of two sections.

First section lists out important points for ease of reference during examination time grouped as:

- Classifications
- Criteria
- Disease
- Grading
- Method
- Operation
- Point
- Procedure
- Repair
- Rule
- Scoring system/Score
- Signs
- Space
- Staging
- Syndromes
- Technique
- Tests
- Triads
- Triangles

Second section contains key-terms/keywords arranged alphabetically according to standard format.

## Classifications



## Criteria



## Disease



## Grading



## Method



## Operation



## Point



## Procedure

## Repair



## Rule



## Scoring system/Score



## Sign



## Space



## Staging



## Syndromes

## Technique



## Tests



## Triads



## Triangles